True False   16. Male and female college students are equally likely to wear seatbelts.

True False   17. Alcohol is an important contributor to both intentional and unintentional injuries.

True False   18. "No pain, no gain" is true for receiving health benefits from exercise.

True False   19. The lower a person's cholesterol, the lower his or her risk of dying.

True False   20. Eating a high-protein diet is a healthy choice.

True False   21. Totally eliminating alcohol from one's life is a healthy choice.

True False   22. People who experience chronic pain have underlying psychological disorders that are the real basis of their pain problem.

True False   23. Only viruses and germs trigger activation of the immune system.

True False   24. African Americans are more likely than European Americans to develop and to die of heart disease.

True False   25. Both positive and negative events may produce stress.

True False   26. Psychologists have found that lack of willpower is the primary reason why smokers cannot quit.

True False   27. Sugar pills (placebos) can boost the effectiveness of both psychological and medical treatments.

True False   28. People with a minor illness are about as likely as people with a serious illness to seek medical treatment.

True False   29. People who live with a smoker have about the same risk for cancer and heart disease as do cigarette smokers.

True False   30. Sick people who have a lot of friends usually live longer than sick people who have no close friends.

The answers to these questions appear on the back endpapers. You can also find an answer key on the website for this book: www.cengagebrain.com.

Health
PSYCHOLOGY

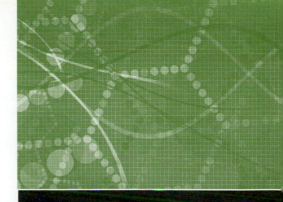

EIGHTH EDITION

Health PSYCHOLOGY

AN INTRODUCTION TO BEHAVIOR AND HEALTH

Linda Brannon

McNeese State University

Jess Feist

McNeese State University

John A. Updegraff

Kent State University

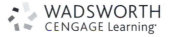

WADSWORTH
CENGAGE Learning·

Australia • Brazil • Japan • Korea • Mexico • Singapore • Spain • United Kingdom • United States

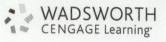

Health Psychology: An Introduction to Behavior and Health, Eighth Edition
Linda Brannon, Jess Feist, and John A. Updegraff

Publisher: Jon-David Hague

Developmental Editor: Ken King

Assistant Editor: Jessica Alderman

Editorial Assistant: Amelia Blevins

Associate Media Editor: Jasmin Tokatlian

Senior Brand Manager: Elisabeth Rhoden

Market Development Manager: Christine Sosa

Art and Cover Direction, Production Management, and Composition: PreMediaGlobal

Manufacturing Planner: Karen Hunt

Rights Acquisitions Specialist: Roberta Broyer

Cover Image: Human intelligence with grunge texture made of cogs and gears: Lightspring; Erythrocyte: Reshavskyi; Female runner silhouette is mirrored below with a soft pastel sunset sky as backdrop: Kovalev Sergey; Fresh fruit and vegetables: stocker1970; Senior African American couple at home: Mark Bowden

For product information and technology assistance, contact us at **Cengage Learning Customer & Sales Support, 1-800-354-9706**

For permission to use material from this text or product, submit all requests online at **www.cengage.com/permissions**. Further permissions questions can be emailed to **permissionrequest@cengage.com.**

Library of Congress Control Number: 2012955709

Student Edition:

ISBN-13: 978-1-133-59307-2

ISBN-10: 1-133-59307-0

Loose-leaf Edition:

ISBN-13: 978-1-133-93430-1

ISBN-10: 1-133-93430-7

Wadsworth
20 Davis Drive
Belmont, CA 94002-3098
USA

Cengage Learning is a leading provider of customized learning solutions with office locations around the globe, including Singapore, the United Kingdom, Australia, Mexico, Brazil, and Japan. Locate your local office at **www.cengage.com/global.**

Cengage Learning products are represented in Canada by Nelson Education, Ltd.

To learn more about Wadsworth, visit **www.cengage.com/wadsworth** Purchase any of our products at your local college store or at our preferred online store **www.cengagebrain.com.**

Printed in the United States of America
1 2 3 4 5 6 7 17 16 15 14 13

Brief Contents

PART 1   Foundations of Health Psychology

Chapter 1   Introducing Health Psychology   1
Chapter 2   Conducting Health Research   18
Chapter 3   Seeking and Receiving Health Care   40
Chapter 4   Adhering to Healthy Behavior   58

PART 2   Stress, Pain, and Coping

Chapter 5   Defining, Measuring, and Managing Stress   87
Chapter 6   Understanding Stress, Immunity, and Disease   120
Chapter 7   Understanding and Managing Pain   143
Chapter 8   Considering Alternative Approaches   172

PART 3   Behavior and Chronic Disease

Chapter 9   Behavioral Factors in Cardiovascular Disease   201
Chapter 10   Behavioral Factors in Cancer   231
Chapter 11   Living With Chronic Illness   253

PART 4   Behavioral Health

Chapter 12   Smoking Tobacco   282
Chapter 13   Using Alcohol and Other Drugs   310
Chapter 14   Eating and Weight   341
Chapter 15   Exercising   372

PART 5   Looking Toward the Future

Chapter 16   Future Challenges   397

Glossary   418

References   424

Name Index   481

Subject Index   509

Contents

Preface   xv

About the Authors   xxi

PART 1   Foundations of Health Psychology

1 Introducing Health Psychology   1

Real-World Profile of Angela Bryan   2

The Changing Field of Health   3

Patterns of Disease and Death   3

WOULD YOU BELIEVE . . . ? College Is Good for Your Health   7

Escalating Cost of Medical Care   8

What Is Health?   9

WOULD YOU BELIEVE . . . ? It Takes More Than a Virus to Give You a Cold   10

IN SUMMARY   11

Psychology's Relevance for Health   12

The Contribution of Psychosomatic Medicine   12

The Emergence of Behavioral Medicine   13

The Emergence of Health Psychology   13

IN SUMMARY   14

The Profession of Health Psychology   14

The Training of Health Psychologists   15

The Work of Health Psychologists   15

IN SUMMARY   16

Answers   16

Suggested Readings   17

2 Conducting Health Research   18

CHECK YOUR BELIEFS   19

Real-World Profile of Sylvester Colligan   19

The Placebo in Treatment and Research   20

Treatment and the Placebo   20

Research and the Placebo   22

WOULD YOU BELIEVE . . . ? Prescribing Placebos May Be Considered Ethical   22

IN SUMMARY   23

Research Methods in Psychology   24

Correlational Studies   24

Cross-Sectional and Longitudinal Studies   25

Experimental Designs   25

Ex Post Facto Designs   26

IN SUMMARY   27

Research Methods in Epidemiology   27

Observational Methods   28

Randomized Controlled Trials   29

Natural Experiments   30

Meta-Analysis   30

An Example of Epidemiological Research: The Alameda County Study   30

IN SUMMARY   31

Becoming an Informed Reader of Health-Related Research on the Internet   32

Determining Causation   33

The Risk Factor Approach   33

Cigarettes and Disease: Is There a Causal Relationship?   33

IN SUMMARY   35

Research Tools   35

The Role of Theory in Research   35

The Role of Psychometrics in Research   36

IN SUMMARY   37

Answers   37

Suggested Readings   39

3 Seeking and Receiving Health Care   40

CHECK YOUR HEALTH RISKS   41

Real-World Profile of Lance Armstrong   41

Seeking Medical Attention   42

Illness Behavior   43

The Sick Role   48

IN SUMMARY   48

Seeking Medical Information From Nonmedical Sources   49

Lay Referral Network   49

The Internet   49

Receiving Medical Care   50

Limited Access to Medical Care   50

Choosing a Practitioner   51

Being in the Hospital   53

WOULD YOU BELIEVE . . . ? Hospitals May Be a Leading Cause of Death   54

IN SUMMARY   56

Answers   57

Suggested Readings   57

4 Adhering to Healthy Behavior   58

CHAPTER

CHECK YOUR HEALTH RISKS   59

Real-World Profile of Nathan Rey   59

Issues in Adherence   60

What Is Adherence?   60

How Is Adherence Measured?   60

How Frequent Is Nonadherence?   61

What Are the Barriers to Adherence?   62

IN SUMMARY   63

What Factors Predict Adherence?   63

Severity of the Disease   64

Treatment Characteristics   64

Personal Factors   65

Environmental Factors   66

Interaction of Factors   68

IN SUMMARY   68

Why and How Do People Adhere to Healthy Behaviors?   68

Continuum Theories of Health Behavior   68

IN SUMMARY   74

Stage Theories of Health Behavior   74

IN SUMMARY   80

The Intention–Behavior Gap   80

Behavioral Willingness   80

Implementational Intentions   81

IN SUMMARY   81

WOULD YOU BELIEVE . . . ? Text Messages Can Help Turn Intentions Into Action   82

Improving Adherence   82

Becoming Healthier   84

IN SUMMARY   84

Answers   85

Suggested Readings   86

PART 2   Stress, Pain, and Coping

5 Defining, Measuring, and Managing Stress   87

CHAPTER

CHECK YOUR HEALTH RISKS   88

Real-World Profile of Lindsay Lohan   88

The Nervous System and the Physiology of Stress   89

The Peripheral Nervous System   89

The Neuroendocrine System   90

Physiology of the Stress Response   94

IN SUMMARY   95

Theories of Stress   95

Selye's View   95

Lazarus's View   97

IN SUMMARY   98

Measurement of Stress   98

Methods of Measurement   99

Reliability and Validity of Stress Measures   100

IN SUMMARY   101

Sources of Stress   101

Cataclysmic Events   101

Life Events   102

Daily Hassles   103

WOULD YOU BELIEVE . . . ? Vacations Relieve Work Stress ... But Not For Long   106

IN SUMMARY   107

Coping With Stress   107

Personal Resources That Influence Coping   107

**WOULD YOU BELIEVE . . . ? Pets May Be
Better Support Providers Than People   110**

Personal Coping Strategies   110

IN SUMMARY   112

**Behavioral Interventions for Managing
Stress   112**

Relaxation Training   112

Becoming Healthier   113

Cognitive Behavioral Therapy   113

Emotional Disclosure   115

IN SUMMARY   117

Answers   118

Suggested Readings   119

**6   Understanding Stress, Immunity,
and Disease   120**

CHAPTER

**Real-World Profile of Lindsay Lohan—
Continued   121**

Physiology of the Immune System   121

Organs of the Immune System   121

Function of the Immune System   122

Immune System Disorders   124

IN SUMMARY   127

Psychoneuroimmunology   127

History of Psychoneuroimmunology   127

Research in Psychoneuroimmunology   128

**WOULD YOU BELIEVE . . . ? Pictures of
Disease Are Enough to Activate the Immune
System   128**

Physical Mechanisms of Influence   130

IN SUMMARY   131

Does Stress Cause Disease?   131

The Diathesis–Stress Model   131

Stress and Disease   132

**WOULD YOU BELIEVE . . . ? Being a Sports Fan
May Be a Danger to Your Health   135**

Stress and Psychological Disorders   138

Becoming Healthier   141

IN SUMMARY   141

Answers   142

Suggested Readings   142

**7   Understanding and Managing
Pain   143**

CHAPTER

CHECK YOUR EXPERIENCES   144

Real-World Profile of Aron Ralston   145

Pain and the Nervous System   145

The Somatosensory System   146

The Spinal Cord   146

The Brain   147

**WOULD YOU BELIEVE . . . ? Emotional and
Physical Pain Are Mainly the Same in the
Brain   148**

Neurotransmitters and Pain   149

The Modulation of Pain   149

IN SUMMARY   150

The Meaning of Pain   150

Definition of Pain   151

The Experience of Pain   151

Theories of Pain   154

IN SUMMARY   157

The Measurement of Pain   157

Self-Reports   157

Behavioral Assessments   159

Physiological Measures   159

IN SUMMARY   160

Pain Syndromes   160

Headache Pain   161

Low Back Pain   161

Arthritis Pain   162

Cancer Pain   162

Phantom Limb Pain   163

IN SUMMARY   164

Managing Pain   164

Medical Approaches to Managing Pain   164

Behavioral Techniques for Managing Pain   166

IN SUMMARY   169

Answers   170

Suggested Readings   171

8 Considering Alternative
Approaches   172

CHAPTER

CHECK YOUR BELIEFS   173
Real-World Profile of Norman Cousins   173
Alternative Medical Systems   174
Traditional Chinese Medicine   175
Ayurvedic Medicine   176

IN SUMMARY   176
Alternative Practices and Products   177
Chiropractic Treatment   177
Massage   177
Diets, Supplements, and Natural Products   178

IN SUMMARY   179
Mind–Body Medicine   179
Meditation and Yoga   180
Becoming Healthier   181
Qi Gong and Tai Chi   181
Energy Healing   182
**WOULD YOU BELIEVE . . . ? Religious
Involvement May Improve Your Health   183**
Biofeedback   183
Hypnotic Treatment   184

IN SUMMARY   185
**Who Uses Complementary and Alternative
Medicine?   185**
Culture, Ethnicity, and Gender   185
Motivations for Seeking Alternative Treatment   187

IN SUMMARY   187
How Effective Are Alternative Treatments?   187
Alternative Treatments for Anxiety, Stress, and
Depression   188
Alternative Treatments for Pain   189
Alternative Treatments for Other Conditions   192
Limitations of Alternative Therapies   195
Integrative Medicine   197

IN SUMMARY   198
Answers   199
Suggested Readings   200

PART 3   Behavior and Chronic
Disease

9 Behavioral Factors in Cardiovascular
Disease   201

CHAPTER

CHECK YOUR HEALTH RISKS   202
Real-World Profile of President Bill Clinton   203
The Cardiovascular System   203
The Coronary Arteries   205
Coronary Artery Disease   205
Stroke   207
Blood Pressure   207

IN SUMMARY   210
**The Changing Rates of Cardiovascular
Disease   210**
Reasons for the Decline in Death Rates   210
Heart Disease Throughout the World   211

IN SUMMARY   212
Risk Factors in Cardiovascular Disease   212
Inherent Risk Factors   213
Physiological Conditions   215
**WOULD YOU BELIEVE . . . ? A Floss a Day May
Keep Cardiovascular Disease Away?   217**
Behavioral Factors   217
**WOULD YOU BELIEVE . . . ? Chocolate May
Help Prevent Heart Disease   219**
Psychosocial Factors   219

IN SUMMARY   223
Reducing Cardiovascular Risks   224
Before Diagnosis: Preventing First Heart
Attacks   224
Becoming Healthier   227
After Diagnosis: Rehabilitating Cardiac Patients   227

IN SUMMARY   229
Answers   229
Suggested Readings   230

10 Behavioral Factors in Cancer   231

CHAPTER

CHECK YOUR HEALTH RISKS   232
Real-World Profile of Steve Jobs   232
What Is Cancer?   233
The Changing Rates of Cancer Deaths   233

Cancers With Decreasing Death Rates 234

Cancers With Increasing Incidence and Mortality Rates 236

IN SUMMARY 236

Cancer Risk Factors Beyond Personal Control 236

Inherent Risk Factors for Cancer 237

Environmental Risk Factors for Cancer 238

IN SUMMARY 239

Behavioral Risk Factors for Cancer 239

Smoking 239

Diet 242

Alcohol 243

Sedentary Lifestyle 245

Ultraviolet Light Exposure 245

WOULD YOU BELIEVE . . . ? Cancer Prevention Prevents More Than Cancer 245

Sexual Behavior 246

Psychosocial Risk Factors in Cancer 247

IN SUMMARY 247

Living With Cancer 247

Problems With Medical Treatments for Cancer 248

Adjusting to a Diagnosis of Cancer 248

Social Support for Cancer Patients 249

Psychological Interventions for Cancer Patients 250

IN SUMMARY 250

Answers 251

Suggested Readings 251

11 Living With Chronic Illness 253

Real-World Profile of President Ronald Reagan 254

The Impact of Chronic Disease 255

Impact on the Patient 255

Impact on the Family 256

IN SUMMARY 257

Living With Alzheimer's Disease 257

WOULD YOU BELIEVE . . . ? Using Your Mind May Help Prevent Losing Your Mind 259

Helping the Patient 260

Helping the Family 260

IN SUMMARY 261

Adjusting to Diabetes 262

The Physiology of Diabetes 262

The Impact of Diabetes 264

Health Psychology's Involvement With Diabetes 265

IN SUMMARY 266

The Impact of Asthma 266

The Disease of Asthma 267

Managing Asthma 268

IN SUMMARY 269

Dealing With HIV and AIDS 269

Incidence and Mortality Rates for HIV/AIDS 270

Symptoms of HIV and AIDS 272

The Transmission of HIV 272

Psychologists' Role in the HIV Epidemic 274

Becoming Healthier 276

IN SUMMARY 277

Facing Death 277

Adjusting to Terminal Illness 277

Grieving 278

IN SUMMARY 279

Answers 279

Suggested Readings 280

PART 4 Behavioral Health

12 Smoking Tobacco 282

CHECK YOUR HEALTH RISKS 283

Real-World Profile of President Barack Obama 283

Smoking and the Respiratory System 284

Functioning of the Respiratory System 284

What Components in Smoke Are Dangerous? 285

IN SUMMARY 287

A Brief History of Tobacco Use 287

Choosing to Smoke 288

Who Smokes and Who Does Not? 289

Why Do People Smoke? 291

CHAPTER

CHAPTER

IN SUMMARY   295

Health Consequences of Tobacco Use   296

Cigarette Smoking   296

WOULD YOU BELIEVE . . . ? Smoking Is Related to Mental Illness   298

Cigar and Pipe Smoking   298

Passive Smoking   299

Smokeless Tobacco   300

IN SUMMARY   300

Interventions for Reducing Smoking Rates   300

Deterring Smoking   300

Quitting Smoking   301

Who Quits and Who Does Not?   303

Relapse Prevention   304

IN SUMMARY   304

Effects of Quitting   305

Quitting and Weight Gain   305

Becoming Healthier   305

Health Benefits of Quitting   306

IN SUMMARY   308

Answers   308

Suggested Readings   309

13 Using Alcohol and Other Drugs   310

CHECK YOUR HEALTH RISKS   311

Real-World Profile of Charlie Sheen   311

Alcohol Consumption—Yesterday and Today   312

A Brief History of Alcohol Consumption   312

The Prevalence of Alcohol Consumption Today   314

IN SUMMARY   316

The Effects of Alcohol   316

Hazards of Alcohol   317

Benefits of Alcohol   320

IN SUMMARY   321

Why Do People Drink?   322

The Disease Model   323

Cognitive-Physiological Theories   325

The Social Learning Model   326

IN SUMMARY   327

Changing Problem Drinking   328

Change Without Therapy   328

Treatments Oriented Toward Abstinence   328

Controlled Drinking   330

The Problem of Relapse   330

IN SUMMARY   331

Other Drugs   331

Health Effects   331

WOULD YOU BELIEVE . . . ? Brain Damage Is Not a Common Risk of Drug Use   332

Becoming Healthier   333

Drug Misuse and Abuse   336

Treatment for Drug Abuse   337

Preventing and Controlling Drug Use   338

IN SUMMARY   339

Answers   339

Suggested Readings   340

14 Eating and Weight   341

CHECK YOUR HEALTH RISKS   342

Real-World Profile of Kirstie Alley   342

The Digestive System   343

Factors in Weight Maintenance   344

Experimental Starvation   345

Experimental Overeating   346

IN SUMMARY   347

Overeating and Obesity   347

What Is Obesity?   347

Why Are Some People Obese?   350

WOULD YOU BELIEVE . . . ? You May Need a Nap Rather Than a Diet   352

How Unhealthy Is Obesity?   353

IN SUMMARY   354

Dieting   355

Approaches to Losing Weight   356

Is Dieting a Good Choice?   359

IN SUMMARY   359

Eating Disorders   360

Anorexia Nervosa   361

Bulimia   365

Binge Eating Disorder   367

Becoming Healthier   367

CHAPTER

CHAPTER

IN SUMMARY   369

Answers   369

Suggested Readings   370

15 Exercising   372

CHECK YOUR HEALTH RISKS   373

Real–World Profile of Tara Costa   373

Types of Physical Activity   374

Reasons for Exercising   374

Physical Fitness   375

Weight Control   375

IN SUMMARY   376

Physical Activity and Cardiovascular Health   377

Early Studies   377

Later Studies   378

Do Women and Men Benefit Equally?   379

Physical Activity and Cholesterol Levels   379

IN SUMMARY   380

Other Health Benefits of Physical Activity   380

Protection Against Cancer   380

Prevention of Bone Density Loss   381

Control of Diabetes   381

Psychological Benefits of Physical Activity   381

WOULD YOU BELIEVE . . . ? It's Never Too Late—or Too Early   382

IN SUMMARY   385

Hazards of Physical Activity   385

Exercise Addiction   387

Injuries From Physical Activity   388

Death During Exercise   389

Reducing Exercise Injuries   390

IN SUMMARY   390

How Much Is Enough but Not Too Much?   390

Improving Adherence to Physical Activity   391

Becoming Healthier   392

IN SUMMARY   394

Answers   395

Suggested Readings   395

PART 5   Looking Toward the Future

16 Future Challenges   397

Real-World Profile of Dwayne and Robyn   398

Challenges for Healthier People   399

Increasing the Span of Healthy Life   400

Reducing Health Disparities   401

WOULD YOU BELIEVE . . . ? Health Literacy Can Improve by "Thinking Outside the Box"   403

IN SUMMARY   405

Outlook for Health Psychology   405

Progress in Health Psychology   405

Future Challenges for Health Care   405

Will Health Psychology Continue to Grow?   411

IN SUMMARY   411

Making Health Psychology Personal   412

Understanding Your Risks   412

What Can You Do to Cultivate a Healthy Lifestyle?   414

Increase Your Health Literacy   415

IN SUMMARY   416

Answers   416

Suggested Readings   417

Glossary   418

References   424

Name Index   481

Subject Index   509

Preface

Health is a far different phenomenon today than it was just a century ago. Most serious diseases and disorders now result from people's behavior. People smoke, eat unhealthily, do not exercise, or cope ineffectively with the stresses of modern life. As you will learn in this book, psychology—the science of behavior—is increasingly relevant to understanding physical health. *Health psychology* is the scientific study of behaviors that relate to health enhancement, disease prevention, safety, and rehabilitation.

The first edition of this book, published in the 1980s, was one of the first undergraduate texts to cover the then-emerging field of health psychology. Now in this eighth edition, *Health Psychology: An Introduction to Behavior and Health* remains a preeminent undergraduate textbook in health psychology.

The Eighth Edition

This eighth edition retains the core aspects that have kept this book a leader throughout the decades: (1) a balance between the science and applications of the field of health psychology and (2) a clear and engaging review of classic and cutting-edge research on behavior and health.

The eighth edition of *Health Psychology: An Introduction to Behavior and Health* has five parts. Part 1, which includes the first four chapters, lays a solid foundation in research and theory for understanding subsequent chapters and approaches the field by considering the overarching issues involved in seeking medical care and adhering to health care regimens. Part 2 deals with stress, pain, and the management of these conditions through conventional and alternative medicine. Part 3 discusses heart disease, cancer, and other chronic diseases. Part 4 includes chapters on tobacco use, drinking alcohol, eating and weight, and physical activity. Part 5 looks toward future challenges in health psychology and addresses how to apply health knowledge to one's life to become healthier.

What's New?

In this edition, we bring a fresh new voice to the writing team: John A. Updegraff. John earned his PhD from one of the top health psychology programs in the United States. He is an influential researcher in health psychology, an acclaimed psychology instructor, and an expert in the areas of health behavior and stress. John brings his passion, knowledge, and (occasional) humor to this revision, so the textbook remains current, accurate, and a delightful read for instructors and students.

The present edition also reorganizes several chapters to better emphasize the theoretical underpinnings of health behavior. For example, Chapter 4 focuses on adherence to healthy behavior and presents both classic and contemporary theories of health behavior, including recent research on the "intention–behavior gap." Readers of the eighth edition will benefit from the most up-to-date review of health behavior theories—and their applications—on the market.

The eighth edition also features new boxes on important and timely topics such as

- How to evaluate the quality of research reported on the Internet
- How the redesign of nutrition labels may improve your health literacy
- How text messaging can help increase your physical activity
- Why your doctor might *ethically* prescribe ineffective medical treatments to you
- Why taking vacations can have unexpected effects on your stress levels
- Why social rejection can feel physically painful
- Why pets may be the best social support providers
- Why you should floss your teeth more (hint: it has nothing to do with cavities or bad breath)
- Why pictures of guns stimulate your immune system

Other new or reorganized topics within the chapters include

- Several new Real-World Profiles, including Steve Jobs, Barack Obama, Tara Costa, Charlie Sheen, Kirstie Alley, and Lance Armstrong

- Expanded discussion of training and employment opportunities for health psychologists in Chapter 1
- Discussion of publication bias and CONSORT guidelines for reporting of clinical trials in Chapter 2, to help students better evaluate health psychology research
- New section on seeking medical information from nonmedical sources such as the Internet in Chapter 3
- Technological advances in assessing adherence in Chapter 4
- Contemporary models of health behavior, such as the health action process approach and the "intention–behavior gap," are now presented in Chapter 4
- A streamlined presentation of life events scales, focusing only on the most widely used measures in Chapter 5
- New discussion of the role of stress in weakening people's responses to vaccination in Chapter 6
- New discussion of acceptance and commitment therapy as a psychological intervention for pain management in Chapter 7
- Reorganization of Chapter 8 to highlight the types of complementary and alternative medicine (CAM) that people use most often, and the latest evidence on the effectiveness of CAM
- Up-to-date findings from the 52-nation INTER-HEART study on heart attack risk factors in Chapter 9
- New information on the role of human papillomavirus (HPV) in cancer in Chapter 10
- A streamlined presentation of the history of the HIV epidemic in Chapter 11
- A streamlined presentation of the physiology of the respiratory system in Chapter 12
- Greater emphasis on the similarities between alcohol and other drugs of abuse in Chapter 13, including the common brain pathways that all drugs may activate and the similarities among treatment approaches
- Updated information in Chapter 14 on binge eating, which will appear as a disorder in DSM-V
- New section on the links between physical activity and cognitive functioning in Chapter 15
- New organization of the section about physical activity interventions, to better distinguish the different approaches to intervention and their effectiveness
- Chapter 16 includes a new discussion of how technological and medical advances create opportunity for health psychologists

What Has Been Retained?

In this revision, we retained the most popular features that made this text a leader over the past two decades. These features include (1) "Real-World Profiles" for each chapter, (2) chapter-opening questions, (3) a "Check Your Health Risks" box in most chapters, (4) one or more "Would You Believe …?" boxes in each chapter, and (5) a "Becoming Healthier" feature in many chapters. These features stimulate critical thinking, engage readers in the topic, and provide valuable tips to enhance personal well-being.

Real-World Profiles   Millions of people—including celebrities—deal with the issues we describe in this book. To highlight the human side of health psychology, we open each chapter with a profile of a person in the real world. Many of these profiles are of famous people, whose health issues may not always be well-known. Their cases provide intriguing examples, such as Barack Obama's attempt to quit smoking, Lance Armstrong's delays in seeking treatment for cancer, Steve Jobs' fight with cancer, Halle Berry's diabetes, Charlie Sheen's substance abuse, Kirstie Alley's battles with her weight, and "Biggest Loser" Tara Costa's efforts to increase physical activity. In the eighth edition, we also introduce a profile of a celebrity in the world of health psychology, Dr. Angela Bryan, to give readers a better sense of the personal motivation and activities of health psychologists.

Questions and Answers   In this text, we adopt a *preview, read, and review* method to facilitate student's learning and recall. Each chapter begins with a series of *Questions* that organize the chapter, preview the material, and enhance active learning. As each chapter unfolds, we reveal the answers through a discussion of relevant research findings. At the end of each major topic, an *In Summary* statement recaps the topic. Then, at the end of the chapter, *Answers* to the chapter-opening questions appear. In this manner, students benefit from many opportunities to engage with the material throughout each chapter.

Check Your Health Risks   At the beginning of most chapters, a "Check Your Health Risks" box personalizes material in that chapter. Each box consists of several health-related behaviors or attitudes that readers should check before looking at the rest of the chapter. After checking the items that apply to them and then becoming familiar with the chapter's material, readers will develop a more research-based understanding of their health risks. A special "Check Your Health Risks" appears inside the front cover of the book. Students should complete this exercise before they read the book and look for answers as they proceed through the chapters (or check the website for the answers).

Would You Believe ...? Boxes We keep the popular "Would You Believe ...?" boxes, adding nine new ones and updating those we retained. Each box highlights a particularly intriguing finding in health research. These boxes explode preconceived notions, present unusual findings, and challenge students to take an objective look at issues that they may have not have evaluated carefully.

Becoming Healthier Embedded in most chapters is a "Becoming Healthier" box with advice on how to use the information in the chapter to enact a healthier lifestyle. Although some people may not agree with all of these recommendations, each is based on the most current research findings. We believe that if you follow these guidelines, you will increase your chances of a long and healthy life.

Other Changes and Additions

We have made a number of subtle changes in this edition that we believe make it an even stronger book than its predecessors. More specifically, we

- Deleted several hundred old references and exchanged them for more than 600 recent ones
- Reorganized many sections of chapters to improve the flow of information
- Added several new tables and figures to aid students' understanding of difficult concepts
- Highlighted the biopsychosocial approach to health psychology, examining issues and data from a biological, psychological, and social viewpoint
- Drew from the growing body of research from around the world on health to give the book a more international perspective
- Recognized and emphasized gender issues whenever appropriate
- Retained our emphasis on theories and models that strive to explain and predict health-related behaviors

Writing Style

With each edition, we work to improve our connection with readers. Although this book explores complex issues and difficult topics, we use clear, concise, and comprehensible language and an informal, lively writing style. We write this book for an upper-division undergraduate audience, and it should be easily understood by students with a minimal background in psychology and biology. Health psychology courses typically draw students from a variety of college majors, so some elementary material in our book may be repetitive for some students. For other students, this material will fill in the background they need to comprehend the information within the field of health psychology.

Technical terms appear in **boldface type**, and a definition usually appears at that point in the text. These terms also appear in an end-of-book glossary.

Instructional Aids

Besides the glossary at the end of the book, we supply several other features to help both students and instructors. These include stories of people whose behavior typifies the topic, frequent summaries within each chapter, and annotated suggested readings.

Within-Chapter Summaries

Rather than wait until the end of each chapter to present a lengthy chapter summary, we place shorter summaries at key points within each chapter. In general, these summaries correspond to each major topic in a chapter. We believe these shorter, frequent summaries keep readers on track and promote a better understanding of the chapter's content.

Annotated Suggested Readings

At the end of each chapter are three or four annotated suggested readings that students may wish to examine. We chose these readings for their capacity to shed additional light on major topics in a chapter. Most of these suggested readings are quite recent, but we also selected several that have lasting interest. We include only readings that are intelligible to the average college student and that are accessible in most college and university libraries.

Instructor's Manual With Test Bank

This edition of *Health Psychology: An Introduction to Behavior and Health* is accompanied by a comprehensive instructor's manual. Each chapter begins with a *lecture outline*, designed to assist instructors in preparing lecture material from the text. Many instructors are able to lecture strictly from these notes; others can use the lecture outline as a framework for organizing their own lecture notes.

A test bank of nearly 1,200 *multiple-choice test items* makes up a large section of each chapter of the instructor's manual. The authors, in conjunction with Amber Emanuel of Kent State University, wrote these test items. Some items are factual, some are conceptual, and others ask students to apply what they have learned. These test items will reduce instructors' work in preparing tests. Each item, of course, is marked with the correct answer. The test items are also available electronically on ExamView.

We also include *True–false questions* and *essay questions* for each chapter. The true–false questions include answers, and each essay question has an outline answer of the critical points.

Each chapter also includes *suggested activities*. These activities vary widely—from video recommendations to student research to classroom debates. We have tried to include more activities than any instructor could feasibly assign during a semester to give instructors a choice of activities.

With so many electronic resources available to students these days, we wanted to include a *Exploring Health on the Web* activity. In this section, we suggest online activities, including websites that are relevant to each chapter. This activity expands the electronic resources students may use to explore health-related topics.

Instructor's Resource CD-ROM

Transparencies include art from the text, as well as several physiology video clips and animations in Microsoft® PowerPoint®.

Text Companion Website

This website contains practice quizzes, web links, the text's glossary, flashcards, and more for each chapter of the text.

Acknowledgments

We would like to thank the people at Cengage Learning for their assistance. Ken King served as development editor for this edition, as he did for the first edition. The symmetry of this situation is especially pleasing. His skill, support, sharp eye, and well-timed prods helped us produce a better book. We also thank the rest of the Cengage editorial team, including publisher Jon-David Hague and editorial assistant Travis Holland for their guidance and help throughout the process. Others who worked on the eighth edition include: Jessica Alderman, assistant editor; Mary Stone and Gunjan Chandola, project managers; Kristine Janssens, permissions manager; Susan Buschhorn, image licensing manager; Brenda Carmichael, design director; Christine Sosa, market development manager; Elisabeth Rhoden, senior brand manager; Jasmin Tokatlian, associate media editor; Karen Hunt, manufacturing planner; and Roberta Broyer, rights acquisitions specialist.

We also are indebted to a number of reviewers who read all or parts of the manuscript for this and earlier editions. We are grateful for the valuable comments of the following reviewers:

Silvia M. Bigatti, Indiana University

Bette Ackerman, Rhodes College

Dale V. Doty, Monroe Community College

Michael B. Madson, University of Southern Mississippi

Mary McNaughton-Cassill, University of Texas at San Antonio

Sangeeta Singg, Angelo State University

Elizabeth Stern, Milwaukee Area Technical College

Joel Hughes, Kent State University

Samantha D. Outcalt, Indiana University, Purdue University Indianapolis

Elizabeth Thyrum, Millersville University

Linda notes that authors typically thank their spouses for being understanding, supportive, and sacrificing, and her spouse, Barry Humphus, is no exception. He made contributions that helped to shape the book and provided generous, patient, live-in, expert computer consultation and tech support that proved essential in the preparation of the manuscript. In addition, Drs. Futoshi Kobayashi and Grant Rich have been so kind as to send their advice and information, which were helpful in updating this edition. Linda also acknowledges the huge debt to Jess Feist and his contributions to this book. Although he did not work on this or the previous edition, his work and words remain as a guide and inspiration for her and for John.

John also thanks his wife, Alanna, for her encouragement to take on this project and support throughout the process. John also thanks his two young children for always asking about the book, even though they didn't comprehend most of what he told them about it. Thanks also go to the graduate students in his research lab (Brian Don, Amber Emanuel, Kristel Gallagher, Cristina Godinho, Scout McCully, and Chris Steinman) for offering a slightly younger generation's perspective on the material. Lastly, John thanks all of his past undergraduate students for making health psychology such a thrill to teach. This book is dedicated to them and to the future generation of health psychology students.

About the Authors

Linda Brannon is a professor in the Department of Psychology at McNeese State University in Lake Charles, Louisiana. Linda joined the faculty at McNeese after receiving her doctorate in human experimental psychology from the University of Texas at Austin.

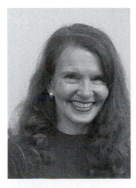

Jess Feist is Professor Emeritus at McNeese State University. He joined the faculty after receiving his doctorate in counseling from the University of Kansas and stayed at McNeese until he retired in 2005. Jess and Linda have each been selected to receive the annual Distinguished Faculty Award from McNeese State University.

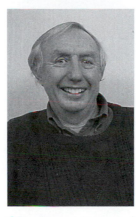

In the early 1980s, Linda and Jess became interested in the developing field of health psychology, which led to their coauthoring the first edition of this book. They watched the field of health psychology emerge and grow, and the subsequent editions of the book reflect that growth and development.

Their interests converge in the area of health psychology but diverge in other areas of psychology. Jess carried his interest in personality theory to his authorship of *Theories of Personality*, coauthored with his son Greg Feist. Linda's interest in gender and gender issues led her to publish *Gender: Psychological Perspectives*, which is in its sixth edition.

John A. Updegraff is a professor of social and health psychology in the Department of Psychology at Kent State University in Kent, Ohio. John received his PhD in Social Psychology at University of California, Los Angeles, under the mentorship of pioneering health psychologist Shelley Taylor. John then completed a postdoctoral fellowship at University of California, Irvine, prior to joining the faculty at Kent State.

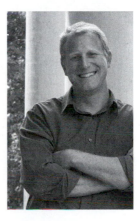

John is an expert in the areas of health behavior, health communication, stress, and coping, and is the recipient of multiple research grants from the National Institutes of Health. His research appears in the field's top journals.

John stays healthy by running the roads and trails near his home, and by running after his two small children. John is also known for subjecting students and colleagues to his singing and guitar playing (go ahead, look him up on YouTube).

CHAPTER 1

Introducing Health Psychology

CHAPTER OUTLINE

- **Real-World Profile of Angela Bryan**
- *The Changing Field of Health*
- *Psychology's Relevance for Health*
- *The Profession of Health Psychology*

QUESTIONS

This chapter focuses on three basic questions:

1. How have views of health changed?

2. How did psychology become involved in health care?

3. What type of training do health psychologists receive, and what kinds of work do they do?

Real-World Profile of
ANGELA BRYAN

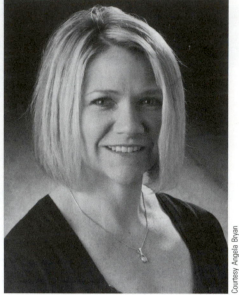

Courtesy Angela Bryan

Health psychology is a relatively new and fascinating field of psychology. Health psychologists examine how people's lifestyles influence their physical health. In this book, you will learn about the diverse topics, findings, and people who make up this field.

First, let's introduce you to Angela Bryan, a health psychologist from the University of Colorado Boulder. Angela develops interventions that promote healthy behavior such as safe sex and physical activity. Angela has won several awards for her work, including a recognition that one of her interventions is among the few that work in reducing risky sexual behavior among adolescents ("Safe on the Outs"; CDC, 2011c).

As an adolescent, Angela thought of herself as a "rebel" (Aiken, 2006), perhaps an unlikely start for someone who now encourages people to maintain a healthy lifestyle. It was not until college that Angela discovered her passion for health psychology. She took a course in social psychology, which explored how people make judgments about others. Angela quickly saw the relevance for understanding safe sex behavior. At this time, the HIV/AIDS epidemic was peaking in the United States, and condom use was one action people could take to prevent the spread of the HIV virus. Yet, people often resisted proposing condoms to a partner, due to concerns such as "What will a partner think of me if I say that a condom is needed?" Angela sought out a professor to supervise a research project on perceptions of condom use in an initial sexual encounter.

Angela continued this work as a Ph.D. student at Arizona State University, where she developed a program to promote condom use among college women. In this program, Angela taught women skills for proposing and using condoms. This work was not always easy. She recalls, "I would walk through the residence halls on my way to deliver my intervention, with a basket of condoms in one arm and a basket of zucchinis in the other. I can't imagine what others thought I was doing!"

Later, she expanded her work to populations at greater risk for HIV, including incarcerated adolescents, intravenous drug users, HIV+ individuals, and truck drivers in India. She also developed an interest in promoting physical activity.

In all her work, Angela uses the biopsychosocial model, which you will learn about in this chapter. Specifically, she identifies the biological, psychological, and social factors that influence health behaviors such as condom use. Angela's interventions address each of these factors.

Angela's work is both challenging and rewarding. She works on a daily basis with community agencies, clinical psychologists, neuroscientists, and exercise physiologists. She uses rigorous research methods to evaluate the success of her interventions. More recently, she has started to examine the genetic factors that determine whether a person will respond to a physical activity intervention.

What is the most rewarding part of her work? "When the interventions work!" she says. "If we can get one kid to use a condom or one person with a chronic illness to exercise, that is meaningful."

In this book, you will learn about the theories, methods, and discoveries of health psychologists such as Angela Bryan. As you read, keep in mind this piece of advice from Angela: "Think broadly and optimistically about health. A health psychologist's work is difficult, but it can make a difference."

The Changing Field of Health

"We are now living well enough and long enough to slowly fall apart" (Sapolsky, 1998, p. 2).

The field of health psychology developed relatively recently—the 1970s, to be exact—to address the challenges presented by the changing field of health and health care. A century ago, the average **life expectancy** in the United States was approximately 50 years of age, far shorter than it is now. When people in the United States died, they died largely from infectious diseases such as pneumonia, tuberculosis, diarrhea, and enteritis (see Figure 1.1). These conditions resulted from contact with impure drinking water, contaminated foods, or sick people. People might seek medical care only after they became ill, but medicine had few cures to offer. The duration of most diseases—such as typhoid fever, pneumonia, and diphtheria—was short; a person either died or got well in a matter of weeks. People felt very limited responsibility for contracting a contagious disease because such disease was not controllable.

Life—and death—are now dramatically different than they were a century ago. Life expectancy in the United States is nearly 80 years of age; some countries boast even longer life expectancy. For most citizens of industrialized nations, public sanitation is vastly better than it was a century ago. Vaccines and treatments exist for many infectious diseases. However, improvements in the prevention and treatment of infectious diseases allowed for a different class of disease to emerge as the new century's killers: **chronic diseases**. Heart disease, cancer, and stroke—all chronic diseases—are now the leading causes of mortality in the United States and account for a greater proportion of deaths than infectious diseases ever did. Chronic diseases develop and then persist or recur, affecting people over long periods of time. Every year, over 2 million people in the United States die from chronic diseases, but over 130 million people—almost one out of every two adults—live with at least one chronic disease.

Furthermore, most deaths today are attributable to diseases associated with individual behavior and lifestyle. Heart disease, cancer, stroke, chronic lower respiratory diseases (including emphysema and chronic bronchitis), unintentional injuries, and diabetes are all due in part to cigarette smoking, alcohol abuse, unwise eating, stress, and a sedentary lifestyle. Because the major killers today arise in part due to lifestyle and behavior, people have a great deal more control over their health than they did in the past. However, many people do not exercise this control, so unhealthy behavior is an increasingly important public health problem. Indeed, unhealthy behavior contributes to the escalating costs of health care.

In this chapter, we describe the changing patterns of disease and disability and the increasing costs of health care. We also discuss how these trends change the very definition of what health is and require a broad view of health. This broad view of health is the biopsychosocial model, a view adopted by health psychologists such as Angela Bryan.

Patterns of Disease and Death

The 20th century brought about major changes in the patterns of disease and death in the United States, including a shift in the leading causes of death. Infectious diseases were leading causes of death in 1900, but over the next several decades, chronic diseases such as heart disease, cancer, and stroke became the leading killers.

During the last few years of the 20th century, deaths from some chronic diseases—those related to unhealthy lifestyles and behaviors—began to *decrease*. These diseases include heart disease, cancer, and stroke, which all were responsible for a smaller proportion of deaths in 2005 than in 1990. Why have deaths from these diseases decreased in the last few decades? We will discuss this in greater detail in Chapter 9, but one major reason is that fewer people in the United States now smoke cigarettes than in the past. This change in behavior contributed to some of the decline in deaths due to heart disease; improvements in health care also contributed to this decline.

Death rates due to unintentional injuries, suicide, and homicide have increased in recent years (Kung, Hoyert, Xu, & Murphy, 2008). Significant increases also occurred in Alzheimer's disease, influenza and pneumonia, kidney disease, septicemia (blood infection), and Parkinson's disease. For these causes of death that have recently increased, behavior is a less important component than for those causes that have decreased. However, the rising death rates due to Alzheimer's and Parkinson's disease reflect another important trend in health and health care: an increasingly older population.

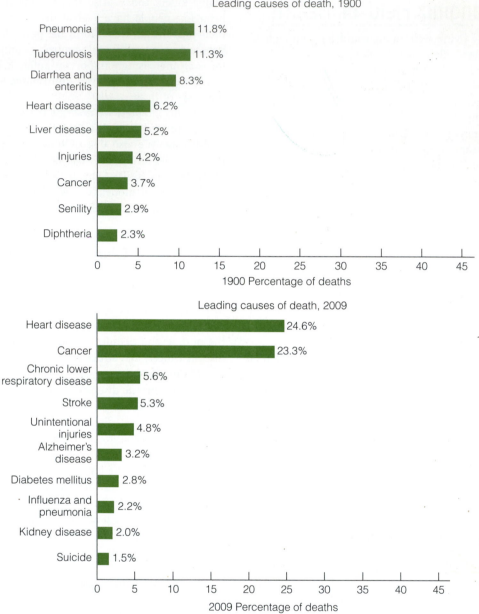

Leading causes of death, 1900

Cause	Percentage
Pneumonia	11.8%
Tuberculosis	11.3%
Diarrhea and enteritis	8.3%
Heart disease	6.2%
Liver disease	5.2%
Injuries	4.2%
Cancer	3.7%
Senility	2.9%
Diphtheria	2.3%

1900 Percentage of deaths

Leading causes of death, 2009

Cause	Percentage
Heart disease	24.6%
Cancer	23.3%
Chronic lower respiratory disease	5.6%
Stroke	5.3%
Unintentional injuries	4.8%
Alzheimer's disease	3.2%
Diabetes mellitus	2.8%
Influenza and pneumonia	2.2%
Kidney disease	2.0%
Suicide	1.5%

2009 Percentage of deaths

FIGURE 1.1 Leading causes of death, United States, 1900 and 2009.

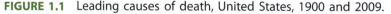

Source: Healthy people, 2010, 2000, by U.S. Department of Health and Human Services, Washington, DC: U.S. Government Printing Office; "Deaths: Final Data for 2009," 2011, by Kochanek, K.D., Xu, J., Murphy, S.L., Miniño, A.M., & Kung, H-C., *National Vital Statistics Reports, 60*(3), Table B.

Age   Indeed, age is an important factor in mortality. Obviously, older people are more likely to die than younger ones, but the causes of death vary among age groups. Thus, the ranking of causes of death for the entire population may not reflect any specific age group and may lead people to misperceive the risk for some ages. For example, cardiovascular disease (which includes heart disease and stroke) and cancer account for about 60% of all deaths in the United States, but they are not the leading cause of death for young people. For individuals between 1 and 44 years of age, unintentional injuries are the leading cause of death, and violent deaths from suicide and homicide rank high on the list (National Center for Health Statistics [NCHS], 2011). Unintentional injuries account for 28% of the deaths in this age group, suicide for almost 10%, and homicide for about 8%. As Figure 1.2 reveals, other causes of death account for much smaller percentages of deaths among adolescents and young adults than unintentional injuries, homicide, and suicide.

For adults 45 to 64 years old, the picture is quite different. Cardiovascular disease and cancer become leading causes of death, and unintentional injuries fall to third place. As people age, they become more likely to die, so the causes of death for older people dominate the overall figures for causes of death. However, younger people show very different patterns of mortality.

Ethnicity, Income, and Disease   Question 2 from the quiz inside the front cover asks if the United States is among the top 10 nations in the world in terms of life expectancy. It is not even close; its rank is 24th among industrialized nations (NCHS, 2011) but 50th among all nations (Central Intelligence Agency [CIA], 2012). Within the United States, ethnicity is also a factor in life expectancy, and the leading causes of death also vary among ethnic groups. Table 1.1 shows the ranking of the 10 leading causes of death for four ethnic groups in the United States. No two groups have identical profiles of causes of death, and some causes do not appear on the list for each group, highlighting the influence of ethnicity on mortality.

If African Americans and European Americans in the United States were considered to be different nations, European America would rank higher in life expectancy than African America—47th place and

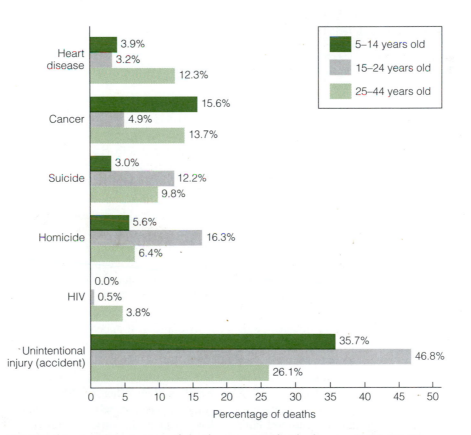

FIGURE 1.2   Leading causes of death among individuals ages 5–14, 15–24, and 25–44, United States, 2007.

Source: Health, United States, 2010, 2010, by National Center for Health Statistics, Hyattsville, MD. Table 27.

TABLE 1.1 Ten Leading Causes of Death for Four Ethnic Groups in the United States, 2007

	European Americans	Hispanic Americans	African Americans	Asian Americans
Heart disease	1	1	1	2
Cancer	2	2	2	1
Chronic lower respiratory disease	3	7	8	7
Stroke	4	4	3	3
Unintentional injuries	5	3	4	4
Alzheimer's disease	6	*	*	10
Diabetes	7	5	5	5
Pneumonia & influenza	8	10	*	6
Kidney disease	9	*	7	9
Suicide	10	*	*	8
Septicemia	*	*	10	*
Chronic liver disease	*	6	*	*
Homicide	*	8	6	*
HIV	*	*	9	*
Conditions originating in perinatal period	*	9	*	*

*Not among the 10 leading causes of death for this ethnic group.

Source: "Deaths: Leading causes for 2007," 2011, by M. Heron, *National Vital Statistics Reports, 59*(8), Tables E and F.

113th place, respectively (CIA, 2012; U.S. Census Bureau [USCB], 2011). Thus, European Americans have a longer life expectancy than African Americans, but neither should expect to live as long as people in Japan, Canada, Iceland, Australia, the United Kingdom, Italy, France, Hong Kong, Israel, and many other countries.

Hispanics have socioeconomic disadvantages similar to those of African Americans (USCB, 2011), including poverty and low educational level. About 10% of European Americans live below the poverty level, whereas 32% of African Americans and 26% of Hispanic Americans do (USCB, 2011). European Americans also have educational advantages: 86% receive high school diplomas, compared with only 81% of African Americans and 59% of Hispanic Americans. These socioeconomic disadvantages translate into health disadvantages (Crimmins, Ki Kim, Alley, Karlamangla, & Seeman, 2007; Smith & Bradshaw, 2006). That is, poverty and low educational level both relate to health problems and lower life expectancy. Thus, some of the ethnic differences in health are due to socioeconomic differences.

Access to health insurance and medical care are not the only factors that make poverty a health risk. Indeed, the health risks associated with poverty begin before birth. Even with the expansion of prenatal care by Medicaid, poor mothers, especially teen mothers, are more likely to deliver low-birth-weight babies, who are more likely than normal-birth-weight infants to die (NCHS, 2011). Also, pregnant women living below the poverty line are more likely than other pregnant women to be physically abused and to deliver babies who suffer the consequences of prenatal child abuse (Zelenko, Lock, Kraemer, & Steiner, 2000).

The association between income level and health is so strong that it appears not only at the poverty level, but also at higher income levels as well. That is, very wealthy people have better health than people who are just, well, wealthy. Why should very wealthy people be healthier than other wealthy people? One possibility comes from the relation of income to educational level, which, in turn, relates to occupation, social class, and ethnicity. The higher the educational level, the less likely people are to engage in unhealthy behaviors such as smoking, eating a high-fat diet, and maintaining a sedentary lifestyle (see Would You Believe …? box). Another possibility is the perception of social status. People's perception of their social standing may differ from their status as indexed by educational, occupational, and income level, and this perception relates to health status more strongly than objective measures (Operario, Adler, & Williams, 2004). Thus, the relationships between health and ethnicity are intertwined with the relationships between health, income, education, and social class.

Changes in Life Expectancy   During the 20th century, life expectancy rose dramatically in the United States and other industrialized nations. In 1900, life expectancy was 47.3 years, whereas today it is more than 77 years (NCHS, 2011). In other words, infants born today can expect, on average, to live more than a generation longer than their great-great-grandparents born at the beginning of the 20th century.

What accounts for the 30-year increase in life expectancy during the 20th century? Question 3 from the quiz inside the front cover asks if advances in medical care were responsible for this increase. The answer is "False"; other factors have been more important than medical care of sick people. The single most important contributor to the increase in life expectancy is the lowering of infant mortality. When infants die before their first birthday, these deaths lower the population's

Would You BELIEVE …? College Is Good for Your Health

Would you believe that attending college is probably good for your health? You may find that difficult to believe, as college seems to add stress, offer opportunities for drug use, and limit the time available for eating a healthy diet, exercising, and sleeping. How could going to college possibly be healthy?

Students may not follow all recommendations for leading a healthy life while they are in college, but people who have been to college have lower death rates than those who have not. This advantage applies to both women and men and to infectious diseases, chronic diseases, and unintentional injuries (NCHS, 2011). Better educated people report fewer daily symptoms and less stress than less educated people (Grzywacz, Almeida, Neupert, & Ettner, 2004).

People who graduate from high school have lower death rates than those who do not, but going to college offers much more protection. For example, people with less than a high school education die at a rate of 575 per 100,000; those with a high school degree die at a rate of 509 per 100,000; but people who attend college have a death rate of only 214 per 100,000 (Miniño, Murphy, Xu, & Kochanek, 2011). That is, people who attend college show a death rate *less than half* that of high school graduates. The benefits of education for health and longevity apply to people around the world. For example, a study of older people in Japan (Fujino et al., 2005) found that low educational level increased the risk of dying. A large-scale study of the Dutch population (Hoeymans, van Lindert, & Westert, 2005) also found that education was related to a wide range of health measures and health-related behaviors.

What factors contribute to this health advantage for people with more education? Part of that advantage may be intelligence, which predicts both health and longevity (Gottfredson & Deary, 2004). In addition, people who are well educated tend to live with and around people with similar education, providing an environment with good health-related knowledge and attitudes (Øystein, 2008). Income and occupation may also contribute (Batty et al., 2008); people who attend college, especially those who graduate, have better jobs and higher average incomes than those who do not, and thus are more likely to have better access to health care. In addition, educated people are more likely to be informed consumers of health care, gathering information on their diseases and potential treatments. Education is also associated with a variety of habits that contribute to good health and long life. For example, people with a college education are less likely than others to smoke or use illicit drugs (Johnston, O'Malley, Bachman, & Schulenberg, 2007), and they are more likely to eat a low-fat diet and to exercise.

Thus, people who attend college acquire many resources that are reflected in their lower death rate—income potential, health knowledge, more health-conscious spouses and friends, attitudes about the importance of health, and positive health habits.

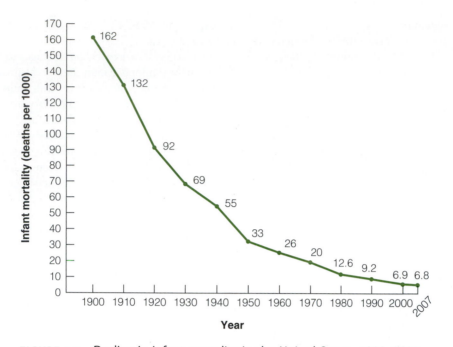

FIGURE 1.3 Decline in infant mortality in the United States, 1900–2007.

Source: Data from *Historical statistics of the United States: Colonial times to 1970*, 1975 by U.S. Bureau of the Census, Washington, DC: U.S. Government Printing Office, p. 60; *Statistical abstract of the United States: 2012* (131st edition), 2011, by U.S. Census Bureau, Washington, DC: U.S. Government Printing Office, Table 116.

average life expectancy much more than do the deaths of middle-aged or older people. As Figure 1.3 shows, infant death rates declined dramatically between 1900 and 1990, but little decrease has occurred since that time.

Prevention of disease also contributes to the recent increase in life expectancy. Widespread vaccination and safer drinking water and milk supplies all reduce infectious disease, which increases life expectancy. A healthier lifestyle also contributes to increased life expectancy, as does more efficient disposal of sewage and better nutrition. In contrast, advances in medical care—such as antibiotics and new surgical technology, efficient paramedic teams, and more skilled intensive care personnel—have played a relatively minor role in increasing adults' life expectancy.

Escalating Cost of Medical Care

The second major change within the field of health is the escalating cost of medical care. In the United States, medical costs have increased at a much faster rate than inflation. Between 1960 and 2005, these costs

represented a larger and larger proportion of the gross domestic product (GDP). Since 1995, the increases have slowed, but medical care costs as a percentage of the GDP have crept up to 15% (Organisation for Economic Co-operation and Development [OECD], 2008). This percentage is greater than in any other country, although several European countries spend about 10% of their GDP on medical care (OECD, 2008). The total yearly cost of health care in the United States increased from $1,067 per person in 1970 to $7,290 in 2007 (NCHS, 2011), a jump of more than 600% and a much faster annual increase than that reported for the years 1960 to 1980.

These costs, of course, have some relationship to increased life expectancy: As people live to middle and old age, they tend to develop chronic diseases that require extended (and often expensive) medical treatment. About 45% of people in the United States have a chronic condition, and they account for 78% of the dollars spent on health care (Rice & Fineman, 2004). People with chronic conditions account for 88% of prescriptions written, 72% of physician visits, and 76% of hospital stays. Even though today's aging population is

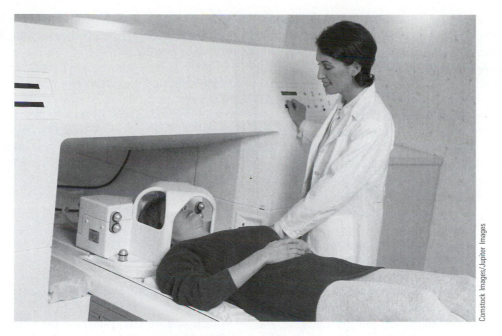

Technology in medicine is one reason for escalating medical costs.

experiencing better health than past generations, their increasing numbers will continue to increase medical costs.

One strategy for curbing mounting medical costs is to limit services, but another approach requires a greater emphasis on the early detection of disease and on changes to a healthier lifestyle and to behaviors that help prevent disease. For example, early detection of high blood pressure, high serum cholesterol, and other precursors of heart disease allow these conditions to be controlled, thereby decreasing the risk of serious disease or death. Screening people for risk is preferable to remedial treatment because chronic diseases are quite difficult to cure and living with chronic disease decreases quality of life. Avoiding disease by adopting a healthy lifestyle is even more preferable to treating diseases or screening for risks. Staying healthy is typically less costly than becoming sick and then getting well. Thus, prevention of disease through a healthy lifestyle, early detection of symptoms, and reduction of health risks are all part of a changing philosophy within the health care field.

What Is Health?

"Once again, the patient as a human being with worries, fears, hopes, and despairs, as an indivisible whole

and not merely the bearer of organs—of a diseased liver or stomach—is becoming the legitimate object of medical interest" (Alexander, 1950, p. 17).

What does it mean to be "healthy"? Question 1 from the quiz at the beginning of the book asks if health is merely the absence of disease. But is health more complex? Is health the presence of some positive condition rather than merely the absence of a negative one?

The **biomedical model** is the traditional view of Western medicine, which defines health as the absence of disease (Papas, Belar, & Rozensky, 2004). This view conceptualizes disease exclusively as a biological process that is an almost mechanistic result of exposure to a specific **pathogen**, a disease-causing organism. This view spurred the development of drugs and medical technology oriented toward removing the pathogens and curing disease. The focus is on disease, which is traceable to a specific agent. Removing the pathogen restores health.

The biomedical model of disease is compatible with infectious diseases that were the leading causes of death 100 years ago. Throughout the 20th century, adherence to the biomedical model allowed medicine to conquer or control many of the diseases that once ravaged humanity. However, when chronic illnesses began to replace infectious diseases as leading cause of death, the biomedical model became inadequate (Stone, 1987).

An alternative model of health exists now, one that advocates a holistic approach to medicine. This holistic model considers social, psychological, physiological, and even spiritual aspects of a person's health. An alternative model must have the power of the old model plus the ability to solve problems that the old model has failed to solve. This alternative model is the **biopsychosocial model**, the approach to health that includes biological, psychological, and social influences. This model holds that many diseases result from a combination of factors such as genetics, physiology, social support, personal control, stress, compliance, personality, poverty, ethnic background, and cultural beliefs. We discuss each of these factors in subsequent chapters. For now, it is important to recognize that the biopsychosocial model has at least two advantages over the older biomedical model: First, it incorporates not only biological conditions but also psychological and social factors, and second, it views health as a positive

condition. The biopsychosocial model can also account for some surprising findings about who gets sick and who stays healthy (see Would You Believe …? box).

According to the biopsychosocial view, health is much more than the absence of disease. A person who has no disease condition is not sick, but this person may not be healthy either. Because health is multidimensional, all aspects of living—biological, psychological, and social—must be considered. This view diverges from the traditional Western conceptualization, but as Table 1.2 shows, other cultures have held different views.

In 1946, the United Nations established the World Health Organization (WHO) and wrote into the preamble of its constitution a modern, Western definition: "Health is a state of complete physical, mental, and social well-being, and not merely the absence of disease or infirmity." This definition clearly affirms that health is a positive state and not just the absence of pathogens. Feeling good is more than not feeling bad, and research in neuroscience has confirmed the difference (Zautra, 2003). The human brain responds in distinctly different

Would You BELIEVE …? It Takes More Than a Virus to Give You a Cold

One of the dirtiest jobs an aspiring health psychologist could probably have is as a research assistant in Sheldon Cohen's laboratory at Carnegie Mellon University. Cohen's assistants sift through the trash of their study participants and search for used, mucous-filled tissues. When such tissues are found, the assistants carefully unfold them, locate the gooey treasures within, and painstakingly weigh their discoveries. These assistants have good reason to rummage for snot: They want an objective measure of just how severely their participants caught the common cold.

Sheldon Cohen and his research team investigate the psychological and social factors that predict the likelihood that a person will succumb to infection. Healthy participants in Cohen's studies receive a

cold or flu virus via a nasal squirt and then get quarantined in a "cold research laboratory"—actually, a hotel room—for a week. Participants also answer a number of questionnaires about psychological and social factors such as recent stress, typical positive and negative emotions, and the size and quality of their social networks. Cohen and his team use these questionnaires to predict who gets the cold and who remains healthy.

Cohen's findings expose the inadequacy of the biomedical approach to understanding infection. Despite the fact that everybody in his studies gets exposed to the same pathogen in exactly the same manner, only a subset gets sick. Importantly, the people who resist infection share similar psychological

and social characteristics. Compared with people who get sick, those who remain healthy are less likely to have dealt with recent stressful experiences (Cohen, Tyrrell, & Smith, 1991), have better sleep habits (Cohen, Doyle, Alper, Janicki-Deverts, & Turner, 2009), typically experience more positive emotion (Cohen, Alper, Doyle, Treanor, & Turner, 2006), are more sociable (Cohen, Doyle, Turner, Alper, & Skoner, 2003), and have more diverse social networks (Cohen, Doyle, Skoner, Rabin, & Gwaltney, 1997).

Thus, it takes more than just exposure to a virus to succumb to a cold or flu bug; exposure to the pathogen interacts with psychological and social factors to produce illness. Only the biopsychosocial model can account for these influences.

TABLE 1.2 Definitions of Health Held by Various Cultures

Culture	Time Period	Health Is
Prehistoric	10,000 BCE	Endangered by spirits that enter the body from outside
Babylonians and Assyrians	1800–700 BCE	Endangered by the gods, who send disease as a punishment
Ancient Hebrews	1000–300 BCE	A gift from God; disease is a punishment from God
Ancient Greeks	500 BCE	A holistic unity of body and spirit
Ancient China	Between 800 and 200 BCE	A state of physical and spiritual harmony with nature
Native Americans	1000 BCE–present	Total harmony with nature and the ability to survive under difficult conditions
Galen in Ancient Rome	130–200 CE	The absence of pathogens, such as bad air or body fluids, that cause disease
Early Christians	300–600 CE	Not as important as disease, which is a sign that one is chosen by God
Descartes in France	1596–1650	A condition of the mechanical body, which is separate from the mind
Western Africans	1600–1800	Harmony achieved through interactions with other people and objects in the world
Virchow in Germany	Late 1800s	Endangered by microscopic organisms that invade cells, producing disease
Freud in Austria	Late 1800s	Influenced by emotions and the mind
World Health Organization	1946	"A state of complete physical, mental, and social well-being"

patterns to positive feelings and negative feelings. Furthermore, this broader definition of health can account for the importance of preventive behavior in physical health. For example, a healthy person is not merely somebody without current disease or disability, but also somebody who behaves in a way that is likely to maintain that state in the future.

IN SUMMARY

In the past century, four major trends changed the field of health care. One trend is the changing pattern of disease and death in industrialized nations, including the United States. Chronic diseases now replace infectious diseases as the leading causes of death and disability. These chronic diseases include heart disease, stroke, cancer, emphysema, and adult-onset diabetes, all of which have causes that include individual behavior.

The increase in chronic disease contributed to a second trend: the escalating cost of medical care.

Costs for medical care rose dramatically between 1970 and 2005, but more recent gains have slowed in relation to the gross domestic product. Much of this cost increase is due to a growing elderly population, innovative but expensive medical technology, and inflation.

A third trend is the changing definition of health. Many people continue to view health as the absence of disease, but a growing number of health care professionals view health as a state of positive well-being. To accept this definition of health, one must reconsider the biomedical model that has dominated the health care field.

The fourth trend, the emergence of the biopsychosocial model of health, relates to the changing definition of health. Rather than define disease as the simple presence of pathogens, the biopsychosocial model emphasizes positive health and sees disease, particularly chronic disease, as resulting from the interaction of biological, psychological, and social conditions.

Psychology's Relevance for Health

Although chronic diseases have biological causes, individual behavior and lifestyle contribute to their development. Because behavior is so important for chronic disease, psychology—the science of behavior—is now more relevant to health care than ever before.

It took many years, however, for psychology to gain acceptance by the medical field. In 1911, the American Psychological Association (APA) recommended that psychology be part of the medical school curriculum, but most medical schools failed to pursue this recommendation. During the 1940s, the medical specialty of psychiatry incorporated the study of psychological factors related to disease into its training, but few psychologists were involved in health research (Matarazzo, 1994). During the 1960s, psychology's role in medicine began to expand with the creation of new medical schools; the number of psychologists who held academic appointments on medical school faculties nearly tripled from 1969 to 1993 (Matarazzo, 1994). By the beginning of the 21st century, psychologists had made significant progress in their efforts to gain greater acceptance by the medical profession (Pingitore, Scheffler, Haley, Seniell, & Schwalm, 2001).

In 2002, the American Medical Association (AMA) accepted several new categories for health and behavior that permit psychologists to bill for services to patients with physical diseases. Also, Medicare's Graduate Medical Education program now accepts psychology internships, and the APA has worked with the World Health Organization to formulate a new diagnostic system for biopsychosocial disorders, the International Classification of Functioning, Disability, and Health (Reed & Scheldeman, 2004). Thus, the role of psychologists in medical settings has expanded beyond traditional mental health problems to include procedures and programs to help people stop smoking, eat a healthy diet, exercise, adhere to medical advice, reduce stress, control pain, live with chronic disease, and avoid unintentional injuries.

The Contribution of Psychosomatic Medicine

The biopsychosocial model accepts that psychological and emotional factors contribute to physical health problems. This notion is not new, as Socrates and

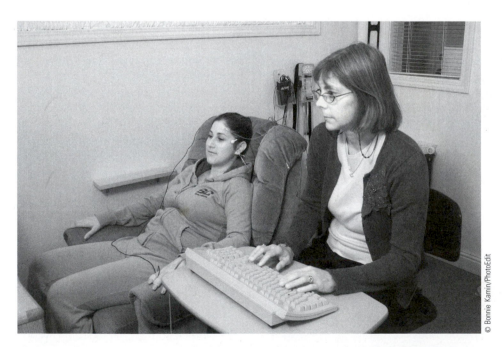

The role of the psychologist in health care settings has expanded beyond traditional mental health problems to include procedures such as biofeedback.

Hippocrates proposed similar ideas. Furthermore, this notion is compatible with the theories of Sigmund Freud, who emphasized the importance of unconscious psychological factors in the development of physical symptoms. However, Freud's methods relied on clinical experience and intuitive hunches, not research.

The search to tie emotional causes to illness drew from Walter Cannon's observation in 1932 that physiological changes accompany emotion (Kimball, 1981). Cannon's research demonstrated that emotions can cause physiological changes that are capable of causing disease. From this finding, Helen Flanders Dunbar (1943) developed the notion that habitual responses, which people exhibit as part of their personalities, relate to specific diseases. In other words, Dunbar hypothesized a relationship between personality type and disease. A little later, Franz Alexander (1950), a onetime follower of Freud, began to see emotional conflicts as a precursor to certain diseases.

These views led others to see a range of specific illnesses as "psychosomatic." These illnesses included such disorders as peptic ulcer, rheumatoid arthritis, hypertension, asthma, hyperthyroidism, and ulcerative colitis. This belief diverged from the biomedical view, which concentrates on the body and ignores the mind. However, the widespread belief in the separation of mind and body—a belief that originated with Descartes (Papas et al., 2004)—led many laypeople to look at these psychosomatic disorders as not being "real" but merely "all in the head." Thus, psychosomatic medicine exerted a mixed impact on the acceptance of psychology within medicine; it benefited by connecting emotional and physical conditions, but it may have harmed by belittling the psychological components of illness. Psychosomatic medicine, however, laid the foundation for the transition to the biopsychosocial model of health and disease (Novack et al., 2007).

The Emergence of Behavioral Medicine

Two new and interrelated disciplines emerged from the psychosomatic medicine movement: *behavioral medicine* and *health psychology*.

The field of **behavioral medicine** developed from a 1977 conference at Yale University. Behavioral medicine is "the interdisciplinary field concerned with the development and integration of behavioral and biomedical science knowledge and techniques relevant to health and illness and the application of this knowledge and these techniques to prevention, diagnosis, treatment and rehabilitation" (Schwartz & Weiss, 1978, p. 250). A key component of this definition is the integration of biomedical science with behavioral sciences, especially psychology. The goals of behavioral medicine are similar to those in other areas of health care: improved prevention, diagnosis, treatment, and rehabilitation. Behavioral medicine, however, attempts to use psychology and the behavioral sciences in conjunction with medicine to achieve these goals. Chapters 3 through 11 cover topics in behavioral medicine.

The Emergence of Health Psychology

At about the same time that behavioral medicine appeared, a task force of the American Psychological Association reported that few psychologists conducted health research (American Psychological Association Task Force, 1976). The report envisioned a future in which psychologists would contribute to the enhancement of health and prevention of disease.

In 1978, with the establishment of Division 38 of the American Psychological Association, the field of **health psychology** officially began. Health psychology is the branch of psychology that concerns individual behaviors and lifestyles affecting a person's physical health. Health psychology includes psychology's contributions to the enhancement of health, the prevention and treatment of disease, the identification of health risk factors, the improvement of the health care system, and the shaping of public opinion with regard to health. More specifically, it involves the application of psychological principles to physical health areas such as controlling cholesterol, managing stress, alleviating pain, stopping smoking, and moderating other risky behaviors, as well as encouraging regular exercise, medical and dental checkups, and safer behaviors. In addition, health psychology helps identify conditions that affect health, diagnose and treat certain chronic diseases, and modify the behavioral factors involved in physiological and psychological rehabilitation. As such, health psychology interacts with both biology and sociology to produce health- and disease-related outcomes (see Figure 1.4). Note that neither psychology nor sociology contributes directly to outcomes; only biological factors contribute directly to physical health and disease. Thus, the psychological and sociological factors that affect

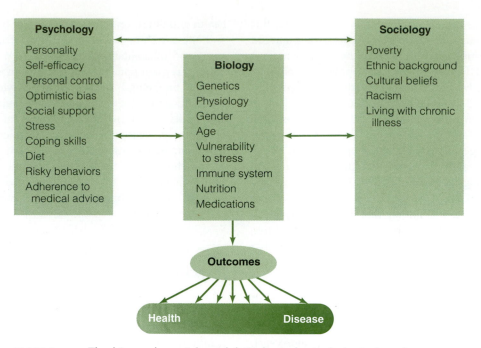

FIGURE 1.4 The biopsychosocial model: Biological, psychological, and sociological factors interact to produce health or disease.

health must "get under the skin" in some way in order to affect biological processes. One of the goals of health psychology is to identify those ways.

With its promotion of the biopsychosocial model, health psychology continues to grow. Clinical health psychology continues to gain recognition in providing health care as part of multidisciplinary teams. Health psychology researchers continue to build a knowledge base that will furnish information about the interconnections among psychological, social, and biological factors that relate to health.

IN SUMMARY

Psychology's involvement in health dates back to the beginning of the 20th century, but at that time, few psychologists were involved in medicine. The psychosomatic medicine movement sought to bring psychological factors into the understanding of disease, but that view gave way to the biopsychosocial approach to health and disease. By the 1970s, psychologists had begun to develop research and treatment aimed at chronic disease and health promotion; this research and treatment

led to the founding of two new fields, behavioral medicine and health psychology.

Behavioral medicine applies the knowledge and techniques of behavioral research to physical health, including prevention, diagnosis, treatment, and rehabilitation. Health psychology overlaps with behavioral medicine, and the two professions have many common goals. However, behavioral medicine is an interdisciplinary field, whereas health psychology is a specialty within the discipline of psychology. Health psychology strives to enhance health, prevent and treat disease, identify risk factors, improve the health care system, and shape public opinion regarding health issues.

The Profession of Health Psychology

Health psychology now stands as a unique field and profession. Health psychologists have their own associations, publish their research in journals devoted to health psychology (*Health Psychology* and *Annals of*

Behavioral Medicine, among others), and acquire training in unique doctoral and postdoctoral programs. In addition, health psychology is becoming recognized within medical schools, schools of public health, universities, and hospitals, and health psychologists work within all of these settings. However, their training occurs within psychology.

The Training of Health Psychologists

Health psychologists are psychologists first and specialists in health second, but the training in health is extensive. People who pursue research in health psychology must learn the topics, theories, and methods of health psychology research. Health psychologists who provide clinical care, known as clinical health psychologists, must learn clinical skills and how to practice as part of a health care team.

Health psychologists usually complete the core courses required of all psychologists and then a program specializing in health psychology. Health psychologists typically receive a solid core of graduate training in such areas as (1) the biological bases of behavior, health, and disease; (2) the cognitive and affective bases of behavior, health, and disease; (3) the social bases of health and disease, including knowledge of health organizations and health policy; (4) the psychological bases of health and disease, with emphasis on individual differences; (5) advanced research, methodology, and statistics; (6) psychological and health measurement; (7) interdisciplinary collaboration; and (8) ethics and professional issues (Belar, 2008). Some health psychologists also seek out training in medical subspecialties such as neurology, endocrinology, immunology, and epidemiology. This training may occur in a doctoral program (Baum, Perry, & Tarbell, 2004), but many health psychologists also obtain postdoctoral training, with at least 2 years of specialized training in health psychology to follow a PhD or PsyD in psychology (Belar, 1997; Matarazzo, 1987). Practicums and internships in health care settings in hospitals and clinics are common components of training in clinical health psychology (Nicassio, Meyerowitz, & Kerns, 2004).

No single discipline in the health care field has the capacity to solve all the problems of health promotion and disease prevention, but the interdisciplinary training of health psychologists equips them to make valuable contributions (Travis, 2001). This interdisciplinary collaboration necessitates skills of cooperation for health psychologists, and their training should prepare them to become part of multidisciplinary teams. Some experts have called for training that equips health psychologists to become primary health care providers in traditional medical settings, including preparation for board certification (McDaniel, Belar, Schroeder, Hargrove, & Freeman, 2002; Tovian, 2004). Thus, training in health psychology is becoming more complex as the work of health psychologists becomes more varied.

The Work of Health Psychologists

Health psychologists work in a variety of settings, and their work setting varies according to their specialty. Some health psychologists such as Angela Bryan are primarily researchers, who typically work in universities or government agencies that conduct research, such as the Centers for Disease Control and Prevention and the National Institutes of Health. Health psychology research encompasses many topics; it may focus on behaviors related to the development of disease or on evaluation of the effectiveness of new interventions and treatments. Clinical health psychologists are often employed in hospitals, pain clinics, or community clinics. Other settings for clinical health psychologists include health maintenance organizations (HMOs) and private practice.

As Angela Bryan's work shows, health psychologists may engage in some combination of teaching, conducting research, and providing a variety of services to individuals as well as private and public agencies. Much of their work is collaborative in nature; health psychologists engaged in either research or practice may work with a team of health professionals, including physicians, nurses, physical therapists, and counselors.

The services provided by health psychologists working in clinics and hospitals fit into several categories. One type of service offers alternatives to pharmacological treatment; for example, biofeedback might be an alternative to analgesic drugs for headache patients. Another type of service is providing behavioral interventions to treat physical disorders, such as chronic pain and some gastrointestinal problems, or to improve the rate of patient compliance with medical regimens. Other clinical health psychologists may provide assessments using psychological and neuropsychological tests, or provide psychological treatment for patients coping with disease. Those who concentrate on prevention and behavior changes are more likely to be employed in health maintenance organizations, school-based prevention programs, or worksite wellness programs. All these organizations use services that trained health psychologists can perform.

Like Angela Bryan, most health psychologists are engaged in several activities. The combination of teaching and research is common among those in educational settings. Those who work exclusively in service delivery settings are much less likely to teach and do research and are more likely to spend the majority of their time providing diagnoses and interventions for people with health problems. Some health psychology students go into allied health profession fields, such as social work, occupational therapy, dietetics, or public health. Those who go into public health often work in academic settings or government agencies and may monitor trends in health issues, or develop and evaluate educational interventions and health awareness campaigns. Health psychologists also contribute to the development and evaluation of wide-scale public health decisions, including taxes and warning labels placed upon healthy products such as cigarettes, and the inclusion of nutrition information on food products and menus.

IN SUMMARY

To maximize their contributions to health care, health psychologists must be both broadly trained in the science of psychology and specifically trained in the knowledge and skills of such areas as neurology, endocrinology, immunology, epidemiology, and other medical subspecialties. Health psychologists with a solid background in generic psychology and specialized knowledge in medical fields work in a variety of settings, including universities, hospitals, clinics, private practice, and health maintenance organizations. They typically collaborate with other health care professionals in providing services for physical disorders rather than for traditional areas of mental health care. Research in health psychology is also likely to be a collaborative effort that may include the professions of medicine, epidemiology, nursing, pharmacology, nutrition, and exercise physiology.

Answers

This chapter has addressed three basic questions:

1. How have views of health changed?

Views of health are changing, both among health care professionals and among the general public. Several trends have prompted these changes, including (1) the changing pattern of disease and death in the United States from infectious diseases to chronic diseases, (2) the increase in medical costs, (3) the growing acceptance of a view of health that includes not only the absence of disease but also the presence of positive well-being, and (4) the biopsychosocial model of health that departs from the traditional biomedical model and the psychosomatic model by including not only biochemical abnormalities but also psychological and social conditions.

2. How did psychology become involved in health care?

Psychology has been involved in health almost from the beginning of the 20th century. During those early years, however, only a few psychologists worked in medical settings, and most were not considered full partners with physicians.

Psychosomatic medicine highlighted psychological explanations of certain somatic diseases, emphasizing the role of emotions in the development of disease. By the early 1970s, psychology and other behavioral sciences were beginning to play a role in the prevention and treatment of chronic diseases and in the promotion of positive health, giving rise to two new fields: behavioral medicine and health psychology.

Behavioral medicine is an interdisciplinary field concerned with applying the knowledge and techniques of behavioral science to the maintenance of physical health and to prevention, diagnosis, treatment, and rehabilitation. Behavioral medicine, which is not a branch of psychology, overlaps with health psychology, a division within the field of psychology. Health psychology uses the science of psychology to enhance health, prevent and treat disease, identify risk factors, improve the health care system, and shape public opinion with regard to health.

3. What type of training do health psychologists receive, and what kinds of work do they do?

Health psychologists receive doctoral-level training in the basic core of psychology, including (1) the biological, cognitive, psychological, and social bases of behavior, health, and disease; (2) advanced research, methodology, and statistics; (3) psychology and health measurement; (4) interdisciplinary collaboration; and (5) ethics and professional issues. In addition, they often receive at least 2 years of postdoctoral work in a specialized area of health psychology.

Health psychologists are employed in a variety of settings, including universities, hospitals, clinics, private practice, and health maintenance organizations. Clinical health psychologists provide services, often as part of a health care team. Health psychologists who are researchers typically collaborate with others, sometimes as part of a multidisciplinary team, to conduct research on behaviors related to the development of disease or to evaluate the effectiveness of new treatments.

Suggested Readings

Baum, A., Perry, N. W., Jr., & Tarbell, S. (2004). The development of psychology as a health science. In R. G. Frank, A. Baum, & J. L. Wallander (Eds.), *Handbook of clinical health psychology* (Vol. 3, pp. 9–28). Washington, DC: American Psychological Association. This recent review of the development of health psychology describes the background and current status of the field of health psychology.

Belar, C. D. (2008). Clinical health psychology: A health care specialty in professional psychology. *Professional Psychology: Research and Practice, 39,* 229–233. Clinical health psychology is the applied branch of health psychology. Cynthia Belar traces the development of this field from the beginning, pointing out the widespread influence of health psychology on research and practice in clinical psychology.

Leventhal, H., Weinman, J., Leventhal, E. A., & Phillips, L. A. (2008). Health psychology: The search for pathways between behavior and health. *Annual Review of Psychology, 59,* 477–505. This article details how psychological theory and research can improve the effectiveness of interventions for managing chronic illness.

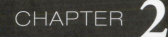

Conducting Health Research

CHAPTER OUTLINE

- **Real-World Profile of Sylvester Colligan**
- *The Placebo in Treatment and Research*
- *Research Methods in Psychology*
- *Research Methods in Epidemiology*
- *Determining Causation*
- *Research Tools*

QUESTIONS

This chapter focuses on five basic questions:

1. What are placebos, and how do they affect research and treatment?

2. How does psychology research contribute to health knowledge?

3. How has epidemiology contributed to health knowledge?

4. How can scientists determine if a behavior causes a disease?

5. How do theory and measurement contribute to health psychology?

☑CHECK YOUR BELIEFS

About Health Research

Check the items that are consistent with your beliefs.

☐ 1. Placebo effects can influence physical as well as psychological problems.

☐ 2. Pain patients who expect a medication to relieve their pain often experience a reduction in pain, even after taking a "sugar pill."

☐ 3. Personal testimonials are a good way to decide about treatment effectiveness.

☐ 4. Newspaper and television reports of scientific research give an accurate picture of the importance of the research.

☐ 5. Information from longitudinal studies is generally more informative than information from the study of one person.

☐ 6. All scientific methods yield equally valuable results, so the research method is not important in determining the validity of results.

☐ 7. In determining important health information, studies with nonhuman subjects can be just as important as those with human participants.

☐ 8. Results from experimental research are more likely than results from observational research to suggest the underlying cause for a disease.

☐ 9. People outside the scientific community conduct valuable research, but scientists try to discount the importance of such research.

☐ 10. Scientific breakthroughs happen every day.

☐ 11. New reports of health research often contradict previous findings, so there is no way to use this information to make good personal decisions about health.

Items 1, 2, 5, and 8 are consistent with sound scientific information, but each of the other items represents a naïve or unrealistic view of research that can make you an uninformed consumer of health research. Information in this chapter will help you become more sophisticated in your evaluation of and expectations for health research.

Real-World Profile of
SYLVESTER COLLIGAN

Sylvester Colligan was a 76-year-old man who had been having trouble with his right knee for 5 years (Talbot, 2000). His doctor diagnosed arthritis but had no treatment that would help. However, this physician told Colligan about an experimental study conducted by Dr. J. Bruce Moseley. Colligan talked to Moseley and reported, "I was very impressed with him, especially when I heard he was the team doctor with the [Houston] Rockets…. So, sure, I went ahead and signed up for this new thing he was doing" (Talbot, 2000, p. 36).

The treatment worked. Two years after the surgery, Colligan reported that his knee had not bothered him since the surgery. "It's just like my other knee now. I give a whole lot of credit to Dr. Moseley. Whenever I see him on the TV during a basketball game, I call the wife in and say, 'Hey, there's the doctor that fixed my knee!'" (Talbot, 2000, p. 36).

Colligan's improvement would not be so surprising, except for one thing: Moseley did not perform surgery on Colligan. Instead, Moseley gave Colligan anesthesia, made some cuts around Colligan's knee that *looked* like surgical incisions, and then sent Colligan on his way home.

Why did Colligan get better? Was Moseley negligent in performing a fake surgery on Colligan? Surprisingly, many people do not view Moseley's treatment as negligent. Moseley and his colleagues (2002) were conducting a study of the effectiveness of arthroscopic knee surgery. This type of procedure is widely performed but expensive, and Moseley had doubts about its effectiveness (Talbot, 2000). So Moseley decided to perform an experimental study that included a placebo as well as a real arthroscopic surgery. A **placebo** is an inactive substance or condition that has the appearance of an active treatment and that may cause participants to improve or change because of their belief in the placebo's efficacy.

Moseley suspected that this type of belief and not the surgery was producing improvements, so he designed a study in which half the participants received sham knee surgery. Participants in this condition received anesthesia and surgical lesions to the knee, but no further treatment. The other half of the participants received standard arthroscopic knee surgery. The participants agreed to be in either group, knowing that they might receive sham surgery. The participants, including Colligan, did not know for several years whether they were in the placebo or the arthroscopic surgery group. Moseley discovered, contrary to widespread belief, that arthroscopic knee surgery provided no real benefits beyond a placebo effect. Those who received the sham surgery reported the same level of knee pain and functioning as those who received the real surgical treatment.

Moseley's findings join those of hundreds of other studies: A belief in the effectiveness of a treatment boosts the treatment's effectiveness. However, this effect presents a problem for researchers like Moseley, who want to determine which effects are due to treatment and which are due to beliefs about the treatment.

This chapter looks at the way scientists work, emphasizing psychology from the behavioral sciences and epidemiology from the biomedical sciences. These two disciplines share some methods for investigating health-related behaviors, but the two areas also have their own unique contributions to scientific methodology. Before we begin to examine the methods that psychologists and epidemiologists use in their research, we need to consider the situation that Sylvester Colligan experienced—improvement due to the placebo effect.

The Placebo in Treatment and Research

As we described in Chapter 1, health psychology involves the application of psychological principles to the understanding and improvement of physical health. The placebo effect represents one of the clearest examples of the link between people's beliefs and their physical health. Like many people receiving treatment, Colligan benefited from his positive expectations; he improved, even though he received a treatment that technically should not have led to improvement.

Most physicians are aware of the placebo effect, and many may even prescribe placebos when no other effective treatments are available (Tilburt, Emanuel, Kaptchuk, Curlin, & Miller, 2008). However, strong placebo effects can pose a problem for scientists trying to evaluate if a new treatment is effective. Thus, the placebo effect may help individuals who receive treatment but complicate the job of researchers; that is, it can have treatment benefits but research drawbacks.

Treatment and the Placebo

The power of placebo effects was nothing new to Moseley, as the potency of "sugar pills" had been recognized for years. Henry Beecher (1955) observed the effects of placebos on a variety of conditions ranging from headache to the common cold. Beecher concluded that the therapeutic effect of the placebo was substantial—about 35% of patients showed improvement! Hundreds of studies have since examined placebo effects. A recent review of this research confirms that placebos can lead to noticeable improvements in health outcomes, especially in the context of pain and nausea (Hróbjartsson & Gøtzsche, 2010). For example, a meta-analysis of migraine headache prevention (Macedo, Baños, & Farré, 2008) shows a placebo effect of 21%. A more recent review (Cepeda, Berlin, Gao, Wiegand, & Wada, 2012) reveals that anywhere from 7% to 43% of patients in pain improve following administration of a placebo, with the likelihood of improvement largely attributable to the type of pain experienced.

Placebo effects occur in many other health conditions aside from pain and nausea. For example, some researchers (Fournier et al., 2010) argue that the placebo effect is responsible for much of the effectiveness of antidepressant drugs, especially among people with mild to moderate symptoms. However, some conditions such as broken bones are not responsive to placebos (Kaptchuk, Eisenberg, & Komaroff, 2002).

The more a placebo resembles an effective treatment, the stronger the placebo effect. Big pills are more effective than little ones, and colored pills work better than white tablets. Capsules work better than tablets, and placebos labeled with brand names work

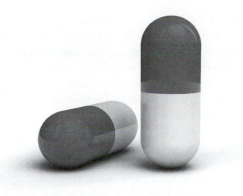

kasiastock/Shutterstock

The more a placebo resembles an effective treatment, the stronger the placebo effect. These sugar pills, which look like real pills, are likely to have strong placebo effects.

better than generics. Two doses provoke a larger placebo response than one dose. An injection is more powerful than a pill, and surgery tends to prompt an even larger placebo response than an injection does. Even cost matters; more expensive placebo pills work better than cheaper pills (Waber, Shiv, Carmon, & Ariely, 2008)!

Both physician and patient expectations also strengthen placebo effects. Physicians who appear positive and hopeful about treatment prompt a stronger response in their patients (Moerman, 2003). Placebo responses also relate to other characteristics of the practitioner, such as his or her reputation, attention, interest, concern, and the confidence the practitioner projects that a treatment will be effective (Moerman & Jonas, 2002). Interestingly, when researchers tell patient-participants that they could be receiving either a placebo or a real treatment—as Moseley told Colligan—placebo effects tend to weaken because the participant is less confident about receiving an effective treatment (Price, Finniss, & Benedetti, 2008). Furthermore, participants do not typically choose which treatment they receive in a research study, which may also weaken the placebo effect. When a person chooses a treatment, placebo effects are stronger (Rose, Geers, Rasinski, & Fowler, 2011).

How and why does the placebo effect occur? Although many people assume that improvements due to placebos are psychologically based—"It's in people's heads"—research suggests that they have both a physical and psychological basis (Benedetti, 2006; Scott

et al., 2008). For example, a placebo analgesic alters levels of brain activity in ways that are consistent with the activity that occurs during pain relief from analgesic drugs (Wager et al., 2004).

Placebos reduce or cure a remarkable range of disorders and symptoms, including insomnia, low back pain, burn pain, headache, asthma, hypertension, and anxiety (Hróbjartsson & Gøtzsche, 2001, 2004). These findings suggest that the underlying physiological mechanisms for placebo responses are the same as for drug treatments (Finniss & Benedetti, 2005). In addition, drugs that block the action of analgesic drugs also block the placebo response to analgesic drugs. Placebos can alter neurotransmitters, hormones, and endorphins, potentially producing a variety of perceptual, behavioral, and physical effects.

Placebos can also produce adverse effects, called the **nocebo effect** (Scott et al., 2008; Turner et al., 1994). Nearly 20% of healthy volunteers given a placebo in a double-blind study experienced some negative effect as a result of the nocebo effect. Sometimes, these negative effects appear as side effects, which show the same symptoms as other drug side effects, such as headaches, nausea and other digestive problems, dry mouth, and sleep disturbances (Amanzio, Corazzini, Vase, & Benedetti, 2009). The presence of negative effects demonstrates that the placebo effect is not merely improvement but includes any change resulting from an inert treatment. Recent research (Scott et al., 2008) shows that the nocebo response also activates specific areas of the brain and acts on neurotransmitters, giving additional support to its physical reality.

Expectancy is a major component of the placebo effect (Finniss & Benedetti, 2005; Stewart-Williams, 2004). People act in ways that they *think* they should. Thus, people who receive treatment without their knowledge do not benefit as much as those who know what to expect (Colloca, Lopiano, Lanotte, & Benedetti, 2004). In addition, culture influences the placebo response. For example, cultures that place greater faith in medical interventions show stronger responses to placebos that resemble a medical intervention (Moerman, 2011). Learning and conditioning are also factors in the placebo response. Through classical and operant conditioning, people associate a treatment with getting better, creating situations in which receiving treatment leads to improvements. Thus, both expectancy and learning contribute to the placebo effect.

When patients' positive expectations increase their chances for improvement, the placebo is a valuable adjunct in treatment. Indeed, in most situations involving medical treatment, patients' improvements may result from a combination of treatment plus the placebo effect (Finniss & Benedetti, 2005). Placebo effects are a tribute to the ability of humans to heal themselves, and practitioners can enlist this ability to help patients become healthier (Ezekiel & Miller, 2001; Walach & Jonas, 2004). Therefore, the placebo effect can be a positive factor in medical and behavioral therapies, as it was for Sylvester Colligan, whose knee improved as a result of sham surgery.

Research and the Placebo

The therapeutic properties of the placebo may be a plus for treatment, but its effects present problems in evaluating treatment effectiveness. For researchers to conclude that a treatment is effective, the treatment must show a higher rate of effectiveness than a placebo. Otherwise, any effects of treatment are probably due only to people's beliefs about the treatment. This standard calls for researchers to use at least two groups in a study: one that receives the treatment and another that receives a placebo. Both groups must have equal expectations concerning the effectiveness of the

treatment. In order to create equal expectancy, not only must the participants be ignorant of who is getting a placebo and who is getting the treatment, but the experimenters who dispense both conditions must also be "blind" as to which group is which. The arrangement in which neither participants nor experimenters know about treatment conditions is called a **double-blind design**. As the Would You Believe …? box points out, this design strategy creates ethical dilemmas.

Psychological treatments such as counseling, hypnosis, biofeedback, relaxation training, massage, and a variety of stress and pain management techniques also produce expectancy effects. That is, the placebo effect also applies to research in psychology, but double-blind designs are not easy to perform with these treatments. Placebo pills can look the same as pills containing an active ingredient, but providers of psychological or behavioral treatments always know when they are providing a sham treatment. In these studies, researchers use a **single-blind design** in which the participants do not know if they are receiving the active or inactive treatment, but the providers are not blind to treatment conditions. In single-blind designs, the control for expectancy is not as complete as in double-blind designs, but creating equal expectancies for participants is usually the more important control feature.

Would You BELIEVE …? Prescribing Placebos May Be Considered Ethical

Cebocap, a capsule available only by prescription, may be a wonder drug. The ingredients in Cebocap can be remarkably effective in relieving a wide range of health problems, with few serious side effects. Yet, Cebocap is not as widely prescribed as it could be. Surprisingly, many people would be upset to learn that their doctor prescribed them with Cebocap.

Cebocap is a placebo pill made by Forest Pharmaceuticals, the same company that manufactures the antidepressants Celexa® and Lexapro®. Why would a physician prescribe

Cebocap, and could it ever be ethical for a physician to do so?

Although it is unclear how often physicians prescribe Cebocap, many doctors already report prescribing treatments that they consider to be placebos, such as vitamins or antibiotics for a viral infection (Tilburt et al., 2008). However, nearly three quarters of doctors who admit to prescribing a placebo describe it simply as "Medicine not typically used for your condition but might benefit you" (Tilburt et al., 2008, p. 3). This is truthful and preserves the active ingredient of

placebos: positive expectations. However, critics of this practice argue that the physician is deceiving the patient by withholding the fact that the treatment has no inherent medical benefit.

Could a placebo still be effective if the provider fully informed the patient about the nature of the treatment? A recent study (Kaptchuk et al., 2010) set out to answer this question, by prescribing placebo pills to patients with irritable bowel syndrome (IBS). IBS is a chronic gastrointestinal disorder, characterized by recurrent abdominal pain. With few other effective treatments available for IBS, many view it as ethically permissible to study the effects of placebos on IBS symptoms.

In one experimental condition of this study, researchers told patients to take placebo pills twice daily, describing them as "made of an inert substance, like sugar pills, that have been shown in clinical studies to produce significant improvement in IBS symptoms through mind-body self-healing processes" (Kaptchuk et al., 2010, p. e15591). Patients in the control condition did not receive any treatment at all. Indeed, the placebo treatment—even when prescribed in this completely transparent manner—led to fewer symptoms, greater improvement, and better quality of life compared with no treatment. Thus, placebos can be both ethically prescribed *and* effective in treatment.

Can placebos be ethically used in research? Typically, clinical researchers do not seek to show that placebos can work. Rather, they seek to show that another treatment performs better than a placebo. Thus, clinical researchers may have to assign patients to an experimental condition that they know does constitute an effective treatment. How do researchers reconcile this ethical difficulty?

Part of the answer to that question lies in the rules governing research with human participants (APA, 2002; World Medical Association, 2004). Providing an ineffective treatment—or any other treatment—may be considered ethical if participants understand the risks fully and still agree to participate in the study. This element of research procedure, known as *informed consent*, stipulates that participants must be informed of factors in the research that may influence their willingness to participate before they consent to participate.

When participants in a clinical trial agree to take part in the study, they receive information about the possibility of getting a placebo rather than a treatment. Those participants who find the chances of receiving a placebo unacceptable may refuse to participate in the study. Sylvester Colligan, who participated in the study with arthroscopic knee surgery, knew that he might be included in a sham surgery group, and he consented (Talbot, 2000). However, 44% of those interviewed about that study declined to participate (Moseley et al., 2002).

Despite the value of placebo controls in clinical research, some physicians and medical ethicists consider the use of ineffective treatment to be ethically unacceptable because the welfare of patients is not the primary concern. This is a valid concern if a patient-participant receives a placebo instead of the accepted standard of care (Kottow, 2007). These critics contend that control groups should receive the standard treatment rather than a placebo, and that placebo treatment is acceptable only if no treatment exists for the condition. Thus, opinion regarding the ethical acceptability of placebo treatment is divided, with some finding it acceptable and necessary for research and others objecting to the failure to provide an adequate standard of treatment.

IN SUMMARY

A placebo is an inactive substance or condition having the appearance of an active treatment. It may cause participants in an experiment to improve or change behavior because of their belief in the placebo's effectiveness and their prior experiences with receiving effective treatment. Although placebos can have a positive effect from the patient's point of view, they are a continuing problem for the researcher. In general, a placebo's effects are about 35%; its effects on reducing pain may be higher, whereas its effects on other conditions may be lower. Placebos can influence a wide variety of disorders and diseases.

Experimental designs that measure the efficacy of an intervention, such as a drug, typically use a placebo so that people in the control group (who receive the placebo) have the same expectations for success as do people in the experimental group (who receive the active treatment). Drug studies are usually double-blind designs, meaning that neither the participants nor the people administering the drug know who receives the placebo and who receives the active drug. Researchers in psychological treatment studies are often not "blind" concerning the treatment, but participants are, creating a single-blind design for these studies.

Research Methods in Psychology

Not long ago, reports of health research appeared mainly in scientific journals, read primarily by physicians. People typically heard of this research from their physicians. Today, diverse outlets—including television, newspapers, and the Internet—publicize the "latest and greatest" health research. However, with this increased publicity comes an increasing problem: Some of this information may not be trustworthy. The news media are in the business of getting people's attention, so news coverage of health information may mislead by focusing on the most sensational findings. And, of course, some commercial advertisements—promoting, for instance, a revolutionary weight loss program or a simple way to stop smoking—may ignore or distort scientific evidence in order to boost sales.

Fortunately, there exists a vast body of health-related information that is relatively objective and free from self-serving claims. This information is produced by researchers trained in the behavioral and biomedical sciences, who typically are associated with universities, research hospitals, and government agencies. Because these women and men use the methods of science in their work, this evidence accumulates gradually over an extended period of time. Dramatic breakthroughs are rare. When scientists are familiar with each other's work, use controlled methods of collecting data, keep personal biases from contaminating results, make claims cautiously, and replicate their studies, evidence is more likely to be evolutionary rather than revolutionary. In contrast, "revolutionary" claims are most often motivated by financial or other personal interests.

How can you discern which findings are the most valid and important? To do so, it is important to know the major ways in health researchers gather and evaluate information. Much health-related information comes from studies conducted by behavioral and biomedical scientists using a variety of research methods. The choice of methods depends in large part on what questions the scientists are trying to answer—it is possible to approach any research topic in a variety of ways.

In this chapter, we use studies of obesity to illustrate common research methods. Obesity is a growing health problem (no pun intended!), both in the United States and in countries around the world (Flegal, Carroll, Kit, & Ogden, 2012; Swinburn et al., 2011). As you will see, findings from each research method add to an understanding of obesity and its relationship to a variety of behaviors and conditions.

When researchers want to identify the factors that predict or are related to either disease or healthy functioning, they use *correlational studies*. When they want to compare people across different age groups, they rely on *cross-sectional studies*. When they desire information on stability or instability of health status or some other characteristic over a period of time, they use *longitudinal studies*. When they wish to compare one group of participants with another, they use either *experimental designs* or *ex post facto designs*. All these methods from the discipline of psychology apply to the field of health.

Correlational Studies

Correlational studies yield information about the degree of relationship between two variables, such as body fat and heart disease. Correlational studies *describe* this relationship and are, therefore, a type of *descriptive research* design. Although scientists cannot determine causal relationships through a single descriptive study, the degree of relationship between two factors may be exactly what a researcher wants to know.

To assess the degree of relationship between two variables (such as body mass index [a measure of overweight] and blood pressure), the researcher measures each of these variables in a group of participants and then calculates the **correlation coefficient** between these measures. The calculation yields a number that varies between −1.00 and +1.00. Positive correlations occur when the two variables increase or decrease together. For example, physical activity and longevity are positively correlated. Negative correlations occur when one of the variables increases as the other decreases, as is the case with the relationship between smoking and longevity. Correlations that are closer to 1.00 (either positive or negative) indicate stronger relationships than do correlations that are closer to 0.00. Small correlations—those less than 0.10—can be *statistically significant* if they are based on a very large number of observations, as in a study with many participants. However, such small correlations, though not random, offer the researcher very little ability to predict scores on one variable from knowledge of scores on the other variable.

Correlation allowed a group of researchers (Heinrich et al., 2008) to study the relationship between neighborhood factors and overweight. The researchers assessed more than 400 residents of housing developments, measuring physical characteristics of the neighborhood and relating those characteristics to obesity. They found a negative correlation (of around −0.35, a

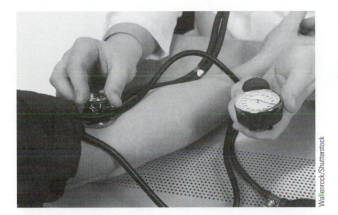

Blood pressure is a risk factor for cardiovascular disease, which means that people with high blood pressure are at increased risk, but not that high blood pressure causes cardiovascular disease.

medium-sized correlation) between neighborhood features that supported physical activity and obesity. That is, people who lived in housing developments that encouraged physical activity were less likely to be obese.

Cross-Sectional and Longitudinal Studies

Some health researchers seek to understand how health problems develop over time. To do this, researchers use two approaches to studying developmental issues. **Cross-sectional studies** are those conducted at only one point in time, whereas **longitudinal studies** follow participants over an extended period. In a cross-sectional design, the investigator studies a group of people from at least two different age groups to determine the possible differences between the groups on some measure, such as food preferences, amount of physical activity, number of calories consumed, percent of calories from fat, or other variable.

Longitudinal studies can yield information that cross-sectional studies cannot because they assess the same people over time, which allows researchers to identify developmental trends and patterns. However, longitudinal studies have one obvious drawback: They take time. Thus, longitudinal studies are more costly than cross-sectional studies and they frequently require a large team of researchers.

Cross-sectional studies have the advantage of speed, but they have a disadvantage as well. Cross-sectional studies compare two or more separate groups of individuals, which make them incapable of revealing information about changes in individuals over a period of time. For example, a cross-sectional study of obesity in children (Reich et al., 2003) found that obesity was progressively more common among children in the second, fifth, and ninth grades compared with standard weight scores. This apparent trend toward increasing levels of overweight in children is distressing because overweight children also showed increases in factors related to the development of heart disease, such as cholesterol levels and blood pressure. However, only a longitudinal study, looking at the same people over a long period of time, can show the developmental trend in overweight and confirm the relationship to heart disease or other disease conditions.

A longitudinal study of overweight and heart disease risks (Freedman, Khan, Dietz, Srinivasan, & Berenson, 2001) confirmed that overweight children not only showed risk factors for heart disease but also retained these risk factors if they remained overweight as adults. By comparing measures taken during childhood to the same measures taken 17 years later, this research showed that 77% of overweight children remained obese as adults, and they tended to retain the risks for heart disease such as high blood pressure and high cholesterol levels. However, normal-weight children who became obese as adults also showed these risks, so being overweight during childhood did not present a special risk—being overweight did.

Experimental Designs

Correlational studies, cross-sectional designs, and longitudinal studies all have important uses in psychology, but none of them can determine causality. Sometimes psychologists want information on the ability of one variable to cause or directly influence another. Such information requires a well-designed experiment.

An experiment consists of a comparison of at least two groups, often referred to as an **experimental group** and a **control group**. The participants in the experimental group must receive treatment identical to that of participants in the control group except that those in the experimental group receive one level of the **independent variable**, whereas people in the control group receive a different level. The independent variable is the condition of interest, which the experimenter systematically manipulates to observe its influence on a behavior or response—that is, on the **dependent variable**. The manipulation of the independent variable is a critical element of experimental design because this manipulation allows researchers to control the situation by choosing and creating the appropriate levels. In addition, good experimental design requires that experimenters assign participants to the experimental or control group randomly to ensure that the groups are equivalent at the beginning of the study.

Often the experimental condition consists of administering a treatment, whereas the control condition consists of withholding that treatment and perhaps presenting some sort of placebo. If the experimental group later shows a different score on the dependent variable than the control group, the independent variable has a cause-and-effect relationship with the dependent variable.

For example, an experimental study assessed the effect of a brief intervention to encourage physical activity among obese adults (Bolognesi, Nigg, Massarini, & Lippke, 2006). The participants were obese adults visiting their family physician. Researchers randomly assigned participants either to the experimental intervention or to a control group for comparison. Physicians delivered a brief counseling concerning physical activity to 48 of the obese patients. A control group of 48 other obese patients received their usual care without any intervention concerning the importance of physical activity. All patients underwent assessments of body mass index (BMI)—a measure of obesity—and abdominal girth measurement. Six months later, the researchers assessed all participants' BMI and abdominal girth. Participants who received the counseling intervention showed lower average BMI and abdominal girth than the control group.

These results suggest that physicians' advice can encourage obese people to become more physically active, which in turn can affect obese people's weight. Such an experimental design allows investigators to speak of causation, or at least of probable causes of changes in weight, because the counseling intervention differed between the two groups and other factors were constant. Figure 2.1 shows a typical experimental design comparing an experimental group with a control group, with counseling as the independent variable and BMI as the dependent variable.

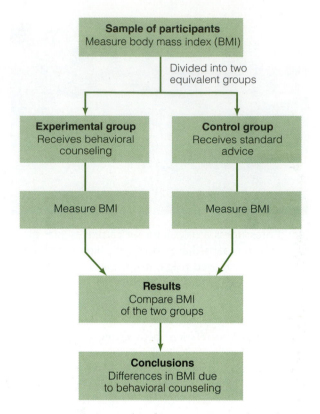

FIGURE 2.1 Example of an experimental method.

Ex Post Facto Designs

Ethical restrictions or practical limitations prevent researchers from manipulating many variables, such as gender, socioeconomic status, death of a loved one, smoking, or sexual behaviors. This means that experiments are not possible with many such variables, but these limitations do not prevent researchers from studying these variables. When researchers cannot manipulate certain variables in a systematic manner, they sometimes rely on ex post facto designs.

An **ex post facto design**, one of several types of quasi-experimental studies, resembles an experiment in some ways but differs in others. Both types of studies involve contrasting groups to determine differences, but ex post facto designs do not involve the manipulation of independent variables. Instead, researchers choose a variable of interest and select participants who already differ on this variable, called a **subject variable** (or *participant variable*). Both experiments and ex post facto studies involve the measurement of dependent variables. For example, researchers might study degree of obesity (subject variable) and food preference (dependent variable) by selecting a group of participants who are obese and choosing a comparison group of people who are normal weight to determine differences in food choices.

The comparison group in an ex post facto design is not an equivalent control group, because these participants were assigned to groups because of their weight rather than by random assignment. Without random assignment, the groups may potentially differ on variables other than weight, such as exercise, diet, cholesterol levels, or smoking. The existence of these other differences means that researchers cannot pinpoint the subject variable as the cause of differences in food preferences between the groups. However, findings about differences in level of food preference between the two groups can yield useful information, making this type of study a choice for many investigations.

Ex post facto designs are quite common in health psychology. For example, a comparison of the eating behavior of obese and normal-weight customers of all-you-can-eat Chinese buffets revealed striking differences that may contribute to weight (Wansink & Payne, 2008). Compared with normal-weight customers, obese customers used larger plates, were more likely to face the buffet, and were more likely to use forks rather than chopsticks. In contrast, normal-weight customers were more likely to browse all the food at the buffet before serving themselves; obese customers were more likely to serve themselves immediately. Normal-weight customers were also more likely to leave food on their plate at the end of dinner, whereas obese customers were not. Although the researchers could not conclude that obesity was the cause of these differences, this ex post facto design does provide useful information about how the eating behaviors of obese individuals may differ from that of normal-weight individuals.

IN SUMMARY

Health psychologists use several research methods, including correlational studies, cross-sectional and longitudinal studies, experimental designs, and ex post facto studies. Correlational studies indicate the degree of association between two variables, but they can never show causation. Cross-sectional studies investigate a group of people at one point in time, whereas longitudinal studies follow the

participants over an extended period of time. Although longitudinal studies may yield more useful results than cross-sectional studies, they are more time consuming and more expensive. With experimental designs, researchers manipulate the independent variable so that any resulting differences between experimental and control groups can be attributed to their differential exposure to the independent variable. Experimental studies typically include a placebo given to people in a control group so that they will have the same expectations as people in the experimental group. Ex post facto studies are similar to experimental designs in that researchers compare two or more groups and then record group differences in the dependent variable, but differ in that the independent variable is preexisting rather than manipulated.

Research Methods in Epidemiology

In addition to contributions from psychology methods, the field of health psychology also profits from medical research, especially the research of epidemiologists. **Epidemiology** is a branch of medicine that investigates factors that contribute to health or disease in a particular population (Beaglehole, Bonita, & Kjellström, 1993; Tucker, Phillips, Murphy, & Raczynski, 2004).

With the increase in chronic diseases during the 20th century, epidemiologists make fundamental contributions to health by identifying the risk factors for diseases. A **risk factor** is any characteristic or condition that occurs with greater frequency in people with a disease than in people free from that disease. That is, epidemiologists study those demographic and behavioral factors that relate to heart disease, cancer, and other chronic diseases (Tucker et al., 2004). For example, epidemiology studies were the first to detect a relationship between the behavior of smoking and heart disease.

Two important concepts in epidemiology are prevalence and incidence. **Prevalence** refers to the proportion of the population that has a particular disease or condition at a specific time; **incidence** measures the frequency of *new cases* during a specified period, usually one year (Tucker et al., 2004). With both prevalence and incidence, the number of people in the population at risk is divided into either the number of people with the disorder (prevalence) or the number of new cases in a particular time frame (incidence). The prevalence of a disorder may be quite different from the incidence of that disorder. For example, the prevalence of hypertension is much greater than the incidence because people can live for years after a diagnosis. In a given community, the annual *incidence* of hypertension might be 0.025, meaning that for every 1,000 people of a given age range, ethnic background, and gender, 25 people per year will receive a diagnosis of high blood pressure. But because hypertension is a chronic disorder, the prevalence will accumulate, producing a number much higher than 25 per 1,000. In contrast, for a disease such as influenza with a relatively short duration (due either to the patient's rapid recovery or to quick death), the incidence per year will exceed the prevalence at any specific time during that year.

Research in epidemiology uses three broad methods: (1) observational studies; (2) randomized, controlled trials; and (3) natural experiments. Each method has its own requirements and yields specific information. Although epidemiologists use some of the same methods and procedures employed by psychologists, their terminology is not always the same. Figure 2.2 lists the broad areas of epidemiological study and shows their approximate counterparts in the field of psychology.

Observational Methods

Epidemiologists use observational methods to estimate the occurrence of a specific disease in a given population. These methods do not show causes of the disease,

but researchers can draw inferences about possible factors that relate to the disease. Observational methods are similar to correlational studies in psychology; both show an association between two or more conditions, but neither can be used to demonstrate causation.

Two important types of observational methods are prospective studies and retrospective studies. **Prospective studies** begin with a population of disease-free participants and follow them over a period of time to determine whether a given condition, such as cigarette smoking, high blood pressure, or obesity, is related to a later condition, such as heart disease or death. For example, the Japan Public Health Center–Based Study (Chei, Iso, Yamagishi, Inoue, & Tsugane, 2008) followed more than 90,000 Japanese adults between ages 40 and 69 for 11 years to determine the risk of high body mass index and weight gain on the development of heart disease. They found that both having a high body mass index and gaining weight during adulthood increased the risk for heart disease, but only among men. Prospective studies such as this one are longitudinal, making them equivalent to longitudinal studies in psychology: Both provide information about a group of participants over time, and both take a long time to complete.

In contrast, **retrospective studies** use the opposite approach: They begin with a group of people already suffering from a particular disease or disorder and then look backward for characteristics or conditions that marked them as being different from people who do not have that problem. This approach has an advantage over prospective studies—it need not take as much time or expense. One retrospective study (Nori Janosz et al., 2008) examined groups of people who had

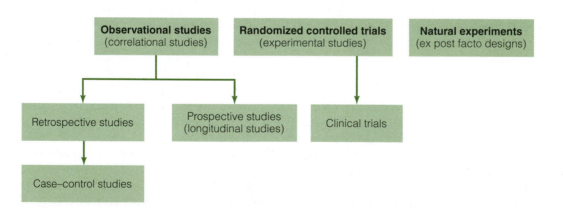

FIGURE 2.2 Research methods in epidemiology, with their psychology counterparts in parentheses.

participated in a behaviorally based weight management program, all of whom had received a diagnosis of Type 2 diabetes. Some of the individuals experienced a resolution of their diabetes through an improvement in their regulation of blood glucose, whereas others continued to have problems with blood glucose regulation. Retrospective studies such as this one are also referred to as **case–control studies** because cases (people who had resolved their diabetes) were compared with controls (people who continued to show symptoms of diabetes). In comparing the two groups, the researchers found several differences, including the amount of weight lost. Those individuals whose diabetes had improved lost about twice as much weight as those who continued to have glucose regulation problems.

Randomized Controlled Trials

A second type of epidemiological research is the randomized controlled trial, which is equivalent to experimental research in psychology. With a randomized controlled trial, researchers randomly assign participants to either a study group or a control group, thus making the two groups equal on all pertinent factors except the variable being studied. (In psychology this would be called the independent variable.) Researchers must also control variables other than those of primary interest to prevent them from affecting the outcome. A randomized controlled trial, as with the experimental method in psychology, must avoid the problem of **self-selection**; that is, it must not let participants choose whether to be in the experimental group or the control group, but rather, it must assign them to groups randomly.

A test of the effectiveness of a lifestyle intervention for overweight adolescent girls (DeBar et al., 2012) assigned participants either to a group that received a 5-month program with nutrition and physical activity components or to a group that received usual care. The random assignment to conditions and the usual-care control group make this study an example of a randomized controlled trial. The results indicated that the teens who received the intervention had lower body mass index scores than those who were in the control condition. These results suggest the potential effectiveness of this approach for weight loss in overweight adolescent girls.

A **clinical trial** is a research design that tests the effects of a new drug or medical treatment. Many clinical trials are randomized controlled trials that feature random assignment and control of other variables, which allow researchers to determine the effectiveness of the new treatment. The study that assessed the effectiveness of the lifestyle intervention for overweight teenagers (DeBar et al., 2012) meets the criteria for a clinical trial; this study included random assignment of participants to conditions, a placebo type of control for expectancy and attention, and an assessment of the program's effectiveness.

Epidemiologists often regard randomized, placebo-controlled, double-blind trials as the "gold standard" of research designs (Kertesz, 2003). This design is commonly used to measure the effectiveness of new drugs, as well as psychological and educational interventions. For example, all drugs approved by the U.S. Food and Drug Administration (FDA) must first undergo extensive clinical trials of this nature, demonstrating that the drug is effective and has acceptable levels of side effects or other risks.

When a controlled clinical trial demonstrates the effectiveness of a new drug or intervention, the researchers often publish and publicize the findings so that others can adopt the treatment. In some cases, a controlled trial may fail to demonstrate the effectiveness of a new intervention. When trials fail to show a treatment to be effective, researchers may be less likely to publish the findings. By some estimates, studies that fail to find an intervention as effective are 3 times less likely to be published (Dwan et al., 2008). Thus, researchers, health care providers, and the public are more likely to learn about research that shows a particular treatment to be effective, but less likely to learn about research that shows the same treatment to be ineffective.

Several safeguards are now in place to help ensure that researchers and health care providers can access all available evidence, rather than just the evidence that supports a treatment. For example, major medical journals require that researchers comply with clear guidelines in reporting results of a clinical trial. These guidelines—known as the Consolidated Standards of Reporting Trials (CONSORT) guidelines (Schulz, Altman, Moher, and the CONSORT Group, 2010)—require researchers to register their clinical trial in a registry *prior* to the start of the study. This database allows anybody to locate all clinical trials conducted on a treatment, not simply the trials that found a treatment to be effective.

Natural Experiments

A third area of epidemiological study is the natural experiment, in which the researcher can only select the independent variable, not manipulate it. Natural experiments are similar to the ex post facto designs used in psychology and involve the study of natural conditions that provide the possibility for comparison.

When two similar groups of people naturally divide themselves into those exposed to a risk or pathogen and those not exposed, natural experiments are possible. Such a situation occurred in 2008 when New York City passed a law requiring restaurants—including all fast food chains like McDonalds, Burger King, and Wendy's—to post the calorie content of food items on the menus (Elbel, Gyamfi, & Kersh, 2011). Newark, a large city just 10 miles west of New York City, did not pass such a law. This natural manipulation of conditions allowed a comparison of food choices of children and adolescents who saw the calorie content of menu items with those who did not, to test the hypothesis that the absence of calorie information encourages children and adolescents to make unhealthy food choices. The results indicated no significant difference in food choices among the young patrons of New York City restaurants compared with Newark restaurants, either before or after the law took effect. Thus, this natural experiment suggested that calorie information does not persuade children and adolescents to make healthier food choices.

This natural experiment differs from case–control studies in that it began by examining all patrons of the restaurants, regardless of their food choices or obesity. This natural experiment differs from randomized controlled trials in that the researchers selected the participants according to their city rather than manipulating who would receive calorie information and who would not. In a true randomized controlled trial, researchers would assign participants to calorie information conditions, but of course, practical considerations make this difficult to do in a busy, big-city fast food restaurant.

Meta-Analysis

As we have seen, researchers use a variety of approaches to study behavior and health-related outcomes. Unfortunately, research on the same topic may not yield consistent findings, putting researchers (and everyone else) in the position of wondering which outcome is valid. Some studies are larger than others, and when it comes to accepting a result, size matters. But sometimes, even large studies furnish results that seem contradictory. However, the statistical technique of **meta-analysis** allows researchers to evaluate many research studies on the same topic, even if the research methods differed. The results from a meta-analysis include a measure of the overall size of the effect of the variable under study. The ability to offer an estimate of the size of an effect is an advantage. If an effect is statistically significant but small, then people should not be encouraged to change their behavior on the basis of such findings; doing so would provide too few benefits. On the other hand, if an effect is large, then working toward change would be beneficial, even if it is difficult.

For example, a group of researchers (Verbeeten, Elks, Daneman, & Ong, 2011) evaluated studies conducted over a period of nearly 20 years to determine the relationship between childhood weight and risk for developing Type 1 diabetes. These researchers included case–control and prospective designs in their meta-analysis. The results indicated that childhood obesity doubles the risk of subsequent Type 1 diabetes. Thus, this meta-analysis allowed researchers to integrate findings from a large number of studies and draw conclusions about the impact of weight on this disease.

An Example of Epidemiological Research: The Alameda County Study

A famous example of an epidemiological study is the Alameda County Study in California, an ongoing prospective study of a single community to identify health practices that may protect against death and disease. As noted earlier, epidemiologists identify risk factors by studying large populations over some period of time and by sifting out behavioral, demographic, or physiological conditions that show a relationship to subsequent disease or death.

In 1965, epidemiologist Lester Breslow and his colleagues from the Human Population Laboratory of the California State Department of Public Health began a survey of a sample of households in Alameda County (Oakland), California. After determining the number of adults living at these addresses, the researchers sent detailed questionnaires to each resident 20 years of age or older. Nearly 7,000 people returned surveys.

Among other questions, these participants answered questions about seven basic health practices: (1) getting 7 or 8 hours of sleep daily, (2) eating breakfast almost every day, (3) rarely eating between meals, (4) drinking alcohol in moderation or not at all, (5) not smoking cigarettes, (6) exercising regularly, and (7) maintaining weight near the prescribed ideal.

At the time of the original survey in 1965, only cigarette smoking had been implicated as a health risk. Evidence that any of the other six practices predicted health or mortality was quite weak. Because several of these practices require some amount of good health, it was necessary to investigate the possibility that original health status might confound subsequent death rates. To control for these possible confounding effects, the Alameda County investigators asked residents about their physical disabilities, acute and chronic illnesses, physical symptoms, and current levels of energy.

A follow-up 5½ years later (Belloc, 1973) revealed that Alameda County residents who practiced six or seven of the basic health-related behaviors were far less likely to have died than those who practiced zero to three. This decreased mortality risk was independent of their 1965 health status, thus suggesting that healthy behaviors lead to lower rates of death.

In 1974, investigators conducted a major follow-up of living participants and also surveyed a new sample to determine whether the community in general had adopted a healthier lifestyle between 1965 and 1974 (Berkman & Breslow, 1983; Wingard, Berkman, & Brand, 1982). The 9-year follow-up determined the relationship between mortality and the seven health practices, considered individually as well as in combination. Cigarette smoking, lack of physical activity, and alcohol consumption were strongly related to mortality, whereas obesity and too much or too little sleep were only weakly associated with increased death rates. As it turned out, skipping breakfast and snacking between meals did not significantly predict mortality.

Moreover, the number of close social relationships also predicted mortality: People with few social contacts were 2½ times more likely to have died than were those with many such contacts (Berkman & Syme, 1979). The Alameda County Study was the first study to uncover a link between social relationships and mortality. As you will learn in the rest of this book, social relationships and social support are important factors in physical health.

If some health practices predict greater risk of *mortality*, then a second question concerns how these same factors relate to *morbidity*, or disease. A condition that predicts death need not also predict disease. Many disabilities, chronic illnesses, and illness symptoms do not inevitably lead to death. Therefore, it is important to know whether basic health practices and social contacts predict later physical health. Do health practices merely contribute to survival time, or do they also raise an individual's general level of health?

To answer this question, researchers (Camacho & Wiley, 1983; Wiley & Camacho, 1980) studied a subset of the original sample of Alameda County participants. In addition to the five health practices that related to mortality, this investigation included a Social Network Index that combined marital status, contacts with friends and relatives, and membership in church and other organizations. Each of the five health behaviors as well as the Social Network Index showed a relationship to changes in health. More specifically, the people with the best health were (1) those who did not smoke; (2) those who drank alcohol, but only moderately; (3) people who slept 7 or 8 hours per night; (4) people who engaged in high levels of physical activity; (5) people at a normal weight; and again (6) people who scored high on the Social Network Index.

IN SUMMARY

Epidemiologists conduct research using designs and terminology that differ from those used by psychology researchers. For example, epidemiologists use the concepts of risk factor, prevalence, and incidence. A risk factor is any condition that occurs with greater frequency in people with a disease than it does in people free from that disease. Prevalence refers to the proportion of the population that has a particular disease at a specific time, whereas incidence measures the frequency of new cases of the disease during a specified period of time.

In order to investigate factors that contribute either to health or to the frequency and distribution of a disease, epidemiologists use research methods that are similar to those used by psychologists, but the terminology varies. Observational studies, which are similar to correlational studies, can be either retrospective or prospective. Retrospective studies begin with a group of people already suffering

Becoming an Informed Reader of Health-Related Research on the Internet

The Internet presents a wealth of useful health information. Over 80% of Internet users turn to the Internet for health information (Pew Internet, 2012). How can you judge the worth of health-related information you read or hear? Here are several questions you should ask yourself as you evaluate health information on the Internet.

1. Who runs the website? Any reputable website should clearly state who is responsible for the information. You can often find this information in an "About Us" section of the website. Often, the website address can also tell you important information. Websites that end in ".gov," ".edu," or ".org" are run by government, educational, or non-for-profit groups. These sites are likely to present unbiased information. In contrast, websites that end in ".com" are run by commercial enterprises and may exist mainly to sell products.

2. What is the purpose of the website? Websites that exist primarily to sell products may not present unbiased information. You should be especially wary of websites that promise "breakthroughs," or try to sell quick, easy, and miraculous cures. Dramatic breakthroughs are rare in science.

3. What is the evidence supporting a claim? Ideally, a website should report information based on studies conducted by trained scientists who are affiliated with universities, research hospitals, or government agencies. Furthermore, websites should include references to these published scientific studies. In contrast, claims supported by testimonials of "satisfied" consumers or from commercial enterprises are less likely to come from scientific research.

4. Is there adequate information available to evaluate the research design of a scientific study? Findings are more reliable if a study uses a large number of participants. If a study suggests that a factor *causes* a particular health outcome, does it use an experimental design with random assignment? Does it control for placebo effects? If the design is prospective or retrospective, did the researchers adequately control for smoking, diet, exercise, and other possible confounding variables? Lastly, is it clear who the participants in a study were? If a study uses a unique population, then the results may only be applicable to similar individuals.

5. How is the information reviewed before it is posted? Most reputable health information will have somebody with medical or research credentials—such as an MD or a PhD—author or review the material.

6. How current is the information? The date of posting or last review should be clear. Scientific knowledge evolves continually, so the best information is up to date.

You can find many of these tips, and others, on the National Institutes of Health website (www.nih.gov). This website, as well as the Centers for Disease Control and Prevention (www.cdc.gov), is an excellent source for the latest scientific information on a wide variety of health topics.

from a disease and then look for characteristics of these people that differ from those of people who do not have the disease; prospective studies are longitudinal designs that follow the forward development of a group of people. Randomized controlled trials are similar to experimental designs in psychology. Clinical trials, a common type of randomized controlled trial, are typically used to determine the effectiveness of new drugs, but they can be used in other controlled studies. Natural experiments, which are similar to ex post facto studies, are used when naturally occurring conditions allow for comparisons. The statistical technique of meta-analysis allows researchers to examine a group of studies that have researched the variable of interest and provide an overall estimate of the size of the effect.

Determining Causation

As noted earlier, both prospective and retrospective studies can identify risk factors for a disease, but they do not demonstrate causation. Obesity is a risk for hypertension, heart disease, diabetes, and kidney disease. Obese people are more likely to develop these conditions than people who are normal weight. However, some people who are not obese—or even overweight—develop heart disease and kidney disease. This section looks at the risk factor approach as a means of suggesting causation and then examines evidence that cigarette smoking *causes* disease.

The Risk Factor Approach

The risk factor approach was popularized by the Framingham Heart Study (Levy & Brink, 2005), a large-scale epidemiology investigation that began in 1948 and included more than 5,000 men and women in the town of Framingham, Massachusetts. From its early years and continuing to the present, this study has allowed researchers to identify such risk factors for cardiovascular disease (CVD) as serum cholesterol, gender, high blood pressure, cigarette smoking, and obesity. These risk factors do not necessarily cause cardiovascular disease, but they relate to it in some way. Obesity, for example, may not be a direct cause of heart disease, but it is generally associated with hypertension, which is strongly associated with cardiovascular disease. Thus, obesity is a risk factor for CVD.

Two types of expression exist for conveying risk: absolute and relative risk. **Absolute risk** refers to the person's chances of developing a disease or disorder independent of any risk that other people may have for that disease or disorder. These chances tend to be small. For example, a smoker's risk of dying of lung cancer during any one year is about 1 in 1,000. When smokers hear their risk expressed in such terms, they may not recognize the hazards of their behavior (Kertesz, 2003). Other ways of presenting the same information may seem more threatening. For example, a male smoker's risk of getting lung cancer in his *lifetime* is much higher, about 15 in 100 (Crispo et al., 2004).

Relative risk (RR) refers to the ratio of the incidence (or prevalence) of a disease in an exposed group to the incidence (or prevalence) of that disease in the unexposed group. The relative risk of the unexposed group is always 1.00. Thus, a relative risk of 1.50 indicates that the exposed group is 50% more likely to develop the disease in question than the unexposed group; a relative risk of 0.70 means that the rate of disease in the exposed group is only 70% of the rate in the unexposed group. Expressed in terms of relative risk, smoking seems much more dangerous. For example, male cigarette smokers have a relative risk of about 23.3 for dying of lung cancer and a relative risk of 14.6 for dying of cancer of the larynx (U.S. Department of Health and Human Services [USDHHS], 2004). This means that, compared with nonsmokers, men who smoke are more than 23 times as likely to die of lung cancer and more than 14 times as likely to die of laryngeal cancer.

The high relative risk for lung cancer among people who have a long history of cigarette smoking may suggest that most smokers will die of lung cancer. However, such is not the case: Most smokers will *not* die of lung cancer. About 39% of male smokers and 40% of female smokers who die of cancer will develop cancer in sites other than the lung (Armour, Woollery, Malarcher, Pechacek, & Husten, 2005). Furthermore, the absolute frequency of death due to heart disease makes a smoker almost as likely to die of heart disease (20% of deaths among smokers) as lung cancer (28% of deaths among smokers). Smokers have a much higher relative risk of dying from lung cancer than cardiovascular disease, but their *absolute risk* of dying from CVD is much more similar.

Cigarettes and Disease: Is There a Causal Relationship?

In 1994, representatives from all the major tobacco companies came before the United States Congress House Subcommittee on Health to argue that cigarettes do not cause health problems such as heart disease and lung cancer. The crux of their argument was that no scientific study had ever proven that cigarette smoking causes heart disease or lung cancer in humans. Technically, their contention was correct because only experimental studies can absolutely demonstrate causation, and no such experimental study has ever been (or ever will be) conducted on humans.

During the past 50 years, however, researchers have used nonexperimental studies to establish a link between cigarette smoking and several diseases, especially cardiovascular disease and lung cancer. Accumulated findings from these studies present an example of how researchers can use those nonexperimental studies to make deductions about a causal relationship. In other words, experimental, randomized, placebo-controlled,

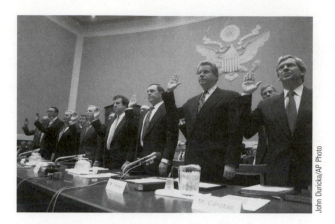

Heads of United States' largest tobacco companies testify before Congress, arguing that no experimental evidence shows that tobacco causes cancer.

double-blind studies are not required before scientists can infer a causal link between the independent variable (smoking) and the dependent variables (heart disease and lung cancer). Epidemiologists draw conclusions that a causal relationship exists if certain conditions are met (Susser, 1991; USDHHS, 2004). Using their criteria, does sufficient evidence exist to infer a cause-and-effect relationship between cigarette smoking and heart disease and lung cancer?

The first criterion is that a *dose–response relationship* must exist between a possible cause and changes in the prevalence or incidence of a disease. A **dose–response relationship** is a direct, consistent association between an independent variable, such as a behavior, and a dependent variable, such as a disease; in other words, the higher the dose, the higher the death rate. A body of research evidence (Bhat et al., 2008; Papadopoulos et al., 2011; USDHHS, 1990, 2004) has demonstrated a dose–response relationship between both the number of cigarettes smoked per day and the number of years one has smoked and the subsequent incidence of heart disease, lung cancer, and stroke.

Second, the prevalence or incidence of a *disease should decline with the removal of the possible cause*. Research (USDHHS, 1990, 2004) has consistently demonstrated that quitting cigarette smoking lowers one's risk of cardiovascular disease and decreases one's risk of lung cancer. People who continue to smoke continue to have increased risks of these diseases.

Third, the *cause must precede the disease*. Cigarette smoking almost always precedes incidence of disease.

(We have little evidence that people tend to begin cigarette smoking as a means of coping with heart disease or lung cancer.)

Fourth, *a cause-and-effect relationship between the condition and the disease must be plausible*; that is, it must be consistent with other data, and it must make sense from a biological viewpoint. Although scientists are just beginning to understand the exact mechanisms responsible for the effect of cigarette smoking on the cardiovascular system and the lungs (USDHHS, 2004), such a physiological connection is plausible. It is not necessary that the underlying connection between a behavior and a disease be known, but it must be a reasonable possibility.

Fifth, *research findings must be consistent*. For more than 50 years, evidence from ex post facto and correlational studies, as well as from various epidemiological studies, has demonstrated a strong and consistent relationship between cigarette smoking and disease. As early as 1956, British researchers Richard Doll and A. B. Hill noted a straight linear relationship between average number of cigarettes smoked per day and death rates from lung cancer. Although a positive correlation such as this is not sufficient to demonstrate causation, hundreds of additional correlational and ex post facto studies since that time yield overwhelming evidence to suggest that cigarette smoking causes disease.

Sixth, the *strength of the association between the condition and the disease must be relatively high*. Again, research has revealed that cigarette smokers have at least a twofold risk for cardiovascular disease and are about 18 times more likely than nonsmokers to die of lung cancer (USDHHS, 2004). Because other studies have found comparable relative risk figures, epidemiologists accept cigarette smoking as a causal agent for both CVD and lung cancer.

The final criterion for inferring causality is the existence of *appropriately designed studies*. Although no experimental designs with human participants have been reported on the relationship between cigarettes and disease, well-designed observational studies can yield the results equivalent to experimental studies (USDHHS, 2004), and a large number of these observational studies consistently reveal a close association between cigarette smoking and both cardiovascular disease and lung cancer.

Because each of these seven criteria is clearly met by the evidence against smoking, epidemiologists are able to discount the argument of tobacco company

TABLE 2.1   Criteria for Determining Causation Between a Condition and a Disease

1. A dose–response relationship exists between the condition and the disease.
2. Removal of the condition reduces the prevalence or incidence of the disease.
3. The condition precedes the disease.
4. A cause-and-effect relationship between the condition and the disease is physiologically plausible.
5. Relevant research data consistently reveal a relationship between the condition and the disease.
6. The strength of the relationship between the condition and the disease is relatively high.
7. Studies revealing a relationship between the condition and the disease are well designed.

representatives that cigarette smoking has not been proven to cause disease. When evidence is as overwhelming as it is in this case, scientists infer a causal link between cigarette smoking and a variety of diseases, including heart disease and lung cancer. Table 2.1 summarizes the criteria for determining causation.

IN SUMMARY

A risk factor is any characteristic or condition that occurs with greater frequency in people with a disease than it does in people free from that disease. Risk may be expressed either in terms of the absolute risk, a person's risk of developing a disease independent of other factors, or the relative risk, the ratio of risk of those exposed to a risk factor compared with those not exposed.

Although the risk factor approach alone cannot determine causation, epidemiologists use several criteria for determining a cause-and-effect relationship between a condition and a disease: (1) A dose–response relationship must exist between the condition and the disease, (2) the removal of the condition must reduce the prevalence or incidence of the disease, (3) the condition must precede the disease, (4) the causal relationship between the condition and the disease must be physiologically plausible, (5) research data must consistently reveal a relationship between the condition and the disease, (6) the strength of the relationship between the condition and the disease must be relatively high, and (7) the relationship between the condition and the disease must be based on well-designed studies. When findings meet all seven of these criteria, scientists can infer a cause-and-effect relationship between an independent variable (such as smoking) and a dependent variable (such as heart disease or lung cancer).

Research Tools

Psychologists frequently rely on two important tools to conduct research: theoretical models and psychometric instruments. Many, but not all, psychology studies use a theoretical model and attempt to test hypotheses suggested by that model. Also, many psychology studies rely on measuring devices to assess behaviors, physiological functions, attitudes, abilities, personality traits, and other variables. This section provides a brief discussion of these two tools.

The Role of Theory in Research

As the scientific study of human behavior, psychology shares the use of scientific methods to investigate natural phenomena with other disciplines. The work of science is not restricted to research methodology; it also involves constructing theoretical models to serve as vehicles for making sense of research findings. Health psychologists have developed a number of models and theories to explain health-related behaviors and conditions, such as stress, pain, smoking, alcohol abuse, and unhealthy eating habits. To the uninitiated, theories may seem impractical and unimportant, but scientists regard them as practical tools that give both direction and meaning to their research.

Scientific **theory** is "a set of related assumptions that allow scientists to use logical deductive reasoning to formulate testable hypotheses" (Feist & Feist, 2006, p. 4). Theories and scientific observations have an inter-active relationship. A theory gives meaning to observa-tions, and observations, in turn, fit into and alter the theory to explain these observations. Theories, then, are dynamic and become more powerful as they expand to explain more and more relevant observations.

Near the beginning of this cycle, when the theoret-ical framework is still rudimentary and not yet suffi-ciently comprehensive to explain a large number of observations, the term **model** is more appropriate than theory. In practice, however, researchers some-times use *theory* and *model* interchangeably.

The role of theory in health psychology is basi-cally the same as it is in any other scientific discipline. First, a useful theory should generate research—both descriptive research and hypothesis testing. The goal of descriptive research is to expand the existing the-ory. This type of research deals with measurement, labeling, and categorization of observations. A useful theory of psychosocial factors in obesity, for example, should generate a multitude of investigations that describe the psychological and social factors related to obesity. On the other hand, hypothesis testing may not expand the theory but, rather, contribute valid data to the body of scientific knowledge. Again, a useful theory of psychosocial factors in obesity should stimulate the formulation of a number of hypotheses that, when tested, produce a greater understanding of the psychological and social condi-tions that relate to the development and maintenance of obesity. Results of such studies would either sup-port or fail to support the existing theory; they ordi-narily do not enlarge or alter it.

Second, a useful theory should organize and explain the observations derived from research and make them intelligible. Unless research data are organized into some meaningful framework, scientists have no clear direction to follow in their pursuit of further knowledge. A useful theory of the psychosocial factors in obesity, for exam-ple, should integrate what researchers know about such factors and allow researchers to frame discerning ques-tions that stimulate further research.

Third, a useful theory should serve as a guide to action, permitting the practitioner to predict behav-ior and to implement strategies to change behavior. A practitioner concerned with helping others change health-related behaviors is greatly aided by a theory of behavior change. For instance, a cognitive therapist will follow a cognitive theory of learning to make

decisions about how to help clients and will thus focus on changing the thought processes that affect cli-ents' behaviors. Similarly, psychologists with other the-oretical orientations rely on their theories to supply them with solutions to the many questions they con-front in their practice.

Theories, then, are useful and necessary tools for the development of any scientific discipline. They gen-erate research that leads to more knowledge, organize and explain observations, and help the practitioner (both the researcher and the clinician) handle a variety of daily problems, such as predicting behavior and helping people change unhealthy practices. Later chap-ters discuss several theoretical models that health psy-chologists use.

The Role of Psychometrics in Research

Health psychologists study a number of phenomena that cannot be described in terms of simple physical measurements, like weight or length. These phenomena include behaviors and conditions such as stress, coping, pain, hostility, eating habits, and personality. To study each of these phenomena, health psychologists must develop new measures that can reliably and validly measure differences between people. Indeed, one of psychology's most important contributions to behav-ioral medicine and behavioral health is its sophisticated methods of measuring important psychological factors in health.

For any measuring instrument to be useful, it must be both *reliable* (consistent) and *valid* (accurate). The problems of establishing reliability and validity are crit-ical to the development of any measurement scale.

Establishing Reliability   The **reliability** of a mea-suring instrument is the extent to which it yields con-sistent results. A reliable ruler, for example, will yield the same measurement across different situations. In health psychology, reliability is most frequently deter-mined by comparing scores on two or more adminis-trations of the same instrument (*test–retest reliability*) or by comparing ratings obtained from two or more judges observing the same phenomenon (*interrater reliability*).

Measuring psychological phenomena is less precise than measuring physical dimensions such as length. Thus, perfect reliability is nearly impossible to come by, and researchers most frequently describe reliability in terms of either correlation coefficients or percentages. The correlation coefficient, which expresses the degree of correspondence between two sets of scores, is the same statistic used in correlational studies. High reliability coefficients (such as 0.80 to 0.90) indicate that participants have obtained nearly the same scores on two administrations of a test. Percentages can express the degree of agreement between the independent ratings of observers. If the agreement between two or more raters is high (such as 85% to 95%), then the instrument should elicit nearly the same ratings from two or more interviewers.

Establishing reliability for the numerous assessment instruments used in health psychology is obviously a formidable task, but it is an essential first step in developing useful measuring devices.

Establishing Validity   A second step in constructing assessment scales is to establish their validity. **Validity** is the extent to which an instrument measures what it is designed to measure. A valid ruler, for example, will tell you an object measures 2 centimeters, but only when that object really does measure 2 centimeters. In the context of a psychological measure such as a stress assessment, for example, a valid stress measure should tell you a person is under high stress, but only when that person experiences high stress.

Psychologists determine the validity of a measuring instrument by comparing scores from that instrument with some independent or outside criterion—that is, a standard that exists independently of the instrument being validated. In health psychology, that criterion can be a physiological measure, like a physiological stress response such as elevated blood pressure. A criterion can also be some future event, such as a diagnosis of heart disease or the development of diabetes. An instrument capable of predicting who will receive such a diagnosis and who will remain disease free has *predictive validity*. For example, scales that measure attitudes about body predict the development of eating disorders. For such a scale to demonstrate predictive validity, it must be administered to participants who are currently free of disease. If people who score high on the scale eventually have higher rates of disease than participants with low scores, then the scale can be said to have predictive validity; that is, it differentiates between participants who will remain disease free and those who will become ill.

IN SUMMARY

Two important tools aid the work of scientists: useful theories and accurate measurement. Useful theories (1) generate research, (2) predict and explain research data, and (3) help the practitioner solve a variety of problems. Accurate psychometric instruments are both reliable and valid. *Reliability* is the extent to which an assessment device measures consistently, and *validity* is the extent to which an assessment instrument measures what it is supposed to measure.

Answers

This chapter has addressed five basic questions:

1. **What are placebos, and how do they affect research and treatment?**

A placebo is an inactive substance or condition that has the appearance of an active treatment and that may cause participants to improve or change because of a belief in the placebo's efficacy. In other words, a placebo is any treatment that is effective because patients' expectations based on previous experiences with treatment lead them to believe that it will be effective.

The therapeutic effect of placebos is about 35%, but that rate varies with many conditions, including treatment setting and culture. Placebos, including sham surgery, can be effective in a wide variety of situations, such as decreasing pain, reducing asthma attacks, diminishing anxiety, and decreasing symptoms of Parkinson's disease. Nocebos are placebos that produce adverse effects.

The positive effects of placebos are usually beneficial to patients, but they create problems for researchers attempting to determine the efficacy of a treatment. Experimental designs that measure the effectiveness of a treatment intervention balance that intervention against a placebo so that people in the control (placebo) group have the same expectations as do people in the experimental (treatment intervention) group. Experimental studies frequently use designs in which the participants do not know which treatment condition they are in (*single-blind* design) or in which neither the participants nor the people administering the treatment know who receives the placebo and who receives the treatment intervention (*double-blind* design).

2. How does psychology research contribute to health knowledge?

Psychology has contributed to health knowledge in at least five important ways. First is its long tradition of techniques to change behavior. Second is an emphasis on health rather than disease. Third is the development of reliable and valid measuring instruments. Fourth is the construction of useful theoretical models to explain health-related research. Fifth are various research methods used in psychology. This chapter mostly deals with the fifth contribution.

The variety of research methods used in psychology include (1) correlational studies, (2) cross-sectional studies and longitudinal studies, (3) experimental designs, and (4) ex post facto designs. Each of these makes its own unique contribution to the understanding of behavior and health. Correlational studies indicate the degree of association or correlation between two variables, but by themselves, they cannot determine a cause-and-effect relationship. Cross-sectional studies investigate a group of people at one point in time, whereas longitudinal studies follow the participants over an extended period. In general, longitudinal studies are more likely to yield useful and specific results, but they are more time consuming and expensive than cross-sectional studies. With experimental designs, researchers manipulate the independent variable so that any resulting differences in the dependent variable between experimental and control groups can be attributed to their differential exposure to the independent variable. Ex post facto designs are similar to experimental designs in that researchers compare two or more groups and then record group differences on the dependent variable. However, in the ex post facto study, the experimenter merely selects a subject variable on which two or more groups have naturally divided themselves rather than create differences through manipulation.

3. How has epidemiology contributed to health knowledge?

Epidemiology has contributed the concepts of risk factor, prevalence, and incidence. A risk factor is any characteristic or condition that occurs with greater frequency in people with a disease than it does in people free from that disease. Prevalence is the proportion of the population that has a particular disease at a specific time; incidence measures the frequency of new cases of the disease during a specified time.

Many of the research methods used in epidemiology are quite similar to those used in psychology. Epidemiology uses at least three basic kinds of research methodology: (1) observational studies, (2) randomized controlled trials, and (3) natural experiments. Observational studies, which parallel the correlation studies used in psychology, are of two types: retrospective and prospective. Retrospective studies are usually *case–control studies* that begin with a group of people already suffering from a disease (the cases) and then look for characteristics of these people that are different from those of people who do not have that disease (the controls). Prospective studies are longitudinal designs that follow the forward development of a population or sample. Randomized controlled trials are similar to experimental designs in psychology. In these studies, researchers manipulate the independent variable to determine its effect on the dependent variable. Randomized controlled trials are capable of demonstrating cause-and-effect relationships. The most common type of randomized controlled trial is the clinical trial, which is frequently used to measure the efficacy of medications. Natural experiments, which are similar to ex post facto studies, involve selection rather than manipulation of the independent variable. The statistical technique of meta-analysis allows psychologists and epidemiologists to combine the results of many studies to develop a picture of the size of an effect.

4. How can scientists determine if a behavior causes a disease?

Seven criteria are used for determining a cause-and-effect relationship between a condition and a disease: (1) A dose–response relationship must exist between the condition and the disease, (2) the removal of the condition must reduce the prevalence or incidence of the disease, (3) the condition must precede the disease, (4) the causal relationship between the condition and the disease must be physiologically plausible, (5) research data must consistently reveal a relationship between the condition and the disease, (6) the strength of the relationship between the condition and the disease must be relatively high, and (7) the relationship between the condition and the disease must be based on well-designed studies.

5. **How do theory and measurement contribute to health psychology?**

Theories are important tools used by scientists to (1) generate research, (2) predict and explain research data, and (3) help the practitioner solve a variety of problems. Health psychologists use a variety of measurement instruments to assess behaviors and theoretical concepts. To be useful, these psychometric instruments must be both reliable and valid. Reliability is the extent to which an assessment device measures consistently, and validity is the extent to which an assessment instrument measures what it is supposed to measure.

Suggested Readings

Kertesz, L. (2003). The numbers behind the news. *Healthplan*, *44*(5), 10–14, 16, 18. Louise Kertesz offers a thoughtful analysis of the problems of reporting the findings from health research and gives some tips for understanding findings from research studies, including a definition of some of the terminology used in epidemiology research.

Price, D. D., Finniss, D. G., & Benedetti, F. (2008). A comprehensive review of the placebo effect: Recent advances and current thought. *Annual Review of Psychology*, *59*, 565–590. This article by one of the leading researchers on the topic of placebo effects describes research on how placebos may work to effect cures.

Russo, E. (2004, August 2). New views on mind–body connection. *The Scientist*, *18*(15), 28. This short article describes current research on the placebo and how high-tech methods allow the investigation of brain responses to placebos.

CHAPTER 3

Seeking and Receiving Health Care

CHAPTER OUTLINE

- **Real-World Profile of Lance Armstrong**
- *Seeking Medical Attention*
- *Seeking Medical Information from Nonmedical Sources*
- *Receiving Medical Care*

QUESTIONS

This chapter focuses on three basic questions:

1. What factors are related to seeking medical attention?

2. Where do people seek medical information?

3. What problems do people encounter in receiving medical care?

☑ CHECK YOUR HEALTH RISKS

Regarding Seeking and Receiving Health Care

☐ 1. If I feel well, I believe that I am healthy.

☐ 2. I see my dentist twice yearly for regular checkups.

☐ 3. The last time I sought medical care was in a hospital emergency room.

☐ 4. If I had a disease that would be a lot of trouble to manage, I would rather not know about it until I was really sick.

☐ 5. I try not to allow being sick to slow me down.

☐ 6. If I don't understand my physician's recommendations, I ask questions until I understand what I should do.

☐ 7. I think it's better to follow medical advice than to ask questions and cause problems, especially in the hospital.

☐ 8. When facing a stressful medical experience, I think the best strategy is to try not to think about it and hope that it will be over soon.

☐ 9. When I have severe symptoms, I try to find out as much information as possible about my medical condition.

☐ 10. I believe that if people get sick, it is because they were due to get sick, and there was nothing they could have done to prevent their sickness.

☐ 11. In order not to frighten patients faced with a difficult medical procedure, it is best to tell them that they won't be hurt, even if they will.

Items 2, 6, and 9 represent healthy attitudes or behaviors, but each of the other items relates to conditions that may present a risk or lead you to less effective health care. As you read this chapter, you will see the advantages of adopting healthy attitudes or behaviors to make more effective use of the health care system.

Real-World Profile of
LANCE ARMSTRONG

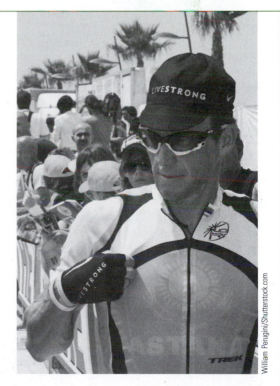

William Perugini/Shutterstock.com

Lance Armstrong was never accustomed to being unhealthy or out of shape. From his teenage years through the age of 25, Lance won numerous triathalons and professional cycling victories, including the 1996 Tour DuPont.

However, his victory in the Tour DuPont worried some of his fans. Instead of pumping his fists in victory as he crossed the finish line, he looked unusually exhausted. His eyes were bloodshot and his face flushed. Later that year, he dropped out of the Tour de France after only 5 days.

Lance later confessed that he did not feel well during that year. He lost energy and suffered from coughs and lower-back pain. When these symptoms appeared, he attributed them to either the flu or a long hard training season. He told himself at the time "Suck it up … you can't afford to be tired" (Jenkins & Armstrong, 2001, "Before and After," paragraph 27).

However, his symptoms did not improve, even after rest from training. One evening, when he developed a sudden and severe headache, Lance attributed it to too many margaritas. His vision started to become blurry, but he attributed that to getting older.

Finally, a symptom emerged that he could not ignore: He began coughing up masses of metallic-tasting blood. After the first instance of this symptom, Lance called a good friend who happened to be a physician. His friend suggested that Lance may only be suffering a cracked sinus. "Great, so it's no big deal," Lance replied, apparently relieved (Jenkins & Armstrong, 2001, "Before and After," paragraph 42).

The next day, Lance awoke to find his testicle swollen to the size of an orange. Rather than contact his doctor immediately, Lance hopped on his bike for another morning training ride. This time, he could not even manage to sit on the seat. Finally—after his symptoms prevented him doing what he loved most and was loved most for—he set up an appointment with a doctor.

That day, in early October 1996, Lance Armstrong learned that he had Stage 3 testicular cancer. Due to his delays in seeking medical attention, Lance's cancer had already spread to his lungs, abdomen, and brain. His doctors gave him only a 40% chance of survival, and he immediately sought treatment for his cancer.

Why did it take so long for Lance Armstrong to seek care for his symptoms? His health was critical to his professional success. He was wealthy, could afford medical care, and had access to personal physicians and team doctors. Still, Lance resisted seeking medical care. He later wrote, "Of course I should have known that something was wrong with me. But athletes, especially cyclists, are in the business of denial. You deny all the aches and pains because you have to in order to finish the race … You do not give in to pain" (Jenkins & Armstrong, 2001, "Before and After," paragraph 21).

From 1996 to 1998, Lance Armstrong underwent chemotherapy and surgery on both his testicles and brain, and eventually his cancer went into remission. He commenced cycling in 1998, and competed in nine subsequent Tour de France competitions. Most importantly, Lance's experience with cancer raised awareness and inspired millions of people worldwide.

Lance Armstrong is one of the lucky few survivors of advanced-stage cancer. His odds of survival would have surely been better had he sought medical care earlier. Why do some people, such as Lance Armstrong, seem to behave unwisely on issues of personal health? Why do others seek medical treatment when they are not ill? Psychologists have formulated several theories or models in the attempt to predict and to make sense of behaviors related to health. This chapter looks briefly at some of these theories as they relate to health-seeking behavior; Chapter 4 examines theory-driven research about people's adherence to medical advice.

Seeking Medical Attention

How do people know when to seek medical attention? How do they know whether they are ill or not? When Lance experienced symptoms that were likely caused by advancing cancer, he tried to ignore them, attributed them to anything but cancer, and consulted friends before making an appointment with a physician. Was Lance unusually reluctant to seek medical care, or was his behavior typical? Deciding when formal medical care is necessary is a complex problem, compounded by personal, social, and economic factors.

Before we consider these factors, we should define three terms: *health*, *disease*, and *illness*. Although the meaning of these concepts may seem obvious, their definitions are elusive. Is health the absence of illness, or is it the attainment of some positive state? In the first chapter, we saw that the World Health Organization (WHO) defines health as positive physical, mental, and social well-being, and not merely as the absence of disease or infirmity. Unfortunately, this definition has little practical value for people trying to make decisions about their state of health or illness, such as Lance's decision about whether to seek medical attention for his cancer-related symptoms.

Another difficulty for many people comes from understanding the difference between disease and illness. People often use these terms interchangeably, but most health scientists differentiate the two. Disease refers to the process of physical damage within the body, which can exist even in the absence of a label or diagnosis. Illness, on the other hand, refers to the experience of being sick and having a diagnosis of sickness. People can have a disease and not be ill. For example, people with undiagnosed hypertension, HIV infection, or cancer all have a disease, but they may appear quite healthy and be completely unaware of their disease. Although disease and illness are separate conditions, they often overlap—for example, when a person feels ill and has also received a diagnosis of a specific disease.

People frequently experience physical symptoms, but these symptoms may or may not indicate a disease. Symptoms such as a headache, a painful shoulder, sniffles, or sneezing would probably not prompt a person to seek medical care, but an intense and persistent stomach pain probably would. At what point should a person decide to seek medical care? Errors in both directions are possible. People who decide to go to the doctor when they are not really sick feel foolish, must pay the bill for an office visit, and lose credibility with people who know about the error, including the physician. If they choose not to seek medical care, they may get better, but they may also get worse; trying to ignore their symptoms may make treatment more difficult and seriously endanger their health or increase their risk of death. A prudent action would seem to be to chance the unnecessary visit, but people (for a variety reasons) are often unable or simply reluctant to go to the doctor.

In the United States and other Western countries, people are not "officially" ill until they receive a diagnosis from a physician, making physicians the gatekeepers to further health care. Physicians not only *determine* disease by their diagnoses but also *sanction* it by giving a diagnosis. Hence, the person with symptoms is not the one who officially determines his or her health status.

Dealing with symptoms occurs in two stages, which Stanislav Kasl and Sidney Cobb (1966a, 1966b) called illness behavior and sick role behavior. **Illness behavior** consists of the activities undertaken by people who experience symptoms but who have not yet

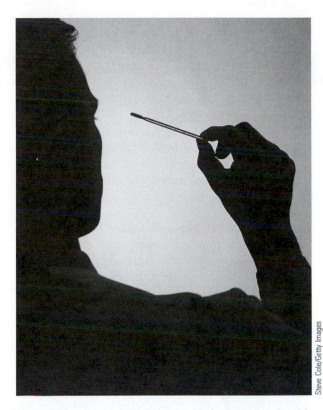

Illness behavior is directed toward determining health status.

Steve Cole/Getty Images

received a diagnosis. That is, illness behavior occurs *before* diagnosis. People engage in illness behaviors to determine their state of health and to discover suitable remedies. Lance Armstrong was engaging in illness behavior when he sought the opinion of his friend, and when he finally made an appointment with a physician. In contrast, **sick role behavior** is the term applied to the behavior of people after a diagnosis, whether from a health care provider or through self-diagnosis. People engage in sick role behavior in order to get well. Lance exhibited sick role behavior when he underwent surgery and chemotherapy, kept medical appointments, took a break from cycling, recovered from his treatments. A *diagnosis*, then, is the event that separates illness behavior from sick role behavior.

Illness Behavior

The goal of illness behavior, which takes place before an official diagnosis, is to determine health status in the presence of symptoms. People routinely experience symptoms that may signal disease, such as chest pain, soreness, or headaches. Symptoms are a critical element in seeking medical care, but the presence of symptoms is not sufficient to prompt a visit to the doctor. Given similar symptoms, some people readily seek help, others do so reluctantly, and still others do not seek help at all. What determines people's decision to seek professional care?

At least six conditions shape people's response to symptoms: (1) personal factors; (2) gender; (3) age; (4) socioeconomic, ethnic, and cultural factors; (5) characteristics of the symptoms; and (6) conceptualization of disease.

Personal Factors   Personal factors include people's way of viewing their own body, their level of stress, and their personality traits. An example comes from people who experience irritable bowel syndrome, an intestinal condition characterized by pain, cramping, constipation, and diarrhea. Stress makes this condition worse. Some people with irritable bowel syndrome seek medical services, whereas many others do not. Interestingly, a person's level of symptoms is *not* the most important reason somebody seeks medical care (Ringström, Abrahamsson, Strid, & Simrén, 2007). Instead, a person typically seeks medical care because of anxiety concerning the condition, coping resources, and level of physical functioning. Those who have adequate resources to cope with the symptoms and feel that the quality of their lives is not too impaired do not seek medical care. These personal factors are more important than the prominence of symptoms in determining who seeks medical care.

Stress is another personal factor in people's readiness to seek care. People who experience a great deal of stress are more likely to seek health care than those under less stress, even with equal symptoms. Those who experience current or ongoing stress are more likely to seek care when symptoms are ambiguous (Cameron, Leventhal, & Leventhal, 1995; Martin & Brantley, 2004). Ironically, other people are *less* likely to view somebody as having a disease if the person also complains about stress. Other people tend to perceive symptoms that coincide with stress as not real. This discounting occurs selectively, with women under high stress judged as less likely to have a physical disease than men in the same circumstances (Martin & Lemos, 2002). This tendency to discount symptoms may be a very important factor in the treatment of women who experience symptoms and for the health care providers who hear their reports.

Personality traits also contribute to illness behavior. In a unique and interesting study headed by Sheldon Cohen (Feldman, Cohen, Gwaltney, Doyle, & Skoner, 1999), investigators inoculated a group of healthy volunteers with a common cold virus to see if participants with different personality traits would report symptoms differently. Participants who scored high on **neuroticism**—that is, those with strong and often negative emotional reactions—generally had high self-reports of illness whether or not objective evidence confirmed their reports. These people also reported more symptoms than other participants, suggesting that people high in the personality trait of neuroticism are more likely to complain of an illness. Additional research confirms the role of neuroticism in the readiness to report physical (and mental) symptoms and to seek medical care (Charles, Gatz, Kato, & Pedersen, 2008; Goodwin & Friedman, 2006).

Gender Differences   In addition to personal factors, gender plays a role in the decision to seek treatment, with women more likely than men to use health care (Galdas, Cheater, & Marshall, 2005). The reasons for this difference are somewhat complex. Women tend to report more body symptoms and distress than men (Koopmans & Lamers, 2007). When asked about their symptoms, men tend to report only life-threatening situations, such as heart disease (Benyamini, Leventhal, & Leventhal, 2000). In contrast, women report not only these symptoms but also non-life-threatening symptoms, such as those from joint disease. Given the same level of symptoms, the female gender role allows women to seek many sorts of assistance, whereas the male gender role teaches men to act strong and to deny pain and discomfort. Research on men with prostate disease (Hale, Grogan, & Willott, 2007) confirms the power of adhering to the male gender role in men's reluctance to seek care. These men were very anxious about their health but were reluctant to seek medical care.

Age   Age is yet another factor that influences people's willingness to seek medical care. Young adults show the greatest reluctance to see a health professional, probably because they feel more indestructible.

As people age, they must decide whether their symptoms are due to aging or the result of disease. This distinction is not always easy, as Lance Armstrong incorrectly attributed his blurred vision to the aging process rather than to the cancer that had already invaded his brain. In general, people tend to interpret problems with a gradual onset and mild symptoms as resulting from age, whereas they are more ready to see problems with a sudden onset and severe symptoms as being more serious. For example, when older patients with symptoms of acute myocardial infarction can attribute these symptoms to age, they tend to delay in seeking medical care. One study (Ryan & Zerwic, 2003) looked at patients who failed to realize that a delay in seeking health care could bring about more severe symptoms as well as increased chance of mortality. Compared with younger and middle-aged patients, these older people were more likely to (1) attribute their symptoms to age, (2) experience more severe and lengthy symptoms, (3) attribute their symptoms to some other disorder, and (4) have had previous experience with cardiac problems. Each of these factors provides information on how older cardiac patients can be treated.

Socioeconomic, Ethnic, and Cultural Factors   People from different cultures and ethnic backgrounds have disparate ways of viewing illness and different patterns of seeking medical care. In the United States, people in higher socioeconomic groups experience fewer symptoms and report a higher level of health than people at lower socioeconomic levels (Matthews & Gallo, 2011; Stone, Krueger, Steptoe, & Harter, 2010). Yet when higher-income people are sick, they are more likely to seek medical care. Nevertheless, poor people are overrepresented among the hospitalized, an indication that they are much more likely than middle- and upper-income people to become seriously ill. In addition, people in lower socioeconomic groups tend to wait longer before seeking health care, thus making treatment more difficult and hospitalization more likely. The poor have less access to medical care, have to travel longer to reach health care facilities that will offer them treatment, and must wait longer once they arrive at those facilities. Thus, poor people utilize medical care less than wealthier people; when poor people do utilize medical care, their illnesses are typically more severe.

Ethnic background is another factor in seeking health care, with European Americans being more likely than other groups to report a visit to a physician. Part of the National Health and Nutrition Examination Survey (Harris, 2001) examined some of the reasons behind these ethnic differences, comparing European Americans, African Americans, and Mexican Americans with Type 2 diabetes on access to and use of health care facilities. Ethnic differences appeared in health insurance coverage as well as in common risk

factors for diabetes and heart disease. Similarly, ethnic differences in insurance coverage account for ethnic differences in the use of dental health care (Doty & Weech-Maldonado, 2003).

A study from the United Kingdom confirmed the notion that culture and ethnic background—not lack of knowledge—are primarily responsible for differences in seeking medical care. In this study (Adamson, Ben-Shlomo, Chaturvedi, & Donovan, 2003), researchers sent questionnaires to a large, diverse group of participants. Each questionnaire included two clinical vignettes showing (1) people experiencing signs of chest pain and (2) people discovering a lump in their armpit. The experimenters asked each participant to respond to the chest pain and the lump in terms of needing immediate care. Results indicated that respondents who were Black, female, and from lower socioeconomic groups were at least as likely as those who were White, male, and from middle- and upper-class groups to make accurate responses to potential medical problems. That is, poor Black women do not lack information about the potential health hazards of chest pain or a lump in the armpit, but they are more likely to lack the resources to respond quickly to these symptoms. Ethnic minorities are also more likely to experience discrimination in their everyday lives, and those who perceive discrimination are less likely to utilize the health care system (Burgess, Ding, Hargreaves, van Ryn, & Phelan, 2008).

Symptom Characteristics   Symptom characteristics also influence when and how people look for help. Symptoms do not inevitably lead people to seek care, but certain characteristics are important in their response to symptoms. David Mechanic (1978) listed four characteristics of the symptoms that determine people's response to disease.

First is the *visibility of the symptom*—that is, how readily apparent the symptom is to the person and to others. Many of Lance Armstrong's symptoms were not visible to others, including his enlarged testes. In a study of Mexican women who had symptoms of possible breast cancer, those whose symptoms were more visible were more likely to seek medical help (Unger-Saldaña & Infante-Castañeda, 2011). Unfortunately, with many diseases such as breast cancer or testicular cancer, the condition may be worse and treatment options more limited once symptoms become visible.

Mechanic's second symptom characteristic was *perceived severity of the symptom*. According to Mechanic, symptoms seen as severe would be more likely to prompt action than less severe symptoms. Lance did not seek immediate medical care partially because he did not see some of his symptoms as serious—he viewed them as the result of the flu or his exhausting training regimen. The perceived severity of the symptom highlights the importance of personal perception and distinguishes between the perceived severity of a symptom and the judgment of severity by medical authorities. Indeed, patients and physicians differ in their perceptions of the severity of a wide variety of symptoms (Peay & Peay, 1998). Symptoms that patients perceive as more serious produce greater concern and a stronger belief that treatment is urgently needed, as a study on women seeking care after experiencing symptoms of heart attack demonstrates (Quinn, 2005). Those women who interpreted their symptoms as indicative of cardiac problems sought care more quickly than women who interpreted their symptoms as some other condition. Thus, perceived severity of symptoms rather than the presence of symptoms is critical in the decision to seek care.

The third symptom characteristic mentioned by Mechanic is the *extent to which the symptom interferes with a person's life*. The more incapacitated the person, the more likely he or she is to seek medical care. Studies on irritable bowel syndrome (Ringström et al., 2007) and overactive bladder (Irwin, Milsom, Kopp, Abrams, & EPIC Study Group, 2008) illustrate this principle; those who seek medical care report a poorer health quality of life than those who do not seek medical care. Lance Armstrong sought attention for his cancer-related symptoms only when they interfered with his ability to ride a bicycle.

Mechanic's fourth hypothesized determinant of illness behavior is the *frequency and persistence of the symptoms*. Conditions that people view as requiring care tend to be those that are both severe and continuous, whereas intermittent symptoms are less likely to generate illness behavior. Severe symptoms—such as coughing up blood, as Lance experienced—prompt people to seek help, but even mild symptoms can motivate people to seek help if those symptoms persist.

In Mechanic's description and subsequent research, symptom characteristics alone are not sufficient to prompt illness behavior. However, if symptoms persist or are perceived as severe, people are more likely to evaluate them as indicating a need for care. Thus, people seek care on the basis of their interpretation of their symptoms, which relates to each person's view of illness.

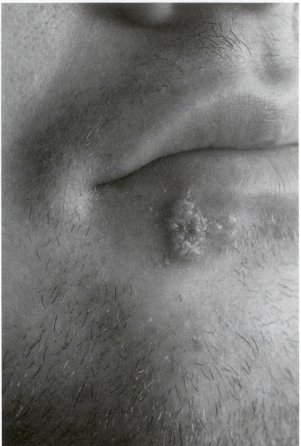

Dani Vincek/Shutterstock.com

People are more likely to seek care for symptoms that are visible to others.

Conceptualization of Disease   Few laypeople are experts in physiology and medicine. Most people are largely ignorant of how their body works and how disease develops. People think about diseases in ways that vary substantially from medical explanations. For example, both children (Veldtman et al., 2001) and college students (Nemeroff, 1995) show inaccurate and incomplete understandings of diseases when they describe diseases they have and how they became ill. Thus, people may seek (or not seek) medical care based on their incomplete and sometimes inaccurate beliefs about health and illness.

What are the important ways in which people conceptualize diseases? Howard Leventhal and his colleagues (Leventhal, Breland, Mora, & Leventhal, 2010; Leventhal, Leventhal, & Cameron, 2001; Martin & Leventhal, 2004) have looked at five components in the conceptualization process: (1) identity of the disease, (2) time line (the time course of both disease and treatment), (3) cause of the disease, (4) consequences of the disease, and (5) controllability of the disease. With each of these components, people's beliefs may not necessarily be accurate. Yet, research shows that these beliefs have important implications for how people seek care and manage a disease.

The *identity of the disease*, the first component identified by Leventhal and his colleagues, is very important to illness behavior. People who have identified their symptoms as a "heart attack" should (Martin & Leventhal, 2004) and do (Quinn, 2005) react quite differently from those who label the same symptoms as "heartburn." As we have seen, the presence of symptoms is not sufficient to initiate help seeking, but the labeling that occurs in conjunction with symptoms may be critical in a person's either seeking help or ignoring symptoms.

Labels provide a framework within which people can recognize and interpret symptoms. In one study, Leventhal and his team gave young adults a blood pressure test and randomly assigned them to receive one of two results: high blood pressure or normal blood pressure (Baumann, Cameron, Zimmerman, & Leventhal, 1989). Compared with the young adults who received results labeled as normal blood pressure, the young adults who received results labeled as high blood pressure were more likely to subsequently report other symptoms related to hypertension. In other words, the label made them report other symptoms that confirmed their diagnosis.

People experience less emotional arousal when they find a label that indicates a minor problem (heartburn rather than heart attack). Initially, they will probably adopt the least serious label that fits their symptoms. For example, Lance Armstrong interpreted headaches as hangovers, and blurred vision as a normal part of aging. Lance—as well as his physician friend—also preferred to interpret his blood-expelling coughs as a sinus problem rather than something more severe. To a large extent, a label carries with it some prediction about the symptoms and time course of the disease, so if the symptoms and time course do not correspond to the expectation implied by the label, the person has to relabel the symptoms. When a swollen testicle became another prominent symptom, Lance quickly realized that the label of a sinus problem did not apply. Thus, the tendency to interpret symptoms as indicating minor rather than major problems is the source of many optimistic self-diagnoses, of which Lance's is an example.

The second component in conceptualizing an illness is the *time line*. Even though a diagnosis usually implies the time course of a disease, people's understanding of the time involved is not necessarily accurate. People with a chronic disorder often view their disease as acute and of short duration. For example, patients with heart disease (a chronic disorder) may see their disease as "heartburn," an acute disorder (Martin & Leventhal, 2004). With most acute diseases, patients can expect a temporary disorder with a quick onset of symptoms, followed by treatment, a remission of symptoms, and then a cure. In fact, people who conceptualize their illness as an acute disorder tend to manage their symptoms better (Horne et al., 2004). Unfortunately, this scenario does not fit the majority of diseases, such as heart disease and diabetes, which are chronic and persist over a lifetime. In a study of adults with diabetes, those who conceptualized their illness as acute rather than chronic managed their illness worse (Mann, Ponieman, Leventhal, & Halm, 2009). However, conceptualizing a chronic disease as time limited may provide patients with some psychological comfort; patients who conceptualize their cancer as chronic report greater distress than those who view the disease as an acute illness (Rabin, Leventhal, & Goodin, 2004).

The third component in conceptualizing an illness is the *determination of cause*. For the most part, determining causality is more a facet of the sick role than of illness behavior because it usually occurs after a diagnosis has been made. But the attribution of causality for symptoms is an important factor in illness behavior. For example, if a person can attribute the pain in his hand to a blow received the day before, he will not have to consider the possibility of bone cancer as the cause of the pain.

Attribution of causality, however, is often faulty. People may attribute a cold to "germs" or to the weather, and they may see cancer as caused by microwave ovens or by the will of God. These conceptualizations have important implications for illness behavior. People are less likely to seek professional treatment for conditions they consider as having emotional or spiritual causes. Culture may also play a role in attributions of causes for diseases. Differences appeared in a study that compared Britons and Taiwanese beliefs about heart disease: Britons were more likely to see heart disease as caused by lifestyle choices, whereas Taiwanese were more likely to see heart disease as caused by worry and stress (Lin, Furze, Spilsbury, & Lewin, 2009). These beliefs may affect how patients care for themselves and manage their disease. Therefore, people's conceptualizations of disease causality can influence their behavior.

The *consequences of a disease* are the fourth component in Leventhal's description of illness. Even though the consequences of a disease are implied by the diagnosis, an incorrect understanding of the consequences can have a profound effect on illness behavior. Many people view a diagnosis of cancer as a death sentence. Some neglect health care because they believe themselves to be in a hopeless situation. Women who find a lump in their breast sometimes delay making an appointment with a doctor, not because they fail to recognize this symptom of cancer but because they fear the possible consequences—surgery and possibly the loss of a breast, chemotherapy, radiation, or some combination of these consequences.

The *controllability* of a disease refers to people's belief that they can control the course of their illness by controlling the treatment or the disease. People who believe that their behaviors will not change the course of a disease are more distressed by their illness and less likely to seek treatment than those who believe that treatment will be effective (Evans & Norman, 2009; Hagger & Orbell, 2003). However, people who are able to control the symptoms of their disease without medical consultation will be less likely to seek professional medical care (Ringström et al., 2007).

In sum, the five beliefs in Leventhal's model predict several important outcomes, including distress, seeking of health care, and disease management. Can changing these beliefs improve health outcomes? A recent study of asthma sufferers suggests that these components can be useful targets for intervention (Petrie, Perry, Broadbent, & Weinman, 2011). In this study, researchers sent some asthma patients periodic text messages that accurately informed the patients of the identity, time line, cause, consequences, and controllability of asthma. Compared with a control group, patients who received the text message intervention reported more accurate beliefs about their asthma, as well as much better management of their condition.

The Sick Role

Kasl and Cobb (1966b) defined sick role behavior as the activities engaged in by people who believe themselves ill, for the purpose of getting well. In other words, sick role behavior occurs after a person receives a diagnosis. Alexander Segall (1997) expanded this concept, proposing that the sick role concept includes three rights or privileges and three duties or

responsibilities. The privileges are (1) the right to make decisions concerning health-related issues, (2) the right to be exempt from normal duties, and (3) the right to become dependent on others for assistance. The three responsibilities are (1) the duty to maintain health along with the responsibility to get well, (2) the duty to perform routine health care management and, (3) the duty to use a range of health care resources.

Segall's formulation of rights and duties is an ideal—not a realistic—conception of sick role behavior in the United States. The first right—to make decisions concerning health-related issues—does not extend to children and many people living in poverty (Bailis, Segall, Mahon, Chipperfield, & Dunn, 2001). The second feature of the sick role is the exemption of the sick person from normal duties. Sick people are usually not expected to go to work, attend school, go to meetings, cook meals, clean house, care for children, do homework, or mow the lawn. However, meeting these expectations is not always possible. Many sick people neither stay home nor go to the hospital, but continue to go to work. People who feel in danger of losing their jobs are more likely to go to work when they are sick (Bloor, 2005), but so did those who experienced good working relationships with their colleagues and were dedicated to their jobs (Biron, Brun, Ivers, & Cooper, 2006). Similarly, the third privilege—to be dependent on others— is more of an ideal than a reflection of reality. For example, sick mothers often must continue to be responsible for their children.

Segall's three duties of sick people all fall under the single obligation to do whatever is necessary to get well. However, the goal of getting well applies more to acute than to chronic diseases. People with chronic diseases will never be completely well. This situation presents a conflict for many people with a chronic disease, who have difficulty accepting their condition as one of continuing disability; instead, they erroneously believe that their disease is a temporary state.

IN SUMMARY

No easy distinction exists between health and illness. The WHO sees health as more than the absence of disease; rather, health is the attainment of positive physical, mental, and social well-being. Curiously, the distinction between disease and illness is clearer. Disease refers to the process of physical damage within the body, whether or not the person is aware of this damage. Illness, on the other hand, refers to the experience of being sick; people can feel sick but have no identifiable disease.

At least six factors determine how people respond to illness symptoms: (1) personal factors, such as the way people look upon their own body; (2) gender—women are more likely than men to seek professional care; (3) age—older people attribute many ailments to their age; (4) ethnic and cultural factors—people who cannot afford medical care are more likely than affluent people to become ill but less likely to seek health care; (5) characteristics of the symptoms—symptoms that interfere with daily activities as well as visible, severe, and frequent symptoms are most likely to prompt medical attention; and (6) people's conceptualization of disease.

People tend to incorporate five components into their concept of disease: (1) the identity of the disease, (2) the time line of the disease, (3) the cause of the disease, (4) the consequences of the disease, and (5) controllability of the disease. If a patient receives a diagnosis of a disease, the diagnosis implies its time course and its consequences. However, people who know the name of their disease do not always have an accurate concept of its time course and consequence and may wrongly see a chronic disease as having a short time course. People want to know the cause of their illness and to understand how they can control it.

After receiving a diagnosis, people engage in sick role behavior in order to get well. People who are sick should be relieved from normal responsibilities and should have the obligation of trying to get well. However, these rights and duties are difficult and often impossible to fulfill.

Seeking Medical Information From Nonmedical Sources

After people notice symptoms that they perceive as being a potential problem, they must decide whether and how to seek help. People's first step in seeking health care, however, is often not to seek help from a doctor. Instead, people often turn to two more easily accessible sources—their lay referral network and the Internet.

Lay Referral Network

When Lance finally decided to seek advice about his symptoms, he did not immediately go to a specialist. Instead, he consulted his friends, one of whom happened to be a physician. Lance's friends were part of his **lay referral network**, a network of family and friends who offer information and advice before any official medical treatment is sought (Friedson, 1961; Suls, Martin, & Leventhal, 1997). Like Lance, most people who seek health care do so as a result of prior conversations with friends and family about symptoms (Cornford & Cornford, 1999). For example, in the study of irritable bowel syndrome (Ringström et al., 2007), about half of those who did not seek medical care sought alternative care or the advice of someone with the same condition. Thus, most people sought help but not necessarily from a physician.

The lay referral network can help a person understand the meaning of symptoms, such as what its label, cause, and cure might be. A lay referral network can also prime a person's perception of symptoms. A woman with chest pain, for example, would react quite differently if her family had a history of heart attacks compared with a history of heartburn. In some cases, people in the lay referral network might advise *against* seeking medical care, particularly if they can recommend simple home remedies or recommend complementary and alternative treatments (see Chapter 8 for a review of complementary and alternative therapies). Thus, people's social networks are often a first source of information and advice on health matters but may not always encourage people to seek traditional medical care (Dimsdale et al., 1979).

The Internet

In recent years, the Internet has become an additional source of information for people who seek information and help with symptoms. Indeed, a majority of Internet users in the United States report using the Internet to search for health information for themselves (Atkinson, Saperstein, & Pleis, 2009). Women and those with higher education are more likely than others to use the Internet for this purpose (Powell, Inglis, Ronnie, & Large, 2011). In fact, public health researchers can use sudden increases in the number of Internet searches about specific disease symptoms to reliably identify outbreaks of infectious diseases in near real time (Ginsberg et al., 2009)!

The Internet is a common source of health information because it satisfies a number of motivations, such as to seek a greater understanding of a health issue, get a second opinion, seek reassurance, and overcome difficulties in getting health information through other sources

(Powell et al., 2011). However, increased access to the Internet opens a vast source of medical information *and* misinformation to the public (Wald, Dube, & Anthony, 2007). One of the challenges that Internet users face is how to distinguish trustworthy websites from those that are simply trying to sell health products. Many people use Wikipedia as a primary source of health information (Laurent & Vickers, 2009), despite the fact that the information on Wikipedia may not be as accurate as other sources. Excellent and credible sources of health information include the Center for Advancing Health website (www.cfah.org) and the National Institutes of Health website (health.nih.gov). Chapter 2 also includes helpful tips on how to identify valid health information on the Internet.

Patients who go to the web for information become more active in their health care, but this knowledge may decrease physicians' authority and change the nature of the physician–patient relationship. When patients bring information to the physician that the physician views as accurate and relevant, then the relationship can benefit (Murray et al., 2003). However, when the patient brings information that is not accurate or relevant, it can deteriorate the relationship and challenge the physician's authority. Many patients are reluctant to bring up Internet health information with their providers out of fear of challenging the provider (Imes et al., 2008). Thus, the Internet is an important source of health information, and patients who do not have access to accurate and relevant information may not be in as good position to be effective users of the medical system (Hall & Schneider, 2008).

Receiving Medical Care

Most people have experience in receiving medical care. In some situations, this experience may be satisfying; in other situations, people face challenges in receiving medical care. These problems include having only limited access to medical care, choosing the right practitioner, and being in the hospital.

Limited Access to Medical Care

The cost of medical care prevents many people from receiving proper treatment and care. This limited access to medical care is more restricted in the United States than in other industrialized nations (Weitz, 2010). Many countries have developed national health insurance or other plans for universal coverage, but the United States has typically resisted this strategy. Hospitalization and complex medical treatments are so expensive that most people cannot afford these services. This situation has led to the rise and development of health insurance, which people may purchase as individuals but more often obtain as part of workplace groups that offer coverage to their members.

Individual insurance tends to be expensive and to offer less coverage, especially for people with health problems, but these individuals may be able to get some insurance as part of a workplace group. Thus, employment is an important factor in access to medical care in the United States. People who are unemployed or whose jobs do not offer the benefit of health insurance are often uninsured, a situation describing about 15% of people in the United States (NCHS, 2011). However, even people with insurance may face barriers to receiving care; their policies often fail to cover services such as dental care, mental health services, and eyeglasses, forcing people to pay these expenses out of their own pockets or forego these services. For insured people who experience a catastrophic illness, coverage may be inadequate for many expenses, creating enormous medical costs. Indeed, medical costs are the underlying cause for over 60% of all personal bankruptcies in the United States (Himmelstein, Thorne, Warren, & Woolhandler, 2009).

The problem of providing medical care for those who cannot afford to pay for these services was a concern throughout the 20th century (Weitz, 2010). In response to these concerns, the U.S. Congress created two programs in 1965—Medicare and Medicaid. Medicare pays hospital expenses for most Americans over the age of 65, and thus few people in this age group are without hospitalization insurance. Medicare also offers medical insurance that those who participate may purchase for a monthly fee, but many expenses are not covered, such as routine dental care. Medicaid provides health care based on low income and physical problems, such as disability or pregnancy. These restrictions make many poor people ineligible; only about half of people living in poverty receive coverage through Medicaid (NCHS, 2011). Children may be eligible for health insurance, even if their parents are not, through the State Children's Health Insurance Program.

People with low incomes struggle to obtain insurance coverage, but even those with insurance may face barriers such as finding a provider who will accept their plan and the out-of-pocket cost of services (Carrillo et al., 2011; DeVoe et al., 2007). The uninsured face more restrictions. These people are less likely to have a regular physician, more likely to have a chronic health problem, and less likely to seek medical care because of the cost (Finkelstein et al., 2011; Pauly & Pagán, 2007). This reluctance has consequences for the management of their diseases. People with chronic diseases and without health insurance have poorly controlled conditions, difficulty in obtaining medications, more health crises, and higher risk of mortality than people with insurance (McWilliams, 2009). In addition, a high proportion of people without insurance may create a spillover effect in which those with insurance experience higher costs and poorer quality of care. Thus, health insurance is an important issue in the access to medical care and plays a role in choosing a practitioner.

Choosing a Practitioner

As part of their attempts to get well, sick people usually consult a health care practitioner. Beginning during the 19th century, physicians became the dominant medical providers (Weitz, 2010). Most middle-class and wealthy people in industrialized nations seek the services of a physician. Toward the end of the 20th century, however, medical dominance began to decline, and other types of health care providers' popularity rose. For example, midwives, nurses, pharmacists, physical therapists, psychologists, osteopaths, chiropractors, dentists, nutritionists, and herbal healers all provide various types of health care.

Some of these sources of health care are considered "alternative" because they provide alternatives to conventional medical care. Almost a third of U.S. residents who seek conventional health care also use some form of alternative health care, and nearly everyone (96%) who uses alternative health care also uses conventional health care (Weitz, 2010). Some people who consult practitioners such as herbal healers do so because these healers are part of a cultural tradition, such as *curanderos* in Latin American culture. However, the recent growth of alternative medicine has come mainly from well-educated people who are dissatisfied with standard medical care and who hold attitudes that are compatible with the alternative care they seek (Weitz, 2010). Well-educated people are more likely to turn to alternative medicine because they are better able to pay for this care, which is less likely to be covered by insurance than conventional care.

People without health insurance are less likely to have a regular health care provider than are those with

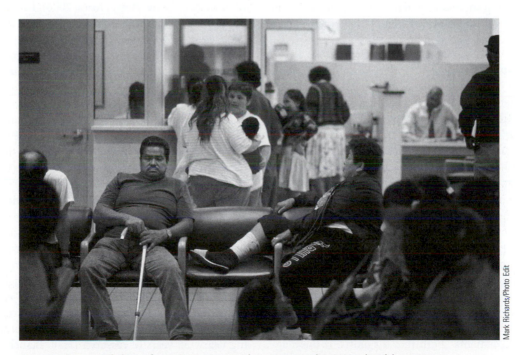

Cost and accessibility of services present barriers to obtaining health care.

Mark Richards/Photo Edit

insurance (Pauly & Pagán, 2007). People who do not have health insurance may receive care from convenient care clinics or hospital emergency rooms, even for chronic conditions. Convenient care clinics offer basic health care, primarily by physicians' assistants and nurse practitioners (Hanson-Turton, Ryan, Miller, Counts, & Nash, 2007). Seeking care through the emergency room may result in people receiving care only after their condition meets the definition of an emergency. Thus, these patients are sicker than they might have been if they had easier access to care. In addition, seeking care from emergency rooms is more expensive and overburdens these facilities, decreasing their ability to provide care to those with acute conditions.

Practitioner–Patient Interaction The interaction between a patient and practitioner is an important consideration in receiving medical care. Practitioners who are successful in forming a working alliance with their patients are more likely to have patients who are satisfied (Fuertes et al., 2007). A satisfying patient–practitioner relationship offers important practical benefits: Satisfied patients are more likely to follow medical advice (Fuertes et al., 2007), more likely to continue to use medical services and obtain checkups, and less likely to file complaints against their practitioners (Stelfox, Gandhi, Orav, & Gustafson, 2005). Important factors in building successful practitioner–patient alliances include verbal communication and the practitioner's personal characteristics.

Verbal Communication Poor verbal communication is perhaps the most crucial factor in practitioner–patient interaction (Cutting Edge Information, 2004). In fact, patients are significantly less likely to follow a practitioner's medical advice when the practitioner communicates poorly (Zolnierek & DiMatteo, 2009). Communication problems may arise when physicians ask patients to report on their symptoms but fail to listen to patients' concerns, interrupting their stories within seconds (Galland, 2006). What constitutes a concern for the patient may not be essential to the diagnostic process, and the practitioner may simply be trying to elicit information relevant to making a diagnosis. However, patients may misinterpret the physician's behavior as a lack of personal concern or as overlooking what patients consider important symptoms. After practitioners have made a diagnosis, they typically tell patients about that diagnosis. If the diagnosis is minor, patients may be relieved and not highly motivated to adhere to (or even listen to) any instructions that may follow. If the verdict is serious, patients may become anxious or frightened, and these feelings may then interfere with their concentration on subsequent medical advice. The patient–practitioner interaction is especially important at this juncture: When patients do not receive information that they have requested, they feel less satisfied with their physician and are less likely to comply with the advice they receive (Bell, Kravitz, Thom, Krupat, & Azari, 2002). However, when patients believe that physicians understand their reasons for seeking treatment and that both agree about treatment, they are more likely to comply with medical advice (Kerse et al., 2004).

For a variety of reasons, physicians and patients frequently do not speak the same language. First, physicians operate in familiar territory. They know the subject matter, are comfortable with the physical surroundings, and are ordinarily calm and relaxed with procedures that have become routine to them. Patients, in contrast, are often unfamiliar with medical terminology (Castro, Wilson, Wang, & Schillinger, 2007); distracted by the strange environment; and distressed by anxiety, fear, or pain (Charlee, Goldsmith, Chambers, & Haynes, 1996). In some cases, practitioners and patients do not speak the same language—literally. Differences in native language present a major barrier to communication (Blanchard & Lurie, 2004; Flores, 2006). Even with interpreters, substantial miscommunication may occur (Rosenberg, Leanza, & Seller, 2007). As a result, patients either fail to understand or to remember significant portions of the information their doctors give them.

The Practitioner's Personal Characteristics A second aspect of the practitioner–patient interaction is the perceived personal characteristics of the physician. When people have the freedom to choose their practitioners, they value technical competence (Bendapudi, Berry, Frey, Parish, & Rayburn, 2006). However, patients have difficulty judging the technical competence of practitioners. Instead, they often base their judgments of technical quality on a practitioner's personal characteristics. Behaviors that differentiate practitioners whom patients rate as providing excellent treatment include being confident, thorough, personable, humane, forthright, respectful, and empathetic. Female physicians are more likely to show these behaviors than male physicians. Two meta-analyses covering nearly 35 years of research (Hall, Blanch-Hartigan, & Roter, 2011; Roter & Hall, 2004) showed that female

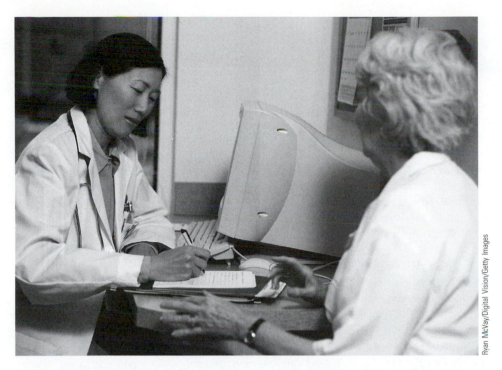

Communication is important for compliance, and female physicians tend to encourage interaction and communication.

physicians were more patient centered, spent 10% more time with patients, employed more partnership behaviors, were more positive in their communication, engaged in more psychosocial counseling, asked more questions, used more emotionally focused talk, and were evaluated more highly by patients than male physicians. Moreover, the patients of female physicians were more likely to disclose more information about their medical symptoms as well as their psychological concerns. This research suggests that when choosing a physician, a person may wish to consider the physician's gender.

Indeed, people are more likely to follow the advice of doctors they see as warm, caring, friendly, and interested in the welfare of patients (DiNicola & DiMatteo, 1984). Alternatively, when patients believe that physicians look down on them or treat them with disrespect, patients are less likely to follow physicians' advice or keep medical appointments (Blanchard & Lurie, 2004).

Being in the Hospital

In serious cases, seeking health care may result in hospitalization. Over the past 30 years, hospitals and the experience of being in the hospital have both changed.

First, many types of surgery and tests that were formerly handled through hospitalization are now performed on an outpatient basis. Second, hospital stays have become shorter. Third, an expanding array of technology is available for diagnosis and treatment. Fourth, patients feel increasingly free to voice their concerns to their physician (Bell, Kravitz, Thom, Krupat, & Azari, 2001). As a result of these changes, people who are not severely ill are not likely to be hospitalized, and people who are admitted to a hospital are more severely ill than those admitted 30 years ago.

Ironically, although managed care has helped control costs through shorter hospital stays, it has not always been in the interest of the patient. Technological medicine has become more prominent in patient care, and personal treatment by the hospital staff has become less so. These factors can combine to make hospitalization a stressful experience (Weitz, 2010). In addition, understaffing and the challenges of monitoring complex technology and medication regimens have created an alarming number of medical mistakes (see Would You Believe …? box).

The Hospital Patient Role   Part of the sick role is to be a patient, and being a patient means conforming to

Would You BELIEVE...? Hospitals May Be a Leading Cause of Death

Would you believe that receiving medical care, especially in an American hospital, can be fatal? Newspaper headlines have painted an alarming picture of the dangers of receiving health care, based on a series of studies. In 1999, a study from the Institute of Medicine made headlines with its findings that at least 44,000—and perhaps as many as 98,000—people die in U.S. hospitals every year as a result of medical errors (Kohn, Corrigan, & Donaldson, 1999). Later reports found even higher numbers of medical mistakes (HealthGrades, 2011; Zhan & Miller, 2003). Although the United States does not recognize medical error as a cause of death, the Washington Post (Weiss, 1999) calculated that medical errors are the fifth leading cause of death in the United States.

Unfortunately, medical errors aren't the only cause of unnecessary deaths of patients in U.S. hospitals. Medication, too, can be fatal. An Institute of Medicine study (Aspden, Wolcott, Bootman, & Cronenwett, 2007) estimated that hospitalized patients experience an average of one medication error per patient per day of hospitalization, resulting in morbidity, mortality, and increased cost of hospitalization. A meta-analysis of studies on adverse drug reactions (Lazarou, Pomeranz, & Corey, 1998) found that, even when prescribed and taken properly, prescription drugs account for between 76,000 and 137,000 deaths each year. This analysis included patients admitted to a hospital for an adverse drug reaction as well as those already in the hospital who suffered a fatal drug reaction. This meta-analysis also estimated the total number of toxic drug reactions among hospitalized patients at more than 2 million. Despite widespread publicity and growing concern, little improvement seems to have occurred during the past 15 years. The medical profession has achieved only limited progress toward solving the problem of medical errors (Leape & Berwick, 2005), and a recent study (HealthGrades, 2011) indicated that medical errors in hospitals have not decreased.

One barrier to correcting the situation comes from the climate of silence and blame that surrounds errors—health care professionals do not want to admit to errors or report colleagues who have made errors because of the blame involved. Rather than silence and blame, Lucian Leape (Leape & Berwick, 2005) suggested that hospitals should be eager to seek information about errors and that analysis should focus on the systems that allow errors rather than the people who make errors.

Interventions may be able to reduce the incidence of medical errors (Woodward et al., 2010). These include patient-focused interventions, such as encouraging patients to state their name to physicians and asking physicians whether they washed their hands. In addition, institutional interventions may also reduce medical errors, such as reducing the number of hours in a typical physician's or nurse's shift and implementing computer systems to better detect potential medication errors. The practice of medicine will never be free of errors, but creating systems that make errors more difficult to commit will improve patient safety and cut hospitalization costs.

the rules of a hospital and complying with medical advice. When a person enters the hospital as a patient, that person becomes part of a complex institution and assumes a role within that institution. That role includes some difficult aspects: being treated as a "nonperson," tolerating lack of information, and losing control of daily activities. Patients find incidents such as waits, delays, and communication problems with staff distressing, and such incidents decrease patients' satisfaction (Weingart et al., 2006).

When people are hospitalized, all but their illness becomes invisible, and their status is reduced to that of a "nonperson." Not only are patients' identities ignored, but their comments and questions may also be overlooked. Hospital procedure focuses on the technical aspects of medical care; it usually ignores patients' emotional needs and leaves them less satisfied with their treatment than patients who are treated as persons, listened to, and informed about their condition (Boudreaux & O'Hea, 2004; Clever, Jin, Levinson, & Meltzer, 2008).

The lack of information that patients experience comes from hospital routine rather than from an attempt to keep information from patients. Most physicians believe that patients should receive full information about their conditions. However, an open exchange of information between patient and practitioner is difficult to achieve in the hospital, where physicians spend only a brief amount of time talking to patients. In addition, information may be unavailable because patients are undergoing diagnostic tests. The hospital staff may not explain the purpose or results of diagnostic testing, leaving the patient without information and filled with anxiety.

Hospitalized patients are expected to conform submissively to the rules of the hospital and the orders of their doctor, thus relinquishing much control over their lives. People tend to manifest heightened physiological responses and to react on a physical level to uncontrollable stimulation more strongly than they do when they can exert some control over their condition. Lack of control can decrease people's capacity to concentrate and can increase their tendency to report physical symptoms.

For the efficiency of the organization, uniform treatment and conformity to hospital routine are desirable, even though they deprive patients of information and control. Hospitals have no insidious plot to deprive patients of their freedom, but this occurs when hospitals impose their routine on patients. Restoring control to patients in any significant way would further complicate an already complex organization, but the restoration of small types of control may be effective. For example, most hospitals now allow patients some choice of foods and provide TV remote controls to give patients the power to select a program to watch (or not watch). These aspects of control are small but possibly important, as we discuss in Chapter 5 (Langer & Rodin, 1976; Rodin & Langer, 1977).

Children and Hospitalization   Few children pass through childhood without some injury, disease, or condition that requires hospitalization, and the hospitalization experience can be a source of stress and anxiety—separation from parents, an unfamiliar environment, diagnostic tests, administration of anesthesia, immunization "shots," surgery, and postoperative pain. Pediatric hospitals often offer some type of preparation program for children. Training children to cope with their fear of treatment presents special problems to health psychologists. Providing children and parents with information about hospital procedures and equipment can be an effective way to decrease anxiety.

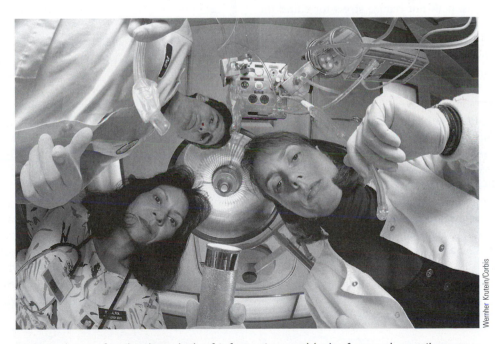

Werhner Krutein/Corbis

Increased use of technology, lack of information, and lack of control contribute to the stress of hospitalization.

Contrary to what many parents may think, reassuring a child is not an effective way to reduce fear in either the child or the parent. In a study with 4- to 6-year-old children who were about to receive preschool immunization shots, researchers (Manimala, Blount, & Cohen, 2000) paired each child with her or his parent and then randomly assigned each dyad to either a distraction group or a reassurance group. Researchers asked the parents of children in the distraction group to distract their child's attention away from the immunization procedure but asked parents of children in the reassurance group to reduce their child's anxiety by reassuring them that they had nothing to fear. Results strongly favored the distraction group, with 3 times as many children in the reassurance group requiring physical restraint. Also, children in the reassurance group showed much more verbal fear then did the other children. An interesting adjunct to these findings involved the training received by parents prior to the immunization process. Those who received training on how to reassure their child expressed a high level of confidence that they could calm their child. Then, after immunization, the reassuring parents not only had problems helping their children, but they also rated themselves as being much more distressed than did the other parents! In turn, parents' distress increases the child's anxiety (Wolff et al., 2009). Reassurance, it seems, does not reduce stress for either the parent or the child.

Another strategy for helping children is modeling—that is, seeing another child cope successfully with a similar stressful procedure. A combination of modeling with a cognitive behavioral intervention and self-talk reduced distress for children who were receiving painful treatments for leukemia (Jay, Elliott, Woody, & Siegel, 1991). Indeed, this intervention was more successful than a drug treatment that included the tranquilizer Valium. A review of interventions for children (Mitchell, Johnston, & Keppel, 2004) indicated that multicomponent programs were generally more effective than single-component programs; providing information and teaching coping skills are both important for children and their parents when faced with hospitalization.

Cost, not effectiveness, is the main problem with intervention strategies to reduce children's distress resulting from hospitalization for specific medical procedures. The trend is toward cost cutting, and all interventions add to medical care costs. Some of these interventions may be cost effective if they reduce the need for additional care or decrease other expenses.

IN SUMMARY

The expense of medical care has led to restricted access for most U.S. residents. People who have medical insurance receive better care and have more choices about their care than people without insurance. Concerns about medical costs led to the creation of two U.S. government programs: Medicare, which pays for hospitalization for those over age 65; and Medicaid, which pays for care for poor people who are aged, blind, disabled, pregnant, or the parents of a dependent child.

Physicians are primary sources of medical care, but alternative sources have become more popular over the past two decades. People without medical insurance often have limitations in securing a regular medical care practitioner. Patients' satisfaction with their providers is an important factor in seeking medical care, as well as adherence to medical advice. Physicians who listen to their patients and are perceived as personable, confident, and empathetic are those who are most likely to be rated as excellent physicians. Female physicians tend to exhibit these characteristics more than male physicians.

Hospitalized patients often experience added stress as a result of being in the hospital. They are typically regarded as "nonpersons," receive inadequate information concerning their illness, and experience some loss of control over their lives. They are expected to conform to hospital routine and to comply with frequent requests of the hospital staff.

Hospitalized children and their parents experience special problems and may receive special training to help them deal with hospitalization. Several types of interventions, including modeling and cognitive behavioral programs, are effective in helping children and their parents cope with this difficult situation.

Answers

This chapter has addressed three basic questions:

1. What factors are related to seeking medical attention?

How people determine their health status when they don't feel well depends not only on social, ethnic, and demographic factors but also on the characteristics of their symptoms and their concept of illness. In deciding whether they are ill, people consider at least four characteristics of their symptoms: (1) the obvious visibility of the symptoms, (2) the perceived severity of the illness, (3) the degree to which the symptoms interfere with their lives, and (4) the frequency and persistence of the symptoms. Once people are diagnosed as sick, they adopt the sick role that involves relief from normal social and occupational responsibilities and the duty to try to get better.

2. Where do people seek medical information?

Prior to seeking medical care and information from the health care system, people often turn to other people and the Internet. The lay referral network is people's family and friends, who often help interpret the meaning of symptoms as well as suggest possible causes and cures. In recent years, the Internet is a common source of health information, although the quality of health information on the Internet varies widely. When patients find accurate and relevant health information, it can benefit the patient–practitioner relationship. However, not all patients have access to health information through the Internet, or are wary of bringing up such information with their providers.

3. What problems do people encounter in receiving medical care?

People encounter problems in paying for medical care, and those without insurance often have limited access to health care. The U.S. government's creation of Medicare and Medicaid has helped people over 65 and some poor people with access to health care, but many people have problems finding a regular practitioner and receiving optimal health care.

Physicians may not have a lot of time to devote to a patient, which may create communication problems that reduce patients' satisfaction. Communication problems include using medical language that is unfamiliar to the patient, as well as focusing on determining and describing a diagnosis rather than allowing the patients to fully describe their concerns.

Although hospital stays are shorter than they were 30 years ago, being in the hospital is a difficult experience for both adults and children. As a hospital patient, a person must conform to hospital procedures and policies, which include being treated as a "nonperson," tolerating lack of information, and losing control of daily activities. Children who are hospitalized are placed in an unfamiliar environment, may be separated from parents, and may undergo surgery or other painful medical procedures. Interventions that help children and parents manage this stressful experience may ease the distress, but cost is a factor that limits the availability of these services.

Suggested Readings

Leventhal, H., Breland, J. Y., Mora, P. A., & Leventhal, E. A. (2010). Lay representations of illness and treatment: A framework for action. In A. Steptoe (Ed.), *Handbook of behavioral medicine: Methods and applications* (pp. 137–154). New York: Springer. This chapter discusses the importance of people's conceptualizations of illness in terms of both health seeking and disease management, but also outlines ways in which illness conceptualizations may be used as targets for intervention.

Martin, R., & Leventhal, H. (2004). Symptom perception and health care–seeking behavior. In J. M. Raczynski & L. C. Leviton (Eds.), *Handbook of clinical health psychology* (Vol. 2, pp. 299–328). Washington, DC: American Psychological Association. This article explores the situations and perceptions that underlie seeking health care, including the difficulty of interpreting symptoms and the theories that attempt to explain this behavior.

Weitz, R. (2010). *The sociology of health, illness, and health care: A critical approach* (5th ed.). Belmont, CA: Cengage. Weitz critically reviews the health care situation in the United States in this medical sociology book. Chapters 10, 11, and 12 provide a description of health care settings and professions, including many alternatives to traditional health care.

CHAPTER 4

Adhering to Healthy Behavior

CHAPTER OUTLINE

- **Real-World Profile of Nathan Rey**
- *Issues in Adherence*
- *What Factors Predict Adherence?*
- *Why and How Do People Adhere to Healthy Behaviors?*
- *The Intention–Behavior Gap*
- *Improving Adherence*

QUESTIONS

This chapter focuses on six basic questions:

1. What is adherence, how is it measured, and how frequently does it occur?

2. What factors predict adherence?

3. What are continuum theories of health behavior, and how do they explain adherence?

4. What are stage theories of health behavior, and how do they explain adherence?

5. What is the intention–behavior gap, and what factors predict whether intentions are translated into behavior?

6. How can adherence be improved?

☑ CHECK YOUR HEALTH RISKS

Regarding Adhering to Healthy Behavior

☐ 1. I believe physical activity is important, but every time I try to exercise I can never keep it up for very long.

☐ 2. If my prescription medicine doesn't seem to be working, I will continue taking it.

☐ 3. I do not need to engage in any planning to change my health habits, as my good intentions always carry me through.

☐ 4. I won't have a prescription filled if it costs too much.

☐ 5. I see my dentist twice a year whether or not I have a problem.

☐ 6. I'm a smoker who knows that smoking can cause heart disease and lung cancer, but I believe that other smokers are much more likely to get these diseases than I am.

☐ 7. I am a woman who doesn't worry about breast cancer because I don't have any symptoms.

☐ 8. I am a man who doesn't worry about testicular cancer because I don't have any symptoms.

☐ 9. People have advised me to stop smoking, but I have never been able to quit.

☐ 10. I frequently forget to take my medication.

☐ 11. When I set a goal to improve my health, I plan out the specific ways and specific situations in which I can act to achieve the goal.

☐ 12. The last time I was sick, the doctor gave me advice that I didn't completely understand, but I was too embarrassed to say so.

Items 2, 5, and 11 represent good adherence beliefs and habits, but each of the other items represents a risk factor for being able to adhere to medical advice. Although it may be nearly impossible to adhere to all good health recommendations (such as not smoking, eating a healthy diet, exercising, and having regular dental and medical checkups), you can improve your health by adhering to sound medical advice. As you read this chapter, you will learn more about the health benefits of adherence, as well as the beliefs and techniques that can improve adherence.

Real-World Profile of
NATHAN REY

Nathan Rey* was a 24-year-old college student who juggled a full course load with a 20-hour-a-week job as an assistant at a legal firm. Nathan enjoyed playing basketball and soccer on the weekends, but his busy work and school life didn't leave him with time to exercise much more than that. His diet consisted of what was easily accessible—mostly sandwiches, fast food, and pizza. Nathan had also been a smoker for years—he usually went through two packs during the workweek, and two packs on the weekends. Although he weighed 25 pounds more than he wanted, he considered himself to be generally healthy.

One Thursday morning, Nathan's father suffered a severe heart attack, requiring a double bypass operation. Nathan's father had coronary heart disease, which was the underlying cause of his heart attack. His heart disease was likely due to years of poor diet and smoking—risk factors that were worsened by a family history of heart disease.

After his father's heart attack, Nathan decided to quit smoking. He had known of the detrimental health effects of smoking, but after his father's heart attack, he learned that the risks could be even worse for people with a family history of heart problems.

Nathan made his first attempt to quit on a Monday. As he would soon discover, weekdays tended to be the easiest days for him to stay away from cigarettes. Weekends, however, were harder because many of his friends also smoked. It was difficult for him to break the pattern established among his friends.

Sometimes, a weekend lapse would strengthen Nathan's commitment to stop for the following week. Other times, a lapse would lead him back to his old habits. Over the next few months, his attempts to quit became too numerous to count. On some of the occasions that he found himself back to smoking, he convinced himself that the health risks of smoking were not that bad after all.

When people like Nathan try to adopt healthy behaviors such as stopping smoking, they often discover that it can be very difficult. Why did it take a scare such as his father's heart attack to convince Nathan to stop smoking? What factors motivated him to quit? Why were his attempts to quit less successful than he had hoped?

*This name has been changed to protect the person's privacy.

Issues in Adherence

Like Nathan, most people in the world value health and want to avoid disease and disability. Nevertheless, many people behave in ways that compromise their health. In Chapter 1, we said that one of the major pathways by which psychological factors influence physical health is through health-related behavior. Why do some people, such as Nathan, seem to behave unwisely on issues of personal health? What explains people's reluctance to believe that their own risky behaviors are dangerous but their willingness to believe that those same behaviors place other people in jeopardy?

For medical advice to benefit a patient's health, two requirements must be met. First, the advice must be valid. Second, the patient must follow this good advice. Both conditions are essential. Ill-founded advice that patients strictly follow may produce new health problems that lead to disastrous outcomes for the adherent patient. On the other hand, excellent advice is worthless if patients do not follow it. As many as 125,000 people in the United States may die each year because they fail to adhere to medical advice, especially by failing to take prescribed medications (Cutting Edge Information, 2004). As two meta-analyses show, adhering to a medical regimen makes a big difference in improvement (DiMatteo, Giordani, Lepper, & Croghan, 2002; Simpson et al., 2006).

In this section, we look at four questions regarding *adherence*: What is adherence? How do researchers measure adherence? How frequently do people fail to adhere? What are common barriers to adherence?

What Is Adherence?

What does it mean to be adherent? We define **adherence** as a person's ability and willingness to follow recommended health practices. R. Brian Haynes (1979)

suggested a broader definition of the term, defining adherence as "the extent to which a person's behavior (in terms of taking medications, following diets, or executing lifestyle changes) coincides with medical or health advice" (pp. 1–2). This definition expands the concept of adherence beyond merely taking medications to include maintaining healthy lifestyle practices, such as eating properly, getting sufficient exercise, avoiding undue stress, abstaining from smoking cigarettes, and not abusing alcohol. In addition, adherence includes making and keeping periodic medical and dental appointments, using seatbelts, and engaging in other behaviors that are consistent with the best health advice available. Adherence is a complex concept, with people being adherent in one situation and nonadherent in another (Ogedegbe, Schoenthaler, & Fernandez, 2007).

How Is Adherence Measured?

How do researchers know the percentage of patients who fail to adhere to practitioners' recommendations? What methods do they use to identify those who fail to adhere? The answer to the first question is that adherence rates are not known with certainty, but researchers use techniques that yield a great deal of information about nonadherence. At least six basic methods of measuring patient adherence are available: (1) ask the practitioner, (2) ask the patient, (3) ask other people, (4) monitor medication usage, (5) examine biochemical evidence, and (6) use a combination of these procedures.

The first of these methods, asking the practitioner, is usually the poorest choice. Physicians generally overestimate their patients' adherence rates, and even when their guesses are not overly optimistic, they are usually wrong (Miller et al., 2002). In general, practitioners' accuracy is only slightly better than chance (Parker et al., 2007).

Asking patients themselves is a slightly more valid procedure, but it is fraught with many difficulties. Self-reports are inaccurate for at least two reasons. First, patients tend to report behaviors that make them appear more adherent than they actually are. Second, they may simply not know their own rate of adherence, as people do not typically pay close attention to their health-related behaviors. Interviews are more prone to these types of errors than asking patients to keep records or diaries of their behavior (Garber, 2004). Because self-report measures have questionable validity, researchers often supplement them with other methods (Parker et al., 2007).

Another method is to ask hospital personnel and family members to monitor the patient, but this procedure also has at least two inherent problems. First, constant observation may be physically impossible, especially with regard to such behaviors as diet, smoking, and alcohol consumption (Observing risky sexual behavior raises clear ethical issues as well!). Second, persistent monitoring creates an artificial situation and frequently results in higher rates of adherence than would otherwise occur. This outcome is desirable, of course, but as a means of assessing adherence, it contains a built-in error that makes observation by others inaccurate.

A fourth method of assessing adherence is to objectively monitor a person's behavior. This may occur by monitoring a patient's medicine usage, such as counting pills or assessing whether patients obtain prescriptions or refills (Balkrishnan & Jayawant, 2007). These procedures seem to be more objective because very few errors are likely to be made in counting the number of pills absent from a bottle or the number of patients who have their prescriptions filled. Even if the required number of pills are gone or the prescriptions filled, however, the patient may not have taken the medication or may have taken it in a manner other than the one prescribed.

The development of electronic technology makes possible more sophisticated methods to monitor adherence. Researchers can assess physical activity by using devices that record physical movement, or by sending surveys to people's mobile phones that ask about physical activity in the past 30 minutes (Dunton, Liao, Intille, Spruijt-Metz, & Pentz, 2011). Researchers can ask patients to send photographs of pill capsules from mobile phones to verify the time when they take their medications (Galloway, Coyle, Guillén, Flower, & Mendelson, 2011). Other methods such as the Medication Event Monitoring System (MEMS) include a microprocessor in the pill cap that records the date and time of every bottle opening and closing, thus yielding a record of usage (assuming that opening the bottle equals using the medication). In addition, this system includes an Internet link that uploads the data stored in the device so that researchers can monitor adherence on a daily or weekly basis. Not surprisingly, assessment by MEMS does not show high consistency with self-reports (Balkrishnan & Jayawant, 2007; Shi et al., 2010). In a study of heart failure patients who were prescribed medications to control their condition, adherence measured by MEMS predicted survival over a 6-month period, but adherence measured by self-report did not (Wu, Moser, Chung, & Lennie, 2008).

Examination of biochemical evidence is a fifth method of measuring adherence. This procedure looks at biochemical evidence, such as analysis of blood or urine samples that reflect adherence, to determine whether the patient behaved in an adherent fashion. For example, researchers can measure the progression of HIV infection with assessments of viral load, a biochemical measure of the amount of the HIV virus in the blood; adherence to HIV medication relates to changes in HIV viral load. Researchers can assess proper management of diabetes by a blood test that gauges the amount of glucose (a sugar) in the blood over a period of months. However, problems can arise with the use of biochemical evidence as a means of assessing adherence because individuals vary in their biochemical response to drugs. In addition, this approach requires frequent medical monitoring that may be intrusive and expensive.

Finally, clinicians can use a combination of these methods to assess adherence. Several studies (Liu et al., 2001; Velligan et al., 2007) used a variety of methods to assess adherence, including interviewing patients, counting pills, electronic monitoring, and measuring biochemical evidence, as well as a combination of all these methods. The results indicate good agreement among pill counts, electronic monitoring, and measuring biochemical evidence but poor agreement between these objective measures and patients' or clinicians' reports. A weakness of using multiple methods of measuring adherence is the cost, but it is an important strategy when researchers need the most accurate evidence to measure adherence.

How Frequent Is Nonadherence?

How common are failures of adherence? The answer to this question depends in part on how adherence is defined, the nature of the illness under consideration, the demographic features of the population, and the methods used to assess adherence. When interest in these questions developed in the late 1970s, David Sackett and John C. Snow (1979) reviewed more than 500 studies that dealt with the frequency of adherence and nonadherence. Sackett and Snow found higher rates for patients' keeping appointments when patients initiated the appointments (75%) than when appointments were scheduled for them (50%). As expected, adherence rates were higher when treatment was meant to cure rather than to prevent a disease. However, adherence was lower for medication taken for a chronic condition over a long period; adherence was around 50% for either prevention or cure.

More recent reviews confirm the problem of nonadherence, estimating nonadherence to medication regimens at nearly 25% (DiMatteo, 2004b). Adherence rates tend to be higher in more recent studies than in older ones, but many of the factors identified in Sackett and Snow's (1979) review continued to be significant predictors of adherence. Medication treatments yielded higher adherence rates than recommendations for exercise, diet, or other types of health-related behavior change. However, DiMatteo's analysis revealed that not all chronic conditions yielded equally low adherence rates. Some chronic conditions, such as HIV, arthritis, gastrointestinal disorders, and cancer, showed high adherences rates, whereas diabetes and pulmonary disease showed lower adherence. Nevertheless, failure to adhere to medical advice is a widespread problem, with one prominent review stating that "effective ways to help people follow medical treatments could have far larger effects on health than any treatment itself" (Haynes et al., 2008; p. 20).

What Are the Barriers to Adherence?

One category of reasons for nonadherence includes all those problems inherent in hearing and heeding physicians' advice. Patients may have financial or practical problems in making and keeping appointments and in filling, taking, and refilling prescriptions. Patients may reject the prescribed regimen as being too difficult, time consuming, expensive, or not adequately effective. Or they may just forget. Patients tend to pick and choose among the elements of the regimen their practitioners offer, treating this information as advice rather than orders (Vermeire, Hearnshaw,

Van Royen, & Denekens, 2001). These patients may stop taking their medication because adherence is too much trouble or does not fit into the routine of their daily lives. Such patients fail to adhere to the prescribed regimen in some ways and so are considered nonadherent.

Patients may stop taking medication when their symptoms disappear. Paradoxically, others stop because they fail to feel better or begin to feel worse, leading them to believe that the medication is useless. Still others, in squirrel-like fashion, save a few pills for the next time they get sick.

Some patients may make irrational choices about adherence because they have an **optimistic bias**—a belief that they will be spared the negative consequences of nonadherence that afflict other people (Weinstein, 1980, 2001). Other patients may be nonadherent because prescription labels are too difficult to read. Visual handicaps that are common among older patients form one barrier. However, even college students may find prescription labels difficult to understand; fewer than half of college students were able to correctly understand prescription labels that had been randomly selected from a pharmacist's records (Mustard & Harris, 1989).

Another set of reasons for high rates of nonadherence is that the current definition of adherence demands lifestyle choices that are difficult to attain. At the beginning of the 20th century, when the leading causes of death and disease were infectious diseases, adherence was simpler. Patients were adherent when they followed the doctor's advice with regard to medication, rest, and so on. Adherence is no longer a matter of taking the proper pills and following short-term advice. The three leading causes of death in the United States—cardiovascular disease, cancer, and chronic obstructive lung disease—are all affected by unhealthy lifestyles. Thus, adherence, broadly defined, currently includes adherence to healthy and safe behaviors as part of an ongoing lifestyle. To be adherent, people must now avoid cigarette smoking, use alcohol wisely or not at all, eat properly, and exercise regularly. In addition, of course, they must also make and keep medical and dental appointments, listen with understanding to the advice of health care providers, and finally, follow that advice. These conditions present a complex array of requirements that are difficult for anyone to fulfill completely. Table 4.1 summarizes some of the reasons patients give for not adhering to medical advice.

TABLE 4.1   Reasons Given by Patients for Not Adhering to Medication Advice

"It's too much trouble."

"I just didn't get the prescription filled."

"The medication was too expensive, so I took fewer pills to make them last."

"The medication didn't work very well. I was still sick, so I stopped taking it."

"The medication worked after only 1 week, so I stopped taking it."

"I have too many pills to take."

"I won't get sick. God will save me."

"I forgot."

"I don't want to become addicted to pills."

"I gave some of my pills to my husband so he won't get sick."

"This doctor doesn't know as much as my other doctor."

"The medication makes me sick."

"I don't like the way that doctor treats me, and I'm not going back."

"I feel fine. I don't see any reason to take something to prevent illness."

"I don't like my doctor. He looks down on people without insurance."

"I didn't understand my doctor's instructions and was too embarrassed to ask her to repeat them."

"I don't like the taste of nicotine chewing gum."

"I didn't understand the directions on the label."

IN SUMMARY

Adherence is the extent to which a person is able and willing to follow medical and health advice. In order for people to profit from adherence, first, the advice must be valid, and second, patients must follow that advice. Inability or unwillingness to adhere to health-related behaviors increases people's chances of serious health problems or even death.

Researchers can assess adherence in at least six ways: (1) ask the physician, (2) ask the patient, (3) ask other people, (4) monitor medical usage, (5) examine biochemical evidence, and (6) use a combination of these procedures. No one of these procedures is both reliable and valid. However, with the exception of clinician judgment, most have some validity and usefulness. When accuracy is crucial, using two or more of these methods yields greater accuracy than reliance on a single technique.

The frequency of nonadherence depends on the nature of the illness. People are more likely to adhere to a medication regimen than to a program that changes health-related behaviors such as diet or exercise. The average rate of nonadherence is slightly less than 25%. To understand and improve adherence, health psychologists seek to understand the barriers that keep people from adhering, including the difficulty of altering lifestyles of long duration, inadequate practitioner–patient communications, and erroneous beliefs as to what advice patients should follow.

What Factors Predict Adherence?

Who adheres and who does not? The factors that predict adherence include personal characteristics and environmental factors that are difficult or impossible to change, such as age or socioeconomic factors. The factors also include specific health beliefs that are more easily modifiable. In this section, we consider the first set of factors, which include: severity of the disease; treatment characteristics, including side effects and complexity of the treatment; personal characteristics, such as age, gender, and personality; and environmental factors such as **social support**, income, and cultural norms. Later in this chapter, we will present major theories of adherence that identify specific beliefs and behavioral strategies that are more easily modifiable through intervention.

Severity of the Disease

Common wisdom suggests that people with severe, potentially crippling, or life-threatening illnesses will be highly motivated to adhere to regimens that protect them against such outcomes. However, little evidence supports this reasonable hypothesis. In general, people with a serious disease are no more likely than people with a less serious problem to adhere to medical advice (DiMatteo, 2004b). What matters in predicting adherence is not the objective severity of a patient's disease but, rather, the patient's *perception* of the severity of the disease (DiMatteo, Haskard, & Williams, 2007). That is, the objective severity of a disease is less closely related to adherence to treatment or prevention regimens than the threat that people perceive from a disease.

Treatment Characteristics

Characteristics of the treatment, such as side effects of a prescribed medication and the complexity of the treatment, also present potential problems for adherence.

Side Effects of the Medication   Early research (Masur, 1981) found little evidence to suggest that unpleasant side effects are a major reason for discontinuing a drug or dropping out of a treatment program. However, more recent research with diabetes medications (Mann, Ponieman, Leventhal, & Halm, 2009) and the complex regimen of HIV medication (Applebaum, Richardson, Brady, Brief, & Keane, 2009; Herrmann et al., 2008) shows that those who experience or have concerns about severe side effects are less likely to take their medications than those who do not have such concerns.

Complexity of the Treatment   Are people less likely to adhere as treatment procedures become increasingly complex? In general, the greater the number of doses or variety of medications people must take, the greater the likelihood that they will not take pills as prescribed

(Piette, Heisler, Horne, & Caleb Alexander, 2006). Researchers observe this relationship between number of doses and adherence across a variety of chronic medical conditions, including diabetes, hypertension, and HIV (Ingersoll & Cohen, 2008; Pollack, Chastek, Williams, & Moran, 2010). For example, people who need to take one pill per day adhere fairly well (as high as 90%), and increasing the dosage to two per day produces little decrease (Claxton, Cramer, & Pierce, 2001). When people must take four doses per day, however, adherence plummets to below 40%; this may be due to people having difficulty fitting medications into daily routines. For example, pills prescribed once a day can be cued to routine activities, such as waking up; those prescribed twice a day can be cued to early morning and late night; and those prescribed three times a day can be cued to meals. Schedules calling for patients to take medication four or more times a day, or to take two or more medications a day, create difficulties and lower adherence rates. Other aspects of a medical regimen can contribute to complexity, such as the need to cut pills in half prior to taking them. In a study of nearly 100,000 patients of Type 2 diabetes, patients who were prescribed the most complex regimen—in terms of both the need to split pills as well as the number of doses per day—showed the lowest rates of adherence (Pollack et al., 2010).

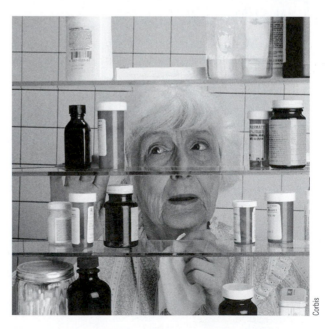

More complex treatments tend to lower compliance rates.

Personal Factors

Who is most adherent, women or men? The young or the old? Are there certain personality patterns that predict adherence? In general, demographic factors such as age and gender show some relationship to adherence, but any of these factors alone is too small to be a good predictor of who will adhere and who will not (DiMatteo, 2004b). Personality was one of the first factors considered in relation to adherence, but other personal factors such as emotional factors and personal beliefs appear more important in understanding adherence.

Age   The relationship between age and adherence is not simple. Assessing adherence among children is difficult because the person whose adherence is important is actually the parent and not the child (De Civita & Dobkin, 2005). As children grow into adolescents, they become more responsible for adhering to medical regimens, and this situation continues throughout adulthood. However, older people may face situations that make adherence difficult, such as memory problems, poor health, and regimens that include many medications (Gans & McPhillips, 2003). These developmental issues contribute to a complex relationship between age and adherence. One study (Thomas et al., 1995) found a curvilinear relationship between age and adherence to colorectal cancer screening. That is, those who adhered best were around 70 years old, with older and younger participants adhering least. Those who are 70 years old may not be the best at adhering to all medical advice, but this result suggests that both older and younger adults, plus children and adolescents, experience more problems with adherence. Other research confirms the problems with these age groups.

Even with caregivers to assist them, children with asthma (Penza-Clyve et al., 2004), diabetes (Cramer, 2004), and HIV infection (Farley et al., 2004) often fail to adhere to their medical regimens. As they grow into adolescence and exert more control over their own health care, adherence problems become even more prominent (DiMatteo, 2004b). Several studies (Miller & Drotar, 2003; Olsen & Sutton, 1998) show that as diabetic children become adolescents, their adherence to recommended exercise and insulin regimens decreases, and conflicts with parents over diabetes management increase. Young adults with these diseases also experience adherence problems (Ellis et al., 2007; Herrmann et al., 2008). Thus, age shows a small but complex relationship with adherence.

Gender   Overall, researchers find few differences in the adherence rates of women and men, but some differences exist in following specific recommendations. In general, men and women are about equal in adhering to taking medication (Andersson, Melander, Svensson, Lind, & Nilsson, 2005; Chapman, Petrilla, Benner, Schwartz, & Tang, 2008), controlling diabetes (Hartz et al., 2006), or keeping an appointment for a medical test (Sola-Vera et al., 2008). However, women are less adherent than men in taking medications to lower cholesterol, but this may be due to the higher prevalence of heart disease among men (Mann, Woodward, Muntner, Falzon & Kronish, 2010). Women may be better at adhering to healthy diets, such as sodium-restricted diets (Chung et al., 2006) and diets with lots of vegetables (Thompson, Yaroch, et al., 2011). Aside from these differences, men and women have similar levels of adherence (DiMatteo, 2004b).

Personality Patterns   When the problem of nonadherence became obvious, researchers initially considered the concept of a nonadherent personality. According to this concept, people with certain personality patterns would have low adherence rates. If this concept is accurate, then the same people should be nonadherent in a variety of situations. However, most evidence does not support this notion. Nonadherence is often specific to the situation (Lutz, Silbret, & Olshan, 1983), and adherence to one treatment program is unrelated to adherence to others (Ogedegbe, Schoenthaler, & Fernandez, 2007). Although there is some evidence that smokers are likely to have the higher rates of nonadherence to other health behaviors compared with nonsmokers (Prochaska, Spring, & Nigg, 2008), people cannot be easily classified as "adherent" and "nonadherent" across many behaviors. Thus, the evidence suggests that nonadherence is not a global personality trait but is specific to a given situation (Haynes, 2001).

Emotional Factors   People who experience stress and emotional problems also have difficulties with adherence. A study that investigated the effects of stressful life events on subsequent exercise adherence (Oman & King, 2000) found that people who experience several stressful events are likely to drop out of an exercise program. Another study found that individuals taking antiretroviral medication for HIV infection who reported high levels of stress were less adherent (Bottonari, Roberts, Ciesla, & Hewitt, 2005; Leserman, Ironson, O'Cleirigh, Fordiani, & Balbin, 2008).

Do anxiety and depression reduce adherence rates? Whereas anxiety has only a small relationship with adherence, depression has a major influence on adherence (DiMatteo, Lepper, & Croghan, 2000). The risk of nonadherence is 3 times greater in depressed patients than in those who are not depressed. More recent studies show that depression relates to lower adherence among people managing chronic illnesses, such as diabetes (Gonzalez et al., 2008; Katon et al., 2010). Given that coping with a chronic illness can increase risk for depression (Nouwen et al., 2010), the link between depression, chronic illness, and adherence is an important public health concern (Moussavi et al., 2007).

Emotional factors clearly present risks, but do some personality characteristics relate to better adherence and improved health? Patients who express optimism and positive states of mind have better physical health (Chida & Steptoe, 2008; Pressman & Cohen, 2005; Rasmussen, Scheier, & Greenhouse, 2009) and are more likely to adhere to their medical regimens (Gonzalez et al., 2004). Furthermore, the trait of **conscientiousness**, one of the factors in the five factor model of personality (McCrae & Costa, 2003), shows a reliable relationship to adherence and improved health. For example, conscientiousness predicts adherence to an overall healthy lifestyle (Bogg & Roberts, 2004; Goodwin & Friedman, 2006). Conscientiousness also relates to slower progression of HIV infection (O'Cleirigh, Ironson, Weiss, & Costa, 2007), and among older adults, conscientiousness relates to greater medication adherence (Hill & Roberts, 2011). Thus, emotional factors and personality traits may present either a risk or an advantage for adherence.

Environmental Factors

Although some personal factors are important for adherence, environmental factors exert an even larger influence. Included in this group of environmental factors are economic factors, *social support*, and cultural norms.

Economic Factors   Of all the demographic factors examined by Robin DiMatteo (2004b), socioeconomic factors such as education and income were the most strongly related to adherence. People with greater income and education tend to be more adherent. Two meta-analyses show that it is income rather than education that relates more strongly to adherence (DiMatteo, 2004b; Falagas, Zarkadoulia, Pliatsika, & Panos, 2008). Difference in income may also explain

some ethnic differences in adherence. For example, Hispanic American children and adolescents have a lower rate of adherence to a diabetes regimen, but this difference disappears after controlling for income differences (Gallegos-Macias, Macias, Kaufman, Skipper, & Kalishman, 2003). Thus, economic factors show a relationship to health; one avenue is through access to health care, and another is through the ability to pay for prescription medications.

In the United States, people without insurance experience difficulties in obtaining access to health care and in follow-up care such as filling prescriptions (Gans & McPhillips, 2003). Many of the people who experience cost concerns have chronic diseases, which often require daily medications over long periods of time (Piette et al., 2006). In a study of Medicare beneficiaries over age 65 (Gellad, Haas, & Safran, 2007), cost concerns predicted nonadherence, and such concerns were more common for African Americans and Hispanic Americans than for European Americans. In another study, people who had been admitted to the hospital for heart disease were more likely to adhere to their medications to reduce cholesterol level during the next year if their insurance plan paid more of the cost of the prescription (Ye, Gross, Schommer, Cline, & St. Peter, 2007). Therefore, how much people must pay for their treatment affects not only access to medical care but also the likelihood that they will adhere to the treatment regimen. These limitations and concerns about costs affect older people and those from ethnic minorities more often than others.

Social Support   **Social support** is a broad concept that refers to both tangible and intangible help a person receives from family members and from friends. A social support network is important for dealing with a chronic disease and for adhering to the required medical regimen (Kyngäs, 2004). Social support networks for adolescents include parents, peers (both those with and without similar conditions), people at school, health care providers, and even pets. In addition, adolescents use technology such as cell phones and computers to contact others and obtain support.

The level of social support one receives from friends and family is a strong predictor of adherence. In general, people who are isolated from others are likely to be nonadherent; those who enjoy many close interpersonal relationships are more likely to follow medical advice. A review of 50 years of research (DiMatteo, 2004a) confirmed the importance of social support for adherence.

Researchers can analyze social support in terms of the variety and function of relationships that people have, as well as the types of support that people receive from these relationships (DiMatteo, 2004a). For example, living with someone is a significant contributor to adherence; people who are married and those who live with families are more adherent than those who live alone. However, simply living with someone is not sufficient—family conflict and partner stress may lead to reductions in adherence (Molloy, Perkins-Porras, Strike, & Steptoe, 2008). Thus, the living situation itself is not the important factor; rather, the support a person receives is the critical issue (DiMatteo, 2004a).

Social support may consist of either practical or emotional support. Practical support includes reminders and physical assistance in adhering. Emotional support includes nurturance and empathy. In studies of both patients recovering from heart problems (Molloy, Perkins-Porras, Bhattacharyya, Strike, & Steptoe, 2008) and adolescents with diabetes (Ellis et al., 2007), practical support was a more important determinant of adherence than emotional support. Thus, social support is an important factor in adherence, and those who lack a support network have more trouble adhering to a medical regimen.

Cultural Norms   Cultural beliefs and norms have a powerful effect not only on rates of adherence but also on what constitutes adherence. For example, if one's family or tribal traditions include strong beliefs in the efficacy of tribal healers, then the individual's adherence to modern medical recommendations might be low. A study of diabetic and hypertensive patients in Zimbabwe (Zyazema, 1984) found a large number of people who were not adhering to their recommended therapies. As might be expected, many of these patients believed in traditional healers and had little faith in Western medical procedures. Thus, the extent to which people accept a medical practice has a large impact on adherence to that practice, resulting in poorer adherence for individuals who are less acculturated to Western medicine, such as immigrants or people who retain strong ties to another culture (Barron, Hunter, Mayo, & Willoughby, 2004).

Failures to adhere to Western, technological medicine do not necessarily indicate a failure to adhere to some other medical tradition. People who maintain a cultural tradition may also retain its healers. For example, a study of Native Americans (Novins, Beals, Moore, Spicer, & Manson, 2004) revealed that many sick people sought the services of traditional healers, sometimes in combination with biomedical services. This strategy of combining treatments might be considered nonadherent by both types of healers.

People who accept a different healing tradition should not necessarily be considered nonadherent when their illness calls for a complex biomedical regimen. Native Hawaiians have a poor record of adherence (Ka'opua & Mueller, 2004), partly because their cultural beliefs are more holistic and spiritual, and their traditions emphasize family support and cohesion. These cultural values are not compatible with those that form the basis of Western medicine. Thus, Native Hawaiians have more trouble than other ethnic groups in Hawaii in adhering to medical regimens to control diabetes and risks for heart disease. The health-related beliefs of Native Hawaiians with heart failure lead them to prefer native healers over physicians (Kaholokula, Saito, Mau, Latimer, & Seto, 2008). However, no differences appear in their rates of adherence to the complex regimen of antiretroviral therapy that helps to control HIV infection, and their cultural value of family support may be a positive factor (Ka'opua & Mueller, 2004).

Cultural beliefs can also increase adherence. For example, older Japanese patients are typically more adherent than similar patients from the United States or Europe (Chia, Schlenk, & Dunbar-Jacob, 2006). The Japanese health care system provides care for all citizens through a variety of services, which creates trust in the health care system. This trust extends to physicians; Japanese patients accept their physicians' authority, preferring to allow physicians to make health care decisions rather than make those decisions themselves. Consistent with this attitude, patients tend to respect the advice they receive from physicians and to follow their orders carefully.

Culture and ethnicity also influence adherence through the treatment that people from different cultures and ethnic groups receive when seeking medical care. Physicians and other health care providers may be influenced by their patients' ethnic background and socioeconomic status, and this influence can affect patient adherence. Physicians tend to have stereotypical and negative attitudes toward African American and low- and middle-income patients (Dovidio et al., 2008; van Ryn & Burke, 2000), including pessimistic beliefs about their rates of adherence. Perceived discrimination and disrespect may contribute to ethnic differences in following physicians' recommendations and keeping appointments (Blanchard & Lurie, 2004).

African Americans (14.1%), Asian Americans (20.2%), and Hispanic Americans (19.4%) reported that they felt discriminated against or treated with a lack of respect by a physician from whom they had received care within the past 2 years. In contrast, only about 9% of European American patients felt that they had been treated with disrespect by their physician. In this study, patients' perception of disrespect predicted lower adherence and more missed medical appointments.

These findings have important implications for physicians and other health care providers whose clientele consists largely of people from different cultural backgrounds. In addition, these findings highlight the importance of interactions between patient and practitioner in adhering to medical advice.

Interaction of Factors

Researchers have identified dozens of factors, each of which shows some relation to adherence. However, many of these factors account for a very small amount of the variation in adhering to medical advice. Some of these factors are statistically significant, but when considered individually, they are poor predictors of who will and who will not adhere (Rietveld & Koomen, 2002). To gain a fuller understanding of adherence, researchers must study the mutual influence of factors that affect adherence. For example, patients' beliefs about the disease are related to adherence, but those beliefs are affected by interactions with physicians, another factor that has been identified as influential for adherence. Thus, many of the factors described earlier are not independent of one another. Many of the factors identified as being related to adherence overlap with and influence other factors in complex ways. Therefore, both researchers and practitioners must understand the complex interplay of factors that affect adherence. Furthermore, many of the factors we have discussed so far are not modifiable. Health psychologists are not only interested in understanding adherence, but also in improving adherence. In the next section, we focus on theories of adherence that identify these potentially modifiable factors.

IN SUMMARY

Several conditions predict poor adherence: (1) side effects of the medication, (2) long and complicated treatment regimens, (3) personal factors such as old or young age, (4) emotional factors such as conscientiousness and emotional problems such as stress and depression, (6) economic barriers to obtaining treatment or paying for prescriptions, (7) lack of social support, and (8) patients' cultural beliefs that the medical regimen is ineffective. Researchers and practitioners need to understand that the factors identified as influencing adherence interact in complex ways.

Why and How Do People Adhere to Healthy Behaviors?

In order to intervene to improve people's adherence, it is critical to identify the potentially modifiable factors that predict adherence. To do this, health psychologists develop theories to understand *why* people make the health decisions they do and *how* they successfully adhere to medical advice. In Chapter 2, we said that useful theories (1) generate research, (2) organize and explain observations, and (3) guide the practitioner in predicting behavior. Theories that successfully identify why people adhere or do not adhere are also useful for practitioners in designing interventions to improve adherence. These theories of health behavior can be classified into continuum theories and stage theories.

Continuum Theories of Health Behavior

Continuum theories were the first class of theories developed to understand health behavior and include the health belief model (Becker & Rosenstock, 1984), self-efficacy theory (Bandura, 1986, 1997, 2001), the theory of planned behavior (Ajzen, 1985, 1991), and behavioral theory. **Continuum theories** are a name given to theories that seek to explain adherence with a single set of factors that should apply equally to all people regardless of their existing levels or motivations for adhering. In other words, continuum theories take a "one size fits all" approach. Stage theories, which we will describe later in this section, take a different approach to explaining adherence, by first classifying people into different stages of behavior change and then identifying the unique variables that predict adherence among people in different stages.

The Health Belief Model   In the 1950s, tuberculosis was a major health problem. The United States Public Health Service initiated a free tuberculosis health-screening program. Mobile units went to convenient neighborhood locations and provided screening X-rays free of charge. Yet, very few people took advantage of the screening program. Why?

Geoffrey Hochbaum (1958) and his colleagues developed the health belief model (HBM) to answer this question. Several versions of the HBM exist; the one that has attracted the most attention is that of Marshall Becker and Irwin Rosenstock (Becker & Rosenstock, 1984).

Like all health belief models, the one developed by Becker and Rosenstock assumes that beliefs are important contributors to health behavior. This model includes four beliefs that should combine to predict health-related behaviors: (1) perceived *susceptibility* to disease or disability, (2) perceived *severity* of the disease or disability, (3) perceived *benefits* of health-enhancing behaviors, and (4) perceived *barriers* to health-enhancing behaviors, including financial costs.

Recall Nathan Rey. You learned about his attempt to stop smoking at the start of this chapter. Each of the health belief model's factors played a part in Nathan's decision to quit smoking. At first, Nathan was unaware of his family history of heart disease and that smoking increases risk of heart disease, so he had low perceived susceptibility. After his father's heart attack, he learned of his susceptibility to heart problems and saw first-hand how severe heart disease can be. This experience also led him to appreciate the health benefits of quitting smoking. At first, Nathan did not recognize the barriers that would make it difficult for him to quit smoking, such as the influence that his friends would have. Thus, according to the health belief model, Nathan should have had a high likelihood of adhering, due to his high perceived susceptibility, high perceived severity, his belief in the benefits of quitting, and little recognition of barriers.

Although the health belief model corresponds with common sense in many ways, common sense does not always predict adherence to health-related behaviors. Nathan had brief periods of success in his attempts to stop smoking, but more difficulty in staying adherent over time.

Nathan's example highlights a limitation of the health belief model. While some interventions based on the health belief model are successful at promoting adherence to relatively simple and infrequent behaviors

such as mammography screening (Aiken et al., 1994), the health belief model does not predict adherence very well. Of the health belief model's four factors, perceived benefits and barriers are the best predictors of behavior, whereas perceived susceptibility and severity are generally weak predictors of behavior (Carpenter, 2010). Similarly, the factors in the health belief model may be more predictive for some groups than for other groups. For example, susceptibility and severity more strongly predict vaccination for African Americans and European Americans than for Hispanic Americans. For Hispanic Americans, barriers more strongly predict vaccination than the other factors (Chen, Fox, Cantrell, Stockdale, & Kagawa-Singer, 2007). These ethnic differences point to the importance of other factors omitted by the health belief model.

The study on influenza vaccination is typical of tests of the health belief model. The components of the model show some relationship to the health-related criterion behavior, but the relationship is weak, and the model seems to be incomplete. Some critics (Armitage & Conner, 2000) argue that the health belief model emphasizes motivational factors too heavily and behavioral factors too little, and thus can never be a completely adequate model of health behavior. One of the biggest limitations of the health belief model, however, is its omission of beliefs about a person's control over a health behavior.

Self-Efficacy Theory   Albert Bandura (1986, 1997, 2001) proposed a social cognitive theory that assumes that humans have some capacity to exercise limited control over their lives. That is, they use their cognitive processes for self-regulation. Bandura suggests that human action results from an interaction of behavior, environment, and person factors, especially cognition. Bandura (1986, 2001) referred to this interactive triadic model as **reciprocal determinism**. The concept of reciprocal determinism can be illustrated by a triangle, with behavior, environment, and person factors occupying the three corners of the triangle and each having some influence on the other two (see Figure 4.1).

An important component of the person factor is **self-efficacy**, defined by Bandura (2001) as "people's beliefs in their capability to exercise some measure of control over their own functioning and over environmental events" (p. 10). Self-efficacy is a situation-specific rather than a global concept; that is, it refers to people's confidence that they can perform necessary

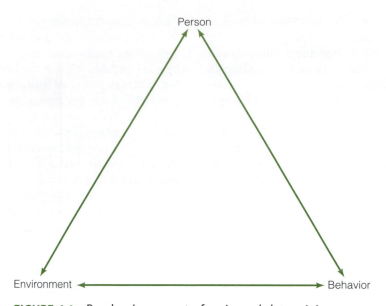

FIGURE 4.1 Bandura's concept of reciprocal determinism. Human functioning is a product of the interaction of behavior, environment, and person variables, especially self-efficacy and other cognitive processes.

Source: Adapted from "The self system in reciprocal determinism," by A. Bandura, 1979, *American Psychologist, 33,* p. 345. Adapted by permission of the American Psychological Association and Albert Bandura.

behaviors to produce desired outcomes in any *particular* situation, such as fighting off a temptation to smoke. Bandura (1986) suggested that self-efficacy can be acquired, enhanced, or decreased in one of four ways: (1) performance, or enacting a behavior such as successfully resisting cigarette cravings; (2) vicarious experience, or seeing another person with similar skills perform a behavior; (3) verbal persuasion, or listening to the encouraging words of a trusted person; and (4) physiological arousal states, such as feelings of anxiety or stress, which ordinarily *decrease* self-efficacy.

According to self-efficacy theory, people's beliefs concerning their ability to initiate difficult behaviors (such as quitting smoking) predict their likelihood of accomplishing those behaviors. People who think they can do something will try and persist at it; people who do not believe they can do something will not try or will give up quickly. Also important in self-efficacy theory are **outcome expectations**, which are people's beliefs that those behaviors will produce valuable outcomes, such as lower risk for heart problems. According to Bandura's theory, the combination of self-efficacy and outcome expectations plays

an important role in predicting behavior. To successfully adhere to a health behavior, people must believe that the behavior will bring about a valuable outcome and that they have the ability to successfully carry out the behavior.

Self-efficacy theory predicts adherence to a variety of health recommendations, including relapse in a smoking cessation program, maintenance of an exercise regimen, adherence to diabetes management, and adherence to HIV medication regimens. For example, a study on self-efficacy and smoking relapse (Shiffman et al., 2000) found that, after an initial lapse, smokers with high self-efficacy tended to remain abstinent, whereas those with waning self-efficacy were likely to relapse. Self-efficacy was the best predictor of completing versus dropping out of an exercise rehabilitation program (Guillot, Kilpatrick, Hebert, & Hollander, 2004) and adhering to an exercise program for cardiac rehabilitation (Schwarzer, Luszczynska, Ziegelmann, Scholz, & Lippke, 2008). One team of researchers (Iannotti et al., 2006) studied diabetes management among adolescents and found self-efficacy to predict better self-management and optimal blood sugar levels. Research with a group of women with AIDS

(Ironson et al., 2005) and women and men with HIV/AIDS (Simoni, Frick, & Huang, 2006) found that self-efficacy related to adherence to taking medications as prescribed and to physical indicators of decreased disease severity. Thus, self-efficacy predicts good adherence and good medical outcomes. For this reason, self-efficacy is now incorporated into nearly all health behavior models. However, one limitation of self-efficacy theory is that it focuses chiefly on self-efficacy as a predictor of behavior but omits other factors that also supply a person with motivation for adherence, such as social pressure.

The Theory of Planned Behavior   Like self-efficacy theory, the theory of planned behavior assumes that people act in ways that help them achieve important goals. The *theory of planned behavior* (Ajzen, 1985, 1991) assumes that people are generally reasonable and make systematic use of information when deciding how to behave; they think about the outcome of their actions before making a decision to engage in a particular behavior. They can also choose not to act, if they believe that an action would move them away from their goal.

According to the theory of planned behavior, the immediate determinant of behavior is the *intention* to act or not to act. Intentions, in turn, are shaped by three factors. The first is a personal evaluation of the behavior—that is, one's *attitude toward the behavior*. One's attitude toward the behavior arises from beliefs that the behavior will lead to positively or negatively valued outcomes. The second factor is one's *perception of how much control* exists over one's behavior (Ajzen, 1985, 1991). Perceived behavioral control is the ease or difficulty one has in achieving desired behavioral outcomes, which reflects both past behaviors and perceived ability to overcome obstacles. This belief in perceived behavioral control is very similar to Bandura's concept of self-efficacy. The more resources and opportunities people believe they have, the stronger their beliefs that they can control their behavior.

The third factor is one's perception of the social pressure to perform or not perform the action—that is, one's *subjective norm*. The focus on subjective norms is a unique aspect of the theory of planned behavior. One's subjective norm is shaped by both one's belief that other people encourage the behavior, as well as one's motivation to adhere to the wishes of others. In predicting behavior, the theory of planned behavior also considers the relative weight of personal attitudes measured against subjective norms.

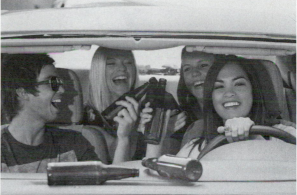

Young adults' perception of social norms can influence their behavior.

Figure 4.2 shows that we can predict a person's behavior from knowledge of a person's (1) attitude toward the behavior, (2) subjective norm, and (3) perceived behavioral control. All three components interact to shape the person's intention to behave.

In predicting whether Nathan would adhere to his motivation to stop smoking, the theory of planned behavior relies on several pieces of information. First, does Nathan believe that quitting smoking will help him achieve his goal of staying healthy? Second, how much does Nathan believe he has control over his ability to stop smoking? Third, how much does Nathan believe that other people want him to stop smoking, and how much does Nathan want to adhere to other people's expectations? The answer to the first question reveals Nathan's attitude toward stopping smoking, the answer to the second question indicates his belief in his control over his smoking behavior, and the answer to the third question suggests the level of social pressure on him to do so. Initially, Nathan's favorable attitudes were in conflict with his subjective norms. Furthermore, as Nathan began to experience failure in his initial attempts to stop smoking, his perceived control likely decreased. Thus, the theory of planned behavior would predict that his intentions to stop smoking would become somewhat mixed, and the prediction of his behavior difficult. Thus, the theory of planned behavior appears to do a decent job at predicting Nathan's difficulties with stopping smoking.

One strength of the theory of planned behavior is that it identifies beliefs that shape behavior. For example, American men consume less fruits and vegetables than American women. This gender difference relates

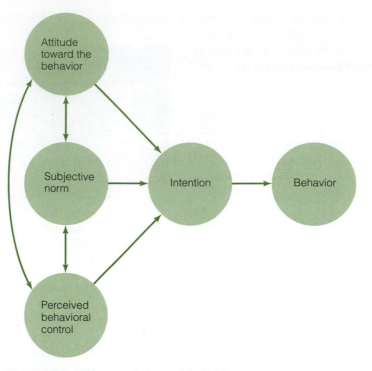

FIGURE 4.2 Theory of planned behavior.

Source: Reprinted from *Organizational Behavior and Human Decision Processes*, 50, I. Ajzen, "The Theory of Planned Behavior", p. 182, Copyright 1991, with permission from Elsevier.

directly to gender differences in components of the theory of planned behavior: Men have less favorable attitudes toward and perceive less control over their ability to eat fruits and vegetables than women do (Emanuel, McCully, Gallagher, & Updegraff, 2012). A study on the topic of premarital sex among Korean university students (Cha, Doswell, Kim, Charron-Prochownik, & Patrick, 2007) also highlights this theory's strengths and weaknesses. In this study, subjective norms were significant predictors for both male and female students. However, perceived behavioral control was a factor only for male students because virginity may be a more deliberate choice for Korean men but not for women (Cha et al., 2007). For females, attitudes were more strongly predictive. Thus, the theory of planned behavior was a good model to explain this behavior, but more so for male students. Similarly, a study of fruit and vegetable consumption found that norms were significant predictors of intentions for African American participants, but not for European American participants (Blanchard et al., 2009), suggesting that cultural differences exist in how much people are motivated by the expectations of close friends and family.

The theory of planned behavior has been useful in guiding the development of Internet-based interventions for a variety of health behaviors (Webb, Joseph, Yardley, & Michie, 2010). A recent meta-analysis of over 200 studies found that the theory of planned behavior was most successful at predicting physical activity and dietary behaviors (McEachan, Conner, Taylor, & Lawton, 2011). In contrast, the theory of planned behavior was less successful at predicting risk-taking behaviors such as speeding, smoking, and alcohol and drug use, as well as screening, safe sex, and abstinence behaviors. What could account for these differences across types of behavior? For the most part, physical activity and diet represent ongoing, individual choices that the theory of planned behavior was designed to predict. Indeed, for these behaviors, the variables of intentions, perceived behavioral control, and attitudes strongly predicted behavior. On the other hand, intentions and perceived behavioral control were less likely to predict risk-taking and sexual behaviors. Across nearly all behaviors, subjective norms were the weakest predictor of behavior, with two exceptions. Subjective norms more strongly predicted behavior for adolescents compared with adults, and subjective norms more strongly predicted risk-taking behaviors than other behaviors. Thus, subjective norms may be especially important in understanding risk-taking behavior among adolescents, a point we will return to later in this chapter.

Thus, the theory of planned behavior does a decent job of predicting adherence to intentional health behavior. However, a number of reviews conclude that the inclusion of additional variables such as past behavior can substantially improve the model's predictive ability (Hagger, Chatzisarantis, & Biddle, 2002; McEachan et al., 2011). Furthermore, even the relationship between intentions and behavior is not as straightforward as the theory of planned behavior would suggest, as we will discuss later in this chapter.

Behavioral Theory   When people begin to engage in a health behavior, behavioral principles may strengthen or extinguish those behaviors. The *behavioral model* of adherence employs the principles of operant conditioning proposed by B. F. Skinner (1953). The key to operant conditioning is the immediate *reinforcement* of any response that moves the organism (person) toward the target behavior—in this case, following medical recommendations. Skinner found that reinforcement, either positive or negative, strengthens the behavior it follows. With **positive reinforcement**, a positively valued stimulus is added to the situation, thus increasing the probability that the behavior will recur. An example of positive reinforcement of adherent behavior would be a monetary payment contingent on a patient's keeping a doctor's appointment. With **negative reinforcement**, behavior is strengthened by the removal of an unpleasant or negatively valued stimulus. An example of negative reinforcement would be taking medication to stop one's spouse from nagging about taking one's medication.

Punishment also changes behavior by decreasing the chances that a behavior will be repeated, but psychologists seldom use it to modify nonadherent behaviors. The effects of positive and negative reinforcers are quite predictable: They both strengthen behavior. However, the effects of punishment are limited and sometimes difficult to predict. At best, punishment will inhibit or suppress a behavior, and it can condition strong negative feelings toward any persons or environmental conditions associated with it. Punishment, including threats of harm, is seldom useful in improving a person's adherence to medical advice.

The behavioral model also predicts that adherence will be difficult, because learned behaviors form patterns or habits that often resist change. When a person must make changes in habitual behavior patterns to take medication, change diet or physical activity, or take blood glucose readings several times a day, the individual often has trouble accommodating a new routine. People need help in establishing such changes, and advocates of the behavioral model also use cues, rewards, and contingency contracts to reinforce adherent behaviors. Cues include written reminders of appointments, telephone calls from the practitioner's office, and a variety of self-reminders. Rewards for adherence can be extrinsic (money and compliments) or intrinsic (feeling healthier). Contracts can be verbal, but they are more often written agreements between practitioner and patient. Most adherence models recognize the importance of incentives in improving adherence.

Support for the behavioral model comes from studies of children with asthma and of people undergoing substance abuse treatment. An interview study (Penza-Clyve, Mansell, & McQuaid, 2004) asked children to identify the strategies that helped them become more adherent. These 9- to 15-year-olds mentioned reminders and social support, but the strategy that they endorsed most strongly was rewards for adhering to their medical regimen. Behavioral principles can also help adults become more adherent. Participants in a Veterans Administration substance abuse treatment program were more likely to complete aftercare and to be abstinent from drugs 1 year later when their program included an aftercare contract, attendance prompts, and reinforcers (Lash et al., 2007).

Critique of Continuum Theories   In Chapter 2, we suggested that a useful theory should (1) generate significant research, (2) organize and explain observations, and (3) help the practitioner predict and change behaviors. How well do continuum theories meet these three criteria?

First, substantial amounts of research apply continuum theories to understanding adherence. The health belief model has prompted the most research, but a body of evidence exists for all these models.

Second, do these models organize and explain health-related behaviors? In general, all these models do better than chance in explaining and predicting behavior. However, the health belief model and the theory of planned behavior address motivation, attitudes, and intentions, but not actual behavior or behavior change (Schwarzer, 2008). Thus, they are only moderately successful in predicting adherence. The theory of planned behavior, however, does a better job than the health belief model and self-efficacy theory in recognizing the social and environmental pressures that influence behavior, in the form of subjective norms.

Another type of challenge comes from the necessity of relying on instruments to assess the various components of the models because such measures are not yet consistent and accurate. The health belief model, for example, might predict health-seeking behavior more accurately if valid measurements existed for each of its components. If a person feels susceptible to a disease, perceives his or her symptoms to be severe, believes that treatment will be effective, and sees few barriers to treatment, then logically that person should seek health care. But each of these four factors is difficult to assess reliably and validly.

Researchers apply these models to a variety of behaviors, including cigarette smoking among elementary school children (Swaim, Perrine, & Aloise-Young, 2007) and Chinese adolescents (Guo et al., 2007), fruit and vegetable consumption among young adults (Blanchard et al., 2009), exercise among bladder cancer survivors (Karvinen et al., 2009), safe sex behavior among HIV-negative drug users (Mausbach, Semple, Strathdee, & Patterson, 2009), and myriad other health-related behaviors. However, a model may have some value for predicting health-seeking behaviors related to one disorder but not to another. Similarly, a theory may relate to health care–seeking behavior but not to prevention behavior or adherence to medical advice, or it may predict the behavior of men but not women. No current theory is comprehensive enough to encompass all these areas.

Finally, do continuum theories allow practitioners to predict and change behavior? One strength of continuum theories is that they identify several beliefs that should motivate *anyone* to change his or her behaviors. Thus, continuum theories have guided the development of "one size fits all" interventions that target these beliefs. Despite these strengths, continuum theories also leave out important psychological factors that predict behavior, such as self-identity and anticipated emotions (Rise, Sheeran, & Hukkelberg, 2010; Rivis, Sheeran, & Armitage, 2009). For example, people who simply think about the regret they might experience if they do not enroll in an organ donation program are more likely to enroll than people who think about all of the beliefs in

the theory of planned behavior combined (O'Carroll, Dryden, Hamilton-Barclay, & Ferguson, 2011).

Lastly, health habits are often very ingrained behaviors and are difficult to change. Indeed, people's past behavior is often a better predictor of their future behavior than any of the beliefs identified in many continuum theories (Ogden, 2003; Sutton, McVey, & Glanz, 1999). Changing people's beliefs about a health behavior may provide motivation, but people often need more concrete steps and skills to translate intention into behavior change (Bryan, Fisher, & Fisher, 2002).

IN SUMMARY

The health belief model includes the concepts of perceived severity of the disease, personal susceptibility, and perceived benefits of and barriers to health-enhancing behaviors. The health belief model has only limited success in predicting health-related behaviors.

Self-efficacy theory emphasizes people's beliefs about their ability to control their own health behaviors. Self-efficacy is one of the most important predictors of health behavior, particularly for behaviors that are relatively difficult to adhere to.

Ajzen's theory of planned behavior focuses on intentional behavior, with the predictors of intentions being attitudes, perceived behavioral control, and subjective norms. Perceived behavioral control and intentions tend to be the strongest predictors of adherence. Subjective norms also predict behavior, but mainly among adolescents and for risk-taking behaviors.

Behavioral theory focuses on reinforcement and habits that must be changed. When a person's attempts to change behavior are met with rewards, it is more likely that those changes will persist. Rewards can be extrinsic (money and compliments) or intrinsic (feeling healthier). Behavioral theory also recognizes the importance of cues and contracts in improving adherence.

Stage Theories of Health Behavior

Stage theories include the transtheoretical model (Prochaska, DiClemente, & Norcross, 1992; Prochaska, Norcross, & DiClemente, 1994), the precaution adoption process model (Weinstein, 1988), and the health action process approach (Schwarzer, 2008). These models of health behavior differ in several important ways from continuum models. Most importantly, stage models propose that people pass through a series of discrete stages as they attempt to change their behavior. In this way, stage models seem to better describe the *processes* by which people change their behavior than continuum models. Stage models also suggest that different variables will be important depending on what stage a person is in. In this way, stage models differ from continuum models, as people in different stages should benefit from different types of interventions. As you will learn in this section of this chapter, interventions based on stage theories typically tailor information to the specific stage that a person is in, rather than employ a "one size fits all" approach.

The Transtheoretical Model   The most well-known stage model is the *transtheoretical model* because it cuts across and borrows from other theoretical models; the *stages-of-change model* is another name for this theory. The transtheoretical model, developed by James Prochaska, Carlo DiClemente, and John Norcross (1992, 1994), assumes that people progress as well as regress through five spiraling stages in making changes in

behavior: precontemplation, contemplation, preparation, action, and maintenance. A smoker's progression through these five stages of change in stopping smoking is illustrated in Figure 4.3.

During the *precontemplation stage*, the person has no intention of stopping smoking. Prior to his father's heart attack, Nathan Rey was likely in the precontemplation stage. In the *contemplation stage*, the person is aware of the problem and has thoughts about quitting, but has not yet made an effort to change. The *preparation stage* includes both thoughts (such as intending to quit within the next month) and action (such as learning about effective quitting techniques, or telling others about intentions). During the *action stage*, the person makes overt changes in behavior, such as stopping smoking or using nicotine replacement therapy. In the *maintenance stage*, the person tries to sustain the changes previously made and attempts to resist temptation to relapse back into old habits. Following his father's heart attack, Nathan quickly progressed from the precontemplation stage to the preparation and action stages.

Prochaska and his associates maintain that a person moves from one stage to another in a spiral rather than a linear fashion and argue that this model captures the time factor of behavior change better than

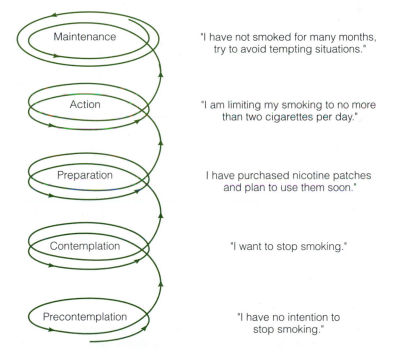

"I have not smoked for many months, try to avoid tempting situations."

"I am limiting my smoking to no more than two cigarettes per day."

I have purchased nicotine patches and plan to use them soon."

"I want to stop smoking."

"I have no intention to stop smoking."

FIGURE 4.3   The transtheoretical model and stages of changing from smoking to stopping smoking.

other models (Velicer & Prochaska, 2008). Relapses propel people back into a previous stage, or perhaps all the way back to the contemplation or precontemplation stages. From that point, the person may progress several times through the stages until completing behavioral change successfully. Thus, relapses are to be expected and can serve as learning experiences that help a person recycle upward through the various stages. Indeed, Prochaska initially developed the transtheoretical model to understand addictive behaviors such as smoking. Nathan appeared to cycle through a number of stages in his attempt to stop smoking.

Prochaska and colleagues (1992, 1994) suggested that people in different stages require different types of assistance to make changes successfully. For example, people in the contemplation and preparation stages should benefit from techniques that raise their awareness of a health problem. In contrast, people in the action and maintenance stages should benefit from strategies that directly address behaviors. Put simply, people in the precontemplation stage need to learn *why* they should change, whereas people in the contemplation and action stages need to learn *how* to change. People in the maintenance stage need help or information oriented toward preserving their changes.

Research tends to supports these contentions. For example, a longitudinal study of adopting a low-fat diet (Armitage, Sheeran, Conner, & Arden, 2004) revealed that people's attitudes and behavior fall into the various stages of the transtheoretical model, and individuals both progress through the stages and regress into earlier stages, much as the model predicts. Furthermore, the interventions that moved people from one stage to another varied by stage. Unfortunately, these researchers found that moving people from the preparation to the action stage was more difficult than other transitions. Thus, the transitions from one stage to another may not be equally easy to influence.

Does the transtheoretical model apply equally to different problem behaviors? A meta-analysis of 47 studies (Rosen, 2000) attempted to answer this question by looking at the model across several health-related issues, including smoking, substance abuse, exercise, diet, and psychotherapy. The results showed that the transtheoretical model worked best for understanding smoking cessation compared with many other health behaviors. For example, in the case of smoking cessation, cognitive processes were more frequently used in deciding to quit, whereas behavioral techniques were more effective during abstinence. However, other reviews of stage-matched interventions for smoking cessation have shown that stage-matched interventions are just as effective as interventions that provide the same information to all people regardless of stage (Cahill, Lancaster, & Green, 2010). Compared with its success in understanding smoking cessation, the transtheoretical model has not been as successful in predicting adherence to other behaviors such as special diets, exercise, or condom use (Bogart & Delahanty, 2004).

The lack of success of stage-matched interventions based on the transtheoretical model may be due to problems with how researchers classify people into stages. For example, the five stages in the transtheoretical model may not represent distinctly different stages (Herzog, 2008). For this reason, some have suggested that stage models with fewer stages may be more accurate and useful (Armitage, 2009). We revisit this point later in this chapter when we describe the health action process approach.

The Precaution Adoption Process Model As described earlier, the health belief model focused on people's beliefs in their personal susceptibility to a health problem. As pointed out by Neil Weinstein (2000), even beliefs about personal susceptibility may change over time in a manner consistent with a stage model. Weinstein's (1988) *precaution adoption process model* assumes that when people begin new and relatively complex behaviors aimed at protecting themselves from harm, they go through several *stages of belief* about their personal susceptibility. People do not move inevitably from lower to higher stages, and they may even move backward, as when a person who has previously considered stopping smoking subsequently abandons the idea.

Weinstein's precaution adoption process model holds that people move through seven stages in their readiness to adopt a health-related behavior (see Figure 4.4). In Stage 1, people have not heard of the hazard and thus are unaware of any personal risk. In Stage 2, they hold an **optimistic bias** regarding their own level of risk; that is, they are aware of the hazard and believe that others are at risk, but they do not believe that they are at risk. Prior to his father's heart attack, Nathan likely held an optimistic bias regarding his own risk for smoking-related health problems. In Stage 3, people acknowledge their personal susceptibility and accept the notion that precaution would be personally effective, but they have not yet decided to take action.

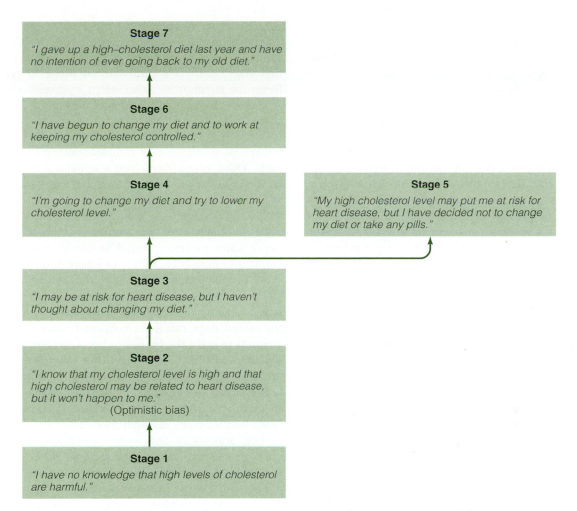

FIGURE 4.4 The seven stages of Weinstein's precaution adoption process model.

Stages 4 and 5 are critical. In Stage 4, people decide to take action, whereas in the parallel Stage 5, people decide that action is unnecessary. Some people who branch off to Stage 5 may later return to Stage 4 and decide to take appropriate action. In Stage 6, people have already taken the precautions aimed at reducing risks. Stage 7 involves maintaining the precaution, if needed. Maintenance would not be necessary in the case of polio vaccination (when one dose provides lifetime immunity), but for smoking cessation or dietary changes, maintenance is essential.

Although Weinstein's notion of optimistic bias generated substantial research, his more global concept of the precaution adoption process model attracted less attention from researchers. Weinstein and his colleagues (Weinstein, Lyon, Sandman, & Cuite, 2003; Weinstein,

Sandman, & Blalock, 2008) hypothesized that barriers to health protective behaviors change from stage to stage. The precaution under investigation encouraged homeowners to test their homes for the presence of radon. Homeowners were classified into those who were undecided about radon testing (Stage 3) and those who had decided to act (Stage 4). The researchers also randomly assigned homeowners to receive either a risk awareness intervention or a low-effort, "how-to-test" intervention. Consistent with the predictions of the precaution adoption process model, homeowners who were undecided about radon testing were more likely to decide to test after receiving the risk awareness intervention compared with the "how-to-test" intervention. For these people, they needed risk information to move to the next stage. In contrast, homeowners who had decided to act were more likely to order a radon testing kit after receiving the "how-to-test" intervention compared with the risk awareness. In other words, they already perceived personal susceptibility, but what they needed were explicit instructions on how to act.

More recent research extends the precaution adoption process model to colorectal cancer screening (Sifri et al., 2010), mammography screening (Costanza et al., 2009), exercise and osteoporosis prevention (Blalock, 2007; Elliott, Seals, & Jacobson, 2007), fruit consumption (de Vet, de Nooijer, Oenema, de Vries, & Brug, 2008), and parents' following recommended safety procedures for protecting young children (Gielen et al., 2007). Each of these behaviors requires that a person become aware of a hazard and move toward taking appropriate action, and the precaution adoption process model seems to capture the variable nature of these beliefs and behaviors better than simpler models.

However, the precaution adoption process model is not without its limitations. First, it is not as extensively researched as other theories. Second, it focuses mainly on how risk perceptions change over time and influence behavior, and does less than other theories to acknowledge other important predictors of behavior. Lastly, like the transtheoretical model, it remains unclear whether the seven stages truly represent different categories, or whether a simpler model would be equally as useful in explaining adherence.

The Health Action Process Approach Schwarzer's (2008) *health action process approach* is a recent model that incorporates some of the most important

aspects of both continuum theories and stage theories. The health action process approach can be viewed as a simplified stage model, with two general stages. In the first stage, called the **motivational phase**, a person forms the intention to either adopt a preventive measure or to change a risk behavior. During the motivational phase, three beliefs are necessary for an intention to form. First, people must perceive a personal risk. Second, people must have favorable outcome expectations. Third, people must have a sense of self-efficacy. In the motivational phase, Schwarzer refers to *action self-efficacy*—or the confidence in one's ability to make the change—as being the important belief. Thus, in many ways the motivational phase of the health action process approach resembles many of the continuum models (as shown in Figure 4.5).

However, simply intending to change a behavior is rarely enough to produce lasting change, as anyone who has failed at a New Year's resolution knows. In the second stage, called the **volitional phase**, a person attempts to make the change to his or her behavior, as well as persist in those changes over time. During the volitional phase, a different set of beliefs and strategies is important. For example, planning is crucial during the volitional phase. To lose weight, a person must make detailed plans for what foods to eat, what foods to buy, and where and when to exercise. However, many people who wish to change their behavior may not realize the importance of planning until they have already failed at their goals.

A large web-based study of German adults (Parschau et al., 2012) reveals the importance of planning in promoting physical activity. Among adults who

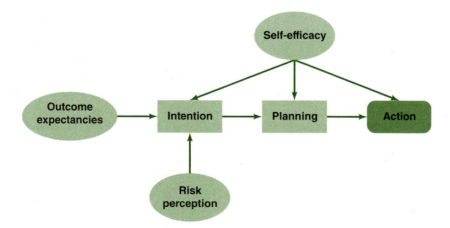

FIGURE 4.5 The health action process approach.
Source: Adapted by permission of Ralf Schwarzer.

intended to exercise but had not yet started, those who engaged in more planning were more likely to be physically active 3 weeks later. However, among the adults who had no intention to exercise, planning had little influence; this finding illustrates the stage-specific role that planning plays in adherence. Planning not only includes detailing the "what, where, and when," but also planning for how to cope with anticipated setbacks. For example, what will a person do if he or she misses an exercise session, or experiences pain when exercising? People who anticipate and plan for such setbacks tend to be more successful and pursuing their health goals (Craciun, Schüz, Lippke, & Schwarzer, 2012; Evers, Klusmann, Ziegelmann, Schwarzer, & Heuser, 2011; Reuter et al., 2010).

Self-efficacy remains an important predictor of behavior in the volitional phase, but different forms of self-efficacy may become critical. In the volitional phase, people must have confidence in both their ability to keep up the behavior (*maintenance self-efficacy*) and to resume the behavior after a lapse (*relapse self-efficacy*). Several studies of exercise show the existence of these different forms of self-efficacy (Rodgers, Hall, Blanchard, McAuley, & Munroe, 2002; Rodgers & Sullivan, 2001). Other studies show that different forms of self-efficacy are important predictors at different stages (Luszczynska & Schwarzer, 2003; Schwarzer & Renner, 2000; Sniehotta, Scholz, & Schwarzer, 2005). For example, among older men recovering from prostate surgery, relapse self-efficacy is the specific belief that predicts who is able to return to an exercise regimen after a lapse (Burkert et al., 2012).

Although the health action process approach is not yet studied as widely as other models, many studies support its propositions. Compared with the health belief model and the theory of planned behavior, the health action process approach does a better job of predicting young adults' intentions to resist unhealthy dieting and to perform breast self-exams (Garcia & Mann, 2003).

Critique of Stage Theories   The transtheoretical model has generated the most research of all stage theories. The precaution adoption process model and the health action process approach have generated less research as they are newer theories.

How well do stage theories organize and explain observations? Of the stage theories, the transtheoretical model is the most complex. It proposes five stages, as well as 10 different processes that could potentially move people from stage to stage. The precaution adoption process model proposes seven stages. As some have noted (Armitage, 2009; Herzog, 2008), this degree of complexity may be unnecessary, as more complex stage models may not explain behavior any better than simpler stage models such as the health action process approach. Furthermore, others question whether people progress from stage to stage in the orderly manner that both the transtheoretical model and the precaution adoption process model suggest (Ogden, 2003). It is not unusual for people to skip a stage or two, which calls into question the validity of these very detailed stage models.

Do stage theories help a practitioner predict and change behavior? One of the strengths of stage models is that they recognize the benefit of tailoring interventions to a person's stage of behavior change. Regarding the transtheoretical model, the evidence is mixed for whether stage-matched interventions are more effective than non-stage-matched interventions. Regarding the health action process approach, there is accumulating evidence for the effectiveness of stage-matched interventions based on the health action process approach for promoting physical activity (Lippke, Schwarzer, Ziegelmann, Scholz, & Schüz, 2010; Lippke, Ziegelmann, & Schwarzer, 2004) and oral health (Schüz, Sniehotta, & Schwarzer, 2007). At this point, most studies of stage models use cross-sectional designs, which make it difficult to observe how an individual changes over time. With all stage models, more longitudinal research is needed to evaluate their validity (Ogden, 2003).

Health psychologists who seek to build valid models for health-related behaviors face challenges. One challenge is that health behavior is often determined by factors other than an individual's beliefs or perceptions. First, they all are unable to accurately account for the many social, economic, ethnic, and demographic factors that also affect people's health behavior. These factors may be harder to change than health beliefs, but they undoubtedly influence behavior. Among such factors are poor interpersonal relationships that keep people away from the health care system and public policies (including laws) that affect health behaviors. In addition, certain health-related behaviors, such as cigarette smoking and dental care, can develop into habits that become so automatic that they are largely outside the personal decision-making process. Other health-producing behaviors, such as dietary changes, may be undertaken for the sake of personal appearance rather than health. All of these factors make it difficult for researchers to create theories of health behavior that account for all of this variability while also keeping the models as simple and parsimonious as possible.

Most of the models postulate some type of barrier or obstacle to seeking health care, and an almost unlimited number of barriers are possible. Often these barriers are beyond the life experience of researchers. For example, barriers for affluent European Americans may be quite different from those faced by poor Hispanic Americans, Africans living in sub-Saharan Africa, or Hmong immigrants in Canada; thus, the health belief model and the theory of planned behavior may not apply equally to all ethnic and socioeconomic groups (Poss, 2000). Models for health-seeking behavior tend to emphasize the importance of direct and personal control of behavioral choices. Little allowance is made for such barriers as racism and poverty.

IN SUMMARY

Stage models of health behavior classify people into different stages of adherence and suggest that progression through each stage is predicted by different sets of variables. Prochaska's transtheoretical model assumes that people spiral through five stages as they make changes in behavior: precontemplation, contemplation, preparation, action, and maintenance. Relapse should be expected, but after relapse, people can move forward again through the various stages.

Weinstein's precaution adoption process model focuses on beliefs of susceptibility and assumes that people go through seven stages of belief. One of the necessary steps is overcoming an *optimistic bias* in people's personal beliefs of susceptibility to a health threat.

Schwarzer's health action process approach proposes only two general stages: the motivational phase and the volitional phase. Planning and specific forms of self-efficacy are thought to be important factors for helping people translate intentions into lasting behavior change.

Stage models suggest that interventions should use a tailored, stage-matched approach, by only addressing the variables relevant in the person's current stage. Thus, the effectiveness of stage-matched interventions depends in part on how well practitioners can classify people into discrete stages. One criticism of the transtheoretical model is that the five stages do not represent discrete stages, and people in different stages may be more similar to each other than the theory suggests. This may explain why there is only mixed support for stage-matched interventions based on the transtheoretical model.

The Intention–Behavior Gap

Stage models acknowledge what many of us already know from our own experiences—that even our best intentions do not always translate into behavior. This "intention–behavior gap" (Sheeran, 2002) is exemplified by people who intend to behave healthily but do not. In this section, we describe models and strategies that help understanding the reasons for this intention–behavior gap, as well as ways to help bridge this gap.

Behavioral Willingness

In some situations, strong social pressures are capable of thwarting the best of intentions. A person may enter into a potential sexual encounter with every intention of using a condom, or embark on a night out on the town with the intent of resisting binge drinking. At some point in the evening, however, the person may forget these intentions altogether. **Behavioral willingness** refers to a person's motivation *at a given moment* to engage in a risky behavior (Gibbons, Gerrard, Blanton, & Russell, 1998). Behavioral willingness reflects more of a reaction to a situation than a deliberate, planned choice. This concept of behavioral willingness has been helpful in understanding a number of adolescent risk-taking behaviors, such as smoking, alcohol use, and lack of safe sex practices (Andrews, Hampson, Barckley, Gerrard, & Gibbons, 2008; Gibbons et al., 1998). In these studies, intention and willingness relate to each other, showing that people with stronger intentions tend to report less of a willingness to engage in risky behaviors "in the moment." However, behavioral willingness is a unique predictor of actual behavior. That is, if you take two people with equally strong intentions to avoid risky behaviors, the person with the greater willingness will most likely be the one whose intentions will ultimately fall short.

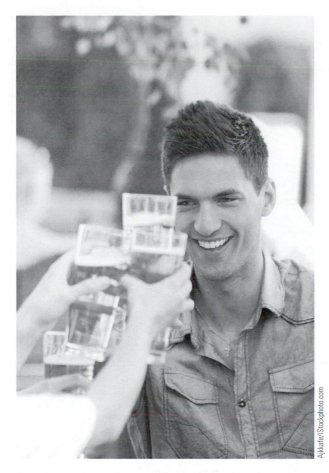

Ajkkafe/iStockphoto.com

People may intend to avoid risky behaviors, but strong social pressures often make them willing to engage in them.

What drives people's willingness to engage in risky behaviors? Many times, people's concern about their social image is what leads to the willingness to engage in risky behavior. When people have positive images of others who engage in risky behaviors, they are more likely to report a willingness to engage in those behaviors (Gibbons et al., 1998). In turn, that willingness can break down the best of intentions.

Implementational Intentions

As emphasized in the health action process approach, planning is an important factor in translating intention into action. A growing body of research shows that short and simple planning exercises can help people adhere to medical advice. **Implementational intentions** are specific plans that people can make that identify not only *what* they intend to do, but also *where*, *when*, and *how*. In essence, implementational intentions connect a situation with the goal that the person wants to achieve. For example, someone who wants to exercise more could form an implementation intention of "I will run 30 minutes immediately after work on Tuesday evening." In this way, implementational intentions go beyond simply the intention of "I plan to exercise more." Over time, it is thought that forming implementational intentions can help make people's pursuit of their goals more automatic.

Indeed, simple implementational intentions exercises are effective in helping people to adhere to a wide variety of health behaviors (see Would You Believe …? box). These include one-time behaviors such as cervical cancer screening (Sheeran & Orbell, 2000) and breast self-exam (Orbell, Hodgkins, & Sheeran, 1997). Implementational intentions also make it more likely that people engage in behaviors that require action over time, such as taking vitamin supplements and medications (Brown, Sheeran, & Rueber, 2009; Sheeran & Orbell, 1999), eating healthily (Armitage, 2004; Verplanken & Faes, 1999), and resisting binge drinking (Murgraff, White, & Phillips, 1996). A meta-analysis of over 20 studies on physical activity confirmed the usefulness of implementational intentions in promoting adherence (Bélanger-Gravel, Godin, & Amireault, 2011).

Why do implementation intentions work? One reason is that they make people less likely to forget their intentions. For example, in a study of cervical cancer screening, 74% of participants scheduled their appointment on the very date they had specified in their implementation intention exercise (Sheeran & Orbell, 2000). Thus, implementational intentions can help turn "intenders" into "actors."

IN SUMMARY

Many people fail to adhere because their intentions do not translate into behavior. For some people, this may occur because of *behavioral willingness*, which represents a person's willingness to engage in risky behaviors at a given moment. Behavioral willingness can put people at risk of nonadherence when strong social pressures exist. People may also not adhere because they do not plan adequately. *Implementational intentions* represent specific plans that link a situation with the enactment of a behavior and can boost adherence to a variety of health behaviors.

Would You BELIEVE...? Text Messages Can Help Turn Intentions Into Action

Text messages help you stay in touch with your family and friends. But did you know that text messages can also help you stay on track with your health goals?

A team of British and Italian psychologists wondered whether text messages could enhance the effects of a planning task for encouraging sedentary young adults to exercise more (Prestwich, Perugini, & Hurling, 2009).

To test this, they had a group of young adults—all of whom were exercising less than three times per week—meet with the researchers. Some of the participants completed an implementational intentions task. In this task, they were asked to think carefully about the types of exercises they wanted to do more frequently and the specific situations in which

they could do these exercises. Then, they created a plan that linked these situations with the exercises, using this form: "When I'm in situation X, then I will do exercise Y." Participants wrote down their plans in sufficient detail to enable them to exercise three times per week for at least 20 minutes each time.

Then, the researchers randomly selected some of the participants to receive text message reminders of their plans over the next 4 weeks. Participants could choose when to receive the texts and what the texts would say. Some participants chose reminders about their specific plans ("go to the gym after class"), whereas some chose reminders that were not about their specific plans ("remember to exercise more").

Who did best in achieving their exercise goals? The participants who received the text messages exercised most often over the following month—but only when they also had completed the implementational intentions task beforehand. Thus, the implementational intentions task and the text messaging reminders acted together to increase people's frequency of exercising. Furthermore, the participants who sent themselves reminders about their specific plans increased their exercise more than those who sent more general reminders about their goals.

So, to keep on track with your health goals, planning is important. But planning and texting together may actually be good for your health!

Improving Adherence

In this chapter, we have surveyed several issues related to adherence, including theoretical models that might explain or predict adherence, techniques for measuring adherence, the frequency of adherence, and factors that relate to adherence. This information, along with knowledge of why some people fail to adhere, can help answer an important question of this chapter: How can adherence be improved?

Methods for improving adherence can generally be divided into (1) educational and (2) behavioral strategies. Educational procedures are those that impart information, sometimes in an emotion-arousing manner designed to frighten the nonadherent patient into becoming adherent. Included with educational strategies are such procedures as health education messages, individual patient counseling with various professional health care providers, programmed instruction, lectures, demonstrations, and individual counseling accompanied by written instructions. Haynes (1976) reported that

strategies that relied on education and threats of disastrous consequences for nonadherence were only marginally effective in bringing about a meaningful change in patients' behaviors; more recent reviews (Harrington, Noble, & Newman, 2004; Schroeder, Fahey, & Ebrahim, 2007) come to similar conclusions. Educational methods may increase patients' knowledge, but behavioral approaches offer a more effective way of enhancing adherence. People, it seems, do not misbehave because they do not know better but because adherent behavior, for a variety of reasons, is less appealing.

Behavioral strategies focus more directly on changing the behaviors involved in compliance. They include a wide variety of techniques, such as notifying patients of upcoming appointments, simplifying medical schedules, providing cues to prompt taking medication, monitoring and rewarding patients' compliant behaviors, and shaping people toward self-monitoring and self-care. Behavioral techniques are typically more effective than educational strategies in improving patient adherence.

Adherence researchers Robin DiMatteo and Dante DiNicola (1982) recommended four categories of behavioral strategies for improving adherence, and their categories are still a valid way to approach the topic. First, various *prompts* can be used to remind patients to initiate health-enhancing behaviors. These prompts may be cued by regular events in the patient's life, such as taking medication before each meal, or they may take the form of telephone calls from a clinic to remind the person to keep an appointment or to refill a prescription. Another type of prompt comes in the form of reminder packaging, which presents information about the date or time that the medication should be taken on the packaging for the medication (Heneghan, Glasziou, & Perera, 2007). In addition, electronic technology can be useful in providing prompts.

A second behavioral strategy proposed by DiMatteo and DiNicola is *tailoring the regimen*, which involves fitting the treatment to habits and routines in the patient's daily life. For example, pill organizers work toward this goal by making medication more compatible with the person's life, and some drug companies are creating medication packaging, called compliance packaging, that is similar to pill organizers in providing a tailored regimen (Gans & McPhillips, 2003). Another approach that fits within this category is simplifying the medication schedule; a review of adherence studies (Schroeder et al., 2007) indicated that this approach was among the most successful in increasing adherence.

Another way to tailor the regimen involves assessing important characteristics of the patient—such as personality or stages of change—and orienting change-related messages to these characteristics (Gans &

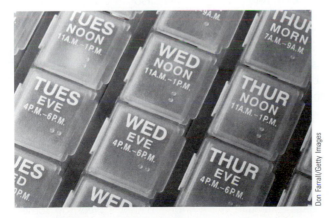

Finding effective prompts helps patients fit medication into their schedules.

Don Farrall/Getty Images

McPhillips, 2003; Sherman, Updegraff, & Mann, 2008). For example, a person in the contemplation stage is aware of the problem but has not yet decided to adopt a behavior (see Figure 4.2). This person might benefit from an intervention that includes information or counseling, whereas a person in the maintenance stage would not. Instead, people in the maintenance stage might benefit from monitoring devices or prompts that remind them to take their medication or to exercise. Applying this approach to the problem of preventing the complications that accompany heart disease, a group of researchers (Turpin et al., 2004) concluded that tailoring adherence programs to patients' previous levels of adherence is critical; patients who are mostly adherent differ from those who are partially adherent or nonadherent. Similar success occurred with a program to help people adhere to lipid-lowering drugs (Johnson et al., 2006). These successes suggest that different stages of readiness to change require different types of assistance to achieve adherence.

A similar way to tailor the regimen involves helping clients resolve the problems that prevent them from changing their behavior. **Motivational interviewing** is a therapeutic approach that originated within substance abuse treatment (Miller & Rollnick, 2002) but has been applied to many other health-related behaviors, including medication adherence, physical activity, diet, and diabetes management (Martins & McNeil, 2009). This technique attempts to change a client's motivation and prepares the client to enact changes in behavior. The procedure includes an interview in which the practitioner attempts to show empathy with the client's situation; discusses and clarifies the client's goals and contrasts them with the client's current, unacceptable behavior; and helps the client formulate ways to change behavior. Reviews indicate that the technique is effective, particularly for motivating people to stop smoking (Lai, Cahill, Qin, & Tang, 2010; Lundahl & Burke, 2009; Martins & McNeil, 2009).

Third, DiMatteo and DiNicola suggested a *graduated regimen implementation* that reinforces successive approximations to the desired behavior. Such shaping procedures would be appropriate for exercise, diet, and possibly smoking cessation programs, but not for taking medications.

The final behavioral strategy listed by DiMatteo and DiNicola is a *contingency contract* (or behavioral contract)—an agreement, usually written, between patients and health care professionals that provides for some kind of reward to patients contingent on their achieving compliance. These contracts may also involve penalties for noncompliance (Gans & McPhillips, 2003). Contingency contracts are most effective when they are enacted at the beginning of therapy and when the provisions are negotiated and agreed upon by patients and providers. Even with these provisions, contracts have not been demonstrated to boost adherence by a great deal (Bosch-Capblanch, Abba, Prictor, & Garner, 2007).

Despite these suggestions, many health care providers put little effort into improving adherence, and adherence rates have improved little over the past 50 years (DiMatteo, 2004a). Evidence indicates that clear instructions about taking medications are the best strategy to boost adherence for short-term regimens (Haynes, McDonald, & Garg, 2002); the instructions work better if they are both verbal and in writing (Johnson, Sandford, & Tyndall, 2007). For long-term regimens, many strategies show some effectiveness, but none offer dramatic improvement (Haynes et al., 2008). Furthermore, the interventions that demonstrate greater effectiveness tend to be complex and costly. Therefore, adherence remains a costly problem, both in terms of the cost in lives and ill health of failures and in terms of the added costs of even marginally effective interventions.

IN SUMMARY

Effective programs to improve compliance rates frequently include cues to signal the time for taking medication, clearly written instructions, simplified medication regimens, prescriptions tailored to the patient's daily schedule, and rewards for compliant behavior. Despite these effective strategies, the problem of nonadherence remains a major challenge for the health psychologist.

Becoming Healthier

You can improve your health by following sound health-related advice. Here are some things you can do to make adherence pay off.

1. Adopt an overall healthy lifestyle—one that includes not smoking, using alcohol in moderation or not at all, eating a diet high in fiber and low in saturated fats, getting an optimum amount of regular physical activity, and incorporating safety into your life. Procedures for adopting each of these health habits are discussed in *Becoming Healthier* boxes in Chapters 12 through 15.

2. Establish a working alliance with your physician that is based on cooperation, not obedience. You and your doctor are the two most important people involved in your health, and the two of you should cooperate in designing your health practices.

3. Another important person interested in your health is your spouse, parent, friend, or sibling. Enlist the support of a significant person or persons in your life. High levels of social support improve one's rate of adherence.

4. Before visiting a health care provider, jot down some questions you would like to have answered; ask the questions and write down the answers during the visit. If you receive a prescription, ask the doctor about possible side effects—you don't want an unanticipated unpleasant side effect to be an excuse to stop taking the medication. Also, be sure you know how long you must take the medication—some chronic diseases require a lifetime of treatment.

5. If your physician gives you complex medical information that you don't comprehend, ask for clarification in language that you can understand. Enlist the cooperation of your pharmacist, who can be another valuable health care provider.

6. Remember that some recommendations (such as beginning a regular exercise program) should be adopted gradually. (If you do too much the first day, you won't feel like exercising again the next day.)

7. Find a practitioner who understands and appreciates your cultural beliefs, ethnic background, language, and religious beliefs.

8. Reward yourself for following your good health practices. If you faithfully followed your diet for a day or a week, do something nice for yourself.

Answers

This chapter addresses six basic questions:

1. **What is adherence, how is it measured, and how frequently does it occur?**

Adherence is the extent to which a person's behavior coincides with appropriate medical and health advice. For people to profit from medical advice, first, the advice must be accurate and, second, patients must follow the advice. When people do not adhere to sound health behaviors, they may risk serious health problems or even death. As many as 125,000 people in the United States die each year because of adherence failures.

Researchers can measure adherence in at least six ways: (1) ask the practitioner, (2) ask the patient, (3) ask other people, (4) monitor use of medicine, (5) examine biochemical evidence, and (6) use a combination of these procedures. Of these, physician judgment is the least valid, but each of the others also has serious flaws; a combination of procedures provides the best assessment.

These different methods of assessment complicate the determination of the frequency of nonadherence. However, an analysis of more than 500 studies revealed that the average rate of nonadherence is around 25%, with people on medication regimens more adherent than those who must change health-related behaviors.

2. **What factors predict adherence?**

The severity of a disease does not predict adherence, but unpleasant or painful side effects of medication do lower adherence. Some personal factors relate to adherence, but a nonadherent personality does not exist. Age shows a curvilinear relationship, with older adults and children and adolescents experiencing problems in adhering to medication regimens, but gender shows little overall effect. Emotional factors such as stress, anxiety, and depression lower adherence, but conscientiousness improves adherence. Personal beliefs are a significant factor, with beliefs in a regimen's ineffectiveness lowering adherence and self-efficacy beliefs increasing adherence.

A person's life situation also affects adherence. Lower income endangers adherence; people are not able to pay for treatment or medications. Higher income levels and greater social support generally increase adherence. Individuals with a cultural background that fails to accept Western medicine are less likely to adhere. Ethnicity may also affect the treatment that patients receive from practitioners, and people who feel discriminated against adhere at lower rates. No one factor accounts for adherence, so researchers must consider a combination of factors.

3. **What are continuum theories of health behavior, and how do they explain adherence?**

Continuum theories of health behavior identify variables that should predict the likelihood a person will adhere to a healthy behavior. Continuum theories propose that the variables should predict adherence in the same manner for all individuals.

The health belief model focuses on people's beliefs in perceived susceptibility to a health problem, perceived severity of the problem, perceived benefits of adhering to a behavior, and perceived barriers to adherence. Self-efficacy theory focuses on beliefs about people's confidence that they can control adherence, as well as their beliefs that adherence will bring about good outcomes. The theory of planned behavior focuses on people's attitudes toward a behavior, their beliefs about subjective norms, and their perceived behavioral control as predictors of intentions.

Continuum theories generate a large amount of research across a wide variety of behaviors and are typically successful at predicting people's motivations to adhere to health behaviors. However, they neglect behavioral factors, so they are often better at predicting people's motivations and intentions than they are at predicting behavior.

4. **What are stage theories of health behavior, and how do they explain adherence?**

Stage theories propose that people progress through discrete stages in the process of changing their behavior, and that different variables will be important depending on what stage a person is in. The transtheoretical model proposes that people progress in spiral fashion through five stages in making changes in behavior—precontemplation, contemplation, preparation, action, and maintenance. People in the earlier stages of contemplation and preparation are thought to benefit more from techniques that raise their awareness of a health problem, such as motivational interviewing. In contrast, people in the later stages of action and maintenance should benefit most from strategies that directly address behaviors.

The precaution adoption process model proposes that people go through seven possible stages of belief about their personal susceptibility. Built into Stage 2 is an optimistic bias, a topic that has been heavily researched.

The health action process approach proposes two stages: a motivational phase and a volitional phase. Perceived susceptibility, self-efficacy, and outcome expectations are the important factors in the motivational phase. Planning and self-efficacy are the important factors in the volitional phase.

The success of stage theories in predicting and changing behavior rests on having accurate and valid methods of assessing a person's stage of behavior change. All theories—continuum and stage theories—are useful for understanding adherence, but limited by their omission of various social, economic, ethnic, and other demographic factors that also affect people's health behavior.

5. **What is the intention–behavior gap, and what factors predict whether intentions are translated into behavior?**

The intention–behavior gap refers to the fact that intentions are imperfect predictors of adherence. Behavioral willingness refers to a person's motivation at a given moment to engage in a risky behavior and is driven largely by social pressures in a specific situation. Poor planning can also explain why intentions are not always translated into behavior. Implementational intentions are effective planning exercises that help people identify the specific situations in which they will perform a specific behavior.

Behavioral theory explains adherence in terms of reinforcement and habits that must be changed. Rewards and reinforcements can help a person to initiate a behavior, as well as maintain it over time. Behavioral theory also recognizes the importance of cues and contracts in improving adherence.

6. **How can adherence be improved?**

Methods for improving adherence can generally be divided into educational and behavioral strategies. Educational methods may increase patients' knowledge, but behavioral approaches are better at enhancing adherence. Strategies for enhancing

adherence fall into four approaches: (1) providing prompts, (2) tailoring the regimen, (3) implementing the regimen gradually, and (4) making a contingency contract. Effective programs frequently include clearly written as well as clear verbal instructions, simple medication schedules, follow-up calls for missed appointments, prescriptions tailored to the patient's daily schedule, rewards for compliant behavior, and cues to signal the time for taking medication.

Suggested Readings

Bogart, L. M., & Delahanty, D. L. (2004). Psychosocial models. In T. J. Boll, R. G. Frank, A. Baum, & J. L. Wallander (Eds.), *Handbook of clinical health psychology: Vol. 3: Models and perspectives in health psychology* (pp. 201–248). Washington, DC: American Psychological Association. This review of models of health-related behaviors critically examines the health belief model and theories of reasoned action and planned behavior. The review is oriented around an evaluation of how well these models predict important health behaviors, including condom use, exercise, smoking, and dieting.

DeCivita, M., & Dobkin, P. L. (2005). Pediatric adherence: Conceptual and methodological considerations. *Children's Health Care, 34*, 19–34. Although this article is oriented toward problems for pediatric adherence, the issues of measurement and discussion of the barriers to adherence apply to any age group.

DiMatteo, M. R. (2004). Variations in patients' adherence to medical recommendations: A quantitative review of 50 years of research. *Medical Care, 42*, 200–209. DiMatteo analyzes more than 500 studies published over a span of 50 years to determine factors that relate to failures in adherence. Her concise summary of these results reveals the relative contribution of demographic factors as well as illness characteristics.

Schwarzer, R. (2008). Modeling health behavior change: How to predict and modify the adoption and maintenance of health behaviors. *Applied Psychology: An International Review, 57*, 1–29. This review outlines the health action process approach, and its application to understanding both the adoption and the maintenance of several health behaviors, such as physical activity, breast self-examination, seat belt use, dietary change, and dental flossing.

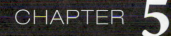

CHAPTER 5

Defining, Measuring, and Managing Stress

CHAPTER OUTLINE

■ Real-World Profile of Lindsay Lohan
■ *The Nervous System and the Physiology of Stress*
■ *Theories of Stress*
■ *Measurement of Stress*
■ *Sources of Stress*
■ *Coping With Stress*
■ *Behavioral Interventions for Managing Stress*

QUESTIONS

This chapter focuses on six basic questions:

1. What is the physiology of stress?

2. What theories explain stress?

3. How has stress been measured?

4. What sources produce stress?

5. What factors influence coping, and what strategies are effective?

6. What behavioral techniques are effective for stress management?

☑CHECK YOUR HEALTH RISKS

Life Events Scale for Students

Has this stressful event happened to you at any time during the last four months? If it has, please check the box next to it. If it has not, leave it blank.

- ☐ Death of a parent (100)
- ☐ Death of your best or very good friend (91)
- ☐ Time in jail (80)
- ☐ Pregnancy, either yourself or being the father (78)
- ☐ Major car accident (car wrecked, people injured) (77)
- ☐ Major personal injury or illness (75)
- ☐ Break-up of parent's marriage/divorce (70)
- ☐ Getting kicked out of college (68)
- ☐ Major change of health in close family member (67)
- ☐ Break-up with boy/girlfriend (65)
- ☐ Major and/or chronic financial problems (63)
- ☐ Parent losing a job (57)
- ☐ Losing a good friend (57)
- ☐ Failing a number of courses (56)

- ☐ Seeking psychological or psychiatric consultation (56)
- ☐ Seriously thinking about dropping out of college (55)
- ☐ Failing a course (53)
- ☐ Major argument with boy/girlfriend (53)
- ☐ Major argument with parents (48)
- ☐ Sex difficulties with boy/girlfriend (48)
- ☐ Beginning an undergraduate program at university (47)
- ☐ Moving away from home (46)
- ☐ Moving out of town with parents (44)
- ☐ Change of job (43)
- ☐ Minor car accident (42)
- ☐ Switch in program within same college or university (37)
- ☐ Getting an unjustified low grade on a test (36)
- ☐ Establishing new steady relationship with partner (35)
- ☐ Minor financial problems (32)
- ☐ Losing a part-time job (31)

- ☐ Vacation with parents (27)
- ☐ Finding a part-time job (25)
- ☐ Family get-togethers (25)
- ☐ Minor violation of the law (e.g., speeding ticket) (24)
- ☐ Getting your own car (21)
- ☐ Vacation alone/with friends (16)

For all of the items you checked, add up the numbers in parentheses next to the items. Healthy undergraduate students, on average, have total scores around 190. Clearly, college students experience stress in their lives. However, as scores increase, so do people's risk of health problems. For example, people with scores of 300 and higher have a very high risk of a serious health change within two years. This chapter explores why stressful life events such as those listed in this checklist can worsen physical health.

Source: Reprinted from *Personality and Individual Differences*, Vol. 20, Issue 6. Clements, K., & Turpin, G., The life events scale for students: Validation for use with British Samples, 747–751, 1996, with permission from Elsevier.

Real-World Profile of
LINDSAY LOHAN

By age 25, Lindsay Lohan had starred in movies that grossed millions of dollars and recorded hit records ("Celebrity Central," 2011). She had also been hospitalized for exhaustion, was treated for alcohol and drug abuse three times, and was arrested several times for driving under the influence of alcohol and for possession of cocaine. She blamed stress and family problems—such as her father's multiple incarcerations—for her behavior: "I hadn't seen my dad; I had a lot of work stress 'cause I was constantly working and never took time to stop" (Silverman, 2008). Lindsay had worked since she was 3 years old, beginning as a child model and becoming a child actor, then a teen movie star and singer. She worked a great deal, but she also partied a lot, using alcohol and drugs. Those behaviors may have also been related to stress.

Although most people find it difficult to accept that people who are wealthy and famous experience stress, research indicates otherwise (Loftus, 1995). Being a celebrity involves stresses that most people do not experience, but those situations are stressful nonetheless. For example, the relentless press coverage that Lindsay Lohan experienced was the type of situation that celebrities rate as stressful. A survey of celebrities found that press coverage was the number one stressor (Loftus, 1995). The type of misbehavior that Lindsay Lohan exhibited is not an unusual reaction to her situation. Indeed, drinking and taking drugs are coping strategies to help manage emotions. Granted, these strategies are neither healthy nor effective, but many people—celebrities and others—often behave similarly.

Stress is a reality of life. The causes of stress are widespread and include major life-changing events such as death of a loved one, unemployment, and disasters such as the terrorist attacks of September 11, 2001, and Hurricane Katrina. Seemingly minor hassles such as relationship breakups and transportation problems can be ongoing sources of stress. Even the rich and famous, such as Lindsay Lohan, experience substantial stress in their lives. This chapter looks at what stress is, how it can be measured, some of the effective and ineffective strategies that people use to cope, and some behavioral management techniques that can help people cope more effectively. Chapter 6 examines the question of whether stress can cause illness and even death. In this chapter, we first look at the physiological bases of stress.

The Nervous System and the Physiology of Stress

The effects of stress on the body result from our nervous system's responses to our environment. The human nervous system contains billions of individual cells called **neurons**, which function electrochemically. Within each neuron, electrically charged ions and the potential for an electrical discharge. The discharge of this potential produces a small electrical current, which travels the length of the neuron. The electrical charge leads to the release of chemicals called **neurotransmitters** that are manufactured within each neuron and stored in vesicles in the neuron. The released neurotransmitters cross the **synaptic cleft**, the space between neurons. These neurotransmitters are the primary ways that neurons communicate with each other.

Billions of neurons make up the nervous system, which is organized in a hierarchy with major divisions and subdivisions. The two major divisions of the nervous system are the **central nervous system (CNS)** and the **peripheral nervous system (PNS)**. The CNS consists of the brain and the spinal cord. The PNS consists of all other neurons, which extend from the spinal cord to all other parts of the body. Figure 5.1 illustrates these divisions and subdivisions of the nervous system.

The Peripheral Nervous System

The peripheral nervous system, that part of the nervous system lying outside the brain and spinal cord, is divided into two parts: the **somatic nervous system** and the **autonomic nervous system (ANS)**. The somatic nervous system primarily serves the skin and the voluntary muscles. The autonomic nervous system primarily serves internal organs and is therefore important in understanding responses to stress.

The ANS allows for a variety of responses through its two divisions: the **sympathetic nervous system** and the **parasympathetic nervous system**. These two subdivisions differ anatomically as well as functionally. They, along with their target organs, appear in Figure 5.2.

The sympathetic division of the ANS mobilizes the body's resources in emergency, stressful, and emotional situations. The reactions include an increase in the rate and strength of heart contractions, increase in rate of breathing, constriction of blood vessels in the skin, a decrease of gastrointestinal activity, stimulation of the sweat glands, and dilation of the pupils in the eyes. Many of these physiological changes serve to direct the flow of blood and oxygen to the skeletal muscles, enabling the organism to mount a quick motor response to a potentially threatening event.

The parasympathetic division of the ANS, on the other hand, promotes relaxation, digestion, and normal growth functions. The parasympathetic nervous system is active under normal, nonstressful conditions. The

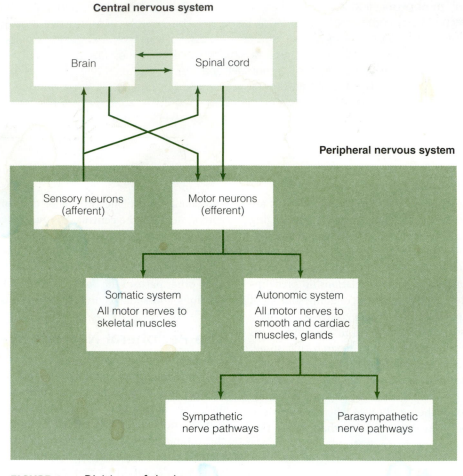

Central nervous system

Brain

Spinal cord

Peripheral nervous system

Sensory neurons
(afferent)

Motor neurons
(efferent)

Somatic system
All motor nerves to
skeletal muscles

Autonomic system
All motor nerves to
smooth and cardiac
muscles, glands

Sympathetic
nerve pathways

Parasympathetic
nerve pathways

FIGURE 5.1   Divisions of the human nervous system.

parasympathetic and sympathetic nervous systems serve the same target organs, but they tend to function reciprocally, with the activation of one increasing as the other decreases. For example, the activation of the sympathetic division reduces the secretion of saliva, producing the sensation of a dry mouth. The activation of the parasympathetic division promotes secretion of saliva.

Neurons in the ANS are activated by neurotransmitters, principally **acetylcholine** and **norepinephrine**. These neurotransmitters have complex effects; each has different effects in different organ systems because the organs contain different neurochemical receptors. In addition, the balance between these two main neurotransmitters, as well as their absolute quantity, is important. Therefore, these two major ANS neurotransmitters can produce a wide variety of responses.

Norepinephrine, as we will describe shortly, plays a number of important roles in the stress response.

The Neuroendocrine System

The **endocrine system** consists of ductless glands distributed throughout the body (see Figure 5.3). The **neuroendocrine system** consists of those endocrine glands that are controlled by and interact with the nervous system. Glands of the endocrine and neuroendocrine systems secrete chemicals known as **hormones**, which move into the bloodstream to be carried to different parts of the body. Specialized receptors on target tissues or organs allow hormones to have specific effects, even though the hormones circulate throughout the body. At the target, hormones may have a direct effect, or they may cause the secretion of another hormone.

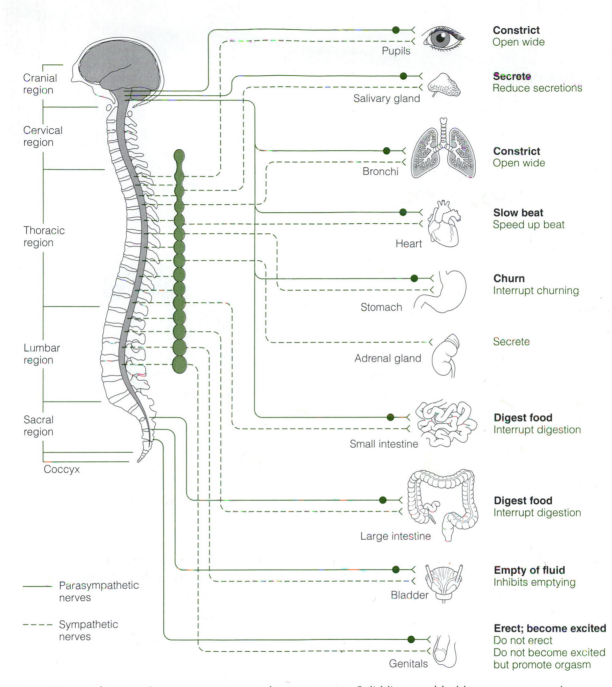

FIGURE 5.2 Autonomic nervous system and target organs. Solid lines and bold type represent the parasympathetic system, whereas dashed lines and lighter type represent the sympathetic system.

The endocrine and nervous systems work closely together because they have several similarities, but they also differ in important ways. Both systems share, synthesize, and release chemicals. In the nervous system, these chemicals are called neurotransmitters; in the endocrine system, they are called hormones. The activation of neurons is usually rapid, and the effect is short term; the endocrine system responds more slowly, and its action persists longer. In the nervous system, neurotransmitters are released by the

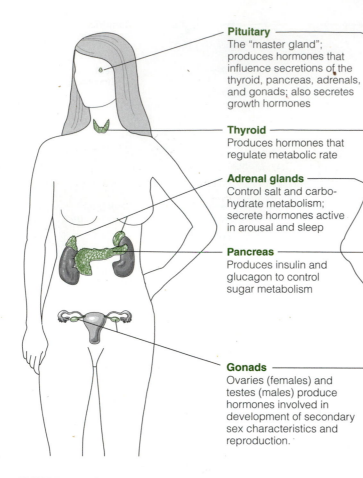

Pituitary
The "master gland";
produces hormones that
influence secretions of the
thyroid, pancreas, adrenals,
and gonads; also secretes
growth hormones

Thyroid
Produces hormones that
regulate metabolic rate

Adrenal glands
Control salt and carbo-
hydrate metabolism;
secrete hormones active
in arousal and sleep

Pancreas
Produces insulin and
glucagon to control
sugar metabolism

Gonads
Ovaries (females) and
testes (males) produce
hormones involved in
development of secondary
sex characteristics and
reproduction.

FIGURE 5.3   Some important endocrine glands.

stimulation of neural impulses, flow across the synaptic cleft, and are immediately either reabsorbed or inactivated. In the endocrine system, hormones are synthesized by the endocrine cells, are released into the blood, reach their targets in minutes or even hours, and exert prolonged effects. The endocrine and nervous systems both have communication and control functions, and both work toward integrated, adaptive behaviors. The two systems are related in function and interact in neuroendocrine responses.

The Pituitary Gland   The **pituitary gland** is located in the brain and is an excellent example of the intricate relationship between the nervous and endocrine systems. The pituitary is connected to the hypothalamus, a structure in the forebrain, and is sometimes referred to as the "master gland" because it produces a number of hormones that affect other glands and prompt the production of yet other hormones.

Of the seven hormones produced by the anterior portion of the pituitary gland, **adrenocorticotropic hormone (ACTH)** plays an essential role in the stress response. When stimulated by the hypothalamus, the pituitary releases ACTH, which in turn acts on the **adrenal glands**.

The Adrenal Glands   The adrenal glands are endocrine glands located on top of each kidney. Each gland is composed of an outer covering, the **adrenal cortex**, and an inner part, the **adrenal medulla**. Both secrete hormones that are important in the response to stress. The **adrenocortical response** occurs when ACTH from the pituitary stimulates the adrenal cortex to release glucocorticoids, one type of hormone. **Cortisol**, the most important of these hormones, exerts a wide range of effects on major organs in the body (Kemeny, 2003). This hormone is so closely associated with stress that the level of cortisol circulating in the blood can be used as an index of stress. Its peak levels appear 20 to 40 minutes after a stressor, allowing time for measurement of this stress hormone. Cortisol can also be assessed in the saliva and urine.

The **adrenomedullary response** occurs when the sympathetic nervous system activates the adrenal medulla. This action prompts secretion of **catecholamines,** a class of chemicals containing norepinephrine and **epinephrine**. Norepinephrine is both a hormone and a neurotransmitter and is produced in many places in the body besides the adrenal medulla. Figure 5.4 shows this adrenomedullary response.

On the other hand, epinephrine (sometimes referred to as adrenaline) is produced exclusively in the adrenal medulla. It is so closely and uniquely associated with the adrenomedullary stress response that it is sometimes used as an index of stress. The amount of epinephrine secreted can be determined by assaying a person's urine, thus measuring stress by tapping into the physiology of the stress response. Like other hormones, epinephrine and norepinephrine circulate through the bloodstream, so their action is both slower and more prolonged than the action of neurotransmitters.

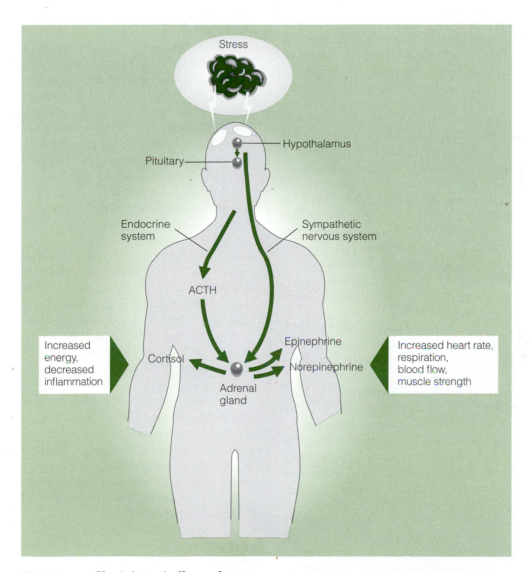

FIGURE 5.4 Physiological effects of stress.

Physiology of the Stress Response

Each of these physiological reactions to stress begins with the perception of stress. That perception results in activation of the sympathetic division of the autonomic nervous system, which mobilizes the body's resources to react in emotional, stressful, and emergency situations. Walter Cannon (1932) termed this configuration of responses the "fight or flight" reaction because this array of responses prepares the body for either option. Sympathetic activation prepares the body for intense motor activity, the sort necessary for attack, defense, or escape. This mobilization occurs through two routes and affects all parts of the body.

One route is through direct activation of the sympathetic division of the ANS (called the adrenomedullary system), which activates the adrenal medulla to secrete epinephrine and norepinephrine (Kemeny, 2003). The effects occur throughout the body, affecting the cardiovascular, digestive, and respiratory systems. The other route is through the **hypothalamic-pituitary-adrenal (HPA)** axis, which involves all of these structures. The action begins with perception of a threatening situation, which prompts action in the hypothalamus. The hypothalamic response is the release of corticotropin-releasing hormone, which stimulates the anterior pituitary (the part of the pituitary gland at the base of the brain) to secrete adrenocorticotropic hormone. This hormone stimulates the adrenal cortex to secrete glucocorticoids, including cortisol. The secretion of cortisol mobilizes the body's energy resources, raising the level of blood sugar to provide energy for the cells. Cortisol also has an anti-inflammatory effect, giving the body a natural defense against swelling from injuries that might be sustained during a fight or a flight. Figure 5.4 shows these two routes of activation.

Together, these physiological reactions to stress prepare the body for a variety of responses that allow adaptation to a threatening situation. **Allostasis** is a term that refers to the body's maintenance of an appropriate level of activation under changing circumstances (McEwen, 2005). Activation of the sympathetic nervous system is the body's attempt to meet the needs of the situation during emergencies. At its optimum in maintaining allostasis, the autonomic nervous system adapts smoothly, adjusting to normal demands by parasympathetic activation and rapidly mobilizing resources for threatening or stressful situations by

sympathetic activation. Not all sympathetic activation leads to health problems, however: Short-term activation of the sympathetic nervous system by physical activity, for example, confers a number of health benefits. Prolonged sympathetic activation creates *allostatic load*, which can overcome the body's ability to adapt. **Allostatic load** represents the "wear and tear" that the body experiences as a result of prolonged activation of physiological stress responses. Allostatic load may be the source of a number of health problems, including weak or dysregulated cortisol production in response to stress, high blood pressure, insulin resistance, fat deposits, and even decline in cognitive abilities over time (Juster, McEwen, & Lupien, 2010; McEwen & Gianaros, 2010). These health problems will be described in greater detail in Chapter 6.

Shelley Taylor and her colleagues (Taylor, 2002, 2006; Taylor et al., 2000) raised objections to the traditional conceptualization of the stress response, questioning the basic notion that people's behavioral responses to stress are necessarily fight-or-flight. These theorists contended that concentrating on men has biased research and theory on stress responses, as fight-or-flight is a more valid description of behavioral responses for men than for women. Although they acknowledge that men's and women's nervous system responses to stress are virtually identical, they argue that women exhibit neuroendocrine responses to stress that differ from men's reactions. They propose that these differences may arise because of the hormone oxytocin, which is released in response to some stressors and linked to a number of social activities such as bonding and affiliation. The effects of oxytocin are especially influenced by estrogen, an interaction that may lay the biological foundation for gender differences in behavioral responses to stress. Taylor and her colleagues propose that women's behavioral responses to stress are better characterized as "tend and befriend" than "fight or flight." That is, women tend to respond to stressful situations with nurturing responses and by seeking and giving social support, rather than by either fighting or fleeing. Indeed, one of the largest gender differences in coping with stress relates to social support seeking: Women seek out the company and comfort of others when stressed more than men (Taylor et al., 2000).

Taylor and her colleagues argued that this pattern of responses arose in women during human evolutionary history and is more consistent with the biological and behavioral evidence than the fight-or-flight conceptualization of stress responses. Although some researchers criticized this view (Geary & Flinn, 2002), recent human research is consistent with the tend-and-befriend view (Taylor, 2006). For example, the patterns of hormone secretion during competition differ for women and men (Kivlinghan, Granger, & Booth, 2005). Furthermore, among women, relationship problems correlate with greater levels of oxytocin in the blood (Taylor et al., 2006; Taylor, Saphire-Bernstein, & Seeman, 2010), confirming a gender difference in responses to stress.

IN SUMMARY

The physiology of the stress response is complex. When a person perceives stress, the sympathetic division of the autonomic nervous system rouses the person from a resting state in two ways: by stimulating the sympathetic nervous system and by producing hormones. The ANS activation is rapid, as is all neural transmission, whereas the action of the neuroendocrine system is slower but longer lasting. The pituitary releases ACTH, which in turn affects the adrenal cortex. Glucocorticoid release prepares the body to resist the stress and even to cope with injury by the release of cortisol. Together the two systems form the physiological basis for allostasis, adaptive responses under conditions of change.

An understanding of the physiology of stress does not completely clarify the meaning of stress. Several models, described next, attempt to better define and explain stress.

Theories of Stress

If you ask people you know whether they are stressed, it is unlikely anyone will ask you what you mean. People seem to know what stress is without having to define it. However, for researchers, *stress* has no simple definition (McEwen, 2005). Indeed, stress has been defined in three different ways: as a stimulus, as a response, and as an interaction. When some people talk about stress, they are referring to an environmental *stimulus*, as in "I have a high-stress job." Others consider stress a physical *response*, as in "My heart races

when I feel a lot of stress." Still others consider stress to result from the *interaction* between environmental stimuli and the person, as in "I feel stressed when I have to make financial decisions at work, but other types of decisions do not stress me."

These three views of stress also appear in different theories of stress. The view of stress as an external event was the first approach taken by stress researchers, the most prominent of whom was Hans Selye. During the course of his research, Selye changed to a more physical response-based view of stress. The most influential view of stress among psychologists is the interactionist approach, proposed by Richard Lazarus. The next two sections discuss the views of Selye and Lazarus.

Selye's View

Beginning in the 1930s and continuing until his death in 1982, Hans Selye (1956, 1976, 1982) made a strong case for the relationship between stress and physical illness and brought this issue to the public's attention. Selye first conceptualized stress as a stimulus and focused his attention on the environmental conditions that produce stress. In the 1950s, he shifted his focus to stress as a response that the organism makes. To distinguish the two, Selye started using the term *stressor* to refer to the stimulus and *stress* to mean the response.

Selye's contributions to stress research included a model for how the body defends itself in stressful situations. According to Selye's model, stress was a nonspecific response: that is, a wide variety of stressors could prompt the stress response, but the response would always be the same.

The General Adaptation Syndrome   Selye coined the term **general adaptation syndrome (GAS)** to refer to the body's generalized attempt to defend itself against a stressor. This syndrome is divided into three stages, the first of which is the **alarm reaction**. During alarm, the body's defenses against a stressor are mobilized through activation of the sympathetic nervous system. Adrenaline (epinephrine) is released, heart rate and blood pressure increase, respiration becomes faster, blood is diverted away from the internal organs toward the skeletal muscles, sweat glands are activated, and the gastrointestinal system decreases its activity.

Selye called the second phase of the GAS the **resistance stage**. In this stage, the organism adapts to the stressor. How long this stage lasts depends on the

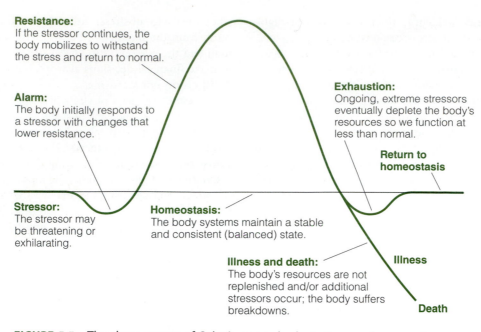

Resistance:
If the stressor continues, the body mobilizes to withstand the stress and return to normal.

Alarm:
The body initially responds to a stressor with changes that lower resistance.

Exhaustion:
Ongoing, extreme stressors eventually deplete the body's resources so we function at less than normal.

Return to homeostasis

Stressor:
The stressor may be threatening or exhilarating.

Homeostasis:
The body systems maintain a stable and consistent (balanced) state.

Illness and death:
The body's resources are not replenished and/or additional stressors occur; the body suffers breakdowns.

Illness

Death

FIGURE 5.5 The three stages of Selye's general adaptation syndrome—alarm, resistance, exhaustion—and their consequences.

Source: An invitation to health (7th ed., p. 40) by D. Hales, 1997, Pacific Grove, CA: Brooks/Cole. From HALES, *Invitation to Health,* 7E. © 1997 Cengage Learning.

severity of the stressor and the adaptive capacity of the organism. If the organism can adapt, the resistance stage will continue for a long time. During this stage, the person gives the outward appearance of normality, but physiologically the body's internal functioning is not normal. Continuing stress will cause continued neurological and hormonal changes. Selye believed that these demands take a toll, setting the stage for what he described as *diseases of adaptation*—diseases related to continued, persistent stress. Figure 5.5 illustrates these stages and the point in the process at which diseases develop.

Among the diseases Selye considered to be the result of prolonged resistance to stress are peptic ulcers and ulcerative colitis, hypertension and cardiovascular disease, hyperthyroidism, and bronchial asthma. In addition, Selye hypothesized that resistance to stress would cause changes in the immune system, making infection more likely.

The capacity to resist stress is finite, and the final stage of the GAS is the **exhaustion stage**. At the end, the organism's ability to resist is depleted, and a breakdown results. This stage is characterized by activation of the parasympathetic division of the autonomic nervous

system. Under normal circumstances, parasympathetic activation keeps the body functioning in a balanced state. In the exhaustion stage, however, the parasympathetic system functions abnormally, causing a person to become exhausted. Selye believed that exhaustion frequently results in depression and sometimes even death.

Evaluation of Selye's View Selye's early concept of stress as a stimulus and his later concentration on the physical aspects of stress influenced stress research. The stimulus-based view of stress prompted researchers to investigate the various environmental conditions that cause people to experience stress and also led to the construction of stress inventories, such as the Life Events Scale for Students that introduces this chapter.

However, Selye's view of the physiology of stress is probably too simplistic (McEwen, 2005). He considered the stress response to all events to be similar, a view that research has failed to confirm. He also believed that the physiological responses to stress were oriented toward maintaining functioning within a narrow range of the optimal level. The concepts of *allostasis* and *allostatic load*, which emphasize the processes of adaptation and change rather than narrow regulation, now replace Selye's view. Allostatic load occurs when many changes are required by presence of chronic stressors. Thus, allostatic load can become overload, resulting in damage and disease. This view of stress is similar to Selye's but shows subtle differences that are more compatible with modern research.

The major criticism of Selye's view is that it largely ignores the situational and psychological factors that contribute to stress. These factors include the emotional component and a person's interpretation of stressful events (Mason, 1971, 1975), which makes Selye's view of stress incomplete in the view of most psychologists. Although Selye's view has had great influence on the popular conception of stress, an alternative model formulated by psychologist Richard Lazarus is more widely accepted among today's psychologists.

Lazarus's View

In Lazarus's view, the interpretation of stressful events is more important than the events themselves. Neither the environmental event nor the person's response defines stress; rather, the individual's *perception* of the psychological situation is the critical factor. For example, a job promotion may represent an opportunity and challenge for one person, but a significant source of stress for another person.

Psychological Factors   Lazarus's emphasis on interpretation and perception differs from that of Selye. This emphasis arose from another difference: Lazarus worked largely with humans rather than nonhuman animals. The ability of people to think about and evaluate future events makes them vulnerable in ways that other animals are not. People feel stressed about situations that would probably not concern an animal, such as employment, plans for the future, or impending deadlines. Humans encounter stresses because they have high-level cognitive abilities that other animals lack.

According to Lazarus (1984, 1993), the effect that stress has on a person is based more on that person's feelings of threat, vulnerability, and ability to cope than on the stressful event itself. For example, losing a job may be extremely stressful for someone who has no money saved or who believes that finding another job will be difficult. Lindsay Lohan, who we introduced at the beginning of this chapter, apparently perceived her

work demands as stressful. Other actors may have experienced her level of employment as a positive event; many actors find unemployment more stressful than working (Loftus, 1995). These examples highlight Lazarus's view that a life event is not what produces stress; rather, it is one's view of the situation that causes an event to become stressful.

Lazarus and Susan Folkman defined psychological stress as a "particular relationship between the person and the environment that is appraised by the person as taxing or exceeding his or her resources and endangering his or her well-being" (1984, p. 19). This definition makes several important points. First, it emphasizes Lazarus and Folkman's interactional or *transactional* view of stress, holding that stress refers to a relationship between person and environment. Second, this definition emphasizes the key role of a person's appraisal of the psychological situation. Third, the definition holds that stress arises when a person appraises a situation as threatening, challenging, or harmful.

Appraisal   According to Lazarus and Folkman (1984), people make three kinds of appraisals of situations: primary appraisal, secondary appraisal, and reappraisal. **Primary appraisal** is not necessarily first in importance, but it is first in time. When people first encounter an event, such as an offer of a job promotion, they appraise the offer in terms of its effect on their well-being. They may view the event as irrelevant, benign-positive, or stressful. Irrelevant events are those that have no implications for a person's well-being, such as a snowstorm in another state. Benign-positive events are those that are appraised as having good implications. A stressful event means that the event is appraised as being harmful, threatening, or challenging. Lazarus (1993) defined *harm* as damage that has already been done, such as an illness or injury; *threat* as the anticipation of harm; and *challenge* as a person's confidence in overcoming difficult demands. Research indicates that the perception of threat or challenge makes a difference for performance; perception of challenge leads to better performance than perception of threat (Gildea, Schneider, & Shebilske, 2007).

After their initial appraisal of an event, people form an impression of their ability to control or cope with harm, threat, or challenge, an impression called **secondary appraisal**. People typically ask three questions in making secondary appraisals. The first is "What options are available to me?" The second is "What is the likelihood that I can successfully apply the necessary strategies to reduce this stress?" The third is "Will this procedure work—that is, will it alleviate my stress?"

When people believe they can successfully change a situation to achieve a positive outcome, stress is reduced. Lindsay Lohan did not have that confidence. She had not found any successful strategy for balancing her work demands with the other aspects of her life. Her father had been convicted of driving under the influence of alcohol and sentenced to prison. Many celebrities anchor their lives around their families, and without that possibility, Lindsay had difficulty finding effective coping strategies.

The third type of appraisal is **reappraisal**. Appraisals change constantly as new information becomes available. Reappraisal does not always result in more stress; sometimes it decreases stress.

Vulnerability   Stress is most likely to be aroused when people are vulnerable—when they lack resources in a situation of some personal importance. These resources may be either physical or social, but their importance is determined by psychological factors, such as perception and evaluation of the situation. An arthritic knee, for example, would produce physical vulnerability in a professional athlete but might be a minor inconvenience to the professional life of someone who works behind a desk.

Lazarus and Folkman (1984) insisted that physical or social deficits alone are not sufficient to produce vulnerability. What matters is whether people consider the situation personally important. Vulnerability differs from threat in that it represents only the *potential* for threat. Threat exists when people perceive that their self-esteem is in jeopardy; vulnerability exists when people's lack of resources creates a potentially threatening or harmful situation. Celebrities remain popular by pleasing people, so their continued fame is always uncertain (Loftus, 1995). Many feel that they are undeserving of their success and, consequently, fear its loss. These situations provide good examples of threat and vulnerability.

Coping   An important ingredient in Lazarus's theory of stress is the ability or inability to cope with a stressful situation. Lazarus and Folkman defined coping as "constantly changing cognitive and behavioral efforts to manage specific external and/or internal demands that are appraised as taxing or exceeding the resources of the person" (1984, p. 141). This definition spells out several important features of coping. First, coping is a

process, constantly changing as one's efforts are evaluated as more or less successful. Second, coping is not automatic; it is a learned pattern of responding to stressful situations. Third, coping requires effort. People need not be completely aware of their coping response, and the outcome may or may not be successful, but effort must have been expended. Fourth, coping is an effort to *manage* the situation; control and mastery are not necessary. For example, most of us make an effort to manage our physical environment by striving for a comfortable air temperature. Thus, we cope with our environment even though complete mastery of the climate is impossible. How well people are able to cope depends on the resources they have available and the strategies they use. We will discuss effective coping strategies later in this chapter.

IN SUMMARY

Two leading theories of stress are those of Hans Selye and Richard Lazarus. Selye, the first researcher to look closely at stress, first saw stress as a stimulus but later viewed it as a response. Whenever animals (including humans) encounter a threatening stimulus, they mobilize themselves in a generalized attempt to adapt to that stimulus. This mobilization, called the general adaptation syndrome, has three stages—alarm, resistance, and exhaustion—and the potential for trauma or illness exists at all three stages.

In contrast, Lazarus held a cognitively oriented, transactional view of stress and coping. Stressful encounters are dynamic and complex, constantly changing and unfolding, so that the outcomes of one stressful event alter subsequent appraisals of new events. Individual differences in coping strategies and in the appraisal of stressful events are crucial to a person's experience of stress; therefore, the likelihood of developing any stress-related disorder varies with the individual. The relationship between stressful events and subsequent health is complex, and any attempt to measure stress and people's attempts to cope with it must also be complex.

Measurement of Stress

Measuring stress is an important part of a health psychologist's job. Researchers must first measure stress in order to understand the effect of stress on disease. This section discusses some of the more widely used methods and addresses the problems involved in determining their reliability and validity.

Methods of Measurement

Researchers have used a variety of approaches to measure stress, but most fall into two broad categories: physiological measures and self-reports (Monroe, 2008). Physiological measures directly assess aspects of the body's physical stress response. Self-reports measure either **life events** or **daily hassles** that a person experiences. Both approaches hold some potential for investigating the effects of stress on illness and health.

Physiological Measures   Physiological measures of stress include blood pressure, heart rate, galvanic skin response, respiration rate, and increased secretion of stress hormones such as cortisol and epinephrine. These physiological measures provide researchers with a window into the activation of the body's sympathetic nervous system and HPA axis.

Another common approach to the physiological measurement of stress is through its association with the release of hormones. Epinephrine and norepinephrine, for example, can be measured in either blood or urine samples and can provide an index of stress (Eller, Netterstrøm, & Hansen, 2006; Krantz, Forsman, & Lundberg, 2004). The levels of these hormones circulating in the blood decrease within a few minutes after the stressful experience, so measurement must be quick to capture the changes. The levels of hormones persist longer in the urine, but factors other than stress contribute to urinary levels of these hormones. The stress hormone cortisol persists for at least 20 minutes, and measurement of salivary cortisol provides an index of the changes in this hormone. A newer method assesses the cortisol in human hair, which represents the body's cortisol production over the preceding 6 months (Kirschbaum, Tietze, Skoluda, & Dettenborn, 2009).

The advantage of these physiological measures of stress is that they are direct, highly reliable, and easily quantified. A disadvantage is that the mechanical and electrical hardware and clinical settings that are frequently used may themselves produce stress. Thus, this approach to measuring stress is useful but not the most widely used method. Self-report measures are far more common.

Life Events Scales   Since the late 1950s and early 1960s, researchers have developed a number of self-report instruments to measure stress. The earliest and best known of these self-report procedures is the Social Readjustment Rating Scale (SRRS), developed by Thomas H. Holmes and Richard Rahe in 1967. The scale is simply a list of 43 life events arranged in rank order from most to least stressful. Each event carries an assigned value, ranging from 100 points for death of a spouse to 11 points for minor violations of the law. Respondents check the items they experienced during a recent period, usually the previous 6 to 24 months. Adding each item's point value and totaling scores yields a stress score for each person. These scores can then be correlated with future events, such as incidence of illness, to determine the relationship between this measure of stress and the occurrence of physical illness.

Other stress inventories exist, including the Life Events Scale for Students (Clements & Turpin, 1996), the assessment that appears as Check Your Health Risks at the beginning of this chapter. College students who check more stress situations tend to use health services more than students who check fewer events.

The Perceived Stress Scale (PSS) (Cohen, Kamarck, & Mermelstein, 1983) emphasizes perception of events. The PSS is a 14-item scale that attempts to measure the degree to which people appraise events in the past

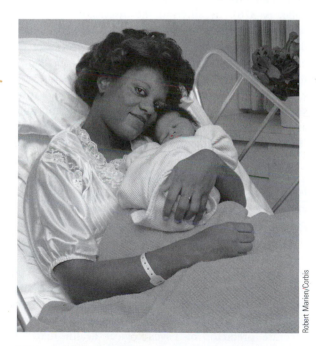

Life events scales also include positive events because such events also require adjustment.

month as being "unpredictable, uncontrollable, and overloading" (Cohen et al., 1983, p. 387). The scale assesses three components of stress: (1) daily hassles, (2) major events, and (3) changes in coping resources. Researchers use the PSS in a variety of situations, such as examining the link between prenatal stress and preterm birth in pregnant women (Glynn, Dunkel Schetter, Hobel, & Sandman, 2008), determining the effectiveness of a relaxation program for elementary teachers (Nassiri, 2005), and predicting burnout among college athletic coaches (Tashman, Tenenbaum, & Eklund, 2010). Its brevity combined with good reliability and validity has led to use of this scale in a variety of research projects.

More recent life events scales include the Weekly Stress Inventory (Brantley et al., 2007; Brantley, Jones, Boudreaux, & Gatz, 1997), which assesses stress over a few weeks or months, and the Stress in General Scale (Stanton, Balzer, Smith, Parra, & Ironson, 2001), designed to measure general work stress.

Everyday Hassles Scales Richard Lazarus and his associates pioneered an approach to stress measurement that looks at daily hassles rather than life events. Daily hassles are "experiences and conditions of daily living that have been appraised as salient and harmful or threatening to the endorser's well-being" (Lazarus, 1984, p. 376). Recall from the discussion of theories of stress that Lazarus views stress as a transactional, dynamic complex shaped by people's *appraisal* of the environmental situation and their *perceived capabilities to cope* with this situation. Consistent with this view, Lazarus and his associates insisted that self-report scales must be able to assess subjective elements such as personal appraisal, beliefs, goals, and commitments (Lazarus, 2000; Lazarus, DeLongis, Folkman, & Gruen, 1985).

The original Hassles Scale (Kanner, Coyne, Schaefer, & Lazarus, 1981) consists of 117 items about annoying, irritating, or frustrating situations in which people may *feel* hassled. These include concerns about weight, home maintenance, crime, and having too many things to do. People also rate the degree to which each item produced stress. The Hassles Scale only modestly correlates with life events, which suggests that these two types of stress are not the same thing. Furthermore, the Hassles Scale can be more accurate predictor of psychological health than life events scales (Lazarus, 1984). A shorter Hassles Scale, developed by the same research team (DeLongis,

Folkman & Lazarus, 1988), is a better predictor than the Social Readjustment Rating Scale of both the frequency and intensity of headaches (Fernandez & Sheffield, 1996) and episodes of inflammatory bowel disease (Searle & Bennett, 2001). Thus, everyday hassles are an important contributor to health problems.

The measurement of everyday hassles also extends to specific situations. For example, the Urban Hassles Index (Miller & Townsend, 2005) measures stressors that commonly affect adolescents in urban environments, and the Family Daily Hassles Inventory (Rollins & Garrison, 2002) targets daily stressors commonly experienced by parents. Thus, researchers have a variety of self-report stress measures to choose from, depending on their purposes and specific populations of study.

Reliability and Validity of Stress Measures

The usefulness of stress measures rests on their ability to predict some established criterion and to do so consistently. For health psychology, the criterion is usually illness or some risk factor for disease. To predict future stress-related illness, these inventories must be both reliable and valid. Reliability is the consistency with which an instrument measures whatever it measures, and validity is the extent to which it measures what it is supposed to measure.

Reliability is the consistency with which an instrument measures whatever it measures. The *reliability* of self-report inventories is frequently determined by the paired-associate method. In the paired-associate method, close associates (usually a spouse) fill out the inventory, answering as if the item applied to their associate. The degree of agreement between the two associates is usually quite high for moderately or severely stressful events (Slater & Depue, 1981) but lower for less stressful experiences (Zimmerman, 1983).

To consider the *validity* of self-report inventories, we must begin with the question "What are these instruments supposed to measure?" At least two approaches to answering this question are possible. First, the scales should accurately represent all of the life events experienced by the respondents. Second, as they are most frequently used, self-report inventories are supposed to measure or predict the incidence of future illness. Let's consider these approaches in more detail.

First, do self-report inventories accurately represent all experiences of stressful life events? Some investigators (Turner & Wheaton, 1995) suggested that many people tend to underreport (omit) life events, whereas other critics contended that sick people over-report life events, providing a kind of justification for their illness. Either overreporting or underreporting decreases the validity of life events measures. Research indicates that life events scales tend to underestimate the stress that African Americans experience (Turner & Avison, 2003).

The second and most useful type of validity for stress inventories is the extent to which they predict future illnesses or disorders. If self-report scales can demonstrate predictive validity, then they will play a valuable role in determining who may be at risk for stress-related illnesses. One problem in measuring the relationship between stress inventories and illness is the confounding of items on the major life events scales with the presence of physical disorders. Being ill can be stressful, of course, but it can also cause problems that appear on the Social Readjustment Rating Scale, such as change in sleeping habits and change in eating habits. Therefore, a high score on the SRRS or other similarly constructed life events scale may be a consequence rather than a cause of illness. However, an analysis of 30 years of research on the SRRS (Scully, Tosi, & Banning, 2000) concluded that the SSRS predicts occurrence of stress-related symptoms, making it a useful tool.

IN SUMMARY

Researchers and clinicians measure stress by several methods, including physiological and biochemical measures and self-reports of stressful events. The most popular life events scale is the Social Readjustment Rating Scale, which emphasizes change in life events. Despite its popularity, the SRRS is a modest predictor of subsequent illness. Lazarus and his associates pioneered the measurement of stress as daily hassles and uplifts. These inventories emphasize the perceived severity and importance of daily events. In general, the revised Hassles and Uplifts Scale is more accurate than the SRRS in predicting future illness.

The prediction of future illness is one measure of validity, or how accurate stress inventories are in their assessment. Another important characteristic of stress measurement is reliability, which is how consistent the measures are. Self-report inventories of stress have only moderate levels of reliability and low levels of validity, and even hassles scales have limited validity for predicting illness.

Sources of Stress

Stress can flow from myriad sources: cataclysmic events with natural or human causes, changes in an individual's life history, and ongoing hassles of daily life. In organizing sources of stress, we follow the model set forth by Richard Lazarus and Judith Cohen (1977), but as these two researchers emphasized, an individual's perception of a stressful event is more crucial than the event itself.

Cataclysmic Events

Lazarus and Cohen defined cataclysmic events as "sudden, unique, and powerful single life-events requiring major adaptive responses from population groups sharing the experience" (p. 91). A number of cataclysmic events, both intentional and unintentional, strike unpredictably in areas around the world. Unintentional major events include such natural disasters as hurricanes, typhoons, fires, tornadoes, floods, earthquakes, and other cataclysmic events that kill large numbers of people and create stress, grief, and fear among survivors. Some of these events, such as hurricanes, typhoons, and floods, are unique and powerful but not necessarily sudden.

Occasionally, stressful events are so powerful that they affect nearly the entire globe, such as the great earthquake and tsunami that devastated large parts of Japan in March 2011, the tsunami in the Indian Ocean in December 2004, and Hurricane Katrina and its aftermath, which destroyed New Orleans and other cities on the Gulf of Mexico in August 2005, followed by hurricane Rita, which devastated southeast Texas and southwest Louisiana about a month later. The physical damage of these natural events was astronomical. More than 200,000 people were killed or missing and countless others left injured, sick, and homeless. Survivors of the Indian Ocean tsunami (Dewaraja & Kawamura, 2006) and residents in the New Orleans area (Weems et al., 2007) experienced symptoms of depression and **posttraumatic stress disorder (PTSD)**. However, several factors moderated or exacerbated these symptoms, such as their feelings of support

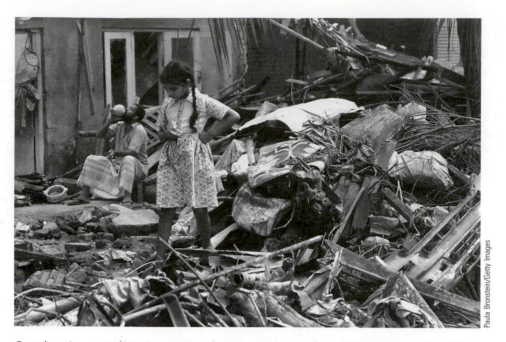

Paula Bronstein/Getty Images

Cataclysmic events require major adaptive responses from large groups of people.

from others, discrimination, and their proximity to the destruction.

Natural disasters can be devastating to huge numbers of people, but they cannot be blamed on any single person or group of persons. In contrast, the 1995 bombing of the Murrah Federal Building in Oklahoma City and the attack on the World Trade Center and the Pentagon on September 11, 2001, were all *intentional* acts. Each was sudden, unique, and powerful, and each required adaptive responses from large numbers of people. Television and the media brought the aftermath of these cataclysmic events into millions of homes, resulting in multitudes of people having similar stress-related experiences.

Several factors contribute to how much stress an event creates, including physical proximity to the event, time elapsed since the event, and the intention of the perpetrators. The September 11 attack on the World Trade Center included all three factors for those living in New York City, creating lingering trauma for people close to the site (Hasin, Keyes, Hatzenbuehler, Aharonovich, & Alderson, 2007). For those not in New York City, stress associated with the attacks began to dissipate within weeks (Schlenger et al., 2002), but other evidence suggests that some people continued to experience negative psychological and physical health effects several years later (Holman et al., 2008;

Richman, Cloninger, & Rospenda, 2008; Updegraff, Silver, & Holman, 2008). The intentional nature of the attacks added to the stress, making these violent events more traumatic than natural disasters.

In summary, cataclysmic events can be either intentional or unintentional, with different effects on stress. Such events strike suddenly, without warning, and people who survive them as well as those who help with the aftermath often see their experience as life altering. Despite the power of cataclysmic events to affect people, researchers have focused more attention on life events as sources of stress (Richman et al., 2008).

Life Events

Major life events—such as experiencing the death of a spouse, getting a divorce, being fired from your job, or moving to a different country—are major sources of stress, but minor life events can also be stressful. Some of the items on the Life Events Scale for Students at the beginning of this chapter are life events, and the popular Holmes and Rahe (1967) Social Readjustment Rating Scale described earlier in this chapter consists of life events.

Life events differ from cataclysmic events in three important ways. Life events and life event scales emphasize the importance of *change*. When events require people to make some sort of change or read-justment, they feel stressed. Positive events such as get-ting married, becoming a parent, and starting a new job all require some adjustment, but negative events such as losing a job, the death of a family member, or being a victim of a violent crime also require adaptation. Unlike cataclysmic events that affect huge numbers of people, stressful life events affect a few people or per-haps only one. Divorce that happens to you can be more profound in changing your life than an earth-quake in a far-off location that affects thousands.

Life events usually evolve more slowly than cata-clysmic events. Divorce does not happen in a single day, and being dismissed from a job is ordinarily pre-ceded by a period of conflict. Crime victimization, however, is often sudden and unexpected. All of these life events produce stress, and subsequent problems are common. For example, divorce may decrease stress between the divorcing partners (Amato & Hohmann-Marriott, 2007) but more often creates short-term and sometimes long-term problems for both the adults and their children (Michael, Torres, & Seeman, 2007). When losing a job results in long-term unemployment, this situation creates a cascade of stressors, including financial problems and family conflict (Howe, Levy, & Caplan, 2004; Song, Foo, Uy, & Sun, 2011). Being the victim of a violent crime "transforms people into vic-tims and changes their lives forever" (Koss, 1990, p. 374). Crime victims tend to lose their sense of invul-nerability, and their risk of PTSD increases (Koss, Bai-ley, Yuan, Herrera, & Lichter, 2003). This risk applies to a variety of types of victimization, and studies have established the risk of PTSD for both children (Sebre et al., 2004) and adults. Even exposure to community violence increases risks for children (Rosario, Salzinger, Feldman, & Ng-Mak, 2008).

Daily Hassles

Unlike life events that call for people to make adjust-ments in their lives, daily hassles are part of everyday life. Living in poverty, fearing crime, arguing with one's spouse, balancing work with family life, living in crowded and polluted conditions, and fighting a long daily com-mute to work are examples of daily hassles. The stress brought on by daily hassles can originate from both the physical and the psychosocial environment.

Daily Hassles and the Physical Environment   Many people associate environmental sources of stress with

urban life. They think of noise, pollution, crowding, fear of crime, and personal alienation as a part of city living. Although these environmental sources of stress may be more concentrated in urban settings, rural life can also be noisy, polluted, hot, cold, humid, or even crowded, with many people living together in a one- or two-room dwelling. Air and water pollution originating in urban or industrial settings may disperse to other, nonurban settings. Nonetheless, the crowding, noise, pollution, fear of crime, and personal alienation more typical of urban living combine to produce what Eric Graig (1993) termed **urban press**. The results from one study (Christenfeld, Glynn, Phillips, & Shrira, 1999) suggested that the combined sources of stress affecting residents of New York City are factors in that city's higher heart attack death rate. Living in a polluted, noisy, and crowded environment creates chronic daily hassles that not only make life unpleasant but may also affect behavior and performance (Evans & Stecker, 2004) and pose a risk to health (Schell & Denham, 2003). Access to a garden or park can diminish this stress; individuals whose living situations include access to such "green spaces" report lower stress (Nielsen & Hansen, 2007) and better self-reported health (van Dil-len, de Vries, Groenewegen, & Spreeuwenberg, 2011).

People tend to deal with problems produced by *pollution* in one of two ways—by ignoring the threat or by concentrating on the impact the pollution will have on them personally (Hatfield & Job, 2001). When neither of these strategies is possible, people may feel threats from environmental pollution, produc-ing stress. For example, a study that examined residents who lived in an area contaminated by industrial pollu-tion showed that these people exhibited significantly more physical and psychological symptoms of stress than did people living in an uncontaminated area (Matthies, Hoeger, & Guski, 2000).

Noise is a type of pollution because it can be a noxious, unwanted stimulus that intrudes into a per-son's environment, but it is quite difficult to define in any objective way. One person's music is another per-son's noise. The importance of subjective attitude toward noise is illustrated by a study (Nivison & End-resen, 1993) that asked residents living beside a busy street about their health, sleep, anxiety level, and atti-tude toward noise. The level of noise was not a factor, but the residents' subjective view of noise showed a strong relationship to the number of their health com-plaints. Similarly, workers who were more sensitive to noise (Waye et al., 2002) showed a higher cortisol level

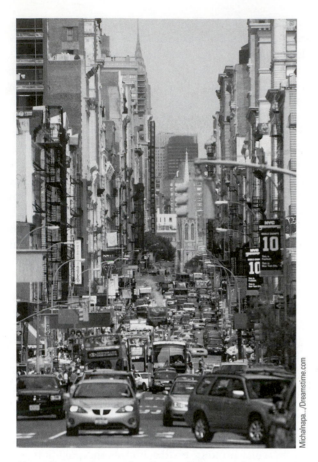

Crowding, noise, and pollution increase the stress of urban life.

A distinction between the concepts of population density and crowding helps in understanding the effects of crowding on humans. In 1972, Daniel Stokols defined **population density** as a *physical* condition in which a large population occupies a limited space. **Crowding**, however, is a *psychological* condition that arises from a person's perception of the high-density environment in which that person is confined. Thus, density is necessary for crowding but does not automatically produce the feeling of being crowded. The crush of people in the lobby of a theater during intermission of a popular play may not be experienced as crowding, despite the extremely high population density. The distinction between density and crowding means that personal perceptions, such as a feeling of control, are critical in the definition of crowding. Crowding in both neighborhoods and residences plays a role in how stressed a person will be (Regoeczi, 2003).

Pollution, noise, and crowding often co-occur in "the environment of poverty" (Ulrich, 2002, p. 16). The environment of poverty may also include violence or the threat of violence and discrimination. On a daily basis, wealthier people experience fewer stressors than poor people (Grzywacz et al., 2004), but even wealthy people are not exempt. The threat of violence and fear of crime are a part of the stress of modern life. Some evidence suggests that community violence is especially stressful for children and adolescents (Ozer, 2005; Rosario et al., 2008). Children who grow up in an environment of poverty experience greater chronic stress and allostatic load, which may contribute to health problems later in life (Matthews, Gallo, & Taylor, 2010). For example, children growing up in lower socioeconomic status households perceive greater threat and family chaos, which are linked to greater cortisol production as they age (Chen, Cohen, & Miller, 2010).

In the United States, poverty is more common among ethnic minorities than among European Americans (USCB, 2011), and discrimination is another type of daily hassle that is often associated with the environment of poverty. However, discrimination is part of the psychosocial environment.

Daily Hassles and the Psychosocial Environment

People's psychosocial environment can be fertile ground for creating daily hassles. These stressors originate in the everyday social environment from sources such as community, workplace, and family interactions.

Discrimination is a stressor that occurs with alarming regularity in a variety of social situations in

and rated a low-frequency noise as more annoying than workers who were less sensitive. Other research demonstrates that noise and vibration affected performance on a cognitive task (Ljungberg & Neely, 2007). However, the most likely health effects of noise are probably hearing loss from the direct influence of exceedingly loud noise rather than an indirect effect produced by increased stress.

Another source of hassles is *crowding*. A series of classic experiments with rats living in crowded conditions (Calhoun, 1956, 1962) showed that crowding produced changes in social and sexual behavior that included increases in territoriality, aggression, and infant mortality and decreases in levels of social integration. These results suggest that crowding is a source of stress that affects behavior, but studies with humans are complicated by several factors, including a definition of crowding.

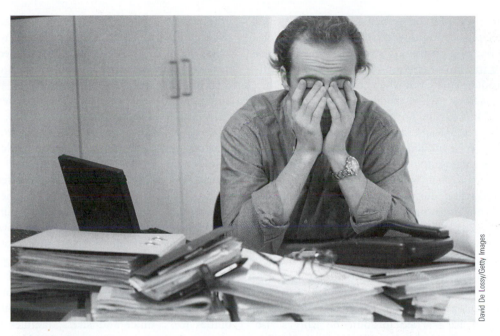

High job demands can produce stress, especially when combined with low levels of control.

the community and workplace for African Americans in the United States (Landrine & Klonoff, 1996), but other ethnic groups (Edwards & Romero, 2008), women, and gay and bisexual men (Huebner & Davis, 2007) also face discrimination. Unfair treatment creates both disadvantage for the individuals discriminated against and a stigma that is stressful (Major & O'Brien, 2005). Discrimination is a source of stress that may increase the risk for cardiovascular disease (Troxel, Matthews, Bromberger, & Sutton-Tyrrell, 2003). A meta-analysis of over 100 studies confirmed this link between perceived discrimination and both mental and physical health problems (Pascoe & Richman, 2009). Furthermore, this review suggests that the link between perceived discrimination and health problems may be attributable to both the activation of physiological stress responses, as well as maladaptive health behaviors that people use to cope with experiences of stigma and discrimination.

Discrimination is not the only stressor that occurs in the workplace—some jobs are more stressful than others. Contrary to some people's assumption, business executives who must make many decisions every day have *less* job-related stress than their employees who merely carry out those decisions. Most executives have jobs in which the

demands are high but so is their level of control, and research indicates that lack of control is more stressful than the burden of making decisions. Lower-level occupations are actually more stressful than executive jobs (Wamala, Mittleman, Horsten, Schenck-Gustafsson, & Orth-Gomér, 2000). Using stress-related illness as a criterion, the jobs of construction worker, secretary, laboratory technician, waiter or waitress, machine operator, farmworker, and painter are among the most stressful. These jobs all share a high level of demand combined with a low level of control, status, and compensation. Middle-level managers such as foremen and supervisors also have highly stressful jobs. They must meet demands from two directions: their bosses and their workers. Thus, they have more than their share of stress (and stress-related illness).

Although it may seem ironic, celebrities such as Lindsay Lohan experience job stress (Loftus, 1995). They are rarely in control of their careers and experience frequent periods of unemployment, creating stress.

High demands and low control combine to produce stress in a variety of work situations for both men and women (Wang, Lesage, Schmitz, & Drapeau, 2008). Men were also affected by lack of job security, whereas creating a balance between work and family life was more stressful for women. High demands and low control also combine with other workplace conditions to increase on-the-job stress. A situation such as working in a noisy environment may not be sufficient to produce stress, but when combined with other workplace factors such as rotating shift work (Cottington & House, 1987), signs of stress appear in both blood pressure and stress hormone production. Stress can even be influenced by whether people find their work engaging or not. People who are engaged and committed to their work environment have lower cortisol production during the workweek compared with those with little engagement in their work (Harter & Stone, 2012). Brief vacations from work may help relieve work-related stress, but this relief does not last as long as people may hope (see Would You Believe …? box).

Stress from trying to balance the roles of worker and family member affects men as well as women. Half of all workers are married to someone who is also employed, creating multiple roles for both women and men (Moen & Yu, 2000). Problems may arise from work stress spilling over into the family or from family conflicts intruding into the workplace (Ilies et al., 2007; Schieman, Milkie, & Glavin, 2009). The differences in men's and women's roles and expectations within the family mean that family and work conflicts influence women and men in different ways. Women often encounter stress because of the increased burden of doing the work associated with their multiple roles as employee, wife, and mother, but overall, these multiple roles offer health benefits (Barnett & Hyde, 2001; Schnittker, 2007).

The positive or negative effects of work and family roles depend on the resources people have available. Partner and family support affects both men and women, but its absence more strongly affects women's health (Walen & Lachman, 2000). Women with children and no partner are especially burdened and, therefore, stressed (Livermore & Powers, 2006). Thus, filling multiple obligations is not necessarily stressful for women, but low control and poor support for multiple roles can produce stress for both men and women. Partners perceive a lack of support as stressful (Dehle, Larsen, & Landers, 2001). Despite the possibilities for conflict and stress, families are a major source of social support, a resource that is important for coping with stress. Celebrities mention the importance of family as an anchoring force in their lives that can decrease their stress (Loftus, 1995). Lindsay Lohan's lack of family support may have contributed to her problems.

Would You BELIEVE …? Vacations Relieve Work Stress … But Not For Long

Summer vacation. Spring break. Winter holiday. Every year, Americans spend millions of dollars on vacations from work and school. Vacations take people away from work and also provide opportunities for fun, travel, and relaxation. But do vacations serve as an effective long-term "intervention" for alleviating work-related stress?

A number of studies attempt to answer this question, and a review of this research yields some surprising results (de Bloom et al., 2009). People experience less stress during a vacation than they did prior to a vacation,

which we expect. Furthermore, in the days following a vacation, people report substantially less stress than they did prior to the vacation. In some cases, vacations may even offer relief from physical health symptoms.

However, this "vacation effect" tends to disappear quickly. Typically, any stress reduction effects of a vacation disappear within 3 to 4 weeks (de Bloom et al., 2009; Kuhnel & Sonnentag, 2011). One study showed the effect to fade within a single week (de Bloom et al., 2010).

This decrease may occur because a person's return to work leaves him or her needing to work extra hours or overtime to "catch up," which increases stress.

Certainly, these findings do not suggest that people should avoid vacations altogether. Instead, they suggest that vacations should not be the only way to cope with work or school-related stress. People can more effectively manage stress by using proven techniques, such as those described at the end of this chapter.

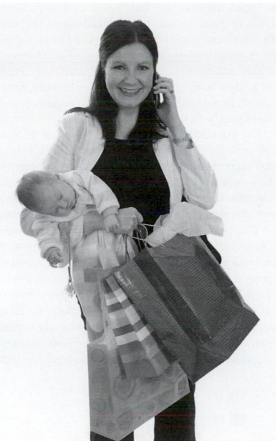

carebott/istock photo

Multiple roles can be a source of stress.

psychosocial environment. Stress from pollution, noise, crowding, and violence combine in urban settings with commuting hassles to create a situation described as *urban press*. Each of these sources of stress may also be considered individually. Noise and crowding are annoyances, but there is some evidence that even low levels of these stressors can prompt stress responses, which suggests that long-term exposure may have negative health consequences. The combination of community stressors such as crowding, noise, and threat of violence is common in poor neighborhoods, creating an environment of poverty.

Daily hassles in the psychosocial environment occur within the situations of the everyday social environment, including community, workplace, and family. Within the community, racism and sexism produce stress for the targets of these types of discrimination. Within the workplace, jobs with high demands and little control create stress, and poor support adds to the stress. Within the family, relationships such as spouse and parent present possibilities for conflict and stress as well as support. In addition, the conflict between family and work demands is a source of stress for many people.

IN SUMMARY

Stress has a number of sources, which can be classified according to the magnitude of the event: cataclysmic events, life events, and daily hassles. Cataclysmic events include natural disasters such as floods and earthquakes and intentional violence such as terrorist attacks.

Life events are events that produce changes in people's lives that require adaptation. Life events may be either negative or positive. Negative life events such as divorce, death of a family member, or crime victimization can produce severe and long-lasting stress.

Daily hassles are everyday events that create repetitive, chronic distress. Some hassles arise from the physical environment; others come from the

Coping With Stress

People constantly attempt to manage the problems and stresses of their lives, and most of these attempts fit into the category of coping. However, the term **coping** is usually applied to strategies that individuals use to manage the distressing problems and emotions in their lives. Coping is an active topic of research: Thousands of studies have explored the personal and situational characteristics that affect coping efforts, as well as the effectiveness of various coping strategies.

Personal Resources That Influence Coping

Lazarus and Folkman (1984) listed *health and energy* as one important coping resource. Healthy, robust individuals are better able to manage external and internal demands than are frail, sick, tired people. A second resource is a *positive belief*: The ability to cope with stress is enhanced when people believe they can successfully bring about desired consequences. This ability is related to a third resource: *problem-solving skills*. Knowledge of anatomy and physiology, for example, can be an important source of coping when receiving information about one's own health from a physician who is speaking in technical terms. *Material resources* are another important means of coping. Having the money to get one's car repaired decreases the stress of having a transmission problem. A fifth coping resource is *social skills*. Confidence in one's ability to get other people to cooperate can be an important source of stress management. Closely allied to this resource is *social support*, listed by Lazarus and Folkman as a sixth coping resource. During the 1980s, evidence emerged suggesting that people who receive support from friends, family members, and health care providers tend to live longer and healthier lives than people who lack support.

Social Support   **Social support** refers to a variety of material and emotional supports a person receives from others. The related concepts of **social contacts** and **social network** are sometimes used interchangeably; both refer to the number and types of people with whom one associates. The opposite of social contacts is **social isolation**, which refers to an absence of specific, meaningful interpersonal relations. People with a high level of social support ordinarily have a broad social network and many social contacts; socially isolated people have neither.

The Alameda County Study (Berkman & Syme, 1979) was the first to establish a strong link between social support and longevity. This study indicated that lack of social support was as strongly linked to mortality as cigarette smoking and a sedentary lifestyle. Figure 5.6 shows that women in all age groups had lower mortality rates than men (as indicated by the height of the bar in the graph). However, for both men and women, as the number of social ties decreased, the death rate increased. In general, participants with the fewest social ties were 2 to 4 times more likely to die than participants with the most social ties. The effects were not uniform for all age groups, but the benefits of social support apply to many age groups, including college students (Hale, Hannum, & Espelage, 2005). Social support related to better

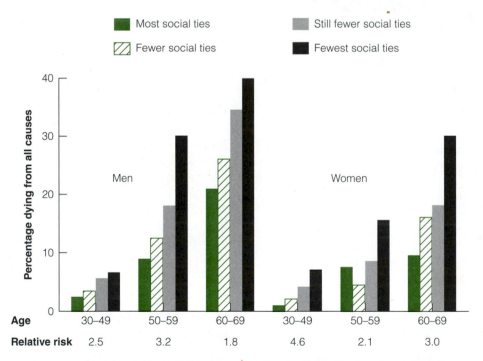

FIGURE 5.6   Social isolation and 9-year mortality in Alameda County, California, 1965–1974.

Source: From "Social Networks, Host Resistance, and Mortality: A Nine-Year Follow-up of Alameda County Residents," by L. F. Berkman & S. L. Syme, 1979, *American Journal of Epidemiology, 109*, p. 190. Copyright © 1979 by the Johns Hopkins University School of Hygiene and Public Health. Reprinted by permission of Oxford University Press.

perceptions of health for college women and fewer physical symptoms for college men.

Social support may influence stress in several ways. For example, stressed individuals may benefit from a support network with members who encourage them to adopt healthier habits, such as stopping smoking, beginning an exercise program, or keeping doctor's appointments. Social support may also help people gain confidence in their ability to handle stressful situations; thus, when they experience stress, they may appraise the stressor as less threatening than do people who have fewer coping resources (Wills, 1998). Another possibility is that social support may alter the physiological responses to stress (DeVries, Glasper, & Detillion, 2003; Kiecolt-Glaser & Newton, 2001). This view, referred to as the *stress-buffering hypothesis*, suggests that social support lessens or eliminates the harmful effects of stress and therefore protects against disease and death. A large epidemiological survey of over 30,000 Americans supports this view (Moak & Agrawal, 2010). For adults who experienced little life stress, social support was not strongly related to their feelings of distress or overall physical health. For those who experienced more life stress, higher levels of social support related to less depression and anxiety, and greater self-reported physical health. Similarly, a meta-analytic review of studies on discrimination and social support found that social support buffered the effects of discrimination on mental health but did not buffer the effects of discrimination on physical health measures such as blood pressure (Pascoe & Richman, 2009). Thus, when social support buffers the effects of stress on physical health, it probably does so by reducing psychological distress.

The positive effects of social support for health are well established (Martin & Brantley, 2004), but some individuals benefit more than others. For example, marriage (or at least happy marriage) would seem to provide excellent social support for both partners, but the benefits of marriage are not equal for women and men—being married benefits men's health more than women's (Kiecolt-Glaser & Newton, 2001). The reason for men's advantage is not clear, but one possibility is that women's role as caregivers puts them in the position of providing more care than they receive. Providing companionship is a positive factor for the caregiver as well as the recipient, but providing help comes at a cost to the helper (Strazdins & Broom, 2007). This situation may describe women's more than men's caregiving and thus the gender difference.

Social support is a significant factor in predicting both the development of disease and the course of chronic disease (Martin & Brantley, 2004). Surprisingly, the stress-buffering benefits of social support are not limited to support provided by humans (see Would You Believe …? box). Furthermore, the benefits of social support are entwined with another factor that influences coping: perceptions of personal control.

Personal Control   A second factor that affects people's ability to cope with stressful life events is a feeling of **personal control**—that is, confidence that they have some control over the events that shape their lives. Both classic and current research confirm the benefits of a sense of control. One classic approach is Julian Rotter's (1966) concept of locus of control, a continuum that captures the extent to which people believe they are in control of the important events in their lives. According to Rotter, people who believe that they control their own lives have an *internal locus of control*, whereas those who believe that luck, fate, or the acts of others determine their lives score high on *external locus of control*. The value of an internal locus of control appeared in a study of people with chronic illness (Livneh, Lott, & Antonak, 2004); those who had adapted well showed a higher sense of control than those who had adapted poorly. Unfortunately, a longitudinal analysis of college students in the United States (Twenge, Liqing, & Im, 2004) showed a movement toward external locus of control over the past 40 years, which may be a danger signal for health.

Ellen Langer and Judith Rodin (1976), who studied older nursing home residents, reported another classic example of the effects of personal control. This research project encouraged some residents to assume more responsibility for and control over their daily lives, whereas others had decisions made for them. The areas of control were fairly minor, such as rearranging furniture, choosing when and with whom to visit in the home, and deciding what leisure activities to pursue. In addition, residents were offered a small growing plant, which they were free to accept or reject and to care for as they wished. A comparison group of residents received information that emphasized the responsibility of the nursing staff, and each of them also received a live plant. Although equal in most other ways, the amount of control made a substantial difference in health. Residents in the responsibility-induced group were happier, more active, and more alert, with a higher level of general well-being. In just

Would You BELIEVE...? Pets May Be Better Support Providers Than People

Sometimes, the best social support may not come from a friend, but instead from "man's best friend." But can pets—such as dogs and cats—really help people cope with stress and improve health?

Nearly 40% of households in the United States own a dog or a cat (Humane Society of the United States, 2011). Pets provide companionship and affection, and in some cases, force their owners to be more physically active. It may be no surprise that among survivors of heart attacks, dog owners are over *8 times* more likely to be alive 1 year after their heart attack than those who do not own a dog (Friedmann & Thomas, 1995).

Can pets also dampen people's physiological responses to stress? In one study, researchers asked adults to perform a series of difficult and painful laboratory stress tasks—including mental arithmetic—while measuring their cardiovascular stress responses (Allen, Blascovich, & Mendes, 2002). Some participants did the tasks alone; some did the tasks in front of a close friend or spouse; others did the tasks in front of a pet dog or cat.

The results are striking. The presence of a pet led to the lowest stress response of all. Surprisingly, the presence of a spouse or friend led to the greatest stress response! Pets, it seems, provide comfort and support, without the possibility of criticism or evaluation. Friends and spouses provide support, too, but they are also more likely to notice someone's poor math skills. In this situation, the support of a trusted pet provides all the benefits of social support without any apparent costs.

Pet support may be especially helpful for people who are sensitive to criticism. For example, a recent study of children with insecure attachment styles shows that those who performed a stressful lab task in the presence of a dog produced significantly lower salivary cortisol than children who completed the task in front of a friendly human (Beetz et al., 2011).

Thus, pets are an excellent source of unconditional social support. Humorist Dave Barry might have said it best: "You can say any foolish thing to a dog, and the dog will give you a look that says, 'My God, you're right! I never would've thought of that!'"

3 weeks, most of the comparison group (71%) had become more debilitated, whereas nearly all the responsibility-induced group (93%) showed some overall mental and physical improvement. An 18-month follow-up of these same residents (Rodin & Langer, 1977) showed that residents in the original responsibility-induced group retained their advantage, and their mortality rate was lower than that of the comparison group.

How do perceptions of control influence health? While there may be many ways in which control buffers stress, one route may be through reductions in potentially harmful physiological responses. A meta-analysis of over 200 studies examined the characteristics of laboratory stress tasks that led to the greatest production of the stress hormone cortisol (Dickerson & Kemeny, 2004). Stress tasks that offered participants very little control—such as completing impossible tasks, performing under extreme time pressures, or exposure to uncontrollable loud noises—led to the largest increases in cortisol production and the longest times to recovery. These results suggest that people who frequently face situations that offer little control may be most likely to suffer the long-term health consequences of prolonged HPA activation.

These studies suggest that lack of control may impair health, and even a minimal amount of control can be beneficial to health. However, the benefits of control may be bound to Western cultures that emphasize individual autonomy and effort. In a comparison of stress and coping among people from Japan and Great Britain (O'Connor & Shimizu, 2002), the Japanese participants reported a lower sense of personal control, but only the British reported that loss of control produced stress. Thus, the benefits of personal control may be restricted to people in Western societies. However, the universal occurrence of stress means that strategies for coping with stress occur in all societies.

Personal Coping Strategies

Psychologists have categorized coping strategies in many ways, but Folkman and Lazarus's (1980) conceptualization of coping strategies as emotion focused or problem focused is the most influential. **Problem-focused coping** is aimed at changing the source of the stress, whereas **emotion-focused coping** is oriented toward managing the emotions that accompany the perception of stress. Both approaches can be effective in making the stressed individual feel better, but the two approaches may not be equally effective in managing the stressful situation.

Several different strategies fall within the emotion-focused and problem-focused categories. For example, taking action to try to get rid of the problem is a problem-focused strategy, but so is making a plan of the steps to take or asking someone to help you in solving the problem. Getting upset and venting emotions is clearly emotion focused, but seeking the company of friends or family for comfort and reassurance and refusing to accept the situation are also strategies oriented toward managing the negative emotions associated with stress.

If an upcoming exam is a source of stress, making (and following) a schedule for studying is a problem-focused strategy. Calling up a friend and complaining about the test or going out to a movie might help manage the distress, but these strategies are almost certainly not effective for dealing with the upcoming test. The problem-focused strategy sounds like a better choice in this case, but emotion-focused coping can be effective in some situations (Folkman & Moskowitz, 2004). When stress is unavoidable, finding a way to feel better may be the best option. For example, a person underdoing an unpleasant dental procedure probably has few options for problem-focused coping, so distancing oneself from unpleasant feelings may be the best way to cope (although avoiding having a necessary procedure would *not* be a wise coping strategy).

A meta-analysis of the effects of coping strategies on psychological and physical health (Penley, Tomaka, & Wiebe, 2002) revealed benefits for some coping strategies but risks for some others. The type of stressor and whether the impact was on psychological or physical health explained the relationships between coping strategies and health outcomes. In general, problem-focused coping contributed to good health, whereas emotion-focused coping strategies contributed to poorer health. For example, people who used emotion-focused and avoidance-oriented coping, such as eating more, drinking, sleeping, or using drugs, reported poorer health. Several recent meta-analyses have confirmed this general pattern of findings—problem-focused coping is better than emotion-focused coping in dealing with chronic stress. Meta-analyses support this advantage in studies focusing on coping with discrimination (Pascoe & Richman, 2009), HIV infection (Moskowitz, Hult, Bussolari, & Acree, 2009), and diabetes (Duangdao & Roesch, 2008).

Problem-focused strategies typically show advantages over emotion-focused approaches because problem-focused coping has the potential to change the situation. Indeed, people are more likely to use problem-focused coping when they appraise a situation as controllable. Among people coping with cancer, those who appraise their situation as a challenge are more likely to use problem-focused coping; those who appraise their situation as harm or loss are more likely to use avoidance coping (Franks & Roesch, 2006). Optimistic people—defined as those who have generally positive expectations for the future—are more likely to employ problem-focused strategies, less likely to use avoidance strategies, and also more likely to adjust their coping strategies to meet the specific demands of the situation (Nes & Segerstrom, 2006).

Additional categories of coping strategies exist (Folkman & Moskowitz, 2004). These include *social coping*, such as seeking support from others, and *meaning-focused coping*, in which the person concentrates on deriving meaning from the stressful experience. For example, people who experience a trauma such as loss of a loved one or a diagnosis of a serious disease often attempt to understand the personal (and often spiritual) meaning within the situation. People who take this approach often succeed (Folkman & Moskowitz, 2000) and in doing so often experience better psychological adjustment (Helgeson, Reynolds, & Tomich, 2006; Updegraff, Silver & Holman, 2008).

Culture exerts a powerful influence on coping, and gender also shows some effects. One might imagine that people who live in cultures that emphasize social harmony would be more likely to use social coping strategies, but such is not the case (Kim, Sherman, & Taylor, 2008). Indeed, Asian Americans are less likely than European Americans to seek social support when coping with stress, largely because of the motivation to maintain harmony with others (Wang, Shih, Hu, Louie, & Lau, 2010). However, another study (Lincoln, Chatters, & Taylor, 2003) found that African Americans were more likely than European Americans to seek social support from their families. Some studies find cross-cultural similarities in coping strategies, and those studies tend to study people in similar situations.

For example, a study of adolescents in seven European nations (Gelhaar et al., 2007) found similarities among coping strategies for adolescents in all of the nations, especially in job-related situations.

Females tend to use social coping strategies more than men (Tamres, Janicki, & Helgeson, 2002). Aside from this difference, research on gender differences in coping tends to find small differences between women's and men's coping strategies when studying individuals in similar situations (Adams, Aranda, Kemp, & Takagi, 2002; Ronan, Dreer, Dollard, & Ronan, 2004; Sigmon, Stanton, & Snyder, 1995) but larger gender differences when studies fail to control for situation (Matud, 2004). Because gender roles vary among cultures, gender and culture may interact to create different situational demands for coping by men and women in various cultures.

IN SUMMARY

Personal resources and a variety of coping strategies allow people to cope with stress in order to avoid or minimize distress. Social support, defined as the emotional quality of one's social contacts, is inversely related to disease and death. In general, people with high levels of social support experience health advantages and lower mortality. People with adequate social support probably receive more encouragement and advice regarding good health practices and may react less strongly to stress, which may buffer them against the harmful effects of stress more than people who are socially isolated.

Adequate feelings of personal control also seem to enable people to cope better with stress and illness. People who believe that their lives are controlled by fate or outside forces have greater difficulty changing health-related behaviors than do those who believe that the locus of control resides with themselves. The classic studies of nursing home residents demonstrated that when people are allowed to assume even small amounts of personal control and responsibility, they seem to live longer and healthier lives.

Coping strategies are classified in many ways, but the distinction between problem-focused coping, which is oriented toward solving the problem, and emotion-focused coping, which is oriented toward managing distress associated with stress, is useful. In addition, meaning-focused coping helps people find underlying meaning in negative experiences. In general, problem-focused coping is more effective than other types, but all types of coping strategies may be effective in some situations. The key to successful coping is flexibility, leading to the use of an appropriate strategy for the situation.

Behavioral Interventions for Managing Stress

In addition to studying stress, psychologists develop techniques that teach people how to manage stress. Some authorities consider these techniques to be part of mind–body medicine and thus part of alternative medicine (Barnes, Bloom, & Nahin, 2008), which is explored in Chapter 8. Other authorities consider that approaches such as relaxation training, biofeedback, and cognitive behavioral therapy have sufficient effectiveness to be part of conventional medicine (Bassman & Uellendahl, 2003).

Relaxation Training

Relaxation training is perhaps the simplest and easiest to use of all psychological interventions, and relaxation may be the key ingredient in other types of therapeutic interventions for managing stress.

What Is Relaxation Training?　During the 1930s, Edmond Jacobson (1938) discussed a type of relaxation he called *progressive muscle relaxation*. With this procedure, patients first receive the explanation that their present tension is mostly a physical state resulting from tense muscles. While reclining in a comfortable chair, often with eyes closed and with no distracting lights or sounds, patients first breathe deeply and exhale slowly. After this, the series of deep muscle relaxation exercises begins, a process described in the Becoming Healthier box. Once patients learn the relaxation technique, they may practice independently or with prerecorded audiotapes at home. Length of relaxation training programs varies, but 6 to 8 weeks and about 10 sessions with an instructor are usually sufficient to allow patients to easily and independently enter a state of deep relaxation (Blanchard & Andrasik, 1985).

Autogenics training is another approach to relaxation. Pioneered by Johannes Schultz during the 1920s

Becoming Healthier

Progressive muscle relaxation is a technique that you may be able to use to cope with stress and pain. Although some people may need the help of a trained therapist to master this approach, others are able to train themselves. To learn progressive muscle relaxation, recline in a comfortable chair in a room with no distractions. You may wish to remove your shoes and either dim the lights or close your eyes to enhance relaxation. Next, breathe deeply and exhale slowly. Repeat this deep breathing exercise several times until you begin to feel your body becoming more and more relaxed.

The next step is to select a muscle group (for example, your left hand) and deliberately tense that group of muscles. If you begin with your hand, make a fist and squeeze the fingers into your hand as hard as you can. Hold that tension for about 10 seconds and then slowly release the tension, concentrating on the relaxing, soothing sensations in your hand as the tension gradually drains away. Once the left hand is relaxed, shift to the right hand and repeat the procedure, while keeping your left hand as relaxed as possible. After both hands are relaxed, go through the same tensing and relaxing

sequence progressively with other muscle groups, including the arms, shoulders, neck, mouth, tongue, forehead, eyes, toes, feet, calves, thighs, back, and stomach. Then repeat the deep breathing exercises until you achieve a complete feeling of relaxation. Focus on the enjoyable sensation of relaxation, restricting your attention to the pleasant internal events and away from irritating external sources of pain or stress. You will probably need to practice this procedure several times to learn to quickly place your body into a state of deep relaxation.

and 1930s in Germany, the technique was refined by Wolfgang Luthe (Naylor & Marshall, 2007). Autogenics training consists of a series of exercises designed to reduce muscle tension, change the way people think, and change the content of people's thoughts. The process begins with a mental check of the body and proceeds with suggestions for relaxation and warmth throughout the body. Advocates contend that practicing autogenics for 10 minutes at least twice a day reduces stress and thus improves health.

How Effective Is Relaxation Training?
Like other psychological interventions, relaxation is effective only if it proves more powerful than a control situation, or placebo. Relaxation techniques generally meet this criterion (Jacobs, 2001). Indeed, relaxation may be an essential part of other interventions such as biofeedback and hypnotic therapies (see Chapter 8).

Relaxation training was a component in a successful stress management program for college students (Iglesias et al., 2005), and children were able to learn and to benefit from relaxation training (Lohaus & Klein-Hessling, 2003). Both progressive muscle relaxation and autogenic training are components in effective treatment programs for such stress-related disorders as depression, anxiety, hypertension, and insomnia (Stetter & Kupper, 2002; McCallie, Blum, & Hood, 2006).

Relaxation techniques also help reduce hormonal stress responses following breast cancer surgery (Phillips et al., 2011) and promote faster healing following gallbladder surgery (Broadbent et al., 2012). Table 5.1 summarizes the effectiveness of relaxation techniques for stress-related problems.

Cognitive Behavioral Therapy

Health psychologists use the same types of interventions for managing stress that they use for other behavior problems, including *cognitive behavioral therapy*. This approach is a combination of *behavior modification*, which arose from the laboratory research on operant conditioning, and *cognitive therapy*, which can be traced to research on mental processes. Cognitive behavioral therapy is more effective than any other approach for stress management.

What Is Cognitive Behavioral Therapy?
Cognitive behavioral therapy (CBT) is a type of therapy that aims to develop beliefs, attitudes, thoughts, and skills to make positive changes in behavior. Like cognitive therapy, CBT assumes that thoughts and feelings are the basis of behavior, so CBT begins with changing attitudes. Like behavior modification, CBT focuses on modifying environmental contingencies and building skills to change observable behavior.

TABLE 5.1   Effectiveness of Relaxation Techniques

Problem	Findings	Studies
1. Stress management for college students	Relaxation is a component in successful stress management.	Iglesias et al., 2005
2. Depression, anxiety, hypertension, and insomnia	Autogenics and progressive muscle relaxation are effective components in programs to manage these disorders.	McCallie et al., 2006; Stetter & Kupper, 2002
3. Laboratory stress	Progressive muscle relaxation produces changes in heart rate, skin conductance, and skin temperature in children.	Lohaus & Klein-Hessling, 2003
4. Stress following surgery for breast cancer	Relaxation training is an important component of a stress management program that lowered women's cortisol levels over a 12-month period.	Phillips et al., 2011
5. Recovery following gallbladder surgery	Relaxation training leads to lower perceived stress and faster wound healing.	Broadbent et al., 2012

An example of CBT for stress management is the stress inoculation program developed by Donald Meichenbaum and Roy Cameron (1983; Meichenbaum, 2007). The procedure works in a manner analogous to vaccination. By introducing a weakened dose of a pathogen (in this case, the pathogen is stress), the therapist attempts to build some immunity against high levels of stress. Stress inoculation includes three stages: conceptualization, skills acquisition and rehearsal, and follow-through or application. The *conceptualization* stage is a cognitive intervention in which the therapist works with clients to identify and clarify their problems. During this overtly educational stage, patients learn about stress inoculation and how this technique can reduce their stress. The *skills acquisition and rehearsal* stage involves both educational and behavioral components to enhance patients' repertoire of coping skills. At this time, patients learn and practice new ways of coping with stress. One of the goals of this stage is to improve self-instruction by changing cognitions, a process that includes monitoring one's internal monologue—that is, self-talk. During the *application and follow-through* stage, patients put into practice the cognitive changes they have achieved in the two previous stages.

Another CBT approach to stress is cognitive behavioral stress management (CBSM; Antoni, Ironson, & Schneiderman, 2007), a 10-week group intervention that shares many features with stress inoculation training. CBSM also works toward changing cognitions concerning stress, enlarging clients' repertoire of coping skills, and guiding clients to apply these skills in effective ways. Other researchers use variations of CBT to investigate the effectiveness of this approach to stress management.

How Effective Is Cognitive Behavioral Therapy?

Research on the efficacy of CBT indicates that it is effective for both prevention and management of stress and stress-related disorders. Furthermore, CBT is effective with a wide variety of clients.

An early meta-analysis (Saunders, Driskell, Johnston, & Sales, 1996) of nearly 40 studies found that stress inoculation training decreased anxiety and raised performance under stress. Stress inoculation training is effective for a range of stressors. For example, one program (Sheehy & Horan, 2004) tested the benefits of stress inoculation training for 1st-year law students to determine if the training helped these students alleviate some of their anxiety and stress. The program succeeded in meeting those goals and also raised grades.

Stress inoculation can also be effective in helping victims of trauma manage their severe distress (Cahill & Foa, 2007). For example, stress inoculation is helpful for crime victims who experience posttraumatic stress disorder (Hembree & Foa, 2003). Researchers adapted stress inoculation therapy for use on the Internet (Litz, Williams, Wang, Bryant, & Engel, 2004), making it available to a larger number of people.

Other varieties of cognitive behavioral therapy are effective for stress management, including cognitive behavioral stress management. This intervention may even help counteract the negative effects of stress by moderating the increased cortisol production that accompanies the stress response (Antoni et al., 2009;

Gaab, Sonderegger, Scherrer, & Ehlert, 2007), an accomplishment that few techniques have achieved (see Chapter 6). One recent study showed that a prenatal cognitive behavior stress management intervention reduced cortisol production of both mothers *and* their infants (Urizar & Muñoz, 2011). However, these effects may not include dramatic improvement in immune functioning. A meta-analysis of cognitive behavioral interventions for people who are HIV positive (Crepaz et al., 2008) revealed significant positive effects for reductions in stress, depression, anxiety, and anger, but immune functioning was less improved. Like stress inoculation programs, cognitive behavioral interventions are also adapted for use on the internet (Benight, Ruzek, & Waldrep, 2008).

Cognitive behavioral stress management also helps those with substance abuse problems manage stress-induced cravings, which could give a boost to substance abuse treatment (Back, Gentilin, & Brady, 2007). Cognitive behavioral therapy is also an effective intervention for posttraumatic stress disorder (Bisson & Andrew, 2007), chronic back pain (Hoffman, Papas, Chatkoff, & Kerns, 2007), and chronic fatigue syndrome (Lopez et al., 2011). Cognitive behavioral techniques are used in workplace stress management, and this approach has demonstrated consistently larger effects than other programs (Richardson & Rothstein, 2008). Furthermore, cognitive behavioral stress techniques can help students improve their performance; a cognitive behavioral stress intervention improved students' motivations and scores on standardized exams (Keogh, Bond, & Flaxman, 2006).

In summary, many studies show that cognitive behavioral therapy interventions are effective for stress management for people with a variety of stress-related problems. Table 5.2 summarizes the effectiveness of cognitive behavioral therapy for stress-related problems.

Emotional Disclosure

Research by James Pennebaker and colleagues (Pennebaker, Barger, & Tiebout, 1989) shows that emotional self-disclosure improves both psychological and physical health. Subsequent research has extended the positive effects of emotional disclosure to a variety of people and settings.

TABLE 5.2   Effectiveness of Cognitive Behavioral Therapy

Problem	Findings	Studies
1. Performance anxiety	Inoculation training reduces performance anxiety and boosts performance under stress.	Saunders et al., 1996
2. Stress of law school	Stress inoculation training decreases stress and increases grades.	Sheehy & Horan, 2004
3. Posttraumatic stress disorder	Inoculation procedures lessen negative effects of posttraumatic stress disorder.	Cahill & Foa, 2007; Hembree & Foa, 2003; Litz et al., 2004
4. Hormonal stress responses	Cognitive behavioral stress management moderates cortisol production during stress response.	Antoni et al., 2009; Gaab et al., 2007; Urizar & Muñoz, 2011
5. Stress, anxiety, depression in people with HIV	Cognitive behavioral therapy improves these symptoms of HIV.	Crepaz et al., 2008
6. Stress-related cravings	Cognitive behavioral stress management decreased cravings.	Back et al., 2007
7. Psychological and physical health symptoms	Cognitive behavioral therapy is an effective treatment.	Bisson & Andrew, 2007; Hoffman et al., 2007; Lopez et al., 2011
8. Workplace stress	Cognitive behavioral therapy is effective.	Richardson & Rothstein, 2008
9. School-related stress	Cognitive behavioral therapy boosts motivation and test performance.	Keogh et al., 2006

What Is Emotional Disclosure? **Emotional disclosure** is a therapeutic technique in which people express their strong emotions by talking or writing about negative events that precipitated those emotions. For centuries, confession of sinful deeds has been part of personal healing in many religious rituals. During the late 19th century, Joseph Breuer and Sigmund Freud (1895/1955) recognized the value of the "talking cure," and **catharsis**—the verbal expression of emotions—became an important part of psychotherapy. Pennebaker took the notion of catharsis beyond Breuer and Freud, by demonstrating the health benefits of talking or writing about traumatic life events.

The general pattern of Pennebaker's research is to ask people to write or talk about traumatic events for 15 to 20 minutes, three or four times a week. Emotional disclosure should be distinguished from emotional expression, which refers to emotional outbursts or emotional venting, such as crying, laughing, yelling, or throwing objects. Emotional disclosure, in contrast, involves the transfer of emotions into language and thus requires a measure of self-reflection. Emotional outbursts are often unhealthy and may add more stress to an already unpleasant situation.

In one of their early studies on emotional disclosure, Pennebaker and colleagues (Pennebaker et al., 1989) asked survivors of the Holocaust to talk for 1 to 2 hours about their war experiences. Those survivors who disclosed the most personally traumatic experiences had better subsequent health than survivors who expressed less painful experiences. Since then, Pennebaker and his colleagues have investigated other forms of emotional disclosure, such as asking people to talk into a tape recorder, write their thoughts privately, or speak to a therapist about highly stressful events. With each of these techniques, the key ingredient is language—emotions must be expressed through language.

The physical and psychological changes in people who use emotional disclosure are typically compared with those of a control group, who are asked to write or talk about superficial events. This relatively simple procedure is responsible for such physiological changes as fewer physician visits, improved immune functioning, and lower rates of asthma, arthritis, cancer, and heart disease. In addition, disclosure has produced psychological and behavioral changes, such as fewer depressive symptoms before taking graduate school entrance exams and better performance on those exams (Frattaroli, Thomas & Lyubomirsky, 2011).

How Effective Is Emotional Disclosure? A substantial number of studies by Pennebaker's team and other researchers demonstrate the effectiveness of disclosure in reducing a variety of illnesses. A review of 146 studies of emotional disclosure found a positive effect on most psychological outcomes and some physical health outcomes (Frattaroli, 2006). This review also identified a number of factors that make emotional disclosure more effective. One of these factors is the amount of stress in a person's life: People who experience more stress benefit from emotional disclosure more than those who experience less stress. Other factors that make emotional disclosure more effective include writing in private, writing for more than 15 minutes, and writing about a stressful event not previously shared with other people. Importantly, the effectiveness of emotional disclosure does not differ based on gender, age, or ethnicity (Frattaroli, 2006).

A notable example of the effect of emotional disclosure on physical health includes an early study that showed that students who disclosed feelings about entering college had fewer illnesses than those who wrote about superficial topics (Pennebaker, Colder, & Sharp, 1990). Despite its emotional basis, a meta-analysis of studies on emotional disclosure (Frisina, Borod, & Lepore, 2004) concluded that this approach is more effective in helping people with physical than psychological problems. Emotional disclosure can reduce symptoms in patients with asthma and arthritis (Smyth, Stone, Hurewitz, & Kaell, 1999) and buffer some of the problems associated with breast cancer among women who perceive low levels of social support (Low, Stanton, Bower, & Gyllenhammer, 2010).

Must the emotional disclosure focus on trauma? Some evidence indicates that when people focus on finding some positive aspect of a traumatic experience, they may accrue even more benefits than when they focus on the negative aspects of the experience. In one study, when participants were led to a less negative interpretation of a traumatic event, they experienced greater benefits than did those whose negative interpretations were validated (Lepore, Fernandez-Berrocal, Ragan, & Ramos, 2004). Other research suggests that when writing about a stressful situation, developing a plan for dealing with the situation (Lestideau & Lavallee, 2007) or focusing on positive aspects of the stressor (Lu & Stanton, 2010) boosts the benefits of expressive writing. These findings extend Pennebaker's research on disclosure by suggesting that people who concentrate on the positive aspects of a traumatic experience or develop a plan to deal with the stressful situation can

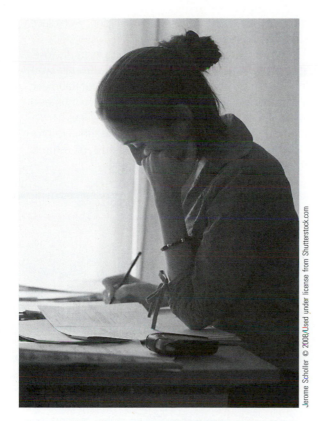

Writing about traumatic or highly stressful events produces physical as well as emotional benefits.

receive health benefits equal or superior to those who simply write about a traumatic life event.

Pennebaker's research adds an effective and easily accessible tool to the arsenal of strategies for managing stress. Indeed, benefits can occur through a program of writing by e-mail (Sheese, Brown, & Graziano, 2004) or through an Internet-based intervention (Possemato, Ouimette, & Geller, 2010). See Table 5.3 for a summary of the effectiveness of self-disclosure through writing or talking.

IN SUMMARY

Health psychologists help people cope with stress by using relaxation training, cognitive behavioral therapy, and emotional disclosure. Relaxation techniques include progressive muscle relaxation and autogenics training. Relaxation approaches have some success in helping patients manage stress and anxiety and are generally more effective than a placebo.

Cognitive behavioral therapy draws upon operant conditioning and behavior modification as well as cognitive therapy, which strives to change behavior through changing attitudes and beliefs. Cognitive behavioral therapists attempt to get patients to think differently about their stress

TABLE 5.3   Effectiveness of Emotional Disclosure

Problem	Findings	Studies
1. General health problems	Holocaust survivors who talked most about their experience had fewer health problems 14 months later.	Pennebaker et al., 1989
2. Performance on graduate entrance exams (GRE, LSAT, MCAT)	Written disclosure about upcoming exam improved performance.	Frattaroli et al., 2011
3. Emotional and physical symptoms	Disclosure associated with better psychological and physical health outcomes.	Frattaroli, 2006; Frisina et al., 2004
4. Anxiety about entering college	Students who disclosed had fewer illnesses.	Pennebaker et al., 1990
5. Asthma, rheumatoid arthritis, and living with cancer	Keeping a journal of stressful events reduces symptoms and improves functioning.	Smyth et al., 1999
6. Emotional and physical symptoms of breast cancer	Disclosure associated with less distress among women with low social support.	Low et al., 2010
7. Emotional and physical symptoms	Focusing on positive aspects of situation produced greater benefits.	Lepore et al., 2004; Lu & Stanton, 2010
8. Emotional and physical symptoms	Focusing on developing a plan produced greater benefits than focusing only on emotions.	Lestideau & Lavallee, 2007
9. Problems in mental and physical health	E-mail and Internet intervention about traumatic events showed benefits.	Possemato et al., 2010; Sheese et al., 2004

Jerome Scholler © 2008/Used under license from Shutterstock.com experiences and teach strategies that lead to more effective self-management.

Stress inoculation and cognitive behavioral stress management are types of cognitive behavioral therapy interventions. Stress inoculation introduces low levels of stress and then teaches skills for coping and application of those skills. Stress inoculation and cognitive behavioral stress management are successful interventions for preventing stress and in treating a wide variety of stress problems, including anxiety and depression in people with HIV, stress cravings in people with substance use

disorders, posttraumatic stress disorder, workplace stress, and school-related stress.

Emotional disclosure calls for patients to disclose strong negative emotions, most often through writing. People using this technique write about traumatic life events for 15 to 20 minutes, three or four times a week. Emotional disclosure generally enhances health, relieves anxiety, and reduces visits to health care providers, and may reduce the symptoms of asthma, rheumatoid arthritis, and cancer.

Answers

This chapter has addressed six basic questions:

1. What is the physiology of stress?

The nervous system plays a central role in the physiology of stress. When a person perceives stress, the sympathetic division of the autonomic nervous system stimulates the adrenal medulla, producing catecholamines and arousing the person from a resting state. The perception of stress also prompts a second route of response through the pituitary gland, which releases adrenocorticotropic hormone. This hormone, in turn, affects the adrenal cortex, which produces glucocorticoids. These hormones prepare the body to resist stress.

2. What theories explain stress?

Hans Selye and Richard Lazarus both proposed theories of stress. During his career, Selye defined stress first as a stimulus and then as a response. Whenever the body encounters a disruptive stimulus, it mobilizes itself in a generalized attempt to adapt to that stimulus. Selye called this mobilization the general adaptation syndrome. The GAS has three stages—alarm, resistance, and exhaustion—and the potential for trauma or illness exists at all three stages. Lazarus insisted that a person's perception of a situation is the most significant component of stress. To Lazarus, stress depends on one's appraisal of an event rather than on the event itself. Whether or not stress produces illness is closely tied to one's vulnerability as well as to one's perceived ability to cope with the situation.

3. How has stress been measured?

Several methods exist for assessing stress, including physiological and biochemical measures and self-reports of stressful events. Most life events scales are patterned after Holmes and Rahe's Social Readjustment Rating Scale. Some of these instruments include only undesirable events, but the SRRS and other self-report inventories are based on the premise that any major change is stressful. Lazarus and his associates pioneered scales that measure daily hassles and uplifts. These scales, which generally have better validity than the SRRS, emphasize the severity of the event as perceived by the person.

Physiological and biochemical measures have the advantage of good reliability, whereas self-report inventories pose more problems in demonstrating reliability and validity. Although most self-report inventories have acceptable reliability, their ability to predict illness remains to be established. For these stress inventories to predict illness, two conditions must be met: First, they must be valid measures of stress; second, stress must be related to illness. Chapter 6 takes up the question of whether stress causes illness.

4. What sources produce stress?

Sources of stress can be categorized as cataclysmic events, life events, and daily hassles. Cataclysmic events include sudden, unexpected events that produce major demands for adaptation. Such events include natural disasters such as earthquakes and hurricanes and intentional events such as terrorist attacks. Posttraumatic stress disorder is a possibility in the aftermath of such events.

Life events such as divorce, criminal victimization, or death of a family member also produce major life changes and require adaptation, but life events are usually not as sudden and dramatic as cataclysmic events. Daily hassles are even smaller and more common, but produce distress. Such daily events may arise from the community, as with noise, crowding, and pollution; from workplace conditions, such as work with high demands and little control; or from conflicts in relationships.

5. What factors influence coping, and what strategies are effective?

Factors that influence coping include social support, personal control, and personal hardiness. Social support, defined as the emotional quality of one's social contacts, is important to a person's ability to cope and to one's health. People with social support receive more encouragement and advice to seek medical care, and social support may provide a buffer against the physical effects of stress. Second, people's beliefs that they have control over the events of their life seem to have a positive impact on health. Even a sense of control over small matters may improve health and prolong life. The factor of personal hardiness includes components of commitment, control, and interpreting events as challenges rather than as stressors.

People use a variety of strategies to cope with stress, all of which may be successful. Problem-focused coping is often a better choice than emotion-focused efforts because problem-focused coping can change the source of the problem, eliminating the stress-producing situation. Emotion-focused coping is oriented toward managing the distress that accompanies stress. Research indicates that most people use a variety of coping strategies, often in combination, and this flexibility is important for effective coping.

6. What behavioral techniques are effective for stress management?

Three types of interventions are available to health psychologists in helping people cope with stress. First, relaxation training can help people cope with a variety of stress problems. Second, cognitive behavioral therapy—including stress inoculation and cognitive behavioral stress management—is effective in reducing both stress and stress-related disorders such as posttraumatic stress disorder. Third, emotional disclosure—including writing about traumatic events—can help people recover from traumatic experiences and experience better psychological and physical health.

Suggested Readings

Kemeny, M. E. (2003). The psychobiology of stress. *Current Directions in Psychological Science*, *12*, 124–129. This concise review furnishes a summary of the physiology of stress, how stress can "get under the skin" to influence disease, and some psychosocial factors that moderate this process.

Lazarus, R. S., & Folkman, S. (1984). *Stress, appraisal, and coping*. New York: Springer. In this classic book, Richard Lazarus and Susan Folkman present a comprehensive treatment of Lazarus's views of stress, cognitive appraisal, and coping. This book also discusses the relevant literature up to that time.

McEwen, B. S. (2005). Stressed or stressed out: What is the difference? *Journal of Psychiatry and Neuroscience*, *30*, 315–318. This brief, readable article summarizes the evolution of the concept of stress, including Selye's work and changes to that framework.

Monroe, S. M. (2008). Modern approaches to conceptualizing and measuring human life stress. *Annual Review of Clinical Psychology*, *4*, 33–52. This readable review describes many of the issues in defining and measuring stress in humans, as well as understanding pathways by which life stress may influence physical health.

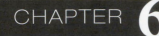
Understanding Stress, Immunity, and Disease

CHAPTER OUTLINE

- **Real-World Profile of Lindsay Lohan—Continued**
- *Physiology of the Immune System*
- *Psychoneuroimmunology*
- *Does Stress Cause Disease?*

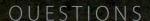

Real-World Profile of
LINDSAY LOHAN—Continued

In Chapter 5, we examined Lindsay Lohan's claim that her drug and alcohol problems were caused by stress. She said that she worked a great deal and failed to take time off for herself. She also talked about unresolved emotional issues with her father that contributed to her coping through drinking and taking drugs, which created problems with work and eventually landed her in rehab (Silverman, 2008). These negative feelings and negative interactions undoubtedly produce stress, and her strategies for coping created major problems in her life, but do they make Lindsay Lohan more vulnerable to illness?

This chapter reviews the evidence relating to stress as a possible cause of disease. In Chapter 5, you learned that stress can influence health-related behaviors, which can increase risk for disease or death. If stress, a psychological factor, can also influence physical disease *directly*, some mechanism must exist to allow this interaction. In this chapter, we will examine how stress can increase risk for health problems through biological processes. We begin with a discussion of the immune system, which protects the body against stress-related diseases and could provide the mechanism for stress to cause disease.

Physiology of the Immune System

Organs of the Immune System

The immune system is spread throughout the body in the form of the **lymphatic system**. The tissue of the lymphatic system is **lymph**; it consists of the tissue components of blood other than red cells and platelets. In the process of vascular circulation, fluid and *leukocytes* (white blood cells) leak from the capillaries, escaping the circulatory system. Body cells also secrete white blood cells. This tissue fluid is referred to as lymph when it enters the lymph vessels, which circulate lymph and eventually return it to the bloodstream.

Lymph circulates by entering the lymphatic system and then reentering the bloodstream rather than staying exclusively in the lymphatic system. The structure of the lymphatic system (see Figure 6.1) roughly parallels the circulatory system for blood. In its circulation, all lymph travels through at least one **lymph node**. The lymph nodes are round or oval capsules spaced throughout the lymphatic system that help clean lymph of cellular debris, bacteria, and even dust that has entered the body.

Lymphocytes are a type of white blood cell found in lymph. There are several types of lymphocytes, the most fully understood of which are T-lymphocytes, or **T-cells**; B-lymphocytes, or **B-cells**; and **natural killer (NK) cells**. Lymphocytes originate in the bone marrow, but they mature and differentiate in other structures of the immune system. In addition to lymphocytes, two other types of leukocytes are granulocytes and monocytes/macrophages. These leukocytes have roles in the nonspecific and specific immune system responses (discussed more fully later).

The **thymus**, which has endocrine functions, secretes a hormone called **thymosin**, which is involved in the maturation and differentiation of the T-cells. Interestingly, the thymus is largest during infancy and childhood and then atrophies during adulthood. Its function is not entirely understood, but the thymus is clearly important in the immune system because its removal impairs immune function. Its atrophy also

At any given moment, you are surrounded by microorganisms such as bacteria, viruses, and fungi. Some of these microorganisms are harmless, but others can endanger your health. The immune system consists of tissues, organs, and processes that protect the body from invasion by such foreign microorganisms (Schindler, Kerrigan, & Kelly, 2002). In addition, the immune system performs housekeeping functions by removing worn-out or damaged cells and patrolling for mutant cells. Once the immune system locates these invaders and renegades, it activates processes to eliminate them. Thus, a well-functioning immune system plays a crucial role in maintaining health.

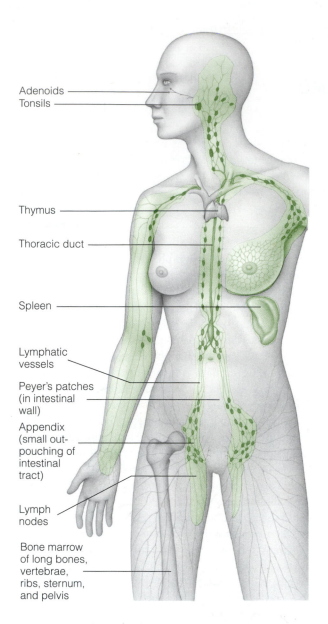

Adenoids

Tonsils

Thymus

Thoracic duct

Spleen

Lymphatic vessels

Peyer's patches (in intestinal wall)

Appendix (small out-pouching of intestinal tract)

Lymph nodes

Bone marrow of long bones, vertebrae, ribs, sternum, and pelvis

FIGURE 6.1 Lymphatic system.

Source: Introduction to microbiology (p. 407), by J. L. Ingraham & C. A. Ingraham. From INGRAHAM/INGRAHAM, Introduction to Microbiology, 1E. © 1995 Cengage Learning.

suggests that the immune system's production of T-cells is more efficient during childhood and that aging is related to lowered immune efficiency (Briones, 2007). The **tonsils** are masses of lymphatic tissue located in the throat. Their function seems to be similar to that of the lymph nodes: trapping and killing invading cells and particles. The **spleen**, an organ near the stomach in the abdominal cavity, is one site where

lymphocytes mature. In addition, it serves as a holding station for lymphocytes as well as a disposal site for worn-out blood cells.

Thus, the organs of the immune system produce, store, and circulate lymph throughout the rest of the body. The surveillance and protection that the immune system offers is not limited to the lymph nodes. Rather, it takes place in other tissues of the body that contain lymphocytes. To protect the entire body, immune function must occur in all parts of the body.

Function of the Immune System

The immune system's function is to defend against foreign substances that the body encounters. The immune system must be extraordinarily effective to prevent 100% of the invading bacteria, viruses, and fungi from damaging our bodies. Few other body functions must operate at 100% efficiency, but when this system performs at some lesser capacity, the person (or animal) becomes vulnerable.

Invading organisms can enter the body in many ways, and the immune system has methods to combat each mode of entry. In general, there are two ways the immune system fights invading foreign substances: general (nonspecific) and specific responses. Both may be involved in fighting an invader.

Nonspecific Immune System Responses To enter the body, foreign substances must first pass the skin and mucous membranes. Thus, these organs and tissues are the body's first line of defense against the outside world. Foreign substances that are able to pass these barriers face two general (nonspecific) mechanisms. One is **phagocytosis**, the attacking of foreign particles by cells of the immune system. Two types of leukocytes perform this function. **Granulocytes** contain granules filled with chemicals. When these cells come into contact with invaders, they release their chemicals, which attack the invaders. **Macrophages** perform a variety of immune functions, including scavenging for worn-out cells and debris, initiating specific immune responses, and secreting a variety of chemicals that break down the cell membranes of invaders. Thus, phagocytosis involves several mechanisms that can quickly result in the destruction of invading bacteria, viruses, and fungi. However, some invaders escape this nonspecific action.

A second type of nonspecific immune system response is **inflammation**, which works to restore tissues that have been damaged by invaders. When an injury occurs, blood vessels in the area of injury dilate, increasing blood flow to the tissues and causing the warmth and redness that accompany inflammation. The damaged cells release enzymes that help destroy invading microorganisms; these enzymes can also aid in their own digestion, should the cells die. Both granulocytes and macrophages migrate to the site of injury to battle the invaders. Finally, tissue repair begins. Figure 6.2 illustrates the process of inflammation.

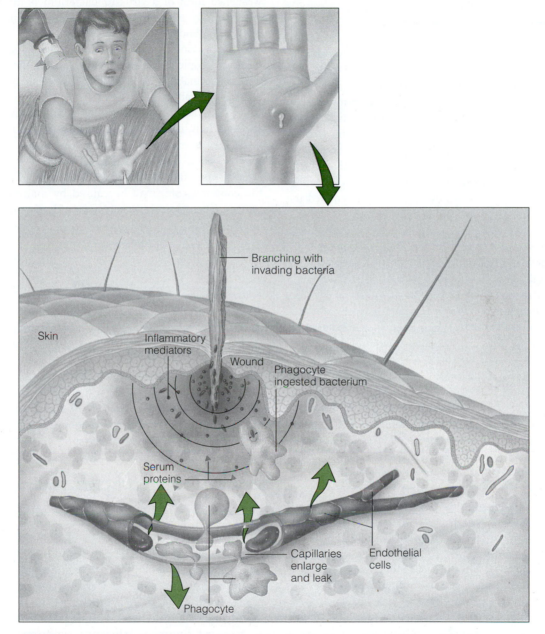

FIGURE 6.2   Acute inflammation is initiated by a stimulus such as injury or infection. Inflammatory mediators, produced at the site of the stimulus, cause blood vessels to dilate and increase their permeability; they also attract phagocytes to the site of inflammation and activate them.

Source: Introduction to microbiology (p. 386), by J. L. Ingraham & C. A. Ingraham. From INGRAHAM/INGRAHAM, Introduction to Microbiology, 1E. © 1995 Cengage Learning.

Specific Immune Systems Responses Specific immune responses are specific to one invader, such as a certain virus or bacteria. Two types of lymphocytes, T-cells and B-cells, carry out specific immune responses. When a lymphocyte encounters a foreign substance for the first time, both the general response and a specific response occur. Invading microorganisms are killed and eaten by macrophages, which present fragments of these invaders to T-cells that have moved to the area of inflammation. This contact sensitizes the T-cells, and they acquire specific receptors on their surfaces that enable them to recognize the invader. An army of *cytotoxic T-cells* forms through this process, and it soon mobilizes a direct attack on the invaders. This process is referred to as *cell-mediated immunity* because it occurs at the level of the body cells rather than in the bloodstream. Cell-mediated immunity is especially effective against fungi, viruses that have already entered the cells, parasites, and mutations of body cells.

The other variety of lymphocyte, the B-cell, mobilizes an indirect attack on invading microorganisms. With the help of one variety of T-cell (the *helper T-cell*), B-cells differentiate into **plasma cells** and secrete **antibodies**. Each antibody is manufactured in response to a specific invader. Foreign substances that provoke antibody manufacture are called **antigens** (for *anti*body *gen*erator). Antibodies circulate, find their antigens, bind to them, and mark them for later destruction. Figure 6.3 shows the differentiation of T-cells and B-cells.

The specific reactions of the immune system constitute the *primary immune response*. Figure 6.4 shows the development of the primary immune response and depicts how subsequent exposure activates the *secondary immune response*. During initial exposure to an invader, some of the sensitized T-cells and B-cells replicate and, rather than go into action, are held in reserve. These *memory lymphocytes* form the basis for a rapid immune response on second exposure to the same invader. Memory lymphocytes can persist for years but will not be activated unless the antigen invader reappears. If it does, then the memory lymphocytes initiate the same sort of direct and indirect attacks that occurred at the first exposure, but much more rapidly. This specifically tailored rapid response to foreign microorganisms that occurs with repeated exposure is what most people consider **immunity**.

This system of immune response through B-cell recognition of antigens and their manufacture of antibodies is called **humoral immunity** because it happens in the bloodstream. The process is especially effective in fighting viruses that have already entered the cells, parasites, and mutations of body cells.

Creating Immunity One widely used method to induce immunity is **vaccination**. In vaccination, a weakened form of a virus or bacterium is introduced into the body, stimulating the production of antibodies. These antibodies then confer immunity for an extended period. Smallpox, which once killed thousands of people each year, was eradicated through the use of vaccination. As a result, people are no longer vaccinated against this disease.

Other vaccines exist for a variety of diseases. They are especially useful in the prevention of viral infections. However, immunity must be created for each specific virus, and thousands of viruses exist. Even viral diseases that produce similar symptoms, such as the common cold, may be caused by many different viruses. Therefore, immunity for colds would require many vaccinations, and such a process has not yet proven practical.

Immune System Disorders

Immune deficiency, an inadequate immune response, may occur for several reasons. For example, it is a side effect of most chemotherapy drugs used to treat cancer. Immune deficiency also occurs naturally. Although the immune system is not fully functional at birth, infants are protected by antibodies they receive from their mothers through the placenta, and infants who breast-feed receive antibodies from their mothers' milk. These antibodies offer protection until the infant's own immune system develops during the first months of life.

In rare cases, the immune system fails to develop, leaving the child without immune protection. Physicians can try to boost immune function, but the well-publicized "children in plastic bubbles" still possess immune deficiency. Exposure to any virus or bacterium can be fatal to these children. They are sealed into sterile quarters to isolate them from the microorganisms that are part of the normal world.

A much more common type of immune deficiency is **acquired immune deficiency syndrome (AIDS)**. This disease is caused by a virus, the human immunodeficiency virus (HIV), which destroys the T-cells and macrophages in the immune system. People infected with HIV may progress to AIDS and become vulnerable to a wide range of bacterial, viral, and malignant

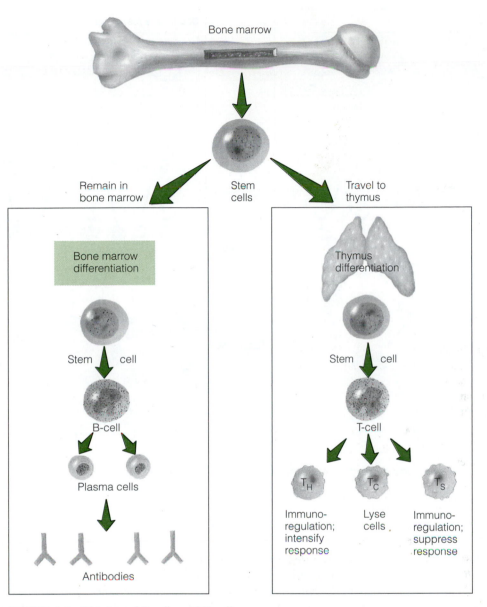

FIGURE 6.3 Origins of B-cells and T-cells.

Source: Introduction to microbiology (p. 406), by J. L. Ingraham & C. A. Ingraham. From INGRAHAM/INGRAHAM, Introduction to Microbiology, 1E. © 1995 Cengage Learning.

diseases. HIV is contagious, but not easily transmitted from person to person. The highest concentrations of the virus are found in blood and in semen. Blood transfusions from an infected person, injection with a contaminated needle, sexual intercourse, and transmission during the birth process are the most common routes of infection. Treatment consists of controlling the proliferation of the virus through antiviral drugs and

management of the diseases that develop as a result of immune deficiency. As of 2012, a combination of antiviral drugs is capable of slowing the progress of HIV infection, but no treatment is yet capable of eliminating HIV from an infected person.

Allergies are another immune system disorder. An allergic response is an abnormal reaction to a foreign substance that normally elicits little or no immune

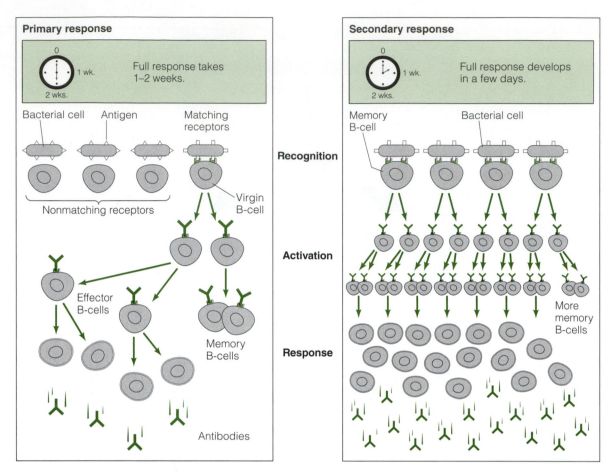

FIGURE 6.4   Primary and secondary immune pathways.

Source: Introduction to microbiology (p. 414), by J. L. Ingraham & C. A. Ingraham. From INGRAHAM/INGRAHAM, Introduction to Microbiology, 1E.
© 1995 Cengage Learning.

reaction. A wide range of substances can cause allergic reactions, and the severity of the reactions also varies widely. Some allergic reactions may be life threatening, whereas others may cause annoyances such as runny noses. Some allergies are treated by introducing regular, small doses of the allergen to desensitize the person and to diminish or alleviate the allergic response. Sometimes, for reasons not well understood, the immune system may attack its own body. This situation occurs with **autoimmune diseases**. Recall that a function of the immune system is to recognize foreign invaders and mark them for destruction. In autoimmune diseases, the immune system loses the ability to distinguish the body from an invader, and it mounts the same vicious attack against itself that it would against an intruder. Lupus erythematosus, rheumatoid arthritis, and multiple sclerosis are autoimmune diseases.

Transplant rejection is not really an immune disorder, but it is a problem caused by the immune system's activity. When a person receives a transplanted organ—such as a heart, kidney, or liver—from another person, the immune system identifies the organ as an invader, because the organ has biochemical markers from the donor that are different from those of its host. Thus, the host's immune system will try to destroy the transplant. In an effort to prevent this reaction, physicians administer drugs that suppress immune system function. This strategy often works, but unfortunately the drugs suppress the patient's entire immune response, leaving the patient vulnerable to infection. To minimize the risk of infection, transplant patients must modify their lifestyle and comply with medical regimens.

IN SUMMARY

If stress can cause disease directly, it can do so only by affecting biological processes (see Figure 1.4). The most likely candidate for this interaction is the immune system, which is made up of tissues, organs, and processes that protect the body from invasion by foreign material such as bacteria, viruses, and fungi. The immune system also protects the body by eliminating damaged cells. Immune system responses can be either nonspecific or specific. The nonspecific response is capable of attacking any invader, whereas specific responses attack one particular invader. Immune system problems can stem from several sources, including organ transplants, allergies, drugs used for cancer chemotherapy, and immune deficiency. The human immunodeficiency virus damages the immune system, creating a deficiency that leaves the person vulnerable to a variety of infectious and malignant diseases.

Psychoneuroimmunology

The previous section described the function of the immune system as well as its tissues, structure, and disorders. Physiologists have traditionally taken a similar approach, studying the immune system as separate from and independent of other body systems. About 30 years ago, however, accumulating evidence suggested that the immune system interacts with the central nervous system (CNS) and the endocrine system. This evidence shows that psychological and social factors can affect the CNS, endocrine system, and immune system. In addition, immune function can affect neural function, providing the potential for the immune system to alter behavior and thought (Maier, 2003). This recognition led to the founding and rapid growth of the field of **psychoneuroimmunology (PNI)**, a multidisciplinary field that focuses on the interactions among behavior, the nervous system, the endocrine system, and the immune system.

History of Psychoneuroimmunology

In the early 1900s, Ivan Pavlov discovered that dogs could be trained to salivate at the sound of a bell. Pavlov showed that, through the process of classical conditioning, environmental events could become automatic triggers of basic physiological processes. Could classical conditioning also influence the functioning of physiological processes as seemingly "invisible" as the immune system?

In 1975, Robert Ader and Nicholas Cohen published a study that investigated this simple question. In doing so, Ader and Cohen showed how the nervous system, the immune system, and behavior could interact—a discovery that essentially created the field of PNI. Ader and Cohen's approach was straightforward and similar to Pavlov's approach: They paired a conditioned stimulus (CS) with an unconditioned stimulus (UCS), to see whether the conditioned stimulus alone would later produce a conditioned response (CR). However, the difference was that Ader and Cohen's conditioned stimulus was a saccharin and water solution that rats drank, and the unconditioned stimulus was the administration of a drug that suppresses the immune system. During the conditioning process, the rats were allowed to drink the saccharin solution and then were injected with the immunosuppressive drug. Much like Pavlov's dogs, the rats quickly associated the two stimuli, such that the rats later showed immune suppression when they were given *only* the saccharine solution! In this groundbreaking study, Ader and Cohen demonstrated that the immune system was subject to the same type of associative learning as other body systems.

Until Ader and Cohen's 1975 report, most physiologists believed that the immune system and the nervous system did not interact, and their results were not immediately accepted (Fleshner & Laudenslager, 2004). After many replications of their findings, physiologists now accept that the immune system and other body systems exchange information in a variety of ways. One mechanism is through **cytokines**, chemical messengers secreted by cells in the immune system (Blalock & Smith, 2007; Maier & Watkins, 2003). One type of cytokine is known as **proinflammatory cytokine** because it promotes inflammation. These cytokines, which include several types of *interleukins*, may underlie a number of states, including feelings associated with sickness, depression, and social withdrawal (Eisenberger, Inagaki, Mashal, & Irwin, 2010; Irwin, 2008; Kelley et al., 2003). This is one example of how the functioning of the immune system may influence psychological states.

The developing knowledge of the connections between the immune and nervous systems spurred researchers to explore the physical mechanisms by which interactions occur. Psychologists began using measures of immune function to test the effects of behavior on the immune system. During the 1980s, the AIDS epidemic focused public attention and research funding on how behavior influences the immune system and therefore health. As a result of this attention, some of the clearest evidence of the role of psychological factors in immune functioning comes from studies of people coping with HIV infection (Chida & Vedhara, 2009). However, researchers in the field of psychoneuroimmunology use a variety of populations and methods to examine the links between psychological factors and the functioning of the immune system (see Would You Believe …? box).

Research in Psychoneuroimmunology

Research in psychoneuroimmunology strives to develop an understanding of the role of behavior in changes in the immune system and the development of disease. To reach this goal, researchers must establish a connection between psychological factors and changes in immune function and also demonstrate a relationship between this impaired immune function and changes in health status. Ideally, research should include all three components—psychological factors such as stress, immune system malfunction, and development of disease—to establish the connection between stress and disease (Forlenza & Baum, 2004). This task is difficult for several reasons.

One reason for the difficulty is the less-than-perfect relationship between immune system malfunction and disease. Not all people with impaired immune systems become ill (Segerstrom & Miller, 2004). Disease is a function of both the immune system's competence and the person's exposure to pathogens, the agents that produce illness. The best approach in PNI comes from longitudinal studies that follow people for a period of time after they (1) experience stress that (2) prompts a decline in

Would You BELIEVE …? Pictures of Disease Are Enough to Activate the Immune System

The ability of the immune system to mount an effective attack against a biological invader is amazing in both its complexity and effectiveness. However, the immune system may have evolved to respond to more than simply pathogens that already entered the body. The immune system may mount defenses against pathogens that the brain *anticipates may soon enter the body.*

Canadian researchers (Schaller, Miller, Gervais, Yager, & Chen, 2010) presented a series of photographs to college student participants. Some participants saw pictures of infectious diseases—such as pox, skin lesions, and sneezing. These pictures were of stimuli that were expected to activate an immune response. Participants in a control group saw pictures of guns,

which were threatening stimuli but were not expected to activate an immune response. Indeed, participants who viewed the pictures of infectious diseases produced significantly more proinflammatory cytokines than participants who viewed the pictures of guns.

An Australian research team (Stevenson, Hodgson, Oaten, Barouei, & Case, 2011) found similar results when they had participants view images intended to induce a feeling of disgust, such as a dead animal, dirty toilet, and a cockroach on a pizza. Compared with participants who viewed neutral or threatening (but not disgusting) images, participants viewing the disgusting images produced greater quantities of the proinflammatory cytokine TNF-a.

Why might such disgusting images stimulate the immune system? While the exact reason is unknown, some researchers suggest the responses may be rooted in evolution. Organisms that mount an immune response when exposed to stimuli that are associated with pathogens may have less likelihood of succumbing to infection when those pathogens eventually enter the body (Schaller et al., 2010). However, such a response may be ineffectual—or even costly—in contexts where disgusting stimuli are not typically followed by exposure to pathogens, for example, when watching a particularly gory horror film.

Taken together, these findings highlight the fascinating links between the brain and the immune system. Pass the popcorn!

immunocompetence and then (3) assess changes in their health status. Few studies included all three components, and most such studies are restricted to non-human animals.

The majority of research in PNI focuses on the relationship between various stressors and altered immune system function. Most studies measure the immune system's function by testing blood samples rather than by testing immune function in people's bodies (Coe & Laudenslager, 2007; Segerstrom & Miller, 2004). Some research concentrated on the relationship between altered immune system function and the development of disease or spread of cancer (Cohen, 2005; Reiche, Nunes, & Morimoto, 2004), but such studies are in the minority. Furthermore, the types of stressors, the species of animals, and the facet of immune system function studied varied, resulting in a variety of findings (Forlenza & Baum, 2004).

Some researchers manipulated short-term stressors such as electric shock, loud noises, or complex cognitive tasks in a laboratory situation; others used naturally occurring stress in people's lives to test the effect of stress on immune system function. Laboratory studies allow researchers to investigate the physical changes that accompany stress, and such studies show correlations between sympathetic nervous system activation and immune responses (Glaser, 2005; Irwin, 2008). This research suggests that sympathetic activation may be a pathway through which stress can affect the immune system. The effect is initially positive, mobilizing resources, but continued stress activates physiological processes that can be damaging.

The naturally occurring stress of medical school exams provides another opportunity to study the relationship between stress and immune function in students (Kiecolt-Glaser, Malarkey, Cacioppo, & Glaser, 1994). A series of studies showed differences in immunocompetence, measured by numbers of natural killer cells, percentages of T-cells, and percentages of total lymphocytes. Indeed, medical students show more symptoms of infectious disease immediately before and after exams. More recent research (Chandrashekara et al., 2007) confirms that anxious students taking exams experience a lowering of immune function, which demonstrates that the effect on immune function is specific to the situation and to the students' psychological state.

Exam stress is typically a short-term stress, but chronic stress has even more severe effects on immune competence. Relationship conflict predicts immune system suppression for couples that experience marital conflict (Kiecolt-Glaser & Newton, 2001). Indeed, marriage is important in immune function and to a wide range of health outcomes (Graham, Christian, & Kiecolt-Glaser, 2006). For example, effects of marital conflict may include poorer response to immunization and slower wound healing (Ebrecht et al., 2004), and lack of partner support may play a role in increased stress during pregnancy, which raises health risk (Coussons-Read, Okun, & Nettles, 2007). However, marital conflict may not always lead to poorer immune response. Partners who deal with conflict with productive communication patterns have immune responses that are less dysregulated by episodes of marital conflict (Graham et al., 2009).

Other chronic stressors also suppress immune function. For example, people who are caregivers for someone with Alzheimer's disease experience chronic stress (see Chapter 11 for more about the disease and the stress of caregiving). Alzheimer's caregivers experience poorer psychological and physical health, longer healing times for wounds, and lowered immune function (Damjanovic et al., 2007; Kiecolt-Glaser, 1999; Kiecolt-Glaser, Marucha, Malarkey, Mercado, & Glaser, 1995). Furthermore, the death of the Alzheimer's patient fails to improve the stressed caregivers' psychological health or immune system functioning (Robinson-Whelen, Tada, MacCallum, McGuire, & Kiecolt-Glaser, 2001). Both caregivers and former caregivers were more depressed and showed lowered immune system functioning, suggesting that this stress continues after the caregiving is over.

The results of meta-analyses of 30 years of studies on stress and immunity (Segerstrom & Miller, 2004) show a clear relationship between stress and decreased immune function, especially for chronic sources of stress. The stressors that exert the most chronic effects have the most global influence on the immune system. Refugees, the unemployed, and those who live in high-crime neighborhoods experience the type of chronic, uncontrollable stress that has the most widespread negative effect on the immune system. Short-term stress may produce changes that are adaptive, such as mobilizing hormone production, but chronic stress exerts effects on many types of immune system response that weaken immune system effectiveness.

Some of the PNI research that most clearly demonstrates the three-way link among stress, immune function, and disease uses stressed rats as subjects, injecting material that provokes an immune system response and observing the resulting changes in immune function and disease (Bowers, Bilbo, Dhabhar, & Nelson, 2008). Some research with human participants also demonstrates the link among stress, immune function, and disease (Cohen, 2005; Kiecolt-Glaser, McGuire, Robles, & Glaser, 2002). For example, healing time after receiving a standardized wound varies, depending on whether the wound occurs during vacation or during exams. Students under exam stress show a decline in a specific immune function related to wound healing; the same students took 40% longer to heal during exams than they did during vacation. Thus, both human and animal research demonstrate that stress can affect immune function and disease processes.

If behavioral and social factors can decrease immune system function, is it possible to *boost* immunocompetence through changes in behavior? Would such an increase enhance health? Researchers have designed interventions aimed at increasing the effectiveness of the immune system—such as hypnosis, relaxation, and stress management—but a meta-analysis of these studies (Miller & Cohen, 2001) indicated only modest effects. Similarly, a meta-analysis of cognitive behavioral interventions for HIV-positive men (Crepaz et al., 2008) showed significant effects for improvements in anxiety, stress, and depression but limited changes in immune system function. However, a 10-week cognitive behavioral stress management intervention for women under treatment for breast cancer led to some improvements in immune measures over a 6-month period (Antoni et al., 2009). Cancer treatment compromises the immune system, so even small improvements may be an advantage for these individuals.

Physical Mechanisms of Influence

How does stress influence the functioning of the immune system? The effects of stress can occur through the relationship of the nervous system to the immune system through two routes—the peripheral nervous system and the secretion of hormones. Evidence exists for connection through both routes. In addition, people who are attempting to cope with stress may behave in ways that affect their immune system negatively, such as missing sleep, drinking alcohol, or smoking (Segerstrom & Miller, 2004).

The peripheral nervous system provides connections to immune system organs such as the thymus, spleen, and lymph nodes. The brain can also communicate with the immune system through the production of *releasing factors*, hormones that stimulate endocrine glands to secrete hormones. These hormones travel through the bloodstream and affect target organs, such as the adrenal glands. (Chapter 5 included a description of these systems and the endocrine component of the stress response.) T-cells and B-cells have receptors for the glucocorticoid stress hormones.

When the sympathetic nervous system is activated, the adrenal glands release several hormones. The adrenal medulla releases epinephrine and norepinephrine, and the adrenal cortex releases cortisol. The modulation of immunity by epinephrine and norepinephrine seems to come about through the autonomic nervous system (Dougall & Baum, 2001).

The release of cortisol from the adrenal cortex results from the release of adrenocorticotropic hormone (ACTH) by the pituitary in the brain. Another brain structure, the hypothalamus, stimulates the pituitary to release ACTH. Elevated cortisol is associated with a number of physical and emotional distress conditions (Dickerson & Kemeny, 2004), and it exerts an anti-inflammatory effect. Cortisol and the glucocorticoids tend to depress immune responses, phagocytosis, and macrophage activation. The nervous system can influence the immune system either through the sympathetic nervous system or through neuroendocrine response to stress.

Communication also occurs in the other direction: The immune system can signal the nervous system by way of cytokines, chemicals secreted by immune system cells (Irwin, 2008; Maier, 2003). Cytokines communicate with the brain, probably by way of the peripheral nervous system. This interconnection makes possible bidirectional interactions of immune and nervous systems and may even enable effects on behavior such as fatigue and depression, which are common symptoms of sickness. Michael Irwin (2008) emphasized the many possibilities for communication between the nervous and immune systems and how behavioral responses are the key to activating processes that influence the immune system. The interrelationship between the nervous system and the immune system makes it possible for each to influence the other to produce the symptoms associated with stress and disease.

Stress may also "get under the skin" by altering health-related behaviors (Segerstrom & Miller, 2004).

For example, people under stress may smoke more cigarettes, drink more alcohol, use illicit drugs, and get less sleep. Each of these behaviors increases risk for a variety of diseases and may influence the immune system in negative ways.

IN SUMMARY

Psychoneuroimmunology research demonstrates that various functions of the immune system respond to both short-term and long-term psychological stress. Researchers are making progress toward linking psychological factors, immune system function, and disease, but few studies have included all three elements.

Some research is successful in linking immune system changes to changes in health status; this link is necessary to complete the chain between psychological factors and disease. In addition to establishing links between psychological factors and immune system changes, researchers attempt to specify the physical mechanisms through which these changes occur. Possible mechanisms include direct connections between nervous and immune systems and an indirect connection through the neuroendocrine system. Chemical messengers called cytokines also allow for communication between immune and nervous system and possible effects on behavior. In addition, stress may prompt people to change their behaviors, adopting less healthy habits that are risk factors for disease.

Does Stress Cause Disease?

Many factors cause disease, and stress may be one of those factors. When considering the link between stress and disease, remember that most people who experience substantial stress do *not* develop a disease. Furthermore, in contrast to other risk factors—such as having high cholesterol levels, smoking cigarettes, or drinking alcohol—the risks conferred by life events are usually temporary. Yet, even temporary stress affects some people more than others.

Why does stress affect some people, apparently causing them to get sick, and leave others unaffected? The diathesis–stress model offers a possible answer to this question.

The Diathesis–Stress Model

The **diathesis–stress model** suggests that some individuals are vulnerable to stress-related diseases because either genetic weakness or biochemical imbalance inherently predisposes them to those diseases. The diathesis–stress model has a long history in psychology, particularly in explaining the development of psychological disorders. During the 1960s and 1970s, the concept was used as an explanation for the development of psychophysiological disorders (Levi, 1974) as well as schizophrenic episodes, depression, and anxiety disorders (Zubin & Spring, 1977).

Applied to either psychological or physiological disorders, the diathesis–stress model holds that some people are predisposed to react abnormally to environmental stressors. This predisposition (diathesis) is usually thought to be inherited through biochemical or organ system weakness, but some theorists (Zubin & Spring, 1977) also consider learned patterns of thought and behavior as components of vulnerability. Whether inherited or learned, the vulnerability is relatively permanent. What varies over time is the presence of environmental stressors, which may account for the waxing and waning of illnesses.

Thus, the diathesis–stress model assumes that two factors are necessary to produce disease. First, the person must have a relatively permanent predisposition to the disease, and second, that person must experience some sort of stress. Diathetic individuals respond pathologically to the same stressful conditions with which most people are able to cope. For people with a strong predisposition to a disease, even a mild environmental stressor may be sufficient to produce an illness episode. For example, a study of symptom stress and depression (Schroeder, 2004) revealed that surgical patients with low coping competence were vulnerable to developing depression in the months following their surgery, whereas patients with better coping skills were less vulnerable to depression. Abuse or maltreatment during childhood may create another source of vulnerability to physical and psychological disorders. As adults, these individuals show increased vulnerability to schizophrenia (Rosenberg, Lu, Mueser, Jankowski, & Cournos, 2007), anxiety and depression (Stein, Schork, & Gelernter, 2008), posttraumatic stress disorder (Storr, Lalongo, Anthony, & Breslau, 2007), and infectious disease (Cohen, 2005). Therefore, personal and psychosocial factors have the power to create vulnerabilities to disorders.

The diathesis–stress model may explain why life event scales (see Chapter 5) are so inconsistent in predicting illness. The number of points accumulated on the Holmes and Rahe Social Readjustment Rating Scale or the number of items checked on the Life Events Scale for Students is only a weak predictor of illness. The diathesis–stress model holds that a person's diathesis (vulnerability) must be considered along with stressful life events in predicting who will get sick and who will stay well; it allows for a great deal of individual variability in who gets sick and who stays well under conditions of stress (Marsland, Bachen, Cohen, & Manuck, 2001).

In this section, we review the evidence concerning the link between stress and several diseases, including headache, infectious disease, cardiovascular disease, diabetes mellitus, premature birth, asthma, and rheumatoid arthritis. In addition, stress shows some relationship to psychological disorders such as depression and anxiety disorders.

Stress and Disease

What is the evidence linking stress to disease? Which diseases have been implicated? What physiological mechanism might mediate the connection between stress and disease?

Hans Selye's concept of stress (see Chapter 5) included suppression of the immune response, and a growing body of evidence now supports this hypothesis through interactions among the nervous, endocrine, and immune systems (Kemeny & Schedlowski, 2007). These interactions are similar to the responses hypothesized by Selye and provide strong evidence that stress could be involved in a variety of physical ailments. Figure 6.5 shows some possible effects.

Several possibilities exist for pathways through which stress could produce disease (Segerstrom & Miller, 2004). Direct influence could occur through the effects of stress on the nervous, endocrine, and immune systems. Because any or all of these systems can create

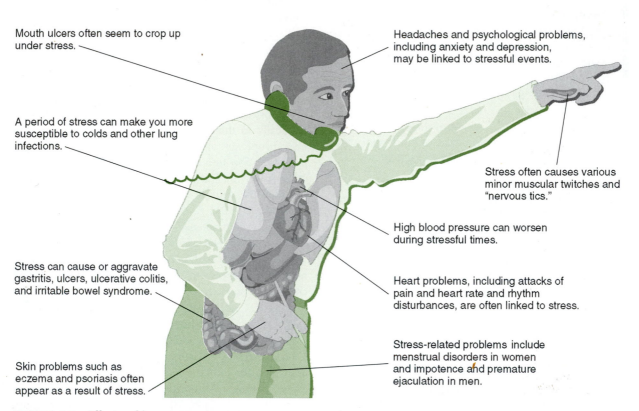

Mouth ulcers often seem to crop up under stress.

A period of stress can make you more susceptible to colds and other lung infections.

Stress can cause or aggravate gastritis, ulcers, ulcerative colitis, and irritable bowel syndrome.

Skin problems such as eczema and psoriasis often appear as a result of stress.

Headaches and psychological problems, including anxiety and depression, may be linked to stressful events.

Stress often causes various minor muscular twitches and "nervous tics."

High blood pressure can worsen during stressful times.

Heart problems, including attacks of pain and heart rate and rhythm disturbances, are often linked to stress.

Stress-related problems include menstrual disorders in women and impotence and premature ejaculation in men.

FIGURE 6.5   Effects of long-term stress.

Source: An invitation to health (7th ed., p. 58), by D. Hales, 1997, Pacific Grove, CA: Brooks/Cole. From HALES, *Invitation to Health*, 7E. © 1997 Cengage Learning.

disease, sufficient physiological foundations exist to provide a link between stress and disease. In addition, indirect effects could occur through changes in health practices that increase risks; that is, stress tends to be related to increases in drinking, smoking, drug use, and sleep problems, all of which can increase the risk for disease. Thus, possibilities exist for both direct and indirect effects of stress on disease. Does the evidence support these hypothesized relationships?

Headaches   Headaches are a common problem; more than 99% of people will experience headaches at some time in their lives (Smetana, 2000). For most people, headaches are an uncomfortable occurrence, but others experience serious, chronic pain. Headache can signal serious medical conditions, but most often the pain associated with the headache is the problem. This source of pain is a major cause of disability (D'Amico et al., 2011). The majority of people who seek medical assistance for headaches experience the same sorts of headaches as those who do not; the difference stems from the frequency and severity of the headaches or from personal factors involved in seeking assistance.

Although more than 100 types of headaches may exist, distinguishing among them is controversial, and the underlying causes for the most common types remain unclear (Andrasik, 2001). Nevertheless, diagnostic criteria have been devised for several types of headaches. The most frequent type is *tension headache*, usually associated with increased muscle tension in the head and neck region. Tension is also a factor in migraine headaches, which are believed to originate in neurons in the brain stem (Silberstein, 2004). Migraines are associated with throbbing pain localized in one side of the head.

Stress is a factor in headaches; people with either tension or vascular headaches name stress as one of the leading precipitating factors (Deniz, Aygül, Koçak, Orhan, & Kaya, 2004; Spierings, Ranke, & Honkoop, 2001). However, a comparison of people with daily headaches and those with infrequent headaches found no difference in stress as measured either by life events or by hassles (Barton-Donovan & Blanchard, 2005), and a study comparing traumatic life events for headache patients found no difference from a comparison group (de Leeuw, Schmidt, & Carlson, 2005). The type of stress that people associate with headaches tends not to be traumatic life events but, rather, daily hassles. Students with chronic or frequent headaches reported more hassles than did students with infrequent

headaches (Bottos & Dewey, 2004). In addition, stressful events precede periods of headache more often than they precede times with no headache (Marlowe, 1998); stress during a headache intensified the attack.

Nash and Thebarge (2006) discussed the ways through which stress might influence headaches. First, stress may be a predisposing factor that influences the development of headaches. Second, stress may act to transform a person who experiences occasional headaches into one who has chronic headaches. Third, stress may worsen headache episodes, magnifying the pain. These routes allow for several possibilities through which stress can contribute to the development of a headache and to chronic headaches. Furthermore, stress may decrease the quality of life for those with headaches.

Infectious Disease   Are people who are under stress more likely than nonstressed individuals to develop infectious diseases such as the common cold? Research suggests that the answer is yes. An early study (Stone, Reed, & Neale, 1987) followed married couples who kept diaries on their own and their spouse's desirable and undesirable daily life experiences. Results indicated that participants who experienced a decline in desirable events or an increase in undesirable events developed somewhat more infectious diseases (colds or flu) 3 and 4 days later. The association was not strong, but this study was the first prospective design to show a relationship between daily life experiences and subsequent disease.

Later studies used a more direct approach, intentionally inoculating healthy volunteers with cold viruses to see who would develop a cold and who would not. Sheldon Cohen and his colleagues (Cohen, 2005; Cohen et al., 1998; Cohen, Tyrrell, & Smith, 1991, 1993) intentionally exposed healthy volunteers to various common cold viruses to determine the role of stress in the development of colds. The results indicated that the higher the person's stress, the more likely it was that the person would become ill.

Cohen and his colleagues (1998) also used the same inoculation procedure to see what types of stressors induce cold symptoms in people exposed to a cold virus. They found that duration of a stressful life event was more important than severity. Acute severe stress of less than 1 month did not lead to the development of colds, but severe chronic stress (more than 1 month) led to a substantial increase in colds. Later research showed that susceptibility varied from individual to individual (Marsland, Bachen, Cohen, Rabin, &

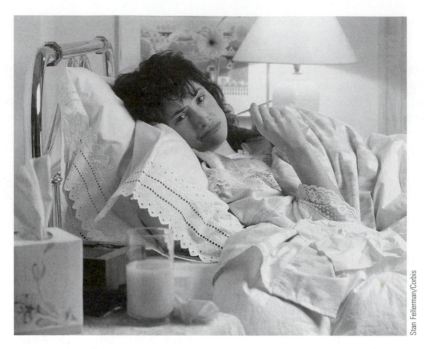

Stan Fellerman/Corbis

Research has shown that stress can influence development of infectious disease.

Manuck, 2002); people who were sociable and agreeable developed fewer colds than others after exposure to a cold virus (Cohen, Doyle, Turner, Alper, & Skoner, 2003). A naturalistic study of stress and colds (Takkouche, Regueira, & Gestal-Otero, 2001) showed that high levels of stress were related to increases in infection. People in the upper 25% of perceived stress were about twice as likely as those in the lowest 25% to get a cold, which suggests that stress may be a significant predictor of developing infectious disease.

Stress may also influence the extent to which vaccinations provide protection against infectious disease. Vaccinations, as you recall, stimulate the immune system to produce antibodies against specific viruses. People under substantial stress—such as caregivers—show weakened antibody production following flu vaccination compared with people under less life stress (Pedersen, Zachariae, & Bovbjerg, 2009). This relationship between stress and weakened response to vaccination suggests it is as apparent among younger adults as it is among older adults. Thus, vaccinations may be less effective in protecting against infectious disease among people who experience stress.

Stress may also affect the progression of infectious disease. Reviews of psychosocial factors in HIV infection (Cole et al., 2001; Kopnisky, Stoff, & Rausch, 2004) explored the effect of stress on HIV infection; they concluded that stress affects both the progression of HIV infection and the infected person's immune response to antiviral drug treatment. HIV is not the only infectious disease that stress influences. The herpes simplex virus (HSV) is transmitted through contact with the skin of an infected person and can cause blisters on the mouth, lips or genitals. Often, these physical symptoms are not present in the infected person but only appear during periodic active outbreaks of HSV. Stress predicts these symptomatic outbreaks of HSV symptoms (Chida & Mao, 2009; Strachan et al., 2011). For example, in a study of women with a sexually transmitted form of HSV, researchers found that experiences of psychosocial distress predicted the onset of genital lesions 5 days later (Strachan et al., 2011). Stress also plays a role in other bacterial, viral, and fungal infections, including pneumonia, hepatitis, and recurrent urinary tract infections (Levenson & Schneider, 2007). Thus, stress is a significant factor in susceptibility, severity, and progression of infection.

Cardiovascular Disease Cardiovascular disease (CVD) has a number of behavioral risk factors, some of which are related to stress. Chapter 9 examines these behavioral risk factors in more detail; in this section we look only at stress as a contributor to CVD. People who have had heart attacks named stress as the cause of their disorder (Cameron, Petrie, Ellis, Buick, & Weinman, 2005), but the relationship is less direct than they imagine. Two lines of research relate stress to CVD: studies that evaluate stress as a precipitating factor in heart attack or stroke, and studies that investigate stress as a cause in the development of CVD.

Evidence for the role of stress as a precipitating factor for heart attack or stroke in people with CVD is clear; stress increases the risks. Stress can serve as a trigger for heart attacks for people with coronary heart disease (Kop, 2003; Sheps, 2007). A large cross-cultural study called the INTERHEART Study compared more than 15,000 people who had experienced a heart attack with almost as many who had not, attempting to identify significant risk factors that held across cultures and continents (Yusuf et al., 2004). This study identified a set of psychological stressors that showed a significant relationship to heart attack, including workplace and home stress, financial problems, major life events in the past year, depression, and external locus of control (Rosengren et al., 2004). These stress factors related to

heart attack and made a substantial contribution to the risk within each population. The individuals who experienced heart attacks may have had long-standing CVD, but stress may also contribute to the development of this disease. However, even positive stress may create a risk for cardiovascular problems (see Would You Believe …? box).

The role of stress in the development of heart disease is indirect but may occur through several routes, including hormone release as a response to stress or as a result of the immune system response (Matthews, 2005). For example, job-related stress (Smith, Roman, Dollard, Winefield, & Siegrist, 2005) and other situations with high demands and low control (Kamarck, Muldoon, Shiffman, & Sutton-Tyrrell, 2007) are implicated in heart disease. One possible route for this effect is through the action of the immune system, which reacts by releasing cytokines, which promote inflammation. This inflammation is a factor in the development of coronary artery disease (Steptoe, Hamer, & Chida, 2007). The action of stress hormones such as the corticoids also affects the development of diseased arteries, exacerbating artery damage and making the development of arterial plaque more likely. These stress-related responses apply to any source of stress, forming an indirect route to heart disease.

Hypertension Although high blood pressure would seem to be the result of stress, no simple relationship exists between stress and blood pressure. Situational

Would You BELIEVE …? Being a Sports Fan May Be a Danger to Your Health

Would you believe that being a sports fan may endanger your health? A week or so before the 2012 Super Bowl, stories appeared in the media suggesting that watching this sports event might present a risk for heart attack. This risk did not stem from the pizza, chips, and beer from Super Bowl parties but from the emotional stress and excitement of the game.

The warnings were not based on research on the dangers of American football but, rather, on the increase in cardiovascular events

during the World Cup Soccer championship held in Germany in 2006 (Wilbert-Lampen et al., 2008). Researchers compared the frequency of cardiac events such as heart attack and cardiac arrhythmia during the month of the World Cup championship with the month before and after the playoffs and found an elevated rate during the playoffs. The incidence of such cardiac events was 3 times higher for men and almost twice as high for women on days when the German team played

compared with days during the comparison period. The risk was greatest during the 2 hours after the beginning of a match. Some evidence suggests that this heightened risk is attributable to stress-induced inflammatory responses (Wilbert-Lampen et al., 2010). The researchers concluded that the stress of watching the matches raised the risk for cardiac problems, especially for individuals who had been identified as having cardiovascular disease.

factors such as noise can elevate blood pressure, but most studies show that blood pressure returns to normal when the situational stimulus is removed. However, a longitudinal study of blood pressure (Stewart, Janicki, & Kamarck, 2006) showed that the time to return to normal blood pressure after a psychological stressor predicted hypertension over 3 years. This response is similar to reactivity.

Reactivity   The idea that some people react more strongly to stress than others is another possibility for the link between stress and cardiovascular disease. This response, called *reactivity*, may play a role in the development of cardiovascular disease if the response is relatively stable within an individual and prompted by events that occur frequently in the individual's life. Many life events can prompt stress responses that include cardiac reactions.

One study showed that reactivity relates to incidence of stroke (Everson et al., 2001). Men with higher systolic blood pressure reactivity were at greater risk for stroke than men with less blood pressure reactivity. In this study, educational level was also a factor that raised the risk of stroke; other studies focused on education, ethnicity, and socioeconomic status as factors in reactivity.

The higher rate of cardiovascular disease for African Americans than for European Americans leads researchers to examine differences in reactivity between these two ethnic groups, as well as the stressors that prompt such reaction. Many African Americans experience a continuous struggle to cope with a variety of stressors that relate to their ethnicity, and this struggle constitutes the type of long-term stressor that poses health threats (Bennett et al., 2004). Beginning during childhood and continuing into adolescence, African Americans show greater reactivity than European Americans (Murphy, Stoney, Alpert, & Walker, 1995); these differences appeared among children as young as 6 (Treiber et al., 1993). In addition, African American children with a family history of cardiovascular disease showed significantly greater reactivity than any other group of children in the study.

Research on the experience of discrimination shows that racist provocations produce reactivity. A study comparing the reactions of African American and European American women (Lepore et al., 2006) showed that African American women who evaluated a stressful situation as racist showed stronger cardiac reactions than women who did not identify the stress as racist. Both European American and African

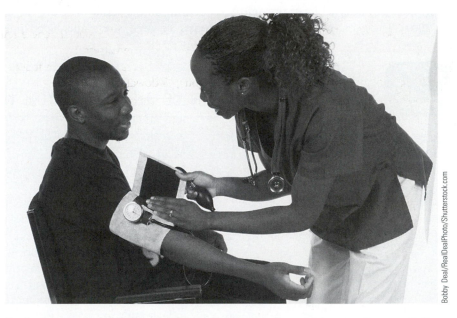

Beginning during childhood, African Americans show higher cardiac reactivity than other ethnic groups, which may relate to their higher levels of cardiovascular disease.

Bobby Deal/RealDealPhoto/Shutterstock.com

American men who viewed a racist film clip experienced a greater increase in blood pressure than they did while viewing emotionally neutral films (Fang & Myers, 2001). Differences exist in reactivity for African Americans and Caribbean Americans, with both showing higher reactivity than European Americans (Arthur, Katkin, & Mezzacappa, 2004). However, Asian Americans showed lower reactivity than European Americans to a laboratory stressor (Shen, Stroud, & Niaura, 2004). This result is consistent with a lower rate of CVD among Asian Americans.

Ulcers

At one time, stress was widely accepted as the cause of ulcers, but during the 1980s, two Australian researchers, Barry Marshall and J. Robin Warren, proposed that ulcers were the result of a bacterial infection rather than stress (Okuda & Nakazawa, 2004). At the time, their hypothesis seemed unlikely because most physiologists and physicians believed that bacteria could not live in the stomach environment with its extreme acidity. Marshall had trouble obtaining funding to research the possibility of a bacterial basis for ulcers.

With no funding for his research and the belief that he was correct, Marshall took matters into his own hands: He infected himself with the bacterium to demonstrate its gastric effects. He developed severe gastritis and took antibiotics to cure himself, providing further evidence that this bacterium has gastric effects. A clinical trial later supported Marshall's hypothesis: Stomach ulcers were less likely to return in patients who received antibiotics compared with patients who received an acid suppressant (Alper, 1993). These findings demonstrated the role that bacterial infection plays in ulcer development. However, the psychological component has not disappeared from explanations for the development and reoccurrence of ulcers because *H. pylori* infection does not seem to account for all ulcers (Levenstein, 2000; Watanabe et al., 2002). This infection is very common and related to a variety of gastric problems, yet most infected people do not develop ulcers (Weiner & Shapiro, 2001). Thus, *H. pylori* infection may create a vulnerability to ulcers, which stress or other psychosocial conditions then precipitate. For example, smoking, heavy drinking, caffeine consumption, and use of nonsteroidal anti-inflammatory drugs all relate to ulcer formation. Stress may be a factor in any of these behaviors, providing an indirect link between stress and ulcer formation in infected individuals. In addition, the hormones and altered immune function associated with the experience of chronic stress may be a more direct link. Therefore, behavioral factors play a role in the development of ulcers, but so does *H. pylori* infection, creating a complex interaction of factors in the formation of ulcers.

Other Physical Disorders

Besides headache, infectious disease, cardiovascular disease, and ulcers, stress is linked to several other physical disorders, including diabetes, premature delivery for pregnant women, asthma, and rheumatoid arthritis.

Diabetes mellitus is a chronic disease that is also related to stress. Two kinds of diabetes mellitus are Type 1, or insulin-dependent, and Type 2, or non-insulin-dependent. Type 1 diabetes usually begins in childhood and requires insulin injections for its control. Type 2 diabetes usually appears during adulthood and can most often be controlled by dietary changes. (The lifestyle adjustments and behavioral management required by diabetes mellitus are discussed in Chapter 11.)

Stress may contribute to the *development* of both types of diabetes. First, stress may contribute directly to the development of insulin-dependent diabetes through the disruption of the immune system, possibly during infancy (Sepa, Wahlberg, Vaarala, Frodi, & Ludvigsson, 2005). Immune system measures at age 1 year indicated that those infants who had experienced higher family stress showed more indications of antibodies consistent with diabetes. Second, a recent epidemiological study of over 55,000 Japanese adults showed that greater perceived stress increased the risk of developing Type 2 diabetes at a 10-year follow-up (Kato, Noda, Inoue, Kadowaki, & Tsugane, 2009). Stress may contribute to the development of Type 2 through its effect on cytokines that initiate an inflammatory process that affects insulin metabolism and produces insulin resistance (Black, 2003; Tsiotra & Tsigos, 2006). Third, stress may contribute to Type 2 through its possible effects on obesity. Research on stress and Type 2 diabetics shows that stress can be a triggering factor and thus play a role in the age at which people develop Type 2 diabetes.

In addition, stress may affect the *management* of diabetes mellitus through its direct effects on blood glucose (Riazi, Pickup, & Bradley, 2004) and through the indirect route of hindering people's adherence with controlling glucose levels (Farrell, Hains, Davies, Smith, & Parton, 2004). Indeed, adherence, discussed in Chapter 4, is a major problem for this disorder.

Stress during pregnancy is the topic of research for both human and nonhuman subjects (Kofman, 2002).

Research with nonhuman subjects conclusively demonstrates that stressful environments relate to lower birth weight and developmental delays, and that infants of stressed mothers show higher reactivity to stress. Research with human participants cannot experimentally manipulate such stressors, so the results are not as conclusive, but studies on stress during pregnancy reveal a tendency for stress to make preterm deliveries more likely and to result in babies with lower birth weights (Dunkel-Schetter, 2011). Both factors contribute to a number of problems for the infants. The importance of type and timing of stress remains unclear, but there is some indication that chronic stress may be more damaging than acute stress, and that stress late in pregnancy is riskier than earlier stress.

Asthma is a respiratory disorder characterized by difficulty in breathing due to reversible airway obstruction, airway inflammation, and increase in airway responsiveness to a variety of stimuli (Cohn, Elias, & Chupp, 2004). The prevalence and mortality rate of asthma is increasing for both European American and African American women, men, and children, but asthma disproportionately affects poor African Americans living in urban environments (Gold & Wright, 2005).

Because inflammation is an essential part of asthma, researchers hypothesize that the proinflammatory cytokines play a fundamental (possibly a causal) role in the development of this disease (Wills-Karp, 2004). The link between stress and the immune system presents the possibility that stress plays a role in the development of this disorder, but stress is also involved in asthma attacks (Chen & Miller, 2007).

Physical stimuli such as smoke can trigger an attack, but stressors, such as emotional events and pain, can also stimulate an asthma attack (Gustafson, Meadows-Oliver, & Banasiak, 2008). Both acute and chronic stress increase the risk of asthma attacks in children with asthma; a population-based study in South Korea (Oh, Kim, Yoo, Kim, & Kim, 2004) found that people who reported more stress were more likely to experience more severe problems with their asthma. Children living in inner-city neighborhoods with parents who have mental problems are at sharply heightened risk (Weil et al., 1999). Even in a laboratory setting, the influence of chronic stress on asthma is evident: Children of low socioeconomic status show greater asthma symptoms following an acute stress task than children of high socioeconomic status (Chen, Strunk, Bacharier, Chan, & Miller, 2010). Thus, stress is a significant factor in triggering asthma attacks.

Rheumatoid arthritis, a chronic inflammatory disease of the joints, may also be related to stress. Although the cause is unknown, rheumatoid arthritis is believed to be an autoimmune disorder in which a person's own immune system attacks itself (Ligier & Sternberg, 2001). The attack produces inflammation and damage to the tissue lining of the joints, resulting in pain and loss of flexibility and mobility. Stress is hypothesized to be a factor in the development of autoimmune diseases through the production of stress hormones and cytokines (Stojanovich & Marisavljevich, 2008).

Stress can make arthritis worse by increasing sensitivity to pain, reducing coping efforts, and possibly affecting the process of inflammation itself. Although it is unclear whether people with rheumatoid arthritis have different cortisol responses to stress than healthy people, there is evidence of greater immune dysregulation among arthritis patients (Davis et al., 2008; de Brouwer et al., 2010). These findings suggest a role for stress in this disease. For example, people with rheumatoid arthritis reported more pain on workdays that were stressful (Fifield et al., 2004). Other factors are important for the development of rheumatoid arthritis, but the stress that results from rheumatoid arthritis brings about negative changes in people's lives and requires extensive coping efforts.

Stress and Psychological Disorders

Stress can put people in a bad mood. For some people, these emotional responses of stress are short lived. For other people, stress may lead to persistent emotional difficulties that can qualify as psychological disorders. Therefore, the study of stress as a factor in psychological disorders parallels other research about stress and disease by adopting the diathesis–stress model. This research concentrates not only on the sources of stress that relate to psychological disorders but also on the factors that create vulnerability.

Mood changes can also lead to changes in immune function. Changes in immune functioning may underlie several psychological disorders (Dantzer, O'Connor, Freund, Johnson, & Kelley, 2008; Harrison, Olver, Norman, & Nathan, 2002). As you will learn, the relationship between stress and psychological disorders may be mediated through processes similar to those involved in other diseases—through the immune system.

Depression   There is clear evidence that stress contributes to the development of depressive symptoms.

Much of the research that focuses on this relationship attempts to answer two questions. First, what factors make some people more vulnerable to depression? Second, what physical mechanisms translate stress into depression? A large body of research attempts to identify the factors that make some people particularly vulnerable to depression.

Ineffective coping may be one source of vulnerability to depression. People who can cope effectively are able to avoid depression, even with many stressful events in their lives. As you will recall from Chapter 5, Richard Lazarus and his colleagues (Kanner et al., 1981; Lazarus & DeLongis, 1983; Lazarus & Folkman, 1984) regarded stress as the combination of an environmental stimulus with the person's appraisal, vulnerability, and perceived coping strength. According to this theory, people become ill not only because they have had too many stressful experiences but also because they evaluate these experiences as threatening or damaging, because they are physically or socially vulnerable at the time, or because they lack the ability to cope with the stressful event.

Another proposal for vulnerability to depression is the "kindling" hypothesis (Monroe & Harkness, 2005). This view holds that major life stress provides a "kindling" experience that may prompt the development of depression. This experience then sensitizes people to depression, and future experiences of stress need not be major to prompt recurrences of depression (Stroud, Davila, Hammen, & Vrshek-Schallhorn, 2011). A meta-analysis of studies on this topic (Stroud, Davila, & Moyer, 2008) showed some support, especially for the hypothesis of stress predicting first episodes of depression.

A negative outlook or the tendency to dwell on problems may exacerbate stress, making people more likely to think in ways that increase depression (Ciesla & Roberts, 2007; Gonzalez, Nolen-Hoeksema, & Treynor, 2003). Rumination—the tendency to dwell on negative thoughts—is one factor implicated in depression. For example, a longitudinal study of Japanese university students (Ito, Takenaka, Tomita, & Agari, 2006) demonstrated that rumination predicted depression. Thus, the tendency to dwell on negative thoughts is one type of vulnerability for depression. Consistent with the diathesis–stress view, more positive ways of thinking or less stress would result in lower risk for depression.

Genetic vulnerability is another type of risk factor for depression. In a longitudinal study of Swedish twins (Kendler, Gatz, Gardner, & Pedersen, 2007), stress was a significant factor in depression, but only under some

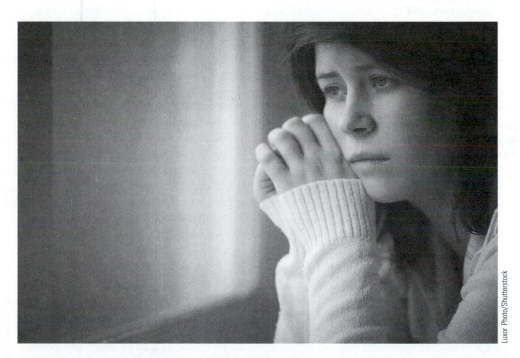

Stress can make people more vulnerable to depression.

Luxor Photo/Shutterstock

circumstances. Stress was more likely to predict earlier compared with later episodes of depression, consistent with the kindling hypothesis. Importantly, stress was also more likely to predict depression for people with low rather than high genetic risk. Another longitudinal study (Caspi et al., 2003) demonstrated the interaction between genes and environment in the development of depression. Individuals who inherited a particular version of a gene pair that is involved with the neurotransmitter serotonin developed depression and suicidal thoughts significantly more frequently than did individuals with a different version of this gene pair, but only when the vulnerable individuals experienced stressful life events. These studies suggest that genes furnish the basis for a vulnerability that interacts with stressful life events to precipitate depression.

Some types of stressful situations produce greater risks for depression than other events. For example, chronic workplace stress is linked to the development of depression, especially for people with low decision-making authority (Blackmore et al., 2007), as is living in a neighborhood where crime and drug use are common (Cutrona et al., 2005). Illness is another type of stress that shows a relationship to depression. Experiencing health problems produces stress both for the sick person and for caregivers. Heart disease (Guck, Kavan, Elsasser, & Barone, 2001), cancer (Spiegel & Giese-Davis, 2003), AIDS (Cruess et al., 2003), and Alzheimer's disease (Dorenlot, Harboun, Bige, Henrard, & Ankri, 2005) are all tied to increased incidence of depression. The relationship between stress and this variety of diseases occurs through the immune system.

Depression that meets the diagnostic criteria for clinical depression (American Psychiatric Association, 2000) is also associated with immune function, with stronger relationships found among older and hospitalized patients. In addition, the more severe the depression, the greater the alteration of immune function. A meta-analysis of depression and immune function (Zorrilla et al., 2001) indicated that depression related to many facets of immune system function, including reduced T-cells and decreased activity of natural killer cells. This link between depression and reduced immune functioning is apparent among women receiving treatment for breast cancer, for whom a healthy immune system is critical in defending against infection (Sephton et al., 2009).

This link between depression and reduced immune functioning may develop when prolonged stress disrupts regulation of the immune system through the action of proinflammatory cytokines (Robles, Glaser, & Kiecolt-Glaser, 2005). The release of proinflammatory cytokines by the immune system (Anisman, Merali, Poulter, & Hayley, 2005; Dantzer et al., 2008) sends a signal to the nervous system, which may generate fatigue, feelings of listlessness, and a loss of feelings of pleasure. Cytokine production increases when people are depressed, and people undergoing treatments that increase the production of certain cytokines also experience symptoms of depression. Thus, several lines of evidence support the role of cytokines in depression. Indeed, the brain may even interpret cytokines as stressors (Anisman et al., 2005), which interact with environmental stressors to increase risk for depression.

Anxiety Disorders Anxiety disorders include a variety of fears and phobias, often leading to avoidance behaviors. Included in this category are such conditions as panic attacks, **agoraphobia**, generalized anxiety, obsessive-compulsive disorders, and posttraumatic stress disorder (American Psychiatric Association, 2000). This section looks at stress as a possible contributor to anxiety states.

One anxiety disorder that, by definition, is related to stress is **posttraumatic stress disorder (PTSD)**. The *Diagnostic and Statistical Manual of Mental Disorders* (4th ed., text revision; American Psychiatric Association, 2000) defines PTSD as "the development of characteristic symptoms following exposure to an extreme traumatic stressor involving direct personal experience of an event that involves actual or threatened death or serious injury" (p. 463). PTSD can also stem from experiencing threats to one's physical integrity; witnessing another person's serious injury, death, or threatened physical integrity; and learning about death of or injury to family members or friends. The traumatic events often include military combat, but sexual assault, physical attack, robbery, mugging, and other personal violent assaults can also trigger posttraumatic stress disorder.

Symptoms of PTSD include recurrent and intrusive memories of the traumatic event, recurrent distressing dreams that replay the event, and extreme psychological and physiological distress. Events that resemble or symbolize the original traumatic event, as well as anniversaries of that event, may also trigger symptoms. People with posttraumatic stress disorder attempt to avoid thoughts, feelings, or conversations about the event and to avoid any person or place that might trigger acute distress. Lifetime prevalence of

PTSD in the general population of the United States is around 7% (Kessler et al., 2005).

However, most people who experience traumatic events do not develop PTSD (McNally, 2003), and researchers have sought to identify the risk factors for PTSD. Initially, PTSD was viewed primarily as a response to combat stress. Now, many types of experiences are considered potential risks for PTSD. People who are the victims of crime (Scarpa, Haden, & Hurley, 2006), terrorist attacks (Gabriel et al., 2007), domestic violence or sexual abuse (Pimlott-Kubiak & Cortina, 2003), and natural disasters (Dewaraja & Kawamura, 2006; Norris et al., 2001) are vulnerable. Personal factors and life circumstances also show a relationship to the development of PTSD (McNally, 2003), such as prior emotional problems, but poor social support and reactions to the traumatic event are more important in predicting who will develop PTSD (Ozer, Best, Lipsey, & Weiss, 2003).

The list of experiences that make people vulnerable to PTSD includes more events experienced by women than by men, and women are more likely to show symptoms of PTSD (Pimlott-Kubiak & Cortina, 2003). Hispanic Americans also seem more vulnerable to PTSD than other ethnic groups (Pole, Best, Metzler, & Marmar, 2005). The disorder is not limited to adults; children and adolescents who are the victims of violence or who observe violence are at increased risk (Griffing et al., 2006). PTSD increases the risk for medical disorders; its effects on the immune system may be the underlying reason. PTSD produces long-lasting suppression of the immune system and an increase in proinflammatory cytokines (Pace & Heim, 2011).

The relationship between stress and other anxiety disorders is less clear, perhaps because of the overlap between anxiety and depression (Suls & Bunde, 2005). Disentangling symptoms of negative affect presents problems for researchers. However, a study conducted in China (Shen et al., 2003) found that people with generalized anxiety disorder reported more stressful life events than did people with no psychological disorder. Furthermore, those with anxiety disorder showed lower levels of some immune system functioning. Thus, stress may play a role in anxiety disorders, and again the route may be through an effect on the immune system.

IN SUMMARY

Much evidence points to a relationship between stress and disease, but the relationship between stressful life events or daily hassles and disease is indirect and complex. The diathesis–stress model is the major framework for understanding the relationship between stress and development of disease. The diathesis–stress model hypothesizes that without some vulnerability, stress does not produce disease;

Becoming Healthier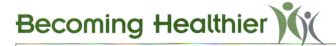

Stress may erode people's good intentions to maintain a healthy lifestyle. Stress may underlie people's decisions to eat an unhealthy diet, smoke, drink, use drugs, miss sleep, or avoid exercise. According to Dianne Tice and her colleagues (Tice, Bratslavsky, & Baumeister, 2001), distressed people tend to behave more impulsively. These researchers showed that when distressed, people do things oriented toward making them feel better, and some of those things are health threatening, such as eating high-fat and high-sugar snacks. Stress is also the rationalization that some people—including Lindsay Lohan—use to smoke (or not quit), have a few drinks, or use drugs.

Some of these indulgences may make people feel better temporarily, but others are poor choices. Maintaining a healthy lifestyle is a better choice. People feel better when they eat a healthy diet, engage in physical exercise, have positive interactions with friends or family, and get enough sleep. Indeed, these steps may be good for your immune system. Social isolation decreases immune function (Hawkley & Cacioppo, 2003), but social support improves its function (Miyazaki et al., 2003), as does getting enough sleep (Lange, Dimitrov, & Born, 2011). So, when you are feeling a lot of stress, try to withstand the temptation to indulge in unhealthy behaviors. Instead, prepare to treat yourself with healthy indulgences, such as time with friends or family, more (rather than less) sleep, or participation in sports or other physical activity.

much of the research on stress and various diseases is consistent with this model. Stress plays a role in the development of several physical disorders, including headache and infectious disease. The evidence for a relationship between stress and heart disease is complex. Stress is not directly responsible for hypertension, but some individuals show higher cardiac reactivity to stress, which may contribute to the development of cardiovascular disease. Experiences of discrimination are also a factor in reactivity. Stress also plays an indirect and minor role in the development of ulcers. Other diseases have a more direct relationship with stress, including diabetes, asthma, and rheumatoid arthritis, as well as some premature deliveries; the influence of stress on the immune system and the involvement of cytokines may underlie all these relationships.

Depression is related to the experience of stressful life events in people who are vulnerable, but not in others. The source of this vulnerability may be genetic, but experiences and attitudes may also contribute to increased vulnerability, especially the experience of abuse or maltreatment during childhood. Posttraumatic stress disorder, by definition, is related to stress, but most people who experience trauma do not develop this disorder. Thus, vulnerability is also a factor for the effect of stress on the development of anxiety disorders.

Answers

This chapter has addressed three basic questions:

1. How does the immune system function?

The immune system consists of tissues, organs, and processes that protect the body from invasion by foreign material such as bacteria, viruses, and fungi. The immune system marshals both a nonspecific response capable of attacking any invader and a specific response tailored to specific invaders. The immune system can also be a source of problems when it is deficient (as in HIV infection) or when it is too active (as in allergies and autoimmune diseases).

2. How does the field of psychoneuroimmunology relate behavior to disease?

The field of psychoneuroimmunology relates behavior to illness by finding relationships among behavior, the central nervous system, the immune system, and the endocrine system. Psychological factors can depress immune function, and some research has linked these factors with immune system depression and severity of physiological symptoms.

3. Does stress cause disease?

Research indicates that stress and illness are related, but as the diathesis–stress model holds, individuals must have some vulnerability for stress to cause disease. Stress is a moderate risk factor for headache and infectious disease. The role of stress in heart disease is complex; reactivity to stress may be involved in hypertension and the development of cardiovascular disease. Most ulcers can be traced to a bacterial infection rather than stress. The experience of stress is one of the many factors that contributes to psychological and mood disorders, but the route through which stress influences the development of these disorders may also be through the immune system.

Suggested Readings

Cohen, S. (2005). Keynote presentation at the eighth International Congress of Behavioral Medicine. *International Journal of Behavioral Medicine, 12*(3), 123–131. Shelton Cohen summarizes his fascinating research on stress and vulnerability to infectious disease.

Irwin, M. R. (2008). Human psychoneuroimmunology: 20 years of discovery. *Brain, Behavior and Immunity, 22*, 129–139. This recent review of the area of psychoneuroimmunology presents an overview of the immune system and the research on the links among psychosocial factors, immune system response, and the development of disease in humans.

Robles, T. F., Glaser, R., & Kiecolt-Glaser, J. K. (2005). Out of balance: A new look at chronic stress, depression, and immunity. *Current Directions in Psychological Science, 14*, 111–115. This short article looks at chronic stress and hypothesizes its relationship to depression through the immune system.

CHAPTER 7

Understanding and Managing Pain

CHAPTER OUTLINE

- **Real-World Profile of Aron Ralston**
- *Pain and the Nervous System*
- *The Meaning of Pain*
- *The Measurement of Pain*
- *Pain Syndromes*
- *Managing Pain*

QUESTIONS

This chapter focuses on five basic questions:

1. How does the nervous system register pain?

2. What is the meaning of pain?

3. How can pain be measured?

☑CHECK YOUR EXPERIENCES

Regarding Your Most Recent Episode of Pain

Nearly everybody experiences pain, but people experience pain in many different ways. The following questions allow you to understand the role pain plays in your life. To complete the exercise, think of the most significant pain that you have experienced within the past month, or if you have chronic pain, make your ratings with that pain problem in mind.

1. How long did your pain persist? _____ hours and _____ minutes

2. If this pain is chronic, how often does it occur?
   - ☐ Less than once a month
   - ☐ Once a month
   - ☐ Two or three times a month
   - ☐ About once a week
   - ☐ Two or three times a week
   - ☐ Daily
   - ☐ Throughout most of every day

3. What did you do to alleviate your pain? (Check all that apply.)
   - ☐ Took a prescription drug
   - ☐ Tried to relax
   - ☐ Did something to distract myself from the pain
   - ☐ Took an over-the-counter drug
   - ☐ Tried to ignore the pain

4. Place a mark on the line below to indicate how serious your pain was.

   Not at all   Unbearable

0	10	20	30	40	50	60	70	80	90	100

5. Place a mark on the line below to indicate how much this pain interfered with your daily routine.

   Not at all   Completely disrupted

0	10	20	30	40	50	60	70	80	90	100

6. During your pain, what did people around you do? (Check all that apply.)
   - ☐ Gave me a lot of sympathy
   - ☐ Did my work for me
   - ☐ Complained when I could not fulfill my normal responsibilities
   - ☐ Ignored me
   - ☐ Relieved me of my normal responsibilities

Completing this assessment will show you something about your own pain experience. Some of the items on this assessment are similar to those on some of the standardized pain scales described in "The Measurement of Pain" later in the chapter.

Real-World Profile of
ARON RALSTON

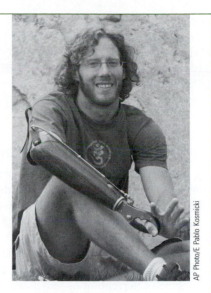

AP Photo/E Pablo Kosmicki

"I smiled as I cut off my arm. I was grateful to be free."—Aron Ralston, 27 years old.

In April 2003, Aron Ralston was hiking alone in a remote area of Utah when an 800-pound boulder dislodged and pinned his right arm against a canyon wall. Aron had not told anybody about his hiking plans, nor did he have a mobile phone with him. With no way to move the boulder, Aron was stranded. After 5 days of trying to free his arm from the boulder, Aron reached a grim realization: he could save his life only if he amputated his arm. With no food or water and little chance of rescue, this was his only option for survival.

To amputate his arm, Aron first used the weight of his body to snap the bones in his forearm. He then used a small, dull pocketknife to cut his flesh, muscles, and tendons. Aron, an experienced out-doorsman, then used his teeth and his other arm to tighten a tourniquet around the stump to stop the profuse blood loss. After freeing himself from the boulder, Aron hiked several more hours until he was eventually rescued.

Did Aron experience pain? Certainly he did. "I wanted to be free. I wanted to be with my family… So it was a case of whatever it took. It was going to hurt. I knew that," Aron said in a later interview. "The pain was irrelevant" (Rollings, 2011).

The complex interplay between the brain and the body is no more apparent than it is in the study of pain. You might think that a life without pain would be wonderful. However, pain plays a necessary and basic role in survival; pain is the body's way of calling attention to injury.

People with the rare genetic disorder called *congenital insensitivity to pain* are not able to feel pain. Because of this condition, these people must be carefully monitored. They often experience serious injuries without any awareness, such as broken bones, bitten tongues, cuts, burns, eye damage, and infections. Many people with this disorder die at a relatively young age, due to health problems that could have been treated if they were only able to heed the warning signs that pain provides.

In other cases, such as with people suffering from chronic pain, pain may exist for no clear reason. In the more extreme cases of phantom limb pain, people experience pain in parts of the body that do not exist! However, for most people, pain is an unpleasant and uncomfortable experience to be avoided whenever possible. Can people's beliefs about pain—such as Aron Ralston's belief that enduring excruciating pain was his only hope for survival—influence their experience of pain? In this chapter, we explore these many mysteries of pain. First, we examine how the nervous system registers pain.

Pain and the Nervous System

All sensory information, including pain, begins with sense receptors on or near the surface of the body. These receptors change physical energy—such as light, sound, heat, and pressure—into neural impulses. We can feel pain through any of our senses, but most of what we think of as pain originates as stimulation to the skin and muscles.

Neural impulses that originate in the skin and muscles are part of the peripheral nervous system (PNS); all neurons outside the brain and spinal cord (the central nervous system, or CNS) are part of the PNS. Neural impulses that originate in the PNS travel toward the spinal cord and brain. Therefore, it is possible to trace the path of neural impulses from the receptors to the brain. Tracing this path is a way to understand the physiology of pain.

The Somatosensory System

The **somatosensory system** conveys sensory information from the body to the brain. All the PNS neurons from the skin's surface and muscles are part of the somatic nervous system. For example, a neural impulse that originates in the right index finger travels through the somatic nervous system to the spinal cord. The interpretation of this information in the brain results in a person's perception of sensations about his or her body and its movements. The somatosensory system consists of several senses, including touch, light and deep pressure, cold, warmth, tickling, movement, and body position.

Afferent Neurons   Afferent neurons are one of three types of neurons—*afferent, efferent,* and *interneurons.* **Afferent** (sensory) **neurons** relay information from the sense organs toward the brain. **Efferent** (motor) **neurons** result in the movement of muscles or the stimulation of organs or glands; **interneurons** connect sensory to motor neurons. The sense organs contain afferent neurons, called **primary afferents**, with specialized receptors that convert physical energy into neural impulses, which travel to the spinal cord and then to the brain, where that information is processed and interpreted.

Involvement in Pain   **Nociception** refers to the process of perceiving pain. The skin is the largest of the sense organs, and receptors in the skin and organs—called **nociceptors**—are capable of responding to various types of stimulation that may cause tissue damage, such as heat, cold, crushing, cutting, and burning.

Some neurons that convey sensory information (including nociception) are covered with **myelin**, a fatty substance that acts as insulation. Myelinated afferent neurons, called A fibers, conduct neural impulses faster than unmyelinated **C fibers** do. In addition, neurons differ in size, and larger ones conduct impulses faster than smaller ones. Two types of A fibers are important in pain perception: the large

A-beta fibers and the smaller **A-delta fibers**. The large, myelinated A-beta fibers conduct impulses more than 100 times faster than small, unmyelinated C fibers (Melzack, 1973). C fibers are much more common; more than 60% of all sensory afferents are C fibers (Melzack & Wall, 1982). A-beta fibers fire with little stimulation, whereas C fibers require more stimulation to fire. Thus, these different types of fibers respond to different stimulation (Slugg, Meyer, & Campbell, 2000). Stimulation of A-delta fibers produces "fast" pain that is sharp or pricking, whereas stimulation of C fibers often results in a slower developing sensation of burning or dull aching (Chapman, Nakamura, & Flores, 1999).

The Spinal Cord

Protected by the vertebrae, the spinal cord is an avenue for sensory information traveling toward the brain and motor information coming from it. The spinal cord also produces the spinal reflexes. Damage to the spinal cord may interrupt the flow of sensory information, motor messages, or both, creating permanent impairment but leaving spinal reflexes intact. However, the most important role of the spinal cord is to provide a pathway for ascending sensory information and descending motor messages.

The afferent fibers group together after leaving the skin and this grouping forms a *nerve.* Nerves may be entirely afferent, entirely efferent, or a mixture of both. Just outside the spinal cord, each nerve bundle divides into two branches (see Figure 7.1). The sensory tracts, which funnel information toward the brain, enter the dorsal (toward the back) side of the spinal cord. The motor tracts, which come from the brain, exit the ventral (toward the stomach) side of the cord. On each side of the spinal cord, the dorsal root swells into a dorsal root ganglion, which contains the cell bodies of the primary afferent neurons. The neuron fibers extend into the **dorsal horns** of the spinal cord.

The dorsal horns contain several layers, or **laminae**. In general, the larger fibers penetrate more deeply into the laminae than the smaller fibers do (Melzack & Wall, 1982). The cells in lamina 1 and especially those in lamina 2 receive information from the small A-delta and C fibers; these two laminae form the **substantia gelatinosa**. Ronald Melzack and Peter Wall (1965) hypothesized that the substantia gelatinosa modulates sensory input information, and subsequent research

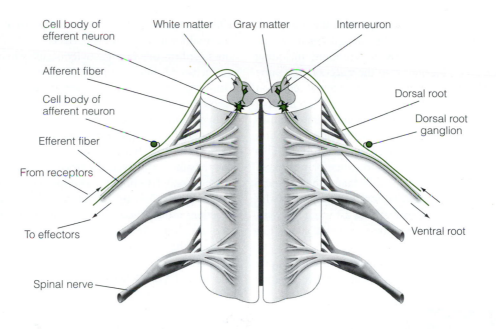

FIGURE 7.1 Cross-section through the spinal cord.

Source: Human physiology: From cells to systems (4th ed.), by L. Sherwood, 2001, p. 164. From SHERWOOD, Human Physiology, 4E. © 2001 Cengage Learning.

shows that they were correct (Chapman et al., 1999). Other laminae also receive projections from A and C fibers, as well as fibers descending from the brain and fibers from other laminae. These connections allow for elaborate interactions between sensory input from the body and the central processing of neural information in the brain.

The Brain

The **thalamus** receives information from afferent neurons in the spinal cord. After making connections in the thalamus, the information travels to other parts of the brain, including the **somatosensory cortex** in the cerebral cortex. The primary somatosensory cortex receives information from the thalamus that allows the entire surface of the skin to be mapped onto the somatosensory cortex. However, not all areas of the skin are equally represented. Figure 7.2 shows the area of the primary somatosensory cortex allotted to various regions of the body. Areas that are particularly rich in receptors occupy more of the somatosensory cortex than those areas that are poorer in receptors. For example, even though the back has more skin, the hands have more receptors, and therefore more area of the brain is devoted to interpreting the

information these receptors supply. This abundance of receptors also means that the hands are more sensitive; hands are capable of sensing stimuli that the back cannot.

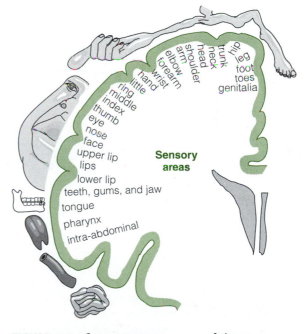

FIGURE 7.2 Somatosensory areas of the cortex.

A person's ability to localize pain on the skin's surface is more precise than it is for internal organs. Internal stimulation can also give rise to sensations, including pain, but the brain does not map the viscera in the same way that it maps the skin, so localizing internal sensation is much less precise. Intense stimulation of internal organs can result in the spread of neural stimulation to the pathways serving skin senses, creating the perception of visceral pain as originating on the skin's surface. This type of pain is called **referred pain**, when pain is experienced in a part of the body other than the site where the pain stimulus originates. For example, a person who feels pain in the upper arm may not associate this sensation with the heart, even though a heart attack can cause this kind of pain.

The development of positron emission tomography (PET) and functional magnetic resonance imaging (fMRI) allows researchers to study what happens in the brain when people experience pain. These techniques confirm that brain activity occurs when nociceptors are activated, but they paint a complex picture of how pain activates the brain (Apkarian, Bushnell, Treede, & Zubieta, 2005). Studies of brain responses to specific pain stimuli show activation in not only many areas of the brain, including the primary and secondary somatosensory cortices, but also the anterior cingulated cortex, the thalamus, and even the cerebellum in the lower part of the brain (Buffington, Hanlon, & McKeown, 2005; Davis, 2000). Adding to the complexity, an emotional reaction usually accompanies the experience of pain, and the brain imaging studies indicate activation in areas of the brain associated with emotion when people experience pain (Eisenberger, Gable, & Lieberman, 2007; see Would You Believe …? box). Thus, brain imaging

Would You BELIEVE...? Emotional and Physical Pain Are Mainly the Same in the Brain

Social rejection is painful. People use phrases such as "emotionally scarred," "slap in the face," "deeply hurt," or "crushed" to describe experiences of social rejection (MacDonald & Leary, 2005). This is as true for English speakers as it is for native speakers of German, Hebrew, Armenian, Cantonese, and Inuktitut.

It may not be a coincidence that people think about social pain in a similar manner to physical pain. Using functional magnetic resonance imaging, Naomi Eisenberger and her colleagues (Eisenberger & Lieberman, 2004; Eisenberger, Lieberman, & Williams, 2003) examined the brain activity of people whose feelings were "hurt" and found that the human brain reacts in similar ways to emotional and physical pain. The participants in this study experienced a virtual-reality, ball-tossing game called "Cyberball" while an fMRI scanner imaged their brains. During the game, the researchers excluded the participants from continuing the game by what participants believed were decisions of two other players. This exclusion represented social rejection, the type of situation in which people get their feelings hurt.

Eisenberger and her colleagues (2003) found that both the anterior cingulate cortex and the right ventral prefrontal cortex became more active during the experience of social exclusion. Importantly, these two regions of the brain also become more active when people experience *physical* pain. Furthermore, the level of activation in the anterior cingulate cortex correlated with the participants' ratings of distress. That is, the experience of social exclusion affected brain activity in a way that was similar to the experience of physical pain, suggesting that the two types of pain are similar in the brain.

If social and physical pain lead to similar patterns of brain activation, could a pill that relieves physical pain also relieve social pain? Acetaminophen—known by the brand name Tylenol—is a pain reliever that acts on the central nervous system. Nathan DeWall and colleagues (DeWall et al., 2010) examined whether acetaminophen would reduce people's reports of social pain. These researchers randomly assigned young adults to take either acetaminophen or a placebo pill daily for 3 weeks. Participants who took the acetaminophen pill reported less social pain over those 3 weeks—such as feeling hurt by being teased—than participants who took the placebo pill! In a follow-up fMRI study, these researchers additionally showed that participants who took acetaminophen prior to being socially excluded during a game of "Cyberball" showed less activity in the anterior cingulate cortex than participants who took a placebo pill.

Thus, there may be many similarities between social pain and physical pain. Will your doctor soon be prescribing two Tylenol as a remedy for both headache *and* heartache?

studies using PET and fMRI do not reveal a "pain center" in the brain. Rather, these studies show that the experience of pain produces a variety of activation in the brain, ranging from the lower brain to several centers in the forebrain.

Neurotransmitters and Pain

Neurotransmitters are chemicals that are synthesized and stored in neurons. The electrical action potential causes the release of neurotransmitters from neurons, which carries neural impulses across the synaptic cleft, the space between neurons. After flowing across the synaptic cleft, neurotransmitters act on other neurons by occupying specialized receptor sites. Each fits a specialized receptor site in the same way that a key fits into a lock; without the proper fit, the neurotransmitter will not affect the neuron. Sufficient amounts of neurotransmitters prompt the formation of an action potential in the stimulated neuron. Many different neurotransmitters exist, and each one is capable of causing an action.

In the 1970s, researchers (Pert & Snyder, 1973; Snyder, 1977) demonstrated that the neurochemistry of the brain plays a role in the perception of pain. This realization came about through an examination of how drugs affect the brain to alter pain perception. Receptors in the brain are sensitive to opiate drugs; that is, some neurons have receptor sites that opiate drugs are capable of occupying and activating. This discovery explained how opiates reduce pain—these drugs fit into brain receptors, modulate neuron activity, and alter pain perception.

The discovery of opiate receptors in the brain raised another question: Why does the brain respond to the resin of the opium poppy? In general, the brain is selective about the types of molecules that it allows to enter; only substances similar to naturally occurring neurochemicals can enter the brain. This reasoning led to the search for and identification of naturally occurring chemicals in the brain that affect pain perception. These neurochemicals have properties similar to those of the opiate drugs (Goldstein, 1976; Hughes, 1975). This discovery prompted a flurry of research that identified more opiate-like neurochemicals, including the **endorphins**, the *enkephalins*, and *dynorphin*. These neurochemicals seem to be one of the brain's mechanisms for modulating pain. Stress, suggestion, and electrical stimulation of the brain can all trigger the release of these endorphins (Turk, 2001). Thus, opiate drugs such as morphine may be effective at relieving pain because the brain contains its own system for pain relief, which the opiates stimulate.

Neurochemicals also seem to be involved in producing pain. The neurotransmitters *glutamate* and *substance P*, as well as the chemicals *bradykinin* and *prostaglandins*, sensitize or excite the neurons that relay pain messages (Sherwood, 2001). Glutamate and substance P act in the spinal cord to increase neural firings related to pain. Bradykinin and prostaglandins are substances released by tissue damage; they prolong the experience of pain by continuing to stimulate the nociceptors.

In addition, proteins produced by the immune system, *proinflammatory cytokines*, also influence pain (Watkins et al., 2007; Watkins & Maier, 2003, 2005). Infection and inflammation prompt the immune system to release these cytokines, which signal the nervous system and produce a range of responses associated with sickness, including decreased activity, increased fatigue, and increased pain sensitivity. Indeed, these cytokines may intensify chronic pain, by sensitizing the structures in the dorsal horn of the spinal cord that modulate the sensory message from the primary afferents (Watkins et al., 2007). Thus, the action of neurotransmitters and other chemicals produced by the body is complex, with the potential to both increase and decrease the experience of pain.

The Modulation of Pain

Research directed toward finding the brain structures involved in pain led to the discovery that one area of the brain, the **periaqueductal gray**, is involved in modulating pain. This brain structure is in the midbrain, close to the center. When it is stimulated, neural activity spreads downward to the spinal cord, and pain relief occurs (Goffaux, Redmond, Rainville, & Marchand, 2007; Sherwood, 2001). Neurons in the periaqueductal gray run down into the reticular formation and the **medulla**, a structure in the lower part of the brain that is also involved in pain perception (Fairhurst, Weich, Dunckley, & Tracey, 2007). These neurons descend into the spinal cord and make connections with neurons in the substantia gelatinosa. The result is that the dorsal horn neurons cannot carry pain information to the thalamus.

The inhibition of transmission also involves some familiar neurotransmitters. Endorphins in the periaqueductal gray initiate activity in this descending inhibitory system. Figure 7.3 illustrates this type of modulation. The substantia gelatinosa contains

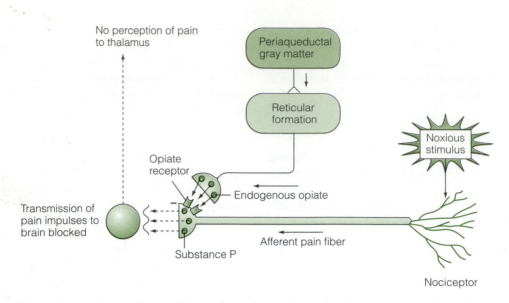

FIGURE 7.3   Descending pathways from the periaqueductal gray prompt the release of endogenous opiates (endorphins) that block the transmission of pain impulses to the brain.

Source: Human physiology: From cells to systems (4th ed.), by L. Sherwood, 2001, p. 181. From SHERWOOD, Human Physiology, 4E. © 2001 Cengage Learning.

synapses that use enkephalin as a transmitter. Indeed, neurons that contain enkephalin seem to be concentrated in the same parts of the brain that contain substance P, the transmitter that activates pain messages (McLean, Skirboll, & Pert, 1985).

These elaborate physical and chemical systems are the body's way of modulating the neural impulses of pain. The value of pain is obvious. Pain after injury is adaptive, furnishing a reminder of injury and discouraging activity that adds to the damage. In some situations, however, pain modulation is also adaptive. When people or other animals are fighting or fleeing, being able to ignore pain can be an advantage. Thus, the nervous system has complex systems that allow not only for the perception but also for the modulation of pain.

cortex includes a map of the skin, with more of the cortex devoted to areas of the body richer in skin receptors. The A-delta and C fibers are involved in pain, with A-delta fibers relaying pain messages quickly and C fibers sending pain messages more slowly.

The brain and spinal cord also contain mechanisms for modulating sensory input and thereby affecting the perception of pain. One mechanism is through the naturally occurring neurochemicals that relieve pain and mimic the action of opiate drugs, which exist in many places in the central and peripheral nervous systems. The second mechanism is a system of descending control through the periaqueductal gray and the medulla. This system affects the activity of the spinal cord and provides a descending modulation of activity in the spinal cord.

IN SUMMARY

The activation of receptors in the skin results in neural impulses that move along afferent pathways to the spinal cord by way of the dorsal root. In the spinal cord, the afferent impulses continue to the thalamus in the brain. The primary somatosensory

The Meaning of Pain

Until about 100 years ago, people thought that pain was a direct consequence of physical injury, and the extent of tissue damage determined the intensity of pain. Near the end of the 19th century, C. A. Strong and others reconceptualized pain. Strong (1895) hypothesized that pain was due to two factors: the sensation and the person's reaction to that sensation. In this view, psychological factors and organic causes were of equal importance. This attention to psychological factors signaled the beginning of a new definition, an altered view of the experience, and new theories of pain.

Definition of Pain

Pain is an almost universal experience. Only those rare people with congenital insensitivity to pain escape the experience of pain. Nevertheless, pain is remarkably difficult to define. Some experts (Covington, 2000) concentrate on the physiology that underlies the perception of pain, whereas others (Wall, 2000) emphasize the subjective nature of pain. These different views reflect the multidimensional nature of pain, which the International Association for the Study of Pain (IASP) has incorporated into its definition. The IASP Subcommittee on Taxonomy (1979, p. 250) defined pain as "an unpleasant sensory and emotional experience associated with actual or potential tissue damage, or described in terms of such damage." Most pain researchers and clinicians continue to agree with this definition.

Another way to understand the meaning of pain is to view it in terms of three stages: acute, chronic, and prechronic (Keefe, 1982). **Acute pain** is the type of pain that most people experience when injured; it includes pains from cuts, burns, childbirth, surgery, dental work, and other injuries. Its duration is normally brief. This type of pain is ordinarily adaptive; it signals the person to avoid further injury. In contrast, **chronic pain** endures over months or even years. This type of pain may be due to a chronic condition such as rheumatoid arthritis, or it may be the result of an injury that persists beyond the time of healing (Turk & Melzack, 2001). Chronic pain frequently exists in the absence of any identifiable tissue damage. It is not adaptive but, rather, can be debilitating and demoralizing and often leads to feelings of helplessness and hopelessness. Chronic pain never has a biological benefit.

Perhaps the most crucial stage of pain is the **prechronic pain** stage, which comes between the acute and the chronic stages. This period is critical because the person either overcomes the pain at this time or develops the feelings of fear and helplessness that can lead to chronic pain. These three stages do not exhaust all possibilities of pain. Several other types of pain exist, the most common of which is **chronic recurrent pain**, or pain marked by alternating episodes of intense pain and no pain. A common example of chronic recurrent pain is headache pain.

The Experience of Pain

The experience of pain is individual and subjective, but situational and cultural factors influence that experience. Henry Beecher, an anesthesiologist, was one of the first researchers to identify the situational influences on the experience of pain. Beecher (1946) observed soldiers wounded at the Anzio beachhead during World War II. Beecher noted that, despite their serious battle injuries, many of these men reported very little pain. What made the experience of pain different in this situation? These men had been removed from the battlefront and thus from the threat of death or further injury, in the same way that Aron Ralston's amputation of his own arm led to his rescue. Under these conditions, the wounded soldiers were in a cheerful, optimistic state of mind. In contrast, civilian patients with comparable injuries experienced much more pain and requested more pain-killing drugs than the soldiers (Beecher, 1956). These findings prompted Beecher (1956) to conclude that "the intensity of suffering is largely determined by what the pain means to the patient" (p. 1609) and that "the extent of wound bears only a slight relationship, if any (often none at all), to the pain experienced" (p. 1612). Finally, Beecher (1957) described pain as a two-dimensional experience consisting of both a sensory stimulus and an emotional component. Other pain researchers came to accept Beecher's view of pain as a psychological and physical phenomenon.

Battle wounds are an extreme example of sudden injury, but people who experience injuries that are more mundane also report variable amounts of pain. For example, most—but not all—people admitted to an emergency room for treatment of injury report pain (Wall, 2000). Pain is more common among people with injuries such as broken bones, sprains, and stabs than among people with injuries to the skin. Indeed, 53% of those with cuts, burns, or scrapes report that they feel no pain for at least some time after their injury, whereas only 28% of those with deep tissue injury fail to feel immediate pain. These individual variations of pain contrast with people who have been tortured, all of whom feel pain, even though their injuries may not be as serious as those of people reporting to an emergency room. People who believe that a

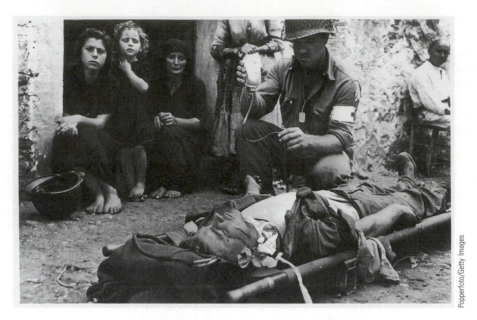

Popperfoto/Getty Images

The experience of pain varies with the situation. Wounded soldiers removed from the front lines may feel little pain despite extreme injuries.

stimulus will be harmful experience more pain than those who have different beliefs about the situation (Arntz & Claassens, 2004). The threat, intent to inflict pain, and lack of control give torture a very different meaning from unintentional injury and thus produce a different pain experience. These variations in pain perception suggest either individual differences, a cultural component for variations in pain-related behaviors, or some combination of these factors.

Individual Differences in the Experience of Pain

Individual factors and personal experience make a difference in the experience of pain. People learn to associate stimuli related to a painful experience with the pain and thus develop classically conditioned responses to the associated stimuli (Sanders, 2006). For example, many people dislike the smell of hospitals or become anxious when they hear the dentist's drill because they have had experiences associating these stimuli with pain.

Operant conditioning may also play an important role in pain by providing a means for acute pain to develop into chronic pain. Pioneering pain researcher John J. Bonica (1990) believed that being rewarded for pain behaviors is a key factor that transforms acute pain into chronic pain. According to Bonica, people who receive attention, sympathy, relief from normal responsibilities, and disability compensation for their injuries and pain behaviors are more likely to develop chronic pain than are people who have similar injury but receive fewer rewards. Consistent with Bonica's hypotheses, headache patients report more pain behaviors and greater pain intensity when their spouses or significant others respond to pain complaints with seemingly helpful responses, such as taking over chores, turning on the television, or encouraging the patient to rest (Pence, Thorn, Jensen, & Romano, 2008).

Despite people's belief in a "pain-resistant" personality, no such thing exists. Some people such as Aron Ralston endure pain with little or no complaint, but nevertheless, they perceive discomfort. They display no sign of their pain because of situational factors, cultural sanctions against the display of emotion, or some combination of these two factors. For example, some Native American, African, and South Pacific island cultures have initiation rituals that involve the silent endurance of pain. These rituals may include body piercing, cutting, tattooing, burning, or beating. To show signs of pain would result in failure, so individuals are motivated to hide their pain. Individuals may withstand these injuries with no visible sign of distress yet react with an obvious display of pain behavior to an unintentional injury in a situation outside the ritual (Wall, 2000). These variations in expressions of pain suggest cultural variations in pain behaviors rather than the existence of a pain-resistant personality.

If a pain-resistant personality does not exist, could there be evidence for a *pain-prone* personality? Research does not support the concept of a pain-prone personality (Turk, 2001). However, people who are anxious, worried, and have a negative outlook tend to experience heightened sensitivity to pain (Janssen, 2002). Fear may be part of this negative outlook; individuals who experience a heightened fear of pain also experience more pain (Leeuw et al., 2007). In addition, people with severe chronic pain are much more likely than others to suffer from some type of psychopathology, such as anxiety disorders or depression (McWilliams, Goodwin, & Cox, 2004; Williams, Jacka, Pasco, Dodd, & Berk, 2006). However, the direction of the cause and effect is not always clear (Gatchel & Epker, 1999). Patients suffering from chronic pain are more likely to be depressed, to abuse alcohol and other drugs, and to suffer from personality disorders. Some chronic pain patients develop these disorders as a result of their chronic pain, but others have some form of psychopathology prior to the beginning of their pain. Thus, individual differences exist in the experience of pain, but cultural and situational factors are more important.

Cultural Variations in Pain Perception   Large culture differences exist in pain sensitivity and the expression of pain behaviors. In addition, cultural background and social context affect the experience (Cleland, Palmer, & Venzke, 2005) and treatment (Cintron & Morrison, 2006) of pain. These differences come from varying meanings that different cultures attach to pain and from stereotypes associated with various cultural groups.

Cultural expectations for pain are apparent in the pain that women experience during childbirth (Callister, 2003; Streltzer, 1997). Some cultures hold birth as a dangerous and painful process, and women in these cultures reflect these expectations by experiencing great pain. Other cultures expect quiet acceptance during the experience of giving birth, and women in those cultures tend not to show much evidence of pain. When questioned about their apparent lack of pain, however, these women reported that they felt pain but that their culture did not expect women to show pain under these circumstances, so they did not (Wall, 2000).

Since the 1950s, studies have compared pain expression for people from various ethnic backgrounds

(Ondeck, 2003; Streltzer, 1997). Some studies have shown differences and others have not, but the studies tend to suffer from the criticism of stereotyping. For example, a stereotype exists of Italians as people who show a lot of emotion. Consistent with this stereotype, studies have found that Italian Americans express more distress and demand more pain medication than "Yankees" (Americans of Anglo-Saxon descent who have lived in the United States for generations), who have a reputation for stoically ignoring pain (Rollman, 1998). These variations in pain behaviors among different cultures may reflect behavioral differences in learning and modeling, differences in sensitivity to pain, or some combination of these factors.

Laboratory studies confirm differences between African Americans and European Americans in sensitivity to painful stimuli. African Americans and Hispanic Americans show higher sensitivity to pain than European Americans (Rahim-Williams et al., 2007). These sensitivities carry over to clinical pain (Edwards, Fillingim, & Keefe, 2001) and chronic pain (Riley et al., 2002); African Americans report higher levels of both. These differences may be due to racial and ethnic differences in endogenous pain modulation as well as differences in coping strategies (Anderson, Green, & Payne, 2009).

Greater sensitivity to pain is doubly unfortunate for African Americans because physicians are more likely to underestimate their pain (Staton et al., 2007) and to prescribe less analgesia than they do for European Americans as outpatients, in hospitals, and in nursing homes, despite similar complaints about pain (Cintron & Morrison, 2006). Hispanics receive similar treatment—less analgesia in many types of medical settings. This discrimination in treatment is a source of needless pain for patients from these ethnic groups.

Gender Differences in Pain Perception   Another common stereotype about pain perception is that women are more sensitive to pain than men (Robinson et al., 2003), and this belief has some research support. Women report pain more readily than men (Fillingim, King, Ribeiro-Dasilva, Rahim-Williams, & Riley, 2009). Women also experience disabilities and pain-related conditions more often than men (Croft, Blyth, & van der Windt, 2010; Henderson, Gandevia, & Macefield, 2008).

One explanation for these gender differences involves gender roles and socialization. A study of

Swedish 9-, 12-, and 15-year-olds (Sundblad, Saartok, & Engström, 2007) showed more frequent reports of pain from girls than boys, and a decrease in pain reports for older boys but an increase among older girls. These changes are consistent with adoption of the male and female gender role; boys may be learning to deny pain, whereas girls are learning that reporting pain is consistent with their gender role. Consistent with this view, men who identify more highly with the male gender role are less likely than other men and less likely than women to report pain in a laboratory experiment (Pool, Schwegler, Theodore, & Fuchs, 2007).

Another explanation for gender differences posits that women may be more vulnerable than men to developing certain pain conditions. Some chronic pain syndromes occur only or mostly in women, such as chronic fatigue syndrome, endometriosis, and fibromyalgia (Fillingim et al., 2009). Sex hormones and gender differences in coping strategies may also contribute to gender differences in sensitivity to musculoskeletal pain (Institute of Medicine, 2011; Picavet, 2010).

However, other research fails to find dramatic differences between men and women. A study on women and men who had dental surgery (Averbuch & Katzper, 2000) reported that more women than men described their pain as severe but found very small differences between pain reports for men and women and no difference in their responses to analgesic drugs. A similar study with adolescents (Logan & Rose, 2004) showed similar results: Girls reported more pain but used no more analgesics than boys. Another study (Kim et al., 2004) found that women reported pain more readily than men in a laboratory situation but showed similar responses to pain associated with oral surgery. One commonality among these studies is that women report higher anxiety and threat related to their experiences of pain, which may be an important factor in gender differences in pain perception (Leeuw et al., 2007).

Theories of Pain

How people experience pain is the subject of a number of theories. Of the several models of pain, two capture the divergent ways of conceptualizing pain: the specificity theory and the gate control theory.

Specificity Theory
Specificity theory explains pain by hypothesizing that specific pain fibers and pain pathways exist, making the experience of pain virtually equal to the amount of tissue damage or injury (Craig, 2003). The

view that pain is the result of transmission of pain signals from the body to a "pain center" in the brain originated with Descartes, who in the 1600s proposed that the body works mechanically (DeLeo, 2006). Descartes hypothesized that the mind works by a different set of principles, and body and mind interact in a limited way. Descartes's view influenced not only the development of a science of physiology and medicine but also the view that pain is a physical experience largely uninfluenced by psychological factors (Melzack, 1993).

Working under the assumption that pain was the transmission of one type of sensory information, researchers tried to determine which type of receptor conveyed what type of sensory information (Melzack, 1973). For example, they tried to determine which type of receptor relayed information about heat, cold, and other types of pain. The attempt failed, as researchers found that some parts of the body (such as the cornea of the eye) contain only one type of receptor, yet those areas feel a full range of sensations. Specificity does exist in the different types of sensory receptors and nerve fibers, such as light touch, pressure, itching, pricking, warmth, and cold (Craig, 2003). Yet, each of these sensations can become painful when intense, so any simple version of specificity theory is not valid.

The Gate Control Theory
In 1965, Ronald Melzack and Peter Wall formulated a new theory of pain, which suggests that pain is *not* the result of a linear process that begins with sensory stimulation of pain pathways and ends with the experience of pain. Rather, pain perception is subject to a number of modulations that can influence the experience of pain. These modulations begin in the spinal cord.

Melzack and Wall hypothesized that structures in the spinal cord act as a gate for the sensory input that the brain interprets as pain. Melzack and Wall's theory is thus known as the **gate control theory** (see Figure 7.4). It has a basis in physiology but explains both sensory and psychological aspects of pain perception.

Melzack and Wall (1965, 1982, 1988) pointed out that the nervous system is never at rest; the patterns of neural activation constantly change. When sensory information from the body reaches the dorsal horns of the spinal cord, that neural impulse enters a system that is already active. The existing activity in the spinal cord and brain influences the fate of incoming sensory information, sometimes amplifying and sometimes decreasing the incoming neural signals. The gate

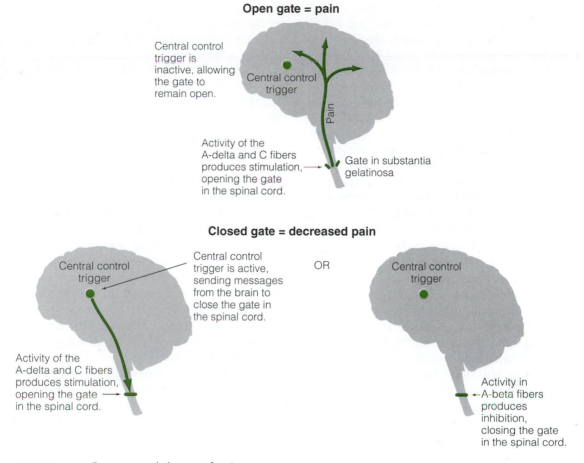

Open gate = pain

Central control trigger is inactive, allowing the gate to remain open.

Central control trigger

Pain

Activity of the A-delta and C fibers produces stimulation, opening the gate in the spinal cord.

Gate in substantia gelatinosa

Closed gate = decreased pain

Central control trigger

Central control trigger is active, sending messages from the brain to close the gate in the spinal cord.

OR

Central control trigger

Activity of the A-delta and C fibers produces stimulation, opening the gate in the spinal cord.

Activity in A-beta fibers produces inhibition, closing the gate in the spinal cord.

FIGURE 7.4   Gate control theory of pain.

control theory hypothesizes that these complex modulations in the spinal cord and in the brain are critical factors in the perception of pain.

According to the gate control theory, neural mechanisms in the spinal cord act like a gate that can either increase (open the gate) or decrease (close the gate) the flow of neural impulses. Figure 7.4 shows the results of opening and closing the gate. With the gate open, impulses flow through the spinal cord toward the brain, neural messages reach the brain, and the person feels pain. With the gate closed, impulses do not ascend through the spinal cord, messages do not reach the brain, and the person does not feel pain. Moreover, sensory input is subject to modulation, depending on the activity of the large A-beta fibers, the small A-delta fibers, and the small C fibers that enter the spinal cord and synapse in the dorsal horns.

The dorsal horns of the spinal cord are composed of several layers (laminae). As described earlier, two of these laminae make up the substantia gelatinosa, which is the hypothesized location of the gate (Melzack & Wall, 1965). Both the small A-delta and C fibers and the large A-beta fibers travel through the substantia gelatinosa, which also receives projections from other laminae (Melzack & Wall, 1982, 1988). This arrangement of neurons provides the physiological basis for the modulation of incoming sensory impulses. Melzack and Wall hypothesized these mechanisms when they formulated the gate control theory, but subsequent research confirms the modulation of afferent messages in the dorsal horns of the spinal cord.

Melzack and Wall (1982) proposed that activity in the small A-delta and C fibers causes prolonged activity in the spinal cord. This type of activity would promote sensitivity, which increases sensitivity to pain. Activity of these small fibers would thus open the gate. On the other hand, activity of the large A-beta fibers produces an initial burst of activity in the spinal cord, followed by inhibition. Activity of these fibers closes the gate. Subsequent research does not confirm this feature of the gate control theory in a clear way (Turk, 2001). Activity of A-delta and C fibers seems to relate to the experience of pain, but under conditions of inflammation, increased activity of A-beta fibers can increase rather than decrease pain.

The gate may be closed by activity in the spinal cord, as well as by messages that descend from the brain. Melzack and Wall (1965, 1982, 1988) proposed the concept of a **central control trigger** consisting of nerve impulses that descend from the brain and influence the gating mechanism. They hypothesized that this system consists of large neurons that conduct impulses rapidly. These impulses from the brain, which cognitive processes can influence, affect the opening and closing of the gate in the spinal cord. That is, Melzack and Wall proposed that the experience of pain is influenced by beliefs and prior experience, and they also hypothesized a physiological mechanism that can account for such factors in pain perception. As we discussed, the periaqueductal gray matter furnishes descending controls (Mason, 2005), which is consistent with this aspect of the gate control theory.

According to the gate control theory, then, pain has not only sensory components but also motivational and emotional components. This aspect of the theory revolutionized conceptualizations of pain (Melzack, 2008). The gate control theory explains the influence of cognitive aspects of pain and allows for learning and experience to affect the experience of pain. Anxiety, worry, depression, and focusing on an injury can increase pain by affecting the central control trigger, thus opening the gate. Distraction, relaxation, and positive emotions can cause the gate to close, thereby decreasing pain. The gate control theory is not specific about how these experiences affect pain, but recent experimental research confirms that factors such as mood indeed influence the extent of pain-related activity in the central nervous system. A team of Japanese researchers experimentally induced participants to experience either a sad, neutral, or positive mood. Following the mood induction, all participants experienced moderately painful electric shocks. Participants in a sad mood showed greater activity in brain regions associated with pain than participants in a neutral or positive mood (Yoshino et al., 2010). Thus, a person's emotional state modulated the amount of pain-related activity in the brain.

Many personal experiences with pain are consistent with the gate control theory. When you accidentally hit your finger with a hammer, many of the small fibers are activated, opening the gate. An emotional reaction accompanies your perception of acute pain. You may then grasp your injured finger and rub it. According to the gate control theory, rubbing stimulates the large fibers that close the gate, thus blocking stimulation from the small fibers and decreasing pain.

The gate control theory also explains how injuries can go virtually unnoticed. If sensory input enters into a heavily activated nervous system, then the stimulation may not be perceived as pain. A tennis player may sprain an ankle during a game but not notice the acute pain because of excitement and concentration on the game. After the game is finished, however, the player may notice the pain because the nervous system functions at a different level of activation and the gate opens more easily.

Although it is not universally accepted, the gate control theory is the most influential theory of pain (Sufka & Price, 2002). This theory allows for the complexities of pain experiences. Melzack and Wall proposed the gate control theory before the discovery of the body's own opiates or of the descending control mechanisms through the periaqueductal gray and the medulla, both of which offer supporting evidence. The gate control theory has been and continues to be successful in spurring research and generating interest in the psychological and perceptual factors involved in pain.

Melzack (1993, 2005) proposed an extension to the gate control theory called the *neuromatrix theory*, which places a stronger emphasis on the brain's role in pain perception. He hypothesized a network of brain neurons that he called the neuromatrix, "a large, widespread network of neurons that consists of loops between the thalamus and cortex as well as between the cortex and limbic system" (Melzack, 2005, p. 86). Normally, the neuromatrix processes incoming sensory information including pain, but the neuromatrix acts even in the absence of sensory input, producing phantom limb sensations. Melzack's neuromatrix theory extends gate control theory but maintains that pain perception is part of a complex process affected not only by sensory input but also by activity of the nervous system and by experience and expectation.

IN SUMMARY

Although the extent of damage is important in the pain experience, personal perception is also important. Pain can be acute, prechronic, or chronic, depending on the length of time that the pain has persisted. Acute pain is usually adaptive and lasts for less than 6 months. Chronic pain continues beyond the time of healing, often in the absence of detectable tissue damage. Prechronic pain occurs between acute and chronic pain. All of these stages of pain appear in pain syndromes, such as headache pain, low back pain, arthritic pain, cancer pain, and phantom limb pain.

Several models seek to explain pain, but specificity theory does not capture the complexity of the pain experience. The gate control theory is the most influential model of pain. This theory holds that mechanisms in the spinal cord and the brain can increase or diminish pain. Since its formulation, increased knowledge of the physiology of the brain and spinal cord has supported this theory. The neuromatrix theory extends the gate control theory by hypothesizing the existence of a set of neurons in the brain that maintain a pattern of activity that defines the self and yet also responds to expectations and to incoming signals such as pain.

The Measurement of Pain

"I have been told to 'suck it up'; I have been asked if I was having trouble at home; I have been accused of being a 'druggy'. I have also found some practitioners who could 'read the tea leaves,' so to speak and TELL ME how much pain I must be in, based on my physical exam."—A person with chronic pain (Institute of Medicine, 2011, p. 59)

Pain, at its core, is a subjective experience. No doctor or other outside observer can know how much pain a patient experiences. The subjective nature of pain presents a great challenge to researchers and clinicians who seek to understand and treat pain. How can clinicians and researchers assess pain most accurately? What are reliable and valid ways of assessing pain, other than asking a person to tell you?

Asking physicians (Marquié et al., 2003; Staton et al., 2007) or nurses (Wilson & McSherry, 2006) to rate their

patients' pain is not a valid approach because these professionals tend to underestimate patients' pain. Asking people to rate their own pain on a scale would seem reliable and valid. Who knows better than patients themselves how much pain they are feeling? However, some pain experts (Turk & Melzack, 2001) have questioned both the reliability and the validity of this procedure, stating that people do not reliably remember how they rated an earlier pain. For this reason, pain researchers have developed a number of techniques for measuring pain, including (1) self-report ratings, (2) behavioral assessments, and (3) physiological measures.

Self-Reports

Self-report pain assessments ask people to evaluate and make ratings of their pain on simple rating scales, standardized pain inventories, or standardized personality tests.

Rating Scales   Simple rating scales are an important part of the pain measurement toolbox. For example, patients may rate the intensity of their pain on a scale from 0 to 10 (or 0 to 100), with 10 being the most excruciating pain possible and 0 being the complete absence of pain. Such numeric ratings showed advantages over other types of self-reports in a comparison of several approaches to pain assessment (Gagliese, Weizblit, Ellis, & Chan, 2005).

A similar technique is the Visual Analog Scale (VAS), which is simply a line anchored on the left by a phrase such as "no pain" and on the right by a phrase such as "worst pain imaginable." Both the VAS and numerical rating scales are easy to use. For some pain patients, the VAS is superior to word descriptors of pain (Rosier, Iadarola, & Coghill, 2002) and numerical ratings (Bigatti & Cronan, 2002). Visual analog scales have been criticized as sometimes being confusing to patients not accustomed to quantifying their experience (Burckhardt & Jones, 2003b) and difficult for those who cannot comprehend the instructions, such as older people with dementia or young children (Feldt, 2007). Another rating scale is the face scales, consisting of 8 to 10 drawings of faces expressing emotions from intense joy to intense pain; patients merely indicate which illustration best fits their level of pain (Jensen & Karoly, 2001). This type of rating is effective with both children and older adults (Benaim et al., 2007). A limitation of each of these rating scales is that they measure only the intensity of pain; they do not tap into patients' verbal description of their pain. Despite this limitation, this approach to pain assessment may be the simplest and most effective for many patients.

Pain Questionnaires Ronald Melzack (1975, p. 278) contended that describing pain on a single dimension was "like specifying the visual world only in terms of light flux without regard to pattern, color, texture, and the many other dimensions of visual experience." Rating scales make no distinction, for example, among pains that are pounding, shooting, stabbing, or hot.

To rectify some of these weaknesses, Melzack (1975) developed the McGill Pain Questionnaire (MPQ), an inventory that provides a subjective report of pain and categorizes it in three dimensions: sensory, affective, and evaluative. *Sensory* qualities of pain are its temporal, spatial, pressure, and thermal properties; *affective* qualities are the fear, tension, and autonomic properties that are part of the pain experience; and *evaluative* qualities are the words that describe the subjective overall intensity of the pain experience.

The MPQ has four parts that assess these three dimensions of pain. Part 1 consists of front and back drawings of the human body. Patients mark on these drawings indicating the areas where they feel pain. Part 2 consists of 20 sets of words describing pain, and patients draw a circle around the one word in each set that most accurately describes their pain. These adjectives appear from least to most painful— for example, *nagging, nauseating, agonizing, dreadful,* and *torturing.* Part 3 asks how the patient's pain has changed with time. Part 4 measures the intensity of pain on a 5-point scale from *mild* to *excruciating.* This fourth part yields a Present Pain Intensity (PPI) score.

The MPQ is the most frequently used pain questionnaire (Piotrowski, 1998, 2007), and a short form of the McGill Pain Questionnaire (Melzack, 1987) preserves the multidimensional assessment and correlates highly with scores on the standard MPQ (Burckhardt & Jones, 2003a). Clinicians use the MPQ to assess pain relief in a variety of treatment programs and in multiple pain syndromes (Melzack & Katz, 2001). The MPQ also exists in 26 different languages (Costa, Maher, McAuley, & Costa, 2009). The short form is growing in use and demonstrates a high degree of reliability (Grafton, Foster, & Wright, 2005). In addition, a computerized, touch-screen administration of this test exists, which shows a high degree of consistency with the paper-and-pencil version (Cook et al., 2004).

The Multidimensional Pain Inventory (MPI), also known as the West Haven–Yale Multidimensional Pain Inventory (WHYMPI), is another assessment tool specifically designed for pain patients (Kerns, Turk, & Rudy, 1985). The 52-item MPI is divided into three sections. The first rates characteristics of the pain, interference with patients' lives and functioning, and patients' moods. The second section rates patients' perceptions of the responses of significant others, and the third measures how often patients engage in each of the 30 different daily activities. Using this inventory allowed researchers (Kerns et al., 1985) to develop 13 different scales that captured different dimensions of the lives of pain patients.

Standardized Psychological Tests In addition to the specialized pain inventories, clinicians and researchers also use a variety of standardized psychological tests in assessing pain. The most frequently used of these tests is the MMPI-2 (Arbisi & Seime, 2006). The MMPI measures clinical diagnoses such as depression, paranoia, schizophrenia, and other psychopathologies. Research from the early 1950s (Hanvik, 1951) found that different types of pain patients could be differentiated on several MMPI scales, and more recent research (Arbisi & Seime, 2006) confirms the use of the MMPI for such assessment. One of the major advantages of using the MMPI-2 for pain assessment is its ability to detect patients who are being dishonest about their experience of pain (Bianchini, Etherton, Greve, Heinly, & Meyers, 2008).

Researchers also use the Beck Depression Inventory (Beck, Ward, Mendelson, Mock, & Erbaugh, 1961) and the Symptom Checklist–90 (Derogatis, 1977) to measure pain. The Beck Depression Inventory is a short self-report questionnaire that assesses depression; the Symptom Checklist–90 measures symptoms related to various types of behavioral problems. People with chronic pain often experience negative moods, so the relationship between scores on psychological tests and pain is not surprising. However, factor analyses of the Beck Depression Inventory with pain patients (Morley, de C. Williams, & Black, 2002; Poole, Branwell, & Murphy, 2006) indicate that pain patients present a different profile than depressed people with no chronic pain. Specifically, chronic pain patients are less likely to endorse negative beliefs about the self than depressed people but are more likely to report behavioral and emotional symptoms of depression. Like the MMPI-2, the Symptom Checklist–90 (McGuire &

Shores, 2001) is also able to differentiate pain patients from those instructed to fake pain symptoms. Thus, these standardized psychological tests may have something to offer in the assessment of pain, including the ability to identify people who may be exaggerating symptoms of pain.

Behavioral Assessments

A second major approach to pain measurement is observation of patients' behavior. Influential researcher Wilbert Fordyce (1974) noted that people in pain often groan, grimace, rub, sigh, limp, miss work, remain in bed, or engage in other behaviors that signify to observers that they may be suffering from pain, including lowered levels of activity, use of pain medication, body posture, and facial expressions. Behavioral observation began as an informal way to assess pain; Fordyce (1976) trained spouses to record pain behaviors, working to obtain a list of between 5 and 10 behaviors that indicate pain for each individual.

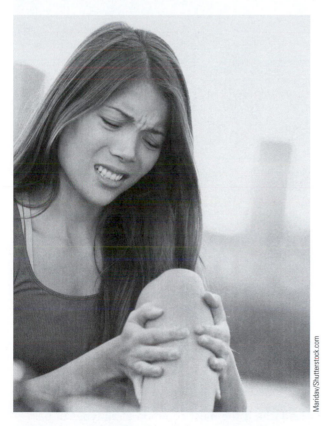

Facial expressions provide a behavioral measure of pain.

Health care professionals tend to underestimate patients' pain (Staton et al., 2007; Wilson & McSherry, 2006) and require extensive training to overcome their bias (Keefe & Smith, 2002; Rapoff, 2003). Another way for health care professionals to assess pain is through the development of behavioral observation into a standardized assessment strategy (Keefe & Smith, 2002). During an observational protocol, pain patients perform a series of tasks while a trained observer records their body movements and facial expressions, noting signs of pain. For example, patients with low back pain may be asked to sit, stand, walk, and recline during a 1- to 2-minute observation. The session may be videotaped to allow other observers to rate pain-related behaviors such as limping and grimacing. This strategy for collecting information yields data about pain behaviors, and analyses confirm that these data are reliable and valid indicators of pain (Keefe & Smith, 2002).

Behavioral observation is especially useful in assessing the pain of people who have difficulty furnishing self-reports—children, the cognitively impaired, and some elderly patients. This approach includes assessments of children's pain (von Baeyer & Spagrud, 2007) and a coding system that allows observers to assess the pain of infants by observing five facial movements and two hand actions (Holsti & Grunau, 2007). Many older patients can report on their pain, but some cannot, and behavioral observation of facial expressions allows an assessment of this difficult group (Clark, Jones, & Pennington, 2004; Lints-Martindale, Hadjistavropoulos, Barber, & Gibson, 2007).

Physiological Measures

A third approach to pain assessment is the use of physiological measures (Gatchel, 2005). Electromyography (EMG), which measures the level of muscle tension, is one of these physiological techniques. The notion behind this approach is that pain increases muscle tension. Attaching the measuring electrodes to the surface of the skin provides an easy way to measure muscle tension, but questions have arisen over the validity of this measurement as a pain indicator. For example, Herta Flor (2001) reported little consistency between self-reports of pain and EMG levels. A meta-analysis of EMG assessment of low back pain (Geisser et al., 2005) indicated that EMG was useful in discriminating those with versus those without low back pain, but EMG alone was not an adequate assessment.

Researchers have also attempted to assess pain through several autonomic indices, including such involuntary processes as hyperventilation, blood flow in the temporal artery, heart rate, hand surface temperature, finger pulse volume, and skin conductance level. Heart rate predicts perceptions of pain, but only for men (Loggia, Juneau, & Bushnell, 2011; Tousignant-Laflamme, Rainville, & Marchand, 2005). In experimental tasks, changes in skin conductance levels correlate with changes in the intensity of a pain stimulus and changes in pain perceptions; however, this method is not well suited for assessing differences between people in clinical pain reports (Loggia et al., 2011). Researchers and clinicians primarily use these physiological assessments with patients who cannot furnish self-reports but more often use behavioral observation of pain-related behaviors for these groups.

More than 30% of the population of the United States (Institute of Medicine, 2011) and almost 20% of those in Europe (Corasaniti, Amantea, Russo, & Bagetta, 2006) experience chronic or intermittent persistent pain. We expect the prevalence of chronic pain in the United States to rise in the upcoming decades due to an aging population and increases in the prevalence of obesity (Croft et al., 2010). In fact, one aim of the United States 2010 Patient Protection and Affordable Care Act is to "increase the recognition of pain as a significant public health problem in the United States."

Chronic pain is categorized according to **syndrome**, symptoms that occur together and characterize a condition. Headache and low back pain are the two most frequently treated pain syndromes, but people also seek treatment for several other common pain syndromes.

IN SUMMARY

Pain measurement techniques fall into three general categories: (1) self-reports, (2) behavioral observation, and (3) physiological measures. Self-reports include rating scales, pain questionnaires such as the McGill Pain Questionnaire and the Multidimensional Pain Inventory, and standardized objective tests such as the Minnesota Multiphasic Personality Inventory and the Beck Depression Inventory. Clinicians who treat pain patients often use a combination of assessments, relying most often on self-report inventories. Behavioral assessments of pain began as informal observation but have evolved into standardized ratings by trained clinicians that are especially useful for individuals, such as young children and people with dementia, who cannot complete self-reports. Physiological measures include muscle tension and autonomic indices such as heart rate, but these approaches are not as reliable or valid as self-reports or behavioral observation.

Pain Syndromes

Acute pain is both a blessing and a burden. The blessing comes from the signals it sends about injury and the reminders it conveys to avoid further injury and allow healing. The burden is that it hurts.

Chronic pain, in contrast, serves no clear purpose—it signals no injury and causes people to live in misery.

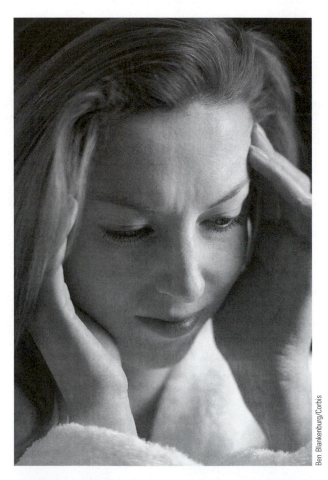

Headache is the most common of all types of pain—more than 99% of people have experienced a headache.

Headache Pain

Headache pain is the most common of all types of pain, with more than 99% of people experiencing headache at some time during their lives (Smetana, 2000), and 16% of people reporting severe headaches in the last 3 months (CDC and NCHS, 2010). Until the 1980s, no reliable classification of headache pain was available to researchers and therapists. Then in 1988, the Headache Classification Committee of the International Headache Society (IHS) published a classification system that standardized definitions of various headache pains (Olesen, 1988). Although the IHS identifies many different kinds of headache, the three primary pain syndromes are migraine, tension, and cluster headaches.

Migraine headaches represent recurrent attacks of pain that vary widely in intensity, frequency, and duration. Originally conceptualized as originating in the blood vessels in the head, migraine headaches are now believed to involve not only blood vessels but also a complex cascade of reactions that include neurons in the brain stem (Corasaniti et al., 2006) and to have a genetic component (Bigal & Lipton, 2008a). The underlying cause and the exact mechanism for producing pain remain controversial. Migraine attacks often occur with loss of appetite, nausea, vomiting, and exaggerated sensitivity to light and sound. Migraine headaches often involve sensory, motor, or mood disturbances. Migraines also exist in two varieties: those with aura and those without aura. Migraines with aura have identifiable sensory disturbances that precede the headache pain; migraines without aura have a sudden onset and an intense throbbing, usually (but not always) restricted to one side of the head. Brain imaging studies indicate that these two varieties of migraine affect the brain in somewhat different ways (Sánchez del Rio & Alvarez Linera, 2004).

The epidemiology of migraine headaches includes gender differences and variations in prevalence around the world. Women are two to three times more likely than men to have migraine headaches, with rates in the United States of 6% to 9% for men and 17% to 18% for women (Lipton et al., 2007; Victor, Hu, Campbell, Buse, & Lipton, 2010). Rates for non-Western countries are lower. For example, between 3% and 7% of people in Africa report migraines (Haimanot, 2002). However, the experience of migraine is similar; men and women who have chronic migraines have similar experiences of symptoms, frequency, and severity (Marcus, 2001). Most migraine patients experience their first headache before age 30 and some before the age of 10. However, the period for the greatest frequency of migraines is between ages 30 and 50 (Morillo et al., 2005). Few patients have a first migraine after age 40, but people who have migraines continue to do so, often throughout their lives.

Tension headaches are muscular in origin, accompanied by sustained contractions of the muscles of the neck, shoulders, scalp, and face, but current explanations (Fumal & Schoenen, 2008) also include mechanisms within the central nervous system. Tension headaches have a gradual onset; sensations of tightness; constriction or pressure; highly variable intensity, frequency, and duration; and a dull, steady ache on both sides of the head. Nearly 40% of the U.S. population experiences tension headaches (Schwartz, Stewart, Simon, & Lipton, 1998), and people with this pain syndrome reported lost workdays and decreased effectiveness at work, home, and school because of their pain.

A third type of headache is the **cluster headache**, a severe headache that occurs in daily or nearly daily clusters (Favier, Haan, & Ferrari, 2005). Some symptoms are similar to those of migraine, including severe pain and vomiting, but cluster headaches are much briefer, rarely lasting longer than 2 hours (Smetana, 2000). The headache occurs on one side of the head, and often the eye on the other side becomes bloodshot and waters. In addition, cluster headaches are more common in men than in women, by a ratio of 2:1 (Bigal & Lipton, 2008b). Most people who have cluster headaches experience episodes of headache, with weeks, months, or years of no headache (Favier et al., 2005). Cluster headaches are even more mysterious than other types of headaches, with no clear understanding of risk factors.

Low Back Pain

As many as 80% of people in the United States experience low back pain at some time, making the problem extensive but not necessarily serious. Most injuries are not permanent, and most people recover (Leeuw et al., 2007). Those who do not recover quickly have a poor prognosis and are likely to develop chronic pain problems. Health care expenditures for these people total more than $90 billion a year in the United States (Luo, 2004). The incidence of low back pain shows some variation for countries around the world (European Vertebral Osteoporosis Study Group, 2004), but this condition produces direct expenses, such as medical care, and indirect costs, such as lost workdays and

disability, affecting people in countries around the world (Dagenais, Caro, & Haldeman, 2008).

Infections, degenerative diseases, and malignancies can all cause low back pain. However, the most frequent cause of low back pain is probably injury or stress resulting in musculoskeletal, ligament, and neurological problems in the lower back (Chou et al., 2007). Pregnancy is also a cause of low back pain, with nearly 90% of pregnant women suffering from the syndrome (Hayes et al., 2000). Aging is yet another factor in back pain, because the fluid content and elasticity of the intervertebral disks decrease as one grows older, and arthritis and osteoporosis become more likely. However, fewer than 20% of back pain patients have a definite identification of the physical cause of their pain (Chou et al., 2007).

Stress and psychological factors most likely play a role not only in back pain but also in all types of chronic pain. Making the transition from the prechronic stage to chronic pain is a complex process, and physiological and psychological processes accompany this progression. Some researchers (Baliki, Geha, Apkarian, & Chialvo, 2008; Corasaniti et al., 2006) focus on physical changes in the nervous system that occur when pain becomes chronic. Other researchers (Leeuw et al., 2007; Sanders, 2006) emphasize psychological factors such as fear, anxiety, depression, a history of trauma and abuse, and reinforcement experiences, all of which are more common among chronic pain patients. However, most chronic pain researchers recognize the role that both physical and psychological factors play in causing and maintaining chronic pain.

Arthritis Pain

Rheumatoid arthritis is an autoimmune disorder characterized by swelling and inflammation of the joints as well as destruction of cartilage, bone, and tendons. These changes alter the joint, producing direct pain, and the changes in joint structure lead to changes in movement, which may result in additional pain through this indirect route (Dillard, 2002). Rheumatoid arthritis can occur at any age, even during adolescence and young adulthood, but it is most prevalent among people 40 to 70 years old. Women are more than twice as likely as men to develop this disease (Theis, Helmick, & Hootman, 2007). The symptoms of rheumatoid arthritis are extremely variable. Some people experience a steady worsening of symptoms, but most

people face alternating remission and intensification of symptoms. Rheumatoid arthritis interferes with work, family life, recreational activities, and sexuality (Pouchot, Le Parc, Queffelec, Sichère, & Flinois, 2007).

Osteoarthritis is a progressive inflammation of the joints that produces degeneration of cartilage and bone (Goldring & Goldring 2007); it affects mostly older people. Osteoarthritis causes a dull ache in the joint area, which worsens with movement; the resulting lack of movement increases joint problems and pain. Osteoarthritis is the most common form of arthritis, which is one of the primary causes of disability in older people, affecting about 50% of those over 70 (Keefe et al., 2002). Older women make up a disproportionate number of those affected. As joints stiffen and pain increases, people with arthritis begin to have difficulties engaging in enjoyable activities and even basic self-care. They often experience feelings of helplessness, depression, and anxiety, which exacerbate their pain.

Fibromyalgia is a chronic pain condition characterized by tender points throughout the body. This disorder also has symptoms of fatigue, headache, cognitive difficulties, anxiety, and sleep disturbances (Chakrabarty & Zoorob, 2007). Although fibromyalgia is not arthritis (Endresen, 2007), some symptoms are common to both, as is a diminished quality of life (Birtane, Uzunca, Tastekin, & Tuna, 2007).

Cancer Pain

More than 13 million people in the United States have a cancer diagnosis (Mariotto, Yabroff, Shao, Feuer, & Brown, 2011). Cancer can produce pain in two ways: through its growth and progression and through the various treatments to control its growth. Pain is present in 44% of all cancer cases and in 64% or more of advanced cases (Institute of Medicine, 2011). Some cancers are much more likely than others to produce pain. Head, neck, and cervical cancer patients experience more pain than leukemia patients (Anderson, Syrjala, & Cleeland, 2001). In addition, treatments for cancer may also produce pain; surgery, chemotherapy, and radiation therapy all produce painful effects. Thus, either the disease or its treatment creates pain for most cancer patients. However, many cancer patients do not get adequate relief from pain. A review of 26 international studies showed that across countries, almost half of cancer patients' pain was untreated (Deandrea, Montanari, Moja, & Apolone, 2008).

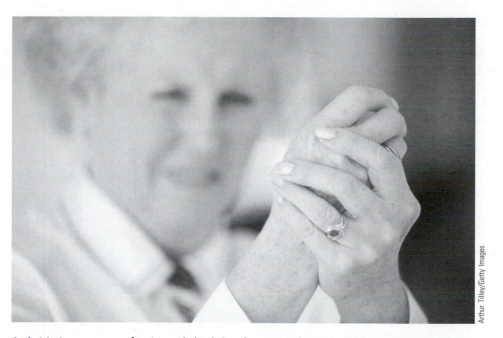

Arthur Tilley/Getty Images

Arthritis is a source of pain and disability for more than 20 million Americans.

Phantom Limb Pain

Just as injury can occur without producing pain, pain can occur in the absence of injury. One such type of pain is **phantom limb pain**, the experience of chronic pain in a part of the body that is missing. Amputation removes the nerves that produce the impulses leading to the experience of pain, but not the sensations. Most amputees experience some sensations from the amputated limb, and many of these sensations are painful (Czerniecki & Ehde, 2003).

Until the 1970s, phantom pain was believed to be rare, with less than 1% of amputees experiencing a painful phantom limb, but more recent research has indicated that the percentage may be as high as 80% (Ephraim, Wegener, MacKenzie, Dillingham, & Pezzin, 2005). The sensations often start soon after surgery as a tingling and then develop into other sensations that resemble actual feelings in the missing limb, including pain. Nor are the sensations of phantom pain limited to limbs. Women who have undergone breast removal also perceive sensations from the amputated breast, and people who have had teeth pulled sometimes continue to experience feelings from those teeth.

Amputees sometimes feel that a phantom limb is of abnormal size or in an uncomfortable position (Melzack & Wall, 1982). Phantom limbs can also produce painful feelings of cramping, shooting, burning, or crushing. These pains vary from mild and infrequent to severe and continuous. Early research suggested that the severity and frequency of the pain decrease over time (Melzack & Wall, 1988); however, subsequent research suggests that phantom pain remains over time (Ephraim et al., 2005). In fact, nearly 75% of amputees who lost a limb over 10 years earlier still report phantom pains (Ephraim et al., 2005). Pain is more likely to occur in the missing limb when the person experienced a great deal of pain before the amputation (Hanley et al., 2007).

The underlying cause of phantom limb pain is the subject of heated controversy (Melzack, 1992; Woodhouse, 2005). Because surgery rarely relieves the pain, some authorities suggest that phantom limb pain has an emotional basis. Melzack (1992) argued that phantom limb sensations arise because of the activation of a characteristic pattern of neural activity, which he called a *neuromatrix*. This neuromatrix pattern continues to operate, even if the neurons in the peripheral nervous system do not furnish input to the brain.

Melzack believed that this pattern of brain activity is the basis for phantom limb sensations, which may include pain, and recent research is consistent with his theory (Woodhouse, 2005). Brain imaging technology allows researchers to investigate patterns of brain activation, and such studies show that the brain is capable of reorganization after injury, producing changes in the nervous system. Such changes are observed in the somatosensory and motor cortex of amputees (Flor, Nikolajsen, & Staehelin Jensen, 2006; Karl, Mühlnickel, Kurth, & Flor, 2004), which is consistent with Melzack's concept of the neuromatrix and its role in phantom limb pain. Therefore, phantom limb pain may arise from changes that occur in both peripheral and central nervous systems after removal of the limb. Rather than compensate for the loss, the nervous system makes changes that are maladaptive, creating pain.

IN SUMMARY

Acute pain may result from hundreds of different types of injuries and diseases, but chronic pain exists as a limited number of syndromes. A few of these syndromes account for the majority of people who suffer from chronic pain. Headache is the most common type of pain, but only some people experience chronic problems with migraine, tension, or cluster headaches. Most people's experience of low back pain is acute, but for some people the pain becomes chronic and debilitating. Arthritis is a degenerative disease that affects the joints, producing chronic pain. Rheumatoid arthritis is an autoimmune disease that may affect people of any age; osteoarthritis is the result of progressive inflammation of the joints that affects mostly older people. Fibromyalgia is a chronic pain condition characterized by pain throughout the body, sleep disturbances, fatigue, and anxiety. Pain is not an inevitable consequence of cancer, but most people with cancer experience pain either as a result of the progression of the disease or from the various treatments for cancer. One of the most puzzling pain syndromes is phantom limb pain, which represents pain that occurs in a missing body part. A majority of people with amputations experience this pain syndrome.

Managing Pain

Pain presents complex problems for management. Treatment for acute pain is usually straightforward because the source of the pain is clear. However, helping people with chronic pain is a challenge because this type of pain exists without obvious tissue damage. Some people achieve relief through medical treatments, and others experience improvement through behavioral management of their pain.

Medical Approaches to Managing Pain

Drugs are the main medical strategy for treating acute pain. Although drugs are also a choice for some chronic pain syndromes, this strategy carries greater risks. Chronic pain that has not responded to drugs may be treated by surgery, which also presents risks.

Drugs **Analgesic drugs** relieve pain without causing loss of consciousness. Hundreds of different analgesic drugs are available, but almost all fall into two major groups: the opiates and the nonnarcotic analgesics (Julien, Advokat, & Comaty, 2010). Both types exist naturally as derivatives of plants, and both have many synthetic variations. Of the two, the opium type is more powerful and has a longer history of use, dating back at least 5,000 years (Melzack & Wall, 1982).

Contemporary opiate painkillers include substances such as morphine, codeine, oxycodone, and hydrocodone (an active ingredient in the drug known as Vicodin). Limitations on using opiate drugs for pain control include the development of both tolerance and dependence. **Tolerance** is the body's decreased responsiveness to a drug. When tolerance occurs, larger and larger doses of a drug are required to bring about the same effect. **Dependence** occurs when the drug's removal produces withdrawal symptoms. Because opiates produce both tolerance and dependence, they are potentially dangerous and subject to abuse.

How realistic are the fears of drug abuse as a consequence of opiate prescription? Do patients become addicted while recovering from surgery? What about the dangers to patients with terminal illnesses? According to one study (Porter & Jick, 1980), the risk of addiction is less than 1%. During the late 1990s, prescriptions for opiate analgesics increased dramatically, and publicity about an epidemic of analgesic abuse fueled the fear that increased prescriptions for these drugs were leading to widespread addiction. Despite increases in opiate use and abuse, the number of chronic pain patients who develop an addiction to opiate pain medications is less than 4% of the number who are prescribed them (Fishbain, Cole, Lewis, Rosomoff, & Rosomoff, 2008).

To date, the best predictor of opiate painkiller abuse is personal history of illegal drug and alcohol use; people who misuse these substances are more likely to also misuse opiate painkillers (Turk, Swanson, & Gatchel, 2008).

The advantages of opiate drugs outweigh their dangers for some people in some situations; no other type of drug produces more complete pain relief. However, their potential for abuse and their side effects make them more suitable for treating acute pain than for managing chronic pain, as there is limited evidence supporting their long-term use for chronic pain (Manchikanti et al., 2011). The opiate drugs remain an essential part of pain management for the most severe, acute injuries, for recovery from surgery, and for terminal illnesses.

Between 1997 and 2007, the use of opiate analgesic drugs increased over 600% (Paulozzi et al., 2012). Much of this increase was for the drugs oxycodone and hydrocodone. Both are opiates with a potential for abuse, which increased during the time when prescriptions increased. Wariness about abuse of these drugs affects both physicians, who are reluctant to prescribe them (Breuer, Fleishman, Cruciani, & Portenoy, 2011), and many patients, who are reluctant to take sufficient doses to obtain relief (Lewis, Combs, & Trafton, 2010). This reluctance applies to all opiate drugs, even for cancer pain (Reid, Gooberman-Hill, & Hanks, 2008). Thus, people with either acute or chronic pain frequently fail to receive sufficient relief.

One procedure that has overcome the undermedication problem is a system of self-paced administration. Patients can activate a pump attached to their intravenous lines and deliver a dose of medication whenever they wish, within well-defined limits. Such systems began to appear in the late 1970s and have since gained wide acceptance because patients tend to use less medication, obtain better pain relief (Sri Vengadesh, Sistla, & Smile, 2005), and experience higher satisfaction (Gan, Gordon, Bolge, & Allen, 2007). Because an intravenous line is necessary for this system of drug delivery, it is most commonly used to control pain following surgery. However, a patient-controlled transdermal delivery system is also available (D'Arcy, 2005). This system allows people to self-administer analgesia through a device about the size of a credit card that adheres to their upper arm. These types of self-administered analgesics help prevent undermedication.

Whereas undermedication may be a problem for cancer pain patients, overmedication is often a problem for patients suffering from low back pain. One team of investigators (Von Korff, Barlow, Cherkin, & Deyo,

1994) grouped primary care physicians according to their low, moderate, or high frequency of prescribing pain medication and bed rest for back pain patients. A 1- and 2-year follow-up found that back pain patients who took less medication and remained active did just as well as those who were told to take more medication and to rest. Another study (Rhee, Taitel, Walker, & Lau, 2007) found that back pain patients who took opiate drugs experienced more frequent health problems such as hypertension, anxiety, depression, and arthritis; in addition, they were more likely to make a visit to a hospital emergency room. Both studies indicated that treatment for these patients was more costly than for patients who took other approaches to managing back pain. Thus, low– back pain patients who use pain medication have poorer outcomes, more health problems, and higher costs than those who do not.

The nonnarcotic analgesics include a variety of nonsteroidal anti-inflammatory drugs (NSAIDs) as well as acetaminophen. Aspirin, ibuprofen, and naproxen sodium appear to block the synthesis of prostaglandins (Julien et al., 2010), a class of chemicals released by damaged tissue and involved in inflammation. The presence of these chemicals sensitizes neurons and increases pain. These drugs act at the site of injury instead of crossing into the brain, but they change neurochemical activity in the nervous system and affect pain perception. As a result of their mechanism of action, NSAIDs do not alter pain perception when no injury is present—for example, in laboratory situations with people who receive experimental pain stimuli.

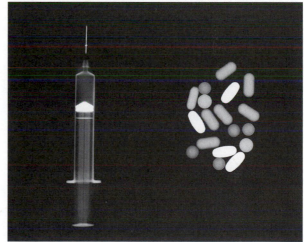

Jim Wehtje/Getty Images

Drugs offer effective treatment for acute pain but are not a good choice to treat chronic pain.

Aspirin and other NSAIDs have many uses in pain relief, including for minor cuts and scratches as well as more severe injuries such as broken bones. But pain that occurs without inflammation is not so readily relieved by NSAIDs. In addition, NSAIDs can irritate and damage the stomach lining, even producing ulcers (Huang, Sridhar, & Hunt, 2002). Aspirin's side effects include the alteration of blood clotting time, and aspirin and other NSAIDs are toxic in large doses, causing damage to the liver and kidneys.

A new type of NSAID, the Cox-2 inhibitor, affects prostaglandins but has lower gastric toxicity. After the approval and heavy marketing of these drugs, their sales skyrocketed, especially among people with arthritis. However, the discovery of increased heart attack risk led to the withdrawal of two Cox-2 inhibitors from the market in the United States and increased caution in the use of this type of NSAID (Shi & Klotz, 2008).

Acetaminophen, another nonnarcotic analgesic, is not one of the NSAIDs. Under brand names such as Tylenol, acetaminophen has become a widely used drug. It has few anti-inflammatory properties but has a pain-relieving capability similar to that of aspirin, though somewhat weaker. Acetaminophen does not have the gastric side effects of aspirin, so people who cannot tolerate aspirin find it a good substitute. However, acetaminophen is not harmless. Large quantities of acetaminophen can be fatal, and even nonlethal doses can do serious damage to the liver, especially when combined with alcohol (Julien et al., 2010).

Analgesic drugs are not the only drugs that affect pain. Antidepressant drugs and drugs used to treat seizures also influence pain perception, and these drugs can be used to treat some types of pain (Maizels & McCarberg, 2005). Antidepressants can be useful in treating low back pain, and some types of anticonvulsant medication can help people with migraine headaches. In addition, other drugs exist that have some ability to prevent migraine headaches (Peres, Mercante, Tanuri, & Nunes, 2006) and to reduce the inflammation that is a damaging part of rheumatoid arthritis (Iagnocco et al., 2008). Similar developments for other chronic pain syndromes would change the lives of millions of people. Unfortunately, even the variety of drugs and strategies for their use are not adequate for many people with chronic pain. Those individuals may consider surgery or other treatments to attain relief.

Surgery Another traditional medical treatment for pain is surgery, which aims to repair the source of the pain or alter the nervous system to alleviate the pain. Low back surgery is the most common surgical approach to pain, but surgery is not an option that physicians recommend until other, less invasive possibilities have failed (van Zundert & van Kleef, 2005).

Surgery can also alter nerves that transmit pain (van Zundert & van Kleef, 2005). This procedure may use heat, cold, or radiofrequency stimulation to change neural transmission and control pain. Complete destruction of nerves is not typically the aim because it can lead to loss of all sensation, which may be more distressing than pain. Another tactic for altering pain through changing nerve transmission involves stimulation of nerves through implanted wires that stimulate rather than damage nerves. Surgery is required for this approach, which involves implanting devices that can deliver electrical stimulation to either the spinal cord or the brain. Activation of the system produces pain relief by activating neurons and by releasing neurotransmitters that block pain. This process does not destroy neural tissue.

Spinal stimulation is a promising technique for controlling back pain (De Andrés & Van Buyten, 2006), but a related type of stimulation, **transcutaneous electrical nerve stimulation (TENS)**, has proven to be less effective. The TENS system typically consists of electrodes that attach to the skin and are connected to a unit that supplies electrical stimulation. Despite some promising early indications of success, TENS has demonstrated only limited effectiveness in controlling pain (Claydon, Chesterton, Barlas, & Sim, 2011).

Surgery has at least two limitations as a treatment for pain. First, it does not always repair damaged tissue, and second, it does not provide all patients with sufficient pain relief. Even those for whom surgery is initially successful may experience a return of pain. That is, surgery is not a successful treatment for many people with chronic back pain (Ehrlich, 2003). Thus, this approach is an expensive but unreliable approach to controlling this pain syndrome (Turk & McCarberg, 2005). Also, surgery has its own potential dangers and possibilities for complications, which lead many pain patients to behavioral approaches for managing their pain.

Behavioral Techniques for Managing Pain

Psychologists have been prominent in devising therapies that teach people how to manage pain, and several behavioral techniques have proven effective with a variety of pain syndromes. These techniques include relaxation training, behavioral therapy, cognitive therapy, and cognitive behavioral therapy. Some authorities consider these techniques to be part of mind–body medicine and thus part of alternative medicine (covered in Chapter 8). Psychologists see these techniques as part of psychology.

Relaxation Training   Relaxation is one approach to managing pain and may be the key ingredient in other types of pain management. *Progressive muscle relaxation* consists of sitting in a comfortable chair with no distractions and then systematic tensing and relaxing of muscle groups throughout the body (Jacobson, 1938). After learning the procedure, people can practice this relaxation technique independently.

Relaxation techniques have been used successfully to treat pain problems such as tension and migraine headache (Fumal & Schoenen, 2008; Penzien, Rains, & Andrasik, 2002), rheumatoid arthritis (McCallie et al., 2006), and low back pain (Henschke et al., 2010). A National Institutes of Health Technology (NIHT) panel evaluated the evidence for progressive muscle relaxation and gave this technique its highest rating in controlling pain (Lebovits, 2007). However, relaxation training typically functions as part of a multicomponent program (Astin, 2004).

Table 7.1 summarizes the effectiveness of relaxation techniques.

Behavioral Therapy   The most prominent behavioral therapy is *behavior modification*, which arose from the laboratory research on operant conditioning. **Behavior modification** is the process of shaping behavior through the application of operant conditioning principles. The goal of behavior modification is to shape *behavior*, not to alleviate *feelings* or *sensations* of pain. People in pain usually communicate their discomfort to others through their behavior—they complain, moan, sigh, limp, rub, grimace, and miss work.

Wilbert E. Fordyce (1974) was among the first to emphasize the role of operant conditioning in the perpetuation of pain behaviors. He recognized the *reward* value of increased attention and sympathy, financial compensation, and other **positive reinforcers** that frequently follow pain behaviors. These conditions create what pain expert Frank Andrasik (2003) called pain traps, situations that push people who experience pain toward developing and maintaining chronic pain. The situations that create chronic pain include attention from family, relief from normal responsibilities, compensation from employers, and medications that people receive from physicians. These reinforcers make it difficult to get better.

Behavior modification works against these pain traps, identifying the reinforcers and training people in the patient's environment to use praise and attention to reinforce more desirable behaviors and to withhold reinforcement when the patient exhibits less desired pain behaviors. In other words, the groans and complaints are now ignored, whereas efforts toward greater physical activity and other positive behaviors are reinforced. Objective outcomes indicate progress, such as the amount of medication taken, absences from work, time in bed or off one's feet, number of pain complaints, physical activity, range of motion, and length of sitting tolerance. The strength of the operant conditioning technique is its ability to increase levels of physical activity and decrease the use of medication—two important targets in any pain treatment regimen (Roelofs, Boissevain, Peters, de Jong, & Vlaeyen, 2002). In addition, this behavioral approach can decrease pain intensity, reduce disability, and improve quality of life (Sanders, 2006; Smeets, Severens, Beelen, Vlaeyen, &

TABLE 7.1   Effectiveness of Relaxation Techniques

Problem	Findings	Studies
1. Tension and migraine headaches	Relaxation helps in managing headache.	Fumal & Schoenen, 2008; Penzien et al., 2002
2. Rheumatoid arthritis	Progressive muscle relaxation is an effective component in programs to manage these disorders.	McCallie et al., 2006
3. Low back pain	Relaxation is effective in programs to treat low back pain.	Henschke et al., 2010
4. Variety of chronic pain conditions	Progressive muscle relaxation is effective according to an NIHT review.	Lebovits, 2007

Knottnerus, 2009). The behavior modification approach does not address the cognitions that underlie and contribute to behaviors, but cognitive therapy focuses on these cognitions.

Cognitive therapy is based on the principle that people's beliefs, personal standards, and feelings of self-efficacy strongly affect their behavior (Bandura, 1986, 2001; Beck, 1976; Ellis, 1962). Cognitive therapies concentrate on techniques designed to change cognitions, assuming that behavior will change when a person alters his or her cognitions. Albert Ellis (1962) argued that thoughts, especially irrational thoughts, are the root of behavior problems. He focused on the tendency to "catastrophize," which escalates an unpleasant situation into something worse. Examples of pain-related catastrophizing might include "This pain will never get better," "I can't go on any longer," or "There is nothing I can do to stop this pain."

The experience of pain can easily turn into a catastrophe, and any exaggeration of feelings of pain can lead to maladaptive behaviors and further exacerbation of irrational beliefs. The tendency to catastrophize is associated with the magnification of pain, both acute (Pavlin, Sullivan, Freund, & Roesen, 2005) and chronic (Karoly & Ruehlman, 2007).

Once irrational cognitions have been identified, the therapist actively attacks these beliefs, with the goal of eliminating or changing them into more rational beliefs. For example, cognitive therapy for pain addresses the tendency to catastrophize, leading people to abandon the belief that their pain is unbearable and will never stop (Thorn & Kuhajda, 2006). Cognitive therapists address these cognitions and work with patients to change them. Rather than concentrate exclusively on thoughts, however, most cognitive therapists working with pain patients address changes in both cognitions and behavior. That is, they practice cognitive behavioral therapy.

Cognitive behavioral therapy (CBT) is a type of therapy that aims to develop beliefs, attitudes, thoughts, and skills to make positive changes in behavior. Like cognitive therapy, CBT assumes that thoughts and feelings are the basis of behavior, so CBT begins with changing attitudes. Like behavior modification, CBT focuses on modifying environmental contingencies and building skills to change observable behavior.

One approach to CBT for pain management is the pain inoculation program designed by Dennis Turk and Donald Meichenbaum (Meichenbaum & Turk, 1976; Turk, 1978, 2001), which is similar to stress inoculation explained in Chapter 5. Pain inoculation includes a cognitive stage, the *reconceptualization* stage, during which patients learn to accept the importance of psychological factors for at least some of their pain and often receive an explanation of the gate control theory of pain. The second stage—*acquisition and rehearsal of skills*—includes learning relaxation and controlled breathing skills. The final, or *follow-through*, phase of treatment includes instructions to spouses and other family members to ignore patients' pain behaviors and to reinforce such healthy behaviors as greater levels of physical activity, decreased use of medication, fewer visits to the pain clinic, or an increased number of days at work. With the help of their therapists, patients construct a posttreatment plan for coping with future pain, and finally, they apply their coping skills to everyday situations outside the pain clinic. A study of laboratory-induced pain (Milling, Levine, & Meunier, 2003) indicated that inoculation training was as effective as hypnosis in helping participants control pain. A study of athletes recovering from knee injury (Ross & Berger, 1996) also found that pain inoculation procedures were effective.

Other CBT programs have demonstrated their effectiveness for a wide variety of pain syndromes. CBT includes strategies for addressing the harmful cognitions that are common among chronic pain patients, such as fear and catastrophizing (Leeuw et al., 2007; Thorn et al., 2007) and a behavioral component to help pain patients behave in ways that are compatible with health rather than illness. Evaluations of CBT for low back pain (Hoffman, Papas, Chatkoff, & Kerns, 2007) indicate its effectiveness for this pain syndrome, and studies of CBT with headache patients (Martin, Forsyth, & Reece, 2007; Nash, Park, Walker, Gordon, & Nicholson, 2004; Thorn et al., 2007) have also demonstrated its benefits. Fibromyalgia patients benefited more from CBT than from a drug treatment (García, Simón, Durán, Canceller, & Aneiros, 2006), and CBT proved beneficial for people with rheumatoid arthritis (Astin, 2004; Sharpe et al., 2001) as well as cancer and AIDS pain (Breibart & Payne, 2001).

Recently, researchers evaluated a form of CBT for pain management called **acceptance and commitment therapy (ACT)**. ACT encourages pain patients to increase acceptance of their pain, while focusing their attention on other goals and activities that they value. This form of therapy may be especially helpful for chronic pain patients, as attempting to directly control pain may lead to distress and disability (McCracken, Eccleston, & Bell, 2005). A recent meta-analysis of 10 studies of chronic pain patients found that ACT led to significant reduction in pain intensity compared with no treatment (Veehof, Oskam, Schreurs, Bohlmeijer, 2010). Thus, ACT may be another good alternative to traditional cognitive behavioral therapy for the management of chronic pain.

In summary, these studies show that behavior modification and cognitive behavioral therapy can be an effective intervention for pain management for people with a variety of pain syndromes. These techniques are among the most effective types of pain management strategies. Table 7.2 summarizes the effectiveness of these therapies and the problems they can treat.

IN SUMMARY

A variety of medical treatments for pain are effective but also have limitations. Analgesic drugs offer pain relief for acute pain and can be of use for chronic pain. These drugs include opiates and nonnarcotic drugs. Opiates are effective in managing severe pain, but their tolerance and dependence properties pose problems for use by chronic pain patients, making health care professionals and patients reluctant to use effective doses. Nonnarcotic drugs such as aspirin, nonsteroidal anti-inflammatory drugs, and acetaminophen are effective in managing mild to moderate acute pain and have some uses in managing chronic pain.

Surgery can alter either peripheral nerves or the central nervous system. Surgical procedures are often a last resort in controlling chronic pain, and procedures that involve destruction of nerve pathways are often unsuccessful. Procedures that allow for stimulation of the spinal cord show more promise in pain management, but transcutaneous electrical nerve stimulation is not an effective method.

Health psychologists help people cope with stress and chronic pain by using relaxation training, behavioral therapy, cognitive therapy, and cognitive

TABLE 7.2   Effectiveness of Behavioral, Cognitive, and Cognitive Behavioral Therapy

Problem	Findings	Studies
1. Increase in pain behaviors	Verbal reinforcement increases pain behaviors.	Jolliffe & Nicholas, 2004
2. Chronic low back pain	Operant conditioning increases physical activity and lowers medication usage; CBT can also be effective.	Roelofs et al., 2002
3. Pain intensity	Behavior modification decreases pain intensity	Sanders, 2006
4. Chronic low back pain	Behavior modification is a cost-effective therapy for reducing disability.	Smeets et al., 2009
5. Catastrophizing the experience of pain	Catastrophizing intensifies acute and chronic pain.	Karoly & Ruehlman, 2007; Pavlin et al., 2005; Thorn & Kuhajda, 2006
6. Laboratory-induced pain	Inoculation training was as effective as hypnosis for pain.	Milling et al., 2003
7. Athletes with knee pain	Pain inoculation reduces pain.	Ross & Berger, 1996
8. Low back pain	CBT was evaluated as effective in a meta-analysis and in a systematic review.	Hoffman et al., 2007
9. Headache pain and prevention	CBT is effective in both management and prevention.	Martin et al., 2007; Nash et al., 2004; Thorn et al., 2007
10. Fibromyalgia	CBT is more effective than drug treatment.	García et al., 2006
11. Rheumatoid arthritis	CBT can relieve some pain.	Astin, 2004; Sharpe et al., 2001
12. Cancer and AIDS pain	CBT helps people cope.	Breibart & Payne, 2000
13. Chronic pain	ACT effective in reducing pain intensity in a meta-analysis	Veehof et al., 2010

behavioral therapy. Relaxation techniques such as progressive muscle relaxation have demonstrated some success in helping patients manage headache pain, postoperative pain, and low back pain. Behavior modification can be effective in helping pain patients become more active and decrease their dependence on medication, but this approach does not address the negative emotions and suffering that accompany pain. Cognitive therapy addresses feelings and thus helps in reducing the catastrophizing that exacerbates pain. Combined with the behavioral components of operant conditioning, cognitive behavioral therapy has demonstrated greater effectiveness than other therapies.

Cognitive behavioral therapy includes pain inoculation therapy, but other combinations of changes in cognitions concerning pain and behavioral strategies for changing pain-related behavior also fit within this category. These approaches have been successful in treating low back pain, headache pain, rheumatoid arthritis pain, fibromyalgia, and the pain that accompanies cancer and AIDS.

Answers

This chapter has addressed five basic questions:

1. **How does the nervous system register pain?**
Receptors near the skin's surface react to stimulation, and the nerve impulses from this stimulation relay the message to the spinal cord. The spinal cord includes laminae (layers) that modulate the sensory message and relay it toward the brain. The somatosensory cortex in the brain receives and interprets sensory input. Neurochemicals and the periaqueductal gray can also modulate the information and change the perception of pain.

2. **What is the meaning of pain?**
Pain is difficult to define, but it can be classified as acute (resulting from specific injury and lasting less than 6 months), chronic (continuing beyond the time of healing), or prechronic (the critical stage between acute and chronic). The personal experience of pain is affected by situational and cultural factors as well as individual variation and learning history. The meaning of pain can also be understood through theories. The leading model is the gate control theory of pain, which takes both physical and psychological factors into account in the experience of pain.

3. **How can pain be measured?**
Pain can be measured physiologically by assessing muscle tension or autonomic arousal, but these measurements do not have high validity. Observations of pain-related behaviors (such as limping, grimacing, or complaining) have some reliability and validity. Self-reports are the most common approach to pain measurement; they include rating scales, pain questionnaires, and standardized psychological tests.

4. **What types of pain present the biggest problems?**
Pain syndromes are a common way of classifying chronic pain according to symptoms. These syndromes include headache pain, low back pain, arthritic pain, cancer pain, and phantom limb pain; the first two are the most common sources of chronic pain and lead to the most time lost from work or school.

5. **What techniques are effective for pain management?**
The techniques that health psychologists use in helping people cope with pain include relaxation training and behavioral techniques. Relaxation training can help people cope with pain problems such as headache and low back pain. Behavioral approaches include behavior modification, which guides people to behave in ways compatible with health rather than pain. Cognitive therapy concentrates on thoughts, guiding pain patients to minimize catastrophizing and fear. Cognitive behavioral therapy combines strategies to change cognitions with behavioral application, which is an especially effective approach for pain control.

Suggested Readings

Baar, K. (2008, March/April). Pain, pain, go away. *Psychology Today*, *41*(2), 56–57. This very brief article provides a summary of psychological factors in pain and the treatments psychologists have used successfully to help people manage pain.

Gatchel, R., Haggard, R., Thomas, C., & Howard, K. J. (2012). Biopsychosocial approaches to understanding chronic pain and disability. In R. J. Moore (Ed.), *Handbook of pain and palliative care* (pp. 1–16). New York: Springer. This chapter walks the reader through the development of major theories of pain, discusses how acute pain can turn into chronic pain, and presents issues in the assessment and management of chronic pain.

Wall, P. (2000). *Pain: The science of suffering*. New York: Columbia University Press. Peter Wall, one of the originators of the gate control theory of pain, tells about his extensive experience in trying to understand this phenomenon. He provides a nontechnical examination of the experience of pain, considering the cultural and individual factors that contribute.

Watkins, L. R., & Maier, S. F. (2003). When good pain turns bad. *Current Directions in Psychological Science*, *12*, 232–236. In this brief article, Watkins and Maier summarize their research on the development of chronic pain, which emphasizes the role of neurochemicals and glia as modulators in the nervous and immune systems' response to injury.

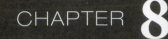
Considering Alternative Approaches

CHAPTER OUTLINE

- **Real-World Profile of Norman Cousins**
- *Alternative Medical Systems*
- *Alternative Practices and Products*
- *Mind–Body Medicine*
- *Who Uses Complementary and Alternative Medicine?*
- *How Effective Are Alternative Treatments?*

QUESTIONS

This chapter focuses on five basic questions:

1. What medical systems represent alternatives to conventional medicine?
2. What practices and products are used in alternative medicine?
3. What is mind–body medicine?
4. Who uses complementary and alternative medicine?
5. What are the effective uses and limitations of alternative treatments?

☑ CHECK YOUR BELIEFS

About Alternative Medicine

Check the items that are consistent with your beliefs.

☐ 1. When I am in pain, I go to the medicine cabinet to find something to alleviate my pain.

☐ 2. I believe that herbal treatments can be as effective as drugs in treating pain.

☐ 3. Drug companies should develop a pill to help people deal with stress.

☐ 4. Stress and pain arise from sources outside the person.

☐ 5. If my pain did not respond to medical treatment, I would be willing to try some alternative approach such as hypnosis or acupuncture.

☐ 6. Too many people take drugs to help them cope with their problems.

☐ 7. I would prefer some alternative to medical treatments for stress and pain problems.

☐ 8. Stress and pain come from an interaction of the person and the situation.

☐ 9. Chiropractic care offers no real benefits.

☐ 10. Alternative treatments cannot be as effective as conventional medical treatments.

☐ 11. Alternative treatments are safer than conventional medical approaches.

☐ 12. I believe that a combination of alternative and conventional medical treatments offers the best approach for pain management.

If you agreed with items 1, 3, 4, 9, and 10, then you probably have a strong belief in conventional medical approaches to treatment, including treatments for stress and pain problems. If you agreed with items 2, 5, 6, 7, 8, 11, and 12, then you show some beliefs that are compatible with alternative and behavioral treatments.

This chapter examines alternative treatments, describes alternative approaches to managing stress and pain, and reviews evidence about the effectiveness of these approaches.

Real-World Profile of
NORMAN COUSINS

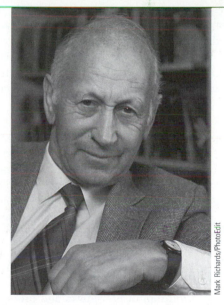

Mark Richards/PhotoEdit

In 1964 Norman Cousins was editor of the influential magazine *Saturday Review* when he was stricken by ankylosing spondylitis, a degenerative, inflammatory disease that affects the connective tissue in the spine. His physician told Cousins that his chances of recovery were 1 in 500 (Cousins, 1979). The treatment involved hospitalization and large doses of anti-inflammatory drugs; Cousins checked into the hospital and began taking the drugs. However, he decided that he could not remain a passive observer in his health care. Furthermore, he began to question the effectiveness of hospital routine, hospital food, seemingly endless tests, and high doses of drugs. Cousins left the hospital.

Cousins's treatment proceeded, but instead of a hospital room, he chose a nice hotel room. Rather than drugs, Cousins prescribed himself a healthy diet, large doses of vitamin C, an optimistic attitude, and a regimen of laughter from episodes of *Candid Camera* and old Marx brothers' movies. His physician was skeptical but agreed to this unusual course of treatment, and to his surprise, Cousins began to improve; eventually, he made a complete recovery. Cousins reported his experience in an article published in 1976 in the *New England Journal of Medicine*, which became the first chapter of his 1979 book, *Anatomy of an Illness As Perceived by the Patient.*

Cousins became a vocal advocate for the power that lies within people to heal themselves. He argued for the necessity of broadening medicine to focus on the patient and including psychological factors in the healing process. By accepting the position of Adjunct Professor of Medical Humanities at the University of California at Los Angeles, Cousins was able to work within conventional medicine to advocate for alternatives to that approach. He spoke and wrote about the possibilities for the healing power of positive emotions until his death in 1990. Cousins helped move medical care from one dominated by the biomedical model based on the concept of pathogens as the underlying cause of disease to a biopsychosocial model that includes social, cultural, and psychological factors.

The biopsychosocial model is an expansion of the biomedical view, but other conceptualizations of illness differ so much from mainstream medicine that they fall into the category of **alternative medicine**, which is a group of diverse medical and health care systems, practices, and products that are not currently considered part of conventional medicine (National Center for Complementary and Alternative Medicine [NCCAM], 2008/2011). Alternatives to conventional medicine come from systems of medicine that arose in different cultures, such as traditional Chinese medicine; from practices that are not yet accepted in mainstream medicine, such as chiropractic treatment and massage therapy; and from products that are not yet recognized as having medicinal value, such as glucosamine or echinacea. These practices and products may be used as alternatives to conventional medicine—for example, when a person seeks chiropractic treatment or massage therapy for back pain rather than take an analgesic drug. However, people usually combine alternative with conventional treatments (Barnes et al., 2008). In such circumstances, the term **complementary medicine** applies—for example, when a person uses both massage and analgesic drugs to control pain. The group of systems, practices, and products is often termed *complementary and alternative medicine (CAM).*

Alternative Medical Systems

The classification of procedures and products as complementary or alternative depends not only on cultural context but also on time period. In the United States 150 years ago, surgery was an alternative treatment not well accepted by established medicine (Weitz, 2010). As surgical techniques improved and evidence began to accumulate that surgery was the best treatment for some conditions, it became part of conventional medicine. More recently, the value of whole-grain diets made the transition from alternative medicine to mainstream medical recommendation when evidence about the health value of high-fiber diets began to accumulate (Hufford, 2003). Some of the techniques that are now classified as CAM will, with research and time, become part of conventional medicine.

Making the transition from CAM to conventional medicine requires a demonstration of the effectiveness of the procedure or substance through scientific research (Berman & Straus, 2004; Committee on the Use of Complementary and Alternative Medicine, 2005). To assist this process, the U.S. Congress created an agency that became the National Center for Complementary and Alternative Medicine, which has provided funding and sponsored research. Beginning in 1992, this agency has sponsored research on CAM in an attempt to determine which of these approaches is effective for what conditions, as well as who uses CAM and for what conditions. Before considering the findings on CAM approaches for managing stress, pain, and other conditions, we will review some of the major CAM approaches and techniques.

The health care most people receive in North America, Europe, and other places around the world comes from physicians, surgeons, nurses, and pharmacists who represent the biomedical system of medicine. Various alternative systems have arisen at different times and places; some have evolved during the same time frame as what we consider to be conventional medicine (NCCAM, 2008/2011). Each of these alternative systems includes a complete theory of disease (and possibly of health as well) and a description of what constitutes appropriate medical practice. In the United States, 4.4% of people have used a treatment based on at least one of these systems (Barnes et al., 2008).

Traditional Chinese Medicine

Traditional Chinese medicine (TCM) originated in China at least 2,000 years ago (Xutian, Zhang, & Louise, 2009) and remains a major treatment approach in China and other Asian countries. The system of TCM holds that a vital force, called *qi* (pronounced "chee" and sometimes written *chi*) animates the body, flowing through channels in the body called *meridians*. These meridians connect parts of the body to each other and to the universe as a whole. If the qi is blocked or becomes stagnant, health impairment and disease can develop. Keeping the qi in balance is important to maintaining and restoring health.

The body exists in a balance between two opposing energies or forces, *yin* and *yang* (Xutian et al., 2009). Yin represents cold, passive, and slow energy, whereas yang is seen as hot, active, and rapid. The two always operate together, and achieving a balance between the two is essential for health; attaining a harmony is ideal. Imbalances may occur through physical, emotional, or environmental events, and thus TCM takes a holistic approach to diagnosis and treatment. Practitioners have a variety of techniques to help individuals revitalize and unblock qi, bring yin and yang into balance, and restore health. These techniques include acupuncture, massage, herbal preparations, diet, and exercise.

Acupuncture became the first component of traditional Chinese medicine to gain widespread publicity in the West in 1971, when *New York Times* journalist James Reston experienced and reported on acupuncture treatment he received in China (Harrington, 2008). Reston had accompanied Secretary of State Henry Kissinger to China as Kissinger worked toward a meeting between Chinese leader Mao Tse-Tung and U.S. President Richard Nixon, who wanted to establish diplomatic relations with China. Reston's story about the success of acupuncture in controlling his postoperative pain captured the interest of many people and led the way toward acupuncture becoming well known as a treatment in alternative medicine. Acupuncture holds an important place in the system of traditional Chinese medicine.

Acupuncture consists of inserting needles into specific points on the skin and continuously stimulating the needles (NCCAM, 2007/2011). The stimulation can be accomplished electrically or by twirling the needles. About 1.4% of people in the United States reported that they have used acupuncture (Barnes et al., 2008). **Acupressure** is a manipulative technique

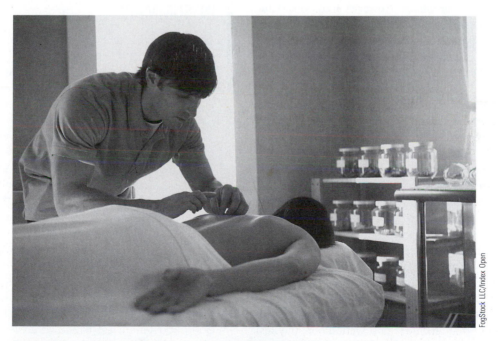

Acupuncture originated within traditional Chinese medicine and has become a popular alternative treatment.

that involves the application of pressure rather than needles to the points used in acupuncture. In the system of traditional Chinese medicine, acupuncture and acupressure help to unblock the flow of qi along the meridians and thus restore health. In addition, massage called *tui na* is used to stimulate or subdue qi. The application of massage is believed to regulate the nervous system, boost immune function, and help flush wastes out of the system.

The *Chinese materia medica* is a reference guide to the use of herbs and herbal preparations in treatment. Herbs such as ginseng and ginger are common, but many other plant, mineral, and even animal preparations are part of herbal remedies. The ingredients are ground into a powder and either made into tea or formed into pills.

Diet and exercise are also part of traditional Chinese medicine. Rather than aim for a diet with a balance of carbohydrates, protein, and fats, recommendations in TCM strive to remedy imbalances in yin and yang by eating certain foods and avoiding others (Xutian et al., 2009). The exercise with therapeutic properties is *qi gong*, which consists of a series of movements and breathing techniques that help with the circulation of qi.

Some of these practices from TCM, such as acupuncture and qi gong, as well as products such as herbal preparations, have been used as alternative treatments for specific problems. However, traditional Chinese medicine consists of an integrated theory of health and disease. Ayurveda is another system of medicine that emphasizes balance.

Ayurvedic Medicine

Ayurveda, or Ayurvedic medicine, is an ancient system that arose in India; the first written texts appeared more than 2,000 years ago (NCCAM, 2005/2009). The term originated in two Sanskrit words, the combination of which means "science of life." The goal of Ayurvedic medicine is to integrate and balance the body, mind, and spirit. These three elements are believed to be an extension of the relationship among all things in the universe. Humans are born in a state of balance, but events can disrupt this balance. When these elements are out of balance, health is endangered; bringing them back into balance restores health.

Ayurvedic practitioners diagnose patients through examinations that include observation of physical characteristics as well as questions about lifestyle and behavior (NCCAM, 2005/2009). Formulating a

treatment plan may require consultation with family members as well as the patient. The goals of treatment are to eliminate impurities and to increase harmony and balance, which are achieved through changes to exercise and diet. These changes may include yoga exercises and special diets or fasting to eliminate impurities in the body. Massage to vital points on the body is also part of Ayurvedic medicine, which provides pain relief and improves circulation. The use of herbs, medicated oils, spices, and minerals is extensive; more than 5,000 products exist in Ayurvedic medicine. Patients may also be directed to change behaviors to reduce worry and increase harmony in their lives, and yoga practice may be part of this element. Less than 1% of people in the United States have sought Ayurvedic treatment, making it much less common than traditional Chinese medicine (Barnes et al., 2008).

Other alternative medical systems include *naturopathy* and *homeopathy*; both arose during the 19th century in Europe and came to North America. Each became prominent and then faded from popularity with the rise of conventional medicine. Neither system has experienced a large increase in popularity in the United States recently (Barnes et al., 2008).

IN SUMMARY

Alternative medicine consists of a group of health care systems, practices, and products that are not currently part of conventional medicine but that people use rather than (alternative medicine) or along with conventional treatments (complementary medicine).

Alternative health care systems include traditional Chinese medicine, Ayurvedic medicine, naturopathy, and homeopathy. TCM and Ayurvedic medicine are ancient; naturopathy and homeopathy arose in the 19th century. Each of these systems presents a theory of health and disease as well as practices for diagnosis and treatment.

TCM holds that the body contains a vital energy called qi; keeping this energy in balance is essential to health. Techniques such as acupuncture and acupressure, herbal remedies, massage (called *tui na*), and the energy-channeling practices of qi gong and tai chi are aimed at achieving this balance. Ayurvedic medicine accepts the notion of vital energy and holds that the integration of body, mind, and spirit is essential to health. Diet and herbal preparations are part of Ayurvedic medicine, and so is exercise, including yoga.

Naturopathy and homeopathy were prominent treatments 100 years ago in the United States, but their popularity declined and has not rebounded.

Alternative Practices and Products

Alternative practices lie outside of conventional medicine but do not constitute entire medical systems. Rather, they consist of practices oriented toward symptom relief or treatment of disease conditions. The most common alternative practices are chiropractic treatment and massage. These practices are among the most popular alternative treatments, accounting for about 17% of CAM usage (Barnes et al., 2008). Natural products are also popular, including fish oil supplements, glucosamine, echinacea, and ginseng. These nonvitamin, nonmineral supplements are among the most commonly used natural products. About 18% of people in the United States have used one or more of these natural products (Barnes et al., 2008). Following specific diets for health improvement (rather than for weight reduction specifically) is less common; about 4% of adults follow one of these diet regimens.

Chiropractic Treatment

Chiropractic was founded by Daniel David Palmer in 1895 (NCCAM, 2007/2010). Palmer believed that manipulation of the spine was the key not only to curing illness but also to preventing it. That focus forms the basis for chiropractic care—performing adjustments to the spine and joints to correct misalignments that underlie health problems. Chiropractic adjustments involve applying pressure with the hands or with a machine that forces a joint to move beyond its passive range of motion. Chiropractors may also use heat, ice, and electric stimulation as part of treatment; they may also prescribe exercise for rehabilitation, dietary changes, or dietary supplements. With these problems corrected, the body can heal itself.

Palmer founded the first chiropractic school in 1896, and chiropractic began to spread in the United States during the early 20th century (Pettman, 2007). Students are accepted into schools of chiropractic training after completing at least 90 hours in undergraduate college courses, focusing on science (NCCAM, 2007/2010). Chiropractic training requires an additional 4 years of study in one of the schools accredited by the Council of Chiropractic Education. The program involves coursework and patient care. All 50 states of the United States license chiropractors after they finish their course of study and undergo board examinations.

Almost from the beginning of chiropractic, physicians attacked the practice, having chiropractors prosecuted for practicing medicine without a license (Pettman, 2007). The American Medical Association waged a bitter battle against chiropractic throughout the mid-20th century, but the chiropractors prevailed. Chiropractic is in the process of becoming integrated into conventional medicine; for example, requests by athletes for chiropractic treatment has encouraged its integration into sport medicine (Theberge, 2008). Chiropractic treatment is also available for clients served through the U.S. Department of Defense and the Department of Veterans Affairs, and efforts to expand this type of coverage are under way ("RAND Corporation," 2011). Indeed, chiropractic treatment has become so well accepted that many insurance plans pay for these services. About 8% of adults, about 4% of children in the United States (Barnes et al., 2008), and about 11% of those in Canada (Park, 2005) used chiropractic within the year before the survey. Back, neck, and headache pain were the most common condition that prompted this treatment (Barnes et al, 2008).

Massage

Chiropractic manipulation focuses on the spine and joints, but massage manipulates soft tissue to produce health benefits. Considered a luxury a few years ago, massage is now recognized as an alternative therapy used to control stress and pain. This approach dates back thousands of years and arose in many cultures (Moyer, Rounds, & Hannum, 2004). Records of massage date back to 2000 B.C.E., and early healers such as Hippocrates and Galen wrote about its benefits. Today, over 8% of adults and 1% of children in the United States have used massage as CAM (Barnes et al., 2008).

Several different types of therapeutic massage exist. Although Per Henrik Ling is often credited, it was

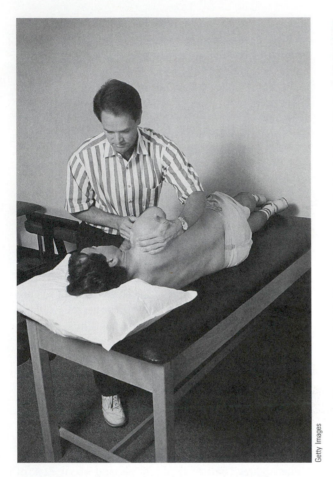

Manipulating the spinal cord or muscles can be effective in helping to relieve pain.

Johan Mezger who developed the massage techniques during the 19th century that became known as Swedish massage (Pettman, 2007). This type of massage uses light strokes in one direction combined with kneading muscles using deeper pressure in the opposite direction to achieve relaxation (NCCAM, 2006/2010a). Originally part of physical therapy and rehabilitation, this approach to massage is now also practiced as an independent therapy for stress and pain management.

Other types of massage come from other systems of medicine, including traditional Chinese medicine, Ayurveda, and naturopathy. Acupressure and *tui na* are both manipulative techniques originating in TCM (Xue, Zhang, Greenwood, Lin, & Story, 2010). Acupressure involves the application of pressure to meridians on the body, with the goal of unblocking the flow of qi. *Shiatsu massage* is the Japanese counterpart of acupressure. *Tui na* is another approach from TCM for allowing the qi to flow freely throughout the body. It may involve pushing the qi along specific meridians using one finger or thumb, which is also similar to shiatsu massage. The rationale for Ayurvedic massage holds that manipulating specific points on the body will channel healing energy within the body. Its practice often involves medicinal oils to decrease friction and to help with the healing. Thus, the practice of massage is common in CAM, arising from several systems and used as an independent healing practice.

Diets, Supplements, and Natural Products

Diet is an important factor in health, and some people follow specific diet plans as a way to improve their health (and also to lose weight). Such diets include vegetarian, macrobiotic, Atkins, Ornish, Zone, or South Beach diets. Less than 4% of people in the United States follow one of these diets (Barnes et al., 2008), and the percentage has decreased over the past 10 years.

All vegetarian diets restrict meat and fish and focus on vegetables, fruits, grains, legumes, seeds, and plant-based oils, but several varieties of vegetarian diets exist (Mayo Clinic Staff, 2008). Lactovegetarian diets allow dairy products, ovolacto vegetarian diets allow dairy products and eggs, whereas vegan diets allow neither dairy nor egg products. Diets that restrict meat and meat products tend to be lower in fat and higher in fiber than other diets, which make them beneficial for people with health problems such as high cholesterol levels. The American Heart Association and the American Cancer Society have recommended limiting meat consumption for health reasons. The American Dietetic Association (Mangels, Messina, & Melina, 2003) has pronounced all three varieties of vegetarian diets capable of furnishing adequate nutrition for people in all stages of development, but vegetarians must plan their meals carefully to assure that they receive adequate protein, calcium, and other nutrients that are plentiful in meat. Those who follow a *macrobiotic diet* must be even more careful than other vegetarians to obtain adequate nutrients (American Cancer Society, 2007) because this diet plan is not only largely vegetarian but also restricts food choices to grains, cereals, cooked vegetables, and a limited amount of fruit and fish.

The Atkins, Pritikin, Ornish, Zone, and South Beach diets vary in terms of the amount of carbohydrates and fats allowed and also vary in their overall goals (Gardner et al., 2007). For example, the Atkins diet program limits carbohydrates but not fat or calories, whereas the Ornish program strives to limit fat intake to 10% of calories, which makes this diet almost entirely vegetarian, difficult to follow, and thus rarely followed (Barnes et al., 2008). The South Beach Diet is a weight loss program that limits both carbohydrates and fats but strives for a nutritionally balanced diet. Between 1% and 2% of adults in the United States follow vegetarian, Atkins, or South Beach diets, making these plans more popular than other dietary regimens.

People also try to maintain or enhance their health by supplementing their diets with a wide variety of vitamins, minerals, herbs, amino acids, extracts, special foods, and other natural products, which may occur along with or as an alternative to adopting a specific diet. In the United States, the Food and Drug Administration regulates natural products as food rather than as drugs; such products are sold without restriction, without evaluations of effectiveness, but with evaluations of safety (NCCAM, 2008/2011).

The practice of supplementing the diet to improve health is ancient, originating in many cultures and in many variations, including Traditional Chinese Medicine (Xue, Zhang, Lin, Da Costa, & Story, 2007) and Ayurveda (NCCAM, 2005/2009) dating back thousands of years. People use vitamin and mineral supplements primarily to preserve their health and to promote wellness, a practice that is so widely used that it does not fall within CAM. Many people also use other nonvitamin, nonmineral supplements to prevent disease or enhance health (Barnes et al., 2008), which does fall within CAM practice. For example, omega-3 fatty acid supplements are used for reducing the risks of cardiovascular disease, echinacea as a treatment for colds and flu, and glucosamine for osteoarthritis ("The Art and Science of Natural Products," 2010). In addition, some people supplement their diets with *functional foods*, components of a normal diet that have biologically active components, such as soy, chocolate, cranberries, and other foods containing anitoxidants. Sales of dietary supplements amount to billions of dollars each year in the United States, and supplements are among the most widely used types of alternative medicine; almost 18% of adults in the United States use such natural products (Barnes et al., 2008).

IN SUMMARY

Alternative practices and products include chiropractic treatments, massage, diets, and dietary supplements. Chiropractic focuses on spinal alignment and the joints, using adjustment techniques to bring the spine back into alignment. Massage is also a manipulation technique, but massage focuses on the soft tissue. Several different types of massage exist, but many share the underlying premise that this type of manipulation helps the body to heal itself. Another common procedure is following a specialized diet. Many diets are oriented toward weight loss or lowering cholesterol levels, such as the Atkins, Ornish, South Beach, or Zone diets; other diets have the goal of improving health, such as vegetarian and macrobiotic diets. People are more likely to supplement their diets with a wide variety of vitamins, minerals, and natural products such as herbs, amino acids, extracts, and special foods to improve health or to treat specific conditions. This approach has become the most commonly used alterative medicine in the United States.

Mind–Body Medicine

Mind–body medicine is the term applied to a variety of techniques that are based on the notion that the brain, mind, body, and behavior interact in complex ways and that emotional, mental, social, and behavioral factors exert important effects on health (NCCAM, 2008/2011). Some of these techniques are associated with psychology and some with conventional medicine, but all share the notion that mind and body represent a holistic system of dynamic interactions. Norman Cousins, whose story began this chapter, was an enthusiastic proponent of this view. However, this conception is not recent; it forms the basis for traditional Chinese medicine, Ayurvedic medicine, and many other systems of traditional and folk medicine. This notion was also prominent in Europe until the 17th century, when French philosopher René Descartes proposed that the mind and the body work according to different principles. Descartes' pronouncement promoted the view that the body functions according to mechanistic principles, which was important in the development of Western medicine but discounted the importance of the mind in physical health.

Those who accept mind–body medicine seek to understand the interaction of mind and body and its relationship to health. Some of the techniques of mind–body medicine come from those systems that propose a holistic view, such as traditional Chinese medicine and Ayurvedic medicine. However, the techniques include not only meditation, tai chi, qi gong, and yoga, which arose within those systems of medicine, but also guided imagery, hypnosis, and biofeedback. A component that is common to most of these practices is deep, controlled breathing, but many people in the United States (12.7%) use deep-breathing exercises alone rather than as a part of other mind–body techniques (Barnes et al., 2008).

Meditation and Yoga

Most approaches to meditation originated in Asian religions, but the mind–body approaches to meditation typically have no religious connotations (NCCAM, 2006/2010b). Many variations of meditation exist, but all involve a quiet location, a specific posture, a focus of attention, and an open attitude. Two prominent types of meditation are transcendental meditation and mindfulness meditation. Over 9% of adults in the United States have practiced meditation (Barnes et al., 2008).

Transcendental Meditation   Transcendental meditation originated in the Vedic tradition in India (NCCAM, 2006/2010b). Participants who practice this type of meditation usually sit with eyes closed and muscles relaxed. They then focus attention on their breathing and silently repeat a sound, such as "om" or any other personally meaningful word or phrase, with each breath for about 20 minutes. Repetition of the single word is intended to prevent distracting thoughts and to sustain muscle relaxation. Meditation requires a conscious motivation to focus attention on a single thought or image along with effort not to be distracted by other thoughts.

Mindfulness Meditation   Mindfulness meditation has roots in ancient Buddhist practice (Bodhi, 2011) but has been adapted as a modern stress reduction practice. In mindfulness meditation, people usually sit in a relaxed, upright posture and focus on any thoughts or sensations as they occur, trying to enhance their own awareness of their perceptions and thought processes in a nonjudgmental way (Kabat-Zinn, 1993). If

unpleasant thoughts or sensations occur, meditators are encouraged not to ignore them, but to let them pass and to concentrate on the breath. By noting thoughts objectively, without censoring or editing them, people can gain insight into how they see the world and what motivates them.

Mindfulness meditation has been adapted into a program of mindfulness-based stress reduction (Kabat-Zinn, 1993). This procedure involves an 8-week course of training, which typically occurs for at least 2 hours per day and may also include an intensive retreat to develop meditation skills. Mindfulness-based stress reduction has been used in a wide variety of settings to help people control anxiety and manage chronic disease and pain conditions. Research into the nature of mindfulness training (Jha, Krompinger, & Baime, 2007) suggests that it improves attention processes by altering the subcomponents of attention such as orienting attention and alerting attention. Additional research (Hölzel et al., 2011) confirms that mindfulness meditation works by altering brain function.

Guided Imagery   Guided imagery shares some elements with meditation, but it also has important differences. In guided imagery, people conjure up a calm, peaceful image, such as the repetitive rhythmic roar of an ocean or the quiet beauty of a pastoral scene. They then concentrate on that image for the duration of a situation, often one that is painful or anxiety provoking. The assumption underlying guided imagery is that a person cannot concentrate on more than one thing at a time. Therefore, imagining an especially powerful or delightful scene will divert attention from the painful experience (see Becoming Healthier box). About 2% of people in the United States have used guided imagery (Barnes et al., 2008).

Yoga   Yoga has its origins in ancient India but is now part of mind–body practice (NCCAM, 2008). It includes physical postures, breathing, and meditation, and its goal is to balance body, mind, and spirit. Of the various schools of yoga, Hatha yoga is the most common in the United States and Europe. The many postures of yoga furnish ways to move and concentrate energy in the body. This concentration of attention on the body permits people to ignore other situations and problems and to live in their bodies in the moment. Controlled breathing fosters relaxation. About 6% of adults and 2% of children in the United States practice yoga (Barnes et al., 2008).

Becoming Healthier

One technique that helps people manage and minimize pain is guided imagery. This technique involves creating an image and being guided (or guiding yourself) through it. The process can be helpful in dealing with both chronic pain and acute pain, such as medical or dental procedures. Those who are not experienced at guided imagery will benefit from having a recorded version of the guided imagery instructions.

To practice guided imagery, choose a quiet place where you will not be disturbed and where you will be comfortable. Prepare for the experience by placing the recording where you can turn it on, seating yourself in a comfortable chair, and taking a few deep breaths. Turn on the player, close your eyes, and follow the instructions you have recorded.

The instructions should include a description of a special place, one that you either imagine or have experienced, where you feel safe and at peace. Tailor the place to fit with your life and experiences—one person's magic place may not be so attractive to another person, so think about what will be appealing to you. Many people enjoy a beach scene, but others like woods, fields, or special rooms. The goal is to imagine somewhere that you will feel relaxed and at peace.

Put instructions on your recording concerning this place and its description. Spend time in this place and experience it in detail. Pay attention to the sights and sounds, but do not neglect the smells and skin senses associated with the place. Spend time imagining each of these sensory experiences, and include instructions to yourself about the feelings. You should feel relaxed and peaceful as you go through this scene. Linger over the details and aim to allow yourself to become completely absorbed in the experience.

Include some instructions for relaxed breathing in your tour of your special place. Your goal is to achieve peace and relaxation that will replace the anxiety and pain that you have felt. As you repeat the guided imagery exercise, you may want to revise the recorded instructions to include more details. The recording should include at least 10 minutes of guided instructions, and your experience and practice may lead you to lengthen it. Eventually, you will not need the recording, and you will be able to use this technique wherever you go.

Qi Gong and Tai Chi

Traditional Chinese medicine includes movement-based approaches to unblock qi and improve health. The basic technique is qi gong (also written *qigong, chi gung*, and *chi gong*), which consists of a series of exercises or movements that are intended to concentrate and balance the body's vital energy (Sancier & Holman, 2004). Its practice promotes relaxation and provides exercise. Tai chi or *tai chi chuan* originated as one of the martial arts but evolved into a set of movements used for therapeutic benefits (Gallagher, 2003).

Qi Gong   Qi gong involves the practice or cultivation (gong) of the qi (energy) by postures and simple movements that channel vital energy and restore balance in the body. It is one of the basic practices of traditional Chinese medicine (Twicken, 2011). One way to view qi gong is as "the manipulation of the regulation of the body, breath, and mind into an integrative whole, with the breath as the key regulator practice to make this happen" (Shinnick, 2006, p. 351). These postures and movements may be practiced individually or integrated into a sequence, called a *form*. Within traditional Chinese medicine, the practice of qi gong increases health and decreases the need for treatments such as acupuncture and herbal remedies.

Although qi gong fits within the philosophy of traditional Chinese medicine, its practice has been adapted to be compatible with Western medicine, under the name *medical qi gong* (He, 2005; Twicken, 2011). Researchers have investigated the physical existence of qi, with claims that the practice of qi gong creates measurable changes in thermal and electrical energy (Shinnick, 2006). Evidence also exists that qi gong training produces changes in the function of the immune system (Lee, Kim, & Ryu, 2005), which allows for a specific route through which qi gong might affect health. The practice of medical qi gong seeks to prevent disease, promote long life, and treat specific disease conditions such as hypertension, diabetes, and heart disease as well as stress and pain. The practice of qi gong is not common in the United States; fewer than

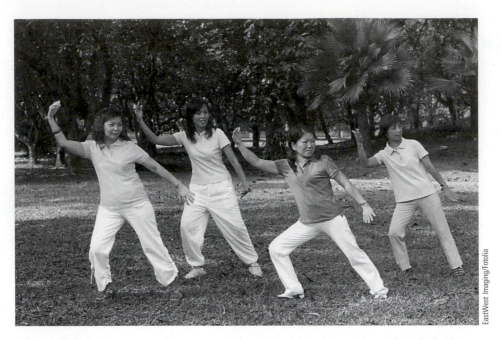

EastWest Imaging/Fotolia

Tai chi chuan is a movement-based technique that produces physical and psychological benefits.

1% of people in the United States have practiced qi gong (Barnes et al., 2008).

Tai Chi Tai chi (or *tai chi chuan*) is one category of qi gong form, which has evolved from a martial art with a long but disputed history. Some advocates trace its history back thousands of years, whereas others point to a history of only several hundred years (Kurland, 2000). The key figures in its development are also the subject of debate, but a commonly cited story involves a Shaolin monk who noticed the struggle between a snake and a crane and adapted their movements to a form of defense. Over time, the practice of tai chi became increasingly popular as a way to promote health, spreading throughout China and around the world. As one of the practices of traditional Chinese medicine, tai chi cultivates balance between the yin and yang energies and thus promotes health.

Tai chi involves slow, gentle movements that shift the weight while the person maintains an upright yet relaxed posture and controlled breathing (NCCAM, 2006/2010c). One movement flows into another, and those who practice tai chi strive to maintain a steady rate of movement while coordinating the breath with the movements, creating a "moving meditation." The history of tai chi includes the development of many different styles, originally perpetuated within families. Currently, the Yang style is the most common in China and among those who practice tai chi as alternative medicine. All of the variations in styles include a set of movements connected together into a sequence, called a form. Tai chi provides moderate intensity aerobic exercise equivalent to brisk walking and a low-impact form of exercise that is appropriate for a wide variety of individuals (Taylor-Piliae, Haskell, Waters, & Froelicher, 2006). Tai chi is more widely practiced in the United States than qi gong, but only 0.4% of adults reported its use (Barnes et al., 2008).

Energy Healing

The view that energy can heal the body or that the body contains vital, healing energy is common to many alternative systems and practices. In traditional Chinese medicine, the techniques of qi gong and *tui na* may be considered ways to channel energy for healing purposes. The Japanese technique of Reiki is another energy healing practice (NCCAM, 2006/2009). This practice originated in Japan in the early 20th century and came to Western cultures in the late 1930s. Reiki appears to be a version of massage, but the concept behind this manipulation is a directing of energy

Would You BELIEVE...? Religious Involvement May Improve Your Health

Beginning with Emile Durkheim (1912–1967) a century ago, social scientists have pondered and debated the health benefits of religious involvement. Millions of people throughout the world find nothing to question—prayer is part of their daily lives, including prayers for their own health and the health of others. Between 2002 and 2007, the use of prayer related to health increased in the United States from 43% to 49% (Wachholtz & Sambamoorthi, 2011). A large majority of people who use prayers for health rated the prayers as helpful (McCaffrey, Eisenberg, Legedza, Davis, & Phillips, 2004), but finding prayer helpful is not the same as being helped by prayers for health. Do people receive measurable health benefits from prayers?

Prayer may influence health through several routes (Breslin & Lewis, 2008). Prayer may prompt a placebo response or distract individuals from unpleasant symptoms of disease. Prayer may increase self-efficacy (Masters & Spielmans, 2007) and thus improve health indirectly. Many religions offer guidelines for behavior such as moderation in lifestyle choices, so people who are religious may practice better health behaviors and thus may be healthier. Another route of influence is through spirituality, which can lead people to enhanced positive mental states that may affect the immune system and thus influence health. In addition, spirituality may allow people to develop feelings of optimism and hope (Ai, Peterson, Tice, Bolling, & Koenig, 2004), providing an additional benefit of prayer. One type of prayer, called centering prayer, may constitute a type of meditation, which has demonstrated its effectiveness in stress and pain relief (Ferguson, Willemsen, & Castañeto, 2010). Thus, prayer may influence health through a variety of routes.

But can the prayers of one person affect the health of others? There is little evidence for the effect of this type of prayer. Meta-analyses (Masters & Spielmans, 2007; Masters, Spielmans, & Goodson, 2005) and a systematic review (Roberts, Ahmed, Hall, & Davison, 2009) indicated that people who were the objects of prayers did not differ significantly from those who were not, either in terms of life expectancy or readmissions to the hospital. Despite widespread beliefs that prayer can affect health directly, when people do not know about the intercession, their health remains the same. However, prayer may affect health indirectly and provide an effective coping mechanism for people with ill health (Wachholtz & Sambamoorthi, 2011).

from the universe through the hands of a practitioner and to the body of the recipient. Practitioners use specific hand postures to channel this healing energy, and people who receive this type of treatment typically experience relaxation and a relief from pain. Energy healing is among the most controversial of alternative treatments; however, one of the most widely used alternative practices fits into this controversial category—prayers for health improvement (see Would You Believe …? box).

Biofeedback

Until the 1960s, most people in the Western world assumed that it was impossible to consciously control physiological processes such as heart rate, the secretion of digestive juices, and the constriction of blood vessels. These biological functions do not require conscious attention for their regulation, and conscious attempts at regulation seem to have little effect. Then, during the late 1960s, a number of researchers began to explore the possibility of controlling biological processes traditionally believed to be beyond conscious control. Their efforts culminated in the development of **biofeedback**, the process of providing feedback information about the status of biological systems. Early experiments indicated that biofeedback made possible the control of some otherwise automatic functions. In 1969, Neal E. Miller reported a series of experiments in which he and his colleagues altered the levels of animals' visceral response through reinforcement. Some subjects received rewards for raising their heart rate and others for lowering it. Within a few hours, significant differences in heart rate appeared. After other investigators demonstrated that biofeedback could be used with humans (Brown, 1970; Kamiya, 1969), interest in this procedure became widespread.

In biofeedback, biological responses are measured by electronic instruments, and the status of those responses is immediately available to the person using the machines. By using biofeedback, a person gains information about changes in biological responses as those responses are taking place. This feedback allows the person to alter physiological responses that cannot be voluntarily controlled without the biofeedback information.

Several types of biofeedback are in clinical use, including electromyography and thermal biofeedback; less than1% of people in the United States reported that they use biofeedback (Barnes et al., 2008). **Electromyograph (EMG) biofeedback** reflects the activity of the skeletal muscles by measuring the electrical discharge in muscle fibers. The measurement is taken by attaching electrodes to the surface of the skin over the muscles to be monitored. The level of electrical activity reflects the degree of tension or relaxation of the muscles. The machine responds with a signal that varies according to that muscle activity. Biofeedback can be used to increase muscle tension in rehabilitation or to decrease muscle tension in stress management. The most common use of EMG biofeedback among CAM users is in the control of low back pain and headaches, however EMG biofeedback is becoming more widely recognized as useful in rehabilitation (Langhorne, Coupar, & Pollock, 2009; Tate & Milner, 2010).

Thermal biofeedback, which may also be used to help people cope with stress and pain, is based on the principle that skin temperature varies in relation to levels of stress. Stress tends to constrict blood vessels, whereas relaxation opens them. Therefore, cool surface skin temperature may indicate stress and tension; warm skin temperature suggests calm and relaxation. Thermal biofeedback involves placing a **thermistor**—a temperature-sensitive resistor—on the skin's surface. The thermistor signals changes in skin temperature, thereby furnishing the information that allows control. The feedback signal, as with EMG biofeedback, may be auditory, visual, or both.

Hypnotic Treatment

Although trancelike conditions are probably older than human history, modern hypnosis is usually traced to the last part of the 18th century, when Austrian physician Franz Anton Mesmer conducted elaborate demonstrations in Paris. Although Mesmer's work was attacked, modifications of his technique, known as *mesmerism*, soon spread to other parts of the world. By the 1830s, mesmerism was being used by some surgeons as an anesthetic during major operations (Hilgard & Hilgard, 1994).

With the discovery of chemical anesthetics, the popularity of hypnosis waned, but during the late 19th century, many European physicians, including Sigmund Freud, employed hypnotic procedures in the treatment of mental illness. Since the beginning of the 20th century, the popularity of hypnosis as a medical and psychological tool has continued to wax and wane. Its present position is still somewhat controversial, but a significant number of practitioners within medicine and psychology are using hypnotherapy to treat health-related problems, especially pain. The technique remains in limited use; less than 1% of people in the United States have used hypnosis (Barnes et al., 2008).

Not only is the use of hypnotic processes still controversial, but the precise nature of hypnosis is also debatable. Some authorities, such as Joseph Barber (1996) and Ernest Hilgard (1978), regard hypnosis as an altered *state* of consciousness in which a person's stream of consciousness is divided or dissociated. Barber argued that hypnotic analgesia works through a process of negative hallucination—not perceiving something that one would ordinarily perceive. To Hilgard, the process of **induction**—that is, being placed into a hypnotic state—is central to the hypnotic process. After induction, the responsive person enters a state of divided or dissociated consciousness that is essentially different from the normal state. This altered state of consciousness allows people to respond to suggestion and to control physiological processes that they cannot control in the normal state of consciousness.

The alternative view of hypnosis holds that it is a more generalized *trait*, or a relatively permanent characteristic of some people who respond well to suggestion (Barber, 1984, 2000). Those who hold this view reject the basic conception that hypnosis is altered consciousness. Rather, they argue that hypnosis is nothing more than relaxation, induction is not necessary, and suggestive procedures can be just as effective without entering a trancelike state.

Research has not resolved this controversy. Brain imaging studies (De Benedittis, 2003; Rainville & Price, 2003) tend to support the view that hypnosis is an altered state of consciousness. However, in a study comparing hypnotic to nonhypnotic suggestion (Milling, Kirsch, Allen, & Reutenauer, 2005), both types were comparably effective. That is, expectancy and suggestion led to a reduction of pain whether participants were hypnotized or not.

IN SUMMARY

Mind–body medicine is a term applied to a variety of techniques that people use to improve their health or treat health problems, including meditation, guided imagery, yoga, qi gong, tai chi, energy healing, biofeedback, and hypnosis. Transcendental meditation directs people to focus on a single thought or sound to achieve relaxation, whereas mindfulness meditation encourages practitioners to focus on the moment, becoming mindful of the details of their current experience. Guided imagery encourages people to create a pleasant scene to achieve relaxation and anxiety relief. Yoga uses physical postures, breathing, and meditation, with the goal of balancing body, mind, and spirit. The movement-based practices of qi gong and tai chi originated in traditional Chinese medicine. Qi gong and tai chi involve postures and movements intended to direct and balance the body's vital energy. Energy healing techniques such as Reiki also work toward directing energy for healing purposes, but this Japanese method of directing healing energy also shares elements with massage.

Biofeedback is the process of providing feedback information about the status of biological systems with the goal of controlling them. Many types of biofeedback exist, but learning to control muscle tension through electromyograph biofeedback and skin temperature through thermal biofeedback have the widest clinical applications. Hypnotic treatment is controversial, with some authorities arguing that it represents an altered state of consciousness that boosts relaxation and suggestibility, whereas others contend that it is a trait of some individuals. In either case, relaxation and suggestibility both have the potential to improve health.

Who Uses Complementary and Alternative Medicine?

People use techniques from complementary and alternative medicine to enhance health, prevent disease, and manage health problems. Many of the techniques from CAM are applicable and widely used in managing anxiety, stress, and pain. Indeed, a great deal of the research funded by the U.S. National Center for Complementary and Alternative Medicine is oriented toward assessing the effectiveness of these approaches for these conditions.

A growing number of people find CAM techniques appealing, and an increasing number of people use them. A comparison of CAM use in 2002 and 2007 in the United States (Barnes et al., 2008) showed increases in the use of several types. The number of people who use natural products such as omega-3 fatty acid supplements, glucosamine, and echinacea has increased, making the category of natural products the most frequently used CAM. Increases also appeared among those who use deep-breathing exercises, meditation, yoga, massage, and chiropractic care. CAM approaches in the category of mind–body medicine increased more than other categories. Table 8.1 shows the most frequently used types of CAM by adults and by children in the United States.

People not only use a variety of CAM techniques, but they also use the techniques for a variety of reasons. However, pain was the most common problem for which adults reported the use of CAM, including back, neck, joint, or arthritis pain (Barnes et al., 2008). The situation suggests that CAM users tend to have conditions that are painful, a suggestion confirmed by other analyses (Ayers & Kronenfeld, 2011; Wells, Phillips, Schachter, & McCarthy, 2010). These people may have some condition that creates pain that has not been addressed through conventional medicine (Freedman, 2011), prompting them to seek alternative care in addition to conventional treatment. Indeed, most adults who use CAM employ the techniques as complementary rather than alternative medicine. This pattern is similar to CAM use in Europe (Rössler et al., 2007), Canada (Foltz et al., 2005), and Israel (Shmueli, Igudin, & Shuval, 2011).

Culture, Ethnicity, and Gender

The use of CAM varies among countries to some extent. In a population study in Australia, 68.9% of people reported using some form of CAM (Xue et al., 2007), indicating a substantially higher level of use than in the United States. In addition, the Australian government has integrated CAM into health care delivery to a greater extent than in most other English-speaking countries (Baer, 2008).

TABLE 8.1   Most Frequently Used CAM Therapies

Technique	Percentage of Adults Who Used This Approach	Percentage of Children (<18 years) Who Used This Approach
Natural products: omega-3 fatty acid supplements, glucosamine, echinacea, ginseng	17.7%	9.2%
Deep-breathing exercises	12.7	5.4
Meditation	9.4	3.0
Chiropractic care	8.6	5.7
Massage	8.3	2.2
Yoga	6.1	4.7
Diet-based therapies: vegetarian, South Beach, Atkins diet	3.6	1.4
Progressive relaxation	2.9	1.3
Guided imagery	2.2	1.5
Any CAM technique	38.3%	11.8%

Source: Data from "Complementary and alternative medicine use among adults and children, United States, 2007," by P. M. Barnes, B. Bloom, & R. L. Nahin, 2008, *National Health Statistics Reports*, no. 12. Hyattsville, MD: National Center for Health Statistics.

In Europe, the percentage of users varies by country. Some countries are similar to the United States, whereas others use CAM as frequently as Australians do (di Sarsina, 2007). The types of treatments and demographics of users are similar among these three geographic areas. Nutritional supplements, massage therapy, meditation, chiropractic treatments, yoga, and acupuncture are among the most popular CAM therapies (Xue et al., 2007).

Within Europe, the availability of CAM varies. In some countries, such as Sweden, the availability is limited; the Swedish health service does not consider offering CAM treatments because of insufficient evidence of their effectiveness (di Sarsina, 2007). In other countries, such as Germany and the United Kingdom, CAM is integrated into medical practice; physicians receive training in CAM and refer patients to CAM practitioners. In countries in which CAM is integrated into the health services, users tend to come from a wider variety of socioeconomic backgrounds than in countries such as the United States, where most CAM users must pay out-of-pocket for such treatment.

In the United States and Canada, CAM use varies with ethnicity, but not in ways that correspond to stereotypes (Keith, Kronenfeld, Rivers, & Liang, 2005; Roth & Kobayashi, 2008). The stereotypical association of CAM with ethnic minorities and recent immigrants is largely incorrect: European Americans are more likely than African Americans or Hispanic Americans to use CAM. Indeed, recent immigrants are *less* likely to use CAM than immigrants who have been in the United States for years (Su, Li, & Pagán, 2008). A similar finding emerged from a study of Asian Americans (Hsiao, Wong, et al., 2006) and Asians in Canada (Roth & Kobayashi, 2008). However, Asian Americans used CAM at higher rates than non-Hispanic European Americans, and Asians in Canada use CAM more frequently than the Canadian population in general. Chinese Americans' usage of CAM tended to correspond to their culture: Chinese Americans were more likely than other Asian Americans to use herbal products (Hsiao, Wong, et al., 2006) and to seek acupuncture treatment (Burke, Upchurch, Dye, & Chyu, 2006). Similar patterns apply to Asians in Canada: Their use of CAM is related to how strongly they identified with Asian culture (Roth & Kobayashi, 2008).

In all ethnic groups and in various countries, individuals who seek CAM tend to be female, well-educated, and in the upper income brackets. In the United States, well-educated European American women are more likely than others to use CAM (Barnes et al., 2008). The willingness of women to use CAM may relate to personal beliefs or health concerns (Furnham, 2007). The importance of personal beliefs and the compatibility of CAM with one's beliefs may explain why some people seek alternative treatments, whereas others do not.

Motivations for Seeking Alternative Treatment

Although culture, ethnicity, and gender each shows a relationship to CAM use, other factors are probably more important. One of those important factors is acceptance of the underlying values of CAM. Research findings suggest that people use CAM when the techniques are compatible with their personal worldviews and concerns about health (Astin, 1998). For example, young men who expressed strong beliefs in science were less likely to use CAM than other people (Furnham, 2007). People who have less faith in conventional medicine and stronger beliefs in the role of attitude and emotion in health are more likely to try CAM. Thus, an openness to different worldviews, an acceptance of the value in holistic treatment, and a belief in the contribution of biopsychosocial factors to health are more typical of CAM users than of those who stay with conventional treatments exclusively.

A person's current health status is also an important predictor of CAM usage. People tend to seek alternative treatments when conventional medicine has not offered relief for their conditions. Those who use CAM may not be dissatisfied with conventional medicine (Astin, 1998); people tend to add alternative treatments to the conventional ones they are using rather than replace conventional treatments with alternative ones. However, individuals who experience chronic health problems that have not responded well to conventional treatments may be open to the possibilities of alternative treatment (Freedman, 2011). Indeed, poor health status is a significant predictor of CAM usage (Barnes et al., 2008). Reasonably enough, people who are unwell and continue to experience distressing symptoms are motivated to find some effective treatment, including alternative medicine. For example, people who received treatment for cancer were substantially more likely to use CAM than those who had not been treated for cancer (Mao, Palmer, Healy, Desai, & Amsterdam, 2011). One analysis (Ayers & Kronenfeld, 2011) indicated that the experience of pain was the best predictor of who had used CAM. However, a survey of CAM users (Nguyen, Davis, Kaptchuk, & Phillips, 2011) indicated that they were more likely than nonusers to rate their health as excellent and to say that their

health had improved over the previous year. This combination of findings suggests that CAM users may be prompted to seek alternative treatments due to some health problem and that they are satisfied with the outcome.

Within both conventional and alternative medicine lie concerns about effectiveness and safety for the various products and practices that fall within CAM. What is the evidence of success for these alternative approaches?

IN SUMMARY

Most people who use CAM use it as a complementary rather than an alternative treatment. People in the United States and other countries use a great variety of CAM products and practices, including natural products, deep-breathing exercises, massage, meditation, chiropractic treatments, and yoga. People in Australia and some European countries use CAM more often than people in the United States, but the assortment of techniques is similar. Ethnicity is a factor in CAM use in the United States, but ethnic stereotypes of recent immigrants' using traditional remedies is incorrect. CAM usage is associated with being female, European American, well educated, and in a high-income bracket. This combination of demographic characteristics also applies to CAM use in Canada, Australia, and some European countries.

People are motivated to use CAM if their worldviews are compatible with the philosophies that underlie CAM—accepting a biopsychosocial view of health rather than a biomedical view. Health status is also a motivation for seeking CAM; people who have health problems that have not responded to conventional treatments may be motivated to seek CAM.

How Effective Are Alternative Treatments?

Alternative treatments are classified as *alternative* because insufficient evidence exists for their effectiveness. Evaluating the effectiveness of alternative treatments has proven to be one of the most controversial areas related to alternative medicine, spurring bitter arguments. Advocates of conventional medicine criticize that little evidence exists for the effectiveness of alternative treatments and that the dangers remain unevaluated (Berman & Straus, 2004; Wahlberg, 2007). According to this view, the only acceptable method of establishing effectiveness is the randomized controlled trial in which participants are assigned randomly to a treatment group or a placebo control group in a double blind design; neither practitioner nor participants know to which treatment condition participants belong.

Using the randomized controlled method of conducting experiments allows researchers to minimize the influence of bias and expectation. Both of these factors are important in evaluating treatment studies (as discussed in Chapter 2). People who have expectations concerning CAM will bring this bias into treatment, which may affect the outcome. For example, a study on acupuncture (Linde et al., 2007) assessed participants' attitudes about the effectiveness of acupuncture at the beginning of the study. The results indicated that those who expressed belief that acupuncture was an effective treatment experienced greater pain relief from an 8-week course of treatment than did those who had lower expectations for success. Although expectations for success boost treatment effectiveness, these expectations are a placebo response rather than a response to the treatment. Thus, those who advocate for randomized placebo-controlled trials have a valid point: This design represents a stringent criterion for evidence of effectiveness.

Unfortunately, many alternative treatments do not lend themselves to placebo control and blinding as easily as drug treatments do. For example, most people who receive a massage, practice meditation, or learn biofeedback training cannot be blind to their treatment, nor can practitioners of massage, biofeedback, or yoga be unaware of the treatment they deliver. Thus, fewer options exist for controlling for expectation in CAM than in research on conventional medicine. When studies lack random assignment, placebo control, and "blinding," advocates of conventional medicine judge these studies to be of lesser quality and thus less convincing. By these standards, CAM is inadequate; the standards that advocates of conventional medicine believe must be met cannot be. Regardless of the number of studies with positive results, treatments that have few randomized controlled trials yield judgments of insufficient evidence to make conclusions of effectiveness in systematic reviews.

Disputing the standard of randomized controlled trials is one strategy that CAM advocates have used to argue that CAM is the target of inappropriate judgments (Clark-Grill, 2007). Indeed, some authorities (Wider & Boddy, 2009) have warned that conducting systematic reviews on CAM treatments requires extra care to achieve a fair evaluation. Another type of objection has come from the argument that conventional medicine has not met the standards that its defenders have required of CAM. Kenneth Pelletier (2002) argued that many of the treatments used in conventional medicine have not submitted this standard of evidence. That is, much of the practice of conventional medicine has not come to be accepted through evidence from randomized controlled trials. Many of the standard treatments in medicine and surgery have evolved through clinical practice and observation of what works rather than through experimental evidence of effectiveness. Indeed, the concept of evidence-based medicine is relatively recent. This standard is being applied to CAM more stringently than to treatments within conventional medicine.

Despite these challenges, CAM researchers strive to conduct research that demonstrates effectiveness and safety; this route allows for greater acceptability of CAM treatments (Shannon, Weil, & Kaplan, 2011). What does the evidence say about alternative treatments? Which have demonstrated that they are effective, and for what conditions?

Alternative Treatments for Anxiety, Stress, and Depression

Many CAM modalities have targeted anxiety, stress, and depression, and some have demonstrated their effectiveness. Meditation is an obvious choice for these conditions, and the research evidence confirms its effectiveness. Brain imaging studies have helped clarify what happens when a person relaxes and meditates. Attention and executive function monitoring are altered in meditation (Manna et al., 2010), and different meditation techniques prompt different patterns of brain activation. In mindfulness meditation, the prefrontal cortex and anterior cingulate cortex show higher levels of activation, and long-term experience with meditation prompts changes in brain structures involved in attention (Chiesa & Serretti, 2010).

Meta-analyses and systematic reviews of mindfulness-based stress reduction (Chisea & Serretti,

2010; Grossman, Niemann, Schmidt, & Walach, 2004; Ivanovski & Malhi, 2007) and mindfulness-based cognitive therapy (Fjorback, Arendt, Ørnbøl, Fink, & Walach, 2011) have evaluated the effectiveness of these techniques, coming to positive conclusions. Mindfulness-based approaches seem to be effective for a wide variety of people and for anxiety, stress-related problems, and prevention of relapse into depression. The analyses also indicated that mindfulness meditation can help not only people with stress-related and anxiety disorders but also people without clinical problems who are seeking better ways to manage the stresses in their lives. Those who practiced the technique more also received greater benefits, indicating a dose–response relationship (Carmody & Baer, 2008).

Studies on transcendental meditation have also been the focus of a systematic review (Krisanaprakornkit, Krisanaprakornkit, Piyavhatkul, & Laopaiboon, 2006), which indicated that this type of meditation is similar to other relaxation modalities in helping people with anxiety disorders. A systematic review of yoga (Chong, Tsunaka, Tsang, Chan, & Cheung, 2011) indicated that yoga also constitutes an effective approach to stress management. Thus, the majority of evidence indicates that meditation and programs that include meditation are effective treatment for managing anxiety and depression.

The movement-based practices of qi gong and tai chi also show stress-reducing effects. A number of physiological measurements indicate that the practice of qi gong reduces stress (Sancier & Holman, 2004) and affects the nervous system in ways that reduce the stress response and improve several chronic illnesses (Ng & Tsang, 2009). A study of older Chinese immigrants at risk for cardiovascular disease showed improvements in mood and stress after practicing tai chi for 12 weeks (Taylor-Piliae et al., 2006). A systematic review of tai chi practice (Wang et al., 2010) indicated a wide range of benefits including relief from anxiety, stress, and depression.

Acupuncture also holds some promise in treating depression. In systematic reviews (Leo & Ligot, 2007; Smith, Hay, & MacPherson, 2010), evaluating the effectiveness of acupuncture for depression was difficult, but results indicated that responses to acupuncture treatment were comparable to the use of antidepressant drugs in relieving symptoms of depression. The possibility also exists that combining acupuncture treatment with medication will lead to a boost in effectiveness (Smith et al., 2010). Yoga has also been used successfully as a complementary treatment for depressed people who did not

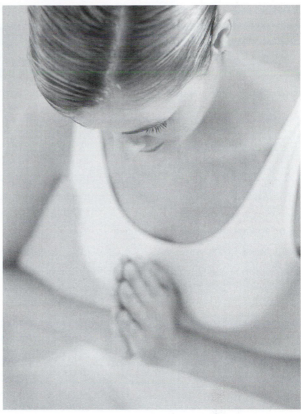

Meditation can help people cope with depression and a variety of stress-related problems.

experience a complete response to antidepressant drugs (Shapiro et al., 2007). Another effective alternative treatment for depression is the herbal remedy Saint-John's wort. A meta-analysis of randomized controlled trials indicated that an extract of this herb alleviates mild to moderate clinical depression, with effectiveness similar to that of antidepressant drugs, but with fewer side effects (Linde, Berner, & Kriston, 2008).

Therefore, a variety of alternative medicine approaches have demonstrated effectiveness in treating anxiety, stress, and depression. Table 8.2 summarizes the evidence for alternative treatments for anxiety, stress, and depression.

Alternative Treatments for Pain

As we discussed in Chapter 7, chronic pain presents problems for those who experience it and for those who attempt to treat it. Conventional medicine often fails to control pain adequately, which motivates

TABLE 8.2   Effectiveness of Alternative Treatments for Anxiety, Stress, and Depression

Problem	Findings	Studies
1. Anxiety and stress	Mindfulness-based stress reduction is effective, according to systematic reviews.	Chiesa & Serretti, 2010; Grossman et al., 2004
2. Relapse into depression	Mindfulness-based cognitive therapy is effective, according to a systematic review.	Fjorback et al., 2011
3. Anxiety disorders and depression	Mindfulness meditation is effective, according to a systematic review.	Ivanovski & Malhi, 2007
4. Stress	Mindfulness-based stress reduction is more effective if practiced more frequently.	Carmody & Baer, 2008
5. Anxiety disorders	Transcendental meditation is comparable to relaxation training, according to a systematic review.	Krisanaprakornkit et al., 2006
6. Anxiety and stress management	Yoga is effective, according to a systematic review.	Chong et al., 2011
7. Stress	Qi gong reduces physiological indicators of stress.	Sancier & Holman, 2004
8. Altering the stress response	Qi gong alters the stress response in ways that are beneficial to several chronic health conditions in older people, according to a systematic review.	Ng & Tsang, 2009
9. Stress and negative mood	Tai chi practice improves stress and mood among older Chinese immigrants.	Taylor-Piliae et al., 2006
10. Anxiety, stress, and depression	Tai chi practice improves these conditions, according to a systematic review	Wang et al., 2010
11. Depression	Acupuncture showed effectiveness comparable to antidepressant drugs in systematic reviews.	Leo & Ligot, 2007; Smith, Hay, & MacPherson, 2010
12. Depression	Yoga is a successful complementary treatment for people taking antidepressants.	Shapiro et al., 2007
13. Depression	Saint-John's wort is as effective as antidepressant drugs and produces fewer side effects, according to a systematic review.	Linde et al., 2008

many people to seek alternative treatments (Ayers & Kronenfeld, 2011; Wells et al., 2010). A variety of alternative treatments have been applied to the problem of pain, but the CAM techniques that are successful in managing pain vary somewhat from those that are effective in managing anxiety, stress, and depression.

Meditation and the related technique of guided imagery received a strong endorsement from a National Institutes of Health Technology panel review, which concluded that these interventions were effective in managing chronic pain (Lebovits, 2007). More recent research (Grant, Courtemanche, Duerden, Duncan, & Rainville, 2010) has determined that experienced meditators' pain sensitivity decreases, including detectable brain changes that underlie this benefit.

Guided imagery has also been described as a best practice for the pain associated with pregnancy and childbirth (Naparstek, 2007). This technique is also effective in managing headaches (Tsao & Zeltzer, 2005) and for reducing postoperative pain in children (Huth, Broome, & Good, 2004) and in older people (Antall & Kresevic, 2004).

Techniques derived from traditional Chinese medicine can also be useful in pain control, including tai chi, qi gong, and acupuncture. Tai chi demonstrated its effectiveness in helping adults with tension headache manage their pain (Abbott, Hui, Hays, Li, & Pan, 2007). A systematic review of studies of qi gong (Lee, Pittler, & Ernst, 2007a) found encouraging evidence regarding its effectiveness in treating chronic pain.

Randomized controlled trials showed that qi gong (Haak & Scott, 2008) and tai chi (Wang et al., 2010) provided relief from pain and improvement in quality of life for people with fibromyalgia.

Acupuncture is better established as a pain treatment than either tai chi or qi gong. A study of the brain changes in connection with acupuncture (Napadow et al., 2007) revealed that participants who received acupuncture, compared with those who received sham acupuncture, showed changes in brain activity that were consistent with decreases in pain perception. Acupuncture also produces complex reactions in the somatosensory system and alters the neurochemistry of the central nervous system, which is likely related to its analgesic effects (Manni, Albanesi, Guaragna, Barbaro Paparo, & Aloe, 2010).

A review of the effectiveness of acupuncture for a variety of pain conditions (Dhanani, Caruso, & Carinci, 2011) indicated that acupuncture has demonstrated positive effects for some pain conditions but not for others. For example, the evidence about benefits of acupuncture is more persuasive for success in treating neck pain than shoulder or elbow pain. Acupuncture is more effective in treating tension-type headache pain than migraine headache pain. The evidence for acupuncture as a treatment for decreasing arthritis knee pain has become more positive as more studies have been conducted and methodology has improved.

Back pain is a common and challenging pain problem, and acupuncture has demonstrated some effectiveness in dealing with this pain syndrome. A meta-analysis of acupuncture for low back pain (Manheimer, White, Berman, Forys, & Ernst, 2005) indicated that this treatment is more effective for short-term relief of chronic back pain than sham acupuncture or no treatment. In a systematic review that considered all types of treatment for back pain (Keller, Hayden, Bombardier, & van Tulder, 2007), acupuncture was among the most effective treatments, although none of the treatments revealed a high degree of effectiveness. This result may point to an answer to some of the confusion concerning the effectiveness of acupuncture (Johnson, 2006): When compared with other treatments, acupuncture may fail to show advantages. When compared to no treatment, the effects may be small. However, none of the available treatment for this condition is very effective. Therefore, acupuncture may be at least as effective a treatment as any for low back pain.

A large-scale research project (Witt, Brinkhaus, Reinhold, & Willich, 2006) examined the benefits of integrating acupuncture into standard medical care for chronic pain. Low back pain, osteoarthritis of the hip and knee, neck pain, and headache were among the types of pain included in treatment. The study found that acupuncture was effective in addition to the benefit obtained from standard medical care. That is, in addition to providing benefits as an alternative treatment, acupuncture was an effective complementary therapy for a variety of pain syndromes.

Massage is another treatment for pain, and a review of massage for all types of chronic pain except cancer pain (Tsao, 2007) indicated varying degrees of effectiveness for different pain syndromes. The strongest evidence of effectiveness came from studies on low back pain (Furlan, Imamura, Dryden, & Irvin, 2008), whereas the evidence for shoulder and headache pain was more modest (Tsao, 2007). A later study (Cherkin et al., 2011) confirmed the benefits for low back pain, and another study (Sherman, Cherkin, Hawkes, Miglioretti, & Deyo, 2009) showed benefits for massage in relieving neck pain. Because of a lack of high-quality studies, a review of massage for musculoskeletal pain (Lewis & Johnson, 2006) failed to reach conclusions concerning effectiveness.

Chiropractic manipulation has also been the subject of systematic review. This type of CAM is most often used for back and neck pain, but a recent review found only small benefits (Rubenstein, van Middlekoop, Assendelft, de Boer, & van Tulder, 2011). However, a review of studies on spinal manipulation for musculoskeletal pain (Perram, 2006) indicated that chiropractic treatment was superior to conventional medical treatment for this type of pain. However, chiropractic manipulation did not appear to be effective in treating tension headaches (Lenssinck et al., 2004), but another review (Haas, Spegman, Peterson, Aickin, & Vavrek, 2010) indicated benefits of spinal manipulation for neck-related headaches.

Early research on the effectiveness of biofeedback (Blanchard et al., 1990) looked promising: Thermal biofeedback with relaxation showed positive results as a treatment for migraine and tension headaches. Later research has painted a less optimistic picture, as biofeedback demonstrated no greater effects than relaxation training in preventing migraine headaches (Stewart, 2004). A meta-analysis of biofeedback studies in the treatment of migraine (Nestoriuc & Martin, 2007) indicated a medium-sized effect, but no such benefit appeared in an assessment of treatment effectiveness for tension-type headache (Verhagen, Damen, Berger, Passchier, & Koes, 2009) or for low back pain (Roelofs, Boissevain, Peters, de Jong, & Vlaeyen, 2002). The added expense associated with providing biofeedback is a drawback for this CAM. On balance, then, biofeedback shows more limited benefits than do some other CAM treatments for pain management.

Hypnotic treatment also has some applications in controlling pain, and the list of pains that are responsive to hypnotic procedures is extensive. A meta-analysis (Montgomery, DuHamel, & Redd, 2000) showed that hypnotic suggestion is equally effective in reducing both experimental pain induced in the laboratory and clinical pain that people experience in the world for about 75% of participants. Research exploring brain activity during hypnosis (Röder, Michal, Overbeck, van de Ven, & Linden, 2007) showed that hypnosis altered the brain response to painful stimulation in areas that underlie both the sensory and emotional responses to pain. Indeed, the effectiveness of hypnosis in managing pain may be its power to change the fear that often accompanies pain (De Benedittis, 2003).

Hypnosis is not equally effective with all types of clinical pain; it is more effective in controlling acute pain than in managing chronic pain (Patterson & Jensen, 2003). Hypnosis is most effective in helping people manage pain associated with invasive medical procedures, postoperative recovery, and burns. For example, research shows that hypnosis was effective in reducing the need for preoperative medication in children (Calipel, Lucaspolomeni, Wodey, & Ecoffey, 2005), in stabilizing the pain of invasive surgical procedures, and in reducing surgery patients' need for analgesic drugs (Lang et al., 2000). Hypnosis is especially effective in relieving gastrointestinal pain in children (Kröner-Herwig, 2009) and appears very effective in managing pain associated with childbirth (Landolt & Milling, 2011). Burns are notoriously difficult to treat because they involve severe pain and suffering. An early review of the effectiveness of hypnosis in treating the pain associated with burns (Van der Does & Van Dyck, 1989) examined 28 studies that used hypnosis with burn patients and found consistent evidence of its benefits. Evidence of those benefits continues to

accrue, and David Patterson (2010) has argued that hypnosis has shown such convincing results that it should no longer be considered alternative medicine.

Although hypnotic treatment is effective with many types of acute pain, chronic pain is a more difficult management issue, and hypnosis is not as successful with chronic pain such as headache and low back pain as it is with acute pain (Patterson & Jensen, 2003). Hypnosis is also more effective with some people than with others. Individual differences in susceptibility to hypnosis are a factor in the analgesic effects of hypnosis—highly suggestible people may receive substantial analgesic benefits from this technique, whereas others receive limited benefits. Thus, hypnosis can be very effective with some people for some pain problems.

Table 8.3 summarizes the effectiveness of CAM treatments for pain. Although the studies on pain management using CAM could benefit from better design, evaluations of the results indicate that several of these techniques work for a variety of pain problems. Conventional medicine has not been very successful for many patients in pain, and the conventional treatments tend to have many side effects, a criticism that is uncommon for CAM and thus an additional benefit.

Fewer side effects are not the only additional benefit to CAM use; a study of participants in several CAM clinical trials for pain (Hsu, BlueSpruce, Sherman, & Cherkin, 2010) identified a range of benefits that occurred in addition to the goals of the trial, including positive changes in emotion, ability to cope, health, and well-being. Thus, CAM treatments have few of the risks of conventional medicine and may have some benefits not assessed in most studies of effectiveness.

Alternative Treatments for Other Conditions

Although anxiety, stress, depression, and pain are the most common problems for which people use CAM, some products and procedures have been found effective for other conditions. Both the products and procedures and the conditions for which they are effective vary widely; CAM has been used to achieve more rapid healing, to lower blood pressure, and to improve balance. For example, use of aloe vera speeds burn wound healing significantly (Maenthaisong, Chaiyakunapruk, Niruntraporn, & Kongkaew, 2007). Although biofeedback is not as effective as other CAM for stress and

TABLE 8.3   Effectiveness of Alternative Therapies for Pain

Problem	Findings	Studies
1. Chronic pain	Meditation is effective, according to a National Institutes of Health Technology panel review.	Lebovits, 2007
2. Pain associated with pregnancy and childbirth	Guided imagery is a best practice for this type of pain. Hypnosis is effective for managing labor and delivery pain.	Naparstek, 2007 Landolt & Milling, 2011
3. Headache pain	Guided imagery is effective in managing headache pain.	Tsao & Zeltzer, 2005
4. Postoperative pain in children	Guided imagery reduces postoperative pain.	Huth et al., 2004
5. Postoperative pain in older people	Guided imagery reduces postoperative pain.	Antall & Kresevic, 2004
6. Tension headache pain in adults	Tai chi was effective in a randomized controlled trial.	Abbott et al., 2007
7. Chronic pain	Qi gong was evaluated as promising in a systematic review.	Lee et al., 2007a
8. Fibromyalgia	Qi gong provided pain relief and lowered distress in a randomized controlled trial. Tai chi provided pain relief and improved quality of life.	Haak & Scott, 2008 Wang et al., 2010
9. Low back pain	Acupuncture is as or more effective than other approaches.	Keller et al., 2007; Manheimer et al., 2005
10. Low back pain, osteoarthritis, neck pain, and headache	Acupuncture was effective as a complementary treatment.	Witt et al., 2006
11. Low back pain, shoulder pain, and headache pain	Massage was effective for low back pain and modestly effective for shoulder and headache pain.	Tsao, 2007
12. Low back pain	Massage can be effective pain relief.	Cherkin et al., 2011
13. Neck pain	Massage can be effective pain relief.	Sherman et al., 2009
14. Musculoskeletal pain	Massage studies are too limited to allow conclusions of effectiveness.	Lewis & Johnson, 2006
15. Back and neck pain	Chiropractic manipulation has only small benefits.	Rubenstein et al., 2011
16. Musculoskeletal pain	Chiropractic manipulation was more effective than conventional medical treatment.	Perram, 2006
17. Tension headache	Chiropractic manipulation was not found effective.	Lenssinck et al., 2004
18. Neck-related headaches	Spinal manipulation showed benefits.	Haas et al., 2010
19. Migraine and tension headache	Thermal biofeedback plus relaxation produced a significant reduction in headache activity.	Blanchard et al., 1990
20. Migraine headache prevention	Thermal biofeedback is comparable to other preventive treatments.	Stewart, 2004
21. Migraine headache treatment	Biofeedback produced a medium-sized effect, according to a systematic review.	Nestoriuc & Martin, 2007

(continued)

TABLE 8.3 Effectiveness of Alternative Therapies for Pain — *Continued*

Problem	Findings	Studies
22. Tension headache treatment	Biofeedback produced no benefit.	Verhagen et al., 2009
23. Low back pain	EMG biofeedback was not effective.	Roelofs et al., 2002
24. Experimental and clinical pain	Hypnotic suggestion is effective for clinical and experimental pain.	Montgomery et al., 2000
25. Fear and anxiety associated with pain	Hypnosis is especially effective.	De Benedittis, 2003
26. Clinical pain	Hypnosis is more effective in controlling acute pain than in managing chronic pain.	Patterson & Jensen, 2003
27. Preoperative distress	Hypnosis reduces preoperative distress better than medication.	Calipel et al., 2005
28. Surgery pain	Self-hypnosis decreases postoperative pain and reduces need for drugs.	Lang et al., 2000
29. Gastrointestinal pain in children	Hypnosis is especially effective.	Kröner-Herwig, 2009
30. Burn pain	Hypnosis is a valuable component in treating severe burn pain.	Patterson, 2010; Van der Does & Van Dyck, 1989

pain, thermal biofeedback is effective in the management of **Raynaud's disease**, a disorder that involves painful constriction of peripheral blood vessels in the hands and feet (Karavidas, Tsai, Yucha, McGrady, & Lehrer, 2006). In addition, biofeedback has demonstrated its usefulness in the rehabilitation of motor abilities after injury and stroke (Langhorne, Coupar, & Pollock, 2009). Hypnosis was found to be effective in controlling nausea and vomiting associated with chemotherapy in children (Richardson et al., 2007). The practice of transcendental meditation has been evaluated as effective in controlling risk factors such as high blood pressure and some of the physiological changes that underlie cardiovascular disease and thus may offer protection (Horowitz, 2010). Yoga may help not only to control some of the risks for Type 2 diabetes (Innes & Vincent, 2007) but also to prevent cardiovascular complications in diabetics. A mindfulness-based meditation program was successful with male and female prisoners in improving mood and decreasing hostility (Samuelson, Carmody, Kabat-Zinn, & Bratt, 2007). This assortment of effective treatments represents many different complementary and alternative interventions, but some systems of alternative medicine have yielded successful treatments for a number of problems.

Traditional Chinese medicine includes acupuncture, qi gong, and tai chi, all of which produce a wide range of effective treatments and other health benefits. For example, acupuncture (Ezzo, Streitberger, & Schneider, 2006) has been found to be effective in controlling nausea and vomiting associated with postoperative symptoms. Also, a systematic review showed that acupuncture was effective in treating insomnia (Chen et al., 2007). Tai chi and qi gong produce improvements in blood pressure and other cardiovascular measures compared to a nonexercise intervention and benefits comparable to other exercise interventions (Jahnke, Larkey, Rogers, & Etnier, 2010). Qi gong practice, however, was not superior to drug treatment for blood pressure treatment (Guo, Zhou, Nishimura, Teramukai, & Fukushima, 2008) but appears to be as effective as drug treatment in managing the risk factors for diabetes such as oral glucose tolerance and blood glucose (Xin, Miller, & Brown, 2007).

Qi gong and the related practice of tai chi seem to have the ability to improve immune system function, which would give these practices the potential for many health benefits. Compared with healthy control participants who did not practice qi gong or tai chi, the immune system response of those who practiced qi gong was enhanced in ways that would resolve inflammation more rapidly (Li, Li, Garcia, Johnson, & Feng, 2005). Older adults who practiced qi gong or tai chi showed an enhanced immune system response to influenza immunization (Yang et al., 2007). Indeed, the immune response was sufficiently strong to produce positive health consequences before immunization. In a randomized controlled trial (Irwin, Pike, Cole, & Oxman, 2003), older adults who practiced tai chi exhibited an enhanced immune response to the herpes zoster (shingles) virus, even before they received the immunization for this virus. Thus, the practice of qi gong and tai chi seems to confer some immune system benefits that have been researched most extensively with older people but may apply to all.

The most common applications of tai chi have been among older people to improve balance and flexibility and to decrease falls. A large body of evidence, including systematic reviews, leads to the conclusion that these practices are successful in reducing fear of falling, improving balance, and in reducing fall rates (Jahnke et al., 2010; Leung, Chan, Tsang, Tsang, & Jones. 2011). Qi gong and tai chi are also beneficial to bone density, which is an important underlying factor in falls among older people (Jahnke et al., 2010). Calcium and vitamin D supplements, another CAM treatment, are also effective in helping people over age 50 retain bone minerals (Tang, Eslick, Nowson, Smith, & Bensoussan, 2007).

Reasoning that the benefits of tai chi for balance and flexibility might apply to individuals with multiple sclerosis and rheumatoid arthritis, researchers have tested those benefits. A systematic review of the research on rheumatoid arthritis (Lee, Pittler, & Ernst, 2007b) found some positive effects for disability, quality of life, and mood but not enough clear evidence to recommend this practice. The study assessing the benefits of tai chi for people with multiple sclerosis was a small one (Mills, Allen, & Morgan, 2000), and thus its findings must be considered as preliminary. However, individuals who practiced tai chi for 2 months experienced improvements in balance, which is a major problem for people with this disorder.

Thus, CAM interventions are effective for a variety of problems. The most persuasive evidence comes from traditional Chinese medicine and from mind–body medicine, but an assortment of products and procedures have demonstrated their effectiveness in randomized controlled trials, in meta-analyses, and in systematic reviews. Table 8.4 summarizes these treatments. Despite some impressive evidence for effectiveness, treatments within complementary and alternative medicine also have limitations.

Limitations of Alternative Therapies

All forms of therapy have limitations, including CAM. One of the primary limitations is the reason any technique is considered *alternative*: the lack of information on its effectiveness. As we have seen, this deficit may be due to the sparseness of research rather than a lack of effectiveness. The growing interest in CAM and the funding for research through the U.S. National Center for Complementary and Alternative Medicine have worked toward solving this problem, revealing that some products and procedures are effective, whereas others are not. Both conventional and alternative treatments are limited by their success for some conditions and not others. However, specific CAM techniques have limitations and even dangers.

Herbal remedies and botanicals are part of many CAM systems, including Ayurvedic medicine, traditional Chinese medicine, naturopathy, and homeopathy. These types of natural products are among the most commonly used CAM approaches (Barnes et al., 2008). Like drug treatments, herbal, botanical, and other natural products carry risks of adverse reactions and interactions with over-the-counter and prescription drugs (Firenzuoli & Gori, 2007; Lake, 2009). Unlike drugs, herbal remedies, dietary supplements, and other natural products are classified as food by the U.S. government, so these products are not evaluated for effectiveness but only for safety. People often consider natural herbs and botanicals to be safe and even if not effective, then at least harmless. Such is not always the case. Sometimes, evidence of dangers accumulates only after these products have been available for some time. Natural products may interact with each other or with prescription or over-the-counter medications, and many people who use natural products fail to inform their physicians of their CAM usage (Lake, 2009).

Massage has many benefits but is not suitable for people with arthritis or other pain problems related to joints, weakened bones, damaged nerves, a tumor, an

TABLE 8.4 Effectiveness of Alternative Treatments for Other Conditions

Problem	Findings	Studies
1. Burn healing	Aloe vera speeds healing.	Maenthaisong et al., 2007
2. Raynaud's disease	Thermal biofeedback is an effective treatment.	Karavidas et al., 2006
3. Rehabilitation of motor abilities after injury or stroke	EMG biofeedback is effective.	Langhorne et al., 2009; Tate & Milner, 2010
4. Nausea and vomiting associated with chemotherapy	Hypnosis is effective in controlling these symptoms.	Richardson et al., 2007
5. Physical reactions related to cardiovascular disease	Transcendental meditation shows beneficial effects.	Horowitz, 2010
6. Risks for Type 2 diabetes	Yoga is effective in controlling risks and in decreasing CVD complications.	Innes & Vincent, 2007
7. Hostility	Mindfulness meditation is effective in moderating hostility among prisoners.	Samuelson et al., 2007
8. Postoperative nausea and vomiting	Acupuncture is effective.	Ezzo et al., 2006
9. Insomnia	Acupuncture is effective.	H. Y. Chen et al., 2007
10. High blood pressure and other responses related to cardiovascular disease	Tai chi and qi gong produce improvements. Qi gong practice lowered blood pressure, but not as much as drugs.	Jahnke et al., 2010 Guo et al., 2008
11. Risk factors for diabetes	Qi gong was effective in lowering risk.	Xin et al., 2007
12. Immune system function	Qi gong altered immune function in ways that decreased inflammation.	Li et al., 2005
13. Immune system function	Qi gong and tai chi enhanced immune system response to influenza vaccination in older adults.	Yang et al., 2007
14. Immune system function	Tai chi practice enhanced older adults' immune system response to herpes zoster before and after immunization.	Irwin et al., 2003
15. Fear of falling, balance, and falls	Tai chi and qi gong practice decreased fear of falling, increased balance, and decreased falls among older adults.	Jahnke et al., 2010; Leung et al, 2011
16. Osteoporosis	Calcium and vitamin D supplements slowed bone mineral loss in people over age 50.	Tang et al., 2007
17. Rheumatoid arthritis	Tai chi showed some positive effects but not enough clear evidence to recommend in a systematic review.	Lee et al., 2007b
18. Multiple sclerosis	Tai chi practice improved balance.	Mills et al., 2000

open wound, or infection, or for people with bleeding disorders or those who are taking blood thinning agents (NCCAM, 2006/2010a). Chiropractic treatment may do harm when applied to individuals with broken bones or infection, and treatment may produce headache or other discomfort (NCCAM, 2007/2010).

Acupuncture and acupressure do not work for everyone. Some people do not respond, some types of manipulation of the needles are more effective than others, and some needle placements work better than others (Martindale, 2001). Needles should be sterile and inserted properly; improper insertion and needles that are not sterile can cause damage and infection (Yamashita & Tsukayama, 2008). However, incidents involving these dangers occur rarely. Tai chi and qi gong are generally safe, but people with severe osteoporosis, sprains, fractures, or joint problems should exercise caution or modify the positions (NCCAM, 2006/2010c). Meditation carries few health risks (NCCAM, 2006/2010b).

People should exercise caution in using any CAM treatment as an alternative to conventional medical care. People who trust alternative approaches and mistrust conventional medicine may fail to seek treatment that could be more effective. For example, yoga may help to control some of the risks for Type 2 diabetes (Innes & Vincent, 2007), but for most people, yoga will not be sufficient to control diabetes. The majority of people who use CAM recognize the limitations of these therapies and use them as additions to conventional medical care. However, many people who use some CAM modality fail to tell their conventional medical practitioner that they are using an alternative as a well as conventional treatment (Lake, 2009). This failure may present risks due to interactions between the two treatments.

Another limitation for CAM is its accessibility. Not everyone who is interested in CAM may be able to find or to afford CAM treatment. Many CAM treatments are limited by the number of qualified practitioners and by their geographic location. For example, acupuncture use increased dramatically between 1997 and 2007 (Nahin, Barnes, Stussman, & Bloom, 2009), but accessibility may remain a problem that limits its use (Burke & Upchurch, 2006). People who used alternative medicine products or procedures are not reimbursed often for the products they purchase or the services they receive (Burke & Upchurch, 2006). The failure to include CAM services in insurance reimbursement is typical in the United States and represents huge out-of-pocket expenditures to CAM users—an estimated $27 billion (Nahin et al., 2009). One way to remove this barrier is to increase the presence of alternative treatments in conventional medical settings. Moving complementary and alternative medicine to group practices, hospitals, and clinics would improve accessibility. This strategy is the focus of integrative medicine.

Integrative Medicine

Integrating conventional and alternative medicine is what Norman Cousins, whose story began this chapter, envisioned for health care and treatment. Cousins's experience with a debilitating disease and cure through a very unorthodox treatment prompted him to work toward changes to conventional medicine. As Cousins said,

> It becomes necessary therefore to create a balanced perspective, one that recognizes that attitudes such as a strong will to live, high purpose, a capacity for festivity, and a reasonable degree of confidence are not an alternative to competent medical attention, but a way of enhancing the environment of treatment. The wise physician favors a spirit of responsible participation by the patients in a total strategy of medical care. (UCLA Cousins Center for Psychoneuroimmunology, 2011, ¶ 1)

One way to overcome the limitations of both conventional medicine and CAM is to integrate them, providing a mixture of both types of treatment, called **integrative medicine** (or *integrative health*). This approach is what most people attempt when they use alternative treatments; few completely reject conventional medicine. Rather, they choose to combine the techniques from each that they believe will help them manage their problem, but they do so on their own rather than under the direction of a health care provider.

Not only do many people who use CAM do so without the guidance of their physician, but they also often do so without informing their physician (Lake, 2009). These people may feel reluctant to discuss their use of alternative treatment with a physician because practitioners of conventional medicine are still skeptical about the efficacy of CAM (Frank, Ratanawongsa, & Carrera, 2010) and thus reluctant to refer patients to practitioners of alternative treatments and even hesitant to enter into collaborative relationships. Integrative medicine requires conventional and alternative medicine practitioners to accept the effectiveness of both approaches and to work together. Both the acceptance and the cooperation present challenges.

Conventional medicine holds different assumptions than alternative medicine, leading to basic differences in the way that practitioners view health and treatment (Lake, 2007). For example, the assumptions of traditional Chinese medicine, chiropractic, and homeopathy have been difficult for many physicians trained in Western medicine to accept. Conventional medical practitioners remain resistant to integrating alternative treatments, including some who are vehemently opposed (Freedman, 2011). Practitioners whose training has not included alternative treatments are more resistant than those who have training in CAM (Hsiao, Ryan, et al., 2006). Students in a variety of professional schools of health care have a great interest in CAM (Song, John, & Dobs, 2007). An increasing number of medical schools include CAM departments and curricula (Frank et al., 2010), but the philosophy of practice and treatment methods and strategies differ (Shannon, Weil, & Kaplan, 2011). In 2009, the U.S. Institute of Medicine sponsored a conference titled "Summit on Integrative Medicine and the Health of the Public" (Ullman, 2010). Those who attended expressed hopes for an integration of conventional and alternative approaches to health and treatment, but they also acknowledged that this integration would require large changes in the medical delivery system.

Integration of care is more common in some areas of practice than others, such as pain treatment, cancer care, and mental health problems. Patients who visit an integrative pain clinic tend to be people with chronic pain problems who have tried many different approaches from conventional medicine and perhaps some from alternative medicine, none of which have been entirely successful. In pain clinics, pain is the problem, and treatment is oriented toward managing it and not the condition that originally caused it. Such a clinic should include health care professionals from several specialties (Dillard, 2002), including (1) a physician trained in neurology, anesthesia, rehabilitation, or psychiatry; (2) a physical rehabilitation expert; (3) a psychiatrist or psychologist; and (4) a chiropractor, massage therapist, or acupuncturist (or all three). This range of health care providers can offer techniques from both conventional and alternative medicine, consult with one another, and tailor the treatment to fit each individual's situation and needs.

Integrative oncology also involves treatment by a team of providers. In addition to conventional treatments for cancer such as chemotherapy, radiation, and surgery, patients may participate in interventions aimed at pain control, stress management, nutrition, and physical activity. Stress management, healthy diet, and exercise represent changes that improve the quality of life for most people, but these lifestyle changes may also affect the progression of cancer (Boyd, 2007). About 26% of cancer patients seek some type of CAM treatment, most often to help with musculoskeletal problems (Lafferty, Tyree, Devlin, Andersen, & Diehr, 2008). Some cancer patients look

to CAM to help them become actively involved in their treatment to "fight" their cancer (Evans et al., 2007). Mindfulness-based stress reduction is useful for individuals with cancer (Smith, Richardson, Hoffman, & Pilkington, 2005), reducing stress and improving mood and sleep quality. Including some type of alternative medicine in conventional cancer treatment has become common in the United States (Cona, 2010). Thus, integrative oncology holds potential for providing a wider range of treatments and improving the quality of life for cancer patients.

Such improvements could apply to many chronic diseases. The growing consumer interest in CAM and the increasing interest in CAM by health care professionals suggest that many people would like the "best of both worlds" by combining conventional medicine with effective treatments from alternative medicine. This pressure may help overcome the barriers to integrative medicine.

IN SUMMARY

For alternative treatments to be accepted by conventional medicine, research evidence must confirm their effectiveness. The standard for this evidence is controversial. Should CAM be held to the standard of effectiveness as demonstrated by randomized controlled trials? Some in conventional medicine say so, but some in alternative medicine argue that most treatments in conventional medicine fail to meet this criterion. Nonetheless, evidence is accruing concerning effectiveness for CAM.

Both transcendental meditation and mindfulness meditation have demonstrated effectiveness for anxiety, and mindfulness-based stress reduction is effective in managing stress. The movement-based practices of qi gong and tai chi are also effective in helping to manage stress. Acupuncture and yoga show some promise of reducing depression, and the herbal remedy Saint-John's wort has also been found to reduce depression.

Guided imagery seems to be an effective intervention in helping people manage several types of pain. Techniques from traditional Chinese medicine have been successful in pain management, including qi gong, tai chi, and acupuncture. Qi gong and tai chi may be good choices for people with chronic pain problems, including headache and fibromyalgia. Acupuncture can be effective for easing low back and neck pain as well as pain from osteoarthritis. Research also indicates that massage is effective for low back pain, neck pain, musculoskeletal pain, and headache; chiropractic manipulation also helps the same set of pain syndromes. However, biofeedback is not as effective as other CAM treatments; biofeedback is similar to relaxation in managing migraine headaches but shows few benefits for treating other types of pain. Hypnosis is effective for a variety of types of pain but is more effective for acute pain such as postsurgical and burn pain than for chronic pain.

Techniques from CAM are also effective for a variety of other conditions, including speeding burn healing (aloe vera), treating insomnia (acupuncture), controlling nausea and vomiting (hypnosis and acupuncture), managing Raynaud's disease (thermal biofeedback), increasing motor movement after stroke (EMG biofeedback), and lowering risk for cardiovascular disease (meditation and qi gong) and diabetes (qi gong). Research has indicated that the practice of qi gong and tai chi can alter

the immune system in beneficial ways, and tai chi improves balance and flexibility and decreases both fear of falling and number of falls in older adults.

Like all treatments, CAM has limitations and even dangers. Some herbal remedies and botanical products may be toxic or may interact with each other or with over-the-counter or prescription drugs. Individuals with some conditions should avoid some treatments; for example, people with weakened bones should be cautious in seeking massage or chiropractic treatment. Another limitation for CAM is its accessibility, in terms of both availability and cost of treatments.

Integrative medicine is the integration of alternative and conventional medicine, which should provide the best of both approaches. The challenges for achieving such integration include melding the two discrepant traditions and training practitioners who will refer patients to each other when appropriate. Two areas in which integrative medicine is advancing most rapidly are pain management and cancer treatment.

Answers

This chapter has addressed five basic questions:

1. **What medical systems represent alternatives to conventional medicine?**
The alternative medical systems include traditional Chinese medicine, Ayurvedic medicine, naturopathy, and homeopathy. TCM and Ayurvedic medicine are ancient; naturopathy and homeopathy arose in the 19th century and gained popularity in the early 20th century. Each of these systems presents a theory of health and disease as well as practices for diagnosis and treatment. All of the alternative systems share the concept of vital energy and the notion that bringing the mind and body together is important to health.

2. **What practices and products are used in alternative medicine?**
Alternative medicine includes a wide variety of practices and products for improving or restoring health. Manipulative techniques include chiropractic and massage; chiropractic manipulation focuses

on adjusting the spine and joints, whereas massage manipulates soft tissue. Energy healing is another alternative practice; the several varieties of energy healing all accept that the body produces or is sensitive to healing energy. Diets such as the Atkins, Ornish, Zone, and South Beach may be undertaken for weight loss or to control risk factors for heart disease or diabetes. Alternative products include dietary supplements such as vitamins and minerals or nonvitamin products such as echinacea, glucosamine, omega-3 fatty acids, and a variety of herbs, extracts, and special foods that may be taken as curatives or preventatives.

3. **What is mind–body medicine?**
Mind–body medicine is the term applied to a variety of techniques that are based on the notion that the brain, mind, body, and behavior interact in complex ways and that emotional, mental, social, and behavioral factors exert important effects on health. These techniques share the view that mind and body form a holistic system of dynamic interaction, with each influencing the other. According to mind–body medicine, overlooking

psychological factors will lead to an incomplete form of health treatment and lose the power that can come from enlisting mind and emotions in treatment. The techniques included within mind–body medicine are meditation, guided imagery, yoga, qi gong, tai chi, biofeedback, and hypnosis.

4. **Who uses complementary and alternative medicine?**

People in high-income nations show an increasing interest and participation in CAM. Countries vary in CAM usage, and within countries, some demographic factors predict CAM use. Australia, Canada, and some European countries show higher percentages of the population seeking CAM treatments than in the United States. Within the United States, ethnicity shows some relationship to CAM use, with European American, well-educated, and upper-income groups using CAM more often than others. In all countries, women are more likely than men to use CAM. Personal attitudes of acceptance of the underlying philosophy of CAM also predict use, as does health status—people who have a persistent health problem that conventional medicine has not helped are more likely to seek alternative treatment.

5. **What are the effective uses and limitations of alternative treatments?**

A variety of techniques are available to help people manage anxiety, stress, depression, pain, and other problems, and an increasing body of research indicates that some alternative treatments are effective in managing these problems. Both transcendental and mindfulness meditation are effective in managing anxiety; mindfulness-based stress reduction helps in coping with stress. Different alternative treatments have been found to be effective in managing various types of pain; no one technique is effective for all pain situations. Chronic pain is difficult to manage using either conventional or alternative treatments. Manipulation techniques such as massage, chiropractic treatment, and acupuncture seem to be as effective as any treatment for the difficult problem of chronic low back pain. The movement-based approaches of qi gong and tai chi show promise of helping to manage headaches and fibromyalgia. In addition, these practices influence

the immune system in beneficial ways that may affect health in a variety of ways. However, their primary therapeutic use is to help older people maintain balance and flexibility. Hypnosis also has benefits for pain control, but these benefits apply more to acute pain than to chronic pain.

Lack of rigorous research has limited evidence concerning the effectiveness of CAM, but that situation is changing. Other limitations are similar to those of treatments in conventional medicine—hazards for some individuals using some treatments and drug interactions arising from the use of herbal treatments or dietary supplements. Availability and cost of treatments are other limitations of CAM.

Suggested Readings

Freedman, D. H. (2011). The triumph of new-age medicine. *The Atlantic, 308*(1), 90–100. This article in a popular magazine explores integrative medicine, interviewing advocates and detractors of alternative approaches to treatment. Through this evaluation, Freedman provides a critique of the current level of medical care in the United States.

Harrington, A. (2008). *The cure within: A history of mind–body medicine*. New York: Norton. Harrington's book takes a social and historical perspective on the status of alternative medicine, weaving together a wide collection of information concerning the interaction between mind and body.

Lake, J. (2007). Philosophical problems in medicine and psychiatry, part II. *Integrative Medicine: A Clinician's Journal, 6*(3), 44–47. This brief article takes a historical and philosophical perspective in explaining the underlying differences in assumptions and worldviews between advocates of conventional and alternative medicine and how these differences present barriers to integrating the two types of medical care.

Shannon, S., Weil, A., & Kaplan, B. J. (2011). Medical decision making in integrative medicine: Safety, efficacy, and patient preference. *Alternative & Complementary Therapies, 17*(2), 84–91. This thoughtful critique of both conventional and alternative medicine details safety and effectiveness concerns that should be used in all types of medicine.

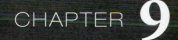
Behavioral Factors in Cardiovascular Disease

CHAPTER OUTLINE

- **Real-World Profile of President Bill Clinton**
- *The Cardiovascular System*
- *The Changing Rates of Cardiovascular Disease*
- *Risk Factors in Cardiovascular Disease*
- *Reducing Cardiovascular Risks*

QUESTIONS

This chapter focuses on four basic questions:

1. What are the structures, functions, and disorders of the cardiovascular system?

2. What are the risk factors for cardiovascular disease?

3. How does lifestyle relate to cardiovascular health?

4. What behaviors allow people to lower their cardiovascular risks?

☑CHECK YOUR HEALTH RISKS

Regarding Cardiovascular Disease

Question	Points
Age	
Are you a man 55 years or older OR woman 65 years or older?	2 if Yes
Smoking	
I never smoked	0
I am a former smoker (last smoked more than 12 months ago)	2
I smoke 1–5 cigarettes per day	2
I smoke 6–10 cigarettes per day	4
I smoke 11–15 cigarettes per day	6
I smoke 16–20 cigarettes per day	7
I smoke more than 20 cigarettes per day	11
Over the past 12 months, what has been your typical exposure to other people's tobacco smoke?	
Secondhand smoke	
Less than 1 hour of exposure per week	0
One or more hours of secondhand smoke exposure per week	2
Other health conditions	
Do you have diabetes mellitus?	6 if Yes
Do you have high blood pressure?	5 if Yes
Have either or both of your biological parents had a heart attack?	4 if Yes
Waist-to-hip ratio	
Less than .873	0
Between .873 and .963	2
Greater than .964	4
Psychosocial factors	
How often have you felt work or home life stress in the last year?	
Never or some periods	0
Several periods of stress or permanent stress	3
During the past 12 months, was there ever a time when you felt sad, blue, or depressed for weeks or more in a row?	3 if Yes
Dietary factors	
Do you eat salty food or snacks one or more times a day?	1 if Yes
Do you eat deep fried foods or snacks or fast foods three or more times a week?	1 if Yes
Do you eat fruit one or more times daily?	1 if No
Do you eat vegetables one or more times daily?	1 if No
Do you eat meat and/or poultry two or more times daily?	2 if Yes
Physical activity	
I am mainly sedentary or perform mild exercise (requiring minimal effort)	2
I perform moderate or strenuous physical activity in my leisure time	0

Source: "Estimating modifiable coronary heart disease risk globally in multiple regions of the world: The INTERHEART modifiable risk score" by C. McGorrian et al. (2011), *European Heart Journal, 32,* Supplementary Table 2.

   This checklist supplies you with your INTERHEART Modifiable Risk Score. The score derives from research on over 30,000 people from 52 different countries and represents the most recent method for calculating heart attack risk. If you score below 9, congratulations: You are at lowest risk for heart attack. If you score above 15, you are at highest risk for heart attack; however, most of these factors are under your control. In this chapter, you will learn why each of these factors increases risk for cardiovascular problems, and how you can decrease your risk.

Real-World Profile of
PRESIDENT BILL CLINTON

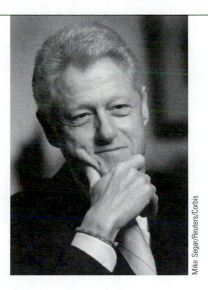

In early September 2004, former President Bill Clinton went to the hospital because he experienced chest pains and shortness of breath (King & Henry, 2004). Soon after, he learned that his coronary arteries were blocked, which led to coronary bypass surgery. Had Clinton not obtained treatment, his chances of a heart attack would have been substantial. Like many people, Clinton did not experience any major symptoms beforehand, so he considered himself fortunate to have a warning of coronary problems. His diagnosis and treatment were opportunities to avoid a heart attack and to gain additional years of healthy life.

Clinton also speculated about the underlying cause of his heart problems. He had a history of heart disease in his family, but he was also fond of high-fat fast food. Clinton's unhealthy diet during his White House years was "legendary" (Templeton, 2008). Clinton had a history of high blood pressure and high cholesterol. All of these factors are risks for heart disease, but Clinton also engaged in some activities that may have protected him against cardiovascular problems. For example, he had been a jogger for years, remaining physically active throughout his presidency and afterward. However, this protective measure was not enough to counter his other risk factors.

Clinton looked healthy, but despite the appearance of health, his coronary arteries were seriously blocked—one more than 90% (Associated Press, 2004). Clinton recovered from his quadruple coronary bypass surgery, but additional surgery was required 6 months later to remove scar tissue (K. Matthews, 2005). Clinton's experience turned him into an advocate for prevention of heart disease (Clinton, 2005). He joined with the American Heart Association to begin an initiative to combat childhood obesity, including urging fast-food restaurants to provide healthier menu choices for children.

In this chapter, we examine the behavioral risks for cardiovascular disease—the most frequent cause of death in the United States and other industrialized nations—and look at Bill Clinton's risk from both inherent and behavioral factors. But first, we describe the cardiovascular system. What is it, and what are methods of measuring how well it functions?

The Cardiovascular System

The **cardiovascular system** consists of the heart, arteries, and veins. The heart is a muscle that, by contracting and relaxing, pumps blood throughout the body. The heart is, essentially, the center of a rapid-transit system that carries oxygen to body cells and removes carbon dioxide and other wastes from cells. Under healthy conditions, the cardiovascular, respiratory, and digestive systems are integrated: The digestive system produces nutrients and the respiratory system furnishes oxygen, both of which circulate through the blood to various parts of the body. In addition, the endocrine system affects the cardiovascular system by stimulating or depressing the rate of cardiovascular activity. Although we will view the cardiovascular system in isolation in this chapter, it does not function that way.

The blood's route through the body appears in Figure 9.1. The entire circuit takes about 20 seconds when the body is at rest, but exertion speeds the process. Blood travels from the right ventricle of the heart

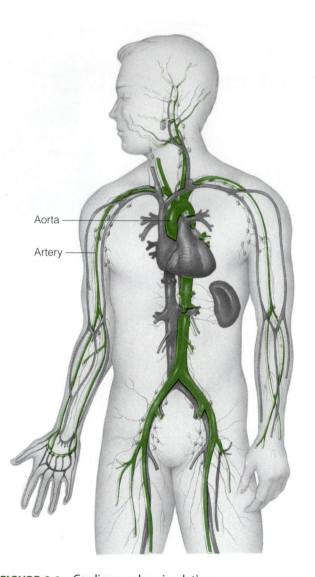

FIGURE 9.1   Cardiovascular circulation.

Source: Introduction to microbiology (p. 671), by J. L. Ingraham & C. A. Ingraham. From INGRAHAM/
INGRAHAM, Introduction to Microbiology, 1E. © 1995 Cengage Learning.

to the lungs, where hemoglobin (one of the components of blood) saturates it with oxygen. From the lungs, oxygenated blood travels back to the left atrium of the heart, then to the left ventricle, and finally out to the rest of the body. The **arteries** carry the oxygenated blood branch into vessels of smaller and smaller diameter, called **arterioles**, and finally terminate in tiny **capillaries** that connect arteries and **veins**. Oxygen diffuses out to body cells, and carbon dioxide and other chemical wastes pass into the blood so they can be

disposed of. Blood that has been stripped of its oxygen returns to the heart by way of the system of veins, beginning with the tiny **venules** and ending with the two large veins that empty into the right atrium, the upper right chamber of the heart.

This section briefly considers the functioning of the cardiovascular system, concentrating on the physiology underlying **cardiovascular disease (CVD)**, a general term that includes coronary artery disease, coronary heart disease, and stroke.

The Coronary Arteries

The coronary arteries supply blood to the heart muscle, the **myocardium**. The two principal coronary arteries branch off from the aorta (see Figure 9.2), the main artery that carries oxygenated blood from the heart. Left and right coronary arteries divide into smaller branches, providing the blood supply to the myocardium.

With each beat, the heart makes a slight twisting motion, which moves the coronary arteries. The coronary arteries, therefore, receive a great deal of strain as part of their normal function. This movement of the heart has been hypothesized to almost inevitably cause injury to the coronary arteries (Friedman & Rosenman, 1974). The damage can heal in two different ways. The preferable route involves the formation of small amounts of scar tissue and results in no serious problem. The second route involves the formation of **atheromatous plaques**, deposits composed of cholesterol and other lipids (fats), connective tissue, and muscle tissue. The plaques grow and calcify into a hard, bony substance that thickens the arterial walls (Kharbanda & MacAllister, 2005). This process also involves inflammation (Abi-Saleh, Iskandar, Elgharib, & Cohen, 2008). The formation of plaques and the resulting occlusion of the arteries are called **atherosclerosis**, shown in Figure 9.3.

A related but different problem is **arteriosclerosis**, or the loss of elasticity of the arteries. The beating of the heart pushes blood through the arteries with great force, and arterial elasticity allows adaptation to this pressure. Loss of elasticity tends to make the cardiovascular system less capable of tolerating increases in cardiac blood volume. Hence, a potential danger exists during strenuous exercise for people with arteriosclerosis.

The formation of arterial plaques (atherosclerosis) and the "hardening" of the arteries (arteriosclerosis) often occur together. Both can affect any artery in the cardiovascular system, but when the coronary arteries are affected, the heart's oxygen supply may be threatened.

Coronary Artery Disease

Coronary artery disease (CAD) refers to damage to the coronary arteries, typically through the processes of atherosclerosis and arteriosclerosis. No clearly visible

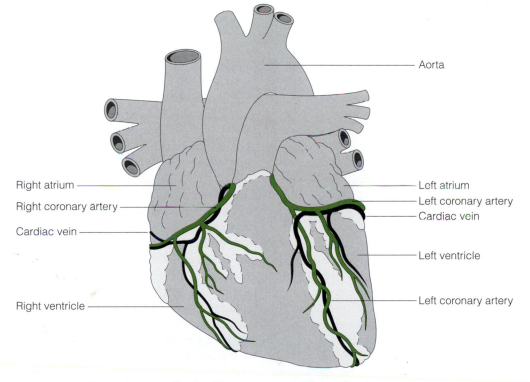

Right atrium

Right coronary artery

Cardiac vein

Right ventricle

Aorta

Left atrium

Left coronary artery

Cardiac vein

Left ventricle

Left coronary artery

FIGURE 9.2   Heart (myocardium) with coronary arteries and veins.

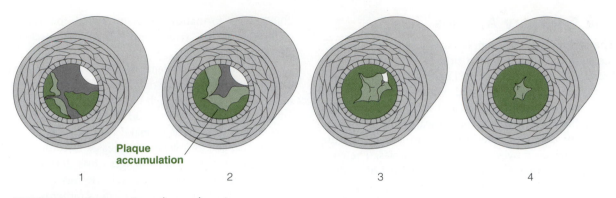

Plaque
accumulation

1   2   3   4

FIGURE 9.3 Progressive atherosclerosis.

outward symptoms accompany the buildup of plaques in the coronary arteries, as Bill Clinton discovered. CAD can develop while a person remains totally unaware of its progress. In CAD, the plaques narrow the arteries and restrict the supply of blood to the myocardium. Deposits of plaque may also rupture and form blood clots that can obstruct an artery. If such an obstruction deprives the heart of oxygen, the heart will not function properly. Restriction of blood flow is called **ischemia**. Bill Clinton's symptoms of chest pain and shortness of breath were likely due to ischemia.

Coronary heart disease (CHD) refers to any damage to the myocardium as a result of insufficient blood supply. Clinton had coronary artery disease, but the disease had not damaged his heart when he experienced symptoms and sought treatment. Thus, Clinton did not yet have coronary heart disease.

Complete blockage of either coronary artery shuts off the blood flow and thus the oxygen supply to the myocardium. Like other tissue, the myocardium cannot survive without oxygen; therefore, coronary blockage results in the death of myocardial tissue, an infarction. **Myocardial infarction** is the medical term for the condition commonly referred to as a heart attack. During myocardial infarction, the damage may be so extensive as to completely disrupt the heartbeat. In less severe cases, heart contractions may become less effective. The signals for a myocardial infarction include a feeling of weakness or dizziness combined with nausea, cold sweating, difficulty in breathing, and a sensation of crushing or squeezing pain in the chest, arms, shoulders, jaw, or back. Rapid loss of consciousness or death may occur, but the victim sometimes remains quite alert throughout the experience. The severity of symptoms depends on the extent of damage to the heart muscle.

In those people who survive a myocardial infarction (more than half do), the damaged portion of the myocardium will not regrow or repair itself. Instead, scar tissue forms at the infarcted area. Scar tissue does not have the elasticity and function of healthy tissue, so a heart attack lessens the capacity of the heart to pump blood efficiently. A myocardial infarction can limit the type and vigor of activities that a person can safely do, prompting some lifestyle changes. The coronary artery disease that caused a first attack can cause another, but future infarctions are not a certainty.

The process of **cardiac rehabilitation** may involve psychologists, who help cardiac patients adjust their lifestyle to minimize risk factors and lessen the chances of future attacks. Because heart disease is the most frequent cause of death in the United States, preventing heart attacks and furnishing cardiac rehabilitation are major tasks for the health care system.

A less serious result of restriction of the blood supply to the myocardium is **angina pectoris**, a disorder with symptoms of crushing pain in the chest and difficulty in breathing—the symptoms Bill Clinton experienced. Angina is usually precipitated by exercise or stress because these conditions increase demand on the heart. Clinton had experienced such symptoms during exercise and was not distressed, but when he had difficulty in breathing and tightness across the chest during his normal activities, he sought medical attention (Clinton, 2005). With oxygen restriction, the reserve capacity of the cardiovascular system is reduced, and heart disease becomes evident. The uncomfortable symptoms of angina rarely last more than a few minutes, but angina is a sign of obstruction in the coronary arteries.

Former President Clinton's symptoms led to a diagnosis of CAD, and his treatment was bypass

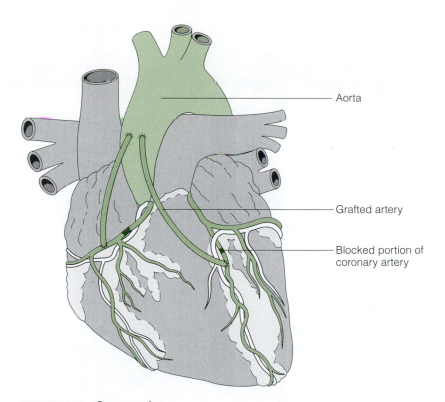

Aorta

Grafted artery

Blocked portion of
coronary artery

FIGURE 9.4   Coronary bypass.

surgery, one of the common treatments for this disorder. This procedure replaces the blocked portion of the coronary artery (or arteries) with grafts of healthy sections of the coronary arteries (see Figure 9.4). Bypass surgery is expensive, carries some risk of death, and may not extend the patient's life significantly, but it is generally successful in relieving angina and improving quality of life, as it has been for Clinton.

Stroke

Atherosclerosis and arteriosclerosis can also affect the arteries that serve the head and neck, thereby restricting the blood supply to the brain. That is, the same disease process that causes CAD and CHD may affect the brain. Any obstruction in the arteries of the brain will restrict or completely stop the flow of blood to the area of the brain served by that portion of the system. Oxygen deprivation causes the death of brain tissue within 3 to 5 minutes. This damage to the brain resulting from lack of oxygen is called a **stroke**, the third most frequent cause of death in the United States. But strokes have other causes as well—for example, a bubble of air (air embolism) or an infection that

impedes blood flow in the brain. In addition, the weakening of artery walls associated with arteriosclerosis may lead to an *aneurysm*, a sac formed by the ballooning of a weakened artery wall. Aneurysms may burst, causing a *hemorrhagic stroke* or death (see Figure 9.5).

A stroke damages neurons in the brain, and these neurons have no capacity to replace themselves. Most commonly, some of the neurons devoted to a particular function (such as speech production) are lost, impairing brain function. The extent of the loss is related to the amount of damage to the area; more extensive damage results in greater impairment. Damage may be so extensive—or in such a critical area—as to bring about immediate death, or damage may be so slight as to go unnoticed.

Blood Pressure

When the heart pumps blood, the force must be substantial to power circulation for an entire cycle through the body and back to the heart. In a healthy cardiovascular system, the pressure in the arteries is not a problem because arteries are quite elastic. In a cardiovascular system diseased by atherosclerosis and

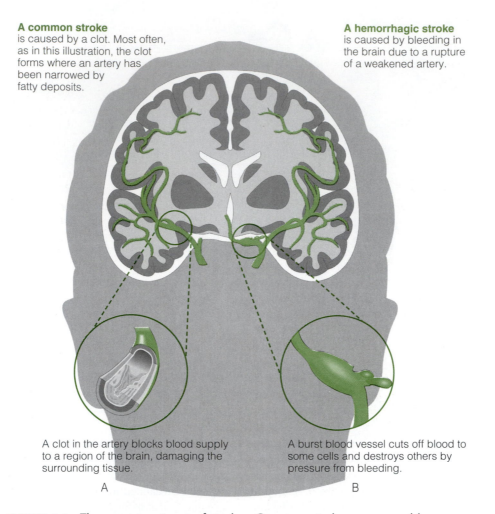

A common stroke
is caused by a clot. Most often, as in this illustration, the clot forms where an artery has been narrowed by fatty deposits.

A hemorrhagic stroke
is caused by bleeding in the brain due to a rupture of a weakened artery.

A clot in the artery blocks blood supply to a region of the brain, damaging the surrounding tissue.

A burst blood vessel cuts off blood to some cells and destroys others by pressure from bleeding.

A   B

FIGURE 9.5   There are two types of strokes: Common strokes are caused by blockage of an artery; hemorrhagic strokes are caused by the bursting of an artery in the brain.

Source: An invitation to health (7th ed., p. 379), by D. Hales, 1997, Pacific Grove, CA: Brooks/Cole. From HALES, Invitation to Health, 7E. ©1997 Cengage Learning.

arteriosclerosis, however, the pressure of the blood in the arteries can produce serious consequences. The narrowing of the arteries that occurs in atherosclerosis and the loss of elasticity that characterizes arteriosclerosis both tend to raise blood pressure. In addition, these disease processes make the cardiovascular system less capable of adapting to the demands of heavy exercise and stress.

Blood pressure measurements are usually expressed by two numbers. The first number represents **systolic pressure**, the pressure generated by the heart's contraction. The second number represents **diastolic pressure**, or the pressure experienced between contractions, reflecting the elasticity of the vessel walls. Both numbers

are expressed in millimeters (mm) of mercury (Hg) because original measurements of blood pressure were obtained by determining how high mercury would rise in a glass column by the pressure of blood in circulation.

Blood pressure elevates through several mechanisms. Some elevations in blood pressure are normal and even adaptive. Temporary activation of the sympathetic nervous system, for example, increases heart rate and also causes constriction of the blood vessels, both of which raise blood pressure. Other elevations in blood pressure, however, are neither normal nor adaptive—they are symptoms of cardiovascular disease.

Millions of people in the United States have **hypertension**—that is, abnormally high blood pressure. This

"silent" illness is the single best predictor of both heart attack and stroke, but it can also cause eye damage and kidney failure (see Figure 9.6). **Essential hypertension** refers to a chronic elevation of blood pressure, which has both genetic and environmental causes (Staessen, Wang, Bianchi, & Birkenhager, 2003). This condition affects one third of people in the United States and other developed countries, for a total of about 76 million in the United States and 1 billion worldwide (Roger et al., 2012; U.S. Department of Health and Human Services [USDHHS], 2003). It is strongly related to aging but also to such factors as African American ancestry, weight, sodium intake, tobacco use, and lack of exercise.

Table 9.1 shows the ranges for normal blood pressure, prehypertension, and Stage 1 and Stage 2 hypertension. Despite beliefs to the contrary, hypertension does not have easily discernible symptoms, so people with hypertension can have dangerously elevated blood pressure and remain completely unaware of their vulnerability to heart attack and stroke.

In younger individuals, high diastolic pressure is most strongly related to cardiovascular risk, but in older individuals, elevated systolic pressure is a better predictor (Staessen et al., 2003). Each 20 mm Hg increase in systolic blood pressure doubles the risk of cardiovascular disease (Roger et al., 2012). Systolic

Eye damage
Prolonged high blood pressure can damage delicate blood vessels on the retina, the layer of cells at the back of the eye. If the damage, known as retinopathy, remains untreated, it can lead to blindness.

Stroke
High blood pressure can damage vessels that supply blood to the brain, eventually causing them to rupture or clog. The interruption in blood flow to the brain is known as a stroke.

Heart attack
High blood pressure makes the heart work harder to pump sufficient blood through narrowed arterioles (small blood vessels). This extra effort can enlarge and weaken the heart, leading to heart failure. High blood pressure also damages the coronary arteries that supply blood to the heart, sometimes leading to blockages that can cause a heart attack.

Damage to artery walls
Artery walls are normally smooth, allowing blood to flow easily. Over time, high blood pressure can wear rough spots in artery walls. Fatty deposits can collect in the rough spots, clogging arteries and raising the risk of a heart attack or stroke.

Kidney failure
Prolonged high blood pressure can damage blood vessels in the kidney, where wastes are filtered from the bloodstream. In severe cases, this damage can lead to kidney failure and even death.

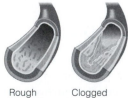

Rough artery walls   Clogged artery

FIGURE 9.6 The consequences of high blood pressure.

Source: An invitation to health (7th ed., p. 370), by D. Hales, 1997, Pacific Grove, CA: Brooks/Cole. From HALES, Invitation to Health, 7E. © 1997 Cengage Learning.

TABLE 9.1 Ranges of Blood Pressure (Expressed in mm of Hg)

	Systolic		Diastolic
Normal	<120	and	<80
Prehypertension	120–139	or	80–89
Stage 1 hypertension	140–159	or	90–99
Stage 2 hypertension	≥160	or	≥100

Source: Adapted from *The seventh report of the joint national committee on prevention, detection, evaluation and treatment of high blood pressure* (NIH Publication No. 03–5233), 2003, by U.S. Department of Health and Human Services (USDHHS). Washington, DC: Author. Table 1.

pressure that exceeds 200 mm Hg presents a danger of rupture in the arterial walls (Berne & Levy, 2000). Diastolic hypertension tends to result in vascular damage that may injure organs served by the affected vessels, most commonly the kidneys, liver, pancreas, brain, and retina.

Because the underlying cause of essential hypertension is complex and not fully understood, no treatment exists that will remedy its basic cause. Treatment tends to be oriented toward drugs or changes in behavior and lifestyle that can lower blood pressure (USDHHS, 2003). Because part of the treatment of hypertension involves behavioral changes, health psychologists play an important role in encouraging such behaviors as controlling weight, maintaining a regular exercise program, and restricting sodium intake. Adherence to these behaviors is important for controlling blood pressure. Unfortunately, adherence to medications is notoriously poor for patients with hypertension.

IN SUMMARY

The cardiovascular system consists of the heart and blood vessels. The heart pumps blood, which circulates throughout the body, supplying oxygen and removing waste products. The coronary arteries supply blood to the heart itself, and when atherosclerosis affects these arteries, coronary artery disease occurs. In this disease process, plaques form within the arteries, restricting the blood supply to the heart muscle. The restriction can cause angina pectoris, with symptoms of chest pain and difficulty in breathing. Blocked coronary arteries can also lead to a myocardial infarction (heart attack). When the oxygen supply to the brain is disrupted, stroke occurs. Stroke can affect any part of the brain

and can vary in severity from minor to fatal. Hypertension—high blood pressure—is a predictor of both heart attack and stroke. Both behavioral and medical treatments can lower hypertension as well as other risk factors for cardiovascular disease.

The Changing Rates of Cardiovascular Disease

The current mortality rate from CVD for people in the United States is lower than it was in 1920. However, between 1920 and 2002, the death rates changed dramatically. Figure 9.7 reveals a sharp rise in CVD deaths from 1920 until the 1950s and 1960s, followed by a decline that continues to the present day. Currently, 34% of all deaths in the United States are from cardiovascular disease (U.S. Census Bureau [USCB], 2011).

In 1920, the rate of deaths due to heart disease was similar for women and men. Overall, the rates of death from CVD remain similar, but the pattern of deaths began to differ when CVD rates began to rise. During the middle of the 20th century, men died from CVD at younger ages than women, creating a gender gap in heart disease.

Reasons for the Decline in Death Rates

The decline in cardiac mortality in the United States is due largely to two causes: improved emergency coronary care and changes in risk factors for CVD (Ford et al., 2007; Wise, 2000). Beginning in the 1960s, many people in the United States began to change their lifestyle. They began to smoke less, be more aware of their

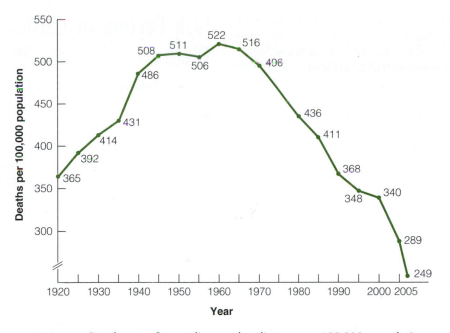

FIGURE 9.7   Death rates for cardiovascular disease per 100,000 population, United States, 1920–2007.

Source: U.S. Public Health Service, *Vital Statistics of the United States*, annual, Vol. I and Vol. II (1900–1970); U.S. National Center for Health Statistics, *Vital Statistics of the United States*, annual (1971–2001); *National Vital Statistics Report*, monthly (2002–2005). Retrieved August 21, 2008, from http://www.infoplease.com/ipa /A0922292.html; *National Vital Statistics Report* (2007). Retrieved April 29, 2012, from http://www.cdc.gov /nchs/data/hestat/cardio2007/cardio2007.pdf

blood pressure, control serum cholesterol, watch their weight, and follow a regular exercise program.

Publicity from two monumental research studies prompted these lifestyle changes. The first was the Framingham Heart Study that began to issue reports during the 1960s, implicating cigarette smoking, high cholesterol, hypertension, a sedentary lifestyle, and obesity as risk factors in cardiovascular disease (Levy & Brink, 2005). The second study was the highly publicized 1964 Surgeon General's report (U.S. Public Health Service [USPHS], 1964), which found a strong association between cigarette smoking and heart disease. Many people became aware of these studies and began to alter their way of living.

Although these lifestyle changes closely parallel declining heart disease death rates, they offer no proof of a causal link between behavior changes and the drop in cardiovascular mortality. During this same period, medical care and technology continued to improve, and many cardiac patients who in earlier years would have died were saved by better and faster treatment. Which factor—lifestyle changes or better

medical care—contributed more to the declining death rate from heart disease? The answer is both. About 47% of the decline in CHD was due to improvements in treatment and 44% to changes in risk factors (Ford et al., 2007). Thus, the declining rate of death from heart disease is due about as much to changes in behavior and lifestyle as it is to improved medical care.

Heart Disease Throughout the World

Heart disease is the leading cause of death, not only in the United States but also worldwide. The total number of deaths from heart disease and stroke accounts for about 30% of all deaths (Mackay & Mensah, 2004). The United States is only one of many high-income Western countries that have seen lifestyle changes and dramatic reductions in cardiovascular deaths among its population (World Health Organization [WHO], 2008b).

In Finland, CVD rates fell more than 70% from the 1970s through the 1990s (Puska, 2002; Puska,

Vartiainen, Tuomilehto, Salomaa, & Nissinen, 1998). Part of this decrease was the result of a countrywide effort to change risk factors. That effort began with a community intervention that targeted an area of Finland with particularly high rates of CVD and attempted to change diet, hypertension, and smoking. This lowering of risk factors was largely responsible for the majority of the reduction (Laatikainen et al., 2005).

In contrast, heart disease has increased in countries that were once part of the Soviet Union (Weidner, 2000; Weidner & Cain, 2003). Since 1990, this epidemic has affected middle-aged men more than other groups, and the gender gap in heart disease is larger in Russia than in any other country. The risk of premature death from heart disease is 4 times greater for a Russian man than for one in the United States. In some countries in Eastern Europe, coronary heart disease accounts for 80% of deaths; the average life expectancy has decreased, and is not expected to increase in the near future. The reasons for this plague of heart disease are not completely understood, but lack of social support, and high levels of stress, smoking, and alcohol abuse are common, and these psychosocial and behavioral differences may underlie the increased rates of CVD (Weidner & Cain, 2003).

Heart disease and stroke are also leading causes of death in developing and underdeveloped countries, where an increase in heart disease and stroke continues (WHO, 2008b). As tobacco smoking, obesity, physical activity, and dietary patterns in these countries become more like those of developed nations, CVD will increase in developing nations. Thus, the worldwide burden of CVD is immense.

IN SUMMARY

Since the mid-1960s, deaths from coronary artery disease and stroke have steadily declined in the United States and most (but not all) other high-income nations. Although some of that decline is a result of better and faster coronary care, lifestyle changes account for 50% or more of this decrease. In low-income countries around the world, the opposite has occurred: Smoking and obesity have increased, and physical activity has decreased. These habits have increased risks for CVD, which will grow in these countries in the coming years.

Risk Factors in Cardiovascular Disease

Research links several risk factors to the development of cardiovascular disease. In Chapter 2, we defined a *risk factor* as any characteristic or condition that occurs with greater frequency in people with a disease than in people free from that disease. The risk factor approach does not identify the cause of a disease. Nor does it allow a precise prediction of who will succumb to disease and who will remain healthy. The risk factor approach simply yields information concerning which conditions are associated—directly or indirectly—with a particular disease or disorder.

The risk factor approach to predicting heart disease began with the Framingham Heart Study in 1948, an investigation of more than 5,000 people in the town of Framingham, Massachusetts (Levy & Brink, 2005). The study was a prospective design; thus, all participants were free of heart disease at the beginning of the study. The original plan was to follow these people for 20 years to study heart disease and the factors related to its development. The results proved so valuable that the study has continued now for more than 50 years and includes both children and grandchildren of the original participants.

At the time of their discovery, medicine had not considered many typical American lifestyle behaviors to be particularly dangerous (Levy & Brink, 2005). Prompted by the growing epidemic of heart disease in the 1950s, the Framingham study revealed that these risk factors are reliably related to the development of heart disease and stroke.

Several large-scale studies followed the Framingham study. These include the Nurses' Health Study, a long-term epidemiological study of women's health that confirms the link between several risk factors and women's risk for cardiovascular disease (Oh, Hu, Manson, Stampfer, & Willett, 2005). The largest study of cardiovascular health to date is the 52-country INTERHEART Study (Yusuf et al., 2004), which matched over 15,000 people who experienced a heart attack with nearly 15,000 similar people who had not. This case–control study examined a host of other potential risk factors, and the extent to which risk factors for cardiovascular disease are similar across countries. Thus, much of our knowledge about the risk factors for major cardiovascular problems comes from the Framingham, Nurses' Health, and INTERHEART studies.

Cardiovascular risk factors include those that are inherent, those that arise from physiological conditions, those that arise from behavior, and a variety of psychosocial factors.

Inherent Risk Factors

Inherent risk factors result from genetic or physical conditions that cannot be readily modified. Although inherent risk factors cannot be changed, people with these risk factors are not necessarily destined to develop cardiovascular disease. Identifying people with inherent risk factors enables these high-risk individuals to minimize their overall risk profile by controlling the things that they can, such as hypertension, smoking, and diet. Inherent risk factors for CVD include advancing age, family history, gender, and ethnic background.

Advancing Age   Advancing age is the primary risk factor for cardiovascular disease as well as for cancer and many other diseases. As people become older, their risk for cardiovascular death rises sharply. Figure 9.8 shows

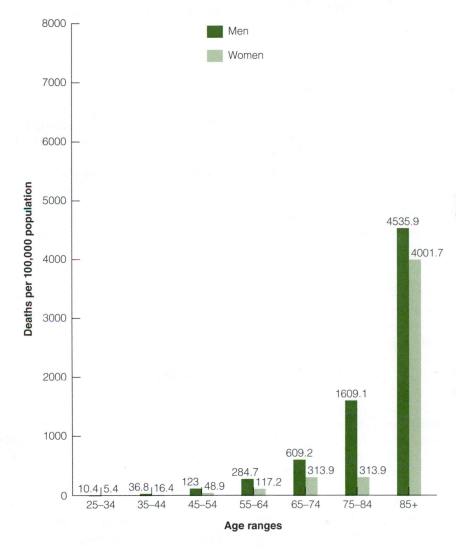

FIGURE 9.8   Cardiovascular disease mortality rates by age and gender, United States, 2008.

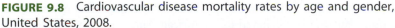

Source: Health United States, 2011, by National Center for Health Statistics, 2012, Hyattsville, MD: U.S. Government Printing Office, pp. 201, 204 Table 30. Retrieved September 17, 2012, from http://www.cdc.gov /nchs/data/hus/hus11.pdf

that for every 10-year increase in age, both men and women more than double their chances of dying of cardiovascular disease. For example, men 85 and older are about 2.7 times as likely to die of cardiovascular disease as men between the ages of 75 and 84, and women 85 and older are about 3.7 times as likely as women 75 to 84 to die from cardiovascular disease.

Family History   Family history is also an inherent risk factor for CVD. People with a history of cardiovascular disease in their family are more likely to die of heart disease than those with no such history. Similarly, people with a parent who has suffered a heart attack are more likely to suffer a heart attack themselves (Chow et al., 2011). Bill Clinton mentioned his family history as a factor that put him at risk for cardiovascular disease. This familial risk is likely to occur through the action of many genes and their interactions with environmental factors in people's lives (Doevendans, Van der Smagt, Loh, De Jonge, & Touw, 2003). Like other inherent risk factors, genes cannot be altered through lifestyle changes, but people with a family history of heart disease can lower their risk by changing their lifestyle.

Gender   Although gender is an inherent risk factor, many behaviors and social conditions are related to gender. Thus, the differing risk for women and men may or may not be inherent.

In 1920, the rate of deaths due to heart disease was similar for women and men. Overall, the rates of death from CVD remain similar, but the pattern of deaths began to differ when CVD rates began to rise. During the middle of the 20th century, men died from CVD at younger ages than women, creating a gender gap in heart disease.

As Figure 9.8 shows, this gender gap continues to exist. Men have a higher rate of death from CVD than women, and this discrepancy shows most prominently during the middle-age years. After that age, the percentage of women's deaths due to CVD increases sharply, and a larger number of older women than older men die of cardiovascular disease; nonetheless, the *rate* of death from CVD remains higher for men.

What factors explain this gender gap? Both physiology and lifestyle contribute (Pilote et al., 2007). Before menopause, women experience a lower rate of CVD than men. At one time, estrogen was believed to furnish protection, but the failure to produce any benefit in a large-scale hormone replacement trial engendered doubt (Writing Group for the Women's Health Initiative Investigators, 2002). A more recent focus is on androgens, including the possibility that these hormones may involve both protections and risks for both men and women (Ng, 2007).

However, lifestyle is responsible for much of the gender gap in heart disease. Across the world, men tend to experience a heart attack at an earlier age than women do, and this difference is explained by men's higher rates of unhealthy lifestyle factors during their younger years (Anand et al., 2008). Furthermore, the gender gap is particularly large in some countries. Russia has the widest gender gap in life expectancy in the world—71 years for women and 58 for men—and most of the discrepancy comes from higher rates of CVD among men (Weidner & Cain, 2003). Russian men's health habits include more smoking and drinking, and they show poorer coping skills for dealing with stress. In other countries, such as Iceland, the gender difference in CVD rate is small (Weidner, 2000). The fact that gender differences in CVD mortality are much greater in some countries than in others suggests that behavioral factors, rather than inherent biological differences, explain the CVD mortality discrepancy between men and women.

Ethnic Background   A fourth inherent risk for cardiovascular disease is ethnic background. In the United States, African Americans have more than a 30% greater risk for cardiovascular death than European Americans, but Native Americans, Asian Americans, and Hispanic Americans have lower rates (CDC/NCHS, 2010). The increased risk for African Americans may be related to social, economic, or behavioral factors rather than to any biological basis, because the INTERHEART Study (Yusuf et al., 2004) indicated that the risk factors for heart disease are the same for people in countries around the world. Thus, ethnic differences in heart disease are likely due to ethnic differences in levels of known risk factors.

African Americans follow that pattern: They have higher levels of risk factors for heart disease than European Americans, Hispanics, Asians, and Native Americans. The strongest risk for African Americans is high blood pressure (Jones et al., 2002), but psychosocial risks such as low income and low educational level also have a major impact (Karlamangla et al., 2005; Pilote et al., 2007). The higher rates of cardiovascular death among African Americans may be due to their higher rate of hypertension. Their higher rate of hypertension may be partly due to greater cardiac reactivity, as a possible result of ongoing experiences of racial discrimination. Even threats of discrimination can raise blood pressure in African Americans (Blascovich, Spencer, Quinn, & Steele, 2001). The tendency to react to stress and threats of stress with increased cardiac reactivity may arise from years of racial discrimination, discrimination most likely to be experienced by dark-skinned people. For example, Elizabeth Klonoff and Hope Landrine (2000) found that dark-skinned African Americans were 11 times more likely than light-skinned African Americans to experience frequent racial discrimination. Thus, racial discrimination seems to be a factor in the increased blood pressure levels among African Americans, but these responses are classified as psychosocial risks that relate to ethnicity rather than as a risk that is inherent in ethnic differences.

Physiological Conditions

A second category of risk factors in cardiovascular disease includes the physiological conditions of hypertension, serum cholesterol level, problems in glucose metabolism, and inflammation.

Hypertension   Other than advancing age, hypertension is the single most important risk factor for cardiovascular disease, yet millions of people with high blood pressure are not aware of their vulnerability. Unlike most disorders, hypertension produces no overt symptoms, and dangerously elevated blood pressure levels commonly occur with no signals or symptoms.

The Framingham Heart Study provided the first solid evidence of the risks of hypertension. More recently, the 52-country INTERHEART Study confirmed the strong link between hypertension and cardiovascular problems across age, gender, ethnicity, and country of residence (Yusuf et al., 2004). As a U.S. government report stated, "The risk between BP and risk of CVD events is continuous, consistent, and independent of other risk factors. The higher the BP, the greater the chance of heart attack, heart failure, stroke, and kidney disease" (USDHHS, 2003, p. 2).

Serum Cholesterol Level   A second physiological condition related to cardiovascular disease is high serum cholesterol level. Cholesterol is a waxy, fat-like substance that is essential for human life as a component of cell membranes. *Serum* or *blood cholesterol* is the level of cholesterol circulating through the bloodstream; this level is related (but not perfectly related) to *dietary cholesterol*, or the amount of cholesterol in

one's food. Dietary cholesterol comes from animal fats and oils but not from vegetables or vegetable products. Although cholesterol is essential for life, too much may contribute to the process of developing cardiovascular disease.

After a person eats cholesterol, the bloodstream transports it as part of the process of digestion. A measurement of the amount of cholesterol carried in the serum (the liquid, cell-free part of the blood) is typically expressed in milligrams (mg) of cholesterol per deciliters (dl) of serum. Thus, a cholesterol reading of 210 means 210 mg of cholesterol per deciliter of blood serum.

However, total cholesterol in the bloodstream is not the best predictor of CVD. Cholesterol circulates in the blood in several forms of **lipoproteins**, which can be distinguished by analyzing their density and function. **Low-density lipoprotein (LDL)** carries cholesterol from the liver to the cells of the body, whereas **high-density lipoprotein (HDL)** carries cholesterol from the tissues back to the liver. The Framingham researchers found that LDL was positively related to cardiovascular disease, whereas HDL was negatively related. Subsequent research supports this relationship. High-density lipoprotein actually seems to offer some protection against CVD, whereas LDL seems to promote atherosclerosis. For these reasons, LDL is sometimes referred to as "bad cholesterol" and HDL as "good cholesterol." Indeed, women's higher levels of HDL may be a partial explanation for the gender gap in heart disease (Pilote et al., 2007).

Total cholesterol (TC) is determined by adding the values for HDL, LDL, and 20% of very low-density lipoprotein (VLDL), also called **triglycerides**. A low ratio of total cholesterol to HDL is more desirable than a high ratio. A ratio of less than 4.5 to 1 is healthier than a ratio of 6.0 to 1; that is, people whose HDL level is about 20% to 22% of total cholesterol have a reduced risk of CVD. Most authorities now believe that a favorable balance of total cholesterol to HDL is more critical than total cholesterol in avoiding cardiovascular disease, and much recent research has focused on lowering LDL via dietary changes or pharmaceuticals known as *statins* (Grundy et al., 2004). Table 9.2 presents the desirable ranges for total cholesterol and each of the subfractions, along with a desirable and an undesirable profile.

Cholesterol is a stronger predictor of cardiovascular problems for young and middle-aged adults, compared with older adults (Psaty et al., 2004; Sacco et al., 2001). Therefore, cholesterol should be a concern

TABLE 9.2   Desirable Ranges for Serum Cholesterol, Along With Examples of Favorable and Risky Profiles

Cholesterol Component	Desirable Range	Good Profile	Risky Profile
HDL cholesterol	>60 mg/dl	70	40
LDL cholesterol	<130 mg/dl	60	180
Triglycerides	<200 mg/dl	150	250
	(20% of VLDL)	30 (= 150 × .20)	50 (= 250 × .20)
Total cholesterol	<200 mg/dl	70 + 60 + 30 = 160	40 + 180 + 50 = 270
Cholesterol/HDL ratio	<4.00	160/70 = 2.28	270/40 = 6.75

through middle age. In contrast, older adults may start to have additional risk factors that obscure the unique influence of cholesterol on cardiovascular risk.

Research on cholesterol suggests several conclusions. First, cholesterol intake and blood cholesterol are related. Second, the relationship between dietary intake of cholesterol and blood cholesterol relates strongly to habitual diet—that is, eating habits maintained over many years. Lowering blood cholesterol level by changing diet is possible, but the process is neither quick nor easy. Third, the ratio of total cholesterol to HDL is probably more important than total cholesterol alone, but lowering LDL is an important goal.

Problems in Glucose Metabolism   A third physiological risk factor for CVD comes from problems with glucose metabolism. The most obvious of such problems is diabetes, a condition in which glucose cannot be taken into the cells because of problems in producing or using insulin. When this situation occurs, glucose remains in the blood at abnormally high levels. People who have juvenile onset (Type 1) diabetes are more likely to develop CVD, and longer-duration problems with glucose metabolism increase the risk (Pambianco, Costacou, & Orchard, 2007). Type 2 diabetes also elevates the risk of CVD (Sobel & Schneider, 2005). (We discuss the risks of diabetes more fully in Chapter 11.)

Many people have problems with glucose metabolism that do not qualify as diabetes but may still create CVD risk. One study (Khaw et al., 2004) showed that people who have problems in glucose metabolism (but not diabetes) had greater risks for CVD development or death than those with normal glucose metabolism. Such problems in glucose metabolism constitute one of the factors in the *metabolic syndrome*, a collection of factors proposed to elevate the risk for CVD (Johnson & Weinstock, 2006). Other components of metabolic

syndrome include excess abdominal fat, elevated blood pressure, and problems with the levels of two components of cholesterol. People with metabolic syndrome are twice as likely to experience cardiovascular health problems than those without the syndrome (Mottillo et al., 2010). In a study testing the components of the metabolic syndrome (Anderson et al., 2004), problems in insulin metabolism more strongly predicted arterial damage than the other components.

Inflammation   As unlikely as it may sound, atherosclerosis results in part from the body's natural inflammatory response. As you learned in Chapter 6, inflammation is a nonspecific immune response. When a tissue is damaged, white blood cells (such as granulocytes and macrophages) migrate to the site of the injury and defend against potential invaders by engulfing them through the process of phagocytosis. When an artery is injured or infected, these white blood cells migrate toward and accumulate on the artery wall. When a person's diet is high in cholesterol, the "diet" of these white blood cells is likewise high in cholesterol. Arterial plaques—the precursors to atherosclerosis—are simply accumulations of cholesterol-filled white blood cells. Inflammation influences not only the development of plaques but also their stability, making them more likely to rupture and cause a heart attack or stroke (Abi-Saleh et al., 2008).

Because chronic inflammation may raise the risk for the development of atherosclerosis (Pilote et al., 2007), factors that produce chronic inflammation may also increase risk for cardiovascular disease. Stress and depression are two factors that may contribute to inflammation (Miller & Blackwell, 2006) and are two known risk factors for cardiovascular disease. Indeed, recent evidence suggests that inflammatory processes

Would You BELIEVE...? A Floss a Day May Keep Cardiovascular Disease Away?

If you look in your medicine cabinet or the bottom of your bathroom drawer, you may discover a new weapon in the fight against cardiovascular disease.

That weapon is dental floss. Like most people, you probably own floss but do not use it regularly. Here is a reason you should start: Flossing not only keeps your teeth and gums healthy, but it may also prevent cardiovascular disease.

Accumulating research draws surprising links between oral health and cardiovascular health. Periodontitis—

or inflammation of the tissues and bones that support the teeth—is a risk factor for cardiovascular disease, independent of other established risk factors (Humphrey, Fu, Buckley, Freeman, Helfand, 2008). Among nonsmokers who previously suffered a heart attack, the presence of periodontitis predicts greater risk of recurrent cardiovascular problems (Dorn et al., 2010). Even a person's frequency of tooth brushing predicts his or her subsequent likelihood of cardiovascular disease (de Oliveira, Watt, & Hamer, 2010).

What explains this connection between oral and cardiovascular health? One possibility is that periodontitis increases the level of systemic inflammation in the body. Another possibility is that the bacteria that cause dental plaque and periodontitis eventually settle on artery walls after they enter the bloodstream. These bacteria then become the target of an inflammatory response, making atherosclerosis more likely.

So blow the dust off that box of dental floss! Your gums—and your heart—will thank you for it.

---

account for some, but not all, of the association between depression and increased risk of cardiovascular mortality (Kop et al., 2010). Metabolic syndrome may also be related to inflammation (Vlachopoulos, Rokkas, Ioakeimidis, & Stefanadis, 2007), suggesting that these conditions interact or have some common pathways for causing damage to the cardiovascular system.

Similarly, any factor that reduces inflammation may reduce risk for cardiovascular disease. For example, aspirin—an anti-inflammatory pain reliever—lowers the risk of heart attack. Thus, the findings about the risks from inflammation explain why taking aspirin lowers the risk of heart attack, and the findings about stress and depression suggest that other behavioral factors may present risks as well as ways to protect against CVD. These findings also help explain why taking care of your teeth and gums may also keep your heart healthy (see Would You Believe … ? box).

Behavioral Factors

Behavioral factors constitute a third risk category for CVD; the most important of these lifestyle factors are smoking, diet, and physical activity. For example, women who do not smoke, eat a diet high in fiber and low in saturated fat, are not overweight, and are physically active have an 80% lower risk for coronary heart disease than other people (Stampfer, Hu,

Manson, Rimm, & Willett, 2000)! Each of these behaviors—smoking, food choice, weight maintenance, and physical activity—is related to CVD.

Smoking   Cigarette smoking is the leading behavioral risk factor for cardiovascular death in the United States, and a major contributor to deaths throughout the world (American Cancer Society, 2012; USDHHS, 2010c). In the United States, cardiovascular deaths due to smoking have begun to decline (Rodu & Cole, 2007). For example, between 1987 and 2002, deaths attributable to smoking declined 41% in men and 30% in women. However, such a decline has not occurred in all parts of the world—smoking continues at higher rates in many other countries than in the United States. Smoking accounts for about 35% of the risk for heart attack worldwide (Yusuf et al., 2004), which translates into more than a million deaths per year.

People who currently smoke are 3 times more likely to suffer a heart attack than people who never smoked (Teo et al., 2006). Fortunately, quitting smoking does reduce the risk of heart attack: Within 3 years of quitting, former smokers are only twice as likely to suffer a heart attack as those who never smoke (Teo et al., 2006). However, the risks of past smoking do not disappear completely, as a small risk for heart attack persists even 20 years after a person quits. However, cardiovascular risks of tobacco remain even when smoke is not inhaled, as the chewing tobacco also increases the risk of heart attack. Passive smoking—or "secondhand" smoking—is not as dangerous as personal tobacco use, but exposure to environmental tobacco smoke raises the risk for cardiovascular disease by about 15% (Kaur, Cohen, Dolor, Coffman, & Bastian, 2004). Thus, tobacco contributes to increased risk for cardiovascular problems in a number of ways.

Weight and Diet   Obesity and diet also increase risk for cardiovascular disease. Although the dangers of obesity seem obvious, the evaluation of obesity as an independent risk for cardiovascular disease is difficult. The main problem is that obesity is related to other risks, such as blood pressure, Type 2 diabetes, total cholesterol, LDL, and triglycerides (Ashton, Nanchahal, & Wood, 2001). A high degree of abdominal fat is a risk factor for heart attack in men (Smith, Ness, et al., 2005), in women (Iribarren, Darbinian, Lo, Fireman, & Go, 2006), and in people worldwide (Yusuf et al., 2005).

The dietary choices that people make may either increase or decrease their chances of developing cardiovascular disease, depending on the foods they eat. Results from two large-scale studies—the Framingham Study (Levy & Brink, 2005) and the INTERHEART Study (Iqbal et al., 2008)—show that diets heavy in saturated fats are positively related to CVD and risk of heart attack. These high-fat foods have an obvious link to serum cholesterol levels, but other nutrients may also affect CVD risks.

For example, sodium intake contributes to high blood pressure (one of the major risks for CVD; Stamler et al., 2003), and some individuals seem to be more sensitive to the effects of sodium intake than others (Brooks, Haywood, & Johnson, 2005). Potassium intake, however, seems to decrease the risk, which brings up the question: Can diet serve as protection against cardiovascular disease? A growing body of results indicates that some diets, and perhaps even some foods, offer protective effects.

Over more than two decades, researchers showed that diets high in fruits and vegetables predict lower CVD risks. The INTERHEART Study, for example, found that people who ate a diet high in fruits and vegetables had a lower risk of heart attack (Iqbal et al., 2008). One analysis of worldwide consumption of fruits and vegetables (Lock, Pomerleau, Causer, Altmann, & McKee, 2005) concluded that if these levels increased to a minimal acceptable level, the rate of

heart disease could be reduced by 31% and stroke by 19%.

A diet high in fish seems to offer some protection against heart disease and stroke (Iso et al., 2001; Torpy, 2006); the protective component is *omega-3 fatty acids*. Fish such as tuna, salmon, mackerel, and other high-fat fish and shellfish are high in this nutrient, but research on the benefits of fish has yielded mixed results. Not all fish meals offer the same protection (Mozaffarian et al., 2005). For example, baked or broiled fish was more beneficial than fried fish in decreasing the risk of stroke in older adults. The American Heart Association recommends at least two servings of fish per week (Smith & Sahyoun, 2005) based on this evidence. That advantage is balanced against the high level of mercury in some fish, which also presents risks.

Do certain vitamins or other micronutrients protect against cardiovascular disease? People who eat diets high in antioxidants such as vitamin E, beta carotene or lycopene, selenium, and riboflavin show a number of health advantages, including lower levels of cardiovascular disease (Stanner, Hughes, Kelly, & Buttriss, 2004). These antioxidants protect LDL from oxidation and thus from its potentially damaging effects on the cardiovascular system. However, research findings do not show that taking supplements of these nutrients is as effective as eating a diet that contains the nutrients in high levels. Such a diet may include some surprising choices (see Would You Believe …? box).

Physical Activity   Across the world, two factors consistently predict higher risk of heart attack: Owning a car and owning a television (Held et al., 2012). These two factors have one thing in common: They both reduce physical activity. The benefits of physical activity in lowering cardiovascular risk are clear and "irrefutable" (Warburton, Nicol, & Bredin, 2006, p. 801; see Chapter 15 for a review of this evidence). Unfortunately, people's jobs have become less physically strenuous, and many individuals do not engage in physical activity in their leisure time, creating large numbers of sedentary people in many industrialized societies.

The risks of inactivity apply to the entire life span. In the United States, children have become less physically active, and their sedentary lifestyle has contributed to their increasing obesity and growing risk for cardiovascular disease (Wang, 2004). At the other end of the age spectrum, women over age 65 showed better health and lower CVD risks when they voluntarily engaged in

Would You BELIEVE...? Chocolate May Help Prevent Heart Disease

Would you believe that chocolate—rather than being bad for you—may contain chemicals that help prevent coronary artery disease? One of the dietary components that seems to offer some protection against artery damage is a class of chemicals called *flavonoids*, which are derived primarily from fruits and vegetables (Engler & Engler, 2006). Several subcategories of flavonoids exist, each with slightly different properties. The subcategory that contains chocolate is the flavonols, which also occur in tea, red wine, grapes, and blackberries. However, all of the subcategories have been linked to health benefits, including growing evidence of the advantages of chocolate.

Not all chocolate contains the same amount of flavonoids, and thus some types of chocolate may offer more protection than others (Engler & Engler, 2006). The processing of the cacao bean, from which chocolate is made, affects the flavonoid content. Dark chocolate contains 2 to 3 times more flavonoids than milk chocolate or Dutch chocolate.

Flavonoids exert their health benefits by reducing oxidation, making them one type of antioxidant. The benefits may occur through effects on the lining of arteries (Engler & Engler, 2006). Flavonoids may be especially effective in protecting arteries against the harmful effects of low-density cholesterol and increase vascular dilation. If flavonoids protect arteries, that mechanism would explain the connection between flavonol intake and lower rates of coronary heart disease mortality (Huxley & Neil, 2003). However, chocolate consumption has also shown cardiovascular benefits in lowering blood pressure and decreasing inflammation, both of which lower risk factors for CVD (Engler & Engler, 2006). This body of research indicates that chocolate consumption may protect against heart disease in a variety of ways.

Chocolate is not the only food that is rich in flavonols. High concentrations of this micronutrient also occur in green and black tea, grapes, red wine, cherries, apples, blackberries, and raspberries. Thus, chocolate may not offer unique health benefits, but legions of chocoholics would testify that its taste is unique. These devotees are overjoyed that a food that was once considered a sin may now offer salvation from heart disease.

exercise (Simonsick, Guralnik, Volpato, Balfour, & Fried, 2005). Sedentary lifestyle also contributes to the metabolic syndrome, the pattern of CVD risks that include overweight, abdominal fat, and blood glucose metabolism problems (Ekelund et al., 2005). Thus, physical inactivity is an important behavioral risk factor for cardiovascular disease.

Psychosocial Factors

A number of psychosocial factors relate to heart disease (Smith & Ruiz, 2002). These factors are education, income, marital status, social support, stress, anxiety, depression, cynical hostility, and anger.

Educational Level and Income   Low socioeconomic status—often assessed by low educational level and low income—are risk factors for cardiovascular disease. For example, in the INTERHEART Study, low socioeconomic status emerged as a risk factor for heart attack (Rosengren et al., 2009). In particular, low education placed people at increased risk for heart attack. In many countries, educational levels are related to ethnicity, but studies in the United States (Yan et al., 2006), Netherlands (Bos, Kunst, Garssen, & Mackenbach, 2005), and Israel (Manor, Eisenbach, Friedlander, & Kark, 2004) examined educational level within ethnic groups. The results showed that, independent of ethnicity, low educational level increased risk for CVD.

What factors link low levels of education to high levels of heart disease? One possibility is that people with low education practice fewer health behaviors than those with higher educational levels; they eat a less healthy diet, smoke, and lead more sedentary lives, which increases their CVD risks factors (Laaksonen et al., 2008). Indeed, in the INTERHEART Study, much of the influence of socioeconomic factors such as education on cardiovascular risk was explained by the modifiable lifestyle factors of smoking, physical activity, diet, and obesity (Rosengren et al., 2009).

Income level is another risk factor for cardiovascular disease; people with lower incomes have higher rates of heart disease than people in the higher income brackets. A report from China (Yu et al., 2000) showed that socioeconomic level—defined as education, occupation, income, and marital status—related to such cardiovascular risk factors as blood pressure, body mass index, and cigarette smoking. This finding is not isolated—many studies show links between socioeconomic status and health, mortality, and cardiovascular disease. A cross-national study (Kim, Kawachi, Hoorn, & Ezzati, 2008) revealed that in societies with a large discrepancy in income levels, individuals in the lower part of the income distribution had higher risk factors for CVD. The effect may occur through income level or social status; evidence exists for both. Income level relates to longevity in the form of a gradient, with higher income predicting longer life (Krantz & McCeney, 2002). Social rank and status have a variety of cardiovascular effects in many species, including humans (Sapolsky, 2004). In addition, research suggests that these socioeconomic cardiovascular risks begin to accumulate during adolescence or even childhood (Karlamangla et al., 2005). Thus, educational level, income, and social status all show effects on the cardiovascular system and on diseases of this system.

Social Support and Marriage   Prospective studies confirm that lacking social support is also a risk for cardiovascular disease (Krantz & McCeney, 2002). This conclusion is consistent with the wide body of research discussed in Chapter 5 that shows the value of social support and the problems that can arise from its absence. Indeed, loneliness during childhood, adolescence, and young adulthood relates to CVD risk factors (Caspi, Harrington, Moffitt, Milne, & Poulton, 2006), and these effects may become more serious with aging (Hawkley & Cacioppo, 2007). For example, older people who had experienced a heart attack were more likely to have another, fatal heart attack if they lived alone (Schmaltz et al., 2007).

Lack of social support may be a factor even more important in the progression of CVD. Studies that measured the progression of blockage of the coronary arteries in women (Wang, Mittleman, & Orth-Gomér, 2005; Wang et al., 2007) found that support at home and at work affected the progression of coronary artery blockage; high stress in either area predicted progressive blockage, whereas satisfactory support in both led to regression of arterial plaques. Another study showed that the number of people in a person's social network related to coronary mortality; CAD patients with only one to three people in their social network were nearly 2 ½ times more likely to die of coronary artery disease than patients with four or more close friends (Brummett et al., 2001). Older men who were more socially involved were less likely to die of CVD than those who were more isolated (Ramsay et al., 2008).

Marriage should provide social support, and in general, married people are at decreased risk for cardiovascular health problems (Empana et al., 2008; Hu et al., 2012). For example, two large population studies—one in France (Empana et al., 2008) and another in China (Hu et al., 2012)—both found that married individuals were less likely to suffer a heart attack than people who were not married. However, the quality of the marital relationship may be a factor. In a 10-year follow-up, married men were almost half as likely to die as unmarried men (Eaker, Sullivan, Kelly-Hayes, D'Agostino, & Benjamin, 2007). For women, the benefits depended on marital communication and quality, with poor communication increasing heart disease risk. Another study (Holt-Lunstad, Birmingham, & Jones, 2008) focused specifically on marriage and also found that marital quality was important; marriage was not beneficial if the individual was dissatisfied with the relationship. However, happily married people received greater benefits in the form of lower blood pressure than single people, even those with a supportive social network.

Spouses (and other sources of social support) may reduce the risk of cardiovascular mortality by providing encouragement for compliance with a healthy lifestyle or a medical regimen or by urging a person to seek medical care (Williams et al., 1992). Sources of social support are usually friends, family, spouses, and even pets (Allen, 2003). Support may also affect CVD

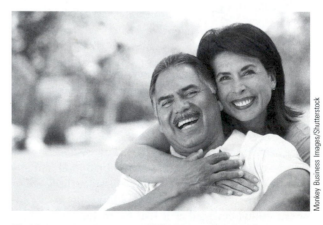

Marriage appears to provide protection against cardiovascular disease.

through its influence on the experience of stress and depression.

Stress, Anxiety, and Depression   Stress, anxiety, and depression relate to cardiovascular disease, but they also relate to each other (Suls & Bunde, 2005). This overlap makes independent assessment of each component difficult. However, a great deal of evidence implicates these factors in cardiovascular disease. For example, the INTERHEART study (Rosengren et al., 2004) revealed that people who had heart attacks also experienced more work and financial stress and more life events than their matched controls. In a large, prospective study of young adults in the United States, increases in work-related stress led to greater incidence of hypertension 8 years later (Markovitz, Matthews, Whooley, Lewis, & Greenlund, 2004).

Anxiety and depression also increase risk for CVD; the evidence for the risks from depression is especially strong. Even after controlling for other risk factors such as smoking and cholesterol, anxiety (Shen et al., 2008) and depression (Goldston & Baillie, 2008; Whang et al., 2009) predict the development of CVD. The risks of depression and anxiety apply not only to the development of CVD but also to its progression, as depression in the year following a heart attack predicts subsequent risk of cardiovascular mortality (Bekke-Hansen, Trockel, Burg, & Taylor, 2012). However, the evidence is stronger for these two negative emotions in the development of CVD (Suls & Bunde, 2005). Indeed, evidence for the beginnings of artery damage appeared in a study of depressed adolescents (Tomfohr, Martin, & Miller, 2008), which is consistent with the long-term damage that accompanies CVD. More evidence about the harm of negative emotions has come from the study of hostility and anger.

Hostility and Anger   Researchers have also found that some types of hostility and anger are risk factors for cardiovascular disease. Much of this research grew out of work on the Type A behavior pattern, originally proposed by **cardiologists** Meyer Friedman and Ray Rosenman (1974; Rosenman et al., 1975), physicians who specialized in heart disease. Friedman and Rosenman may have gotten their inspiration for studying the Type A behavior pattern from a rather unusual source: an upholsterer. On numerous occasions, Friedman and Rosenman paid an upholsterer to repair the fabric on the seats in their waiting room. One day the upholsterer commented that only

the cardiology patients wore out the seats so quickly, with a pattern that suggested they were habitually sitting on the edges of their seats. Years later, Meyer Friedman reported that this was the first time he remembered anybody making a connection between people's behavior patterns and their risk for cardiovascular disease (Sapolsky, 1997).

Friedman and Rosenman described people with the Type A behavior pattern as hostile, competitive, concerned with numbers and the acquisition of objects, and possessed of an exaggerated sense of time urgency. During the early years of its history, the Type A behavior pattern demonstrated promise as a predictor of heart disease, but later researchers were unable to affirm a consistent link between the global Type A behavior pattern and incidence of heart disease. This situation led investigators to consider the possibility that some component of the pattern—rather than the entire pattern—might be a predictor.

Hostility appeared to be the component of Type A that was risky. In 1989, Redford Williams suggested that cynical hostility is especially harmful to cardiovascular health. He contended that people who mistrust others, think the worst of humanity, and interact with others with cynical hostility are harming themselves and their hearts. Furthermore, he suggested that people who use *anger* as a response to interpersonal problems have an elevated risk for heart disease.

Hostility early in life does predict cardiovascular health later in life. In one long-term prospective study, young adults who scored high in hostility had higher levels of coronary calcification—a precursor of atherosclerosis—at a 10-year follow-up than young adults low in hostility (Iribarren et al., 2000). Higher levels of hostility also predicted greater incidence of hypertension at a 15-year follow-up (Yan et al., 2003). In addition to increasing risk for these two precursors to cardiovascular disease, a recent review of over 20 longitudinal studies confirmed hostility as a significant predictor of subsequent cardiovascular disease (Chida & Steptoe, 2009). The cardiovascular health of men, in particular, relates to both hostility as well as another related emotion: anger.

Anger and hostility may seem the same, but they have important differences. Anger is an unpleasant *emotion* accompanied by physiological arousal, whereas hostility is a negative *attitude* toward others (Suls & Bunde, 2005). The *experience* of anger is probably unavoidable and may not present much of a risk. However, the manner in which a person deals with

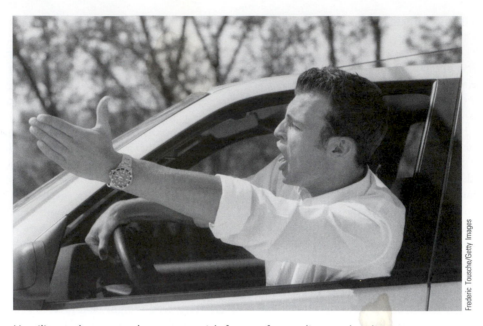

Frederic Tousche/Getty Images

Hostility and expressed anger are risk factors for cardiovascular disease.

anger may be a factor in the development of cardiovascular disease. People may express their anger, including yelling back when someone yells at them, raising their voice when arguing, and throwing temper tantrums. Alternatively, people may suppress their anger, holding in their feelings. Some evidence suggests that either strategy may pose problems.

Anger and Cardiovascular Reactivity One way that the expression of anger might relate to coronary heart disease is through **cardiovascular reactivity (CVR)**, typically defined as increases in blood pressure and heart rate due to frustration, harassment, or any laboratory stress task. Most past research on CVR used laboratory methods in which researchers presented participants with various situations intended to arouse anger and monitored their physiological responses, often using a variety of cardiac measurements such as blood pressure and heart rate. Sometimes, the measurements also included the persistence of such cardiac responses.

In one study using such a procedure (Suarez, Saab, Llabre, Kuhn, & Zimmerman, 2004), African American men showed a stronger blood pressure response than did European American men or women from either ethnic group. This result suggests that the higher prevalence of hypertension among African American men may relate to their tendency to higher reactivity. Another reactivity study (Merritt, Bennett, Williams,

Sollers, & Thayer, 2004) focused on educational level and anger-coping strategies among African American men and found that low educational level and a high-effort style of coping are associated with higher blood pressure reactivity. For African Americans, the experiences of racism constitute a source of anger, and one study (Clark, 2003) connected the perception of racism with blood pressure reactivity. This type of reactivity difference also appeared in a study comparing African American and European American women (Lepore et al., 2006). Thus, reactivity may relate to hypertension among African Americans.

Suppressed Anger If expressing anger can undermine cardiac health for some people, then would it be better to suppress anger? Results from early studies (Dembroski, MacDougall, Williams, Haney, & Blumenthal, 1985; MacDougall, Dembroski, Dimsdale, & Hackett, 1985) and more recent findings (Harburg, Julius, Kaciroti, Gleiberman, & Schork, 2003; Jorgensen & Kolodziej, 2007) suggest that suppressing anger may be more toxic than forcefully expressing anger. One version of suppressed emotion is rumination—repeated negative thoughts about an incident—which tends to increase negative feelings and depression (Hogan & Linden, 2004). Thus, people who suppress their anger but "stew" over their feelings may be using a coping style that puts them in danger. However, expressing anger (and other negative

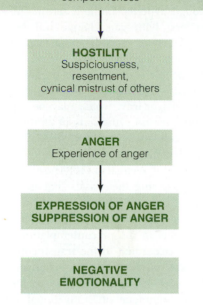

TYPE A BEHAVIOR PATTERN
Concerned with numbers and the acquisition of objects,
exaggerated sense of time urgency,
competitiveness

↓

HOSTILITY
Suspiciousness,
resentment,
cynical mistrust of others

↓

ANGER
Experience of anger

↓

**EXPRESSION OF ANGER
SUPPRESSION OF ANGER**

↓

**NEGATIVE
EMOTIONALITY**

Note: **BOLDFACE** denotes components suggested by
research to be the strongest link to heart disease.

FIGURE 9.9 Evolution from the Type A behavior
pattern to negative emotionality.

emotions) in a forceful way may act as triggers for those
with CVD, precipitating a heart attack or stroke (Suls &
Bunde, 2005).

So when it comes to expressing anger, are you
"Damned if you do, damned if you don't" (Dorr,
Brosschot, Sollers, & Thayer, 2007, p. 125)? How can
people handle anger situations? Aron Siegman (1994)
suggested that people learn to recognize their anger but
to express it calmly and rationally, in a way that will be
likely to resolve rather than escalate a conflict. Indeed,
the manner in which a person expresses anger may
affect cardiovascular health. People who discuss anger
in a way that seeks to resolve a situation have better
cardiovascular health, particular among men (Davidson & Mostofsky, 2010). In contrast, people who justify
their anger by blaming other people have greater long-
term incidence of cardiovascular health problems
(Davidson & Mostofsky, 2010). Thus, it may not be
just the anger that increases risk for cardiovascular problems, but also the additional stress caused by alienat-
ing others with hostile expressions of anger.

It may not be surprising, then, that anger combines
with the negative emotions that accompany anxiety and
depression to present greater risk for the development of
CVD (Bleil, Gianaros, Jennings, Flory, & Manuck, 2008;
Suls & Bunde, 2005). In addition, cynical hostility and
anger relate to each other and may interact with other
risk factors such as high blood pressure to increase a
person's risk for heart disease. Figure 9.9 shows the evolution of the Type A behavior pattern to hostility, to
anger, to the expression or suppression of anger, and
finally to negative emotionality.

IN SUMMARY

Although the causes of cardiovascular disease are
not fully understood, an accumulating body of evidence points to certain risk factors. These factors
include such inherent risks as advancing age, family
history of heart disease, gender, and ethnic background. Other risk factors include physiological conditions such as hypertension, problems in glucose
metabolism, and high serum cholesterol levels.
Other than age, hypertension is the best predictor
of coronary artery disease, and a higher blood pressure equals higher risk for heart disease. Total cholesterol level is also related to coronary artery
disease, but the *ratio* of total cholesterol to high-
density lipoprotein is a more critical risk factor.

Behaviors such as smoking and unwise eating
also relate to heart disease. Cigarette smoking is
associated with increased risk for heart disease
worldwide. Stopping smoking reduces risks, but
deciding to never start smoking is the best choice
for maintaining cardiovascular health. Eating foods
high in saturated fat may lead to obesity, which is a
risk for CVD. Also, consuming low levels of fruits and
vegetables add to one's risk of heart disease.

Psychosocial risk factors related to coronary
artery disease include low educational and income
levels; low levels of social support and marital satisfaction; and high levels of stress, anxiety, and depression. The anger and hostility components descended
from the Type A behavior pattern are independent
risk factors for heart disease. Both the violent expression and the suppression of anger may contribute to
CHD disease. Expressing anger in a soft, calm voice is
a better coping strategy than violently expressing
anger or timidly holding it in.

Reducing Cardiovascular Risks

Psychology's main contribution to cardiovascular health involves changing unhealthy behaviors before these behaviors lead to heart disease. In addition, psychologists may help people who have been diagnosed with heart disease; that is, they often help cardiac rehabilitation patients adhere to an exercise program, a medical regimen, a healthy diet, and smoking cessation.

Before Diagnosis: Preventing First Heart Attacks

What can people do to lower their risks for cardiovascular disease? Ideally, people should prevent CVD by modifying risk factors before the disease process causes damage. A longitudinal study by Jerry Stamler and his colleagues (1999) indicated that prevention is possible—maintaining a low level of risk factors protects against CVD. This study examined young adult and middle-aged men and women in five large cohorts to see if a low-risk profile would reduce both CVD and other causes of mortality. After dividing the participants into risk groups and screening for as long as 57 years, results indicated that low-risk participants had lower rates of death not only from CHD and stroke but also from all causes. Thus, young and middle-aged men and women who can modify CVD risks to attain low-risk profiles will also lower their risk for all-cause mortality and can expect to live 6 to 10 years longer.

The factors examined by Stamler et al. (1999) included smoking, cholesterol levels, and blood pressure—three major risk factors for CVD. However, the importance of maintaining a healthy lifestyle may begin as early as childhood (Beilin & Huang, 2008), when dietary and physical activity patterns are often established, and definitely continues during adolescence, when most smokers begin their habit. Keeping risk factors low can pay substantial dividends in later years (Matthews, Kuller, Chang, & Edmundowicz, 2007). After people acquire high risks from behavioral factors such as smoking and unwise eating, managing those risks is more difficult. As psychologists are frequently concerned with changing behavior, many of their techniques can be helpful in modifying behaviors that place people at risk for developing cardiovascular disease.

The most serious behavioral risk factor is cigarette smoking, a behavior that also contributes to many other disorders, especially lung cancer. For this reason, all of Chapter 12 is devoted to a discussion of tobacco use. Although hypertension and serum cholesterol are not behaviors, both can change indirectly through changes in behavior, making these factors candidates for intervention (Linden, 2000).

Before people cooperate with programs to change their behavior, they must perceive that these behaviors place them in jeopardy, which may be a problem for people who have no symptoms of cardiovascular disease. These individuals may recognize established risk factors in calculating their personal risk, but they often display what Neil Weinstein (1984) called an **optimistic bias** in assessing their risk. That is, they tend to believe that they are immune from the risks that make other people vulnerable. These thoughts place such individuals in the precontemplation or contemplation stage, according to the transtheoretical model, when they are not ready to make changes (Prochaska et al., 1992, 1994; see Chapter 4 for more on this model). The technique of motivational interviewing, for example, challenges people's beliefs with the goal of moving people toward making positive change; this technique was part of a successful program to increase fruit and vegetable consumption (Resnicow et al., 2001). Thus, moving people to the point of making changes in their health habits is a major challenge for health psychologists involved in cardiovascular health.

Reducing Hypertension   Lowering high blood pressure into the normal range is difficult because a number of physiological mechanisms act to keep blood pressure at a set point (Osborn, 2005). Many different feedback systems either raise or lower blood pressure when the body senses that blood pressure is out of the critical range. The body may even perpetuate hypertension by means of these feedback mechanisms, regulating blood pressure to the hypertensive level instead of regulating it into the normal range. Because complex feedback systems work against rather than for the maintenance of appropriate blood pressure, hypertension tends to be difficult to control.

Interventions aimed at hypertension usually try to control blood pressure through antihypertensive drugs that require a physician's prescription. The goal is typically to lower blood pressure to 130/80 mmHg or lower (USDHHS, 2003). Because hypertension presents no unpleasant symptoms and the medications may cause side effects, many patients are reluctant to follow this regimen. (The factors affecting adherence to this and other medical regimens are discussed in Chapter 4.)

Several behaviors relate to both the development and the treatment of hypertension, and these behaviors are also targets of interventions. Obesity correlates with hypertension, and many obese people who lose weight lower their blood pressure into the normal range (Moore et al., 2005). Thus, losing weight is part of blood pressure control. (We discuss strategies for losing weight in Chapter 15.) Hypertensive individuals also typically receive recommendations to restrict sodium intake and make dietary changes (Bhatt, Luqman-Arafath, & Guleria, 2007), The Dietary Approach to Stop Hypertension (DASH) originated as a plan to control hypertension; it includes a diet high in fruits, vegetables, whole grains, and low-fat dairy products as well as other lifestyle changes. Table 9.3 shows a daily menu that adheres to the DASH diet, with both regular and low-sodium options. Not only is the DASH diet

TABLE 9.3   Sample Daily Menu From the DASH Plan, With Regular and Low-Sodium Options

2,300 mg Menu	Sodium	Substitution to Reduce Sodium to 1,500 mg	Sodium
Breakfast			
¾ cup bran flakes cereal	220	¾ cup shredded wheat cereal	1
1 medium banana	1		
1 cup low-fat milk	107		
1 slice whole wheat bread	149		
1 tsp margarine	26	1 tsp unsalted margarine	0
1 cup orange juice	5		
Lunch			
¾ cup chicken salad	179	Remove salt from recipe	120
2 slices whole wheat bread	299		
1 Tbsp Dijon mustard	373	1 Tbsp regular mustard	175
Salad			
½ cup cucumber slices	1		
½ cup tomato wedges	5		
1 Tbsp sunflower seeds	0		
1 tsp Italian dressing, low calorie	43		
½ cup fruit cocktail, juice pack	5		
Dinner			
3 oz roast beef	35		
2 Tbsp fat-free gravy	165		
1 cup green beans	12		
1 small baked potato	14		
1 Tbsp sour cream, fat free	21		
1 Tbsp reduced-fat cheddar cheese	67	1 Tbsp reduced-fat cheddar cheese, low sodium	1

(continued)

TABLE 9.3   Sample Daily Menu From the DASH Plan, With Regular and Low-Sodium Options
      — *Continued*

2,300 mg Menu	Sodium	Substitution to Reduce Sodium to 1,500 mg	Sodium
1 small whole wheat roll	148		
1 tsp margarine	26	1 tsp unsalted margarine	0
1 small apple	1		
1 cup low-fat milk	107		
Snacks			
⅓ cup unsalted almonds	0		
¼ cup raisins	4		
½ cup fruit yogurt, fat free, no added sugar	86		

Source: Adapted from *Your guide to lowering your blood pressure with DASH* (NIH Publication No. 06–4082), 2006, by U.S. Department of Health and Human Services (USDHHS). Washington, DC: Author.

effective in lowering blood pressure, but it also decreases the risk for stroke and CHD in women (Fung et al., 2008). A regular physical activity program is also effective in controlling hypertension, especially in people who have been sedentary (Murphy, Nevill, Murtagh, & Holder, 2007). (We discuss exercise in Chapter 15.) Other techniques for reducing blood pressure include stress management, meditation, and relaxation training, and we discuss these interventions in Chapter 5 and Chapter 8. Thus, a program to control hypertension may have both drug and behavioral components.

Lowering Serum Cholesterol   Interventions aimed at lowering cholesterol levels can include drugs, dietary changes, increased physical activity, or a combination of these components. Eating a diet low in saturated fat and high in fruits and vegetables and maintaining a program of regular physical activity are good strategies for preventing high cholesterol levels, and dietary and exercise interventions are key components in managing high cholesterol levels (USDHHS, 2003). However, once a person develops high cholesterol levels, a prudent diet and physical activity are not likely to lower cholesterol to an acceptable level. Thus, many people with high cholesterol cannot achieve substantially lower cholesterol levels through diet and exercise.

Physicians may prescribe cholesterol-lowering drugs such as the *statin* drugs to patients with high total cholesterol or high LDL levels (Grundy,

2007). These drugs act by blocking an enzyme that the liver needs to manufacture cholesterol. They are especially effective in lowering LDL cholesterol and can reduce risks and improve survival of people at risk for cardiovascular disease (Brugts et al., 2009; Cholesterol Treatment Trialists' [CTT] Collaboration, 2010). Despite their effectiveness, these drugs require a prescription, cost money, and have side effects.

The recommendations for cholesterol lowering are complex. First, relying on drugs to lower cholesterol without behavioral changes is not a good strategy. Behavioral interventions can help both men and women adhere to a regular exercise program as well as a low-fat diet. Such adherence can lower LDL and improve the ratio of total cholesterol to HDL. If lifestyle changes do not lower cholesterol, then drugs are an option, but not before, especially for people with low levels of risk. Second, the ratio of total cholesterol to HDL is more important than total cholesterol. Statins tend to lower LDL rather than raise HDL, but these drugs lower cholesterol and incidence of heart attacks and stroke, making them a good choice for people with very high or resistant cholesterol levels (Cheng, Lauder, Chu-Pak, & Kumana, 2004). Third, people with multiple risks for CVD, such as hypertension, diabetes, or smoking, should consider the task of lowering cholesterol as more urgent than those with fewer risks (Grundy, 2007).

Modifying Psychosocial Risk Factors   Earlier, we discussed research that links psychosocial factors such

Becoming Healthier

1. Learn about your family risk for heart disease. Although you cannot change this risk factor, knowing that you are at high risk can motivate you to change some modifiable risk factors.

2. Have your blood pressure checked. If it is in the normal range, you can keep it that way by exercising, controlling your weight, and moderating alcohol consumption. Also try some of the relaxation techniques discussed in Chapter 8. If your blood pressure is above the normal range (even a little), consult a physician.

3. Know your cholesterol level, but be sure to ask for a complete profile, one that includes measures of both HDL and LDL as well as the ratio of total cholesterol to HDL.

4. If you are a smoker but have failed at prior attempts to quit, keep trying. Many smokers make multiple attempts before quitting successfully.

5. Keep a food diary for at least 1 week. Note the amount of saturated fat as well as fruits and vegetables you eat and the approximate number of calories consumed per day. A heart-healthy diet is low in saturated fat and includes five servings of fruits and vegetables per day.

6. If you are persistently angry and react to anger-arousing events with loud, sudden explosions of anger or if you "stew" over such events, try to change your reactions by expressing your frustrations in a soft, quiet voice.

as stress, anxiety, depression, and anger with cardiovascular disease. The evidence for these risks is sufficiently compelling for some authorities to call for the development of *behavioral cardiology* (Rozanski, Blumenthal, Davidson, Saab, & Kubzansky, 2005), urging cardiologists to screen for psychological risks and to recommend psychological interventions to decrease anxiety and depression and to manage stress and anger. Consistent with this concept, research on people who received angioplasty (Helgeson, 2003) indicated that those who had a more positive outlook about themselves and their future were less likely to experience a recurrence of cardiovascular disease. These results are good news for former president Bill Clinton, whose optimistic outlook was evident even before his cardiac surgery (King & Henry, 2004).

Anger and negative emotions are also a target of intervention, and clinical health psychologists recommend a variety of strategies for coping with hostility, anger, and depression. To reduce the toxic element in anger, perpetually angry people can learn to become aware of cues from others that typically provoke angry responses. They can also remove themselves from provocative situations before they become angry, or they can do something else. In interpersonal encounters, angry people can use self-talk as a reminder that the situation will not last forever. Humor is another potentially effective means of coping with anger (Godfrey, 2004), but it may present its own risks. Sarcastic or hostile humor can incite additional anger, but silliness or mock exaggerations often defuse potentially volatile situations. Relaxation techniques can also be effective strategies for dealing with anger. These techniques can include progressive relaxation, deep-breathing exercises, tension reduction training, relaxing to the slow repetition of the word "relax," and relaxation imagery, in which the person imagines a peaceful scene. Finally, angry people can lower their blood pressure by constructively discussing their feelings with other people (Davidson, MacGregor, Stuhr, Dixon, & MacLean, 2000).

Discussing feelings with a therapist may also benefit people who are depressed, but physicians may not always recognize this problem. Thus, screening for depression among people at risk for CVD is an urgent need (Goldston & Baillie, 2008). Depression is also common among people who experience a heart attack or other CVD event. These individuals may be more willing to undertake changes to avoid another heart attack or stroke.

After Diagnosis: Rehabilitating Cardiac Patients

After people experience a heart attack, angina, or other symptoms of CVD, they sometimes receive a referral to a cardiac rehabilitation program to change their lifestyle and lower risk for a subsequent (and possibly even more serious) event. In addition to survival, the goals of cardiac rehabilitation programs are to help patients deal with psychological reactions to their diagnosis, to return to normal activities as soon as possible, and to change to a healthier lifestyle.

Patients recovering from heart disease, as well as their spouses, often experience a variety of psychological reactions that include depression, anxiety, anger, fear, guilt, and interpersonal conflict. For cardiac patients, the most common psychological reaction to a myocardial infarction is *depression*, which decreases adherence to medication and lifestyle changes (Kronish et al., 2006) and increases the risk of death to 3.5 times that for nondepressed cardiac patients (Guck et al., 2001).

Treating depression among cardiac patients is an important, but difficult problem. Two large-scale interventions sought to treat depression among cardiac patients, through the use of antidepressant medications (Glassman, Bigger, & Gaffney, 2009) or cognitive behavioral therapy (Berkman et al., 2003). Although these trials have some success in treating depression, the antidepressant intervention did not improve survival. The cognitive behavioral intervention improved survival among European American men, but not among ethnic minority men or among women (Schneiderman et al., 2004).

Another common psychological reaction related to depression is *anxiety*. A follow-up study of cardiac rehabilitation patients (Michie, O'Connor, Bath, Giles, & Earll, 2005) showed that those who completed the rehabilitation program continued to make progress not only in lowering their physiological risks but also in lowering their levels of anxiety and depression and increasing their feelings of control. One common source of anxiety among heart patients and their spouses is the resumption of sexual activity. The probable source of this anxiety is concern about the elevation of heart rate during sex, especially during orgasm. However, sexual activity poses little threat to cardiac patients. Also, male CAD patients who take Viagra do not have an elevated risk of subsequent heart problems, but this drug may interact in dangerous ways with drugs for hypertension that such patients may be taking (Jackson, 2004).

Cardiac rehabilitation programs usually include components to help patients stop smoking, eat a low-fat and low-cholesterol diet, control weight, moderate alcohol intake, learn to manage stress and hostility, and adhere to a prescribed medication regimen. Also, cardiac patients frequently participate in a graduated or structured exercise program in which they gradually increase their level of physical activity. In other words, the same lifestyle recommendations for avoiding a first cardiovascular event also apply to survivors of myocardial infarction, coronary artery bypass graft surgery, and stroke. In addition, cardiac patients are often encouraged to join a social support group, participate in health education programs, and allow support from their primary caregiver. Some research (Clark, Whelan, Barbour, & MacIntyre, 2005) indicated that cardiac patients rated such social support and being with others who shared the same problem as the most valuable aspects of the program.

Dean Ornish and his colleagues (1998) devised a comprehensive cardiac rehabilitation program with diet, stress management, smoking cessation, and physical activity components in an effort to *reverse* heart patients' coronary artery damage. Although similar to the interventions that attempt to alter risk factors, this program was more comprehensive and imposed more stringent modifications, especially with regard to diet. The Ornish program recommends that cardiac patients reduce their consumption of fat to only 10% of their total caloric intake, which necessitates a careful vegetarian diet with no added fats from oils, eggs, butter, or nuts. An evaluation of the program included a control group that received a typical cardiac rehabilitation program along with the experimental group of participants on the Ornish program.

Early research on the benefits of the program painted a slightly more optimistic picture of its benefits than later research. After 1 year of the program, Ornish and his colleagues (1990) found that 82% of patients in the treatment group showed a regression of plaques in the coronary arteries. After 5 years, this program produced less artery blockage and fewer coronary events. Although a later study (Aldana et al., 2007) failed to confirm the reversal of arterial plaque, it did show that patients on the Ornish program decreased their risk factors to a greater extent than those in a standard cardiac rehabilitation program and decreased their symptoms of angina substantially. The benefits in decreasing angina also appeared in another study (Frattaroli, Weidner, Merritt-Worden, Frenda, & Ornish, 2008), and other research confirms that dietary change can reverse arterial plaque (Shai et al., 2010). The main disadvantage of a program such as the Ornish plan is the difficulty of following such a stringent diet (Dansinger, Gleason, Griffith, Selker, & Schaefer, 2005). No cardiac rehabilitation program can be optimally effective if patients fail to adhere or drop out.

Adherence is a major problem with cardiac rehabilitation programs in general. Less than half of cardiac patients complete their rehabilitation regimen (Taylor, Wilson, & Sharp, 2011). One factor that may influence adherence involves the physician, rather than the patient: Many cardiologists fail to endorse rehabilitation programs, which affects their patients' willingness to participate. Many patients also cite difficulties in finding time for and traveling to a clinic for rehabilitation. However, the same factors that predict the development of cardiovascular disease also predict failure to adhere to rehabilitation: depression, being a smoker, being overweight, and having a high cardiovascular risk profile (Taylor et al., 2011). Thus, the patients who are most in need of intervention may be least likely to adhere. When used as intended, many different rehabilitation programs are effective, including brief interventions (Fernandez et al., 2007) and at-home rehabilitation programs (Dalal, Zawada, Jolly, Moxham, & Taylor, 2010).

A meta-analysis of studies on the effectiveness of two components of cardiac rehabilitation programs (Dusseldrop, van Elderen, Maes, Meulman, & Kraaj, 1999) found that heart disease patients who followed a health education and stress management program had a 34% reduction in cardiac mortality and a 29% reduction in recurrence of a heart attack. Exercise-based cardiac rehabilitation programs are also effective in reducing cardiac mortality and heart attack recurrence (Lawler, Filion, & Eisenberg, 2011). Exercise may present some risks for cardiac patients, but the benefits far outweigh the risks. For example, a graded exercise program can enhance patients' self-efficacy for increasing levels of activity (Cheng & Boey, 2002) as well as increase self-esteem and physical mobility (Ng & Tam, 2000). After a diagnosis of heart problems, exercise programs have three main goals (Thompson, 2001). First, exercise can maintain or improve functional capacity; second, it can enhance a person's quality of life; and third, it can help prevent recurrent heart attacks. Thus, cardiac rehabilitation programs are an effective but underused strategy.

IN SUMMARY

Health psychologists contribute to reducing risks for a first cardiovascular incident as well as to rehabilitating people who have already been diagnosed with CVD. Many of the risks for CVD relate to behaviors, such as smoking, diet, physical activity, and management of negative emotions. Combinations of lifestyle change and drugs are effective in lowering hypertension and cholesterol level, two important risks for CVD. In addition, health psychologists can help people modify negative emotions such as anxiety, depression, and anger, all of which are risks for CVD and often occur in patients after heart attacks. Health psychologists also strive to keep cardiac patients in rehabilitation and boost their levels of physical activity.

Answers

This chapter has addressed four basic questions:

1. What are the structures, functions, and disorders of the cardiovascular system?

The cardiovascular system includes the heart and blood vessels (veins, venules, arteries, arterioles, and capillaries). The heart pumps blood throughout the body, delivering oxygen and removing wastes from body cells. Disorders of the cardiovascular system include (1) coronary artery disease, which occurs when the arteries that supply blood to the heart become clogged with plaque and restrict the blood supply to the heart muscle; (2) myocardial infarction (heart attack), which is caused by blockage of coronary arteries; (3) angina pectoris, which is a nonfatal disorder with symptoms of chest pain and difficulty in breathing; (4) stroke, which occurs when the oxygen supply to the brain is disrupted; and (5) hypertension (high blood pressure), which is a silent disorder but a good predictor of both heart attack and stroke. Heart attack and stroke account for more than 30% of deaths in the United States.

2. What are the risk factors for cardiovascular disease?

Beginning with the Framingham study, researchers identified a number of cardiovascular risk factors. These factors include (1) inherent risk, (2) physiological risks, (3) behavioral and lifestyle risks, and (4) psychosocial risks. Inherent risk factors, such as advancing age, family history, gender, and ethnicity, are not modifiable, but people with inherent risk can alter their other risks to lower their chances of developing heart disease.

The two primary physiological risk factors are hypertension and high cholesterol, and diet can play a role in controlling each of these. Behavioral factors in CVD include smoking, a diet high in saturated fat and low in fiber and antioxidant vitamins, and low physical activity level. Psychosocial risks include low educational and income levels; lack of social support; and persistently high levels of stress, anxiety, and depression. In addition, hostility and both loud, violent expressions of anger and suppression of anger elevate risk slightly.

3. How does lifestyle relate to cardiovascular health?

Lifestyle factors such as cigarette smoking, unwise eating, and a sedentary lifestyle all predict cardiovascular health. During the past three decades, deaths from heart disease have steadily decreased in the United States; perhaps as much as 50% of that drop is a result of changes in behavior and lifestyle. During this same time period, millions of people have quit smoking, altered their diet to control weight and cholesterol, and begun an exercise program.

4. What behaviors allow people to lower their cardiovascular risks?

Both before and after a diagnosis of heart disease, people can use a variety of approaches to reduce their risks for CVD. Drugs, sodium restriction, and weight loss all can control hypertension. Drugs, diet, and exercise also can lower cholesterol levels. Lowering the ratio of total cholesterol to HDL is probably a better idea, but the statin type of cholesterol-lowering drugs tends to lower LDL, which can also be beneficial. Also, people can learn to manage stress more effectively, enter therapy to improve depression, and learn to manage anger to avoid loud, quick outbursts and to express their frustrations in a soft, slow manner.

Suggested Readings

Holt-Lunstad, J., Birmingham, W., & Jones, B. Q. (2008). Is there something unique about marriage? The relative impact of marital status, relationship quality, and network social support on ambulatory blood pressure and mental health. *Annals of Behavioral Medicine, 35,* 239–244. This journal article gives a technical analysis of social support, considering the notion that good marriages provide the best type of support.

Levy, D., & Brink, S. (2005). *A change of heart: How the Framingham Heart Study helped unravel the mysteries of cardiovascular disease.* New York: Knopf. This report on the Framingham Heart Study includes not only the fascinating history of this project but also the major findings from the study and tips for maintaining heart health.

Miller, G. E., & Blackwell, E. (2006). Turning up the heat: Inflammation as a mechanism linking chronic stress, depression, and heart disease. *Current Directions in Psychological Science, 15,* 269–272. This brief article reviews the concept of inflammation and its risks while attempting to build a model that integrates stress and depression into an explanation for the development of heart disease.

Yusuf, S., Hawken, S., Ôunpuu, S., Dans, T., Avezum, A., Lanas, F., et al. (2004). Effect of potentially modifiable risk factors associated with myocardial infarction in 52 countries (the INTERHEART study): Case-control study. *Lancet, 364,* 937–952. The INTERHEART Study identified nine factors that predicted most of the variance in heart attack deaths in countries throughout the world. This report details the study and presents the relative contributions of each of the nine.

CHAPTER 10

Behavioral Factors in Cancer

CHAPTER OUTLINE

- **Real-World Profile of Steve Jobs**
- *What Is Cancer?*
- *The Changing Rates of Cancer Deaths*
- *Cancer Risk Factors Beyond Personal Control*
- *Behavioral Risk Factors for Cancer*
- *Living With Cancer*

QUESTIONS

This chapter focuses on five basic questions:

1. What is cancer?

2. Are cancer death rates increasing or decreasing?

3. What are the inherent and environmental risk factors for cancer?

4. What are the behavioral risk factors for cancer?

5. How can cancer patients be helped in coping with their disease?

✔CHECK YOUR HEALTH RISKS

Regarding Cancer

1. Someone in my immediate family (a parent, sibling, aunt, uncle, or grandparent) developed cancer before age 50.

2. I am African American.

3. I have never had a job where I was exposed to radiation or hazardous chemicals.

4. I have never been a cigarette smoker.

5. I am a former smoker who quit during the past 5 years.

6. I have used tobacco products other than cigarettes (such as chewing tobacco, a pipe, or cigars).

7. My diet is low in fat.

8. My diet includes lots of smoked, salt-cured, or pickled foods.

9. I rarely eat fruits or vegetables.

10. My diet is high in fiber.

11. I have light-colored skin, but I like to get at least one nice tan every year.

12. I have had more than 15 sexual partners during my life.

13. I have never had unprotected sex with a partner who was at high risk for HIV infection.

14. I am a woman over age 30 who has not given birth to a child.

15. I have at least two alcoholic drinks every day.

16. I exercise on a regular basis.

Each of these topics is either a known risk factor for some type of cancer or has the potential to protect against it. Items 3, 4, 7, 10, 13, and 16 describe situations that may offer some protection against cancer. If you checked none or only a few of these items and a large number of the remaining items, your risk for some type of cancer is higher than people who checked different items. Behaviors related to smoking and diet (items 4–10) place you at a greater risk than other behaviors, such as item 15 (alcohol).

Real-World Profile of
STEVE JOBS

Featureflash/Shutterstock.com

In 2003, Steve Jobs and his company Apple were revolutionizing the technology world. The iPod, unveiled a year and a half earlier, changed how the world listened to music. Jobs and his team started developing the iPhone and the iPad, two products that would similarly revolutionize the mobile phone and computer industries. Steve Jobs—a charismatic, perfectionistic, and demanding workaholic—had already appeared on the cover of *Time* magazine four times. Apple's worth steadily mounted.

In this same year, during a CT scan to look for kidney stones, Steve's doctors noticed something unexpected on his pancreas. The diagnosis soon became islet cell neuroendocrine pancreatic cancer, a rare form of one of the deadliest of cancers. With a low survival rate for conventional treatments, people diagnosed with pancreatic cancer often try alternative therapies. Steve initially refused his doctors' suggestions for surgery, saying, "I really didn't want them to open up my body" (Isaacson, 2011, "Cancer," ¶ 6).

Jobs first tried a variety of alternative treatments, including a vegan diet, acupuncture, herbal remedies, and even a psychic. After delaying standard medical treatment for 9 months, Steve finally relented to surgery. By then, the cancer had already spread to other parts of his body. Steve then sought the most advanced treatments for his condition, which included radiation therapy and a liver transplant. The treatments and transplant took a physical toll with Steve becoming increasingly gaunt.

In August 2011, he resigned from Apple for health reasons. Two months later, Steve Jobs died of respiratory failure due to complications arising from advanced pancreatic cancer.

Steve Jobs' battle with cancer lasted a total of 8 years, far longer than his initial prognosis. Steve's wealth afforded him the best medical treatments, which may have extended his life. However, he later came to regret his decision to delay initial surgery. Why did Steve initially reject treatment for his cancer? What issues did Steve likely cope with in his battle against cancer? Was Steve's "fighting spirit" something that helped him live for so long after his diagnosis? We will explore these questions in this chapter, but first, we need to define what cancer is.

What Is Cancer?

Cancer is a group of diseases characterized by the presence of new cells that grow and spread beyond control. During the 19th century, the great physiologist Johannes Muller discovered that tumors, like other tissues, consisted of cells and were not formless collections of material. However, their growth seemed unrestrained by the mechanisms that control other body cells.

The finding that tumors consist of cells did not shed light on what causes their growth. During the 19th century, the leading theory of cancer was that a parasite or infectious agent caused the disorder, but researchers could find no such agent. Because of this failure, the mutation theory arose, holding that cancer originates because of a change in the cell—a mutation. The cell continues to grow and reproduce in its mutated form, and the result is a tumor.

Cancer is not unique to humans; all animals get cancer, as do plants. Indeed, any cell that is capable of division can transform into a cancer cell. In addition to the diverse *causes* of cancer, many different *types* exist. However, different cancers share certain characteristics, the most common of which is the presence of **neoplastic** tissue cells, which have nearly unlimited growth that robs the host of nutrients and that yields no compensatory beneficial effects. All true cancers share this characteristic of neoplastic growth.

Neoplastic cells may be **benign** or **malignant**, although the distinction is not always easy to determine. Both types consist of altered cells that reproduce true to their altered type. However, benign growths tend to remain localized, whereas malignant tumors tend to spread and establish secondary colonies. The tendency for benign tumors to remain localized usually makes them less threatening than malignant tumors, but not all benign tumors are harmless. Malignant tumors are much more dangerous because they invade and destroy surrounding tissue and may also move, or **metastasize**, through blood or lymph and thus spread to other sites in the body.

The most dangerous characteristic of tumor cells is their autonomy—that is, their ability to grow without regard to the needs of other body cells and without being subject to the restraints of growth that govern other cells. This unrestrained tumor growth makes cancer capable of overwhelming its host, damaging other organs or physiological processes, or using nutrients essential for body functions. The tumor then becomes a parasite on its host, gaining priority over other body cells.

Malignant growths fall into four main groups: carcinomas, sarcomas, leukemias, and lymphomas. **Carcinomas** are cancers of the epithelial tissue, cells that line the outer and inner surfaces of the body, such as skin, stomach lining, and mucous membranes. **Sarcomas** are cancers that arise from cells in connective tissue, such as bone, muscles, and cartilage. **Leukemias** are cancers that originate in the blood or blood-forming cells, such as stem cells in the bone marrow. These three types of cancers—carcinomas, sarcomas, and leukemias—account for more than 95% of malignancies. The fourth type of cancer is **lymphoma**, a cancer of the lymphatic system, which is one of the rarer types of cancer.

Although some people may have a genetic predisposition to cancer, people almost never inherit the disease. Behavior and lifestyle are primary contributors to cancer, making it possible for the rates of cancer to change over relatively short periods.

The Changing Rates of Cancer Deaths

For the first time on record, the death rate from cancer in the United States declined during the 1990s. This trend ended a century-long increase in cancer deaths that peaked in 1993, when cancer mortality was more than 3 times higher than in 1900. Figure 10.1 shows an increase in total cancer death rates in the United States from 1900 to 1990 and then a gradual decline. The decrease is significant—more than 22% for men and more than 15% for women since 1990 (Siegel, Naishadham, & Jemal, 2012).

Why did cancer death rates drop? At least two explanations are possible. First, the decline might be

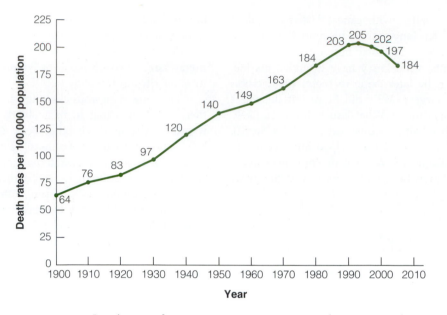

FIGURE 10.1 Death rates from cancer per 100,000 population, United States, 1900–2005.

Source: Data from *Historical statistics of the United States: Colonial times to 1970, Part 1* (p. 68) by U.S. Bureau of the Census, 1975, Washington, DC: U.S. Government Printing Office; *Statistical abstract of the United States, 2008* (127th edition), by U.S. Census Bureau, (2007). Washington, DC: U.S. Government Printing Office; Cancer statistics, 2008, by A. Jemal et al., 2008, CA: *Cancer Journal for Clinicians, 58,* 71–96.

due to improved treatment that prolongs the life of cancer patients. We can test the validity of this explanation by examining the difference between cancer incidence and cancer deaths. If incidence remained the same or even increased while deaths declined, then better treatment would account for the drop in cancer deaths. However, the evidence does not support this hypothesis, as both cancer incidence and cancer deaths declined during the 1990s (Siegel et al., 2012). Some of that decrease is attributable to the lower incidence of certain cancers, such as lung cancer in men, and some of it is due to improved early detection and treatment, such as the decline in deaths from prostate and breast cancer. Thus, better treatment regimens play a role in the recent decrease in cancer rates, but people are developing cancer less often than they did over a decade ago. In the United States, for example, people are smoking much less and eating a healthier diet than they did 40 years ago. Because lifestyle factors such as smoking, diet, and physical inactivity account for about two thirds of all cancer deaths in the United States (American Cancer Society [ACS], 2012), improvements in these areas should result in lower rates of cancer.

Cancers With Decreasing Death Rates

Cancer of the lungs, breast, prostate, and colon/rectum account for about half of all cancer deaths in the United States, and mortality rates for each of these sites are currently declining.

Lung cancer accounts for about 14% of all cancer cases, but 28% of all cancer deaths—figures that reveal the deadliness of lung cancer. Between 1990 and 2008, mortality due to lung cancer in the United States declined for men but not for women (ACS, 2012; see Figures 10.2 and 10.3). Figure 10.2 shows that lung cancer mortality for women rose dramatically from 1965 to 1995, but since that time death rates have been almost level. In Europe, this pattern is somewhat similar, with lung cancer mortality for men declining since 1990; however, lung cancer mortality for women continues to rise (Ferlay, Parkin, & Steliarova-Foucher, 2010). Because cigarette smoking is the primary cause of lung cancer deaths, the current decline in women's smoking rates in the United States should eventually effect a decrease in lung cancer mortality for women.

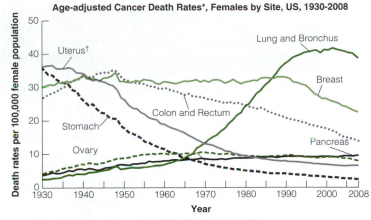

Age-adjusted Cancer Death Rates*, Females by Site, US, 1930-2008

* Per 100,000, age adjusted to the 2000 US standard population.
† Uterus cancer death rates are for uterine cervix and uterine corpus combined.

NOTE: Due to changes in ICD coding, numerator information has changed over time. Rates for cancer of the lung and bronchus, colon and rectum, and ovary are affected by these coding changes.

SOURCE: US Mortality Data 1960 to 2008, US Mortality Volumes 1930 to 1959, National Center for Health Statistics, Centers for Disease Control and Prevention.

American Cancer Society, Surveillance Research, 2012

FIGURE 10.2   Cancer death rates for selected sites, women, United States, 1930–2008.

Source: Adapted with permission from the American Cancer Society. *Cancer Facts and Figures 2012.* Atlanta: American Cancer Society, Inc.

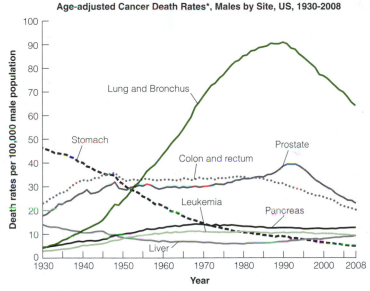

Age-adjusted Cancer Death Rates*, Males by Site, US, 1930-2008

* Per 100,000, age adjusted to the 2000 US standard population.

NOTE: Due to changes in ICD coding, numerator information has changed over time. Rates for cancer of the liver, lung and bronchus, and colon and rectum are affected by these coding changes.

SOURCE: US Mortality Data 1960 to 2008, US Mortality Volumes 1930 to 1959, National Center for Health Statistics, Centers for Disease Control and Prevention.

American Cancer Society, Surveillance Research, 2012

FIGURE 10.3   Cancer death rates for selected sites, men, United States, 1930–2008.

Source: Adapted with permission from the American Cancer Society. *Cancer Facts and Figures 2012.* Atlanta: American Cancer Society, Inc.

Other than prostate cancer, *breast cancer* has the highest incidence (but not death rate) of any cancer in the United States, accounting for about 29% of cancer cases among women. Men also develop breast cancer, but women account for 99% of all new cases. The incidence of female breast cancer increased from 1980 to 2001 but then began to decline. One factor that may be involved in this decline is the decrease in the number of postmenopausal women using hormone replacement therapy, some types of which were linked to breast cancer (Siegel et al., 2012). The decline in the breast cancer death rate is due mainly to improvements in early detection and treatment.

Prostate cancer has the highest incidence of cancer among men in the United States, but again, it does not have the highest mortality rate—about twice as many men die each year from lung cancer as from prostate cancer. In 2012, the number of men diagnosed with prostate cancer was higher than the number of women diagnosed with breast cancer (Siegel et al., 2012). As with breast cancer incidence, new cases of prostate cancer increased sharply during the 1980s when prostate-specific antigen (PSA) screening was first introduced. From 2000 to 2012, however, the number of new cases—about 29% of all cancer cases in men—declined significantly.

Colorectal cancer is the second leading cause of cancer deaths in the United States and other developed countries, exceeded only by lung cancer. However, in the United States, both the incidence and the mortality rates of colorectal cancer are decreasing. Incidence and mortality rates vary widely by ethnic background, with African Americans more likely to receive a diagnosis of and die from colorectal cancer than either Hispanic Americans or European Americans (Siegel et al., 2012). Although the incidence of colorectal cancer increased slightly until about 1985, the mortality rate has been declining since about 1945 (see Figures 10.2 and 10.3).

Death rates from *stomach cancer* have dropped from being the leading cause of cancer deaths for both women and men to having a very low mortality rate. As we discuss later, modern refrigeration and fewer salt-cured foods probably account for most of the decrease in stomach cancer.

Cancers With Increasing Incidence and Mortality Rates

In general, incidence rates for the four leading cancers—lung, breast, prostate, and colorectal—are declining, especially for men. However, not all cancer rates are decreasing. Several cancers have increased in recent years (Siegel et al., 2012).

Liver cancer, like lung cancer, is quite lethal, with a death rate (3.6%) nearly twice as high as its incidence rate (1.7%). This cancer is the only type that is increasing among both women and men, and both incidence and death rates are higher for minorities compared with European Americans (Siegel et al., 2012). As mentioned, lung cancer continues to show a slight increase among women but a continuing decline among men. Melanoma, a potentially fatal form of skin cancer, is increasing among both men and women. Cancer of the esophagus is increasing among men yet falling among women.

IN SUMMARY

Cancer is a group of diseases characterized by the presence of neoplastic cells that grow and spread without control. These new cells may form benign tumors, which tend to remain localized, or malignant tumors, which may metastasize and spread to other organs.

After more than a century of rising mortality rates, cancer deaths are declining. This decrease is most evident among the four cancers that cause most cancer deaths—lung, breast, prostate, and colorectal cancers. Since 1992, incidence and death rates among men for these four cancers have declined at a slow but steady pace, whereas women have not experienced the same magnitude of decrease. The leading cause of cancer deaths for both women and men continues to be lung cancer. The incidence of breast cancer among women and prostate cancer among men is much higher than the incidence of lung cancer, but lung cancer kills far more people in the United States than does either breast cancer or prostate cancer.

Cancer Risk Factors Beyond Personal Control

Most risk factors for cancer result from personal behavior, especially cigarette smoking. However, some factors are largely beyond personal control; these factors include both inherent and environmental risks.

Inherent Risk Factors for Cancer

Inherent risks for cancer include genetics and family history, ethnic background, and age. Many people attribute their risk of cancer to these factors, especially genetics. A survey ("Practical Nurse," 2008) indicated that 9 out of 10 people overestimated the genetic risk, and 60% of people named genetics as the primary risk for cancer. Does their perception agree with the research? How important are genetic and other inherent risk factors such as ethnicity and age?

Ethnic Background   Compared with European Americans, African Americans fare more poorly; they have a greater incidence of most cancers, and mortality is higher in almost every category (Siegel et al., 2012). However, Hispanic Americans, Asian Americans, and Native Americans have lower rates than either African Americans or European Americans for all cancer sites combined, as well as for the four most common cancers (Siegel et al., 2012). These discrepancies are most likely due to behavioral and psychosocial factors rather than to biology. For example, although Asian Americans generally have lower total cancer death rates than European Americans, they have a much higher mortality rate for stomach and liver cancer. Both cancers are caused by behavioral and environmental factors. Stomach cancer is strongly influenced by diet and chronic infection by the *Helicobacter pylori* bacteria, whereas liver cancer is strongly influenced by infection with the hepatitis C virus (Siegel et al., 2012). Thus, behavioral factors may account for these ethnic differences.

Minority status plays a greater role in survival of cancer than it does in cancer incidence. For cancer sites with a low mortality level, the discrepancy between incidence and mortality widens with ethnic background. With breast cancer, for example, European American women have a higher incidence rate than African American women, but African American women are more likely to die from this cancer (Siegel et al., 2012).

How does minority status contribute to cancer outcomes—that is, length of survival and quality of life? Although Hispanic Americans, African Americans, Native Americans, and Asian Americans develop many cancers at a lower rate than European Americans, their diagnoses tend to come at a later stage of their cancers (Siegel et al., 2012). This difference affects survival; later diagnoses tend to lead to more advanced disease, more difficulty in treatment, and lower survival

rates. An examination of survival differences between African Americans and European Americans (Du, Meyer, & Franzini, 2007) showed that controlling for socioeconomic factors erased the difference in survival rates, which suggests that social and economic factors create the disparity.

Advancing Age   The strongest risk factor for cancer—and many other diseases—is advancing age. The older people become, the greater their chances of developing and dying of cancer. Figure 10.4 shows a steep increase in cancer mortality by age for both men and women, but especially for men.

Cancer is also the second leading cause of death among children between ages 1 and 14 (exceeded only by unintentional injuries; Siegel et al., 2012). Cancers that are most common among children include leukemia, cancers of the brain and nervous system, and non-Hodgkin's lymphoma. Testicular cancer is also an exception to the general rule concerning age: The highest risk for this cancer occurs during young adulthood. These cancers are likely to have some genetic component.

Family History and Genetics   The first evidence of a genetic component for cancer came from the Nurses' Health Study (Colditz et al., 1993), which showed that

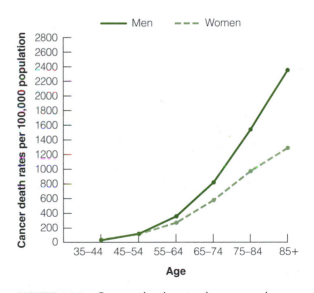

FIGURE 10.4 Cancer death rates by age and gender, United States, 2009.

Source: Data from *Health United States, 2011* (Table 32), by National Center for Health Statistics, 2012, Hyattsville, MD: U.S. Government Printing Office.

women whose mothers received a breast cancer diagnosis before age 40 were more than twice as likely to develop breast cancer. A sister with breast cancer also doubled the risk, and having both a sister and a mother with breast cancer increased a woman's risk about 2 ½ times. This research has progressed to the identification of specific genes involved in breast cancer, the *BRCA 1* and *BRCA 2* genes. These genes protect against cancer by providing the code for a protective protein (Paull, Cortez, Bowers, Elledge, & Gellert, 2001). Women who have a mutated form of *BRCA 1*, which does not allow that protective protein to develop, are as many as 7 times more likely to develop breast cancer as women with the healthy form of this gene. Mutations in *BRCA 1* and *BRCA 2* have also been implicated in the development of breast cancer in men and pancreatic cancer in both women and men (Lynch et al., 2005). This gene does not create a certainty of developing cancer, but people with the mutation have a sharply increased risk.

The form of breast cancer involving *BRCA 1* and *BRCA 2* is responsible for no more than 10% of breast cancer, and the other cancers associated with *BRCA* are even less likely to arise from a gene mutation. Thus, many genes for breast cancer remain unidentified, and most of the risk for developing breast cancer comes from other sources (Oldenburg, Meijers-Heijboer, Cornelisse, & Devilee, 2007).

Across all cancers, only 5% to 10% percent are due to inherited genetic mutations (ACS, 2012), with breast, ovarian, prostate, and colorectal cancers being the types of cancer most likely to arise from inherited genetic mutations (Baker, Lichtenstein, Kaprio, & Holm, 2005). The search for single genes that underlie the development of cancer has been largely unsuccessful (Hemminki, Försti, & Bermejo, 2006). Instead, researchers have identified configurations of genes that seem to lead to vulnerabilities for specific cancers. Furthermore, some cancers may arise from a complex interaction between genetic vulnerability and behavioral risk factors. For example, some evidence suggests that women with the *BRCA 2* mutation may be at a greater risk of alcohol-induced breast cancer compared with women without the *BRCA 2* mutation (Dennis et al., 2011). Therefore, despite the widespread publicity about genetic causes of cancer, genes play a fairly minor role in the development of cancer; environmental and behavioral factors are much more important.

Environmental Risk Factors for Cancer

Environmental risk factors for cancer include exposure to risks such as radiation and asbestos and to pollutants such as pesticides, herbicides, motor exhaust, and other chemicals (Miligi, Costantini, Veraldi, Benvenuti, & Vineis, 2006). In addition, arsenic, benzene, chromium, nickel, vinyl chloride, and various petroleum products are possible contributors to a number of cancers (Boffetta, 2004; Siemiatycki et al., 2004).

Longtime exposure to asbestos can increase risk for lung cancer, depending on the type of asbestos and the frequency and duration of exposure. A study in Sweden (Gustavsson et al., 2000) examined the possible carcinogenic effects of asbestos as well as diesel exhaust, motor exhaust, metals, welding fumes, and other environmental conditions that some workers encounter on the job. The results showed that workers with exposure to environmental carcinogens had about a 9% additional chance of developing lung cancer compared with people without exposure to these conditions. A 25-year longitudinal study of asbestos workers in China (Yano, Wang, Wang, Wang, & Lan, 2001) reported that male asbestos workers, compared with other workers, had 6.6 times the likelihood of developing lung cancer, and 4.3 times the likelihood of developing any cancer.

Exposure to radiation is also a risk. Nuclear power plant workers exposed to high levels of radiation showed elevated risks for leukemia and cancers of the rectum, colon, testicles, and lung (Sont et al., 2001). Living in a community with a nuclear power plant, however, seems to present no elevated risk; the observed rate of cancer in such communities is similar to that of other communities (Boice, Bigbee, Mumma, & Blot, 2003). The radioactive gas radon also presents increased risks for lung cancer, both for miners who are exposed and for people who live in homes with high levels of this type of radiation (Krewski et al., 2006).

Some infections and chronic inflammation also present elevated risks for cancers. Infection with the bacterium *Helicobacter pylori* is widespread throughout the world and increases the risk for gastric ulcers as well as gastric cancer (McColl, Watabe, & Derakhshan, 2007). Hepatitis infection is a risk for liver cancer. Chronic inflammation is a factor in the development of bladder cancer (Michaud, 2007) and possibly in prostate cancer (De Marzo et al., 2007). However, infection and inflammation may be more attributable to behavior than to environmental exposure.

IN SUMMARY

Inherent risks for cancer include ethnic background, advancing age, and family history and genetics. African Americans have higher cancer incidence and death rates than European Americans, but people from other ethnic backgrounds have a lower incidence. These differences are due not to biology but to differences in socioeconomic status, which is related both to the incidence of cancer and to 5-year survival with the disease.

The strongest risk factor for cancer—as well as many other diseases—is advancing age. As a person gets older, the risk for cancer increases. Furthermore, men have an even greater increase than women.

Although cancer seldom develops because of a single gene, family history and genetic predisposition play a role in the development of some cancers, especially prostate and breast cancer. A woman who has a mother or sister with breast cancer has a two- to threefold higher chance of developing the disease, and mutations of the *BRCA 1* and *BRCA 2* genes place people at elevated risk for breast and pancreatic cancer. However, genetic factors play a relatively small role in the development of cancer.

Environmental risks also contribute to cancer incidence and deaths. Pollutants, pesticides, radiation exposure, and infections increase the risk for various cancers. Workers exposed to asbestos and radiation are at increased risk, as are people living in homes with high levels of radon.

Behavioral Risk Factors for Cancer

Cancer results from an interaction of genetic, environmental, and behavioral conditions, most of which are still not clearly understood. As with cardiovascular diseases, however, several behavioral cancer risk factors are clear. Recall that risk factors are not necessarily *causes* of a disease, but they do predict the likelihood that a person will develop or die from that disease. Most risk factors for cancer relate to personal behavior and lifestyle, especially smoking and diet. Other known behavioral risks include alcohol, physical inactivity, exposure to ultraviolet light, sexual behavior, and psychosocial factors.

Smoking

"If nobody smoked, 1 of every 3 cancer deaths in the United States would not happen." (United States Department of Health and Human Services [USDHHS], 2010, p. 7)

The vast majority of smoking-related cancer deaths are from lung cancer, but smoking is also implicated in deaths from many other cancers, including leukemia and cancers of the stomach, bladder, upper digestive tract, esophagus, colon, and prostate (Batty et al., 2008). Smoking also increases risk for cancers of the larynx, pharynx, oral cavity, sinuses, cervix, pancreas, liver, and kidney (Gandini et al., 2008). There is not a consistent relationship between smoking and breast cancer, but women who smoke throughout adolescence may increase their risk for this type of cancer (Ha et al., 2007). The risk of cigarette smoking also applies to other countries around the world; smoking is the single largest risk for cancer mortality worldwide (Danaei, Vander Hoorn, Lopez, Murray, & Ezzati, 2005). Thus, it is a misconception that smoking causes only lung cancer. Figure 10.5 shows all the types of cancer associated with tobacco use.

What Is the Risk?   Sufficient evidence exists for epidemiologists to conclude a causal relationship exists between cigarette smoking and lung cancer. Chapter 2 includes a review of that evidence and explains how epidemiologists can infer causation from nonexperimental studies. The strong relationship between smoking and lung cancer becomes apparent when observing the way lung cancer rates track smoking rates. About 25 to 40 years after smoking rates began to increase for men, lung cancer rates started a steep rise; about 25 to 40 years after cigarette consumption decreased for men, lung cancer death rates for men began to drop (see Figure 10.6). Women's smoking has declined more gradually, and so have their lung cancer mortality rates.

The strong relationship holds when analyzed by income. Low-income men smoke more than high-income men, and they have a higher lung cancer mortality rate; low-income women smoke a little less than

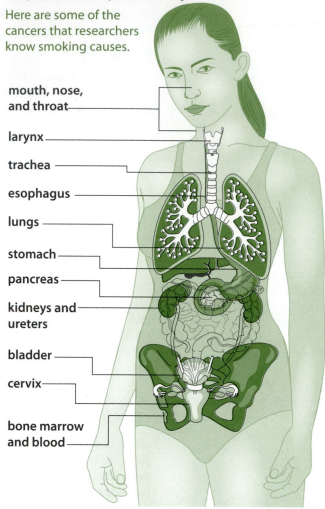

Smoking can cause cancer almost anywhere in your body.

Here are some of the cancers that researchers know smoking causes.

mouth, nose, and throat

larynx

trachea

esophagus

lungs

stomach

pancreas

kidneys and ureters

bladder

cervix

bone marrow and blood

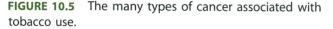

FIGURE 10.5   The many types of cancer associated with tobacco use.

Source: Adapted from U.S. Department of Health and Human Services. A Report of the Surgeon General: How Tobacco Smoke Causes Disease: What It Means to You. U.S. Department of Health and Human Services, Centers for Disease Control and Prevention, National Center for Chronic Disease Prevention and Health Promotion, Office of Smoking and Health, 2010.

high-income women, and they have a slightly lower rate of lung cancer mortality (Weir et al., 2003). The dose–response relationship between cigarette smoking and lung cancer and the close tracking of smoking rates and lung cancer rates provide compelling evidence for a causal relationship between smoking and the development of lung cancer.

How high is the risk for lung cancer among cigarette smokers? The United States Department of Health and Human Services (USDHHS, 2004) estimated the relative risk of death for male smokers at about 23.3, meaning that men who smoke are *23.3 times more likely to die of lung cancer* than men who have never smoked. The risk that cigarette smokers have of dying

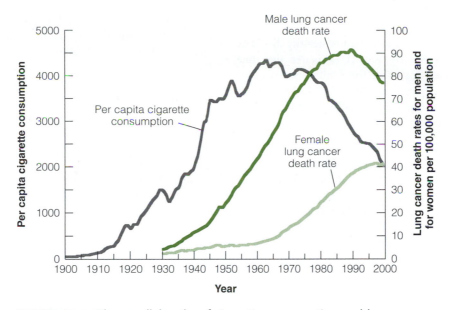

FIGURE 10.6   The parallel paths of cigarette consumption and lung cancer deaths for men and women, United States, 1900–2000.

Source: Data from *Health United States, 2011* (Table 32), by National Center for Health Statistics, 2012, Hyattsville, MD: U.S. Government Printing Office.

of lung cancer is the strongest link between any behavior and a major cause of death.

Cigarette smoking is not the only form of tobacco use that increases risk for cancer. Smoking cigars or using smokeless tobacco—also known as "chew," "spit," or "snuff" tobacco—also increases likelihood of death from several forms of cancer, including laryngeal, oral, esophageal, and pancreatic cancer (ACS, 2012). As we discuss in greater detail in Chapter 12, there is no safe way to use tobacco products.

In addition to tobacco use, such factors as polluted air, socioeconomic level, occupation, ethnic background, and building material in one's house all link to lung cancer. Each of these has an additive or possibly a **synergistic effect** with smoking, so studies of different populations may yield quite different risk factor rates, depending on the combination of risks that cigarette smokers have in addition to their risk as a smoker. For example, Chinese men who smoke have an elevated risk for lung cancer that increases with exposure to smoke from burning coal, a common practice for household heating and cooking in China (Danaei et al., 2005).

What Is the Perceived Risk?   Despite their heightened vulnerability to cancer, many smokers do not perceive that their behavior puts them at risk. They show what Neil Weinstein (1984) referred to as an *optimistic bias* concerning their chances of dying from cigarette-related causes. Both smokers and nonsmokers acknowledge that smoking is a health risk. Despite knowledge to the contrary, both high school smokers (Tomar & Hatsukami, 2007) and adult smokers (Peretti-Watel et al., 2007) believe that, unlike other smokers, they will somehow escape the deadly effects of cigarette smoking. The adult smokers expressed the belief that smoking is dangerous at some level—but not at the level of their consumption.

This tendency to deny personal risk may be stronger in countries where smoking is more prevalent and attitudes toward smoking are more lenient. Denmark is such a country, and Danish people are more likely to deny personal risk than Americans (Helweg-Larsen & Nielsen, 2009). This denial of risk is all the more surprising when considering that, compared with the United States, Denmark has *higher* rates of mortality due to tobacco-related diseases such as lung cancer, oral cancer, cardiovascular disease, and chronic obstructive pulmonary disease (World Health Organization [WHO], 2010). Thus, optimistic biases are common and may be tied to the cultural prevalence and acceptability of smoking.

Diet

Another risk factor for cancer is an unhealthy diet. The American Cancer Society (2012) estimates that one third of all cancer deaths in the United States are a result of dietary choices and sedentary lifestyle. Poor dietary practices are associated with a wide variety of cancers, and good choices decrease the risks.

Foods That May Cause Cancer   Some foods are suspected of being **carcinogenic**—that is, of causing cancer, almost always because of contaminants or additives (Abnet, 2007). "Natural" foods lack preservatives, which can result in high levels of bacteria and fungi. A long list of bacteria and fungi present risks for stomach cancer. The sharp decline in this cancer is due in part to increased refrigeration during the last 75 years and to lower consumption of salt-cured foods, smoked foods, and foods stored at room temperature (see Figures 10.2 and 10.3). Aflatoxin is a fungus that grows on improperly stored grains and peanuts; exposure to this toxin increases the risk for liver cancer (World Cancer Research Fund/American Institute for Cancer Research [WCRF/AICR], 2007). However, food additives used as preservatives can also be carcinogenic, and toxic chemicals produced by various industries can work their way into the environment and into foods, as in the case of dioxin. Thus, both foods that lack preservatives and those with preservatives may present some risk.

In Chapter 9, we saw that dietary fat is an established risk for cardiovascular disease; a number of studies have shown that dietary fat is also a risk for cancer, especially colon cancer (Murtaugh, 2004). However, a high-fat diet is a stronger risk for cardiovascular disease than it is for cancer. Much of the research on dietary fat and cancer centers on breast cancer and suggests that dietary fat is a modest but reliable risk factor for this cancer (Freedman, Kipnis, Schatzkin, & Potischman, 2008). A high-fat diet also contributes to high cholesterol levels, which appeared as a risk factor for testicular cancer in men—raising the risk 4.5 times (Dobson, 2005).

Consumption of preserved meat (such as ham, bacon, and hot dogs) raises the risk of colorectal cancer (Williams & Hord, 2005). A possible risk associated with red meat is the method of cooking; charred, smoked, or overcooked red meats may be a factor in this risk (Alaejos, González, & Afonso, 2008), and salt-cured or heavily salted meats also raise risks for stomach cancer (WCRF/AICR, 2007).

A stronger risk for colorectal cancer comes not from any specific dietary component but from overweight and obesity (WCRF/AICR, 2007; Williams & Hord, 2005). Obesity accounts for 14% to 20% of all cancer-related deaths (ACS, 2012). Obesity is strongly related to cancer of the esophagus, breast (in postmenopausal women), endometrium, and kidney. Abdominal fat is a risk not only for cardiovascular disease but also for cancer of the pancreas, endometrium, and kidney. Although eating several specific types of food increases the risk for cancers, a diet that leads to overweight or obesity is more of a risk.

Foods That May Protect Against Cancer   If specific foods and overall diet can increase the risk for cancer, might some dietary measures offer protection? One team of researchers has calculated that if people around the world were to eat an adequate amount of fruits and vegetables, as many as 2.6 million deaths per year would be eliminated (Lock, Pomerleau, Causer, Altmann, & McKee, 2005). The same researchers estimated that this fruit and vegetable-rich diet might reduce the incidence of stomach cancer by 19%, esophageal cancer by 20%, lung cancer by 12%, and colorectal cancer by 2%. Consistent with this analysis, another review (Williams & Hord, 2005) concluded that the evidence is strong for a high-fiber diet as protective for colorectal cancer.

Despite these known benefits of a diet high in fiber and rich in fruits and vegetables, it remains unclear whether specific nutrients protect against the development or proliferation of cancer. This lack of clarity may be due to the research methods used to investigate dietary components. For example, population studies showed that people in countries with a high-fiber diet experienced lower rates of colorectal cancer than people in countries with a low-fiber diet. This result prompted research using the case–control method in which people who eat a high-fiber diet were compared with those who eat a low-fiber diet (see Chapter 2 for a description of this method). Such studies involve fewer people than population studies, so small effects of fiber in the diet may not be clear using this approach. Alternatively, other differences between the two groups may contribute to the effect of fiber in the diet, making a clear conclusion difficult. If case–control studies indicate that the nutrient has a positive effect, which they have for fiber and colorectal cancer (WCRF/AICR, 2007), researchers then perform experimental studies.

The randomized clinical trial is an experimental method that is the best method for detecting differences between groups. For dietary studies, however, this method has drawbacks (Boyd, 2007). Such studies are experimental, involving the manipulation of a factor—in this case a dietary component. Half the participants receive the component, and half do not, creating a clear comparison. However, the exposure is typically short term; few clinical trials last longer than a few years, and most have limited follow-ups. Eating a high-fiber diet for 2 years may not provide sufficient exposure to have an impact on the development of colorectal cancer, which develops over years. Or participants may need to ingest nutrients during childhood or adolescence for maximum benefit, but most studies include only adult participants. In addition, randomized clinical trials usually isolate a nutrient and provide that nutrient through supplements rather than through broad changes to the diet. Taking supplements often fails to produce the benefits of eating a diet high in the same nutrients. Thus, the benefits of specific nutrients may be complex, and randomized clinical trials may miss some of those important benefits.

These limitations have restricted researchers from coming to conclusions about the cancer-preventive benefits of many nutrients. An extensive review of the evidence (WCRF/AICR, 2007) was able to place several nutrients into the category of *probable* (but not *convincing*) evidence for benefits. **Beta-carotene** is one of the carotenoids, a form of vitamin A found abundantly in foods such as carrots and sweet potatoes. Eating a diet rich in carotenoids probably lowers the risk of cancer of the mouth, larynx, pharynx, and lungs; high beta-carotene intake has a similar benefit for the risk of cancer of the esophagus, as does a diet rich in vitamin C. People who eat foods high in folate, one of the B vitamins, probably decrease their chances of developing pancreatic cancer. Evidence for any protective power for these nutrients is weaker for other types of cancer.

Evidence concerning selenium intake is somewhat stronger (Williams & Hord, 2005). **Selenium** is a trace element found in grain products and in meat from grain-fed animals. It enters the food chain through the soil, but not all soils throughout the world contain equal amounts of selenium. In excess, selenium is toxic, but in moderate amounts, it provides some protection against colon and prostate cancers. Foods with high levels of selenium protect against colon cancer in laboratory rats (Finley, Davis, & Feng, 2000), and selenium supplements

can significantly reduce cancer incidence, but only in men (Bardia et al., 2008). Calcium has received a great deal of publicity for its benefit in preventing bone mineral loss, but it may also offer some protection against colorectal cancer (WCRF/AICR, 2007).

Thus, an evaluation of the extensive research suggests that some nutrients can protect against some cancers, but the evidence of a protective effect is stronger concerning overall diet and maintaining close to ideal body weight. A healthy diet includes lots of fruits and vegetables, whole grains, legumes, nuts, fish and seafood, and low-fat dairy products; the amount of preserved and red meat, saturated fat, salt-cured foods, and foods made of highly processed ingredients is low. This description fits with the concept of a Mediterranean-type diet, emphasizing a plant-based diet with a variety of foods that people can adopt as part of a healthy lifestyle (Williams & Hord, 2005). Another element of the Mediterranean diet is alcohol—but in limited amounts.

Alcohol

Alcohol is not as strong a risk factor for cancer as either smoking or eating an imprudent diet. Nevertheless, alcohol does increase risk for cancers of the mouth, esophagus, breast, and liver (WCRF/AICR,

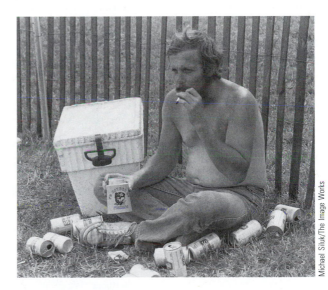

Risks from smoking, drinking, and sun exposure can have a synergistic effect, multiplying the chances of developing cancer.

2007). The liver has primary responsibility for detoxifying alcohol. Therefore, persistent and excessive drinking often leads to cirrhosis of the liver, a degenerative disease that curtails the organ's effectiveness. Cancer is more likely to occur in cirrhotic livers than in healthy ones (WCRF/AICR, 2007), but alcohol abusers are likely to die of a variety of other causes before they develop liver cancer.

Does drinking alcohol cause breast cancer? Current evaluations of the research indicate that the evidence is convincing (WCRF/AICR, 2007). The risk varies by exposure; women who consume three or more drinks per day have a moderate to strong risk for breast cancer, and women who consume as little as one to two drinks daily have some risk (Singletary & Gapstur, 2001). The risk is not equal in all countries. In the United States, about 2% of breast cancer cases can be attributed to alcohol, but in Italy, where alcohol intake is considerably higher, as many as 15% of breast cancer cases may be due to drinking. Table 10.1 summarizes the risks and

TABLE 10.1   Diet and Its Effects on Cancer

Type of Food	Findings of Increased Risk	Studies
"Natural" foods with no preservatives	Grains and peanuts may be contaminated with aflatoxin, which is carcinogenic. Spoiled food increases risk for stomach cancer.	Abnet, 2007
Foods high in preservatives High-fat diet	Preservatives can be carcinogenic. Contributes to colon cancer Modest risk for breast cancer High cholesterol level is a strong risk for testicular cancer.	Abnet, 2007 Murtaugh, 2004 Freedman et al., 2008 Dobson, 2005
Consumption of preserved meats and red meat	Increases the risk for colorectal cancer, especially if meat is smoked or charred	WCRF/AICR*, 2007; Williams & Hord, 2005
Overweight and obesity	Strong link to colorectal, esophageal, breast, endometrial, and kidney cancer Abdominal fat is a risk for cancer of the pancreas, endometrium, and kidney.	WCRF/AICR, 2007; Williams & Hord, 2005
Alcohol	Raises the risk of cancers of the mouth, esophagus, breast, and liver, especially heavy drinking and drinking combined with smoking	WCRF/AICR, 2007

Type of Food	Findings of Decreased Risk	Studies
Diet rich in fruits and vegetables	Could reduce worldwide rates of stomach cancer by 19%, esophageal cancer by 20%, lung cancer by 12%, and colorectal cancer by 2%	Lock et al., 2005
Diet rich in fiber	Protects against colon cancer	Williams & Hord, 2005
Diet high in carotenoids, including beta-carotene	Probably lowers the risk of cancer of the mouth, larynx, pharynx, and lungs Diets high in beta-carotene (but not supplements) lower the risk for cancer of the esophagus.	WCRF/AICR, 2007
Vitamin C	Probably lowers the risk of cancer of the esophagus	WCRF/AICR, 2007
Diet high in folate	Probably lowers the risk of pancreatic cancer	WCRF/AICR, 2007
Selenium	Protects against colon cancer in laboratory rats Reduces risk of several types of cancer in men	Finley et al., 2000 Bardia et al., 2008
Calcium	May protect against colon cancer.	WCRF/AICR, 2007
Summary	Overall diet and healthy weight are more strongly related to cancer than any one dietary component.	WCRF/AICR, 2007; Williams & Hord, 2005

*World Cancer Research Fund/American Institute for Cancer Research

benefits of specific dietary choices and alcohol consumption.

Alcohol has a synergistic effect with smoking, so people who both smoke and drink heavily have a risk for certain cancers exceeding that of the two independent risk factors added together. People who both drink and smoke and who have a family history of esophageal, stomach, or pharynx cancers have an increased risk for cancers of the digestive tract (Garavello et al., 2005). These data suggest that people who both drink heavily and smoke could substantially reduce their chances of developing cancer by giving up either smoking or drinking. Quitting both, of course, would reduce the risk still more.

Sedentary Lifestyle

A sedentary lifestyle increases the risk for some types of cancer, including cancers of the colon, endometrium, breast, lung, and pancreas (WCRF/AICR, 2007). Thus, physical activity can reduce risks for these cancers. There is strong evidence of the beneficial effect of physical activity for colon, endometrial, and breast cancer (in women after menopause); the evidence is less clear for lung and pancreatic cancer and for breast cancer in premenopausal women. Some studies (Bernstein, Henderson, Hanisch, Sullivan-Halley, & Ross, 1994; Thune, Brenn, Lund, & Gaard, 1997) suggest that women who begin a physical activity program when they are young and who continue to exercise 4 hours a week greatly reduce their risk for breast cancer. This age-sensitive effect may make the overall benefit of exercise difficult to determine for premenopausal women.

Another indirect benefit of physical activity for cancer risk is its relationship with body weight. Physical activity is important for maintaining a healthy body weight and a favorable level of body fat, both of which increase risk for a number of cancers. Thus, some form of vigorous physical activity can lower cancer risk in several ways. The benefits (and potential risks) of physical activity are discussed more fully in Chapter 15. (See Would You Believe …? box to learn more about how physical activity, in addition to other cancer-prevention behaviors, reduces risk for many causes of death.)

Ultraviolet Light Exposure

Exposure to ultraviolet light, particularly from the sun, is a well-known cause of skin cancer, especially for

Would You BELIEVE...? Cancer Prevention Prevents More Than Cancer

With one out of three cancer-related deaths attributable to smoking, your best way to avoid cancer is to avoid smoking. But how much do other cancer prevention behaviors matter, such as keeping a normal weight, maintaining a healthy diet, staying physically active, and drinking only in moderation (if at all)?

A recent study (McCullough et al., 2011) investigated this simple question. In the early 1990s, this research team from the American Cancer Society surveyed over 100,000 nonsmoking, older adults and asked them about their weight and height, diet, physical activity, and alcohol use. From these questions, the researchers computed a score representing the extent of adherence to the existing American Cancer Society guidelines for cancer prevention. Nearly 15 years later, the research team consulted the National Death Registry to obtain answers to two additional, important questions: Was the person dead, and if so, what was the cause of death?

One finding may not be surprising: Respondents who were the most adherent to cancer prevention guidelines had a *30% lower risk of cancer-related death* than those who were the least adherent. Thus, adhering to all the other behaviors conferred a clear benefit in preventing cancer.

However, the cancer prevention behaviors prevented much more than just cancer. The most adherent respondents had a *48% lower risk of death by cardiovascular disease* than the least adherent respondents. Taking all causes of death together, the most adherent respondents had a *42% lower risk of all-cause mortality*, compared with the least adherent respondents. Of all the behaviors this research team examined, maintaining a normal weight was the component most strongly tied to mortality.

Thus, by avoiding tobacco and following these other cancer prevention recommendations, you can reduce your odds of untimely death by nearly half! Excellent odds, indeed.

light-skinned people (WCRF/AICR, 2007). Both cumulative exposure and occasional severe sunburn relate to subsequent risk of skin cancer. Since the mid-1970s, the incidence of skin cancer has risen in the United States. However, because this form of cancer has a low mortality rate, it has only slightly affected total cancer mortality statistics. Not all skin cancers, however, are harmless. One form, malignant melanoma, is often deadly. Malignant melanoma is especially prevalent among light-skinned people exposed to the sun.

Although we associate skin cancer with a behavioral risk (voluntary exposure to the sun over a long period), there also is a strong genetic component (Pho, Grossman, & Leachman, 2006). Light-skinned, fair-haired, blue-eyed individuals are more likely than dark-skinned people to develop skin cancer, and much of the damage occurs with sun exposure during childhood (Dennis et al., 2008). During the past 50 years, the relationship between melanoma mortality rates and geographic latitude has gradually decreased; residence in areas of the United States with high ultraviolet radiation is no longer a risk factor for melanoma but remains a risk for other types of skin cancer (Qureshi, Laden, Colditz, & Hunter, 2008). Fair-skinned people should avoid prolonged and frequent exposure to the sun by taking protective measures, including using sunscreen lotions and wearing protective clothing.

People should also avoid indoor tanning beds, which increase risk for melanoma. An international comprehensive review of research found a 75% increase in melanoma risk among people who used tanning beds in their teenage and young adult years (International Agency for Research on Cancer [IARC], 2007). Furthermore, a dose–response relationship exists: As people's frequency of tanning bed use increases, so does risk for melanoma (Lazovich et al., 2010).

Not all exposure to sunlight is detrimental to health. Vitamin D derives from sun exposure and also contributes to lower rates of several types of cancer, including cancers of the breast, colon, prostate, ovary, lungs, and pancreas (Ingraham, Bragdon, & Nohe, 2008). However, the level of vitamin D necessary to protect against cancer seldom comes from diet alone. Therefore, low levels of exposure to ultraviolet light can be a healthy means of supplying vitamin D. How much sun exposure is enough but not too much? In addition to the usual dietary supply of vitamin D, as little as 5 to 10 minutes of sun exposure of the arms and legs or the arms, hands, and face two or three times a week seems sufficient (Holick, 2004). Alternatively, dietary supplementation can provide vitamin D and its protective benefits (Ingraham et al., 2008).

Sexual Behavior

Some sexual behaviors also contribute to cancer deaths, especially cancers resulting from acquired immune deficiency syndrome (AIDS). Two common forms of AIDS-related cancers are Kaposi's sarcoma and non-Hodgkin's lymphoma. **Kaposi's sarcoma** is a malignancy characterized by soft, dark blue or purple nodules on the skin, often with large lesions. The lesions can be so small at first as to look like a rash but can grow to be large and disfiguring. Besides covering the skin, these lesions can spread to the lung, spleen, bladder, lymph nodes, mouth, and adrenal glands. Until the 1980s, this type of cancer was quite rare and was limited mostly to older men of Mediterranean background. However, AIDS-related Kaposi's sarcoma occurs in every age group and in both men and women. Not all people with AIDS are equally susceptible to this disease; gay men with AIDS are much more likely to develop Kaposi's sarcoma than are people who developed AIDS as a result of injection drug use or heterosexual contact (Henke-Gendo & Schulz, 2004).

In **non-Hodgkin's lymphoma,** rapidly growing tumors spread through the circulatory or lymphatic system. Like Kaposi's sarcoma, non-Hodgkin's lymphoma can occur in AIDS patients of all ages and both genders. However, most people with non-Hodgkin's lymphoma do *not* have AIDS. The greatest risk for AIDS-related cancers continues to be unprotected sex with an HIV-positive partner.

Exposure to another sexually transmitted virus—the human papillomavirus, or HPV—increases risk for two types of cancer: cervical cancer and oral cancer. HPV is necessary for the development of cervical cancer (Baseman & Koutsky, 2005; Danaei et al., 2005). The rates of HPV infection are high, especially for sexually active young people (Datta et al., 2008). Thus, women who have had many sex partners and those whose first sexual intercourse experience occurred early in life are most vulnerable to cervical cancer because these behaviors expose them to HPV. Men's sex practices can also increase female partners' likelihood of getting cervical cancer. When men have multiple sex partners, specifically with women who have had many sex partners, their female sex partners are at increased risk of cervical cancer.

HPV is a cause of some oral cancers as well. In the last 20 years, the proportion of oral cancers associated with HPV increased dramatically, from 16% in the late 1980s to 73% in the early 2000s (Chaturvedi et al., 2011). By some estimates, new diagnoses of HPV-related oral cancer will exceed that of cervical cancers by the year 2020 (Chaturvedi et al., 2011). Furthermore, HPV-related oral cancer is twice as common in men as women (Chaturvedi, Engels, Anderson, & Gillison, 2008). Oral HPV is likely spread through oral sex, and oral HPV infections are more likely to persist among smokers (D'Souza & Dempsey, 2011). Thus, sexual behavior—in combination with tobacco use—can substantially increase the likelihood of oral cancers.

Men's sexual practices can also increase the risk of prostate cancer. Karin Rosenblatt and her associates (Rosenblatt, Wicklund, & Stanford, 2000) found a significant positive relationship between prostate cancer and lifetime number of female sex partners (but not male sex partners), early age of first intercourse, and prior infection with gonorrhea. However, they found no risk for prostate cancer associated with lifetime frequency of sexual intercourse.

Psychosocial Risk Factors in Cancer

Since the days of the Greek physician Galen (A.D. 131–201), people have speculated about the relationship between personality traits and certain diseases, including cancer. However, that speculation does not match the findings from scientific research. For example, a prospective study from the Swedish Twin Registry (Hansen, Floderus, Frederiksen, & Johansen, 2005) found that neither extraversion nor neuroticism—as measured by the Eysenck Personality Inventory—predicted an increased likelihood of cancer.

This study and its findings are fairly typical of attempts to relate psychosocial factors to cancer incidence and mortality. During the past 30 or 40 years, a number of researchers investigated the association between a variety of psychological factors and cancer development and prognosis. Some studies have identified various personality factors that seemed to relate to the development of cancer, but large-scale studies and reviews of the topic (Aro et al., 2005; Garssen, 2004; Levin & Kissane, 2006; Stürmer, Hasselbach, & Amelang, 2006) have found only weak association between any psychosocial factor and cancer. Factors that show the strongest relationship come from negative emotionality and the tendency to repress (rather than express) emotion. However, these traits show a stronger relationship to response to a diagnosis of cancer than to the development of cancer.

IN SUMMARY

Cigarette smoking is the leading risk factor for lung cancer. Although not all cigarette smokers die of lung cancer and some nonsmokers develop this disease, clear evidence exists that smokers have a greatly increased chance of developing some form of cancer, particularly lung cancer. The more cigarettes per day people smoke and the more years they continue this practice, the more they are at risk.

The relationship between diet and the development of cancer is complex, with some types of food presenting dangers for the development of cancer and others offering some protection. "Natural" foods avoid the risk of preservatives but increase the likelihood of other toxins. A high-fat diet is related to colon and breast cancer, but a diet that produces overweight or obesity is a risk for a variety of cancers, including colorectal, esophageal, breast (in postmenopausal women), endometrial, and kidney cancer. Some dietary components can protect against cancer, including fruits, vegetables, and other high-fiber foods. The evidence for specific nutrients in foods is less persuasive, and taking supplements generally offers no protection.

Alcohol is probably only a weak risk factor for cancer. Nevertheless, it has a synergistic effect with cigarette smoking; when the two are combined, the total relative risk is much greater than the risks of the two factors added together. Lack of physical activity and high exposure to ultraviolet light are additional risk factors for cancer. Also, certain sexual behaviors, such as number of lifetime sex partners, relate to cervical, oral, and prostate cancer as well as to cancers associated with AIDS.

In general, psychosocial factors show only weak relationships to cancer incidence. Negative affect and repression of emotion may contribute to the development of cancer, but the relationship is not strong.

Living With Cancer

As Steve Jobs did in 2003, more than a million Americans receive a diagnosis of cancer each year (ACS, 2012). Most of these people receive their diagnosis with feelings of fear, anxiety, and anger, partly because they fear the disease and partly because current cancer treatments produce unpleasant effects for many cancer patients. Steve Jobs, for example, refused surgery for his pancreatic cancer for almost a year because of fears surrounding the treatment. Psychologists assist patients in coping with their emotional reactions to a cancer diagnosis, provide **social support** to patients and families, and help patients prepare for the negative side effects of some cancer treatments.

Problems With Medical Treatments for Cancer

Nearly all medical treatments for cancer have negative side effects that may add stress to the lives of cancer patients, their friends, and their families. The three most common therapies are also the three most stressful: surgery, radiation, and chemotherapy. In recent years, some **oncologists** have added hormonal treatment and immunotherapy to their arsenal of treatment regimens, but these newer treatments are generally not yet as effective as surgery, radiation, or chemotherapy.

Surgery is a common treatment recommendation when cancerous growth has not yet metastasized and when physicians have some confidence that the surgical procedure will be successful in making the tumor more manageable. Cancer patients who undergo surgery are likely to experience distress, rejection, and fears, and they often receive less emotional support than other surgery patients. These reactions are especially likely for patients with breast cancer (Wimberly, Carver, Laurenceau, Harris, & Antoni, 2005) and prostate cancer (Couper, 2007) because of the sexual implications of their surgery. Postsurgery stress and depression lead to lower levels of immunity, which may prolong recovery time and increase vulnerability to other disorders (Antoni & Lutgendorf, 2007). Observers noted a marked decline in Steve Jobs' appearance following his liver transplant surgery in 2009, due possibly to both the cancer as well as compromised immune functioning (Lauerman, 2011).

Radiation also has severe side effects. Many patients who receive radiation therapy anticipate their treatment with fear and anxiety, dreading loss of hair, burns, nausea, vomiting, fatigue, and sterility. Most of these outcomes occur, so patients' fears are not unreasonable. However, patients are seldom adequately prepared for

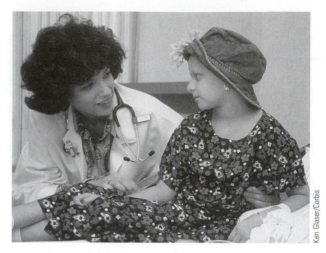

Negative side effects of chemotherapy such as hair loss add to the stress of cancer patients.

their radiation treatments, and thus their fears and anxieties may exaggerate the severity of these side effects.

Chemotherapy has some of the same negative side effects as radiation, and these side effects often precipitate stressful reactions in cancer patients. Cancer patients treated with chemotherapy experience some combination of nausea, vomiting, fatigue, loss of coordination, decreased ability to concentrate, depression, weight change, loss of appetite, sleep problems, and hair loss. Not only do these negative effects create problems in adjusting to a diagnosis of cancer, but patients' expectations of the negative effects of chemotherapy (Olver, Taylor, & Whitford, 2005) and their beliefs about the nature of the disease (Thuné-Boyle, Myers, & Newman, 2006) contribute to distress and adjustment.

Adjusting to a Diagnosis of Cancer

Adjusting to a diagnosis of cancer is a challenge for everyone, but some people have more difficulties than others. Others, like Steve Jobs, may appear to ultimately cope well with a cancer diagnosis. Did Steve's personality—often described as confident and excessively optimistic—play a role in his adjustment to cancer?

Factors that predict a poor reaction to a diagnosis of cancer are the same factors that show some relationship to the development of cancer—negative affect and social inhibition (Verma & Khan, 2007). If negative affect is a problem for adjustment, then optimism should be an advantage, and research generally supports this hypothesis. Optimism is strongly related to adjusting well to a diagnosis of cancer (Carver et al., 2005), but its relationship to long-term outcome is less clear (Segerstrom, 2005, 2007). This difference may arise from the difficulty of the task of adjusting to cancer treatment or from miscalculations on the part of optimists concerning the course and outcome of their treatments (Winterling, Glimelius, & Nordin, 2008). When outcomes are disappointing, optimists may find adjustment more difficult than those who have more realistic expectations. However, while being optimistic predicts better subsequent physical health among people coping with cancer (Rasmussen, Scheier, & Greenhouse, 2009), the strength of this relationship is very small.

These findings are consistent with reviews of research on a "fighting spirit," which reflects an optimistic outlook, a belief that a cancer is controllable, and the use of active coping strategies. While a fighting spirit predicts better adjustment in early-stage cancer (O'Brien & Moorey, 2010), it appears to confer no advantage for long-term survival (Coyne & Tennen, 2010). This conclusion led one research team to advise, "People with cancer should not feel pressured into adopting particular coping styles to improve survival or reduce the risk of recurrence" (Petticrew, Bell, & Hunter, 2002, p. 1066).

After diagnosis, people with cancer show a variety of responses and different trajectories in adjusting and functioning over the course of their treatment and afterward (Helgeson, Snyder, & Seltman, 2004). Most cancer survivors report improvement in their functioning over time, but some long-term survivors attribute problems with low energy, pain, and sexual functioning to their cancers (Phipps, Braitman, Stites, & Leighton, 2008). Even 8 years after cancer, survivors report some problems, which are much more likely to be physical complications than psychological problems (Schroevers, Ranchor, & Sanderman, 2006).

The same emotional factors that enhance the survival of heart disease patients may not be similarly helpful to cancer patients. That is, the calm expression of emotion that may be good advice for cardiovascular patients may not be a good choice for cancer patients; expression of emotion seems to be a better strategy. For example, for children (Aldridge & Roesch, 2007) and for men coping with prostate cancer (Roesch et al., 2005), use of emotion-focused coping did not present the disadvantages that this strategy typically does (see Chapter 5 for a discussion of coping strategies).

Expression of both positive and negative emotions can be beneficial (Quartana, Laubmeier, & Zakowski, 2006). However, expressing some negative emotions may do more harm than good (Lieberman & Goldstein, 2006); expressing anger seems to lead to a better adjustment, whereas expressing fear and anxiety related to lower quality of life and higher depression. Being able to express emotions and being guided to do so in the most helpful manner requires appropriate social support.

Social Support for Cancer Patients

Social support can help cancer patients adjust to their condition, but the type and timing of support play a role in how helpful it is. For recently diagnosed individuals, health care providers can supply information and help with decision making, which such patients rate as supportive and useful (Arora, Rutten, Gustafson, Moser, & Hawkins, 2007). Cancer survivors may receive emotional support from family and friends, which also can be helpful. In the context of breast cancer, women with greater structural social support—that is, with larger social support networks—have slower cancer progression than women with less structural social support (Nausheen, Gidron, Peveler, & Moss-Morris, 2009). Social support is an important factor for men as well, as prostate cancer survivors who perceive more available social support from others manifest greater emotional well-being over time (Zhou et al., 2010). Unfortunately, not all social support attempts by friends and family are beneficial for people with cancer. Sometimes partners' attempts to protect spouses from the reality of their illness are not helpful (Hagedoorn et al., 2000). Thus, social support from families may or may not provide the type of support people with cancer need. Many people with cancer turn to support groups or therapists to provide emotional support.

Professionals such as psychologists, nurses, or oncologists may lead support groups, but often these groups consist of other individuals who are cancer survivors. Some studies indicate that some people profit from support groups more than others. For example, women with breast cancer who lacked adequate marital support profited more from peer group support than from support of their partners, whereas women with strong support from their partners had poorer adjustments when they participated in a peer discussion group (Helgeson, Cohen, Schulz, & Yasko, 2000). A systematic review of the value of peer support groups for cancer survivors (Hoey, Ieropoli, White, & Jefford,

2008) indicated that such groups could be but were not always helpful. In general, face-to-face support delivered by an individual and Internet groups demonstrated the best outcomes, but all types of groups can be effective for some individuals.

Psychological Interventions for Cancer Patients

Psychologists have used both individual and group techniques to help cancer patients cope with their diagnosis. To be effective, an intervention should accomplish at least one of two objectives: It should improve emotional well-being, increase survival time, or both. To what extent do psychological interventions succeed at these two objectives?

Two reviews (Edwards, Hulbert-Williams, & Neal, 2008; Manne & Andrykowski, 2006) conclude that psychological interventions generally yield short-term benefits in helping cancer patients manage the distress related to their condition. Furthermore, some psychological interventions for women with breast cancer improve physiological outcomes, such as cortisol responses and measures of immune functioning (McGregor & Antoni, 2009).

Some psychological interventions focus on cognitive behavioral stress management skills, while others focus on providing social support and an opportunity to express emotions. There is evidence that each of these types of interventions improves some outcomes (Edwards et al., 2008). For example, a program that targeted emotional regulation (Cameron, Booth, Schlatter, Ziginskas, & Harman, 2007) indicated success. However, this emphasis may not be the best approach for everyone. As one research team asked, "Does one size fit all?" (Zimmerman, Heinrichs, & Baucom, 2007, p. 225). This question highlights the need to match the characteristics and needs of people with cancer to a psychotherapy, support, educational, or multicomponent program that will be effective for each person.

Although psychological interventions can improve short-term emotional adjustment, there is less evidence that psychological interventions prolong the life span of people with cancer. The possibility that interventions could have such an effect arose when David Spiegel and colleagues (Spiegel, Bloom, Kraemer, & Gottheil, 1989) conducted a multicomponent intervention to help breast cancer patients adjust to the stressful aspects of their disease and their treatment. Not only was the intervention

successful in managing pain, anxiety, and depression, but also the women in the intervention group lived longer than those in the comparison group. That finding prompted researchers to examine how psychosocial and CAM (complementary and alternative medicine) interventions might prolong the life of those with cancer (see Chapter 8 for a discussion of integrative cancer treatments). Plausible mechanisms include the effect on the immune system and improvements in functioning that allow cancer patients to adhere to their medical treatment regimen (Antoni & Lutgendorf, 2007; Spiegel, 2004; Spiegel & Geise-Davis, 2003).

However, the basic finding that psychosocial interventions prolong life is now in question. Although one recent psychological intervention with women with early-stage breast cancer significantly reduced risk for recurrence and death at an 11-year follow-up (Andersen et al., 2008), large-scale reviews find little evidence that psychological interventions reliably extend survival time for breast cancer patients (Edwards, Hailey, & Maxwell, 2004; Smedslund & Ringdal, 2004). Despite a plausible mechanism for such action and despite the hope that such a benefit is possible (Coyne, Stefanek, & Palmer, 2007), little evidence exists at this point that psychological interventions prolong the life of those with cancer (Edwards et al., 2008). Thus, the value of psychological interventions lies mainly in improving the *quality* rather than the quantity of a cancer patient's life.

IN SUMMARY

After people receive a cancer diagnosis, they typically experience fear, anxiety, depression, and feelings of helplessness. The standard medical treatments for cancer—surgery, chemotherapy, and radiation—all have negative side effects that often produce added stress and discomfort. These side effects include loss of hair, nausea, fatigue, sterility, and other negative conditions. Receiving social support from family and friends, joining support groups, and receiving emotional support through psychological interventions probably help some people with cancer to increase psychological functioning, decrease depression and anxiety, manage pain, and enhance quality of life. Little evidence exists that psychotherapy can increase survival time.

Answers

This chapter has addressed five basic questions:

1. What is cancer?

Cancer is a group of diseases characterized by the presence of new (neoplastic) cells that grow and spread beyond control. These cells may be either benign or malignant, but both types of neoplastic cells are dangerous. Malignant cells are capable of metastasizing and spreading through the blood or lymph to other organs of the body, thus making malignancies life threatening.

2. Are cancer death rates increasing or decreasing?

Cancer is the second leading cause of death in the United States, accounting for about 23% of deaths. During the first nine and a half decades of the 20th century, cancer death rates in the United States rose threefold, but since the mid-1990s, death rates have begun to decline, especially for cancers of the lung, colon and rectum, breast, and prostate—the four leading sites for cancer deaths in the United States. Currently, lung cancer death rates for women are beginning to level off and may soon begin to decline.

3. What are the inherent and environmental risk factors for cancer?

The uncontrollable risk factors for cancer include family history, ethnic background, and advancing age. Family history is a factor in many types of cancer; inheritance of a mutated form of a specific gene increases the risk of breast cancer two- to threefold. Ethnic background is also a factor; compared with European Americans, African Americans have a significantly higher rate of mortality from cancer, but other ethnic groups have lower rates. Advancing age is the single most powerful mortality risk for cancer, but age is also the leading risk for death from cardiovascular and other diseases. Environmental exposure to airborne pollutants, radiation, and infectious organisms constitute significant risks for cancer if the exposure is heavy and prolonged.

4. What are the behavioral risk factors for cancer?

More than half of all cancer deaths in the United States have been attributed to either smoking or unwise lifestyle choices, such as diet and exercise. Smoking cigarettes raises the risk of lung cancer by a factor of 23, but smoking also accounts for other cancer deaths.

The relationship between diet and cancer is complex; diet can increase or decrease the risk for cancer. Toxins and contaminants in food raise the risks, but a diet high in fruits, vegetables, whole grains, low-fat dairy products, beans, and seeds and low in fat, red meat, processed meat, and salt tends to be associated with lowered risk for a variety of cancers. A diet that leads to overweight or obesity raises the risk. Alcohol is not as strong a risk for cancer as diet, but combining alcohol with smoking sharply increases the risk. A sedentary lifestyle also presents a risk, especially for breast cancer. Exposure to ultraviolet light and sexual behaviors can increase the risks for various cancers. Research has also revealed a weak link between negative affect and depression and cancer.

5. How can cancer patients be helped in coping with their disease?

Cancer patients usually benefit from social support from spouse, family, and health care providers, but the type and timing of support affect its benefits. Support groups offer another type of support that is beneficial to some cancer patients, especially in allowing the expression of emotion. Therapists can use cognitive behavioral methods to assist cancer patients in coping with some of the negative aspects of cancer treatments and adjusting to their disease, thus increasing the quality of life for cancer patients, but no evidence exists that psychosocial factors can increase survival time.

Suggested Readings

American Cancer Society. (2012). *Cancer facts and figures 2012*. Atlanta, GA: American Cancer Society. This yearly publication provides extensive, updated information about cancer in the United States with some international comparisons.

Antoni, M. H., & Lutgendorf, S. (2007). Psychosocial factors in disease progression in cancer. *Current Directions in Psychological Science*, *16*, 42–46. This brief article focuses on the influence of psychosocial factors and how these factors may affect the biology of cancer.

Danaei, G., Vander Hoorn, S., Lopez, A. D., Murray, C. J. L., & Ezzati, M. (2005). Causes of cancer in the world: Comparative risk assessment of nine behavioural and environmental risk factors. *Lancet, 366,* 1784–1793. For those who want an international perspective, this article examines nine behavioral and environmental factors and traces the differing rates of cancer in countries throughout the world related to these factors.

U.S. Department of Health and Human Services. (2010). *A report of the Surgeon General: How tobacco smoke causes disease: What it means to you.* Atlanta, GA: U.S. Department of Health and Human Services and Centers for Disease Control and Prevention. This short and engaging article details, in easy-to-understand language, the pathways by which tobacco increases risk for several types of cancer, as well as a multitude of other health problems.

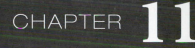
Living With Chronic Illness

CHAPTER OUTLINE

- **Real-World Profile of President Ronald Reagan**
- *The Impact of Chronic Disease*
- *Living With Alzheimer's Disease*
- *Adjusting to Diabetes*
- *The Impact of Asthma*
- *Dealing With HIV and AIDS*
- *Facing Death*

QUESTIONS

This chapter focuses on six basic questions:

1. What is the impact of chronic disease on patients and families?

2. What is the impact of Alzheimer's disease?

Real-World Profile of
PRESIDENT RONALD REAGAN

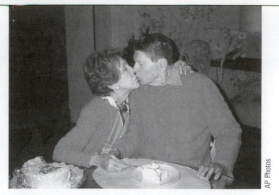

After Ronald Reagan was diagnosed with Alzheimer's disease, his wife, Nancy, learned how to cope with the consequences of living with this chronic illness.

On September 30, 1983, President Ronald Reagan declared the month of November 1983, to be National Alzheimer's Disease Month. At the time, researchers knew little about the prevalence of Alzheimer's disease. Today, we know that one in eight older Americans has Alzheimer's disease. Eleven years after Reagan declared National Alzheimer's Disease Month, he revealed to the world that he had been diagnosed with Alzheimer's disease (Alzheimer's Organization, 2004).

During the decade between the announcement of his Alzheimer's disease and his death on June 5, 2004, Reagan and his family experienced the same stresses and frustrations that millions of families endure when a family member is chronically ill. For daughter Maureen, her first realization that something was wrong with her father came in 1993, when he could not remember making one of his favorite movies (Ellis, 2004). Soon afterward, Reagan noticed that he sometimes felt disoriented. His wife, Nancy, however, said that she noticed no problems at all and was "dumbfounded" when her husband received the Alzheimer's diagnosis. Experts have commented (in Ellis, 2004) that the tendency to overlook problems is common among those closest to the patients—it's easy to deny serious problems when they present subtle symptoms.

As Reagan's symptoms became worse, Nancy was faced with the reality of his symptoms and her increasing loneliness (Ellis, 2004). Despite their resources and fame, Nancy felt isolated, a typical experience for those who are caregivers for Alzheimer's patients. She wrote, "But no one can really know what it's like unless they've traveled this path—and there are many right now traveling the same path I am. You know that it's a progressive disease and that there's no place to go but down, no light at the end of the tunnel. You get tired and frustrated, because you have no control and you feel helpless" (Reagan, 2000, p. 184).

Unlike the other millions of cases of Alzheimer's disease, Ronald Reagan's case stirred public interest, and his family's activism spurred research initiatives. The United States Congress passed a bill known as the Ronald Reagan Alzheimer's Breakthrough Act of 2005, which provided increased funding for Alzheimer's disease research, more help for caregivers, and greater efforts in public education and prevention. Alzheimer's disease is one of the **chronic diseases** that has increased in frequency and will continue to do so, unless research finds a cure or preventive.

Chronic diseases cause 7 in 10 deaths each year in the United States, and almost half of adults live with at least one chronic illness (Centers for Disease Control and Prevention [CDC], 2009). Chronic illness also affects children, with 10% to 15% having some chronic physical health problem (Bramlett & Blumberg, 2008). This chapter looks at the consequences of living with chronic illnesses such as Alzheimer's disease, diabetes, asthma, and AIDS. These and other chronic illnesses share many elements. The diseases vary in physiology, but the emotional and physical adjustments, the disruption of family dynamics, the need for continued medical care, and the necessity of self-management also apply to such chronic diseases as arthritis, heart disease, cancer, kidney disease, multiple sclerosis, head injury, and spinal cord injury.

The Impact of Chronic Disease

Chronic disease places an enormous physical and emotional burden on a patient, as well as a patient's family. Some theorists describe the diagnosis of a chronic illness as a crisis (Moos & Schaefer, 1984). Other theorists suggest that people pass through several stages in their adjustment to chronic disease, but as we will learn, there is little support for stage models of adjustment to chronic disease. Instead, adjustment seems to be a dynamic process influenced by many factors, including the characteristics of the disease, such as rapidity of progress; characteristics of the individual, such as a dispositional optimism; and characteristics of the person's social environment, such as social support. Thus, adjustment to chronic disease is a variable process, and many individual factors shape how people adjust and adapt to a chronic illness (Parker, Schaller, & Hansmann, 2003).

Impact on the Patient

Adapting to chronic disease includes dealing with the symptoms of the disease, managing the stresses of treatment, living as normal a life as possible, and facing the possibility of death. Adjustment to some chronic diseases is more difficult than others because of symptom severity and the demands of coping with symptoms. However, some chronic illnesses may influence quality of life less than healthy people imagine (Damschroder, Zikmund-Fisher, & Ubel, 2005). Research that evaluated the functioning of large groups of patients with a variety of chronic illnesses (Arnold et al., 2004; Heijmans et al., 2004) found similarities and differences among people with different chronic diseases. For some chronic diseases, such as hypertension and diabetes, people reported levels of functioning similar to those with no chronic disease. However, people with heart disease, rheumatoid arthritis, and cancer experienced more intrusive symptoms than did those with hypertension, asthma, or diabetes. Indeed, the psychological functioning appears to matter more than physical functioning in determining the quality of life of chronic disease patients, highlighting the important role of adaptation and coping (Arnold et al., 2004). Using a variety of coping strategies allows people to deal with the stresses of chronic disease (Heijmans et al., 2004); however, active coping strategies tend to produce better results than avoidant strategies (Stanton, Revenson, & Tennen, 2007).

Receiving treatment for chronic diseases also requires adaptation. Interactions with the health care system are likely to create frustrations and problems for people with chronic illness (Parchman, Noel, & Lee, 2005). When patients must interact with the health care system, they tend to feel deprived not only of their sense of competence and mastery but also of their rights and privileges. That is, sick people begin to feel like "nonpersons" and to experience loss of personal control and threats to self-esteem (Stanton et al., 2007).

Developing and maintaining relationships with health care providers also present challenges, for both patients and practitioners. The medical system and people's experience of illness both focus on acute conditions. This experience may lead sick people to believe in the power of modern medicine and to be optimistic about cures. Physicians and other health care workers usually share this attitude (Bickel-Swenson, 2007), which may create a positive climate of trust and optimism for their treatment. Conversely, people with a chronic illness may have a hopeless and even helpless attitude toward their condition—modern medicine can offer them no cure. Health care professionals, too, tend to orient themselves toward providing cures. When they cannot do so, they may feel less positive about those whom they cannot cure (Bickel-Swenson, 2007; Turner & Kelly, 2000). These feelings can create a difficult climate for treatment, with patients questioning and resisting health care providers, and providers feeling frustrated and annoyed with patients who fail to follow treatment regimens and do not get better. Fortunately, younger physicians may be less likely to hold such negative attitudes (Lloyd-Williams, Dogra, & Petersen, 2004), which will benefit treatment and may help to counteract the growing difficulty in negotiating the U.S. health care system experienced by people with chronic conditions.

People with chronic diseases often adopt a number of coping strategies to deal with their illness. A variety of strategies can be successful, but some work better in certain situations. For example, avoidance-oriented coping, such as denial or ignoring the problem, is typically a less effective strategy than problem-focused strategies, such as planning and information seeking (Livneh & Antonak, 2005; Stanton et al., 2007). However, when events are uncontrollable, avoidance coping may be effective in easing negative emotions; when events are controllable, this strategy would be a very poor choice.

Physicians often feel inadequately prepared to help patients deal with these emotional reactions (Bickel-Swenson, 2007; Turner & Kelly, 2000). Such deficits have led to two types of supplements: psychological interventions and support groups. For many chronic illnesses, health psychologists have created interventions that emphasize the management of emotions such as anxiety and depression. Support groups also address emotional needs by providing emotional support to patients or family members who must confront an illness with little chance of a cure. These services supplement conventional health care and help chronically ill patients maintain compliance with the prescribed regimen and sustain a working relationship with health care providers. Reviews of studies dealing with the effectiveness of psychosocial interventions with cancer patients (Osborn, Demoncada, & Feuerstein, 2006) and their families (Barlow & Ellard, 2004) indicate that cognitive behavioral interventions provide effective assistance in helping people cope with chronic diseases.

A major impact of chronic illness involves the changes that occur in how people think of themselves; that is, the diagnosis of a chronic disease changes self-perception. Chronic illness and treatment force many patients to reevaluate their lives, relationships, and body image (Livneh & Antonak, 2005). Being diagnosed with a chronic illness represents a loss (Murray, 2001), and people adapt to such losses through a process of grieving (Rentz, Krikorian, & Keys, 2005). Finding meaning in the experience of loss is more extensive than grieving, but developing an understanding of the meaning of the loss is a common part of coping with chronic disease. Some chronically ill people never move past the grief (Murray, 2001). Other people reconstruct the meaning of their lives in positive ways.

People with chronic diseases often find some positive aspect to their situation (Folkman & Moskowitz, 2000). Part of healthy adjustment is accepting the changes that disease brings, but some research (Fournier, de Ridder, & Bensing, 2002) found that positive expectancies and even unrealistic optimism were advantages in coping with chronic disease. As Annette Stanton and her colleagues (2007, p. 568) summarized, "A disease that disrupts life does not preclude the experience of joy." Thus, some people manage to experience personal growth through loss and grief (Hogan & Schmidt, 2002), which relates to less depression and greater well-being (Helgeson, Reynolds, & Tomich, 2006). This outcome applies not only to patients with chronic diseases but also to their families and caregivers.

Impact on the Family

Illness requires adaptation not only for patients but also for their families. Families may react with grief and feel loss during the sick person's lifetime because families see the person's loss of abilities and sometimes the sense of self.

Involving family members in psychosocial interventions benefits the well-being of both the patient (Martire, Schulz, Helgeson, Small, & Saghafi, 2010) and the family member (Martire, Lustig, Schulz, Miller, & Helgeson, 2004). However, some interventions may be more effective than others. For example, interventions that emphasize communication and interactions—especially those affecting health—provide greater benefits for patients than interventions with other components (Martire & Schulz, 2007). People with chronic illness also benefit from a type of support described as "invisible" (Bolger et al., 2000). This type of interaction may be easier to manage when a partner is not ill; a sick partner needs help, but being the obvious recipient of assistance makes that support stressful as well as helpful. Therefore, chronic illness presents difficulties even to well-intentioned, caring partners.

Although the rates of childhood diseases declined dramatically in the 20th century, a significant number of children still experience chronic diseases (Brace, Smith, McCauley, & Sherry, 2000). The majority of these illnesses are relatively minor, but many children experience severe chronic conditions such as cancer, asthma, rheumatoid arthritis, and diabetes—conditions that limit mobility and activity. These illnesses bring changes in the lives of the entire family. Parents and siblings try to "normalize" family life while coping with therapy for the sick child (Knafl & Deatrick, 2002). However, parents may experience shock, grief, and anger. Such parents face the task of providing support and care, plus the adjustments that chronically ill patients face in finding meaning in the experience of illness. Siblings also face challenges in adjusting to the illness of a family member, tending to notice the differences between their families and "normal" families and feeling some combination of sympathy for and resentment of their sick sibling (Waite-Jones & Madill, 2008a).

For adults, the changes that come with illness can alter their relationships and redefine their identity, but for children who are sick, illness can be even more distressing and disruptive. For some children, the restrictions that come with chronic illness are very difficult, leading to isolation, depression, and distress, whereas other children cope more effectively (Melamed, Kaplan, & Fogel, 2001). Younger children may have difficulty understanding the nature of their disease, and older children and adolescents may resent the restrictions that their disease imposes. Health care providers and parents can help these children make adjustments by offering alternative or modified activities.

Families of sick children face problems similar to couples: They must continue their relationships and manage the problems of caregiving (Knafl & Deatrick, 2002). A child who is ill requires a great deal of emotional support, most of which is supplied by mothers. These efforts can leave mothers so drained that they have little emotional energy left for their husbands, which can leave husbands feeling abandoned and excluded from the family. Fathers tend to cope by concealing their distress and through avoidance, which is seldom an effective coping strategy (Waite-Jones & Madill, 2008b).

zFamilies can follow several recommendations to facilitate adjustment to a chronic disease. Families can try to be flexible and establish a routine that is as close to normal as they can manage (Knafl & Deatrick, 2002). One example of this would be to put the disease into the background and focus on the ways in which the sick child is similar to other children and other family members. Magnifying the ways that the disease makes the child different and focusing on the changes to family routine tend to lead to poorer adaptations. Families should find ways to meet sick children's needs without reinforcing their anxiety and depression (Brace et al., 2000). Like individuals with chronic illness, families tend to make a better adjustment if they focus on finding meaning and some positive aspect in their situation (Ylvén, Björck-Åkesson, & Granlund, 2006).

IN SUMMARY

Chronic diseases bring changes that require adaptation for both the person with the disease and family members. Chronically ill patients must manage their symptoms, seek appropriate health care, and adapt to the psychological changes that occur in this situation. Health care professionals may neglect the social and emotional needs of chronically ill patients, attending instead to their physical needs. Health psychologists and support groups help provide for the emotional needs associated with chronic illness. The adaptations that occur may lead to prolonged feelings of loss and grief or to changes that constitute personal growth.

Living With Alzheimer's Disease

Alzheimer's disease, a degenerative disease of the brain, is a major source of impairment among older people (Mayeaux, 2003). This disease varies in prevalence among countries but remains a major source of cognitive disability in both industrialized and developing countries. Medical researchers identified the brain abnormalities that underlie Alzheimer's disease in the late 19th century. In 1907, a German physician, Alois Alzheimer, reported on the relationship between autopsy findings of neurological abnormalities and psychiatric symptoms before death. Shortly after his report, other researchers began to call the disorder *Alzheimer's disease.*

The disease can be diagnosed definitively only through autopsy, but brain imaging technology is capable of diagnosing Alzheimer's disease with close to 90% accuracy (Vemuri et al., 2008). In addition, Alzheimer's patients show behavioral symptoms of cognitive impairment and memory loss that may lead to a provisional diagnosis (Mayeaux, 2003). During autopsy, a microscopic examination of the brain reveals "plaques" and tangles of nerve fibers in the cerebral cortex and hippocampus. These tangles of nerve fibers are the physical basis for Alzheimer's disease.

The biggest risk factor for Alzheimer's disease is age; the incidence of Alzheimer's disease rises sharply with advancing age. The prevalence of Alzheimer's disease is low for those under age 75—about 9% of people in this age group (Fitzpatrick et al., 2004; Lindsay, Sykes, McDowell, Verreault, & Laurin, 2004). However, the percentage of affected individuals doubles about every 5 years, so that by age 85, almost 50% of individuals exhibit signs of Alzheimer's disease. The increase seems not to continue at the same rate; people in their 90s who have not developed signs of the disease are not nearly as likely to do so as people between ages 65 and 85 (Hall et al., 2005). The high number of people over 85 years old who have symptoms of probable Alzheimer's disease presents a pessimistic picture for the aging population in many industrialized and some developing countries, where Alzheimer's seems destined to become a large public health problem (Haan & Wallace, 2004).

The underlying mechanisms in the development of the disease are not yet completely understood, but two different forms of the disease exist: an early-onset version that occurs before age 60 and a late-onset version that occurs after age 60. The early-onset type is quite rare, representing fewer than 5% of all Alzheimer's patients (Bertram & Tanzi, 2005). Early-onset Alzheimer's may arise from a genetic defect, and at least three different genes on chromosomes 1, 14, and 21 contribute.

The late-onset type has symptoms similar to the early-onset type but begins after age 60, as President Reagan's disease did. Susceptibility to this version of the disease also has a genetic component related to apolipoprotein ε, a protein involved in cholesterol metabolism (Bertram & Tanzi, 2005; Ertekin-Taner, 2007). One form of apolipoprotein, the ε4 form, affects accumulation of the amyloid ε protein, which forms the building blocks for amyloid plaque (Selkoe, 2007). This plaque seems to constitute the underlying pathology for Alzheimer's disease. The risk increases about 3 times for individuals who have one ε4 gene and about 15 times for individuals who have two. Older adults who do not have Alzheimer's disease but who carry the ε4 variant of this gene show lower levels of cognitive functioning than those with other variants of the gene (Small, Rosnick, Fratiglioni, & Bäckman, 2004). The ε2 form of the gene may actually offer some protection against Alzheimer's disease.

These genetic factors increase a person's susceptibility to Alzheimer's disease, rather than guarantee it. A variety of environmental and behavioral factors also play a role in the development of Alzheimer's disease, interacting with the genetics of the disease. For example, having a stroke increases the risk, and so does head injury (Pope, Shue, & Beck, 2003). These risks may apply more strongly to people who carry the ε4 form of the gene for apolipoprotein. Type 2 diabetes increases the risk for Alzheimer's disease, but the combination of ε4 apolipoprotein and diabetes raises the risk more than 5 times (Peila, Rodriguez, & Launer, 2002). The process of inflammation is also a risk for Alzheimer's, as it is for cardiovascular disease (Martins et al., 2006). This risk may accrue throughout life, with increased risk for people who experience prolonged bouts of inflammation, even during young or middle adulthood (Kamer et al., 2008). Fat intake during middle adulthood also increases the risk (Laitinen et al., 2006), but high cholesterol during older age has no relationship (Reitz et al., 2008). Physical activity—a protective risk factor for many other health problems—also appears to protect against the subsequent development of Alzheimer's disease (Qiu, Kivipelto, & von Strauss, 2011).

Research into risk factors for Alzheimer's disease also reveals some protective factors. Cognitive activity decreases the risk, so people whose jobs demand a high level of cognitive processing are less likely to develop Alzheimer's disease than others with less cognitively demanding jobs (see Would You Believe …? box). Low levels of alcohol consumption cut the risk in half in one study (Ruitenberg et al., 2002). Regular doses of nonsteroidal anti-inflammatory drugs (NSAIDs) also appear to decrease the risk, especially for people who carry the ε4 form of the apolipoprotein gene (Szekely et al., 2008). Therefore, it is possible to modify the genetic risk through this behavior. Many of the risks for Alzheimer's disease overlap with those for cardiovascular disease and cancer, and so do the protective factors. That is, a healthy lifestyle may offer protection for a range of disorders. Table 11.1 presents a summary of these risks and protective factors.

TABLE 11.1   Risks and Protective Factors for the Development of Alzheimer's Disease

Risks	Protective Factors
Age—over age 65 presents increasing risk	
Inheriting apolipoprotein ε4	Inheriting apolipoprotein ε2
Stroke, head injury, or diabetes, especially for those who carry apolipoprotein ε4	
Inflammation	Taking anti-inflammatory drugs (NSAIDs)
High-fat diet during middle adulthood	
Low levels of education	Higher levels of education
Cognitively undemanding job	Cognitively demanding job
	Low-to-moderate alcohol intake
A sedentary lifestyle	Many forms of physical activity, including walking

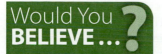

Would You BELIEVE...? Using Your Mind May Help Prevent Losing Your Mind

Although age and genetics contribute to the risk of developing Alzheimer's disease, not everyone of the same age or even with the same genes is at equal risk. Your intelligence, education, job, and even your television viewing habits also contribute to the risk.

People with more education have a lower risk of developing Alzheimer's disease. Because education and IQ are strongly related, separating the protective effect of education is not easy, but one study (Pavlik, Doody, Massman, & Chan, 2006) estimated that IQ score, not educational level, was a better predictor of the progression of Alzheimer's disease. This result suggests that being intelligent offers some protection against this disease. Other research, however, hints that being intelligent is by no means the whole story.

What you do with your mind may be more important than how intelligent you are in combating Alzheimer's disease. For example, the complexity of people's jobs affects the risk. In a study of pairs of twins, in which one twin had Alzheimer's disease and the other did not (Andel et al., 2005), a distinguishing feature was the complexity of work performed by the unaffected twins. Because the study involved twins, genetic factors could not have played a role. The results indicated that those whose work involved more complexity, in terms of tasks with people or data, were likely to be unaffected by the disorder. A study of nearly 1,000 Swedish adults also confirmed this finding (Karp et al., 2009), suggesting that using your mind is protective. Would you also believe that retirement—which, for many people might mean stopping a cognitively complex job—may also increase the risk of cognitive decline? One recent study suggests that it does (Roberts, Fuhrer, Marmot, & Richards, 2011).

Rest assured, working throughout your retirement years is not the only solution to preventing Alzheimer's disease, as work complexity is not the only type of mental activity that may offer protection. A study of leisure time activities (Lindstrom et al., 2005) found that leisure activities during middle age could be protective or risky. People who participated in intellectually stimulating leisure and social activities were at lower risk of Alzheimer's disease during their older years, whereas those who watched television were at increased risk. Indeed, each additional daily hour of television viewing raised the risk. So, using your mind during young and middle age may protect against the development of Alzheimer's disease later in life—presenting another case of "use it or lose it."

Because the symptoms of Alzheimer's include a number of behavior problems that are also symptoms of psychiatric disorders, the disease can be difficult to diagnose. These symptoms occur in a majority of people with Alzheimer's disease (Weiner, Hynan, Bret, & White, 2005). In addition to memory loss, behavioral symptoms include agitation and irritability, sleep difficulties, delusions such as suspiciousness and paranoia, inappropriate sexual behavior, and hallucinations. People with Alzheimer's disease are more likely than others to engage in dangerous behavior (Starkstein, Jorge, Mizrahi, Adrian, & Robinson, 2007). Even individuals with mild Alzheimer's disease show psychiatric symptoms similar to those with more severe cases (Shimabukuro, Awata, & Matsuoka, 2005). These behavioral symptoms can be the source of much distress to patients as well as to their caregivers, and more severe behavioral symptoms predict shorter survival times (Weiner et al., 2005).

The most common psychiatric problem among Alzheimer's patients is depression, with as many as 20% of patients exhibiting symptoms of clinical depression (van Reekum et al., 2005). Depression may even precede the development of Alzheimer's disease, serving as a risk factor. The experience of negative mood is especially common among people in the early phases of the disease and in early-onset Alzheimer's. Those who retain awareness of their problems find their deterioration distressing and respond with feelings of helplessness and depression.

The memory loss that characterizes Alzheimer's patients may first appear in the form of small, ordinary failures of memory, which represent the early stages of the disease (Morris et al., 2001). This memory loss progresses to the point that Alzheimer's patients fail to recognize family members and forget how to perform even routine self-care; former President Reagan experienced these losses. In the early phases of the disease, patients are usually aware of their memory failures, as Reagan was, making this symptom even more distressing.

The common symptoms of paranoia and suspiciousness may also relate to cognitive impairments. Alzheimer's patients may forget where they have put belongings and, because they cannot find their possessions, accuse others of taking them. However, suspicious and accusatory behaviors are not limited to misplaced belongings. Verbal aggression occurs in about 37% of Alzheimer's patients and physical aggression in about 17% (Weiner et al., 2005).

Although difficulties in staying asleep are common among older adults, Alzheimer's patients have even more severe problems than their peers (Tractenberg, Singer, & Kaye, 2005). As a result, these patients tend to wander at all times of the day and night. This behavior can disturb those who sleep in the same house and provide opportunities for patients to injure themselves. Incontinence is also very common in patients with advanced cases of Alzheimer's disease. A pattern of behavioral symptoms, such as Ronald Reagan exhibited, is a strong indication of Alzheimer's disease and the only means of diagnosis before autopsy.

Helping the Patient

At present, Alzheimer's disease remains without a cure. However, incurability and untreatability are two different things; the physical symptoms and other accompanying disorders of Alzheimer's disease are treatable. Although researchers seek to develop drugs that prevent the disease, the primary focus of treatment is the use of drugs to slow its progress. Treatment approaches include drugs for delaying the progression of cognitive deficits and neuroleptic drugs for reducing agitation and aggression. Unfortunately, a systematic review (Seow & Gauthier, 2007) indicated that the drugs that target cognitive deficits offer only modest benefits. For some patients, these drugs slow the progress of the disease by months or even a few years, but they do not stop or cure it. One drug (donepezil) slows the loss of neurons in the hippocampus, the brain location critical for formation of new memories. This finding explains why this drug is effective for some Alzheimer's patients in delaying cognitive losses. Another drug (mematine) may improve cognitive measures and overall functioning. In addition, some researchers (Langa, Foster, & Larson, 2004) have found some benefits of statin drugs, typically prescribed for cardiovascular patients, in slowing the dementia associated with Alzheimer's disease.

Behavioral approaches can be helpful for people with Alzheimer's disease. These approaches include sensory stimulation and reality orientation to help Alzheimer's patients retain their cognitive abilities. Several reviews (Hulme, Wright, Crocker, Oluboyede, & House, 2010; O'Connor, Ames, Gardner, & King, 2009; Verkaik, Van Weert, & Francke, 2005) indicated that a few programs demonstrate effectiveness. Those that show the most promise are programs that provide pleasant stimulation, such as music, aromatherapy, exposure to sunlight, and muscle relaxation training, and programs that concentrate on cognitive skills and problem solving. Music therapy may be more useful than other types of sensory stimulation (Svansdottir & Snaedal, 2006), and is the one approach that most consistently benefits Alzheimer's patients (Hulme et al., 2010; O'Connor et al., 2009; Verkaik et al., 2005). A meta-analysis of programs to develop cognitive skills (Sitzer, Twamley, & Jeste, 2006) indicates that such programs can be helpful in improving memory, verbal and visual learning, and activities of daily living. In addition, caregivers can manage behavior problems of Alzheimer's patients through improvements in communication and modification of the environment to help decrease confusion and manage problem behaviors (O'Connor et al., 2009; Yuhas, McGowan, Fontaine, Czech, & Gambrell-Jones, 2006). For example, locking exit doors may prevent wandering. For those who get lost in their own homes, labeling the doors can be helpful.

Although none of these treatments can cure Alzheimer's disease, most will help control undesirable behaviors and alleviate some of the distressing symptoms of the disease. Any treatment that can delay symptoms of Alzheimer's disease can make a significant difference in the number of cases and in the costs of management (Haan & Wallace, 2004). In the early phases of Alzheimer's disease, both patients and their families are distressed by its symptoms, but as the patient worsens and loses awareness, the stress of Alzheimer's becomes more severe for the family. The burden of caregiving is one factor in the decision to have a family member institutionalized (Mausbach et al., 2004), which adds to the cost of this disease.

Helping the Family

As with other chronic illnesses, Alzheimer's disease affects not only patients but also family members, who bear the burden of caregiving. Some of the distressing symptoms can make caregiving difficult—caring for a spouse or parent who may be abusive and no longer recognizes you is a very difficult task. Cognitive impairments lead to changes in behavior that may make the affected one no longer seem like the same person.

Caregiving affects families in industrialized and developing countries similarly: Caring for a family member with a dementing disease such as Alzheimer's creates a burden for families (Prince, 2004). This burden is emotional and practical. The problems of taking care of an Alzheimer's patient require time, demand new skills, and greatly disrupt family routine.

In the United States (Cancian & Oliker, 2000) and around the world (Prince, 2004), the caregiver role is occupied mostly by women. In a study of those providing care for older family members with memory impairments (Chumbler, Grimm, Cody, & Beck, 2003), almost 70% were women; daughters were about twice as likely as spouses to be providing such care. Unfortunately, the anger and suspiciousness that are common symptoms of Alzheimer's disease are more distressing to female than to male caregivers (Bédard et al., 2005), so that women tend to feel more burdened by providing care than men do. Their tasks may be burdensome indeed. A survey of Alzheimer's caregivers (Georges et al., 2008) indicated that these tasks may occupy more than 10 hours a day when the recipients of care are late-stage dementia patients.

The chronic stress of caregiving makes these family members of interest to psychoneuroimmunologists, who study how chronic stress affects the immune system. Janice Kiecolt-Glaser and her colleagues (Kiecolt-Glaser, McGuire, Robles, & Glaser, 2002) have studied Alzheimer's caregivers and found that they experience poorer physical and psychological health and poorer immunological function than people of similar age who are not caregivers. Also, the level of impairment of the Alzheimer's patient is directly related to the level of distress in the caregiver (Robinson-Whelen, Tada, MacCallum, McGuire, & Kiecolt-Glaser, 2001); that is, the more impaired the patient, the more distressed the caregiver. Furthermore, their distress does not decrease when their caregiving ends (Aneshensel, Botticello, & Yamamoto-Mitani, 2004). Thus, caregiving imposes severe burdens, extending even after the death of the Alzheimer's patient.

Caregivers now have more assistance available to them. For example, programs now exist to help people develop the skills they will need to be effective caregivers for someone with Alzheimer's disease (Paun, Farran, Perraud, & Loukissa, 2004). Caregivers do not feel so overwhelmed when they have the knowledge and skills to perform the necessary tasks. Reviews of such educational interventions (Coon & Evans, 2009; Gallagher-Thompson & Coon, 2007) indicate that this approach is successful in reducing stress and depression and improving self-efficacy and well-being. Support groups can also be sources of information about caring for patients and about community resources that provide respite care. Many support groups exist to provide information and emotional support for caregivers. In addition, the Internet can be a source of support. Online and telephone-based services provide support to caregivers who have difficulty obtaining assistance from other sources (Glueckauf, Ketterson, Loomis, & Dages, 2004; Wilz, Schinkothe, & Soellner, 2011).

Alzheimer's caregivers frequently experience feelings of loss for the relationship that they once shared with the patient; these feelings of loss may begin with a partner's diagnosis (Robinson, Clare, & Evans, 2005). Making sense of dementia and adjusting to the loss is a strain for partner and family. However, only 19% of those caring for someone with Alzheimer's disease reported only strains (Sanders, 2005); most found positive aspects to their caregiving, such as feelings of mastery and personal and spiritual growth. In most ways, Nancy Reagan was more fortunate than the typical caregiver. She was able to hire others to help her provide care for her husband, but she and the Reagan family felt helpless and frustrated as they saw the former president progressively losing abilities (Ellis, 2004). Nancy said that she needed and appreciated the support of the many people who sent letters. Nancy's feelings of isolation and frustration were typical of caregivers for Alzheimer's patients, but Nancy and the Reagan family struggled to find meaning in their experience. One way that they did so was by becoming activists in the effort to find a cure or prevention for Alzheimer's disease.

IN SUMMARY

Alzheimer's disease is a progressive, degenerative disease of the brain that affects cognitive functioning, especially memory. Other symptoms include agitation and irritability, paranoia and other delusions, sleep disorders, wandering, depression, and incontinence. These symptoms are also indicative of some psychiatric disorders, making Alzheimer's disease difficult to diagnose and distressing to both patients and caregivers.

Increasing age is a risk factor for Alzheimer's disease, with as many as half the people over 85 exhibiting symptoms. Both genetics and environment seem to play a role in development of the disease; both early- and late-onset varieties exist.

At this point, treatment is largely oriented toward slowing the progress of the disease, managing the negative symptoms, and helping family caregivers cope with the stress. Drug treatments intended to slow the progress of the disease have limited effectiveness but help some people. Management of symptoms can include providing sensory and cognitive stimulation to slow cognitive loss and changing the environment to make care less difficult. Training and support are also desirable for those who provide care to Alzheimer's patients because caregivers are burdened by the demands of caring for someone with this disease.

Adjusting to Diabetes

In 1989, actress Halle Berry had a role in a television sitcom and was working longer, harder hours than she ever had (Siegler, 2003). She had no opportunity to rest when she was tired or to eat a candy bar when she felt that her blood glucose level was low. Berry has **diabetes mellitus**, and her failure to take care of herself caused her to go into a coma that lasted 7 days. Despite that terrifying experience, Berry says that she left the hospital feeling better than she had in years. She sees the experience as a "wake-up call" that forced her to attend to her health. Now she is very careful about her diet, exercise, and stress. She regulated her blood glucose level by taking insulin, but in October 2007, Berry announced that she had cured herself of diabetes through a healthy diet and no longer took insulin (Goldman, 2007). Her remarks caused a furor because Berry had been diagnosed with Type 1 diabetes, for which there is no cure; if she no longer requires insulin injections, then her diabetes was really Type 2 all along. Her diagnosis, behavior, and even her misunderstanding of her disease illustrate some of the challenges presented by diabetes.

The Physiology of Diabetes

Before examining the psychological issues in the management of diabetes, let's look more closely at the physiology of the disorder. The **pancreas**, located below the

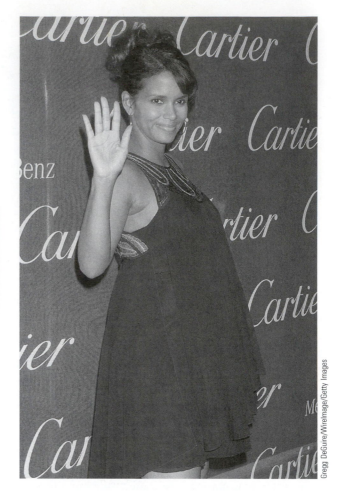

Actress Halle Berry has followed a diet and exercise regimen to control her diabetes and managed to have a healthy pregnancy.

stomach, produces different types of secretions. The **islet cells** of the pancreas produce several hormones, two of which, glucagon and insulin, are critically important in metabolism. **Glucagon** stimulates the release of glucose and therefore acts to elevate blood sugar levels. The action of **insulin** is the opposite. Insulin decreases the level of glucose in the blood by causing tissue cell membranes to open so glucose can enter the cells more freely. Disorders of the islet cells result in difficulties in sugar metabolism. Diabetes mellitus is a disorder caused by insulin deficiency. If the islet cells do not produce adequate insulin, sugar cannot move from the blood to the cells for use. Lack of insulin prevents the body from regulating blood sugar level. Excessive sugar accumulates in the blood and also appears in abnormally high levels in the urine. When

Halle Berry went into a coma in 1989, she thought she was going to die, and she might have. Both coma and death are possibilities for uncontrolled diabetes.

The two types of diabetes mellitus are (1) insulin-dependent diabetes mellitus (IDDM), also known as Type 1 diabetes, and (2) non-insulin-dependent diabetes mellitus (NIDDM), also known as Type 2 diabetes. Type 1 diabetes is an autoimmune disease that occurs when the person's immune system attacks the insulin-making cells in the pancreas, destroying them (Permutt, Wasson, & Cox, 2005). This process usually occurs before age 30 and leaves the person without the capability to produce insulin and thus dependent on insulin injections. Type 1 diabetes was Halle Berry's diagnosis when she fell into a coma; her age and symptoms were consistent with Type 1 diabetes, but that diagnosis may have been incorrect. People with Type 1 diabetes do not recover from this disease.

Halle Berry received a diagnosis of Type 1 diabetes and followed the demands and restrictions of that regimen for years, including insulin injections, daily exercise with a personal trainer, and a low-fat/low-carbohydrate diet with lots of vegetables, fish, and chicken but few fruits and sweets. In 2007, Berry announced that she had "weaned" herself off insulin and now considered herself to have Type 2 diabetes (Goldman, 2007). Medical experts said that she was mistaken; no one can make a transition from Type 1 to Type 2 diabetes. It is likely that her initial diagnosis was mistaken and that she always had Type 2 diabetes.

Type 2 diabetes is the most common type of diabetes, representing 90% to 95% of all diagnosed cases of diabetes (CDC, 2011c). Until a few years ago, Type 2 diabetes was called *adult-onset diabetes* because it typically developed in people past the age of 30. However, Type 2 diabetes increasingly appears among children and adolescents, accounting for at least 33% of diabetes cases among this age group (Ludwig & Ebbeling, 2001). This trend appears not only in the United States but also in developed countries throughout the world (Malecka-Tendera & Mazur, 2006). For both children and adults, Type 2 diabetes affects ethnic minorities disproportionately, and those who develop this disease are often overweight, sedentary, and poor (Agardh, Allebeck, Hallqvist, Moradi, & Sidorchuk, 2011; CDC, 2011c). The characteristics of both types of diabetes are shown in Table 11.2. A third type of diabetes is *gestational diabetes*, which develops in some women during pregnancy. Gestational diabetes ends when the pregnancy is completed, but the disorder complicates pregnancy and presents a risk for the development of Type 2 diabetes in the future (Reader, 2007).

The management of all types of diabetes requires lifestyle changes in order for the person to adjust to the disease and to minimize health complications. Diabetes requires daily monitoring of blood sugar levels and relatively strict compliance with both medical and lifestyle regimens to regulate blood sugar. Like other chronic diseases, diabetes can be controlled but not cured.

In addition to the danger of coma, the inability to regulate blood sugar often causes people with diabetes to have a host of other health problems. Oral or injected insulin can control the most severe symptoms

TABLE 11.2 Characteristics of Type 1 and Type 2 Diabetes Mellitus

Type 1	Type 2
Onset occurs before age 30	Onset may occur during childhood or adulthood
Patients are often normal weight or underweight	Patients are often overweight
Patients experience frequent thirst and urination	Patients may or may not experience frequent thirst and urination
Caused primarily by genetic factors	Caused by both lifestyle factors (poor diet, low physical activity, obesity) and genetic factors
Has no socioeconomic correlates	Affects more poor than middle-class people
Management involves insulin injections and dietary change	Management involves physical activity and dietary change, medication, and sometimes insulin injections
Carries risk of kidney damage	Carries risk of cardiovascular damage
Accounts for 5% of diabetics	Accounts for 90%–95% of diabetics

of insulin deficiency but does not mimic the normal production of insulin. People with diabetes still experience elevated levels of blood sugar, which may lead to the development of (1) damage to the blood vessels, leaving diabetics prone to cardiovascular disease (diabetics are twice as likely as other people to have hypertension and to develop heart disease); (2) damage to the retina, leaving diabetics at risk for blindness (diabetics are 17 times as likely to go blind as nondiabetics); and (3) kidney diseases, leaving diabetics prone to renal failure. In addition, diabetics, compared with nondiabetics, have double the risk of cancer of the pancreas (Huxley, Ansary-Moghaddam, de González, Barzi, & Woodward, 2005).

The Impact of Diabetes

The diagnosis of any chronic disease produces an impact on patients for two reasons: First, the emotional reaction to having a lifelong incurable disease, and second, the lifestyle adjustments required by the disease. For diabetes that begins during childhood, both children and their parents must come to terms with the child's loss of health (Lowes, Gregory, & Lyne, 2005) and the management of the disorder, which includes careful restrictions in diet, insulin injections, and recommendations for regular exercise. Dietary restrictions include careful scheduling of meals and snacks as well as adherence to a set of allowed and disallowed foods.

Diabetics must test their blood sugar levels at least once (and possibly several times) a day, drawing a blood sample and using the testing equipment correctly. The results guide diabetics to appropriate levels of insulin. Injections are the standard mode of administration for Type 1 diabetics, and the daily (or more frequent) injections can be a source of fear and stress. Alternative modes of testing and insulin administration are desirable because drawing blood samples and taking injections are painful, and diabetics tend to perform less testing and fewer injections than would be optimal in managing their blood sugar.

Alternatives to finger-prick testing are available, but their accuracy is not as good as that of standard testing. Other modes of insulin administration exist, including external or implanted insulin pumps. Pumps are appropriate for some individuals, including children and adolescents, providing more stable blood glucose levels (Pickup & Renard, 2008). Although blood glucose testing and insulin administration are

critically important, these aspects of diabetes care present difficulties for most diabetics.

Non-insulin-dependent (Type 2) diabetes often does not require insulin injections, but this type of diabetes does require lifestyle changes and oral medication. African Americans, Hispanic Americans, and Native Americans are at higher risk for Type 2 diabetes than are European Americans (CDC, 2011c), and being overweight is a risk for all groups. Indeed, gaining weight increases, and losing weight decreases, the risk for Type 2 diabetes (Black et al., 2005). Even bariatric surgery, a medical treatment for extreme obesity, resolves Type 2 diabetes in a majority of diabetics who undergo the procedure (Buchwald et al., 2009). More frequently, the components of treatment for Type 2 diabetes are behavioral methods for weight loss and a healthy diet.

Type 2 diabetics must deal with dietary restrictions and attend to their schedule of oral medication. Diabetes often affects sexual functioning in both men and women, and diabetic women who become pregnant often have problem pregnancies. Halle Berry announced that she was pregnant in 2007 (Bonilla, 2007). Although Halle Berry said that she felt some fear in connection with her pregnancy, she expressed a great deal more optimism and joy. Her fame and wealth allowed her to obtain excellent medical care, and her faithful adherence to her diabetes care helped minimize the potential complications; she gave birth to a healthy baby girl in 2008.

Type 2 diabetes is more likely to cause circulatory problems, leaving these individuals prone to cardiovascular problems, which is their leading cause of death. Both women (Hu et al., 2000) and men (Lotufo et al., 2001) with Type 2 diabetes are at dramatically increased risk for death from all causes, but especially from cardiovascular disease.

Some diabetics deny the seriousness of their condition and ignore the need to restrict diet and take medication. Others acknowledge the seriousness of their problems but believe that the recommended regimen will be ineffective (Skinner, Hampson, & Fife-Schaw, 2002). Others become aggressive; they either direct their aggression outward and refuse to comply with their treatment regimen or turn their aggression inward and become depressed. Finally, many diabetics become dependent and rely on others to take care of them, thus taking no active part in their own care. All these reactions can interfere with the management of blood sugar levels and lead to serious health complications, including death.

Health Psychology's Involvement With Diabetes

Health psychologists seek to both research and treat diabetes (Gonder-Frederick, Cox, & Ritterband, 2002). Psychologist Richard Rubin became head of the American Diabetes Association in 2006, and he emphasized the role of psychology: "I want more and more people to understand that behavior and emotion play a part in diabetes and how that affects human and economic outcomes" (quoted in Dittmann, 2005, p. 35).

Researchers have concentrated on the effect of stress on glucose metabolism, the ways that diabetics understand and conceptualize their illness, the dynamics of families with diabetic children, and the factors that influence patient compliance with medical regimens. Health psychologists orient their efforts toward improving adherence to medical regimens so diabetics can control their blood glucose levels and minimize health complications.

Stress may play two roles in diabetes: as a possible cause of diabetes and as a factor in the regulation of blood sugar in diabetics. To examine the role of family stress in the development of diabetes, a team of researchers (Sepa, Wahlberg, Vaarala, Frodi, & Ludvigsson, 2005) followed a large group of infants for the first year of their lives, measuring family stress and taking blood samples to test for signs of the autoimmune response that underlies Type 1 diabetes. Indeed, stress predicted the development of this response. However, a prospective study with Native Americans (Daniels, Goldberg, Jacobsen, & Welty, 2006) found no relationship between stress during adulthood and subsequent development of Type 2 diabetes.

Clearer evidence exists showing that stress affects glucose metabolism and control among diabetics. A meta-analytic review shows that having a stress-prone personality and experiencing stressful events both predict poorer metabolic control (Chida & Hamer, 2008). A study of people with Type 2 diabetes (Surwit et al., 2002) showed that adding a stress management component to diabetes education has a small but significant effect on blood sugar levels. Depression is another factor that affects diabetics and worsens blood glucose control (Lustman & Clouse, 2005). Thus, negative emotions can adversely affect diabetes, and interventions to manage stress and depression can be a worthwhile (and cost-effective) component for diabetes management programs.

Social support appears to be particularly important for metabolic control, as poor social support is the psychosocial factor most strongly tied to poor diabetes management (Chida & Hamer, 2008). Support from family and friends may promote greater glucose monitoring and physical activity, whereas support from health professionals may increase meal plan adherence (Khan, Stephens, Franks, Rook, & Salem, 2012; Rosland et al., 2008). Among Latinos with Type 2 diabetes, the availability of support from sources such as family, friends, health care providers, and the community together predicted better illness management and lower depression (Fortmann, Gallo & Philis-Tsimkias, 2011). However, support need not come from face-to-face contact with another person to be helpful. For example, several recent interventions use text messaging to provide supportive information to help patients' metabolic control. These interventions are generally effective, for both adolescents and adults (Krishna & Boren, 2008; Liang et al., 2011). For example, supportive text-messaging interventions have improved metabolic control among children and adolescents with Type 1 diabetes in Scotland (Franklin, Waller, Pagliari, & Greene, 2006) and Austria (Rami, Popow, Horn, Waldhoer, & Schober, 2006).

Health psychologists also research diabetic patients' understanding of their illness and how that understanding affects their behavior. Both patients and health care workers assume that patients understand the disease and recognize the symptoms of high and low blood glucose levels. These assumptions are not always true. For example, people's perception of the risk of developing diabetes is neither accurate nor based on their existing risk factors, even for physicians (Walker, Mertz, Kalten, & Flynn, 2003). Rather, having a close friend or family member with diabetes was a circumstance that raised the perception of vulnerability (Montgomery, Erblich, DiLorenzo, & Bovbjerg, 2003). Perceptions also affect how people with diabetes care for themselves. Their conceptualizations of diabetes affect their coping behavior (Searle, Norman, Thompson, & Vedhara, 2007). For example, belief in the consequences of diabetes predicted the use of problem-focused coping strategies, and those who believed they were able to control their diabetes were more likely to use their medication.

Inaccurate beliefs can have a significant impact on self-care. In a study of the interrelationships among beliefs, personality characteristics, and self-care behavior among diabetics (Skinner et al., 2002), beliefs emerged as the most important component. The perceived effectiveness of the treatment regimen predicted all aspects of diabetes self-care. This finding emphasizes the importance of diabetes education in building adherence to the diet, exercise, and medication regimen that is necessary to control blood glucose levels.

Complete adherence to the medication and lifestyle regimen is rare (Cramer, 2004). As Chapter 4 explored, a number of factors relate to poor adherence, and diabetes combines several of these factors. First, complexity makes adherence more difficult, and second, making lifestyle changes is more difficult than taking medication. Diabetics must do both. Third, they must also perform blood sugar testing several times a day, even when they feel well. Fourth, their adherence will not cure the disease, and serious complications may be years away. Thus, poor adherence is common, and improving adherence is of primary concern to psychologists involved in providing care for diabetics.

The role of health psychology in diabetes management is likely to expand because behavioral components are important in controlling blood glucose levels. Indeed, lifestyle changes can prevent the development of diabetes in individuals who exhibit blood glucose tolerance problems (Gillies et al., 2007). For example, a lifestyle intervention conducted in China (Li et al., 2008) showed a remarkable reduction in long-term incidence of Type 2 diabetes. Diabetic adults who participated in a 6-year, group-based diet and exercise intervention reported significantly lower incidence of diabetes during the course of the intervention, as well as at a 20-year follow-up. A behavioral component can add to the effectiveness of educational programs for diabetic patients. Education alone is not adequate in helping diabetics follow their regimen (Rutten, 2005; Savage, Farrell, McManus, & Grey, 2010). Because situational factors such as stress and social pressure to eat the wrong foods affect adherence, programs with a behavioral skills training component might be a valuable addition to diabetes management training. A program that fostered feelings of control (Macrodimitris & Endler, 2001) improved diabetics' adherence to diet, exercise, and blood glucose testing, and another program (Rosal et al., 2005) used a cognitive behavioral framework to increase self-management skills in low-income, Spanish-speaking diabetics. In sum, psychosocial interventions show promise in helping diabetics stick to their management regimen (Savage et al., 2010).

IN SUMMARY

Diabetes mellitus is a chronic disease that results from failure of the islet cells of the pancreas to manufacture sufficient insulin, affecting blood glucose levels and producing effects in many organ systems. Type 1 diabetes is an autoimmune disease that typically appears during childhood; Type 2 diabetes also affects children but is more typical of people over age 30. People with diabetes must maintain a strict regimen of diet, exercise, and insulin supplements to avoid the serious cardiovascular, neurological, and renal complications of the disorder.

As with other chronic diseases, a diagnosis of diabetes mellitus produces distress for both patients and their families. Health psychologists study adjustment to the disorder and compliance with the necessary lifestyle changes. Few people with diabetes adhere to all aspects of blood glucose testing, medication, diet, and exercise that minimize the risks of health complications. Skills-training programs show some success in helping diabetics manage their disorder, but health care professionals need to find ways to encourage the development of responsibility and self-management in order to put diabetics in charge of their own health.

The Impact of Asthma

Seeing David Beckham out of breath is not unusual. The international star of soccer, a sport that requires remarkable aerobic fitness, is renowned for his two-decade long career that includes the most World Cup appearances for any player on the English national team.

In 2009, a photographer caught David Beckham out of breath on the sidelines of a soccer field, but this time it *was* unusual. David Beckham was using an asthma inhaler. Until that day, the sports world did not realize that David Beckham suffered from asthma, as he had since he was a small boy. After this photograph surfaced to the public, Beckham revealed that he takes medicine regularly to control his condition. Despite the challenges that any person with asthma faces, David Beckham remains optimistic about his health, saying "I've played 65 games a season for the last 20 years, so it doesn't affect the future" (*Daily Mail*, 2009).

The number of people with asthma grew throughout the 1980s and into the 1990s in the United States

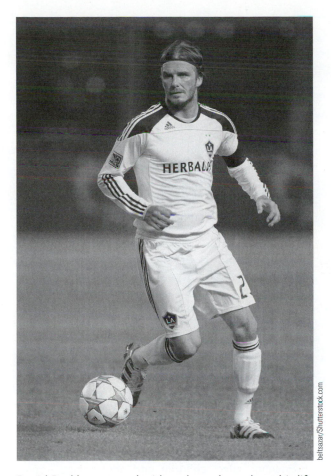

David Beckham coped with asthma throughout his life and soccer career.

but began to decrease by the late 1990s (American Lung Association, 2007). About 23 million adults in the United States have asthma (7.7%), but the rate is highest for children and adolescents between 5 and 17 years old. For all age groups, the rates are higher for African Americans than for other ethnic groups. The death rate from asthma is not high, and that mortality rate has decreased in recent years, but asthma is the largest cause of disability among children and the leading cause of missed school days, making it a serious health problem in the United States.

The Disease of Asthma

Asthma is a chronic inflammatory disease that causes constriction of the bronchial tubes, preventing air from passing freely. People experiencing an asthma attack will wheeze, cough, and have trouble breathing; such an attack can be fatal. At other times they appear to be fine, but the underlying inflammation remains (Cohn, Elias, & Chupp, 2004).

Asthma shares some features with chronic obstructive lung diseases (COLD) such as chronic bronchitis and emphysema, but asthma also differs in some ways (Barnes, 2008). All of these conditions involve inflammation, though not to the same extent or through the same immune system mechanisms. But the most important difference is that people with COLD experience constant problems, whereas people with asthma may go for long periods of time without any problems in breathing.

The cause of asthma is not understood. Indeed, asthma may not be one disease but rather a number of diseases that share symptoms yet have differences in underlying pathologies (Wenzel, 2006). Until recently, experts believed that asthma was an allergic reaction to substances in the environment, but several newer explanations involve more complex reactions of the immune system (Cohn et al., 2004; Renz, Blümer, Virna, Sel, & Garn, 2006). One view holds that a genetic vulnerability makes some infants' immune systems respond with an allergic reaction to substances in the environment that other infants' immune systems encounter without problems. This *diathesis–stress model* is a variation on the traditional view that asthma is an allergic reaction triggered by environmental allergens. These allergens include an assortment of common substances such as tobacco smoke, household dust (along with dust mites), cockroaches, animal dander, and environmental pollutants. People with the vulnerability who are exposed to the substance to which they are sensitive develop asthma; those who are not exposed fail to develop asthma or show such mild symptoms that they are not diagnosed.

Another view, called the *hygiene hypothesis*, holds that asthma is a result of the cleanliness that has become common in modern societies (von Hertzen & Haahtela, 2004). Infants have undeveloped immune systems, and in hygienic environments they encounter too little dirt and too few bacteria, leaving their immune systems underprepared to deal with these substances. Exposure then leads to overresponsiveness, which produces inflammation; this inflammation forms the basis for asthma. Support for this hypothesis comes from studies of children in rural Central Europe (Ege et al., 2011). Children who grew up on farms had greater exposure to bacteria and fungi than children who did not grow up on farms. Consistent with the hygiene hypothesis, greater exposure to microbes related to decreased risk of asthma. A refinement of the hygiene hypothesis (Martinez, 2001) combines elements of genetic vulnerability and early exposure to substances in the environment that influence immune system development to either sensitize or protect children from asthma and allergic conditions.

Both of these views (and the combination) are consistent with some of the evidence about asthma. Support for the genetic vulnerability view comes from a study of the Hutterites, a religious group that immigrated to the United States from Europe in the 1870s (Shell, 2000). Symptoms of asthma are very uncommon among the Hutterites, who nevertheless show high rates of the type of inflammation that characterizes asthma. The rural, farming lifestyle of these people puts them into contact with few of the triggers for asthma attacks, leaving these vulnerable individuals without serious symptoms. However, the children of parents from underdeveloped countries who immigrate to industrialized countries tend to have asthma at rates similar to those of other children in the industrialized country (von Hertzen & Haahtela, 2004). That is, the combination of genetic vulnerability, underdevelopment of the immune system, and exposure to triggers results in asthma.

As the hygiene hypothesis suggests, asthma is more common in developed countries that emphasize cleanliness and a hygienic environment for infants. For example, asthma is less common in rural China than in the United States, Sweden, Australia, and New Zealand (von Hertzen & Haahtela, 2004). However, within the United States, asthma is more common in the urban inner city, where air pollution is more common, and high levels of air pollution increase the risk of developing asthma (Islam et al., 2007). In addition, asthma varies with ethnicity, and African Americans are more vulnerable than people from other ethnic groups (American Lung Association, 2007).

Other risk factors for asthma include sedentary lifestyle and obesity (Gold & Wright, 2005). People take few deep breaths when they are sedentary, which may be the link between lack of exercise and asthma. In addition, staying indoors exposes people to some of the allergens that provoke asthma attacks. The link between asthma and obesity is significant: Obese people are 2 to 3 times more likely to have asthma than nonobese people. Psychological factors also show a relationship with the development of asthma (Chida,

Hamer, & Steptoe, 2008), serving as predictors of its development and appearing as a result of living with the disease. Depression is a specific psychological factor that relates to asthma (Strine, Mokdad, Balluz, Berry, & Gonzalez, 2008). Although the factors related to the development of asthma are complex and not completely understood, the triggers for attacks are better known.

Triggers are substances or circumstances that cause the development of symptoms, provoking the narrowing of the airways that causes difficulty in breathing. The substances include allergens such as mold, pollen, dust and dust mites, cockroaches, and animal dander; infections of the respiratory tract; tobacco or wood smoke; and irritants such as air pollutants, chemical sprays, or other environmental pollution (Harder, 2004). The circumstances include exercise and emotional reactions such as stress or fear. Any of these substances and experiences may provoke an attack, but most people with asthma are sensitive to only a few. Identifying an individual's triggers is part of managing asthma.

Managing Asthma

Managing asthma shows some similarities (and similar problems) to managing diabetes. Both disorders require frequent contact with the health care system, can be life threatening, affect children and adolescents, impose restrictions on lifestyle, and pose substantial adherence problems (Elliott, 2006). People with diabetes may manage their blood sugar levels so that they have no symptoms, but even with careful management, people with asthma have attacks. The underlying inflammation of the bronchial tract is always present, but a person with asthma may go for weeks or months without an attack. Minimizing attacks is the primary goal of managing asthma. Daily attention to symptoms and status improves the chances of avoiding attacks, and behaviors are critical.

Managing asthma requires a variety of medications as well as learning personal triggers and avoiding them (Courtney, McCarter, & Pollart, 2005). To decrease the chances of an attack, people with asthma must take medication, which is usually an anti-inflammatory corticosteroid or some other medication that decreases the respiratory inflammation that underlies asthma. These drugs require daily attention and have unpleasant side effects, such as weight gain and lack of energy. The schedule may be very complicated, and as Chapter 4 detailed, complexity decreases compliance with medical regimens. The side effects also contribute to problems in adherence. Thus, adherence to their preventive medication is a major problem for people with asthma, especially for children and adolescents (Asthma Action America, 2004; Elliott, 2006).

When people with asthma have an attack, they have trouble breathing or cannot breathe. Gasping for breath, they either use a bronchodilator to inhale medication that relieves the symptoms or go to a hospital emergency room for treatment (Asthma Action America, 2004). If used improperly, bronchodilators produce a type of "high," and asthma experts believe that most people with asthma rely on bronchodilators too much and on preventive medication too little. More than 20% of people with asthma use their inhalers improperly, decreasing the effectiveness of this important device (Molimard & Le Gros, 2008). Relying on emergency rooms for managing asthma is an expensive choice and contributes to rising medical costs.

A large-scale survey (Asthma Action America, 2004) revealed widespread misunderstandings and misperceptions concerning asthma among parents and other caregivers. Misunderstandings included what underlies the condition and what constitutes adequate management; misperceptions included the frequency of children's symptoms. People with asthma also hold incorrect beliefs about the disease (Elliott, 2006). For example, they may believe that asthma is not a serious disease or that it is an intermittent disease that does not require daily care. All of these misperceptions may affect appropriate care.

Boosting self-care and increasing adherence to medication regimens are major goals for improving asthma care. A number of interventions have targeted these goals, with some success. Many of these interventions have been oriented toward education for people with asthma, assuming that when people understand the severity of the disease and the steps that are necessary to manage it, they will adhere. Research does not support those assumptions; interventions that are basically educational may increase knowledge but are not very successful in changing behavior (Bussey-Smith & Rossen, 2007; Coffman, Cabana, Halpin, & Yelin, 2008). However, a text-messaging intervention that delivered asthma information that was tailored to young adults' beliefs was effective in improving adherence (Petrie, Perry, Broadbent, & Weinman, 2012). Interventions with a behavioral component, such as developing self-care

(Guevara, Wolf, Grum, & Clark, 2003) or providing a written action plan (Bhogal, Zemek, & Ducharme, 2006), tend to be more successful. Adhering to the medication and behavioral regimen to control this disorder is a challenge for people with asthma, but behavioral interventions represent a promising strategy for helping them take their medication and avoid situations that precipitate attacks.

IN SUMMARY

Asthma is a chronic disease that involves inflammation of the bronchial tubes, which leads to difficulties in breathing. Substances such as smoke or allergens and situations such as fear can trigger attacks that have symptoms of coughing, wheezing, and choking. The cause for the inflammation that underlies asthma remains unknown, but theories include a genetic component and an overreaction of the immune system that occurs in hygienic environments.

Asthma usually develops during childhood, and children and adolescents experience problems in coping with their disease. People with asthma need to take medication to decrease the chances of attacks and identify their triggers so as to avoid them. The complex schedule of medications and their unpleasant side effects contribute to adherence problems. A major goal of treatment is to help people with asthma take medication to prevent attacks rather than rely on inhaled medications to stop symptoms or use hospital emergency room assistance. Behavioral strategies to increase compliance and self-management skills have shown some success.

Dealing With HIV and AIDS

Earvin "Magic" Johnson was the best basketball player in the world when he retired in 1991 (Beacham, 2011). That retirement came as a surprise, but his announcement that he was HIV positive was more so. Johnson learned of his HIV infection through a routine physical examination. Until that announcement, most people considered HIV infection to be a disease of gay European Americans, and Johnson was neither. Johnson's openness about his HIV status helped to change public opinion about this disease, and his celebrity status enabled him to raise money for HIV research and education. More than 20 years after his diagnosis, Johnson remains healthy and is an advocate for increasing minority participation in clinical trials. He attributes his continued health to someone who participated in a clinical trial for the many drugs developed to treat HIV infection (Gambrill, 2008).

AIDS is a disorder in which the immune system loses its effectiveness, leaving the body defenseless against bacterial, viral, fungal, parasitic, cancerous, and other opportunistic diseases. Without the immune system, the body cannot protect itself against the many organisms that can invade it and cause damage. (For a more complete discussion of the immune system and its function, see Chapter 6.) The danger from AIDS comes from the opportunistic infections that start when the immune system no longer functions effectively. In this way, AIDS is similar to the immune deficiency in children who have been born without immune system organs and are susceptible to a variety of infections.

AIDS is the result of exposure to a contagious virus, the **human immunodeficiency virus (HIV)**. So far, researchers have discovered two variants of the human immunodeficiency virus: HIV-1, which causes most AIDS cases in the United States; and HIV-2, which is responsible for most AIDS cases in Africa, although some HIV-2 cases have appeared in the United States. The progression from HIV infection to AIDS varies, and people such as Magic Johnson who are HIV positive may remain free of AIDS symptoms for many years.

Incidence and Mortality Rates for HIV/AIDS

AIDS appears to be a relatively new disease, first recognized in 1981 and identified in 1983. The disease originated in Africa in a virus that affects monkeys (Moore, 2004). Nobody knows how and when the virus came to infect humans. The first confirmed case of AIDS appeared in the Congo in 1959, but the disease was very limited. During the 1960s, the disease spread to Haiti and from there to other places in North America and the world (Gilbert et al., 2007). Both the number of new cases and the number of deaths from AIDS spread during the 1980s.

In the mid-1990s, death rates from AIDS declined sharply in the United States, but only recently has the rate begun to level worldwide (UNAIDS, 2010). AIDS remains among the leading causes of death in the world, and the leading cause of death in Africa. According to one estimate (Lamptey, 2002), AIDS is the deadliest plague in history. Almost 40 million people were infected by 2001; when those people die, HIV will surpass the number of people killed by the bubonic plague in the 14th century. About 2.6 million people acquire HIV infection each year, which represents a decline in the rate of infection but also poses a number that extends this plague (UNAIDS, 2010). No effective vaccine yet exists (Callaway, 2011), but drugs now extend the lives of people who are infected (UNAIDS, 2010).

In 1992, the Centers for Disease Control and Prevention (CDC, 1992) revised its definition of HIV infection so that incidence figures from 1992 and subsequent years are not directly comparable to earlier figures. The number of cases in 1992 appears to rise sharply (see Figure 11.1), but this count includes a large backlog of people who in previous years would not have been classified as having AIDS. As Figure 11.1 shows, AIDS cases reported each year (incidence) began a steady decline after 1992.

Despite these declines, HIV and AIDS disproportionately affect minority ethnic groups in the United States, especially by the epidemics affecting heterosexuals and injection drug users. As Magic Johnson points out (Beacham, 2011), African Americans are the largest segment of the U.S. population with HIV. Although African Americans represent only 14% of the U.S. population, they account for 44% of all new HIV infections (CDC, 2011a). This ethnic disparity is particularly strong among women, with 57% of new diagnoses among women in 2009 occurring in African American women (CDC, 2011a). Hispanic Americans are also disproportionately affected by HIV, with 2009 new infection rate nearly 3 times as high as that of European Americans. Figure 11.2 shows the percentages of men and women of different ethnic backgrounds infected with HIV.

Age is also a factor in HIV infection. Young adults are more likely to acquire an HIV infection than other age groups, largely due to their risky behaviors, lack of information about HIV, and lack of power to protect themselves from unsafe sex (Mantell, Stein, & Susser, 2008). For example, in the United States, 39% of all new HIV infections are among adolescents and young adults aged 15–29 (CDC, 2011b). Recent analyses indicate that this situation is improving, at least in Africa. People over age 50 are less likely to acquire an infection

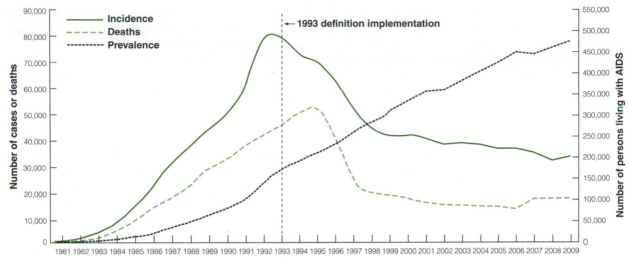

FIGURE 11.1   Incidence, prevalence, and deaths from AIDS cases by year, United States, 1981–2009.

Source: "Update, AIDS—United States, 2000," by R. M. Klevens & J. J. Neal, 2002, *Morbidity and Mortality Weekly Report*, vol. 51, no., 27, p. 593; *HIV/AIDS Surveillance Report, 2002,* by Centers for Disease Control and Prevention, 2004, vol. 14; *HIV/AIDS Surveillance Report, 2006,* by Centers for Disease Control and Prevention, 2008, vol. 18; *HIV/AIDS Surveillance Report, 2010,* by Centers for Disease Control and Prevention, 2012, vol. 22.

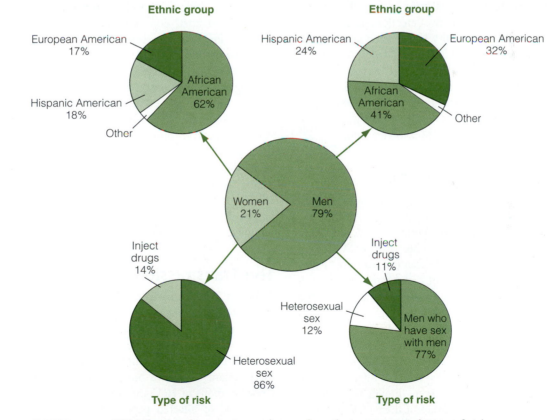

FIGURE 11.2   HIV infection for women and men, by ethnic group and type of risk.

Source: HIV/AIDS Surveillance Report, 2010, by Centers for Disease Control and Prevention, 2012, vol. 22 (Tables 1b and 3b).

than younger adults, but when infected, they tend to develop AIDS more rapidly and to get more opportunistic infections (CDC, 2008).

Incidence of HIV infection increased rapidly in the United States from 1981 to 1995 and then began to decrease (Torian, Chen, Rhodes, & Hall, 2011). Mortality from AIDS dropped even more. Between 1993 and 1998, AIDS diagnoses decreased by 45%, but AIDS deaths decreased by 63%. One reason the number of deaths from AIDS has declined is that HIV-infected individuals now live longer. People diagnosed with AIDS in 1984 had an average survival time of 11 months (Lee, Karon, Selik, Neal, & Fleming, 2001), but more effective treatment lengthened the life expectancy of individuals who are HIV-positive. Magic Johnson is an example of this increased life expectancy; Johnson has lived more than 20 years since his diagnosis.

The number of people living with AIDS (prevalence) continues to increase, as Figure 11.1 shows, but combinations of antiretroviral drugs have changed the course of HIV infection, drastically slowing the progression of infection and prolonging lives (UNAIDS, 2010). This increased survival time is a result of more effective drug therapies, early detection, and lifestyle changes. Giving up unhealthy habits such as smoking, drinking alcohol, and taking illicit drugs; becoming more vigilant about their health; and exercising more control over their treatment can help infected persons live longer and healthier lives (Chou, Holzemer, Portillo, & Slaughter, 2004). An optimistic attitude also contributes to longevity (Moskowitz, 2003).

Symptoms of HIV and AIDS

Typically, HIV progresses over a decade or more from infection to AIDS, but the progression varies. During the first phase of HIV infection, symptoms are not easily distinguishable from those of other diseases. Within a week or so of infection, people may (or may not) experience symptoms consisting of fever, sore throat, skin rash, headache, and other symptoms that resemble the flu (Cibulka, 2006). This phase lasts from a few days to 4 weeks, followed typically by a period that may last as long as 10 years, during which infected people are asymptomatic or experience only minimal symptoms. During this time, the immune systems of infected people gradually become destroyed, even though the infected individuals may remain unaware of their HIV status.

People who go untreated usually progress to symptoms, which is the beginning of HIV disease (Cibulka, 2006). Early symptomatic HIV disease occurs when a person's CD4+ T-lymphocyte cell count drops and the person's immune system becomes less able to fight infections. When the CD4+ count falls to 200 or less per cubic millimeter of blood (healthy people have a CD4+ count of 1,000), the person has AIDS. As their immune system loses its defensive capacities, people with early symptomatic HIV disease become susceptible to various opportunistic infections that a healthy immune system would resist. They may experience weight loss, persistent diarrhea, white spots in the mouth, painful skin rash, fever, and persistent fatigue.

As the supply of CD4+ T-lymphocytes depletes, the immune system loses an important mechanism for fighting infections within cells. The diseases associated with HIV are caused by a variety of agents, including viruses, bacteria, fungi, and parasites. The HIV virus damages or kills the part of the immune system that fights *viral* infections, leaving no way for the body to fight HIV. But HIV does not destroy the antibodies that the immune system has already manufactured, so the immune system response that occurs through antibodies circulating in the blood remains intact. Therefore, HIV disease does not often cause a person to develop, for example, infections with the bacterium that causes strep throat or the virus that causes influenza. Most HIV-infected people have antibodies to fight against these common agents.

As their CD4+ count falls to the level defining AIDS, people are subject to lung, gastrointestinal, nervous system, liver, bone, and brain damage from infections from otherwise rare organisms, which leads to such diseases as *Pneumocystis carinii* pneumonia, Kaposi's sarcoma, tuberculosis, and toxoplasmic encephalitis. Symptoms include greater weight loss, general fatigue, fever, shortness of breath, dry cough, purplish bumps on the skin, and AIDS-related dementia.

The Transmission of HIV

Although HIV is an infectious organism with a high fatality rate, the virus is not easily transmitted from person to person. The main routes of infection are from person to person during sex, from direct contact with blood or blood products, and from mother to child during pregnancy, birth, or breastfeeding (UNAIDS, 2007). Concentrations of HIV are especially high in the semen and blood of infected people. Therefore, contact with infected semen or blood is a risk. Other body fluids do not contain such a high concentration of HIV, making contact with saliva, urine, or tears much less of a risk. No evidence exists that any sort of casual contact spreads the infection. Eating with the same utensils or plates or drinking from the same cup as someone who is infected does not transmit HIV, nor does touching or even kissing someone who is infected. Insect bites do not spread the virus, and even being bitten by someone who is infected is not likely to infect the person who is bitten.

People most at risk for HIV infection are those affected by causes of the four epidemics: male–male sexual contact, injection drug use, heterosexual contact, and transmission from mother to baby. Each of the groups reflected by these four epidemics experiences somewhat different risks.

Male–Male Sexual Contact

In the early years of AIDS, men who had sex with men made up the majority of AIDS cases in North America and Western Europe. Male–male sexual contact is still the leading source of HIV infection in the United States. This mode of transmission declined during the 1990s but has increased slightly during the past few years; it now accounts for more than half of HIV transmissions in the United States (Prejean et al., 2001).

Among gay and bisexual men, unprotected anal intercourse is an especially risky behavior, particularly for the receptive partner. Anal intercourse can easily damage the delicate lining of the rectum, so the receptive person is at high risk if his partner is infected with HIV. The damaged rectum makes an excellent route for the virus to enter the body, and infected semen has a high concentration of HIV. Unprotected oral sex with an infected partner is also a risky practice because HIV can enter the body through any tiny cut or other lesion in the mouth.

Condom use became common among gay men, but as treatment became more effective, gay men became less concerned with contracting HIV (Kalichman et al., 2007), and a subculture of gay men are attracted to unprotected anal intercourse, despite their knowledge of its dangers (Shernoff, 2006). Using alcohol or other drugs contributes to the decision to have unprotected sex (Celentano et al., 2006). In addition, the Internet has become a meeting place for men who want to have casual sex with other men, and these encounters are less likely to include condoms than other types of meetings (Garofalo, Herrick, Mustanski, & Donenberg, 2007). Thus, risky sexual behaviors continue to put men who have sex with men in danger of HIV exposure.

Injection Drug Use

Another high-risk behavior is the sharing of unsterilized needles by injection drug users, a practice that allows the direct transmission of blood from one person to another. Injection drug use is the second most frequent source of HIV infection in the United States (CDC, 2008) and accounts for about 32% of HIV cases among women in the United States. However, in other parts of the world—such as Asia, Thailand, Pakistan, and India—injection drug use fuels the HIV epidemic (UNAIDS, 2010). Some injection drug users engage in this behavior in certain situations—for example, when intoxicated or when there is no immediate access to sterile drug equipment. Some evidence (Heimer, 2008) indicates that relatively small-scale needle exchange programs can be effective in controlling HIV infection in a variety of communities.

Transmission through injection drug use accounts for a greater percentage of infected African Americans and Hispanic Americans than European Americans (CDC, 2008). Also, a higher percentage of infected women than men are exposed to the virus through this route. Several behavioral factors relate to HIV infection for women who inject drugs, including the number of sex partners and whether they have traded sex for money or drugs. These behaviors increase the chances for transmission through heterosexual sex.

Heterosexual Contact

Heterosexual contact is the leading source of HIV infection in Africa (UNAIDS, 2007), but in the United States, heterosexual sex accounts for about 30% of cases (CDC, 2008). African Americans and Hispanic Americans are disproportionately represented among those infected through heterosexual contact, and women from these two ethnic backgrounds are in greater danger than men from heterosexual contact.

This gender asymmetry comes from ease of transmission during sexual intercourse. Although men are susceptible to HIV through sexual contact with women, male-to-female transmission is 8 times more likely than female-to-male transmission. Despite women's greater likelihood of infection through heterosexual sex, they tend to see their sexual partners as safer than men do (Crowell & Emmers-Sommers, 2001).

Trust and confidence in one's partner in a heterosexual relationship may be unfounded and result in HIV infection. One study (Crowell & Emmers-Sommers, 2001) questioned HIV-positive individuals, and found many that reported a high level of trust in their past sexual partners. Another study (Klein,

Elifson, & Sterk, 2003) found that women who perceived themselves to be at some risk behaved in ways that raised their risks, but half of women who felt no risk still engaged in at least some risky behaviors. Thus, people's overly trusting view of partners and failure to accept the possibility of risks lead to unprotected sex. Regular use of condoms may provide a high level of safety for heterosexual men and women, but many young heterosexual couples use condoms more as a means of preventing pregnancy than of preventing HIV (Bird, Harvey, Beckman, & Johnson, 2000).

Transmission During the Birth Process Another group at risk for HIV infection is children born to HIV-positive women. This transmission tends to occur during the birth process. Breastfeeding can also transmit the virus (Steinbrook, 2004). Children infected with HIV during the birth process suffer a variety of developmental disabilities, including intellectual and academic impairment, psychomotor dysfunction, and emotional and behavioral difficulties (Mitchell, 2001). In addition, many of these children are born to mothers who ingested drugs during pregnancy and thus are put at further risk for developmental difficulties.

Most individuals who are HIV positive are within their reproductive years, and knowledge of HIV-positive status does not necessarily deter people from reproduction (Delvaux & Nostlinger, 2007). Both HIV-positive women and men may wish to have children, and the family traditions of some Asian cultures push couples toward decisions to reproduce (Ko & Muecke, 2005). With people who are HIV positive, reproduction is a risk for the child. Semen carries HIV that can transmit to the fetus, and transmission during the birth process is likely unless the HIV-positive mother undergoes antiretroviral therapy. Therefore, seeking prenatal counseling and care are critically important for HIV-positive women and men who wish to start a pregnancy. Early prenatal care can reduce the risk of transmission from mother to child to about 1%.

Psychologists' Role in the HIV Epidemic

From the beginning of the AIDS epidemic, psychologists have played an important role in combating the spread of infection (Kelly & Kalichman, 2002). During the early years of the epidemic, psychologists contributed to both primary and secondary prevention efforts. Primary prevention includes changing behavior to

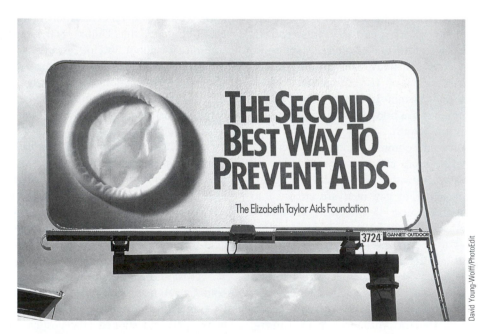

Psychologists have been involved in primary prevention for HIV infection, such as promoting condom use.

decrease HIV transmission. Secondary prevention includes helping people who are HIV positive to live with the infection, counseling people about HIV testing, helping patients deal with social and interpersonal aspects of the disease, and helping patients adhere to their complex treatment program. Much of the improvement in length of survival of HIV-infected patients rests with the effectiveness of drug treatments, highly active antiviral therapy (HAART). This treatment consists of a combination of pills that must be taken on a strict schedule, making adherence a challenge. Psychologists' knowledge concerning adherence to medical regimens is now relevant to managing HIV infection.

Encouraging Protective Measures Except for infants born to HIV-infected mothers, most people have some control in protecting themselves from the human immunodeficiency virus. Fortunately, HIV is not easily transmitted from person to person, making casual contact with infected persons a low risk. Health care workers who participate in surgery, emergency care, or other procedures that bring them into contact with blood should be careful to prevent infected blood from entering their body through an open wound. For example, dentists and dental hygienists wear protective gloves, and health care workers should adhere to a set of standard protective measures.

Although some risks are specific to certain professions, most people infected with HIV acquired the virus through sexual behavior or by sharing contaminated needles. People can protect themselves against infection with HIV by changing those behaviors that are high risks for acquiring the infection—namely, having unprotected sexual contact or sharing needles with an infected person. Limiting the number of sex partners, using condoms, and avoiding shared needles are three behaviors that will protect the largest number of people from HIV infection. However, for people who engage in these risk behaviors, they are very difficult to change. A variety of factors contribute to this difficulty.

One factor that makes behavior change difficult is perception of risk. Most people in the United States do not perceive that they are at risk for HIV infection, and they are correct (Holtzman, Bland, Lansky, & Mack, 2001). That is, most adults do not engage in the behaviors that are primary HIV risks. However, some people are at risk and fail to perceive that risk accurately. For example, young men who have sex with men reported overly optimistic beliefs about their risk

(MacKellar et al., 2007), as did college students in Nigeria (Ijadunola, Abiona, Odu, & Ijadunola, 2007). Their misperceptions play a role in their continued risky behavior, and culture is an important influence in sexual risk behaviors.

Cultures in which male dominance is supported by social custom or religion and in which women have little access to economic resources also have high rates of heterosexually transmitted HIV, such as countries in sub-Saharan Africa, the Caribbean, and Latin America (UNAIDS, 2007). When women are financially dependent on men and have limited access to economic resources, they may have little control over sexual encounters or even be vulnerable to forced or coerced sex. Thus, they may be unable to negotiate condom use, which increases their risk for infection. These dangers also apply to women in the United States. A study of HIV-positive African American women (Lichtenstein, 2005) confirmed the presence of abuse and dominance as factors in these women's HIV infection, and a large study of young adults found that alcohol use and violence contribute to HIV transmission (Collins, Orlando, & Klein, 2005).

Helping People With HIV Infection People who believe they may be infected with HIV, as well as those who know that they are, can benefit from various psychological interventions. People who engage in high-risk behaviors may have difficulty deciding whether to be tested for HIV, and psychologists can provide both information and support for these people. Individuals from several high-risk groups have not been tested for HIV, including (1) a significant minority of gay and bisexual men, (2) a significant minority of injection drug users, and (3) a larger proportion of heterosexual men and women with multiple partners and inconsistent use of condoms (Awad, Sagrestano, Kittleson, & Sarvela, 2004). Indeed, many people who are HIV positive have not been tested and thus do not know their HIV status.

The decision to get an HIV test has both benefits and costs to the individual, but testing is considered essential to the control of HIV infection (Janssen et al., 2003). Far too many people undergo testing after their disease progresses and treatment options are less effective; a prominent part of Magic Johnson's campaign targets early testing and services for people whose tests indicate infection. Early testing for those who are HIV positive allows early treatment, which will prolong their lives and will permit them to find ways to reduce or eliminate behaviors that place others at risk.

The costs of being tested include all the problems of arranging a health care visit, plus the distress that comes with the potential for bad news. Currently, HIV testing is not part of routine health examinations, and individuals must seek testing (Clark, 2006). At least 25% of those with HIV infection are unaware of their status because they have not sought testing. In addition, many people who agree to testing never take steps to learn the results. Alternatives to the standard testing procedure, such as rapid results testing and at-home testing, increase the likelihood of learning one's HIV status (Hutchinson, Branson, Kim, & Farnham, 2006).

Learning of HIV-positive status is a traumatic event that can lead to anxiety, depression, anger, and distress. The ongoing experience of coping with HIV likewise can lead to these emotional responses, which have clear implications for disease progression. A review of over 30 prospective studies of people living with HIV concluded that emotional distress predicts a variety of indicators of HIV disease progression, including lower levels of CD4+ cells, AIDS symptoms

and diagnosis, and even mortality due to AIDS (Chida & Vedhara, 2009). People's coping styles also relate to adjustment and disease progression. For example, people who take direct action to cope, maintain a positive outlook, and express emotions tend to have better physical health (Moskowitz, Hult, Bussolari, & Acree, 2009). In contrast, people who deny their illness and use disengagement coping methods such as alcohol or drug use have faster disease progression and worse physical health (Chida et al., 2009; Moskowitz et al., 2009). Some of these coping strategies may matter more in certain contexts. For example, taking direct action to cope appears to benefit physical health when it occurs soon after HIV diagnosis (Moskowitz et al., 2009). Receiving support both from health care professionals and from family and friends also leads to better psychological adjustment (Moskowitz et al., 2009; Reilly & Woo, 2004).

Interventions tailored to the person's specific situation and needs have advantages over less personalized programs (Moskowitz & Wrubel, 2005). Cognitive behavioral and stress management interventions are generally effective in reducing the anxiety, depression,

Becoming Healthier

1. If you have a chronic illness, understand your condition and form a cooperative relationship with health care professionals. However, take charge of its management yourself; you are the person most affected by your condition.

2. If you are the primary caregiver for someone who is chronically ill, don't ignore your own health—both physical and psychological. Regularly schedule some time for yourself.

3. If you have Type 1 diabetes, don't try to hide your illness from your friends. Although you have a chronic disease, you can live a long and productive life, but you must adhere faithfully to a lifelong regimen that includes diet,

insulin injection, and regular exercise. If you live with someone with diabetes, offer social and emotional support and encourage that person to stick with required health practices.

4. Know your blood sugar level. Type 2 diabetes can develop at any age, and this disorder may have few symptoms.

5. If you have asthma, try to minimize attacks and use of dilators. Concentrate on taking preventive medication and knowing your triggers to avoid attacks.

6. Protect yourself against HIV infection. The most common mode of transmission is sexual, and condoms make sex safer.

7. If you are the primary caregiver for someone with a terminal

chronic disease such as AIDS or Alzheimer's disease, seek social and emotional support through groups specifically convened to offer such support. Take breaks from caregiving, allowing others to assume those responsibilities for a while.

8. If you have a chronic disease or if you are the caregiver for someone with such a disease, use the Internet to gain information and support. A wide variety of websites offer information, and online support groups are available for all disorders. Do not use these websites as a substitute for health care but allow these resources to supplement your knowledge and support.

and distress of those who are HIV positive and improve their quality of life (Crepaz et al., 2008; Scott-Sheldon, Kalichman, Carey, & Fielder, 2008). Some cognitive behavioral stress management interventions also report beneficial effects on physiological health outcomes (Antoni et al., 1991, 2000); however, most interventions do not (Scott-Sheldon et al., 2008).

Psychologists can also help HIV patients adhere to the complex medical regimens designed to control HIV infection (Simoni, Pearson, Pantalone, Marks, & Crepaz, 2006), particularly those patients who have the greatest difficulty with adherence (Amico, Harman, & Johnson, 2006). HAART consists of a combination of antiretroviral medications; patients often take other drugs to combat side effects of the antiretroviral drugs as well as drugs to fight opportunistic infections. These regimens may include as many as a dozen drugs, all of which require precise timing. When patients do not follow the schedule, the effectiveness diminishes. Psychologists can help patients adhere to this schedule as well as facilitate their self-management skills. For example, the technique of motivational interviewing appeared to be successful in helping with the scheduling aspect of HAART adherence (DiIorio et al., 2008).

Another aspect of adjustment to HIV infection is finding meaning in the experience and developing the potential for growth and positive experiences. People with AIDS and their caregivers often succeed in finding positive experiences in their lives. In two studies (Milam, 2004; Updegraff, Taylor, Kemeny, & Wyatt, 2000), over half of individuals with HIV or AIDS had experienced positive changes, and in another study (Folkman & Moskowitz, 2000), more than 99% of AIDS patients and caregivers were able to recall a positive experience. The search for positive meaning may even influence the course of HIV infection by affecting CD4 count (Ickovics et al., 2006). This quest for positive meaning is common to the experience of many people with chronic illness (Updegraff & Taylor, 2000), and this attitude may also appear in those who are dying.

IN SUMMARY

Acquired immune deficiency syndrome is the result of depletion of the immune system after infection with the human immunodeficiency virus. When the immune system fails to defend the body, a number of diseases may develop, including bacterial, viral, fungal, and parasitic infections that are uncommon in people who have functioning immune systems.

The modes of transmission of HIV are behavioral, with receptive anal intercourse and the sharing of needles for intravenous drug injection the two behaviors that have spread the infection to the most people in the United States. Unprotected heterosexual contact with an infected partner accounts for a larger proportion of people with HIV worldwide. The number of babies infected with HIV has decreased because antiretroviral drug therapies sharply decrease transmission from an infected mother during the birth process.

Psychologists use a variety of interventions to help patients reduce high-risk behaviors, cope with their illness, manage their symptoms, and adhere to the complex drug regimens that improve survival. In addition, psychologists have provided counseling services for those seeking to be tested and for those whose tests reveal infection. These programs not only encourage protective behaviors but also emphasize the role of positive health in combating AIDS.

Facing Death

Over the last century, life expectancy has increased. People do not necessarily expect a long life, but they prefer it, saying that a life of about 85 years is about right (Lang, Baltes, & Wagner, 2007). However, people also want to have control over the end of their lives, including when and how they die. This desire is consistent with the concept of "the good death," which consists of physical comfort, social support, appropriate medical care, and attempts to minimize psychological distress for the dying person and the family (Carr, 2003). What do we know about the issues that people deal with when they are dying and how people adjust to losing a loved one?

Adjusting to Terminal Illness

The experience of a "good death" is possible for many. Most of the leading causes of death in the United States and other industrialized countries are chronic diseases such as cardiovascular disease, cancer, chronic lower respiratory disease, Alzheimer's disease, kidney disease, chronic liver disease, and HIV infection. These diseases are often fatal, but death is not sudden, giving people and their families an opportunity to adjust. Even if the chronic disease does not signal terminal illness, the diagnosis entails loss and thus the need to adapt (Murray, 2001).

A common perception is that people go through several predictable stages of adaptation to a terminal illness. This perception was popularized by Elizabeth Kübler-Ross (1969). Kübler-Ross's stages included denial, anger, bargaining, depression, and acceptance. Denial is a failure to accept the validity or the severity of the diagnosis; people use this defense mechanism to deal with the anxiety they experience when they learn of their condition (Livneh & Antonak, 2005). Anger is another emotional reaction, and bargaining often takes the form of trying to negotiate a better outcome, either with God or with health care personnel. Depression is a common response of those who come to understand the progression of their disease, followed by acceptance of the situation.

Was Kübler-Ross correct? While it is true that people react to a terminal diagnosis with reactions such as denial, anger, bargaining, depression, and acceptance, there is no evidence that people respond in a set pattern (Schulz & Aderman, 1974). Nor is there any evidence that people *should* experience these reactions in a set pattern. Instead, people diagnosed with chronic diseases and people with terminal illness usually exhibit a range of negative reactions, but they may also experience positive responses oriented around growth and finding meaning in their situation.

A more useful conceptualization of adaptation to terminal illness is the notion of the dying role (Emanuel, Bennett, & Richardson, 2007). This role is an extension of the sick role, which we described in Chapter 3. Like the sick role, the dying role includes certain privileges and responsibilities and can take many forms, both healthy and unhealthy. Three key elements are involved: practical, relational, and personal. The practical element includes the tasks that people need to arrange at the end of their lives, such as arranging financial matters and making plans for medical care as the disease progresses. The relational element involves reconciling the dying role with other roles, such as caregiver, spouse, and parent. This reconciliation may be difficult: The dying role is not automatically compatible with these other roles, so the dying person must work to find ways to integrate these roles. The personal element involves "finishing one's life story" (Emanuel et al., 2007, p. 159). This element may prompt people to reexamine their life while thinking about its end and to derive new meaning from it. This new meaning may constitute a reintegration (Knight & Emanuel, 2007), or some less healthy outcome may occur.

Barriers to a good adjustment include institutional impediments and lack of access to palliative care. Institutional barriers occur when people cannot assume the dying role because health care professionals keep them in the sick role, even though it is inappropriate (Emanuel et al., 2007). Medical care is so oriented toward cures that accepting death may be difficult for medical practitioners. Appropriate care, such as hospice care or support for home care, may be unavailable, forcing people to stay in a hospital that may not serve their needs. Concentrating on the physical aspects of dying does not allow people to work toward the social and personal tasks from which they may derive a feeling of completion and reintegration.

Entry into the dying role typically meets with loss and grief (Emanuel et al., 2007). The person faces the loss of physical abilities, social relationships, and the experiences of continued life. People imagine that those in this situation are frightened of dying, but research involving people with terminal illnesses indicates otherwise (McKechnie, Macleod, & Keeling, 2007). Instead, the concerns of the dying revolve around anxiety—over their condition, whether they would be able to complete planned activities, and provisions for managing their comfort during the last stages of their disease. Because their disease imposes physical limitations on their activities, they feel unable to "live until they died" (McKechnie et al., 2007, p. 367).

Grieving

Loss and grief are also common to bereavement, making the reactions and processes of adaptation applicable to family and friends after the death of a loved one (Murray, 2001). Thus, a diagnosis of chronic illness, awareness of a terminal condition, and loss of a loved one provoke similar reactions, with similar possibilities for outcomes. That is, bereavement may result in caregivers' experiencing worsened symptoms or improvements (Aneshensel et al., 2004) and, eventually, growth (Hogan & Schmidt, 2002).

The similarities between those who are dying and those who are bereaved have led to similar theories of adaptation, including a stage theory of bereavement with stages of disbelief, yearning, anger, depression, and then acceptance. As with Kübler-Ross's stage theory of adaptation to dying, there is little evidence to support a stage theory of bereavement (Maciejewski, Zhang, Block, & Prigerson, 2007). People exhibit some, none, or all of these reactions. A potentially better way to describe people's reactions to bereavement is to acknowledge that some people react differently to bereavement than others. One study of over 400 German adults' reactions to bereavement (Mancini, Bonanno, & Clark, 2011) identified four different profiles of responses. Most adults exhibited a response called *resiliency*, characterized by stable levels of well-being from before a loss to 4 years after a loss of a loved one. Only 21% of the adults showed a response called *acute-recovery*, characterized by a drop in well-being at the time of loss, followed by a graduate return to normal. About 15% of adults showed *chronic low levels* of well-being that were relatively unaffected by bereavement. Surprisingly, about 5% of adults showed *improvement*, with levels of well-being that increased in the years following the death of a loved one. (Incidentally, those who showed improvement were more likely to have gained income as a result of their loss.) Clearly, people's responses to bereavement are varied and do not fit neatly into a stage model.

Bereavement typically includes negative emotions, and people have difficulty accepting such emotions as normal. Even among health care professionals, the grieving process may seem abnormal when people exhibit strong negative reactions or their feelings persist for a time considered too lengthy. Thoughts of lost loved ones and longings for their company can persist for many years (Camelley, Wortman, Bolger, & Burke, 2006). Experts suggest that it is these people who may benefit the most from psychological intervention (Mancini, Griffin, & Bonanno, 2012). In contrast, psychological intervention may have little to no benefit among people who do not show persistent and elevated levels of distress.

Even the terminology used by mental health professionals carries negative connotations. People who are adapting to the loss of a loved one are referred to as *recovering*, which implies that these individuals will go back to "normal" and that their grief reactions signal psychological problems. This tendency to "pathologize" the bereavement process should be avoided (Tedeschi & Calhoun, 2008). Some grief responses may present problems for adaptation, but like the process of adapting to chronic and terminal illness, grieving offers the promise of transformative and spiritual growth (Tedeschi & Calhoun, 2006). Thus, all three processes share essential elements.

IN SUMMARY

Facing death requires adjustment for the person who is dying and for the family. Although the process of stages of acceptance has gained popular appeal, no research supports this view. Instead, people who are dying experience a variety of negative reactions that may be better conceptualized as a role with practical, relationship, and personal elements. Some people are able to work through challenges and have access to the facilities to experience a "good death," allowing them to die without pain but with social support, appropriate medical care, and minimal psychological distress. Their adaptation may leave them with a sense of completion and even transcendence. Growth is also a possibility for those who grieve for loved ones, but the bereaved also face a process of adjustment that includes negative emotions. A wide variety of emotional responses follow bereavement, but no research suggests that people pass through predictable stages of grief. The negative emotions that are involved in grieving should not be seen as abnormal; resolving grief may take years, but this process also offers the promise of positive change.

Answers

This chapter has addressed six basic questions:

1. ## What is the impact of chronic disease on patients and families?

Long-term chronic illnesses bring about a transition in people's lives, requiring adaptations to live with symptoms and receive medical care, changing relationships, and pushing people toward a reevaluation of themselves. Support groups and programs designed by health psychologists help people cope with the emotional problems associated with chronic illness, problems that traditional medical care often overlooks. Chronic diseases may be terminal, which forces people to consider their impending death.

2. What is the impact of Alzheimer's disease?

Alzheimer's disease damages the brain and produces memory loss, language problems, agitation and irritability, sleep disorders, suspiciousness, wandering, incontinence, and loss of ability to perform routine care. The most common form of Alzheimer's disease occurs through a genetic vulnerability combined with environmental risks. Age is the main risk, with the prevalence doubling for every decade after age 65. Lifestyle factors relate to the development of Alzheimer's disease, making prevention a possibility. Medical treatments are being developed, but the main management strategies consist of interventions to allow patients longer periods of functioning, and counseling and support groups for family members, who frequently experience more stress than the patient.

3. What is involved in adjusting to diabetes?

Diabetes, both insulin-dependent (Type 1) and non-insulin-dependent (Type 2), requires changes in lifestyle that include monitoring and adherence to a treatment regimen. Treatments include insulin injections for Type 1 diabetics and adherence to careful dietary restrictions, scheduling of meals, avoidance of certain foods, regular medical visits, and routine exercise for all diabetics. Health psychologists are involved in helping diabetics learn self-care to control the dangerous effects of their condition.

4. How does asthma affect the lives of people with this disease?

Inflammation of the bronchial tubes is the underlying basis for asthma. Combined with this inflammation, triggering stimuli or events cause bronchial constriction that produces difficulty in breathing. Asthma may be fatal, and it is the leading cause of disability among children. The origin of this process is not understood, but medication can control the inflammation and decrease the risk of attacks. People with asthma are faced with a complex medication regimen that they must follow to decrease the risk of attacks.

5. How can HIV infection be managed?

Infection with the human immunodeficiency virus depletes the immune system, leaving the body vulnerable to acquired immune deficiency syndrome and a variety of opportunistic infections. HIV epidemics affect four different populations in the United States: (1) men who have sex with men, (2) injection drug users, (3) heterosexuals, and (4) children born to HIV-positive mothers. Psychologists are involved in the HIV epidemic by encouraging protective behaviors, counseling infected people to help them cope with living with a chronic disease, and helping patients adhere to complex medical regimens that have changed HIV infection to a manageable chronic disease.

6. What adaptations do people make to dying and grieving?

People tend to react to the knowledge that they have a terminal illness with a variety of negative emotions, and the process of grieving also includes negative emotions. Contrary to popular conceptualizations, however, these reactions do not progress through a pattern of stages. Instead, dying may be conceptualized as a role that includes practical, relational, and personal elements that people encounter in their process of adaptation. Grieving can also be conceptualized as a process with negative emotions but also with the possibility of growth.

Suggested Readings

Asthma Action America. (2004). *Children and asthma in America*. Retrieved August 29, 2008, from http://www.asthmainamerica.com/frequency.html. This comprehensive survey details the impact of asthma on the lives of children and their caregivers, examining the misperceptions about the disease, the available treatments, and recommendations for more effective strategies to deal with this disease.

DeBaggio, T. (2002). *Losing my mind: An intimate look at life with Alzheimer's*. New York: Free Press. When former newspaper writer Thomas DeBaggio began to recognize symptoms of Alzheimer's disease at age 57, he decided to write about his experience of "losing his mind." The result is a moving account of Alzheimer's disease from an insider's point of view.

Stanton, A. L., & Revenson, T. A. (2011). Adjustment to chronic disease: Progress and promise in research. In H. Friedman (Ed.), *The Oxford handbook of health psychology* (pp. 241–268). This chapter examines the growing body of longitudinal research on adjustment to chronic illness, exploring the important risk and protective factors that affect the process.

UNAIDS. (2010). *UNAIDS report on the global AIDS epidemic, 2010.* Geneva: Joint United Nations Programme on HIV/AIDS. This comprehensive report details the status of HIV infection worldwide and in each geographic area, analyzing the nature of the epidemic in each region and the progress that has been made in controlling the disease.

CHAPTER 12

Smoking Tobacco

CHAPTER OUTLINE

- **Real-World Profile of President Barack Obama**
- *Smoking and the Respiratory System*
- *A Brief History of Tobacco Use*
- *Choosing to Smoke*
- *Health Consequences of Tobacco Use*
- *Interventions for Reducing Smoking Rates*
- *Effects of Quitting*

QUESTIONS

This chapter focuses on five basic questions:

1. How does smoking affect the respiratory system?

2. Who chooses to smoke and why?

3. What are the health consequences of tobacco use?

4. How can smoking rates be reduced?

5. What are the effects of quitting?

☑ CHECK YOUR HEALTH RISKS

Regarding Tobacco Use

Check the items that apply to you.

☐ 1. I have not smoked more than 100 cigarettes in my life.

☐ 2. I have probably smoked between 100 and 200 cigarettes in my life, but I have not smoked at all in more than 5 years and have no desire to do so.

☐ 3. I currently smoke more than 10 cigarettes a day.

☐ 4. I currently smoke more than two packs of cigarettes a day.

☐ 5. I am a smoker who believes that the health risks of smoking have been exaggerated.

☐ 6. I am a smoker who believes that smoking is probably harmful, but I plan to stop smoking before those effects can harm me.

☐ 7. I don't smoke cigarettes, but I do smoke at least one cigar a day.

☐ 8. I don't smoke cigarettes, but I do smoke my pipe at least once a day.

☐ 9. I smoke cigars because I believe that they carry a very low risk for any health problems.

☐ 10. I smoke a pipe because I believe that pipe smoking is safer than cigarettes.

☐ 11. I live with someone who smokes inside the dwelling.

☐ 12. I use smokeless tobacco (chewing tobacco) on a daily basis.

Except for the first two statements, each of these items represents a health risk from tobacco products, which account for about 443,000 deaths a year in the United States, mostly from heart disease, cancer, and chronic lower respiratory disease. Count your checkmarks for the last 10 items to evaluate your risks. As you read this chapter, you will see that some of these items are riskier than others.

Real-World Profile of
PRESIDENT BARACK OBAMA

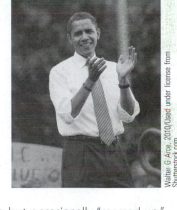

Walter G Arce, 2010/Used under license from Shutterstock.com

United States President Barack Obama quit smoking after years of struggling to break the habit ("Michelle Obama," 2011). Obama began smoking when he was a teenager and escalated into a heavy smoker. When he decided to run for the office of U.S. President, he promised his wife Michelle that he would quit, but he relapsed into smoking during his campaign. During a press conference President Obama held after he had signed an antismoking law, Obama admitted that he had lapsed and had begun occasional smoking ("Obama Admits," 2008). He said that he struggled to refrain from smoking but occasionally "messed up."

Obama's occasional smoking continued during the first 2 years of his presidency, but in February, 2011, First Lady Michelle Obama announced that the President had not smoked a cigarette for almost a year ("Michelle Obama," 2011). President Obama felt the pressure to quit from a number of sources, including the continued urging from his health-conscious wife, the knowledge that his smoking provided a poor role model to his children (and to other young people), and the urgings of his physician to quit for the sake of his health.

The President's struggle to become a nonsmoker was typical of the more than a million former smokers in the United States. He began smoking as a teenager, escalated his smoking as a young adult, wanted to quit, made repeated attempts to do so, and finally succeeded.

Smoking is the most preventable cause of death in the world. In the United States, 443,000 people die every year from tobacco use (U.S. Department of Health and Human Services [USDHHS], 2010c). It's quite easy to read through the number 443,000, but let's see if we can personalize it. *Each year in the United States*, smoking kills enough people to wipe out half the population of Montana. More people die every year from smoking than live within the city limits of Atlanta. Stated differently, an average of 1,213 people die *every day* in the United States from tobacco-related causes. Throughout the world, the death total is almost 6 million people per year (American Cancer Society, 2012), which is equivalent to the population of Denmark. Later, we summarize the various risks from cigarette, cigar, and pipe smoking, as well as from other tobacco products, including the dangers of passive smoking and smokeless tobacco. This chapter also includes information on the prevalence of smoking, the reasons why people smoke, and some methods of preventing and reducing smoking. First, however, we briefly review the effects of smoking on the respiratory system, the body system most immediately affected by smoking.

Smoking and the Respiratory System

Respiration takes oxygen into the body and expels carbon dioxide. This process draws air deep into the lungs, which routinely introduces a variety of particles into the lungs. Thus, smoking provides a pathway for lung damage and disease.

Functioning of the Respiratory System

The exchange of oxygen and carbon dioxide occurs deep in the lungs. To get air into the lungs, the **diaphragm** and the muscles between the ribs (intercostal muscles) contract, increasing the volume within the chest. As the space inside the chest increases, the pressure within the chest falls below atmospheric pressure, forcing air into the lungs.

Figure 12.1 illustrates where air goes on its way to the lungs. The nasal passages, pharynx, larynx, trachea, bronchi, and bronchioles conduct air into the lungs. These passages have little ability to absorb oxygen, but in the process of inhalation, the air is warmed, humidified, and cleansed. Millions of alveoli, located at the ends of the bronchioles, are the site of oxygen and carbon dioxide exchange. Air rich in oxygen is drawn into the lungs and reaches the alveoli, where an exchange of carbon dioxide and oxygen occurs in the capillaries that surround each alveolus. The blood, now oxygen rich, travels back to the heart and is pumped out to all areas of the body.

Air is an excellent medium for the introduction of foreign matter into the body. Airborne particles potentially move into the lungs with every breath. Protective mechanisms in the respiratory system, such as sneezing and coughing, expel some dangerous particles. Noxious stimulation in the nasal passages may activate the sneeze reflex, whereas stimulation in the lower respiratory system promotes the cough reflex.

Several respiratory disorders are of interest to health psychologists. All kinds of smoke, as well as other types of air pollution, increase mucus secretion in the respiratory system but decrease the activity of the respiratory system's protective mechanisms, thus making the system vulnerable to problems. As mucus builds up, people cough to get rid of it, but coughing may also irritate the bronchial walls. Irritation and infection of the bronchial walls may damage the respiratory system and destroy tissue in the bronchi. The formation of scar tissue in the bronchi, irritation or infection of bronchial tissue, and coughing are characteristics of **bronchitis**, one of several *chronic lower respiratory diseases* (previously called chronic obstructive pulmonary disease or COPD) that are the third leading cause of death in the United States.

Acute bronchitis is caused by infection and usually responds quickly to antibiotics. When the irritation persists and the mechanism underlying the illness continues, it can become a chronic problem. Cigarette smoke is the major cause of chronic bronchitis, but environmental air pollution and occupational hazards may also underlie chronic bronchitis.

The most common of the chronic lower respiratory diseases is **emphysema**, which occurs when scar tissue and mucus obstruct the respiratory passages, bronchi lose their elasticity and collapse, and air is trapped in the alveoli. The trapped air breaks down the alveolar walls, and the remaining alveoli become enlarged. Both damaged and enlarged alveoli have reduced surface area for the exchange of oxygen and carbon dioxide. Damage also obstructs blood flow to the undamaged alveoli, and so the respiratory system becomes restricted. The loss of efficiency in the

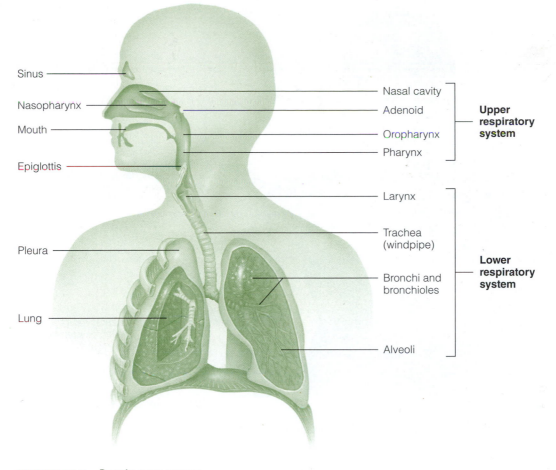

Sinus

Nasopharynx

Mouth

Epiglottis

Pleura

Lung

Nasal cavity

Adenoid

Oropharynx

Pharynx

Upper respiratory system

Larynx

Trachea (windpipe)

Bronchi and bronchioles

Lower respiratory system

Alveoli

FIGURE 12.1   Respiratory system.

Source: Introduction to microbiology (p. 525), by J. L. Ingraham & C. A. Ingraham. From INGRAHAM/INGRAHAM, Introduction to Microbiology, 1E. © 1995 Cengage Learning.

respiratory system means that respiration delivers a limited amount of oxygen. People with emphysema experience problems with breathing and usually cannot exercise strenuously.

Chronic bronchitis, emphysema, and lung cancer are all diseases of the respiratory system associated with the inhalation of irritating, damaging particles such as smoke. Figure 12.2 shows how smoke can damage the lungs, producing bronchitis and emphysema. Cigarette smoking is of particular interest to health psychologists because it is a voluntary behavior that people can avoid, whereas air pollution and occupational hazards are social problems that may be harder for people to avoid. Thus, smoking is the target for much negative publicity and for interventions for change. But what specifically makes inhaled smoke dangerous?

What Components in Smoke Are Dangerous?

The processed tobacco in cigarettes contains at least 4,000 compounds; at least 60 of these are known carcinogens—substances that are capable of causing cancer. All of these compounds are potentially involved in the development of disease, but cigarette smoke is a complex mixture (USDHHS, 2010c). Analyzing the process through which cigarette smokes causes lung damage is difficult and not yet fully understood. However, nicotine is the pharmacological agent that underlies addiction to cigarette smoking. What are the effects of nicotine in the body?

Nicotine is a stimulant drug, an "upper," which affects both the central and peripheral nervous systems

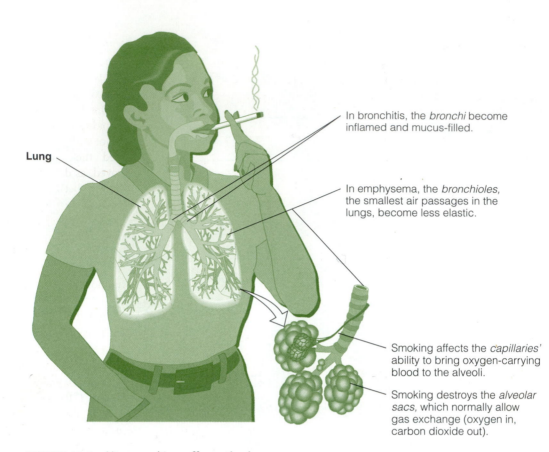

Lung

In bronchitis, the *bronchi* become inflamed and mucus-filled.

In emphysema, the *bronchioles,* the smallest air passages in the lungs, become less elastic.

Smoking affects the *capillaries'* ability to bring oxygen-carrying blood to the alveoli.

Smoking destroys the *alveolar sacs,* which normally allow gas exchange (oxygen in, carbon dioxide out).

FIGURE 12.2 How smoking affects the lungs.

Source: An invitation to health (7th ed., p. 493) by D. Hales, 1997, Pacific Grove, CA: Brooks/Cole. From HALES, Invitation to Health, 7E. © 1997 Cengage Learning.

(USDHHS, 2010c). Certain central nervous system receptor sites are specific for nicotine; that is, the brain responds to nicotine, as it does to many drugs. But smoking is a particularly effective means of delivering drugs to the brain. Nicotine, for example, can be found in the brain 7 seconds after having been ingested by smoking—twice as fast as via intravenous injection. The half-life of nicotine, the time it takes to lose half its strength, is 30 to 40 minutes. Addicted smokers rarely go more than this length of time between "fixes."

When nicotine is delivered to the brain, it occupies receptor sites and affects the release and metabolism of several neurotransmitters, including acetylcholine, epinephrine, norepinephrine, glutamate, and dopamine (USDHHS, 2010c). The overall action is to increase cortical arousal. In addition, smoking releases beta-endorphins, the brain's natural opiates. The pleasurable effects of smoking may be

due to the release of these neurotransmitters. Nicotine also increases the metabolic level and decreases appetite, which explains the tendency for smokers to be thinner than nonsmokers. However, nicotine may not be the main culprit responsible for the dangerous health effects of smoking; other dangerous compounds exist in tobacco.

The term *tars* describes the water-soluble residue of tobacco smoke condensate, which contains a number of compounds identified or suspected as carcinogens. Although tobacco companies have reduced the level of tars in cigarettes, no level is safe. Nevertheless, as tar levels go down, death rates from smoking-related diseases also go down. However, experienced smokers who smoke low-nicotine cigarettes tend to increase their rate of smoking and to inhale low-nicotine smoke more deeply, thus exposing themselves to more of the dangerous tars.

Additional by-products of tobacco smoke may also pose health risks. **Acrolein** and **formaldehyde** belong to a class of irritating compounds called **aldehydes**. Formaldehyde, a demonstrated carcinogen, disrupts tissue proteins and causes cell damage. **Nitric oxide** and **hydrocyanic acid** are gases generated in smoking tobacco that affect oxygen metabolism and therefore could be dangerous. Because tobacco companies do not provide the public with specific information about the content of cigarettes, consumers may not be fully informed about the potential health risks posed by smoking (USDHHS, 2010c).

IN SUMMARY

The respiratory system allows oxygen to be taken into the lungs where an exchange with carbon dioxide occurs at the level of the alveoli. Along with air, other particles can enter the lungs; some of these particles can be harmful. Cigarette smoke can cause damage to the lungs, and smokers are prone to bronchitis, an inflammation of the bronchi. Cigarette smoke contributes heavily to the development of chronic lower respiratory diseases, such as chronic bronchitis and emphysema.

Several chemicals, either within the tobacco itself or produced as a by-product of smoking, can cause organic damage. Although nicotine in large doses is extremely toxic, its precise harmful effects on the average smoker are difficult to assess. This difficulty exists because the level of nicotine in commercial cigarettes varies with the level of tars, another class of potentially hazardous substances. Thus, determining what specific components of smoke connect to which sources of illness and death is difficult.

A Brief History of Tobacco Use

When Christopher Columbus and other early European explorers arrived in the Western hemisphere, they found that the Native Americans had a custom considered odd by European standards: The natives carried rolls of dried leaves, which they set afire and then "drank" the smoke. The leaves were, of course, tobacco. Those early European sailors tried smoking, liked it, and soon became quite dependent on it. Although Columbus disapproved of his sailors' tobacco use, he quickly recognized that "it was not within their power to refrain from indulging in the habit" (Kluger, 1996, p. 9). Within a century, smoking and the cultivation of tobacco spread around the world, and no country where people have learned to use tobacco has ever successfully barred the habit (Brecher, 1972).

The popularity of the smoking habit grew rapidly among Europeans, but it was not without its detractors. Elizabethan England adopted the use of tobacco, although Elizabeth I disapproved, as did her successor, James I. Another prominent Elizabethan, Sir Francis Bacon, spoke against tobacco and the hold it exerted over its users. Many objections to tobacco were of a similar nature—namely, that people who became addicted to it often spent money on tobacco even though they could not afford it. Because of its scarcity, tobacco was expensive; in London in 1610, it sold for an equal weight of silver.

In 1633, the Turkish Sultan Murad IV decreed the death penalty for subjects who were caught smoking. He then conducted "sting" operations on the streets of his empire and beheaded those people who were caught using tobacco (Kluger, 1996). From the early Romanoff Empire in Russia to 17th-century Japan, the penalties for tobacco use were also severe. Still the habit spread. In the Spanish colonies, smoking by priests during Mass became so prevalent that the Catholic Church forbade it. In 1642 and again in 1650, tobacco was the subject of two formal papal bulls, but in 1725, Pope Benedict XIII annulled all edicts against tobacco—he liked to use snuff, which is ground tobacco.

Over the centuries, tobacco has been used in a variety of forms, including cigarettes, cigars, pipes, and snuff. Although some soldiers smoked cigarettes during the U.S. Civil War, cigarette use was not popular until the 20th century. During that time, many men considered cigarette smoking rather effeminate. Ironically, cigarette smoking was not socially acceptable for women either; thus, few women smoked during the 19th century. Cigarette smoking became more popular when ready-made cigarettes came on the market during the 1880s.

In 1913, the development of the "blended" cigarette—a mixture of air-cured Burley and Turkish varieties of tobacco with flue-cured Virginia tobacco—aided the widespread adoption of cigarette smoking. This blending process created a cigarette with a pleasing flavor and aroma that was also easy to inhale. Cigarette smoking increased in popularity during World War I, and during the 1920s, the age of the "flapper," cigarette smoking started to gain popularity among women.

From the time of Columbus until the mid-19th century, tobacco had many detractors, but the objections came from those who damned it on moral, social, xenophobic, or economic grounds rather than for scientific or medical reasons (Kluger, 1996). The tobacco industry continued to grow despite (or perhaps because of) the fact that many in authority condemned the use of tobacco. It was not until the mid-1960s that people began to recognize the scientific evidence on the dangerous consequences of smoking. Indeed, during the 1940s and 1950s, it was common for physicians to smoke and to recommend the practice to their patients as a method of relaxation and stress reduction. Tobacco companies, of course, encouraged this thinking and used a variety of techniques to increase smoking rates. Besides multiple advertising approaches, they provided free cigarettes to soldiers during World War II and continued to give away free samples after the war. At that time, only a few people suspected that smoking might have negative health consequences, so the choice to smoke was a common one.

Choosing to Smoke

Unlike many health hazards, smoking is a voluntary behavior, with each person choosing to smoke or not to smoke. What factors have influenced this choice?

Several historical and social events in the United States have accompanied the increasingly popular choice not to smoke. First was the 1964 report of the Surgeon General of the United States that spelled out the adverse effects of smoking on health (U.S. Public Health Service [USPHS], 1964). Other events included placing a warning of the potential danger of cigarettes on each cigarette package, banning cigarette advertising on television, designating public buildings and spaces as smoke free, increasing the price of cigarettes, removing cigarette machines from public places, requiring identification for the purchase of cigarettes, and designing and implementing programs aimed at deterring smoking and encouraging quitting. Coincidental with these and other programs, smoking rates in the United States declined. The highest rate of per capita cigarette consumption was in 1966, 2 years after the first Surgeon General's report on the dangers of smoking. Figure 12.3

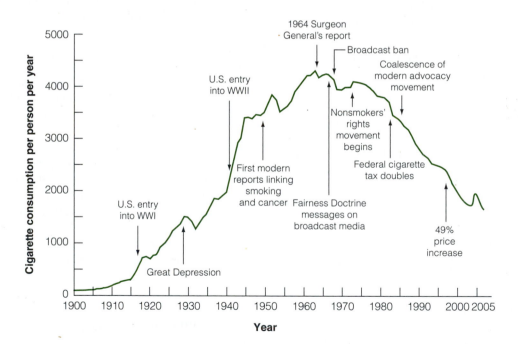

FIGURE 12.3 Cigarette consumption per person 18 and over, United States, 1900–2007.

Sources: "Surveillance for Selected Tobacco Use Behaviors—United States, 1900–1994," by G. A. Givovino et al., 1994, *Morbidity and Mortality Weekly Report*, *43*, No. SS-3, pp. 6–7; National Center for Health Statistics, 2001, *Health, United States 2001*, Hyattsville, MD: U.S. Government Printing Office. "Trends in Tobacco Use," by American Lung Association, Research and Program Services, Epidemiology and Statistics Unit, 2011, Table 2. Retrieved September 27, 2011 from www.lung.org/finding-cures/our-research/trend-reports/Tobacco-Trend-Report.pdf

shows a significant decrease in the per capita consumption of cigarettes in the United States since the Surgeon General's report; it also shows historical events that may have increased or decreased the per capita consumption of cigarettes.

Who Smokes and Who Does Not?

Currently, slightly more than 21% of adults in the United States are classified as smokers, a percentage that is half of the 42% who smoked in 1965 (National Center for Health Statistics [NCHS], 2011). The number of former smokers has declined recently as the number of never-smokers has increased (see Figure 12.4); President Barack Obama is now among that group of former smokers.

How Do Smokers Differ From Nonsmokers? Smokers differ from nonsmokers in gender, ethnicity, age, occupation, educational level, and a variety of other factors. By gender, about 23.5% of adult men and 17.9% of adult women in the United States are current smokers

(Centers for Disease Control and Prevention [CDC], 2010b). From 1965 to about 1985, the quit rate was higher for men than it was for women, thus producing a sharper decline in the number of men who smoked. During the past 20 years, the quit rates for women and men have been nearly identical, with both genders showing a small decline in smoking rates and a slightly higher smoking rate for men than for women.

As for ethnic groups, American Indians (including Alaska Natives) have the highest rate of cigarette consumption (about 24%), and Asian Americans have the lowest percentage of smokers (fewer than 11%) (NCHS, 2011). Perhaps because many longtime smokers die of cigarette-related causes, smoking prevalence is lowest for people age 65 and older, with about 7% of older people classified as smokers. Despite the high cost of cigarettes, people living below the poverty level have higher smoking rates (30%) than those who are wealthier (about 14%). Even for those who are not poor, smoking is inversely related to personal net wealth—smokers are poorer than nonsmokers, and poorer smokers are less likely

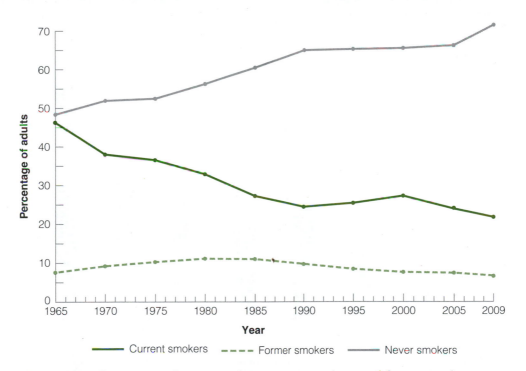

FIGURE 12.4 Percentage of never smokers, current smokers, and former smokers among adults, United States, 1965–2009.

Source: "Trends in tobacco use," by American Lung Association, Research and Program Services, Epidemiology and Statistics Unit, 2011, Table 2. Retrieved September 27, 2011 from www.lungusa.org/finding-cures/our-research/trend-reports/Tobacco-Trend-Report.pdf. Used with permission © 2012 American Lung Association.

to quit and more likely to relapse than higher-income smokers (Kendzor et al., 2010).

Finally, level of education is a good predictor of smoking rates: the higher the level of education, the lower the rate of smoking (CDC, 2010b). In the United States, for example, only 5.6% of people with a graduate (master's or doctoral) degree are current smokers, whereas more than 49% of people with a General Education Diploma (GED) are current smokers (CDC, 2010b). This difference appears even before students enter college—college-bound high school students smoke at lower rates than those who do not plan to attend college (Johnston, O'Malley, Bachman, & Schulenberg, 2011). Figure 12.5 shows the inverse relationship between level of smoking and level of education in the United States.

The inverse relationship between level of education and level of smoking holds true for most, but not all, segments of European society. This pattern appeared in a large sample of people in Germany (Schulze & Mons, 2006), but a more complex pattern appeared in a study involving nine European countries (Schaap, van Agt, & Kunst, 2008). The relationship of smoking and education was stronger among younger people, whereas occupational status was more influential among older people in Northern Europe. The pattern was more varied for residents of Southern Europe, but education remained a predictor of smoking.

Smoking Rates Among Young People

President Barack Obama started smoking when he was a teenager ("Barack Obama Quits," 2011), which makes him similar to most smokers. In a survey of risky behaviors, about 12% of ninth-grade boys and 15% of ninth-grade girls smoked at least once in the previous month (Eaton et al., 2010). Figure 12.6 shows slightly different patterns of smoking for female and male students, with male students increasing their levels of smoking throughout high school. By the time students reach 12th grade, about 8% of the boys and 6% of the girls are frequent smokers.

Many adolescents begin to experiment with smoking during middle school and high school, but adolescence is probably not the time that young people adopt a consistent pattern of smoking. This pattern is usually established after age 18 and may consist of being a nonsmoker, a light smoker, an occasional smoker, or a heavy smoker. Recall that President Obama began

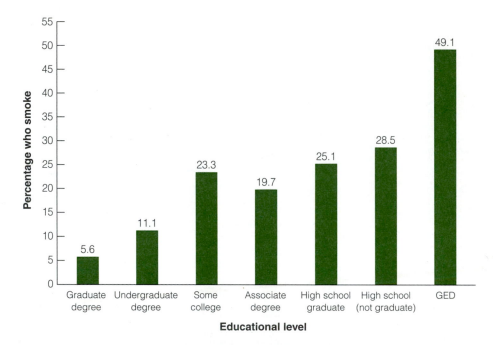

FIGURE 12.5 Percentage of persons 18 and older who are smokers, by educational level, United States, 2009.

Source: "Vital signs: Current smoking among adults aged >18 years–United States, 2009," by S.R. Dube, A. McClave, C. James, R. Caramello, R Kaufmann, & T. Pechacek, 2010, *Morbidity & Mortality Weekly Report 59, 35*, p. 1137.

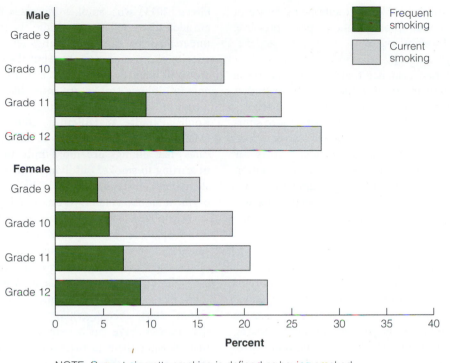

NOTE: Current cigarette smoking is defined as having smoked cigarettes on 1 or more days of the 30 days preceding the survey; frequent cigarette smoking is defined as having smoked cigarettes on 20 or more of the 30 days preceding the survey.

FIGURE 12.6   Current cigarette smoking among high school students by gender, frequency, and grade level, United States, 2009.

Source: "Youth Behavior risk surveillance—United States, 2009," by D. K. Eaton et al., 2010, *Morbidity and Mortality Weekly Reports Surveillance Summaries, 59* (SS-5), Table 28.

smoking as a teenager and escalated his smoking, becoming a heavy smoker during young adulthood.

Compared with students, much less attention has been given to young adults 18 to 24. In Canada, the highest rate of smoking is among young adults (Hammond, 2005). That finding is partially consistent with data from the United States: Rates for 18- to 24-year-old men are high (about 28%), but young women's smoking has decreased at a rate similar to other age groups (to about 16%).

Why Do People Smoke?

Despite widespread publicity linking cigarette smoking to a variety of health problems, millions of people continue to smoke. This situation is puzzling because many smokers themselves acknowledge the potential dangers of their habit. Let us divide the question of

why people smoke into two separate ones: Why do people begin to smoke, and why do they continue?

Answers to the first question are difficult because most young people are aware of the hazards of smoking, and many of them become ill from their first attempt at smoking. The best answer to the second question seems to be that different people smoke for different reasons, and the same person may smoke for different reasons in different situations.

Why Do People Start Smoking?   Most young people are aware of the hazards of smoking (Waltenbaugh & Zagummy, 2004) and how much disapproval the habit carries (Johnston et al., 2011), yet thousands of them begin to smoke each year. Many of these young people have an optimistic bias, believing that the dangers do not apply to them. In addition to this optimistic bias, researchers have examined at least four explanations for why people begin smoking despite being aware of the dangers: genetic predisposition, peer pressure, advertising, and weight control.

Genetics   The first evidence that smoking has some genetic component appeared in the 1950s from studies on twins (Pomerleau & Kardia, 1999). These studies indicated that identical twins tended to be more similar than fraternal twins in their choice to smoke or not. More recent research implicates genetic factors for smoking initiation, nicotine dependence, and cessation success (Furberg et al., 2010). A large number of genes have been identified that affect smoking behavior, mostly through the effect of genes on neurotransmitters in the brain (Ju Wang & Li, 2010).

One neurotransmitter has been implicated in smoking (and other addictions) more strongly than others: dopamine. This neurotransmitter is important in the brain's reward system. Some genetic variations involving dopamine reception and transport seem to increase vulnerability to begin and continue smoking (Clague, Cinciripini, Blalock, Wu, & Hudmon, 2010; Laucht et al., 2008).

A great deal of evidence indicates that smoking has heritable components, and evidence concerning specific genes and gene location is beginning to appear. Thus, genetic variations increase some people's vulnerability to become and remain smokers. However, the research on genetics also confirms the importance of environmental influences. In a longitudinal study of smoking initiation that controlled for genetic relatedness (Slomkowski, Rende, Novak, Lloyd-Richardson, & Niaura, 2005), both genetics and social environment contributed to smoking initiation: Adolescents who reported a closer connection to smoking siblings were more likely to become smokers. These results highlight the interaction between social and genetic factors in the initiation of smoking.

Social Pressure   Teenagers tend to be sensitive to social pressure, and having friends, parents, or siblings who smoke increases the chances that a teen will smoke (Vitória, Salgueiro, Silva, & De Vries, 2009). Teenagers may be encouraged to smoke and to continue smoking by peers who offer them cigarettes, but overt pressure is not necessary—young people may begin to smoke to fit in with a social group (Stewart-Knox et al., 2005). However, the behavior of friends is important; having a close childhood friend (Bricker et al., 2006) or a romantic partner (Kennedy, Tucker, Pollard, Go, &

Green, 2011) who smokes increases the chances that an adolescent will try smoking. As President Obama understood, parents and siblings who smoke may not encourage a teenager to start, but they furnish a model that is influential. Thus, teens in families in which parents or siblings smoke are more likely to do so than teens in nonsmoking families (O'Loughlin, Karp, Koulis, Paradis, & DiFranza, 2009). Some evidence (Mercken, Candel, Willems, & de Vries, 2007) indicates that siblings are more influential than parents in starting to smoke. But living with a smoker—even a stepparent—increases the risk that an adolescent will begin to smoke (Fidler, West, van Jaarsvelt, Jarvis, & Wardle, 2008).

People are not the only source of modeling for smoking; movies and other media can provide a source of social pressure. A growing body of evidence implicates the influence of movies in beginning smoking. John Pierce and his colleagues (Distefan, Pierce, & Gilpin, 2004; Pierce, 2005) examined the influence that movies have on young adolescents and found that viewing their favorite movie stars smoking on film influences these teens. In a longitudinal study with a representative sample of adolescents in the United States (Wills, Sargent, Stoolmiller, Gibbons, & Gerrard, 2008), viewing smoking in movies appeared to influence positive attitudes about smoking and to prompt affiliating with friends who smoked. Both attitudes and friends who smoke relate to smoking initiation. A systematic review of media influence on smoking (Nunez-Smith et al., 2010) found a strong association between media exposure and smoking.

The influence of smoking in movies extends to young people in countries other than the United States (although the movies that portray smoking are mostly from the United States). In a study of German children between ages 10 and 17 (Hanewinkel & Sargent, 2007), viewing movies with portrayals of smoking influenced the initiation and continuation of smoking. Thus, the social environment provides many sources that may influence young people to smoke or to decline; advertising is also part of that environment.

Advertising   In addition to social pressure, tobacco companies use advertising as a means of getting teenagers interested in smoking. John Pierce and associates (Pierce, Distefan, Kaplan, & Gilpin, 2005) studied how adolescents may become susceptible to advertising by dividing 12- to 15-year-old adolescents who had never smoked into two groups: committed never-smokers

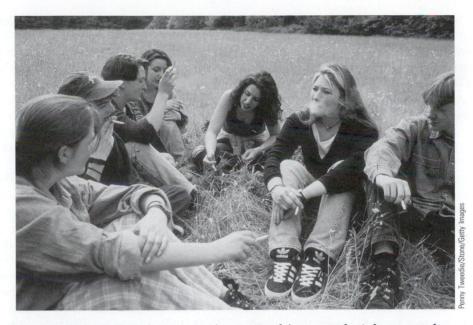

Penny Tweedie/Stone/Getty Images

Acceptance into a social group can be a powerful source of reinforcement for adolescents, increasing the pressure to begin smoking.

who showed no interest in smoking, and susceptible never-smokers who reported some interest in smoking. An important difference between the two groups was curiosity. Committed never-smokers who lacked curiosity tended to pay little attention to tobacco ads and were unlikely to begin smoking. Thus, curiosity may be a critical ingredient in adolescents' decision to smoke or not to smoke. Advertising that arouses curiosity can be an effective means of marketing any product, including cigarettes.

Several longitudinal studies and a systematic review indicate that advertising boosts smoking, especially among young people. One longitudinal study (Henriksen, Schleicher, Feighery, & Fortmann, 2010) focused on the influence of cigarette advertising in stores and found that adolescents who often visited stores with prominent cigarette advertising were significantly more likely to begin smoking than adolescents who visited such stores less often. Another longitudinal study (Gilpin, White, Messer, & Pierce, 2007) showed that adolescents who had a favorite cigarette advertisement or were willing to use cigarette promotional items were more likely to be smokers 3 and 6 years later. The systematic review (Paynter & Edwards, 2009) evaluated the influence of advertising that appears where cigarettes are sold and concluded that such advertising not only makes it more likely that young people will begin

to smoke but also contributes to more purchases among smokers and to relapses among those who have quit.

If prosmoking advertising is effective, can antismoking advertising be effective as well? Antismoking media campaigns can be effective, but probably not as effective as advertising to promote smoking. A mass media antismoking campaign (Flynn et al., 2010) showed little effect. Another study found that both antismoking and prosmoking advertising can be effective, but the antismoking messages were not strong enough to counteract the prosmoking appeals (Weiss et al., 2006). Thus, antismoking advertising is not yet sufficiently effective to be an antidote to tobacco company advertising.

Weight Control   Many girls and some boys begin smoking because they believe it will help them control their weight. A longitudinal study with Dutch adolescents (Harakeh, Engels, Monshouwer, & Hanssen, 2010) showed that weight concerns were positively related to smoking initiation. Smoking also appeared as a weight control strategy in another study (Fulkerson & French, 2003), which showed a more widespread effect—only young African American women were immune from this tactic. This study also showed that young men were willing to use smoking for weight control, with Native American and Asian American men adopting this strategy more often than young men from other ethnic groups.

Young women who were dieting reported that they used smoking as a strategy to lose weight (Jenks & Higgs, 2007). Adolescent smokers who wanted to lose weight were likely not only to use smoking as a strategy but also to use other unhealthy dieting strategies, such as diet pills or laxatives (Johnson, Eaton, Pederson, & Lowry, 2009). Thus, smoking is a choice for losing weight among young people, and this risky practice is associated with other risky weight control behaviors.

Why Do People Continue to Smoke? Different people smoke for different reasons, including being addicted to nicotine, receiving positive and negative reinforcement, having an optimistic bias, and fearing weight gain.

Addiction Once people begin to smoke, they quickly become dependent. The Centers for Disease Control and Prevention (CDC, 1994) surveyed smokers 10 to 22 years old and found that nearly two thirds of those who had smoked at least 100 cigarettes during their lifetime reported that "It's really hard to quit," but only a small number of those who had smoked fewer than 100 lifetime cigarettes gave this response. In addition, nearly 90% of participants who smoked more than 15 cigarettes a day found quitting to be very hard. These results suggest that people will become dependent on smoking and have great difficulty quitting once they have smoked about 100 cigarettes or have increased their cigarette consumption to more than 15 per day. These results are consistent with President Obama's smoking—his smoking escalated, and he became an addicted smoker who had a great deal of difficulty quitting.

When addicted smokers are restricted to low-nicotine cigarettes, they smoke more cigarettes to compensate for the scarcity of nicotine they are receiving. An early study by Stanley Schachter (1980) manipulated the amount of nicotine in cigarettes supplied to heavy, long-duration smokers. The participants smoked 25% more low-nicotine than high-nicotine cigarettes and took more puffs from low-nicotine cigarettes. A more recent study (Strasser, Lerman, Sandborn, Pickworth, & Feldman, 2007) performed a similar manipulation and obtained similar results—smokers compensate when they smoke lower-nicotine cigarettes.

Addicted smokers not only are aware of smoking but also are keenly conscious of the fact when they are

not smoking. They usually know how long it has been since their last cigarette and how long it will be before their next one. Addicted smokers never leave home or office without first checking their supply of cigarettes. They often keep several extra packs available in case of emergency. These smokers will be willing to smoke bad-tasting cigarettes, whereas smokers whose focus is pleasure or relaxation will not (Leventhal & Avis, 1976).

Nicotine addiction, however, does not explain why some people are light smokers and others smoke heavily. In addition, if nicotine were the only reason for smoking, then other modes of nicotine delivery should substitute fully for smoking. A variety of nicotine delivery systems exist, including patches, gum, nasal spray, inhalers, and lozenges, which means that smokers may receive nicotine in other (less dangerous) ways. However, other delivery methods are not as satisfactory as cigarettes to smokers (Hughes, 2003; Sweeney, Fant, Fagerstrom, McGovern, & Henningfield, 2001). Indeed, smokers rated cigarettes with tobacco from which the nicotine has been removed as more satisfying and relaxing than nicotine inhalers (Barrett, 2010). Although nicotine may play a role in the reason people continue to smoke, this research indicates that nicotine addiction is not the entire story of continuing to smoke.

Positive and Negative Reinforcement A second reason why people continue to smoke is that they receive either positive or negative reinforcement, or both. Behaviors are positively reinforced when they are followed immediately by a pleasant or pleasurable event. The smoking habit is strengthened by such positive reinforcers as pleasure from the smell of tobacco smoke, feelings of relaxation, and satisfaction of manual needs.

Negative reinforcement may also account for why some people continue to smoke (USDHHS, 2010c). Behaviors are negatively reinforced when they are followed immediately by the removal of or lessening of an unpleasant condition. After smokers become addicted, they must continue to smoke to avoid the aversive effects of withdrawal; that is, when addicted smokers begin to feel tense, anxious, or depressed after not smoking for some period of time, they can remove these unpleasant symptoms by smoking another cigarette.

Examinations of smokers' motivations are consistent with both types of reinforcement. Smokers attending a cessation clinic (McEwen, West, & McRobbie, 2008) rated relief from stress and boredom as their top two reasons for smoking; these reasons were similar among deployed military personnel (Poston et al., 2008). Relief from an unpleasant emotion meets the definition of negative reinforcement. Smokers also reported pleasure and enjoyment as reasons for smoking (McEwen et al., 2008), which fit into the category of positive reinforcement.

Optimistic Bias   In addition to addiction and reinforcement, many people continue to smoke because they have an **optimistic bias** that leads them to believe that they personally have a lower risk of disease and death than do other smokers (Weinstein, 1980). For example, when asked about their chances of living to be 75 years old, people who had never smoked and those who were former and light smokers estimated fairly accurately (Schoenbaum, 1997). Heavy smokers, on the other hand, greatly overestimated their chances of living to age 75.

Neil Weinstein (2001) reviewed research on smokers' recognition of their vulnerability to harm and found strong support for the hypothesis that smokers tend to have an optimistic bias. That is, smokers do not perceive that they are at the same level of risk as other smokers. Indeed, smokers acknowledged the risk of cardiovascular disease, lung cancer, and emphysema that accompanies smoking (Waltenbaugh & Zagummy, 2004), but applied that risk to other smokers more than to themselves. Also, smokers in four countries showed an optimistic bias by rating the brand of cigarettes that they smoked as less likely to cause disease than other brands (Mutti et al., 2011). Thus, smokers tend to maintain an optimistic bias concerning their vulnerability to smoking-related dangers, which contributes to their continued smoking.

Fear of Weight Gain   Adolescents are not the only age group using cigarette smoking as a means of weight control. Adults, too, often continue to smoke for fear of weight gain. In a later section, we examine the validity of those concerns, but here we look at the magnitude of fears concerning weight gain.

Concern about weight gain extends to a wide range of smokers, but concern varies with age, gender, and ethnicity. Weight control is a factor that may influence some young people to begin smoking (Harakeh et al., 2010), and this concern continues during young adulthood (Koval, Pedersen, Zhang, Mowery, & McKenna, 2008). In addition, weight concern plays a role in adults' choice to continue smoking (Sánchez-Johnsen, Carpentier, & King, 2011).

Gender is an even stronger predictor of who uses smoking for weight control. For example, college-age women with body image problems were more likely to be smokers than women without such body image problems (Stickney & Black, 2008). A study of African American and White American women and men (Sánchez-Johnsen et al., 2011) revealed weight concern as a factor in continuing to smoke for all groups, but women (and especially White women) were more concerned than men of either ethnicity. A study of women with strong weight concerns (King, Saules, & Irish, 2007) indicated that such women were much more likely to smoke (37.5%) compared with women without strong weight concerns (22%). Should women with high weight concerns quit smoking, their concerns may increase; normal-weight women who were ex-smokers expressed higher concerns over their weight than normal-weight women who had never smoked (Pisinger & Jorgensen, 2007). These results point to a factor of weight concern, which some people attempt to manage through choosing to smoke and to whom quitting presents a threat.

IN SUMMARY

The rate of smoking in the United States has declined since the mid-1960s, but that decline has stalled. Presently, about 18% of adult women and 23% of adult men in the United States meet the definition of smoker. Ethnic background is a factor in smoking for both adolescents and adults, with Native Americans having the highest smoking rate, followed by African Americans, European Americans, Hispanic Americans, and Asian Americans. Currently, educational level is a better predictor of smoking status than gender, with highly educated people smoking at a much lower rate than those with less education.

Reasons for smoking can be divided into questions concerning why people begin to smoke and why they continue to smoke. Most smokers begin as teenagers, at a time when they are very vulnerable to peer pressure. Genetics may play a role in beginning to smoke, but social factors such as friends, siblings, and parents who smoke; advertising; and weight concerns also influence smoking initiation. The question about why people continue is a difficult one because people smoke for a variety of reasons. Nearly every smoker in the United States is familiar with the potential dangers of smoking, but many do not relate those hazards to themselves; that is, their knowledge of the dangers of smoking is attenuated by an optimistic bias. For many people, smoking reduces stress, anxiety, and depression and therefore provides negative reinforcement. Some people smoke because they are addicted to the nicotine in tobacco products, and others continue to smoke because they are concerned about weight gain.

Health Consequences of Tobacco Use

Tobacco use is responsible for more than 443,000 deaths yearly in the United States, or more than 1,200 deaths a day (USDHHS, 2010c), and almost 6 million per year worldwide (American Cancer Society, 2012). All forms of tobacco use have health consequences, but smoking cigarettes is the most common and thus the most hazardous. Those hazards include cardiovascular disease, cancer, chronic lower respiratory disease, and a variety of other disorders.

Cigarette Smoking

Cigarette smoking is the single deadliest behavior in the history of the United States (and possibly the world), and it is the largest preventable cause of death and disability. In Chapter 2, we discussed how scientists have found evidence to support the criteria for establishing a cause-and-effect relationship between smoking and several diseases, even though experimental research is not possible with human participants. Evidence for the harmful effects of tobacco use began to emerge as early as the 1930s, and by the 1950s, the relationship between cigarette smoking and cancer, cardiovascular disease, and chronic lower respiratory disease was well established (USDHHS, 2010c). These diseases remain the three leading causes of death in the United States, and cigarette smoking contributes to all three.

Smoking and Cancer Cancer is the second leading cause of death in the United States but the leading cause of smoking-related deaths. Smoking plays a role in the development of a long list of cancers, especially

lung cancer. Sufficient evidence exists to conclude that smoking is a causal factor in cancers of the lip, pharynx, esophagus, pancreas, larynx, trachea, urinary bladder, kidney, cervix, and stomach (USDHHS, 2010c). Both female and male smokers have an extremely high risk of dying from cancer, with men's relative risk being about 23.3 times that of nonsmokers. This risk is the strongest link established to date between any behavior and a major cause of death.

From 1950 to 1989, lung cancer deaths rose sharply, a trend that lagged about 20 to 25 years behind the rapid rise in cigarette consumption. During the mid-1960s, cigarette consumption began to drop sharply, and then about 25 to 30 years later, lung cancer deaths among men began to decline. Figure 10.6 (see Chapter 10, page 241) shows the close tracking of men's and women's deaths from lung cancer and the rise and fall of cigarette consumption in the United States. This is strong circumstantial evidence for a causal link between smoking and lung cancer.

Could other factors, including environmental pollutants, be responsible for the rapid rise in lung cancer deaths before 1990? Evidence from a prospective study (Thun, Day-Lally, Calle, Flanders, & Heath, 1995) strongly suggested that neither pollution nor any other nonsmoking factor was responsible for the increase in lung cancer deaths from 1959 to 1988. Another piece of evidence against smoking is data showing that lung cancer deaths for smokers rose significantly during this period, whereas lung cancer deaths among nonsmokers remained about the same (USDHHS, 1990), indicating that indoor/outdoor pollution, radon, and other suspected carcinogens had little effect on increases in lung cancer mortality. These results, along with those from earlier epidemiological studies, strongly suggest that cigarette smoking is the primary contributor to lung cancer deaths.

Smoking and Cardiovascular Disease Cardiovascular disease (CVD),including both heart disease and stroke, is the leading cause of death in the United States. Until the mid-1990s, the largest number of smoking-related deaths resulted from cardiovascular disease, but these deaths declined, whereas those from cancer have not declined so rapidly. Now, CVD is the second largest cause of tobacco-related deaths.

What is the level of risk for cardiovascular disease among people who smoke? In general, research suggests that the risk is at least doubled (USDHHS, 2010c). The risk is slightly higher for men than for women, but both male and female smokers have a significantly increased chance of both fatal and nonfatal heart attack and stroke.

What biological mechanism might explain the association between smoking and cardiovascular disease? Smoking damages the inner wall of arteries and speeds the formation of plaque within the arteries (USDHHS, 2010c). Smoking is also related to formation of blood clots along the walls of arteries, which is a dangerous complication to artery damage. In addition, smoking is related to inflammation, not only in the lungs but also within the entire body; growing evidence implicates the role of inflammation in the development of artery disease. Smoking has also been implicated in harmful changes in lipid metabolism, so smoking may be linked to unfavorable cholesterol levels. Smoking also decreases the availability of oxygen to the heart muscle while at the same time increasing demand for oxygen by the heart. The exact mechanisms through which these reactions occur are becoming clearer (USDHHS, 2010c). Nicotine itself has been implicated, and carbon monoxide is also a suspect. Thus, smoking produces a variety of physiological reactions that increase the risks for CVD.

Smoking and Chronic Lower Respiratory Disease

Chronic lower respiratory disease includes a number of respiratory and lung diseases; the two most deadly are emphysema and chronic bronchitis. These diseases are relatively rare among nonsmokers; most of those afflicted have been exposed to passive smoking from a spouse who smokes.

In summary, the three leading causes of death in the United States are also the three principal smoking-related causes of death. The U.S. Public Health Service has estimated that about half of all cigarette smokers eventually die from their habit (USDHHS, 1995).

Other Effects of Smoking　In addition to cancer, cardiovascular disease, and chronic lower respiratory disease, a number of other problems have been linked to smoking. For example, as many as 1,000 people die each year in the United States from fires begun by cigarettes (USDHHS, 2004). In England, cigarettes and materials related to smoking (such as lighters) were the most common cause of fire fatalities for both adults and children (Mulvaney et al., 2009). Drinking alcohol interacts with smoking cigarettes to magnify the risk of fires and burns, but of course, smoking by itself contributes more to those fires than drinking by itself.

Smoking also relates to diseases of the mouth, pharynx, larynx, esophagus, pancreas, kidney, bladder, and cervix (USDHHS, 2004). Smokers also have more than their share of periodontal disease (Bánóczy & Squier, 2004) and multiple sclerosis (Hernán et al., 2005), which may be related to the effects of smoking on inflammation and the immune system (Gonçalves et al., 2011). Smoking is also related to diminished physical strength, poorer balance, impaired neuromuscular performance (Nelson, Nevitt, Scott, Stone, & Cummings, 1994) and a variety of injuries, including motor vehicle crashes (Wen et al., 2005). Smokers are also more likely than nonsmokers to commit suicide (Miller, Hemenway, & Rimm, 2000), to develop acute respiratory disease such as pneumonia (USDHHS, 2004), to experience problems with cognitive functioning (Sabia, Marmont, Dufouil, & Singh-Manoux, 2008), and to suffer from macular degeneration (Jager, Mieler, & Miller, 2008). Smoking also relates to a variety of mental illnesses (see Would You Believe …).

Women who smoke experience risks specific to their gender. Some research (Kiyohara & Ohno, 2010) has indicated that female smokers may be more vulnerable to lung cancer than male smokers. Smoking at least one pack of cigarettes a day places women at double the risk for cardiovascular disease and a tenfold risk of dying from chronic lower respiratory disease. Female smokers have an increased risk of fertility problems, miscarriages, preterm delivery, birth defects, and low-birth-weight infants (USDHHS, 2010c). Pregnant women who smoke double their chances of delivering a stillborn infant, and they almost triple their risk of having an infant who dies during the first year of life (Dietz et al., 2010). Children and adolescents who smoke have slower growth of lung function and begin to lose lung function at earlier ages than those who do not smoke (USDHHS, 2004).

Male smokers also experience some specific risks from their habit. Smoking not only may make men look older and less attractive (Ernster et al., 1995), but it also increases their chances of experiencing erectile dysfunction (USDHHS, 2004).

In any given year, at least 14% of smokers and former smokers will experience a chronic disease (Kahende, Woollery, & Lee, 2007), and half of smokers will die of smoking-related causes (American Cancer Society, 2012). The negative effects are not limited to individual smokers. Society, too, pays a price. Smoking-related illnesses and economic losses cost the people of the United States $226 billion annually (American

Would You BELIEVE...? Smoking Is Related to Mental Illness

Most people know that smoking is a risk for a variety of physical illnesses, but smoking is also related to mental illness. Indeed, people who smoke are as much as 3 times more likely to have been diagnosed with psychiatric disorders than nonsmokers (McClave, McKnight-Eily, Davis, & Dube, 2010). This increased risk for mental illness applies to a number of diagnoses, and the more serious disorders are more strongly associated with smoking. (The rate of smoking in the United States is about 21%, so anything higher represents an elevation.) About 34% of people with phobic fears (a relatively minor type of mental disorder) smoke, but almost 60% of those who have been diagnosed with schizophrenia (a very serious mental disorder) are smokers. People who are depressed also have elevated smoking rates (Strong et al., 2010), as do individuals with personality disorders (Zvolensky, Jenkins,

Johnson, & Goodwin, 2011). Nor does the relationship between smoking and mental illness begin during adulthood: It appears during adolescence (Lawrence, Mitrou, Sawyer, & Zubrick, 2010). As the severity of the mental illness increases, so does the smoking rate (Dixon et al., 2007). In addition, people with a diagnosis of multiple mental disorders have increased chances of being heavy smokers (McClave et al., 2010).

Being a heavy smoker creates severe nicotine dependence, which means that people with serious mental disorders experience an increased risk of health problems, but they also encounter even more than typical difficulties in quitting (Tsoi, Porwal, & Webster, 2010). One possibility for the problems in quitting comes from the medication that people with schizophrenia and bipolar disorder take to control their symptoms. These drugs affect brain chemistry, perhaps

in ways that influence nicotine receptors in the brain, making people who take these medications more vulnerable to nicotine's effects and possibly more resistant to quitting. The evidence for this position is not very strong (Matthews, Wilson, & Mitchell, 2011), and other possibilities for the relationship between smoking and mental illness exist. One possibility is that people with mental illness use smoking as a form of self-medication to help them cope with their disorder. Or, the social environment of those with mental disorders may encourage and support continuing smoking rather than quitting.

Despite the barriers, some people with serious mental disorders manage to quit (Dickerson et al., 2011). However, smokers with mental disorders experience increased chances for the dangers for smoking and present a difficult challenge for smoking cessation treatment.

Cancer Society, 2012). These costs, of course, are not limited to smokers—they affect everyone who pays health insurance premiums and everyone who pays for lost worker productivity. Smokers obviously cannot legitimately argue that their smoking habit affects only themselves; their habit costs society as much as it costs individual smokers.

Cigar and Pipe Smoking

Are cigar and pipe smoking as hazardous as cigarette smoking? People from Australia, Canada, the United Kingdom, and the United States expressed the opinion that smoking cigars or pipes is less hazardous than smoking cigarettes (O'Connor et al., 2007). The tobacco used in pipes and cigars differs somewhat from the tobacco used to make cigarettes, but pipe and cigar tobacco is similarly carcinogenic.

Whereas male, cigarette-only smokers have a risk for lung cancer of about 23 times that of nonsmokers, cigar and pipe smokers' risk is elevated only about 5 times that of nonsmokers (Henley, Thun, Chao, & Calle, 2004). Thus, the beliefs of lower risk for cigar and pipe smokers are correct. However, cigar and pipe smokers experience reduced lung function and increased airflow obstruction (Rodriguez et al., 2010), but these smokers' life expectancy is not lowered as drastically as those who smoke cigarettes (Streppel, Boshuizen, Ocké, Kok, & Kromhout, 2007). Heavy cigarette smoking produced a reduction in life expectancy of 8.8 years, whereas cigar or pipe smoking decreased life expectancy by 4.7 years. The diseases that kill cigar and pipe smokers are the same as those that increase the mortality of cigarette smokers—heart disease, chronic lower respiratory disease, and a variety of cancers. These findings suggest that cigar and pipe smoking may be less hazardous than cigarettes, but they are not safe.

The dangers of pipe smoking are of increasing concern with the spread of water pipe smoking (Maziak, 2011). This practice is common in the Middle East among adults, but within the past decade, its popularity has spread around the world. The practice has become especially popular among young people. In the United States, between 6% and 34% of adolescents with Middle Eastern background and between 5% and 17% of adolescents with other ethnic backgrounds smoke tobacco in water pipes. Authorities are concerned that this trend may forecast a new worldwide tobacco epidemic.

Passive Smoking

Many nonsmokers find the smoke of others to be a nuisance and even irritating to their eyes and nose. This annoying exposure still occurs commonly but less often than in the past (Kaufmann et al., 2010), decreasing from 52% of nonsmokers in 1999 to about 40% in 2008. This decline occurred in all age, ethnic, and gender groups.

But is **passive smoking**, also known as **environmental tobacco smoke (ETS)** or secondhand smoke more than annoying—is it harmful to the health of nonsmokers? In the 1980s, some evidence began to accrue that passive smoking might be a health hazard. Specifically, passive smoking has been linked to lung cancer, breast cancer, heart disease, and a variety of respiratory problems in children.

Passive Smoking and Cancer   The effect of passive smoking on lung and other cancers is difficult to determine because of problems in assessing the intensity and duration of exposure. Research has focused on workplace exposure and nonsmokers who live in households with a smoker. In general, the more environmental tobacco smoke people are exposed to and the longer the exposure, the higher the risk for cancer.

People whose jobs expose them to high levels of smoke have an increased risk of lung cancer mortality. One review (Siegel & Skeer, 2003) described such jobs cleverly as the "5 B's"—bars, bowling alleys, billiard halls, betting establishments, and bingo parlors. Long-time employees of these establishments had up to 18 times higher nicotine concentrations than people who worked in restaurants, residences, and offices. A meta-analysis that drew from studies worldwide (Stayner et al., 2007) found that exposed workers showed a 24% increase in lung cancer. For workers whose exposure was heavy, the risk of lung cancer was doubled.

Nonsmokers who live in a household with a smoker are also exposed to cigarette smoke unless the smoker refrains from smoking indoors, which is true for an increasing number of smokers. Indeed, the restriction on places where smokers are allowed to smoke is a major factor in the decrease in exposure to environmental tobacco smoke (Kaufmann et al., 2010). A meta-analysis of cancer risk in nonsmoking wives on three continents (Taylor, Najafi, & Dobson, 2007) revealed that risk increased between 15% and 31%, depending on geographic location. Therefore, evidence from both types of individuals exposed to cigarette smoke show that this exposure increases their risk of cancer.

Passive Smoking and Cardiovascular Disease
Although the effect of environmental exposure to tobacco smoke exerts a modest increase in risk for cancer, its effects on cardiovascular disease are substantial. Exposure to smoke prompts some of the same physiological reactions as smoking—inflammation, formation of blood clots, and changes to the lining of arteries—which increases the risks for heart disease (Venn & Britton, 2007). A meta-analysis of studies (Enstrom & Kabat, 2006) showed that the excess risk of heart disease for passive smokers is about 25%, a risk similar to the risk for stroke (Lee & Forey, 2006). However, even this small elevation of risk for heart disease translates into thousands of deaths each year from passive smoking, but this large number is only about one tenth of the number of those who die from active smoking.

Passive Smoking and the Health of Children   Infants and young children are more likely to be exposed to tobacco smoke and are more vulnerable to the hazards of tobacco smoke than adults (Kaufmann et al., 2010). The hazards can begin even before babies are born and extend into childhood. For example, smoke exposure increases the risks of sudden infant death syndrome (SIDS). Other health problems for children include decreased lung function, increased risk for chronic lower respiratory disease, and triggering of asthma attacks. In general, the negative effects of environmental tobacco smoke diminish as children age, but school-age children exposed to passive smoking have more than their share of wheezing, missed school days, and weaker lung function volume.

In summary, passive smoking is a health risk for lung cancer, cardiovascular disease, and many health problems of children. In general, the greater the exposure, the greater is the risk.

Smokeless Tobacco

Smokeless tobacco includes snuff and chewing tobacco, forms of tobacco that were more popular during the 19th century than at present. Currently, European American and Hispanic American male adolescents use smokeless tobacco more than any other segment of the U.S. population (Eaton et al., 2010), but smokeless forms of tobacco use are common among adolescents and young men in some areas of the world, especially in the eastern Mediterranean region (Warren et al., 2008). Although many of the young people who use smokeless forms of tobacco acknowledge that it carries risks, they tend to believe that it is safer than smoking.

The belief that smokeless tobacco is safer than smoking has been a factor in its increased use throughout North America and parts of Europe. In some sense, this belief is correct; smokeless tobacco does not carry as high a risk for disease as smoking does (Colilla, 2010), but tobacco is still a toxin and a carcinogen with health risks. The evidence is not sufficiently strong to support a causal link, but the use of smokeless tobacco is associated with increased mortality from oral, pancreatic, and lung cancer as well as cardiovascular disease. The use of smokeless tobacco as a substitute for smoking is questionable; adolescents who begin to use smokeless tobacco are more likely to begin smoking than those who do not try this form of tobacco (Severson, Forrester, & Biglan, 2007). The risks of using smokeless tobacco are not as great as those associated with smoking cigarettes; nevertheless, chewing tobacco presents some health hazards.

IN SUMMARY

The health consequences of tobacco use are multiple and serious. Smoking is the number one cause of preventable mortality in the world. Smoking causes about 443,000 deaths a year in the United States, mostly from cancer, cardiovascular disease, and chronic lower respiratory disease. But smoking also carries a risk for nonfatal diseases and disorders such as periodontal disease, loss of physical strength, infertility among women, respiratory disorders, cognitive dysfunction, erectile dysfunction, and macular degeneration.

Many nonsmokers are bothered by the smoking of others, and rightfully so—many of these nonsmokers also have an excess risk of respiratory disease from passive smoking. Research suggests that environmental tobacco smoke raises the risk for lung cancer only slightly but boosts deaths from cardiovascular disease much more. However, children are the most serious victims of passive smoking; their risk for respiratory disorders is increased substantially.

Like cigars and pipes, smokeless tobacco is not as dangerous as cigarette smoking. Teenagers who use smokeless tobacco tend to believe that this form of tobacco is much safer than cigarette smoking, but no level of exposure to tobacco is safe.

Interventions for Reducing Smoking Rates

Although smoking rates are declining in many high-income nations, smoking rates are increasing in middle- and lower-income nations, which will prompt an increase in smoking-related diseases throughout the world (World Health Organization [WHO], 2008a). Thus, the need to reduce smoking rates has become a worldwide goal. Interventions designed to reduce smoking rates can be divided into those that deter people (usually adolescents) from beginning and those that encourage current smokers to stop.

Deterring Smoking

Information alone is not an effective way to change behavior, and this generalization applies to deterring smoking. Nearly every teenager in the United States (and many other parts of the world) knows that smoking is dangerous to health, yet almost 20% of high school students in the United States smoke at least once a month (Eaton et al., 2010).

Choosing to smoke does not occur because children or adolescents lack information about the dangers of tobacco; they receive many messages about the dangers of smoking through antismoking media messages (Weiss et al., 2006), health officials, and concerned parents. By the time adolescents are 14 years old, they pay little attention to health warnings, making such warnings worthless (Siegel & Biener, 2000). Thus, information about the health dangers of smoking does not create successful prevention programs (Flay, 2009). Deterring smoking is a challenge that requires more and different types of interventions.

The most common approach to preventing children from beginning to smoke is through school-based programs, which vary in terms of who delivers the antismoking message, length of intervention, and age of the target students. The most common such program is Project D.A.R.E., which is oriented to drug use but also includes tobacco. This intervention includes antidrug use messages delivered by police officers, typically once a week for a school semester. Evaluations of this program (West & O'Neal, 2004) have revealed that it is not effective in deterring smoking or other drug use. However, other programs have shown more success (Dobbins, DeCorby, Manske, & Goldblatt, 2008). The elements of more successful, school-based programs use interactive delivery rather than only informational lectures, build students' refusal skills and elicit a commitment not to smoke, include at least 15 sessions that stretch into high school, integrate smoking prevention into a comprehensive health education program, and provide prevention messages in the community as well as by parents and through media messages (Flay, 2009). A systematic review of mass media campaigns aimed at young people (Brinn, Carson, Esterman, Chang, & Smith, 2010) indicated that these programs can be effective, and the more media are involved and the longer the messages persist, the more effective the campaign. Unfortunately, the evidence is more impressive for short-term than for long-term effectiveness (Dobbins et al., 2008). Prevention researcher Brian Flay (2009) argued that the elements that build very successful short-term results (listed in the preceding text) can also help with extending prevention effectiveness. Deterring children and adolescents from smoking is not an easy task—nor is giving up smoking.

Quitting Smoking

A second method of reducing smoking rates is for current smokers to quit. Although quitting smoking is not easy, millions of Americans have done so during the past 50 years. As a result, there are now more former smokers in the United States than there are current

smokers—about 23% are former smokers and about 21% are current smokers. Figure 12.4 indicates that the decline in smoking rates is due not only to fewer people starting to smoke but also to increased cessation rates.

Nevertheless, many barriers to quitting exist. One barrier is smoking's addictive quality. Most people who both smoke and drink alcohol consider smoking to be the more difficult habit to break. People seeking treatment for alcohol or drug dependence who also smoked were asked which would be more difficult to quit—their problem substance or tobacco (Kozlowski et al., 1989). A majority of these people reported that cigarettes would be more difficult to quit.

Despite the difficulties of quitting, many smokers have quit on their own, and others have done so with the assistance of pharmacological approaches, psychological interventions, and community-wide antismoking campaigns.

Quitting Without Therapy   Most people who have quit smoking have done so on their own, without the aid of formal cessation programs. In the United States, about 44% of smokers try to quit each year, and about 64% of those people used no cessation treatment (Shiffman, Brockwell, Pillitteri, & Gitchell, 2008). Who are the smokers most likely to quit on their own?

In an important study on unaided quitting, Stanley Schachter (1982) surveyed two populations: The psychology department at Columbia University and the resident population of Amaganset, New York. Schachter found a success rate of more than 60% for both groups, with an average abstinence length of more than 7 years. Surprisingly, nearly a third of the heavy smokers who quit said they had no problems in quitting. Schachter interpreted the high success rate, even for heavy smokers, as evidence that quitting may be easier than the clinic evaluations indicate. He suggested that people who attend clinic programs are, for the most part, those who have failed in attempts to quit on their own, and research on the use of smoking cessation treatment (Shiffman et al., 2008) confirmed this reasoning. In addition, Schachter hypothesized that the clinic success rates of 20% to 30% represent success for each program, with those who fail in one program going on to another, in which they may also have about a 20% to 30% quit rate. Smokers who try to quit on their own largely succeed and never attend a clinic. Thus, people who attend clinics are self-selected on the basis of previous failure. These people, therefore, do not represent the general population of smokers, and failure rates based on clinic populations may be too high. Quitting on one's own is possible.

Using Pharmacological Approaches   People who have not been able to quit on their own may seek help from outside sources, including some type of drug to help them quit. Currently, several pharmacological approaches are available, including nicotine replacement therapy and the drugs varenicline (Chantix) and bupropion (Zyban).

Nicotine replacement includes gum, inhalers, lozenges (tablets), patches, and spray. This approach works by releasing small doses of nicotine into the body. Smokers work toward weaning themselves from larger doses to smaller ones until they are no longer dependent on nicotine. How effective are these nicotine replacement therapies? Large-scale analyses of well-designed studies (Hughes, 2009; Stead, Perera, Bullen, Mant, & Lancaster, 2008) examined studies with various types of nicotine replacement therapy and concluded that this form of treatment is successful, with higher quit rates for nicotine replacement than for no treatment or placebos. President Obama used nicotine gum when he was trying to quit during his first presidential campaign ("Michelle Obama," 2011). Indeed, campaign aides kept a supply of nicotine gum with them to help Obama refrain from smoking, and his physician advised him to continue to use this strategy in his efforts to quit.

The drugs varenicline and bupropion are also effective treatments (Cahill, Stead, & Lancaster, 2011). These drugs work by affecting brain chemistry to decrease withdrawal symptoms and to make smoking less reinforcing. Varenicline may be somewhat more effective than bupropion (but also much more expensive), and both are similar in effectiveness to nicotine replacement. Like all drug treatments, these pharmacological treatments have side effects, most of which are not serious; all of the side effects are less dangerous than continuing to smoke. Unfortunately, the same positive results may not occur for adolescent smokers using one of these pharmacological approaches. A meta-analysis (Kim et al., 2011) found no significant effect for these approaches for adolescents. Adding other components may boost the effectiveness of all pharmacological interventions for adults, and adolescents may require some other approach to quit smoking.

Receiving a Psychological Intervention   Psychological approaches aimed at smoking cessation typically

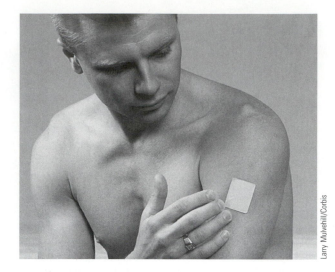

Nicotine replacement can help smokers with symptoms of withdrawal, but the effectiveness is higher when combined with behavioral techniques.

include a combination of strategies, such as behavior modification, cognitive behavioral approaches, contracts made by smoker and therapist in which the smoker agrees to stop smoking, group therapy, social support, relaxation training, stress management, "booster" sessions to prevent relapse, and other components.

Most psychologists working with smoking cessation problems begin with some implicit or explicit theory, such as one or more of the models we discussed in Chapter 4. For example, many researchers have adopted James Prochaska's stages-of-change model. In this model, smokers at the *precontemplation* stage have no intention to quit and, therefore, are not yet good candidates for psychological interventions. When smokers are at this level, a technique such as motivational interviewing may help them move to the *contemplation* stage, at which they are aware of the problem and may consider quitting sometime in the future. Indeed, a systematic review of research using motivational interviewing for smoking cessation (Heckman, Egleston, & Hofmann, 2010) showed that this approach is successful. However, a systematic review of stage-based approaches to smoking cessation (Cahill, Lancaster, & Green, 2010) failed to find an advantage for tailoring a cessation program to smokers' stage of readiness for change. Successful elements of a cessation program work without such adaptations.

Both individual and group counseling can be successful in helping some people quit smoking.

Psychologists, physicians, and nurses can be effective providers, but effectiveness is positively related to the amount of contact between client and therapist. For example, receiving advice from a physician to quit produces an increase in cessation (Stead, Bergson, & Lancaster, 2008), but some types of physician advice are more effective. When physicians phrase their messages to prepare smokers to quit rather than give information about the dangers of smoking, smokers are more likely to accept these messages (Gemmell & DiClemente, 2009). However, face-to-face contact is not necessary; people may receive effective assistance through computer-based or web-based formats (Myung, McDonnell, Kazinets, Seo, & Moskowitz, 2009).

Programs that include more sessions tend to be more effective than programs with fewer sessions. For example, counseling and behavioral programs of smoking cessation are successful for individuals who have experienced heart attacks when these programs are of sufficient duration (Barth, Critchley, & Bengel, 2008). The most effective programs include both a counseling component and a pharmacological component. Each of these elements is effective, and the combination of the two improves outcomes (Hughes, 2009; Stead, Perera, et al., 2008).

Participating in a Community Campaign People also stop smoking as a result of a health campaign that covers their entire community. Such health campaigns are not new. More than two centuries before anyone campaigned against the dangers of cigarette smoking, Cotton Mather used pamphlets and oratory to persuade the people of Boston to accept smallpox inoculations (Faden, 1987). Today, community programs exist throughout the world, a growing number of which have the goal of creating smoke-free environments (WHO, 2009). Such campaigns are typically sponsored by government agencies or by large corporations as an intervention designed to improve the health of large numbers of people. A systematic review of studies on smoke-free workplaces (Fichtenberg & Glantz, 2002) indicated that this strategy not only reduces the number of cigarettes that workers smoke but also decreases the prevalence of smoking, creating a low-cost approach to reducing smoking rates. Another effective community or national strategy to decrease smoking is raising the price of cigarettes, which affects smokers' willingness to purchase cigarettes.

The percentage of people who change behavior as a result of a community or media health campaign is usually quite small, but if the message reaches millions of people, then the approach is successful. For example, an intervention in Vermont and New Hampshire (Secker-Walker et al., 2000) used random-digit dialing to contact female smokers and to encourage them to quit. After 4 years, the quit rate was higher in the two intervention counties than in two matched comparison counties—24% versus 21%. This difference may seem small, but it represents hundreds of women who might not have quit otherwise. A systematic review of media campaigns (Bala, Strzeszynski, & Cahill, 2008) indicated that such campaigns have been successful in decreasing smoking rates, increasing quitting, and on other measures of cessation success. Thus, attempting to reach large numbers of people through media campaigns can be a successful strategy.

Who Quits and Who Does Not?

Who is successful at quitting, and who is not? Investigators have examined several factors that may answer this question, including age, gender, educational level, quitting other drugs, and weight concern (which we discuss in a later section). Age shows a relation to quitting. In general, younger smokers, especially those who smoke at a high level, are more likely to continue smoking than older smokers (Ferguson, Bauld, Chesterman, & Judge, 2005; Hagimoto, Nakamura, Morita, Masui, & Oshima, 2010).

Are men more likely than women to quit smoking? More men have quit smoking than women, leading to the hypothesis that women find quitting more difficult. Some evidence supports this hypothesis (Torchalla, Okoli, Hemsing, & Greaves, 2011), possibly because female smokers who try to quit have more obstacles to overcome. For example, women do not respond as favorably to pharmacological treatments. In addition, women tend to use smoking to manage stress, anxiety, and depression, to which they are more vulnerable. Losing a coping strategy presents difficulties; people who use smoking as a coping strategy are less likely to quit than those who smoke for pleasure (Ferguson et al., 2005). It has been proposed that women experience more severe symptoms of cessation, but some research has indicated no gender differences in severity of symptoms (Weinberger, Krishnan-Sarin, Mazure, & McKee, 2008) or in success at quitting (Ferguson et al., 2005). However, people who experience severe symptoms tend to be less successful at quitting, as are those who live with a smoker.

Women are also less likely to receive social support for quitting, and a supportive social network is helpful in quitting. Unfortunately, only about 24% of smokers in the United States who tried to quit reported that they experienced social support (Shiffman et al., 2008). Cessation programs are more effective in maintaining abstinence when spouses of participants are trained to offer support to the partner who is trying to quit.

Does the lower rate of smokers among those with higher levels of education apply to quitting as well? Research that drew participants from 18 European countries (Schaap et al., 2008) suggested an affirmative answer. In this comparison across countries, more highly educated smokers were more likely to quit, including both women and men in all age groups.

Finally, do smokers who abuse alcohol and other drugs find it harder to give up cigarettes? Those who work in addictions treatment have long recognized the strong relationship between smoking and drinking, and the dominant view for many years was that addressing drinking problems was more urgent than smoking cessation for people who used both substances. That belief has been reevaluated; the dangers of smoking are recognized as important to address in treatment. In addition, research (Nieva, Ortega, Mondon, Ballbé, & Gual, 2011) indicates that people are capable of quitting both smoking and drinking simultaneously.

Relapse Prevention

The problem of relapse is not unique to smoking. Relapse rates are quite similar among people who have quit smoking, given up alcohol, and stopped using heroin (Hunt, Barnett, & Branch, 1971). For those who endeavor to quit, some do succeed in quitting or cutting down, but 22% go back to smoking at a higher rate than before their quit attempt (Yong, Borland, Hyland, & Siahpush, 2008).

The high rate of relapse after smoking cessation treatment prompted G. Alan Marlatt and Judith Gordon (1980) to examine the relapse process itself. For some people who have been successful in quitting, one cigarette precipitates a full relapse, complete with feelings of total failure. Marlatt and Gordon termed this phenomenon the **abstinence violation effect**. They incorporated strategies into their treatment to cope with patients' despair when they violate their intention to remain abstinent. By training patients that one "slip" does not constitute a relapse, Marlatt and Gordon's technique buffers them against a full-blown relapse. Slips are common even among people who will eventually quit (Yong et al., 2008). Thus, a single slip should not discourage people from continuing their efforts to stop smoking.

Self-quitters have very high relapse rates, as many as two thirds of smokers who quit on their own relapse after only 2 days (Hughes et al., 1992); 75% resume smoking within 6 months (Ferguson et al., 2005). A systematic review of relapse prevention (Agboola, McNeill, Coleman, & Leonardi Bee, 2010) indicated that self-help materials were effective in fighting relapse after a year for these former smokers. However, the relapse rate slows drastically after 1 year of abstinence (Herd, Borland, & Hyland, 2009), so former smokers may not be in great need of assistance past that time.

Behavioral relapse prevention techniques are most effective in the short term, between 1 and 3 months after quitting (Agboola et al., 2010), but this time is when former smokers are more vulnerable to the stress and cravings that are important in prompting relapse (McKee et al., 2011). Pharmacological treatment can be effective to prevent relapse within the important first year after quitting (Agboola et al., 2010). Thus, different approaches may be effective at different times, and researchers must work toward understanding both smoker and treatment characteristics to develop more effective ways to prevent the common problem of relapse.

IN SUMMARY

Smoking rates can be reduced either by prevention or by quitting. Providing young people with information on the dangers of smoking is not an effective strategy, and many of the school-based prevention programs have limited effects. Some of the programs are more effective when they are interactive, teach social skills to refuse smoking, and are well-integrated into the school health curriculum and the wider community. Such programs are more effective than simpler, more limited programs.

How can people quit smoking? Most people who attempt to quit do so without seeking any type of program for help, but some try pharmacological treatments or psychological interventions, whereas others are exposed to media and community campaigns to decrease smoking. Because giving up nicotine may result in withdrawal symptoms, many successful cessation programs include some form of nicotine replacement, such as a patch or gum, or a drug that affects the brain chemistry involved in smoking. Both types are more effective than a placebo or no treatment, and so are several drugs. A second approach to quitting is behavioral programs, which can be effective. Another approach to reducing smoking rates involves large-scale community programs, which usually include antitobacco mass media campaigns. If even a small percentage of people exposed to such campaigns stop smoking, this change can translate into thousands of people giving up tobacco. Some studies have found that men are more likely to be successful at quitting than women. Well-educated people are also more likely to quit than less educated ones. Many people are able to quit for months or even a year, but the problem of relapse remains a challenge. Programs aimed at relapse prevention have not demonstrated the degree of success that is needed; relapse remains a serious problem for those who quit smoking.

Effects of Quitting

When smokers quit, they experience a number of effects, almost all of which are positive. However, one possible negative effect is weight gain.

Quitting and Weight Gain

Many smokers fear weight gain if they give up smoking; this fear applies to men (Clark, Decker, et al., 2004) as well as women (King, Matacin, White, & Marcus, 2005). Are such concerns justified? Several factors need to be examined when considering the health benefits of quitting smoking and adding weight.

The weight gain associated with quitting is quite modest for most people who have stopped smoking, but that weight gain may make a difference in the health benefits associated with quitting. A study on the overall benefits of smoking cessation (Chinn

Becoming Healthier

1. If you do not smoke, don't start. College students are still susceptible to the pressure to smoke if their friends are smokers. The easiest way to be a nonsmoker is to stay a nonsmoker.
2. If you smoke, don't fool yourself into believing that the risks of smoking do not apply to you. Examine your own optimistic biases regarding smoking. Do not imagine that smoking low-tar and low-nicotine cigarettes makes smoking safe. Research indicates that these cigarettes are about as risky as any others.
3. Understand that cutting down is better than continuing to smoke at a high rate, but you will not receive the health benefits of quitting unless you quit.
4. If you smoke, try to quit. Even if you feel that quitting will be difficult, make an attempt to quit. If your first attempt is not successful, try again. Keep trying until you quit. Research indicates that people who keep trying are very likely to succeed.
5. If you have tried to quit on your own and have failed, look for a program to help you. Remember that not all programs are equally successful. Research indicates that the most effective programs combine some psychological techniques with some form of pharmacological treatment.
6. The best cessation programs allow for some individual tailoring to meet personal needs. Try different techniques until you find one that works for you.
7. If you are trying to quit smoking, find a supportive network of friends and acquaintances to help you stop and to boost your motivation to quit. Avoid people who try to sabotage your attempts to quit, and be cautious in going to places or engaging in activities that have a high association with smoking.
8. Cigar smoking has undergone a resurgence in popularity. Cigar and pipe smoking are not as dangerous as cigarette smoking, but remember that no level of smoking is safe.
9. Even if you do not smoke, remember that no level of tobacco exposure is safe. Exposure to environmental tobacco smoke is not nearly as dangerous as smoking, but it is not safe either. Smokeless tobacco use carries a number of health risks.
10. If you smoke, do not expose others to your smoke. Young children are especially vulnerable, and smoking parents can minimize the risks of respiratory disease in their children by keeping smoke away from them.

et al., 2005) found that some of the respiratory benefits of quitting were offset by weight gain.

When people quit smoking, the variation in weight gain is large. Some people experience increased appetite as a symptom of nicotine withdrawal (John, Meyer, Rumpf, Hapke, & Schumann, 2006), which leads to eating more. Unfortunately, overweight ex-smokers are more likely to gain a great deal more weight than normal-weight ex-smokers (Lycett, Munafò, Johnstone, Murphy, & Aveyard, 2011). However, weight gain following smoking cessation is often fairly modest—about 6 pounds for women and about 11 for men (Reas, Nygård, & Sørensen, 2009). In addition, the weight gain may be temporary; former smokers may be heavier within a few years of quitting, but 5 years after quitting, former smokers' weight is similar to those who never smoked. Therefore, even former smokers who gain weight tend to lose the weight they have gained.

Physical activity for ex-smokers can curtail weight gain. For example, research on female smokers (Prapavessis et al., 2007) revealed that women who increased their level of exercise and used nicotine replacement after quitting smoking gained less weight than women who quit but did not become more physically active. Similarly, a study with men (Froom et al., 1999) found that those who stopped smoking had a slight increase in body mass index, but men who were active in sports gained less than sedentary ex-smokers. Although maintaining close to ideal weight and quitting smoking are both desirable, the extra weight gained by former smokers does not negate the health benefits of quitting smoking. Quitting smoking is much more beneficial to health than maintaining a lower weight (Taylor, Hasselblad, Henley, Thun, & Sloan, 2002).

Health Benefits of Quitting

Can smokers reduce their all-cause mortality by quitting smoking? An extensive review (Critchley & Capewell, 2003) compared a large group of smokers who continued to smoke with another large group who were able to stop smoking. The result: Smokers who quit reduced their all-cause mortality by 36%. The authors saw this reduction in mortality as solid evidence that quitting smoking can decrease the rate of mortality. To receive these health benefits, however, smokers must quit and not just cut down the number of cigarettes smoked (Pisinger & Godtfredsen, 2007).

Two important questions for smokers considering quitting are: (1) can smokers regain some of their life expectancy by quitting, and (2) how long must ex-smokers remain abstinent before they reverse the detrimental effects of smoking? The 1990 report of the Surgeon General (USDHHS, 1990) summarized studies on the health benefits of quitting for different levels and durations of smoking, and researchers in other countries (Bjartveit, 2009; Dresler, Leon, Straif, Baan, & Secretan, 2006; Gielkens-Sijstermans et al., 2010; Hurley & Matthews, 2007) have conducted similar analyses. The results of all reviews have been consistent: Quitting improves a range of risks for health problems produced by smoking. The earlier analysis indicated that former light smokers (fewer than 20 cigarettes a day) who were able to abstain for 16 years had about the same rate of mortality as people who had never smoked. Figure 12.7 shows that after more than 15 years of abstinence, women's mortality risk decreased substantially. Figure 12.8 shows that men's mortality risk reduces steadily for up to 16 years.

Longtime smokers who quit reduce their chances of dying from heart disease much more rapidly than they lower their risk of death from lung cancer. The risk of lung cancer remains elevated for 10 years or longer, especially among men. Thus, men who quit smoking for 30 years reduce their risk of both cardiovascular disease and lung cancer, but their risk for lung cancer remains substantially higher than that of men who have never smoked. Women also reduce their risks by quitting, and the younger they are when they quit, the less likely they will be to die of lung cancer (Zhang et al., 2005). Quitting at younger ages also lowers the risk of cardiovascular disease events (Mannan, Stevenson, Peeters, Walls, & McNeil, 2011).

These studies suggest that by quitting smoking, both male and female smokers can reduce their risk of cardiovascular disease to that of nonsmokers, although their elevated risk of lung and other cancers declines much more slowly. Thus, never starting to smoke is healthier than quitting, but quitting, though seldom easy, can pay off.

How much does quitting matter? For the average male and female smokers who are free of heart disease, eating a diet with no more than 10% of calories from saturated fat would extend their lives somewhere between 3 days and 3 months (Grover, Gray-Donald, Joseph, Abrahamowicz, & Coupal, 1994). By contrast, quitting smoking at age 35 would add 7 to 8 years to life expectancy. Smokers who quit earlier realize even greater extension of life expectancy, and in addition, smokers who quit also add years of healthy life, not just years of life (Hurley & Matthews, 2007).

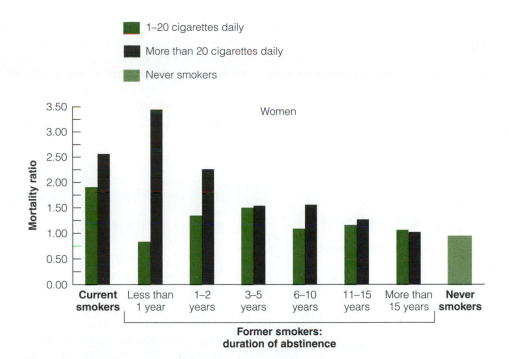

FIGURE 12.7   Overall mortality ratios for female current and former smokers compared with never smokers, by duration of abstinence.

Source: The health benefits of smoking cessation: A report of the Surgeon General (p. 78), by U.S. Department of Health and Human Services, 1990, DHHS Publication No. CDC 90–8416, Washington, DC: U.S. Government Printing Office.

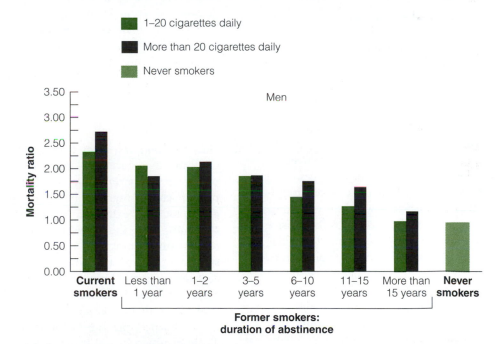

FIGURE 12.8   Overall mortality ratios for male current and former smokers compared with never smokers, by duration of abstinence.

Source: The health benefits of smoking cessation: A report of the Surgeon General (p. 78), by U.S. Department of Health and Human Services, 1990, DHHS Publication No. CDC 90–8416, Washington, DC: U.S. Government Printing Office.

IN SUMMARY

Many smokers fear that if they stop smoking, they will gain weight, and they may, but most people do not gain a lot of weight. For most smokers, excessive weight is less risky than continuing to smoke.

On a more positive note, stopping smoking improves health and extends life expectancy. Some evidence suggests that 16 years after quitting, former smokers' all-cause mortality rate returns to that of nonsmokers, although they may continue to have an excess risk for cancer mortality.

Answers

This chapter has addressed five basic questions:

1. How does smoking affect the respiratory system?

The respiratory system allows for the intake of oxygen and the elimination of carbon dioxide. Cigarette smoke drawn into the lungs eventually damages the lungs. Chronic bronchitis and emphysema are two chronic pulmonary diseases related to smoking. Tobacco contains several thousand compounds, including nicotine, and smoke exposes smokers to tars and other compounds that contribute to heart disease and cancer.

2. Who chooses to smoke and why?

About 21% of all U.S. adults smoke, slightly more are former smokers, and a little more than half have never smoked. Slightly more men than women smoke, but gender is not as important as educational level as a predictor of smoking—higher education is associated with lower smoking rates. Most smokers start as adolescents, and genes contribute to both initiation and nicotine dependence. Additional motivation comes from peers, parents, siblings, positive media images, and advertising. Smoking is part of a risk-taking, rebellious style that is consistent with the way some adolescents want to see themselves. No conclusive answer exists for why people continue to smoke, but the addictive properties of nicotine play a role, especially for some smokers. Smokers may derive positive reinforcement such as relaxation or stress reduction from smoking, or they may receive negative reinforcement from relief of withdrawal symptoms. Other smokers, especially young women, may use smoking as a weight control strategy.

3. What are the health consequences of tobacco use?

Smoking is the number one cause of preventable death in the United States, causing about 443,000 deaths a year, mostly from cancer, cardiovascular disease, and chronic lower respiratory disease. Smoking also carries a risk of nonfatal diseases and disorders such as periodontal disease, loss of physical strength and bone density, respiratory disorders, cognitive dysfunction, erectile dysfunction, and macular degeneration. Passive smoking does not contribute substantially to death from cancer but does contribute to cardiovascular deaths. Environmental tobacco smoke also raises young children's risk of respiratory disease and even death. Cigar or pipe smoking is less risky than cigarette smoking, but these forms of smoking are not safe. Smokeless tobacco is probably somewhat safer than cigarette smoking, but the use of smokeless tobacco is associated with increased rates of oral cancer and periodontal disease and may be related to coronary heart disease.

4. How can smoking rates be reduced?

One way to reduce smoking rates is to prevent people from starting. Such programs are often part of school programs, but to be effective, programs must be extensive, build students' refusal skills, and lead them toward a commitment to refrain from smoking. Most people who quit smoking do so on their own without any formal cessation program, but relapse is a big problem for these smokers. Pharmacological treatment may take the form of nicotine replacement or drugs that influence nicotine's effects in the brain. These pharmacological treatments can be a useful component in smoking cessation but even more successful when combined with behavioral interventions. Psychological counseling can also be effective in helping people quit, especially in the early phase of quitting. Mass media or community-based campaigns that reach thousands or even millions of smokers are successful in helping some smokers quit.

5. What are the effects of quitting?

Many smokers fear weight gain upon quitting, and a modest gain (6 to 11 pounds) is common. Nevertheless, gaining weight is not as hazardous to a person's health as continuing to smoke. Quitting improves health and extends life, but returning to the risk level of nonsmokers takes years, and most ex-smokers will retain some elevated risk for lung cancer unless they quit smoking when they were young. Indeed, quitting while young is a health advantage.

Suggested Readings

Corrigan, P. W. (2004). Marlboro man and the stigma of smoking. In S. Gilman & Z. Xun (Eds.), *Smoke: A global history of smoking* (pp. 344–354). London: Reaktion Books. More than 50 years ago, the Marlboro man was introduced to the smoking world as a virile yet cool cowboy. The image was unmistakably masculine, and advertising was oriented around that image. In this article, Patrick Corrigan writes about the social stigma of smoking and why Marlboro country is not the place to be.

Hughes, J. R. (2009). How confident should we be that smoking cessation treatments work? *Addiction, 104*(10), 1637–1640. In an attempt to counter the pessimism concerning the difficulty of quitting, smoking cessation authority John Hughes offers evidence that several types of cessation programs are effective. Although Hughes focuses on pharmacological treatments, he evaluates the range of treatment options and finds reason for optimism.

Kennedy, D. P., Tucker, J. S., Pollard, M. S., Go, M.-H., & Green, H. D. (2011). Adolescent romantic relationships and change in smoking status. *Addictive Behaviors, 36*(4), 320–326. These findings highlight the importance of social relationships for initiating and quitting smoking by focusing on romantic relationships among adolescents, revealing that romantic partners can be good and bad influences. This research also takes other social factors into account, thus reviewing the complex social environment of smoking initiation.

World Health Organization (WHO). (2008). *The WHO report on the global tobacco epidemic, 2008*. Geneva, Switzerland: World Health Organization. This extensive report details tobacco use around the world and offers interesting contrasts between smoking in the United States and other countries.

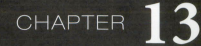

CHAPTER **13**

Using Alcohol and Other Drugs

CHAPTER OUTLINE

- **Real-World Profile of Charlie Sheen**
- *Alcohol Consumption—Yesterday and Today*
- *The Effects of Alcohol*
- *Why Do People Drink?*
- *Changing Problem Drinking*
- *Other Drugs*

QUESTIONS

This chapter focuses on six basic questions:

1. What are the major trends in alcohol consumption?

2. What are the health effects of drinking alcohol?

✔CHECK YOUR HEALTH RISKS

Regarding Alcohol and Drug Use

Check the items that apply to you.

☐ 1. I have had five or more alcoholic drinks in 1 day at least once during the past month.

☐ 2. I have had five or more alcoholic drinks on the same occasion on at least 5 different days during the past month.

☐ 3. When I drink too much, I sometimes don't remember a lot of the things that happened.

☐ 4. I sometimes ride with a driver who has been drinking.

☐ 5. On at least one occasion during the past year, I drove a motor vehicle after having an alcoholic drink.

☐ 6. I rarely have more than two drinks in 1 day.

☐ 7. I do not drive when I am intoxicated, but I have driven an automobile after drinking.

☐ 8. I sometimes play sports or go swimming after drinking.

☐ 9. Some of my friends or family have told me that I drink too much.

☐ 10. I have tried to cut down on my drinking, but I never seem to succeed.

☐ 11. At least once in my life, I tried to completely quit drinking, but I was not successful.

☐ 12. I believe that the best way to enjoy many activities (such as a dance or a football game) is to drink alcohol.

☐ 13. After waking up with a hangover, I sometimes have a drink to feel better.

☐ 14. There are some activities that I perform better after drinking.

☐ 15. I have consumed fewer than 10 alcoholic drinks in my lifetime.

Most of these items represent a health risk related to using alcohol by increasing risk for diseases and unintentional injuries. However, agreeing with item 6 probably reflects a healthy pattern of consumption for many people, but agreeing with item 15 is not necessarily a healthy choice for everyone. As you read this chapter, you will learn that some of these items are riskier than others.

Real-World Profile of
CHARLIE SHEEN

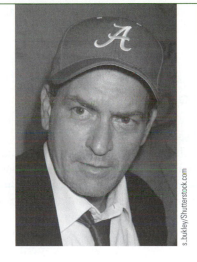

s_bukley/Shutterstock.com

The list of celebrities who have experienced alcohol and drug problems is long, but few have such an extensive history or made such a flamboyant impression as Charlie Sheen. Since the 1990s, Sheen has experienced problems with alcohol and drugs that have landed him in legal trouble and in rehabilitation clinics ("Charlie Sheen," 2011). Beginning in December, 2010 and escalating through March, 2011, Sheen became the center of media attention that focused on Sheen's erratic behavior, which seemed to be fueled by alcohol and drugs.

Sheen's work as the principal actor on a popular television comedy reportedly began to suffer from his drug abuse, and he was the center of well-publicized incidents involving hotel rooms, cocaine, alcohol, porn stars, violence, and the neglect of his children (D. Brown, 2011). Unlike other celebrities who have behaved badly under the influence of drugs, Sheen was not apologetic and did not enter rehab voluntarily. Instead, he began to give interviews during which he proclaimed his invincibility and bragged about how much crack cocaine he used. Some clinical psychologists began to speculate that perhaps Sheen's seemingly uncontrolled behavior might be the result of a mental disorder in addition to his drug abuse. The two problems are not an unusual combination.

Sheen's drug use has been extreme but not entirely unusual. Many people who abuse drugs combine illicit drugs with alcohol and experience health problems, relationship issues (and even domestic violence), legal difficulties, and financial problems due to their substance use. Those drug abusers also tend to have trouble in acknowledging their personal responsibility and recognizing how unacceptable their behavior is; that is, they deny the problem, just as Charlie Sheen did.

Sheen's wealth and fame has protected him from some of the potential consequences of his misbehavior, but ironically, that wealth and fame present risks for drug abuse; children of wealthy families are at higher risk for drug use and abuse than children from middle-class families (Luthar & Latendresse, 2005). Like Charlie Sheen, alcohol abuse seems to create more problems than other drugs, but his use of illicit drugs was far from typical.

Alcohol Consumption— Yesterday and Today

Alcohol is more widely consumed than other drugs, not only in the United States but also in many other countries (Edwards, 2000), and its use both presents problems and raises questions. Charlie Sheen's drinking caused serious problems, but is all alcohol consumption dangerous? What does alcohol do in the body, and what are its risks? What drinking patterns present problems? This chapter includes answers to these questions, but first we examine the history of drinking, which reveals different attitudes about alcohol use in the past.

A Brief History of Alcohol Consumption

The history of alcohol cannot be traced easily; it was discovered worldwide and repeatedly, dating back before recorded history. Producing beverage alcohol requires no sophisticated technology: The yeast that is responsible for producing alcohol is airborne, and fermentation occurs naturally in fruits, fruit juices, and grain mixtures. Even ancient cultures used beverage alcohol (Anderson, 2006). Ancient Babylonians discovered both wine (fermented grape juice) and beer (fermented grain), as did the ancient Egyptians, Greeks, Romans, Chinese, and Indians. Pre-Columbian tribes in the Americas also used fermented products.

Ancient civilizations also discovered drunkenness, of course. In several of those countries, such as Greece, drunkenness was not only allowed but also practically required on certain occasions, but these occasions were limited to festivals. This pattern resembles present-day practices in the United States, where drunkenness is condoned at some parties and celebrations. Most societies condone drinking alcohol but prohibit drunkenness or restrict it to certain occasions.

Distillation was discovered in ancient China and refined in 8th-century Arabia. Because the process is somewhat complex, the use of distilled spirits did not become widespread until they were commercially manufactured. In England, fermented beverages were by far the most common form of alcohol consumption until the 18th century, when England encouraged the proliferation of distilleries to stimulate commerce. Along with cheap gin came widespread consumption and widespread drunkenness. However, intoxication from distilled spirits was confined mostly to the lower and working classes; the rich drank wine, a less intoxicating beverage that was imported and thus expensive.

In colonial America, drinking was much more prevalent than it is today. Men, women, and children all drank, and it was considered acceptable for all to do so. This practice may not be consistent with our present-day image of the Puritans, but nevertheless, the Puritans did not object to drinking. Rather, they considered alcohol one of God's gifts. Indeed, in those years, alcohol was often safer than unpurified water or milk, so the Puritans had a legitimate reason to condone the consumption of alcoholic beverages. Drunkenness, however, was not acceptable. The Puritans believed that alcohol, like all things, should be used in moderation. Therefore, the Puritans established severe prohibitions against drunkenness but not against drinking.

The 50 years following U.S. independence marked a transition in the way early Americans thought about alcohol (Edwards, 2000). A dedicated, vocal minority came to consider liquor a "demon" and to argue for total abstention from its use. A similar movement arose in Britain. Initially, this attitude was limited to the upper and upper-middle classes, but later, abstention came to be an accepted doctrine of the middle class and people who aspired to join the middle class. Intemperance in drinking alcohol thus became associated with the lower classes, and "respectable" people, especially women, were expected not to be heavy drinkers.

Temperance societies proliferated throughout the United States during the mid-1800s. However, the name is not quite accurate. The societies did not promote *temperance*—that is, the moderate use of alcohol. Rather, they advocated *prohibition*, the total abstinence from alcohol. Temperance societies held that liquor weakens inhibitions; loosens desires and passions; causes a large percentage of crime, poverty, and broken homes; and is powerfully addicting, so much so that even an occasional drink would put one in danger. Figure 13.1 shows a dramatic decrease in per capita alcohol consumption in the United States after 1830, a decrease due directly to the spread of this movement.

In response to the growing temperance movement, both the demographics and the location of drinking changed. Rather than being consumed in a family setting or a respectable tavern, alcohol became increasingly confined to saloons, which were patronized largely by urban industrial workers (Popham, 1978); drinking became associated with the lower and working classes. Portrayed by the temperance movement as the personification of evil and moral degeneracy, saloons served as a focus for growing prohibitionist sentiment.

Prohibitionists were finally victorious in 1919 with the ratification of the 18th Amendment to the Constitution of the United States. This amendment outlawed the manufacture, sale, or transportation of alcoholic beverages, and per capita consumption fell drastically (as Figure 13.1 shows). The amendment was not popular and created a large illegal market for alcohol; in 1934, the 21st Amendment repealed the 18th Amendment, and Prohibition ended. Figure 13.1 shows that after the repeal of Prohibition, alcohol consumption rose sharply. Although the current per capita consumption of alcohol is considerably higher than during Prohibition, it is less than half the rate reached during the first three decades of the 19th century.

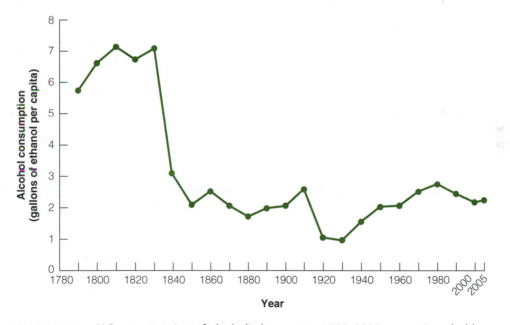

FIGURE 13.1   U.S. consumption of alcoholic beverages, 1790–2005, ages 15 and older.

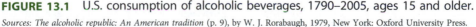

Sources: The alcoholic republic: An American tradition (p. 9), by W. J. Rorabaugh, 1979, New York: Oxford University Press. Copyright 1979 by Oxford University Press. Also, *Apparent per capita ethanol consumption for the United States, 1850–2005*, retrieved July 21, 2008, from http://www.niaaa.nih.gov/Resources/DatabaseResources/QuickFacts/AlcoholSales/consum01.html

The Prevalence of Alcohol Consumption Today

About two thirds of adults in the United States are classified as current drinkers (defined as having had at least 12 drinks during one's lifetime and 1 drink during the past year), about half are regular drinkers, about 10% engage in binge drinking (5 or more drinks on the same occasion at least once per month), and a little more than 5% are heavy drinkers (more than 14 drinks per week for men or 7 per week for women) (NCHS, 2011). The drinking rates shown in Figure 13.2 reflect a leveling of a 20-year decline in alcohol consumption in the United States. Worldwide, about 2 billion people are current drinkers, which represent about half of the adult population (Anderson, 2006).

The frequency of drinking and the prevalence of heavy drinking are not equal for all demographic groups in the United States. As Figure 13.3 shows, drinking varies by ethnicity. European Americans tend to have higher rates of drinking than other ethnic groups (NCHS, 2011). Rates of binge and heavy drinking also vary with ethnicity. Native Americans have the highest rates of these drinking patterns, and Asian Americans have the lowest.

Age is another factor in drinking. Adults 25 to 44 have the highest rates of drinking, but young adults

aged 18 to 24 have the highest rates of binge drinking and heavy drinking. Slightly more than a third of drinkers aged 18 to 24 are binge drinkers (NCHS, 2011), but they may later become more moderate drinkers. This increasing and then decreasing frequency of binge drinking among young people is one pattern that appeared in a study on adolescent binge drinkers (Tucker, Orlando, & Ellickson, 2003). However, many other patterns occur for binge drinking. A study of binge drinking adolescents in Great Britain (Viner & Taylor, 2007) indicated that their pattern of drinking predicted problem drinking in adulthood.

Binge drinking can lead to a variety of hazards (especially for inexperienced drinkers), including intoxication, poor judgment, and impaired coordination. Certain situations promote binge drinking, and college students are at particular risk, not only in the United States but also in Australia, Europe, and South America (Karam, Kypri, & Salamoun, 2007). College men face risks concerning alcohol use when they try to "man up" and match some representation of masculine norms such as risk taking, being the "playboy," and drinking to the point of intoxication (Iwamoto, Cheng, Lee, Takamatsu, & Gordon, 2011). Men in fraternities are especially at risk; these organizations hold social norms that promote these attitudes and behaviors. However, drinking patterns tend to change when individuals are no longer affiliated. Thus, college drinking habits are not predictors of drinking problems after graduation (Jackson, Sher, Gotham, & Wood, 2001). For young people, however, binge drinking is a persistent problem that creates many hazards for the leading causes of death in this age group—unintentional injury, homicide, and suicide (Panagiotidis, Papadopoulou, Diakogiannis, Iacovides, & Kaprinis, 2008).

Among adolescents 12 to 17, current use of alcohol dropped dramatically after the legal age for buying alcohol was raised to 21. In 1985, more than 40% of the adolescents in this age group were current users, but by 1992, only 20% were current drinkers. The rate has drifted downward slightly since the late 1990s (Johnston et al., 2011). Binge drinking, however, is common among high school and college students. Among male high school seniors, for example, the binge drinking rate is 28%, and it is 18% for female high school seniors. Although these rates may not seem large, all of these students are drinking illegally. However, reaching the legal age for drinking—one's 21st birthday celebration—is a major occasion for a drinking binge that often prompts the highest level of

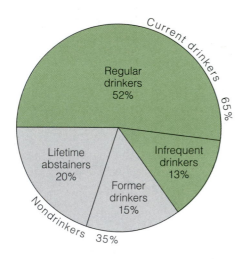

FIGURE 13.2 Types of drinkers, adults, United States, 2009.

Source: Health, United States, 2010 (2011), Table 64, by National Center for Health Statistics, Hyattsville, MD: U.S. Government Printing Office.

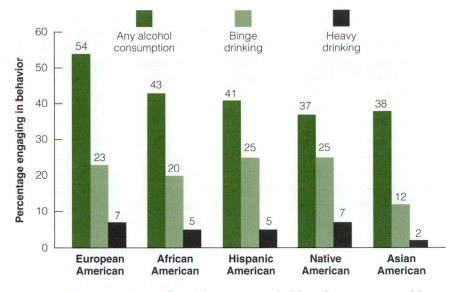

FIGURE 13.3 Percentage of people age 12 and older who report monthly alcohol use, binge drinking, and heavy drinking, by ethnic group, United States, 2010.

Source: SAMHSA, 2011, *Results from the 2010 National Survey on Drug Use and Health: Summary of National Findings*, NSDUH Series H-41, HHS Publication No. (SMA) 11-4658, Table 2.42B. Rockville, MD: Substance Abuse and Mental Health Services Administration. Retrieved September 30, 2011 from http://oas.samhsa.gov/NSDUH/2k10NSDUH/tabs/Sect2peTabs1to42.htm#Tab2.242B

drinking in which the celebrant has ever engaged (Rutledge, Park, & Sher, 2008).

When the rate for drinking among young people began to decline, authorities speculated that illicit drugs may be replacing alcohol as preferred substances. However, the evidence for this hypothesis is not clear. The Monitoring the Future Project (Johnston et al., 2011) found that the decreases in illicit drug use parallel the decrease in alcohol use rather than rise in compensation as drinking decreases. One exception to this trend as been marijuana use: In recent years, marijuana has replaced alcohol as the drug most widely used among high school students.

Alcohol consumption rates are lowest among older adults (Substance Abuse and Mental Health Services Administration [SAMHSA], 2010). Some people decrease their alcohol consumption as soon as they leave college with its social situations and pressures to drink. However, alcohol intake is inversely related to age—older ages are associated with lower levels of drinking. The general trend toward decreased alcohol consumption with increasing age may be a result of people quitting or of drinkers reducing the amount they drink.

Gender and educational level are also related to alcohol consumption. Men are more likely than women to be current drinkers (71% to 60%), binge drinkers (33% to 15%), and heavy drinkers (6% to 4.5%) (NCHS, 2011). These percentages suggest that men have more problems with binge and heavy drinking than do women. Educational level is another predictor of drinking behavior. In Chapter 12, we saw that the more education people have, the less likely they are to smoke cigarettes. With alcohol, however, the reverse is true: The more years of schooling, the greater the likelihood that people will drink alcohol. In 2009, about 68% of college students were defined as current drinkers, compared with only 35% of people who failed to graduate from high school (SAMHSA, 2010). After graduation, however, individuals with a college education are less likely to be binge or heavy drinkers than any other educational group (SAMHSA, 2010). High school dropouts are more likely to be heavy drinkers and to develop drinking problems when they reach their 30s (Muthen & Muthen, 2000).

These patterns of alcohol consumption are not unique to the United States, but amount and patterns of alcohol consumption vary internationally. Across the world, between 18% and 90% of men drink, and between 1% and 81% of women drink (Anderson, 2006). Some countries, such as the United States, Canada, and the Scandinavian countries, associate alcohol with a restricted number of occasions, whereas other countries, such as France, Italy, and Greece, integrate alcohol into daily life (Bloomfield, Stockwell, Gmel, & Rehn, 2003). Drinking is more common in the latter countries, but intoxication is more common in the former. However, more numerous drinking occasions tend to be related to more numerous problems related to drinking, regardless of the pattern (Kuntsche, Plant, Plant, Miller, & Gabriel, 2008).

IN SUMMARY

People have been consuming alcohol since before recorded history, and people have probably abused alcohol for almost as long. In most ancient societies—as well as modern societies—alcohol in moderation was condoned, but drunkenness and alcohol abuse were condemned.

Alcohol consumption per capita reached a peak in the United States during the first three decades of the 19th century. From about 1830 to 1850, consumption dropped dramatically due to the efforts of early prohibitionists. Presently, alcohol consumption in the United States is stable: About half of adults are current regular drinkers, 10% are binge drinkers, and 5% are heavy drinkers. European Americans have higher rates of alcohol consumption than Hispanic Americans and African Americans; adults 21 to 44 consume more than other age groups; and college graduates are much more likely to be drinkers than high school dropouts, who nevertheless are more likely to be heavy drinkers later in their lives. Drinking attitudes and patterns also vary among countries.

The Effects of Alcohol

Essentially the same thing happens to alcohol when you drink it as when you do not—it turns to vinegar (Goodwin, 1976). In the body, two enzymes turn alcohol into vinegar, or acetic acid. The first enzyme, **alcohol dehydrogenase**, is located in the liver and has no other known function except to metabolize alcohol. Alcohol dehydrogenase breaks down alcohol into aldehyde, which is a very toxic chemical. The second enzyme, **aldehyde dehydrogenase**, converts aldehyde to acetic acid.

The process of metabolizing alcohol produces at least three health-related outcomes: (1) an increase in lactic acid, which correlates with anxiety attacks; (2) an increase in uric acid, which causes gout; and (3) an increase of fat in the liver and in the blood.

The specific alcohol used in beverages is called **ethanol**. Like other alcohols, ethanol is a poison. But cases of alcohol poisoning are not common and almost always involve inexperienced drinkers who have drunk very large amounts of distilled liquor in a very short time. Otherwise, ingesting beverage alcohol is self-limiting: Intoxication usually yields to unconsciousness, preventing lethal poisoning.

Men and women are not equally affected by drinking alcohol. One factor is the difference in body weight; a 120-pound person will be more strongly affected by 3 ounces of alcohol than a 220-pound person. But body weight is not the only factor in this gender difference. Given the same blood alcohol level, men's brains are more strongly affected than women's brains (Ceylan-Isik, McBride, & Ren, 2010). However, women's stomachs tend to absorb alcohol more efficiently, producing higher blood alcohol levels with less drinking (Bode & Bode, 1997). Thus, women and men have different physiological responses to alcohol, some of which may make women more vulnerable to the effects of alcohol.

Among the problems associated with drinking are alcohol's ability to produce tolerance, dependence, withdrawal, and addiction. Although these concepts apply to many drugs, their application to alcohol is necessary in evaluating alcohol's potential hazards.

Tolerance is a term applied to the effects of a drug when, with continued use, more and more of the drug is required to produce the same effect. Drugs with high tolerance potential may be dangerous because people who build up tolerance need to take more of the drug to produce the effect they want and expect. If this amount is progressively larger, any dangerous effects or side effects of the drug will become more of a hazard. Alcohol is a drug with generally moderate tolerance potential, but it seems to affect people differentially. For some, heavy use of alcohol for an extended period is required before noticeable tolerance begins to develop. For others, tolerance can develop within a week of moderate daily consumption. With increased tolerance comes an increased risk of the physical damage that alcohol can cause.

Dependence is separate from tolerance, and it, too, is a term that can be applied to many drugs. Dependence occurs when a drug becomes so incorporated into the functioning of the body's cells that it becomes necessary for "normal" functioning. If the drug is discontinued, the body's dependence on that drug becomes apparent and **withdrawal** symptoms develop. These symptoms are the body's signs that it is adjusting to functioning without the drug. Dependence and withdrawal are physical symptoms connected to drug use. Generally, withdrawal symptoms are the opposite of the drug's effects. Because alcohol produces mostly depressant effects, withdrawal from it produces symptoms of restlessness, irritability, and agitation.

Many drugs produce notoriously unpleasant withdrawal, and alcohol is one of the worst. How difficult the process will be depends on many factors, including the length of use and the degree of dependence. In some cases, withdrawal from alcohol can be life threatening through effects on the cardiovascular system (Bär et al., 2008) and requires careful management (Mayo-Smith et al., 2004). Usually the first symptom to appear is tremor—the "shakes." In those severely addicted, **delirium tremens** occurs, with hallucinations, disorientation, and possibly convulsions. The withdrawal process usually lasts between 2 days and a week. The physical dangers are so severe that the process is often completed in a special facility devoted to alcohol treatment.

Tolerance and dependence are independent properties. A drug may produce tolerance but not dependence; also, a person can develop dependence on a drug that has little or no tolerance potential. However, some drugs have both a tolerance and dependence potential. Tolerance and dependence are not inevitable consequences of taking drugs (Zinberg, 1984), and alcohol is a good example. Not everyone who drinks alcohol does so with sufficient frequency and in sufficient quantity to develop a tolerance, and most drinkers do not become dependent.

The combination of dependence and withdrawal is sometimes described as **addiction**, but laypeople (Chassin, Presson, Rose, & Sherman, 2007) and experts (Pouletty, 2002) tend to use different definitions. Element of craving for the substance and compulsive use are part of everyone's definition, but adolescents emphasize the cravings in their conceptualization, whereas adults focus on the compulsive use of the substance in their view of addiction (Chassin et al., 2007). More consistent with adults' definitions, experts

distinguish addiction from dependence by considering the compulsive behavior and damage done to people's life through this behavior—"loss of control of drug use or the compulsive seeking and taking of drugs despite adverse consequences" (Pouletty, 2002, p. 731). Some experts even differentiate drug abuse from addiction, defining abuse as excessive and harmful use, even if the person is not dependent or addicted. Thus, considering the properties of a drug such as alcohol includes tolerance, dependence, addiction, and abuse, each of which is separable from the others.

Some people speak of "psychological" dependence or addiction, but this term is not equivalent to dependence on a drug such as alcohol. Many behaviors become part of one's habitual manner of responding. Giving up the activity is accomplished only through much difficulty because the person has become habituated to it. Psychological dependence could be extended to many behaviors that are difficult to change, such as gambling, overeating, jogging, or even watching television, some of which may seem to meet the criterion of compulsive behavior that signals addiction. Whether this conceptualization is valid remains controversial; so the term *addiction* should be used with caution.

Hazards of Alcohol

Alcohol produces a variety of hazards, both direct and indirect. *Direct hazards* are the harmful physical effects of alcohol itself, exclusive of any psychological, social, or economic consequences. Individuals with severe alcohol problems have more than twice the mortality risk as those with no alcohol problems (Fichter, Quadflieg, & Fischer, 2011). *Indirect hazards* are the harmful consequences that result from psychological and physiological impairments produced by alcohol. Both direct and indirect hazards contribute to an increased mortality rate for heavy drinkers (Standridge, Zylstra, & Adams, 2004).

Direct Hazards Alcohol affects many organ systems in the body, but liver damage is the main health consideration for long-term, heavy drinkers because the liver is mainly in charge of detoxifying alcohol. The oxidation that occurs during alcohol metabolism may be toxic, destroying cell membranes and causing liver damage (Reuben, 2008). With prolonged heavy drinking, scarring occurs, and this scarring is typically followed by **cirrhosis**, or the accumulation of nonfunctional scar tissue in the liver. Cirrhosis is an irreversible condition and a major cause of death among alcoholics. Not all alcoholics develop liver cirrhosis, and people with no history of alcohol abuse may also develop the condition, but cirrhosis has a significant association with heavy alcohol use in countries around the world (Mandayam, 2004) and is one of the leading causes of death in the United States.

Prolonged heavy drinking is also implicated in the development of a neurological dysfunction called Korsakoff syndrome (also known as Wernicke-Korsakoff syndrome). Korsakoff syndrome is characterized by chronic cognitive impairment, severe memory problems for recent events, disorientation, and an inability to learn new information. Alcohol is related to the development of this syndrome through its interference with the absorption of thiamin, one of the B vitamins. Heavy drinkers can experience thiamin deficiency, which is worsened by their typically poor nutrition (Stacey & Sullivan, 2004). Alcohol accelerates the progression of thiamin-related brain damage, and when this process has started, vitamin supplements do not reverse the progression. Moreover, most alcoholics do not receive treatment until the process is at an irreversible stage. Although heavy, prolonged drinking is a risk factor for neurological damage (Harper & Matsumoto, 2005), light to moderate consumption does not seem to lead to cognitive impairment. Indeed, research suggests that light to moderate drinkers are less likely to develop dementia, including Alzheimer's disease (Collins, 2008).

Alcohol affects the cardiovascular system, but the effects may not all be negative. (The next section looks at the possible positive effects of moderate alcohol consumption on cardiovascular functioning.) Chronic heavy drinking or periodic heavy (binge) drinking, however, does have a direct and harmful effect on the cardiovascular system (Rehm et al., 2010; Standridge et al., 2004). In large doses, alcohol reduces oxidation of fatty acids (the heart's primary fuel source) in the myocardium. The heart directly metabolizes ethanol, producing fatty-acid ethyl esters that impair functioning of the energy-producing structures of the heart. Alcohol can also depress the myocardium's ability to contract, which can lead to abnormal cardiac functioning. Thus, heavy drinking is related to hypertensive and ischemic heart disease as well as hemorrhagic stroke (Rehm et al., 2010).

Heavy drinking also increases the risk for a wide variety of other diseases (Rehm et al., 2010). The list includes cancers of the mouth, pharynx, esophagus, colon, rectum, liver, and breast. In addition, heavy drinking is associated with increased risk for tuberculosis, seizure disorder, diabetes mellitus, and pneumonia.

Alcohol has a direct and hazardous effect on pregnancy and the developing fetus in two basic ways. First, alcohol consumption reduces fertility; women who are heavy drinkers are at increased risk for infertility (Eggert, Theobald, & Engfeldt, 2004). Women who are chronic heavy users of alcohol experience amenorrhea, cessation of the menstrual cycle, which may be caused either by cirrhosis or by a direct effect of alcohol on the pituitary or the hypothalamus. Other possibilities include alcohol's effects on hormone production and regulation and interference with ovulation.

The second direct, hazardous effect of excessive drinking during pregnancy is the increased risk of developmental problems for the fetus, such as congenital malformations of the respiratory and musculoskeletal systems, which produces *fetal alcohol spectrum disorders* (Baumann, Schild, Hume, & Sokol, 2006; Rehm et al., 2010). The most severe form is **fetal alcohol syndrome (FAS)**, which affects many infants of mothers who drank heavily during pregnancy, especially those who binge drink. Some tissues in the embryo, such as neurons, are especially sensitive to alcohol, and exposure causes problems in the developing embryo. These problems in development produce specific facial abnormalities, growth deficiencies, central nervous system disorders, and cognitive deficiencies. Indeed, fetal alcohol spectrum disorders are the leading cause of mental retardation in the world (Murthy, Kudlur, George, & Mathew, 2009). Although heavy drinking is the main contributor to fetal alcohol syndrome, heavy smoking, stress, and poor nutrition are also involved, and combinations of these factors are not unusual in heavy drinkers.

What about moderate and even light drinking during pregnancy? Light to moderate drinking is not likely to cause fetal alcohol syndrome unless binge drinking is involved, but any level of alcohol exposure affects developing embryos. Even light drinking increases the risk for miscarriages and stillbirths (Kesmodel, Wisborg, Olsen, Henriksen, & Secher, 2002), and binge drinking during pregnancy produces deficits in cognitive functioning (Bailey et al., 2004) and increases the frequency of psychological problems (O'Leary et al., 2010). Even small amounts of alcohol, especially during the early months of pregnancy, may have direct and hazardous effects on the developing fetus (Baumann et al., 2006; Goldsmith, 2004). Unfortunately, over

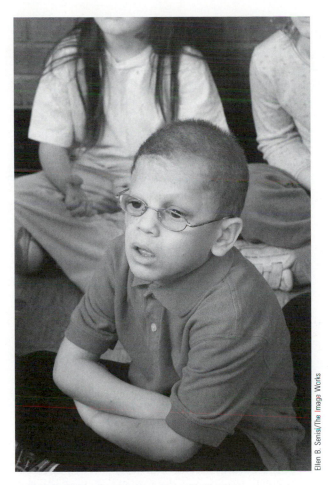

Facial abnormalities, growth deficiencies, central nervous system disorders, and mental retardation are symptoms of fetal alcohol syndrome.

Ellen B. Sensi/The Image Works

20% of women of childbearing age in the United States fit the pattern of risky drinking (NCHS, 2011).

Indirect Hazards
Despite the many direct hazards of drinking alcohol, the indirect hazards are even more common. Most of the indirect dangers arise from alcohol's effects on aggression, judgment, and attention. Alcohol also affects coordination and alters cognitive functioning in ways that contribute to increased chances of unintentional injury not only to the drinker but also to others (Rehm et al., 2010).

The most frequent and serious indirect hazard of alcohol consumption is the increased likelihood of unintentional injuries, the fourth leading cause of death in the United States, the leading cause of death for people under age 45, and a leading cause of death

and injury worldwide (Rehm et al., 2010). A dose–response relationship exists between alcohol consumption and unintentional fatal injuries; that is, the greater the number of drinks consumed per occasion, the greater the incidence of fatalities from unintentional injuries. As many as 32% of fatal unintentional injuries throughout the world involve alcohol.

Motor vehicle crashes account for the largest number of alcohol-related fatalities. In the United States, more than 44,000 people die each year from injuries resulting from motor vehicle crashes, and about 40% of those deaths (about 17,000 per year) are related to alcohol-impaired driving (Yi, Chen, & Williams, 2006). The National Survey on Drug Use and Health (SAMHSA, 2010) found that alcohol-impaired driving was most frequent among young people 21 to 25 years old, with about 25% reporting this behavior. However, 17% of 18- to 20-year-olds—who are not yet old enough to purchase alcohol legally—also said they had driven after drinking. European Americans are more likely to drive after drinking than other ethnic groups, and men are about twice as likely as women to do so. These impaired drivers are not necessarily heavy or binge drinkers; half of the drivers involved in crashes who had used alcohol were nonproblem drinkers—who became problems when they drove after drinking (Voas, Roman, Tippetts, & Durr-Holden, 2006)

For some drinkers, alcohol consumption can also lead to more aggressive behavior. Both laboratory experiments and crime statistics have shown a relationship between alcohol and aggression, but the effect does not apply to everyone. Trait anger (the disposition to experience and respond with anger) is an important factor. Not surprisingly, men with moderate or high trait anger behaved more aggressively than men with lower levels of anger (Parrott & Zeichner, 2002). However, trait anger combined with alcohol prompted these men to administer longer and higher levels of shock than their sober counterparts and provoked both women and men to engage in more aggressive verbal exchanges (Eckhardt & Crane, 2008). Alcohol may not be the underlying cause of partner violence, but it intensifies the violence (Graham, Bernards, Wilsnack, & Gmel, 2011). Jealousy combined with alcohol predicted intimate partner violence (Foran & O'Leary, 2008). Thus, some people are more likely than others to become aggressive under the influence of alcohol. Charlie Sheen's history of violence toward his wives and girlfriends is consistent with these research results.

Alcohol is also related to suicidal ideation and suicide attempts (Schaffer, Jeglic, & Stanley, 2008). Research indicates that alcohol use has a higher relationship to suicide attempts than other drug use (Rossow, Grøholt, & Wichstrøm, 2005).

Similarly, alcohol is related to crime. Two early studies (Mayfield, 1976; Wolfgang, 1957) indicated that either the victim or the perpetrator, or both, had been drinking in two-thirds of the homicides studied. Recent research (Felson & Staff, 2010) has confirmed this relationship and extended the findings to assaults, including sexual assaults, as well as robbery and burglary. Not only are people who commit homicides likely to be drinking, but consuming alcohol also relates to increased chances of being a crime victim. These relationships, however, do not demonstrate that alcohol causes crime. Most crimes are committed by people who are not problem drinkers, and the majority of alcohol abusers do not commit violent crimes. Thus, the relationship between alcohol and crime is complex (Dingwall, 2005).

Finally, drinking alcohol can influence people's decision making. A study of group decision making (Sayette, Kirchner, Moreland, Levine, & Travis, 2004) showed that when group members had been drinking, the decision was riskier than when the group members were completely sober. Alterations also appear on the individual level and in nonproblem drinkers, who experienced problems in factoring several variables into a decision-making situation after drinking (George, Rogers, & Duka, 2005). Unfortunately, drinking also impairs drinkers' recognition that their decision-making capacity is impaired (Brumback, Cao, & King, 2007).

Impairment and risky decisions can be dangerous in sexual situations. For example, young men who were intoxicated expressed more interest in having unprotected sex with an attractive woman than comparable men who were not intoxicated, even when reminded of the risk (Lyvers, Cholakians, Puorro, & Sundram, 2011). Other research indicates that people who have been drinking are more likely than others to be involved in forced sexual experiences, either as victim or as perpetrator (Testa, Vazile-Tamsen, & Livingston, 2004). Thus, drinking conveys a variety of risks.

Benefits of Alcohol

Is it possible that drinking might be good for you? This question was raised as a result of several early studies

(Room & Day, 1974; Stason, Neff, Miettinen, & Jick, 1976) that reported a U-shaped or J-shaped relationship between alcohol consumption and mortality. In other words, light to moderate drinkers (one to five drinks per day) seemed to have the best prospects for longer life, whereas both heavy drinkers and nondrinkers had the greater risk. As unlikely as this possibility sounds, a great deal of later research has supported these findings—light or moderate drinking seems positively related to both reduced mortality and lower risk of many diseases (Holahan et al., 2010; Hvidtfelt et al., 2010).

An analysis of the benefits of drinking (Rehm, Patra, & Taylor, 2007) indicated that the benefits outweigh the risks for some people, whereas others are more at risk from drinking. Pattern of drinking and age are critical factors in drinking's dangers. Binge drinking brings intoxication and dangerous impairments of judgment and coordination. Thus, binge drinking is a dangerous practice that makes the risks outweigh the any potential benefits. In addition, the benefits of drinking do not appear among young people but begin during middle age (Klatsky & Udaltsova, 2007; Rehm et al., 2007). Older people are less likely to binge drink than younger people and also, drinking tends to reduce coronary heart disease, which is the leading cause of death for older people.

Reduced Cardiovascular Mortality   When researchers initially investigated the benefits of drinking, they discovered overall lower mortality for people who drank at light to moderate levels (Holahan et al., 2010; Klatsky & Udaltsova, 2007). This advantage appeared first among men, but women who are light drinkers also show lower mortality rates (Baer et al., 2011). This reduction in mortality is due mostly to lower heart disease deaths (Klatsky, 2010; Mukamal, Chen, Rao, & Breslow, 2010) and applies to people in cultures around the world.

The research evidence does not show as strong a protection against stroke as it does against heart disease (Patra et al., 2010; Rehm et al., 2010). Indeed, drinking increases risk of hemorrhagic stroke, those strokes caused by rupture of a blood vessel that bleeds into the brain. However, people who drink at light to moderate levels derive some protection against ischemic strokes, those strokes caused by restriction of blood supply to the brain. Ischemic strokes are more common than hemorrhagic strokes; thus, the protection offered by drinking lowers the rate of death due to strokes. Another cardiovascular disorder, peripheral vascular disease, is also lower among drinkers.

The health benefits of drinking have been controversial, mostly because drinking carries unquestionable hazards. However, a Canadian study (Rehm et al., 2007) calculated the risk-to-benefit ratio, revealing that the benefits outweigh the risks for middle-aged and older people who are light to moderate drinkers and who do not binge drink. For younger drinkers, the risks make drinking an unwise choice. Overall, drinking presents more risks than benefits to the population (Danaei et al., 2009). People who provide treatment for those with drinking problems find it difficult to recommend drinking to anyone, and skepticism has lingered in the form of questioning the methodology and validity of the multitude of studies that have found benefits in drinking. However, one study that attempted to control for these errors (Holahan et al., 2010) found that, even with these flaws discounted, light to moderate drinking provided health benefits compared with heavy drinking or abstaining. During the time that some researchers were questioning the validity of the benefits, others were working toward understanding the physiology of a protective effect.

That search has resulted in findings that alcohol produces changes in the course of atherosclerosis, the disease condition that underlies most CVD (Mochly-Rosen & Zakhari, 2010). Alcohol alters cholesterol, raising specific subfractions of high-density lipoprotein that are beneficial and reducing the tendency to form blood clots. In addition, alcohol affects insulin sensitivity and inflammation (Mukamal et al., 2005; Rimm & Moats, 2007). All of these actions may work toward reducing CVD, thus offering the beginnings of a plausible mechanism through which drinking could decrease heart disease.

Other Benefits of Alcohol Cardiovascular disease is not the only condition that is lower among middle-aged and older drinkers. Chances of developing Type 2 diabetes are lower among light to moderate drinkers than among those who abstain (Hendriks, 2007). Alcohol affects glucose tolerance and insulin resistance, which makes this effect comprehensible. The role of alcohol in cholesterol metabolism and its effect on bile acids suggest that drinkers may be at lowered risk for gallstones (Walcher et al., 2010). Epidemiological research bears out this conjecture: Moderate drinkers experienced gallstones at about half the rate of those who did not drink.

Alcohol also has some effect on *H. pylori*, a bacterium that infects the gastrointestinal system and is involved in gastritis, ulcer development, and possibly gastric cancers. People who drink have lower concentrations of this bacterium in their digestive tracts (Gao, Weck, Stegmaier, Rothenbacher, & Brenner, 2010). (See Chapter 6 for a discussion of *H. pylori* and ulcer formation.) Reductions in the levels of this infection may decrease risk for ulcer formation and digestive tract cancers.

Some surprising evidence suggests that drinking may protect against cognitive deficits (Collins, 2008; Lobo et al., 2010). This effect is unexpected because heavy drinking is associated with Korsakoff syndrome, which produces memory problems and other cognitive deficits. However, drinking seems to relate to decreased risk for Alzheimer's disease, the most common form of dementia associated with advancing age. As Chapter 11 explained, Alzheimer's disease is a devastating degenerative brain disorder, and few protective measures have been identified. This intriguing finding offers hope of a way to combat this disease in an aging population.

For all of the diseases for which alcohol has shown some protective effect, the amount of alcohol and the pattern of drinking are important factors (Klatsky, 2010). At high levels of drinking, alcohol becomes a risk. Binge drinking, even occasionally, fails to convey the protections of light to moderate drinking and produces several of the risks. Individual differences are important in calculating who may benefit from drinking how much. Women gain the protective effects of alcohol at lower levels of drinking than men and feel the hazards at lower levels. In addition, the benefits of drinking do not appear among young people but begin during middle age (Klatsky & Udaltsova, 2007); young people are safer and healthier when they do not drink.

Drinking offers more health benefits than hazards for some people. However, those people who do not drink probably should not start, and those who do drink regularly (about half the people in the United States) should strive to keep their drinking at low levels of consumption and avoid binge drinking in order to experience the health benefits.

IN SUMMARY

Alcohol consumption has both harmful and beneficial effects on health. In addition, it has some negative indirect effects on society that reach beyond an individual's physical health. The direct hazards of prolonged and heavy drinking include cirrhosis of the liver, an increased risk for some cancers, and a brain dysfunction called Korsakoff syndrome. In addition, heavy drinking during pregnancy increases the risk of fetal alcohol spectrum disorders, the most serious of which is fetal alcohol syndrome, a serious disorder that often includes growth deficiencies and severe mental retardation. Alcohol is also a risk factor for many types of violence, both intentional and unintentional. The level of alcohol consumption necessary to increase the risk is not as high as the level necessary to produce legal intoxication, but the more heavily people drink, the more likely it is that they will be involved in accidents and violent crimes. Finally, alcohol consumption may also lead to poor decisions.

The principal positive aspect of alcohol consumption is its buffering effect against coronary heart disease and peripheral vascular disease, but these benefits accrue only in middle-aged and older individuals. Other health benefits may include lowered risks for diabetes, gallstones, *H. pylori* infection, and Alzheimer's disease, but heavy or binge drinking increases these risks.

Why Do People Drink?

Investigators trying to understand drinking and alcohol abuse have proposed several models to explain behavior related to alcohol consumption. These models go beyond the pharmacological effects of alcohol and even beyond the research findings to integrate and explain drinking. To be useful, a model for drinking behavior must address at least three questions. First, why do people start drinking? Second, why do most people maintain moderate rather than excessive drinking levels? Third, why do some people drink so much that they develop serious problems?

Until the 19th century, drinking was well accepted in the United States and Europe; this attitude makes drinking the norm, thus requiring no explanation. However, drunkenness was unacceptable under most circumstances, leaving drunkenness in need of some explanation. Two models arose during that time to explain drunkenness: the moral model and the medical model (Rotskoff, 2002).

The moral model appeared first, holding that people have free will to choose their behaviors, including excessive drinking. Thus, those who do so are either sinful or morally lacking in the self-discipline necessary to moderate their drinking. The moral model of alcoholism began to fade in the late 19th century with the growing prominence of medical approaches to problems. Unacceptable behaviors that were formerly cast as moral problems became medical problems and, thus, subject to scientific explanation and medical treatment. However, many people and even some alcoholism treatment staff still take a moralistic view of excessive drinking (Palm, 2004).

The medical model of alcoholism conceptualized problem drinking as symptomatic of underlying physical problems, and the notion that alcoholism is hereditary grew from this view. The first form of this hypothesis took the view that a "constitutional weakness" ran in families and that this weakness produced alcoholics.

Problem drinking does run in families, but the relative contributions of heredity and environment remain the subject of heated debates. Most authorities agree that both genetic and environmental influences play a role in shaping alcohol abuse (Ball, 2008). Children of problem drinkers are more likely than children of nonproblem drinkers to abuse alcohol as well as other drugs. Perhaps genetics played a role in Charlie Sheen's alcohol and drug use; his father, Martin Sheen, went through his own battle with drinking problems ("Martin Sheen," 2008), but his brother, Emilio Estevez, seems to have no such problems.

How can investigators learn about the relative effects of environment and heredity on the development of problem drinking? Researchers have taken several approaches, including the degree of agreement in drinking behavior between twins or between adopted children and parents (Foroud, Edenberg, & Crabbe, 2010). Twin studies ordinarily involve measuring the degree of agreement between pairs of identical twins compared with the amount of agreement between pairs of fraternal twins. If identical twins are more similar to each other than fraternal twins are, the reason points to genetics. Indeed, research generally shows a closer concordance of problem drinking for identical twins than for fraternal twins. This greater concordance between identical twins supports the idea of some genetic component in alcohol abuse.

A second test of a hereditary factor in alcohol abuse is the study of adopted children (Ball, 2008). Adoption studies investigate the frequency of alcohol abuse in adoptees whose biological parent was alcoholic. Results from several large-scale studies using this approach also indicate a genetic component in problem drinking. Both types of studies indicate a stronger role for genetics in the problem drinking of men than of women.

Genes do not determine drinking. Indeed, genes do not produce any behavior. Genes govern protein synthesis, and a number of steps intervene between genes and behavior. Research has begun to explore the molecular basis of how genes affect drinking.

One effect of genes on alcohol metabolism is fairly well understood, but this type of inheritance *protects against* rather than creates a vulnerability for problem drinking. When individuals inherit a gene variant that results in deficient activity of aldehyde dehydrogenase (one of the enzymes that metabolizes alcohol), they experience an unpleasant "flushing" reaction when they drink (Foroud et al., 2010). This gene configuration is more common among people of Asian ancestry than other ethnic groups, and people with this pattern develop problem drinking far less often than others do.

Alcohol metabolism offers various possibilities for creating a vulnerability to problem drinking. The functioning of neurotransmitters in the brain, such as dopamine, GABA, and serotonin, is affected by genetics and has also been linked to alcohol's effects (Foroud et al., 2010; Köhnke, 2008). A specific genetic susceptibility to problem drinking may lie in a variant of the genes that are involved with alcohol dehydrogenase, which is the other enzyme involved in alcohol metabolism (Tolstrup, Nordestgaard, Rasmussen, Tybjærg-Hansen, & Grønbæk, 2008). According to this view, the speed of alcohol metabolism is related to drinking more, and variants of this gene affect that speed. However, problem drinking will not be traced to one gene pair; hundreds of genes are likely involved (Foroud et al., 2010). In addition, researchers accept the importance of a person's environment in drinking; they expect that the search for the genetic contributions to problem drinking will reveal multiple gene locations that underlie a vulnerability to problem drinking rather than a genetic determination of alcoholism. That is, researchers are looking for genetic, biological, and environmental factors that contribute to problem drinking.

The Disease Model

The disease concept of alcoholism is a variation of the medical model, holding that people with problem drinking have the disease of alcoholism. Throughout history, isolated attempts have been made to describe alcohol intoxication as a disease brought about by the physical properties of alcohol. This view became increasingly popular beginning in the late 1930s and early 1940s. It was accepted by the American Medical Association in 1956 and remains the dominant view in psychiatric and other medically oriented treatment programs in the United States (Lee, Lee, Lee, & Arch, 2010). The disease model is less influential in psychologically based treatment programs and in treatment programs in Canada, Europe, and Australia.

The disease model of alcoholism was elevated to scientific respectability by the pioneering work of Jellinek (1960), who described several different types of alcoholism and their characteristics. The two most common types are **gamma alcoholism**, or loss of control once drinking begins, and **delta alcoholism**, or the inability to abstain. Any model that conceptualizes alcoholism as an incurable unitary disorder is too simplistic, even if it includes different varieties of alcoholism.

The Alcohol Dependency Syndrome   Dissatisfaction with Jellinek's disease model led Griffith Edwards and his colleagues (Edwards, 1977; Edwards & Gross, 1976; Edwards, Gross, Keller, Moser, & Room, 1977) to advocate the alcohol dependency syndrome, which rejects the term *alcoholism*, substituting the term *alcohol dependency syndrome*. Rather than assert that alcoholics experience loss of control, Edwards and his colleagues proposed that those who are alcohol dependent have *impaired control*, suggesting that people drink heavily because, at certain times and for a variety of reasons, they do not exercise control over their drinking. The seven elements of the alcohol dependency syndrome appear in Table 13.1. This concept has influenced the "official" one that forms the basis for a diagnosis of substance abuse dependency, based on the *Diagnostic and Statistical Manual of Mental Disorders* (American Psychiatric Association, 2000), and, with slight changes, will appear in the upcoming revision of this manual.

Evaluation of the Disease Model   Despite the widespread acceptance of the disease model of alcoholism, the concept has only limited research support—the basis for the disease of alcoholism has not been identified. This model fails to address our first question: Why do people begin to drink? Its answer to the second question about why some people continue to drink at

TABLE 13.1 Elements of the Alcohol Dependency Syndrome

Element	Behaviors Associated With This Element
Narrowing of drinking repertoire	Drinking the same beverage at the same time of day
Salience of drink-seeking behavior	Drinking begins to take precedence over other behaviors.
Increased tolerance for alcohol	Drinkers become accustomed to performing daily tasks with high blood alcohol levels.
Withdrawal symptoms	Restlessness, irritability, and agitation
Avoiding withdrawal symptoms	Additional drinking
Personal awareness of the need to drink	Drinkers acknowledge their need to drink.
Reinstatement of dependence after abstinence	Drinkers who have quit become dependent more rapidly when they begin to drink again; the development of dependence is inversely related to severity of prior dependence.

Source: "Alcohol Dependence: Provisional Description of a Clinical Syndrome" by G. Edwards & M. M. Gross, 1976, *British Medical Journal, 1*(6017), 1058–1061.

moderate levels is hardly adequate: People who are not alcoholic do not develop a dependence on alcohol.

One key concept in the disease model is loss of control or impaired control—the inability to stop or moderate alcohol intake once drinking begins. This concept has been difficult to define specifically, and research has not been consistent concerning its influence (Martin, Fillmore, Chung, Easdon, & Miczek, 2006). G. Alan Marlatt and his colleagues (Marlatt, Demming, & Reid, 1973; Marlatt & Rohsenow, 1980)

have conducted experiments suggesting that many effects of alcohol, including impaired control, are due more to expectancy than to any pharmacological effect of alcohol. Their experimental design, called the balanced placebo design, included four groups, two of which expected to be given alcohol and two of which did not. Two groups actually received alcohol, and two did not. Figure 13.4 shows all four combinations.

Using the balanced placebo design, several studies (Marlatt et al., 1973; Marlatt & Rohsenow, 1980)

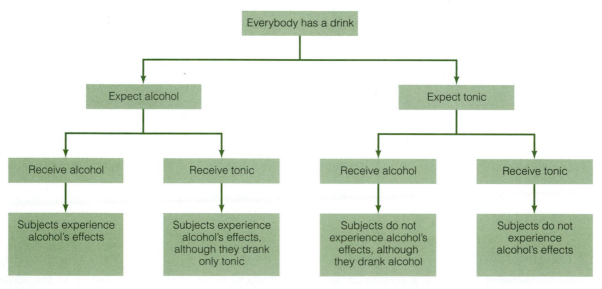

FIGURE 13.4 Balanced placebo design used in experiments on expectancy and alcohol effects.

showed that people who think they have received alcohol behave as though they have (whether they have or not). Even for those who had been in treatment for problem drinking, expectancy appeared to be the controlling factor in the craving for alcohol and in the amount consumed. These findings suggest that expectancy plays an important role in loss of control and craving for alcohol. A meta-analysis of studies on alcohol expectancy (McKay & Schare, 1999) confirmed that expectancy plays an important role in alcohol's effects.

Some investigators (Peele, 2007; Quinn, Bodenhamer-Davis, & Koch, 2004) have criticized the disease model of alcohol, arguing that it does not adequately consider environmental, cognitive, and affective determinants of abusive drinking; that is, in its emphasis on the physical properties of alcohol, the disease model neglects the cognitive and social learning aspects of drinking.

Cognitive-Physiological Theories

Of the various alternatives to the disease model, several emphasize the combination of physiological and cognitive changes that occur with alcohol use. Rather than hypothesize that alcohol use and misuse are based only on the chemical properties of alcohol, these models contend that the cognitive changes experienced by drinkers also contribute to drinking behavior.

The Tension Reduction Hypothesis   As the name suggests, the tension reduction hypothesis (Conger, 1956) holds that people drink alcohol because of its tension-reducing effects. This hypothesis has much intuitive appeal because alcohol is a sedative drug that leads to relaxation and slowed reactions.

Despite its consistency with popular belief, experimental studies have furnished limited support for the tension reduction hypothesis. Studies that have manipulated tension or anxiety to observe their effects on participants' readiness to consume alcohol have yielded contradictory results; some participants experience tension reduction, whereas others do not (Kambouropoulos, 2003). In more naturalistic settings (Frone, 2008; Moore, Sikora, Grunberg, & Greenberg, 2007), factors other than stress and tension have been found to relate to drinking. One factor that complicates assessment of the tension reduction hypothesis is expectancy. When people expect to experience tension reduction, they tend to get what they expect. A large-scale study in Germany (Pabst, Baumeister, & Kraus, 2010) found

that tension reduction is one of the effects that drinkers expect. Thus, tension reduction is one of many effects that may occur as a result of drinking, but expectancy may be more important than alcohol in these effects.

The realization that alcohol's effects on physiological processes are not simple led to a reformulation of the tension reduction hypothesis. A group of researchers at Indiana University (Levenson, Sher, Grossman, Newman, & Newlin, 1980; Sher, 1987; Sher & Levenson, 1982) discovered that high levels of alcohol consumption decrease the strength of responses to stress. They labeled this decrease the *stress response dampening (SRD) effect*. People who had been drinking did not respond as strongly as nondrinking participants to either physiological or psychological stressors. People whose personality profile suggested a high risk of developing problem drinking showed the strongest SRD effect, and those whose profile indicated a low risk showed a weaker effect (Sher & Levenson, 1982). This stress response–dampening effect appears in some drinkers but not in others (Zack, Poulos, Aramakis, Khamba, & MacLeod, 2007) and more strongly at higher levels of intoxication (Donohue, Curtin, Patrick, & Lang, 2007). In addition, stress response dampening tends to occur in social drinking situations, suggesting that some drinkers may use alcohol as a way to manage their stress responses (Armeli et al., 2003). However, neither the original tension reduction hypothesis nor stress response dampening provides a general explanation for drinking, especially for initiating drinking.

Alcohol Myopia   Claude Steele and his colleagues (Steele & Josephs, 1990) have developed a model of alcohol use and abuse based on alcohol's psychological and physical properties. This model hypothesizes that alcohol use creates effects on social behaviors that they term *alcohol myopia*, "a state of shortsightedness in which superficially understood, immediate aspects of experience have a disproportionate influence on behavior and emotion, a state in which we can see the tree, albeit more dimly, but miss the forest altogether" (Steele & Josephs, 1990, p. 923). According to this view, alcohol blocks out insightful cognitive processing and alters thoughts related to the self, stress, and social anxiety.

Part of alcohol myopia is drunken excess, the tendency for those who drink to behave more excessively. This tendency appears as increased aggression, friendliness, sexiness, and many other exaggerated behaviors. Tendencies to behave in such extreme ways are usually inhibited, but when people drink, they experience less inhibition, and their behavior becomes more extreme.

Another aspect of alcohol myopia is self-inflation, a tendency to inflate self-evaluations. When asked to rate the importance of 35 trait dimensions for their real and ideal selves, drunken participants rated themselves higher on traits that were important to them and on which they had rated themselves low when sober (Banaji & Steele, 1989). Thus, drinking allowed participants to see themselves as better than they did when they were not drinking, confirming the ability of alcohol to inflate a person's self-evaluation.

A third aspect of alcohol myopia is drunken relief (Steele & Josephs, 1990); that is, people who drink tend to worry less and pay less attention to their worries. When consumed in large quantities, alcohol alone may produce drunken relief, but it can also affect behavior in smaller quantities. For example, women with low self-esteem who drank alcohol interacted more with a flirtatious man after drinking than did similar women who had not been drinking and more than women with high self-esteem (Monahan & Lannutti, 2000). This finding suggests that drunken relief is not an effect entirely of alcohol but of alcohol in combination with other factors.

The alcohol myopia model has quite a bit of research support. Intoxicated people tend to analyze information at a more superficial level, are more susceptible to distraction (Ortner, MacDonald, & Olmstead, 2003), and recall fewer details of a situation they have experienced (Villalba, Ham, & Rose, 2011) than people who have not been drinking. For example, people playing an online gambling game became less focused on suggestions concerning how to maximize their winnings after they started drinking (Phillips & Ogeil, 2007).

In addition, alcohol myopia has offered a framework for interpreting a number of changes in sexual behavior that occur after drinking. A review of the research on high-risk sexual behavior and alcohol (Griffin, Umstattd, & Usdan, 2010) indicated that college students' sexual decision making is affected by intoxication. Drinking leads people to focus on specific cues in the environment, which can lead to either more or less risky decisions. For example, when intoxicated men or women focus on their sexual feelings, they tend to be more willing to engage in risky sex than those who are not intoxicated. When similarly intoxicated people's attention is focused on the perils of risky sex, they tend to be less likely to engage in risky sex than

those who are sober. That is, drinkers' tendency to process information in a limited way is influenced by what cues are present rather than by a general tendency for disinhibition. Thus, many studies offer strong research support for this model.

The Social Learning Model

The social learning model provides an explanation for why people begin to drink, why they continue to drink in moderation, and why some people drink in a harmful manner. This model conceptualizes drinking as learned behavior, acquired in the same manner as other behaviors.

According to social learning theory, people begin to drink for at least three reasons. First, the taste of alcohol and its immediate effects may bring pleasure (positive reinforcement); second, drinking may allow a person to escape from an unpleasant situation (negative reinforcement); and third, the person may learn to drink through observing others (modeling). Research offers support for each of these possibilities.

First, research from countries around the world (Bergmark & Kuendig, 2008) found positive expectations for alcohol consumption. The reasons for drinking among college students in the United States (Read, Wood, & Capone, 2005) and in the United Kingdom (Orford, Krishnan, Balaam, Everitt, & van der Graaf, 2004) also support the role of positive reinforcement, revealing that interpersonal factors, such as social interaction and mood enhancement, are key reasons for drinking. For individuals who do not drink, social influences are also important; lifetime abstainers tended to report that they had no interest in drinking or that their religion or upbringing influenced them to abstain (Bernards, Graham, Kuendig, Hettige, & Obot, 2009).

Second, modeling and social pressure were found to be related to increases in drinking during college, and students who were heavier drinkers put themselves in situations to receive different pressures than did students who drank less (Orford et al., 2004), which relates to the influence of modeling. A combination of modeling and expectancies of the effects of alcohol is the mechanism hypothesized to underlie the transmission of drinking from parents to children (Campbell & Oei, 2010). People who are heavy drinkers also tend to associate with other people who have similar drinking patterns. Thus, modeling offers explanations for both the initiation of drinking and the tendency of some people to drink to excess.

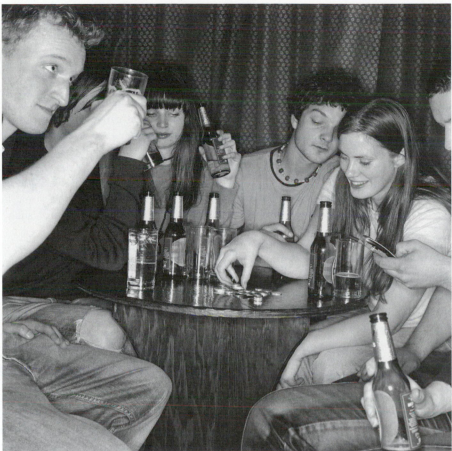

Image Source/Getty Images

College social gatherings may encourage binge drinking.

A third explanation for excessive drinking offered by the social learning model is based on the principles of negative reinforcement. Dropping alcohol levels creates discomfort, and ingesting more alcohol relieves this discomfort. This process fits with the definition of negative reinforcement and provides another explanation for continuing to drink (Lowman, Hunt, Litten, & Drummond, 2000).

Social learning theory provides an explanation for why people start drinking, why some continue to drink in moderation, and why others become problem drinkers. In addition, social learning theory suggests a variety of treatment techniques to help people overcome excessive drinking habits. The treatment rationale holds that if drinking behavior is learned, then it can be unlearned or relearned, with either abstinence or moderation as a goal of therapy.

IN SUMMARY

The question of why people drink has three components: (1) why do people begin drinking? (2) why do some people drink in moderation? (3) why do others drink to excess? Theories of drinking behavior should be able to offer explanations in response to each of these questions. This section discussed three theories or models, each of which has some potential explanatory ability. The disease model assumes that people drink excessively because they have the disease of alcoholism. One variation of the disease model—the alcohol dependency syndrome—assumes that alcohol-dependent people have impaired control and drink heavily for a variety of reasons. Cognitive-physiological models, including the tension reduction hypothesis and alcohol myopia, propose that people drink because alcohol produces alterations in cognitive function that allow them to escape tension or process information differently. Social learning theory hypothesizes that people acquire drinking behavior the same way that they learn other behaviors—that is, through positive or negative reinforcement and modeling. All three models offer some explanation of why some people continue to drink, but only social learning theory addresses all three components of drinking.

Changing Problem Drinking

Despite a decline in the percentage of drinkers in the United States, an increasing number of people seek help for problem drinking; almost 3 million people received treatment for alcohol use in 2009 (SAMHSA, 2010). Men outnumber women by a ratio of 2 to 1. Women are more reluctant than men to seek treatment, and they may also seek treatment from sources that specialize in mental health treatment rather than alcohol treatment (Walter et al., 2003). Outpatient treatment is more common than inpatient treatment, but the most common form of treatment is attendance at a self-help group (SAMHSA, 2010). Private, for-profit facilities emphasize inpatient treatment, but these programs may have benefits that are limited to people with the most serious problems, and the costs are much higher. Cost is a factor in treatment; almost half of those who needed but failed to receive treatment cited cost not covered by insurance as the most important factor (SAMHSA, 2010). Although adequate treatment is important for changing drinking behavior, some individuals with drinking problems are able to quit without formal treatment (Hodgins, 2005; Scarscelli, 2006).

Change Without Therapy

Some problems (and some diseases) disappear without formal treatment, and problem drinking is no exception. When a disease disappears without treatment, the term **spontaneous remission** is used to describe the cure. Many authorities in the field of problem drinking prefer the term *unassisted change* or *natural recovery* to describe a switch from problem to nonproblem drinking. Even these terms may be somewhat misleading because people who change their drinking patterns may have the help and support of many people, including family members, employers, and friends, but not a formal therapy program. Changes of this type do occur (Scarscelli, 2006). In a study of individuals diagnosed as alcohol dependent (Dawson et al., 2005), only 25% were still in that category 1 year later; 18% were abstinent, and another 18% had moderated their drinking to nonproblem levels. Heavy drinkers who change their drinking behavior may be those who are less dependent (Cunningham, Blomqvist, Koski-Jännes, & Cordingley, 2005); others may need professional help or the assistance of traditional groups such as Alcoholics Anonymous.

Presently, nearly all treatment programs in the United States are oriented toward abstinence, but programs in other countries may be oriented toward harm reduction rather than abstinence and allow for the possibility that some problem drinkers can moderate their alcohol intake.

Treatments Oriented Toward Abstinence

All formal treatments—even those that permit the possibility of resuming drinking—seek immediate abstinence as their goal. This section examines several treatment programs aimed at total and permanent abstinence.

Alcoholics Anonymous Alcoholics Anonymous (AA) is one of the most widely used alcohol treatment programs, and it is often a component in other treatment programs. Founded in 1935 by two former alcoholics, AA has become the best known of all approaches to problem drinking. The organization follows a very strict version of the disease model and combines it with an emphasis on spirituality that is designed to bring the problem drinker into the group to receive support and mentoring from others who have experienced similar problems.

To adhere to the AA doctrine, a person must maintain total abstinence from alcohol. Part of the AA philosophy is that those who are in need of joining AA can never drink again; problem drinkers are addicted to alcohol and have no power to resist it. According to AA, alcoholics never recover but are always in the process of recovering. They will be alcoholics for life, even if they never take another drink.

AA and other 12-step programs have attained a high level of acceptance, attracting large numbers of people. Each year, over 2 million people in the United States attend a self-help program such as AA for drinking problems (SAMHSA, 2010). A majority of those individuals—perhaps as many as 75%—attend AA meetings (Magura, 2007).

The anonymity offered to those who attend AA meetings presents barriers to researchers wishing to conduct studies on the effectiveness of this program. A systematic evaluation (Ferri, Amato, & Davoli, 2006) found that the experimental evidence for the effectiveness of AA is lacking. Experimentation would involve randomly assigning participants to attend AA or some other option, which is not how most treatment occurs. Instead, people choose to attend a program, and for some people with drinking problems, AA is helpful. Indeed, AA helps people who attend to form social networks of nondrinkers, which can be helpful in replacing harmful social connections that may encourage drinking (Kelly, Stout, Magill, & Tonigan, 2011). For others, the AA 12-step program with its "one-size-fits-all approach" is not helpful (Buddie, 2004, p. 61), and many drop out of AA. Alternative self-help organizations predate the development of AA and continue to proliferate around the world (White, 2004). Organizations such as Secular Organization for Sobriety, Women for Sobriety, SMART Recovery, Rational Recovery, and Moderation Management offer the value of support and group discussions with different philosophies than AA; for example, some do not insist on the goal of lifetime abstinence. Online groups available through the Internet offer easier access, making the benefits of group support more accessible.

Psychotherapy   Nearly as many psychotherapeutic techniques have been used to treat alcohol abuse as there are psychotherapies. Research has demonstrated that many approaches are not very effective in helping problem drinkers, whereas other techniques are much more so (Huebner & Kantor, 2010; Kaner et al., 2007). Many varieties of behavioral therapy exist, and those therapies tend to be more effective than less directive approaches such as education about alcohol or counseling (Miller, Wilbourne, & Hettema, 2003; Witkiewitz, & Marlatt, 2010). Brief interventions are becoming more popular and can also be effective (Kaner et al., 2007). These techniques are designed to change motivation and may last for only a few hours, and this brevity offers advantages.

An example of both a brief intervention and one oriented toward changing motivation is motivational interviewing (Miller & Rollnick, 2002). Therapists using motivational interviewing convey their empathy with the client's situation and help clients resolve their ambivalence about their problem behavior. This process is designed to move clients toward change, making this approach a directive type of psychological intervention. Linking motivational interviewing to the transtheoretical model (see Chapter 4) provides a framework for understanding and promoting behavioral change. Reviews of motivational interviewing (Lundahl, Kunz, Brownell, Tollefson, & Burke, 2010; Rubak, Sanboek, Lauritzen, & Christensen, 2005) have revealed this type of brief intervention to be effective in decreasing problem drinking. In addition to the behavioral approaches that can be effective, some chemical treatments can also be useful in controlling problem drinking.

Chemical Treatments   Many treatment programs for problem drinking include administering drugs that interact with alcohol to produce a range of unpleasant effects. **Disulfiram** (Antabuse) is one such drug. Taken alone, this drug produces a few unpleasant effects, but in combination with alcohol, the unpleasant effects are severe—flushing of the face, chest pains, a pounding heart, nausea and vomiting, sweating, headache, dizziness, weakness, difficulty in breathing, and a rapid decrease in blood pressure. The rationale behind the use of these drugs is to produce an aversion to drinking by building up an association between drinking and the unpleasant consequences. This process, called **aversion therapy**, applies to the use of disulfiram as well as other methods that involve aversive conditioning. Getting people to take a drug that will make them sick if they drink is a challenge, and disulfiram is only modestly successful in treating problem drinkers (Krishnan-Sarin, O'Malley, & Krysta, 2008).

An alternative drug treatment is naltrexone, a drug that attaches to opiate receptors in the brain and prevents their activation. Its action for drinkers may be to decrease the reward that comes from drinking (Mann, 2004). A systematic review of studies on naltrexone as a treatment for alcoholism (Rösner et al., 2010) revealed that the effects were modest but positive. Naltrexone may be more useful in preventing relapse than in other phases of treatment, and the effects may be short-term rather than longer.

Another drug that shows some promise is acamprosate, which acts to affect GABA, one of the brain's neurotransmitters. Its action may decrease craving (Mann, 2004) and increase the chances of achieving abstinence (Carmen, Angeles, Ana, & María, 2004). Similar to the other drugs used to treat drinking, acamprosate has a modest effect. Some research (Mann & Hermann, 2010) has suggested that analyzing the behavioral and biological characteristics of drinkers may allow more tailored therapy that will boost the effectiveness of these drug interventions.

Controlled Drinking

Until the late 1960s, all treatments for problem drinking were aimed at total abstinence. Then something quite unexpected happened. In 1962 in London, D. L. Davies found that 7 of the 93 recovered alcoholics whom he studied were able to drink "normally" (defined as consumption of up to 3 pints of beer or its equivalent per day) for at least a 7-year period following treatment. These moderate drinkers represented fewer than 8% of those Davies studied, but this finding was still remarkable because it opened up the possibility that problem drinkers could successfully return to nonproblem drinking. This finding provoked a controversy that continues today.

Prompted by Davies's results, several studies conducted in the United States (Armor, Polich, & Stambul, 1976; Polich, Armor, & Braiker, 1980) showed that controlled drinking occurred in a small percentage of patients who received treatment oriented toward abstinence. Publicity about this study produced a wave of criticism from those holding the position that alcoholics can never drink again, and this controversy became more heated when researchers began to design treatment programs with controlled drinking as the goal.

Problem drinkers can become moderate drinkers. Some problem drinkers in abstinence-oriented treatment programs become moderate drinkers (Miller, Walters, & Bennett, 2001; Sobell, Cunningham, & Sobell, 1996), and some who quit on their own moderate their drinking (Dawson et al., 2005). Despite the evidence concerning controlled drinking, most treatment centers in the United States have resisted the possibility that former problem drinkers can learn to moderate their use of alcohol and stick to the goal of abstinence. This attitude does not extend to other countries; in England, Wales, and Scotland, nearly all treatment centers accept continued drinking among those who have experienced drinking problems. The goal is to reduce the harm that often accompanies

drinking rather than eliminate drinking itself (Heather, 2006; Rosenberg & Melville, 2005).

The thought of being able to continue drinking is appealing to most drinkers, including those whose drinking is problematic. Thus, controlled drinking appeals to many with drinking problems (Kosok, 2006). This appeal is one reason for the creation of a self-help group oriented toward moderating drinking, called Moderation Management. This group includes face-to-face and online meetings, and research on this approach (Hester, Delaney, & Campbell, 2011) showed that both formats can reduce problem drinking. Many of those who are affiliated with Moderation Management have not sought other assistance for their drinking problems, perhaps because other available treatment is abstinence oriented (Hodgins, 2005).

The Problem of Relapse

Problem drinkers who successfully complete either an abstinence-oriented or a moderation-oriented treatment program do not necessarily maintain their goals. As we saw with smoking, people who complete a treatment program usually improve quite a bit, but the problem of relapse is substantial. Interestingly, the time course and rate of relapse are similar for those who complete treatment programs for smoking, alcohol abuse, or opiate abuse (Hunt et al., 1971). Most relapses occur within 90 days after the end of the program. At 12 months after the end of treatment, only about 35% of those completing the programs remain abstinent. These similarities may be attributable to the underlying brain mechanisms involved in habitual drug use, which share some similarities regardless of differences in the pharmacological properties of the drug (Camí & Farré, 2003).

A growing view in treatment holds that alcohol abuse is a chronic illness that requires continuing care (McKay & Hiller-Sturmhöfel, 2010). Thus, treatment programs should include provisions for follow-up care to address relapse. Many inpatient treatment programs make such provisions through the requirement that participants attend AA meetings, which provide a supportive environment that discourages drinking and thus deters relapse (Huebner & Kantor, 2011).

Most behavior-based treatment regimens include training for relapse prevention, taking the view that a relapse occurs in a complex environment with many sources of influence. Understanding those sources and knowing how to cope with their influence is critical; behavior change is not quick or easy (Witkiewitz &

Marlatt, 2010). As discussed in Chapter 12, relapse prevention training is aimed at changing cognitions so that the addict comes to believe that one slip does *not* equal total relapse. Programs that focus on long-term goals and incorporate relapse prevention into their regimen tend to have the highest rates of success (McLellan, Lewis, O'Brien, & Kleber, 2000), but if lifetime abstinence is the goal, many relapse prevention programs do not have a high rate of success (Miller et al., 2003). However, if the standard is improvement and a lower level of problems caused by drinking, then relapse is not as common; as many as 60% of people who complete a treatment program achieve this level of success.

IN SUMMARY

Despite a decline in the percentage of drinkers in the United States, the number of people seeking help for their drinking problems has continued to grow. Many problem drinkers are able to quit without therapy; others seek formal treatment programs. Traditional alcohol treatment programs—such as Alcoholics Anonymous, the most widely sought treatment—are oriented toward abstinence. Many problem drinkers are not able to achieve this goal; only about 25% of problem drinkers are abstinent 1 year after treatment. Drinking levels typically drop substantially, however, and so do alcohol-related problems.

Some behavioral programs are successful, including brief interventions such as motivational interviewing; these brief interventions are becoming more common. Chemical treatments such as the drugs disulfiram, naltrexone, and acamprosate have been used to curb alcohol consumption, and all show modest levels of success.

Controlled drinking may be a reasonable goal for some problem drinkers. However, this goal is very controversial, and many abstinence-oriented therapists do not consider controlled drinking a viable alternative, which may keep some problem drinkers from seeking therapy.

With all alcohol treatment approaches, relapse has been a persistent problem. Most relapses occur within 3 months after the end of treatment, and after 12 months, only 25% of those who complete programs are still abstinent. Relapse training has become a common component of behaviorally oriented programs, but the goal of sustained abstinence is a difficult one.

Other Drugs

Illicit drugs have created many serious problems in the United States, but these problems are mainly social and are not major threats to physical health. The effects of smoking cigarettes, drinking alcohol, eating unwisely, and remaining sedentary are responsible for over 60% of deaths in the United States; deaths attributable to illicit drug use account for less than 2% (Kochanek, Xu, Murphy, Miniño, & Kung, 2011). Even one death from illicit drugs, of course, is too many, but both legal and illegal drug use can have negative consequences.

Researchers are beginning to understand how drugs function in the brain to alter mood and behavior. Alcohol and other drugs produce effects on neurotransmitters, the chemical basis of neural transmission. Several neurotransmitters are involved in drug actions, including GABA, glutamate, serotonin, and norepinephrine (López-Moreno, González-Cuevas, Moreno, & Navarro, 2008), but the neurotransmitter **dopamine** is especially important (Young, Gobrogge, & Wang, 2011). Dopamine may be the most important neurotransmitter in a brain subsystem that relays messages from the ventral tegmental area in the midbrain to the nucleus accumbens in the forebrain. Researchers have known for years that this area is involved in the brain's experience of reward and pleasure. However, the actions of many drugs seem to be common to the same system, including these two brain structures as well as the hippocampus, amygdala, and forebrain (López-Moreno et al., 2008). That is, drugs seem to activate the brain circuits that underlie reward. Indeed, experiences such as gambling may activate the same brain mechanisms (Martin & Petry, 2005).

Psychoactive drugs do not all act in the same way in this subsystem, but all affect the availability of neurotransmitters, especially dopamine. Alterations of these neurotransmitters produce temporary changes in brain chemistry but rarely damage neurons. Changing the brain's chemistry carries risks, but brain damage is not a health effect associated with most drugs (see Would You Believe …?).

Health Effects

Even though most drugs do not damage neurons, both legal and illegal drugs pose potential health hazards. However, illegal drugs present certain risks not found with legal drugs, regardless of pharmacological effects.

Would You BELIEVE...? Brain Damage Is Not a Common Risk of Drug Use

Despite the vivid media images of a brain "fried" by drug use, most psychoactive drugs do not cause damage to the nervous system. Indeed, some of the drugs that can most wreck a person's life are among the *least* likely to damage the brain. For example, opiate drugs such as heroin, morphine, oxycodone, and hydrocodone produce both tolerance and dependence. Repeated use of these drugs results in compulsive drug taking and a pattern of use in which social relationships and responsibilities become unimportant. People who are dependent on opiate drugs usually experience major problems, but brain damage is not among them.

Like other psychoactive drugs, opiates cross the blood–brain barrier, where they occupy receptors for endorphins, the body's own analgesics (Julien, Advokat, & Comaty, 2010). Thus, these drugs are compatible with the brain's existing neurochemistry, so they occupy these receptors without causing damage. Their repeated use produces a host of physiological effects, some of which can be dangerous, but damage to the nervous system is unlikely.

Marijuana also acts by occupying brain receptors for neurochemicals called endocannabinoids (Pope, Mechoulam, & Parsons, 2010). The discovery of these neurochemicals suggested that the brain makes its own marijuana-like chemicals and also explained some of the actions that marijuana takes in the brain. Marijuana also produces a wide variety of physiological and behavioral effects, some of which may be dangerous. However, those effects do not include damage to neurons in the brain. Indeed, recent research (Pope et al., 2010) has suggested that endocannabinoids may exert protective effects in the nervous system.

Both publicity and public service announcements have decried the dangers of the drug Ecstasy, but the research that formed the basis for these claims was withdrawn by the researcher because of inaccuracies (Holden, 2003). Use of Ecstasy may not pose the risk to life that some feared, but the drug is not without dangers (Halpern et al., 2011). However, the only evidence that implicates this drug in neural damage comes from combinations with alcohol or stimulants, and then only as a possibility (Gouzoulis-Mayfrank & Daumann, 2006).

However, some drugs do carry risks of damage to the nervous system. Those risks typically occur with heavy, long-term use to those who fit into the category of abusers. For example, the potential for brain damage as a result of extended alcohol abuse is well known (Harper & Matsumoto, 2005). Some evidence has also suggested that the abuse of stimulants such as cocaine (Rosenberg, Grigsby, Dreisbach, Busenbark, & Grigsby, 2002) and amphetamines (Chang et al., 2002) produces toxic neurological effects. The evidence for brain damage from the use of household solvents is strong (Rosenberg et al., 2002). These chemicals act to alter consciousness not through changes to neurotransmitters but through oxygen restriction to the brain, so, of course, these substances cause brain damage.

The greatest risks from drug use are not neurological damage but rather the ability of these drugs to alter perception, decision making, and coordination. These effects increase the risk for unintentional injuries, which are a far more likely result than brain damage.

Illegal drugs may be sold as one drug when they are actually another, buyers have no assurance as to dosage, and illegally manufactured drugs may have impurities that can be dangerous chemicals themselves. In addition, the sources of illegal drugs can be dangerous people. Legal drugs are free from these risks, but they are not harmless and not always safe.

All drugs have potential hazards, but drugs termed *safe* are tested by the U.S. Food and Drug Administration (FDA) and defined as safe when potential benefits outweigh potential hazards. Many drugs, such as antibiotics, have been approved although they produce severe side effects in some people. The more potentially beneficial a drug, the more likely it is to be labeled *safe* despite unpleasant side effects.

The FDA classifies drugs into five categories, based on their potential for abuse and their potential medical benefits. Table 13.2 summarizes this schedule, presents the restrictions on availability, and gives examples of drugs in each category. This classification has evolved somewhat haphazardly over the past 100 years and represents legislative and social convention rather than scientific findings.

TABLE 13.2   FDA Drug Schedules, Restrictions, and Examples of Drugs in Each Category

Schedule	Description	Restriction on Availability	Examples
I	High abuse potential; no medical uses	Not legally available	LSD, marijuana, heroin
II	High abuse potential; medical uses	Prescription only	Morphine, oxycontin, barbiturates, amphetamines, cocaine
III	Moderate or low dependence; medical uses	Prescription only	Codeine, some tranquilizers
IV	Low dependence, low abuse potential; medical uses	Prescription only	Phenobarbital, most tranquilizers
V	Less abuse potential than drugs in Schedule IV	Over the counter	Aspirin, antacids, antihistamines, and others

A classification of drugs based on the action of the drugs would be more useful and can be accomplished by forming major classifications according to the effects of the drugs. Such a classification would have major sections for sedatives, stimulants, hallucinogens, marijuana, and anabolic steroids. **Sedatives** are drugs that induce relaxation and sometimes intoxication by lowering the activity of the brain, the neurons, the muscles, and the heart, and even by slowing the metabolic rate (Julien et al., 2010). The types of drugs within the major category include **barbiturates, tranquilizers, opiates**, and alcohol. In low doses, these drugs tend to make people feel relaxed and even euphoric. In high doses, they cause loss of consciousness and can result in coma and death as a result of their inhibitory effect on the brain center that controls respiration. These risks represent the most common hazards of sedative use. Table 13.3 shows the types of

Becoming Healthier

1. Avoid binge drinking—that is, drinking five or more drinks on any one occasion. There are no health benefits associated with binge drinking, and there are many risks.
2. Avoiding alcohol may not be the healthiest choice for middle-aged and older individuals, but if you do not drink and are comfortable with that choice, do not start drinking. If you are younger than 40, drinking is not likely to confer health benefits.
3. Occasional drinking—either light or heavy—presents some risks but does not convey many benefits. The pattern that confers the most benefits is daily (or almost daily) light drinking.
4. One or two drinks per day can impair judgment and coordination. These dangers are the biggest risk of alcohol consumption, and people who drink should find ways to manage this risk.
5. Do not drive, operate machinery, or swim after drinking.
6. Do not escalate your drinking; keep to one or two drinks per day (not an average of one or two).
7. The safest level of alcohol for pregnant women is none.
8. If one or both of your parents experienced drinking problems, you may be at elevated risk. Manage this risk by moderating your drinking.
9. If you have an extremely pleasant experience with any drug (including alcohol) the first time you try it, be aware that future use of this drug may present problems for you.
10. Don't combine drugs; drugs in combination are more dangerous than taking one drug.
11. Drugs that produce dependence are more dangerous than those that do not. Be aware and cautious about using such drugs, including alcohol and nicotine as well as opiates, barbiturates, and amphetamines.
12. Illegal drugs, even those without tolerance or dependence potential, can be dangerous because they are illegal.

TABLE 13.3   Summary of Characteristics of Psychoactive Drugs

Name	Tolerance	Dependence	Effects	Risks
Sedatives/Depressants				
Barbiturates	Yes	Yes	Relaxes, intoxicates	Unconsciousness, coma, death
Tranquilizers	Yes	Yes	Relaxes, intoxicates	Altered judgment, impaired coordination, coma
Opiates Opium derivatives; oxycodone; hydrocodone	Yes	Yes	Produces analgesia, euphoria, sedation	Coma, respiratory arrest, death
Alcohol	Yes	Yes	Relaxes, intoxicates	Impaired judgment and coordination, unconsciousness
Stimulants				
Caffeine	Yes	Yes	Increased alertness, reduced fatigue	Increased nervousness
Cocaine	Yes	Yes	Euphoria, suppressed appetite	Heart arrhythmia, heart attack
Amphetamines (methamphetamine, crystal meth)	Yes	Yes	Produces alertness, reduces fatigue	Heart attack, feelings of paranoia, increased violence
Nicotine (tobacco products)	Yes	Yes	Increases alertness, decreases appetite, elevates blood pressure	Increased heart disease and cancer
Hallucinogens				
Ecstasy (MDMA)	No	No	Produces feelings of well-being	Temperature regulation problems
LSD	No	No	Produces perceptual distortions, intoxicates	Altered perception and judgment
Marijuana				
Marijuana	No	Yes	Relaxes, intoxicates	Impaired judgment, coordination, respiratory problems (if smoked)
Steroids				
Anabolic steroids	Yes	No	Builds muscles, increases blood pressure, reduces immune system functioning	Testicular atrophy, increased aggression, lowered immune function

drugs that fit into this category, their effects, and their risks.

Stimulants are another main category of psychoactive drugs. All drugs in the stimulant category tend to produce alertness, reduce feelings of fatigue, elevate mood, and decrease appetite, including caffeine, nicotine, amphetamines, and cocaine. Caffeine, found in coffee, tea, and many types of sodas, is so widely consumed that many people do not think of it as a drug, but it produces the effects typical of stimulant drugs. **Amphetamines** are a class of powerful stimulant drug that includes methamphetamines and crystal methamphetamine that are often abused because of their mood-altering effects. Another stimulant drug, **cocaine**, is extracted from the coca plant. Cocaine is sold in powder form and as crack cocaine, which can be smoked. Using cocaine in combination with alcohol enhances the dangers of each drug by producing a third chemical, *cocaethylene* (Hearn et al., 1991). This chemical is hazardous (Huq, 2007) and may boost the user's risk for cardiac problems (Tacker & Okorodudu, 2004). Table 13.3 also summarizes these drugs and their characteristics.

Methylenedioxymethamphetamine (MDMA)—Ecstasy—is a derivative of methamphetamine, but people use it for its mild hallucinogenic effects, including feelings of peace and empathy with others. These feelings come from a massive release of the neurotransmitter *serotonin*, which depletes the supply of serotonin, but this depletion tends to be temporary (Buchert et al., 2004). Other hallucinogenic drugs such as lysergic acid diethylamide (LSD), mescaline, and psilocybin exert more complex effects on neurotransmitters, but serotonin is also involved in the effects of these drugs (Halberstadt & Geyer, 2011).

Marijuana has some hallucinogenic properties but lacks most other characteristics of hallucinogens. The intoxicating ingredient in marijuana, delta-9-tetrahydrocannabinol (THC), comes from the resin of the *Cannabis sativa* plant. The brain contains receptors for cannabinoids in many locations, which results in a variety of effects from ingesting marijuana, including altered thought processes, memory impairment, feelings of relaxation and euphoria, increased appetite, and impaired coordination (Nicoll & Alger, 2004). Its potential for serious health consequences is still debated, but few authorities regard it as a major health risk. However, its effects on cognition, judgment, and coordination boost the risk of unintentional injuries. In addition, users who smoke marijuana face increased

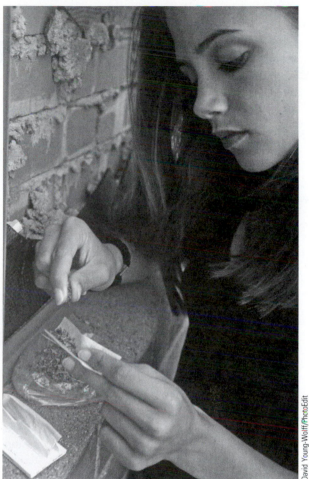

David Young-Wolff/*PhotoEdit*

Marijuana is the most commonly used illicit drug, particularly among adolescents and young adults.

risks for respiratory problems and lung cancer (Kalant, 2004). Despite potential benefits for some users, marijuana possession is against U.S. federal law. Nevertheless, a growing number of states have passed "medical marijuana" laws that allow access to marijuana.

Anabolic steroids (ASs) are synthetic hormones used to enhance athletic performance (King & Pace, 2005). The effects of anabolic steroids include thickening of the vocal cords, enlargement of the larynx, increase of muscle bulk, and decrease of body fat. These last two properties make ASs attractive to athletes, bodybuilders, and people who wish to alter their appearance. Unfortunately, use of anabolic steroids can upset the chemical balance in the body, produce toxicity, and shut off the body's production of its own steroids, leaving the person more susceptible to stress and

TABLE 13.4   Lifetime, Past Year, and Past Month Use of Various Drugs, Including Nonmedical Use of Legal Drugs, Persons Aged 12 Years and Older, United States, 2009

Drug	Lifetime Use	Use During Past Year	Use During Past Month
Alcohol	82.8%	66.8%	51.9%
Cigarettes	64.6	27.5	23.3
Smokeless tobacco	17.8	4.8	3.4
Sedatives	3.4	0.3	0.1
Tranquilizers	8.6	2.2	0.8
Heroin	1.5	0.2	0.2
Pain relievers	13.9	4.9	2.1
Stimulants	8.7	1.2	0.5
Cocaine	14.5	1.9	0.7
Crack cocaine	3.3	0.4	0.2
Marijuana	41.5	11.3	6.6
LSD	9.4	0.3	0.1
Ecstasy	5.7	1.1	0.3

Source: Results from the 2009 National Survey on Drug Use and Health: National Findings, by Substance Abuse and Mental Health Services Administration, 2010. List of Tables Containing Prevalence Estimates and Sample Sizes. Retrieved July 4, 2011, from http://www.oas.samhsa.gov/NSDUH/2k9NSDUH/tabs/TOC.htm, Tables 1.1B, 2.1B.

infection and altering reproductive functioning. In addition, behavioral problems include aggression, euphoria, mood swings, distractibility, and confusion. Table 13.3 presents a summary of anabolic steroids and other psychoactive drug characteristics.

How common is the use of these illicit drugs? Is drug use increasing or decreasing? Illicit drug use in the United States has varied over the past 40 years, reaching a peak in the late 1970s, followed by a decline in the 1980s (SAMHSA, 2010). Another increase occurred in the early 1990s and another decrease in the late 1990s. This overall pattern is similar across age groups, but levels of use are not: Young people use illicit drugs more often than older people. Indeed, trends in drug use among high school students often predict societal drug use several years later (Johnston et al., 2011).

Illicit drug use has varied little overall within the past decade, with fluctuations from year to year and from drug to drug (SAMHSA, 2010). (The use of alcohol and nicotine has also varied, but the percentage of people who use these legal drugs is higher than those who use illicit drugs.) Marijuana remains the most commonly used illicit drug, with levels of use far above any other type of illicit drug. The next most

commonly used classification is the nonmedical use of therapeutic drugs such as painkillers (oxycontin, hydrocodone) and methamphetamines. Cocaine use has not increased over the past 10 years, but cocaine remains one of the most commonly used illicit drugs. Ecstasy use has increased slightly, but as Table 13.4 shows, the level of use of these drugs is much lower than marijuana use. The use of these drugs represents occasional use by some people, but others misuse and abuse these drugs.

Drug Misuse and Abuse

Most people believe that some drugs are acceptable and even desirable because of the medical benefits they confer. But all *psychoactive* drugs—drugs that cross the blood–brain barrier and alter mental functioning—pose potential health risks. Most have the capacity for tolerance or dependence (see Table 13.2). Even drugs that are not psychoactive have the potential for unpleasant side effects. For example, penicillin can cause nausea, vomiting, diarrhea, swelling, and skin eruptions. In addition, people who have allergies to penicillin can die from ingesting it. Caffeine, a drug commonly found in coffee and cola drinks, can produce effects that meet the *DSM-IV* criteria of substance dependence. A review of studies on caffeine withdrawal (Juliano & Griffiths, 2004) confirmed this diagnosis—people who habitually consume caffeine experience withdrawal symptoms that include headache, difficulty concentrating, and depressed mood. Thus, all drug use carries some risks.

Almost all drugs that have potential medical or health benefits also have the potential for misuse and abuse. The moderate use of alcohol, for instance, is related to decreased cardiovascular mortality. The *misuse* of alcohol—defined as inappropriate but not health-threatening levels of consumption—can result in social embarrassment, violent acts, and injury. And abuse of alcohol—defined as frequent, heavy consumption to the point of addiction—can lead to cirrhosis, brain damage, heart attack, and fetal alcohol syndrome.

Not all individuals who use drugs or alcohol are equally likely to become abusers. Genetic and situational factors contribute to the risks of substance abuse, but another major risk is the presence of psychopathology. Individuals with schizophrenia and bipolar disorder who use illicit drugs tend to have more severe symptoms and to respond more poorly to treatment than individuals with the same disorders who do not use illicit drugs (Ringen et al., 2008).

Treatment for Drug Abuse

Treatment for the use and abuse of illegal drugs is similar to the treatment of alcohol abuse, both in the philosophy and in the administration of treatment (Schuckit, 2000). In the United States and many other countries, the goal of treatment for all types of illegal drug use is total abstinence. In many cases, the programs that treat drug abusers coexist physically (as well as philosophically) with treatment programs for alcohol abuse, and patients who are receiving treatment for their drug problems participate in the same therapy as those who are receiving therapy for their alcohol problems. The philosophy that guides Alcoholics Anonymous led to the development of Narcotics Anonymous, an organization devoted to helping drug users abstain from using drugs. Self-help groups are common components in treating drug abuse, as they are in dealing with alcohol abuse (Margolis & Zweben, 2011).

The reasons for entering drug abuse treatment programs are often similar to those for entering treatment for alcohol abuse, and those reasons are primarily social. The abuse of illegal drugs leads to legal, financial, and interpersonal problems, just as alcohol abuse does. Like alcohol, most illegal drugs produce impairments of judgment that lead to unintentional injury and death, making such injury the leading health risk from drug abuse. The abuse of most illegal drugs does not produce as many direct health hazards as alcohol abuse. However, when health problems occur, they are likely to be major and life threatening. Such crises may precipitate a person's decision to seek treatment or lead family members to enforce treatment. Charlie Sheen has been in treatment for his drug abuse several times, but his father was instrumental in that treatment ("Martin Sheen," 2008). His several stays in inpatient treatment facilities were typical of such facilities in the United States—their goal is complete abstinence, and its philosophy is the same as AA's.

Inpatient treatment programs for drug abuse are strikingly similar to those designed to treat alcohol abuse but differ from such programs in several minor ways. The detoxification phase of inpatient hospitalization is typically shorter and less severe for most types of drug use than it is for alcohol, for which withdrawal can be life threatening. Alcohol is a depressant drug, as are barbiturates, tranquilizers, and opiates. Therefore, all these drugs have similar symptoms during withdrawal, including agitation, tremor, gastric distress, and possibly perceptual distortions (Julien et al., 2010). Stimulants such as amphetamines and cocaine produce different withdrawal symptoms—namely, lethargy and depression. These differences necessitate different medical care during detoxification.

After detoxification, additional care is important for success. Frequently, this continued care comes from joining a support group such as Narcotics Anonymous. Getting substance abusers to attend such groups is a challenge, and the low rate of success for such interventions is a problem. Other interventions show better results. A meta-analysis of psychosocial interventions (Dutra et al., 2008) identified several types as effective, including contingency management and cognitive behavioral therapy. Such interventions were most effective for marijuana use and least effective with those who abused several substances. Unfortunately, relapse prevention interventions were not among the more effective programs.

One similarity between drug and alcohol abuse treatment is the high rate of relapse. As noted earlier, alcohol, smoking, and opiate treatment all share a high rate of relapse (Hunt et al., 1971), and the first 6 months after treatment are critical. To ameliorate this problem, drug treatment programs, like alcohol treatment interventions, typically include some after-care or "booster" sessions, which may consist only of attendance in a support group such as Narcotics Anonymous. A one-size-fits-all approach may not be successful for relapse prevention because people relapse for different reasons (Zywiak et al., 2006). Some people are provoked to relapse by negative feelings, and others cannot withstand cravings, whereas others succumb to social pressure from their drug-using friends. Addressing individual concerns and weaknesses through interventions that are specific to individuals may improve the situation.

Charlie Sheen provides an excellent example of the problem of relapse. He experienced trouble staying in treatment, and after completing the program, he relapsed several times. His behavior in early 2011 was a dramatic example of relapse and resisting treatment for an obvious problem ("Charlie Sheen," 2011).

Preventing and Controlling Drug Use

Chapter 12 presented information on attempts to decrease smoking in children and adolescents by various interventions aimed at discouraging their experimentation with cigarettes and smokeless tobacco. Similar efforts have been applied to the use of alcohol and other drugs (Lemstra et al., 2010; Roe & Becker, 2005; Soole, Mazerolle, & Rombouts, 2008). The prevention attempts aimed at keeping children and adolescents from experimenting with drugs are intended to delay or inhibit the initiation of drug use. As with efforts to prevent smoking (see Chapter 12), those aimed at preventing drug use do not have an impressive success rate. Programs that rely on scare tactics, moral training, factual information about drug risks, and boosting self-esteem are generally ineffective. For example, the popular Drug Abuse Resistance Education (DARE) program has minimal effects (West & O'Neal, 2004).

However, some types of prevention programs are more effective than others. The Life Skills Training program (Botvin & Griffin, 2004) has demonstrated both short-term and longer-term effectiveness. This program teaches social skills, both to resist social pressure to use drugs and to enhance social and personal competence. In addition, some evidence (Springer et al., 2004) indicates that prevention programs that are tailored to be culturally compatible with the targeted groups are more effective than more general programs. Systematic reviews of prevention programs (Lemstra et al., 2010; Roe & Becker, 2005; Soole et al., 2008) have indicated that school programs that are interactive, are intensive, and focus on life skills are more effective than programs that lack these components. Aiming prevention efforts at children between 11 and 13 is most effective, but programs aimed at children and adolescents are not the only approach to controlling drug use.

A more common control technique is to limit availability. This strategy is common in all Western countries through laws that limit legal access to drugs. However, legal restriction of drugs has a number of side effects, some of which create other social problems (Robins, 1995). For example, when the United States legally prohibited the manufacture and sale of alcohol, illegal manufacture and distribution flourished, creating a large criminal enterprise, huge profits, loss of tax revenue, and corruption among law enforcement agencies. Thus, limiting availability has negative as well as positive consequences, and the extent to which this approach should be enacted remains controversial.

Another strategy is control of the harm of drug use. This strategy assumes that people will use psychoactive drugs, sometimes unwisely, but that reducing the health consequences of drug use should be the first priority (Heather, 2006; O'Hare, 2007; Peele, 2002). Rather than take a moralistic stand on drug use, this strategy takes a practical approach to minimizing the dangers of drug use. An example of the *harm reduction strategy* is helping injection drug users exchange used needles for sterile ones, thus slowing the spread of HIV infection. Another example is encouraging the designated driver approach to avoiding vehicle injuries. The controversy surrounding such programs is representative of the debate over the harm reduction strategy. However, a systematic review of harm reduction (Ritter & Cameron, 2006) concluded that the evidence indicates that this approach should be adopted as a policy for illicit drugs. Furthermore, some experts in the field (Lee, Engstrom, & Petersen, 2011) have contended that the approaches oriented toward abstinence are not as incompatible with harm reduction as the controversy suggests. Both approaches may have a place in controlling drug use.

IN SUMMARY

Abuse of alcohol is a serious health problem in most developed nations, but other drugs—including depressants, stimulants, hallucinogens, marijuana, and anabolic steroids—are also potentially harmful to health. Although abuse of these drugs often leads to a number of personal and social problems, their health risks are much less than those associated with cigarettes or alcohol. Treatments for drug abuse are similar to those for alcohol abuse, and programs aimed at prevention are similar to those aimed at preventing smoking. A new strategy called *harm reduction* aims at decreasing the social and health risks of taking drugs by changing drug policies.

Answers

This chapter has addressed six basic questions:

1. What are the major trends in alcohol consumption?

People have consumed alcohol worldwide since before recorded history. Alcohol consumption in the United States reached a peak during the first three decades of the 19th century, dropped sharply during the mid-1800s as a result of the "temperance" movement, and continued at a steady rate until it declined even more during Prohibition. Currently, rates of alcohol consumption in the United States are holding steady after a period of slow decline. About two thirds of adults drink; half are classified as current, regular drinkers, including 10% as binge drinkers and 5% as heavy drinkers. Adult European Americans have higher rates of drinking than members of other ethnic groups, but the patterns of alcohol consumption vary in countries around the world.

2. What are the health effects of drinking alcohol?

Drinking has both positive and negative health effects. Prolonged heavy drinking of alcohol often leads to cirrhosis of the liver and other serious health problems, such as heart disease and brain dysfunction. Moderate drinking may have certain long-range health benefits, including reduced heart disease and lowered probability of developing gallstones, Type 2 diabetes, and Alzheimer's disease, but these advantages apply to middle-aged and older individuals and not younger people. Overall, the risks of alcohol outweigh the benefits.

3. Why do people drink?

Models for drinking behavior should be able to explain why people begin drinking, why some can drink in moderation, and why others drink to excess. The disease model assumes that people drink excessively because they have the disease of alcoholism. Cognitive-physiological models, including the tension reduction hypothesis and alcohol myopia, propose that people drink because alcohol allows them to escape tension and negative self-evaluations. Social learning theory assumes that people acquire drinking behavior through positive or negative reinforcement, modeling, and cognitive mediation.

4. How can people change problem drinking?

Many problem drinkers seem to be able to quit without therapy, and treatment programs are moderately effective in helping people who do not succeed in quitting on their own. About 25% of treated alcoholics are abstinent at the end of 1 year, but many others have decreased their drinking to a level that is no longer a problem. In the United States, most treatment programs are oriented toward abstinence, and those drinkers who do not quit are often considered treatment failures. Alcoholics Anonymous is the most popular treatment program, and it is helpful to some problem drinkers. However, other approaches may be more effective. Brief interventions oriented toward enhancing motivation, such as motivational interviewing, show higher effectiveness. Chemical treatments such as disulfiram, naltrexone, and acamprosate can also be useful components in a treatment program. Controlled drinking remains controversial as a treatment goal, although some problem drinkers are capable of attaining this type of drinking.

5. What problems are associated with relapse?

Relapse is common among heavy drinkers who have quit, although many are able to maintain abstinence or to drink in a controlled manner. Most relapses occur during the first 3 months. After a year, about 65% of all successful quitters have resumed drinking, some in a harmful manner. The knowledge of frequent relapse has led to the creation of follow-up relapse prevention treatment.

6. What are the health effects of other drugs?

Other drugs—including depressants, stimulants, hallucinogens, marijuana, and anabolic steroids—have had some medical use, but they are also potentially harmful to health. The principal problems from most of these drugs are social, but the use of any drug brings physical risks, which may include coma, heart attack, or respiratory failure. Treatments for drug abuse are similar to those for alcohol abuse, and programs aimed at prevention are similar to those aimed at preventing smoking.

Suggested Readings

Heather, N. (2006). Controlled drinking, harm reduction and their roles in the response to alcohol-related problems. *Addiction Research and Theory*, *14*, 7–18. Heather discusses the controlled drinking controversy, presenting the difference between the harm reduction approach that is common in Europe and the strategy of decreasing drug/alcohol use to a controlled level.

Lee, P. R., Lee, D. R., Lee, P., & Arch, M. (2010). 2010: U.S. drug and alcohol policy, looking back and moving forward. *Journal of Psychoactive Drugs*, *42*(2), 99–114. This article provides an examination of the history of drug and alcohol policy that can lead to an understanding of U.S. laws and policies that govern alcohol and drugs. The efforts to control these substances and the treatment options and their availability are also included.

Nestler, E. J., & Malenka, R. C. (2004, March). The addicted brain. *Scientific American*, *290*, 78–85. This article details the brain mechanisms that underlie reward and addiction, pointing out the commonalities among all compulsive drug use.

Rehm, J., Baliunas, D., Borges, G. L. G., Graham, K., Irving, H., Kehoe, T., et al. (2010). The relation between different dimensions of alcohol consumption and burden of disease: An overview. *Addiction, 105*(5), 817–843. This review presents a comprehensive view of the harm that alcohol does in creating disease. The analysis includes an examination of the pathways through which alcohol creates disease and the patterns of drinking that are most dangerous.

Witkiewitz, K., & Marlatt, G. A. (2004). Relapse prevention for alcohol and drug problems. *American Psychologist*, *59*, 224–235. Witkiewitz and Marlatt present a revised model for understanding the complexities of the relapse process and suggest more effective ways to combat this too common problem.

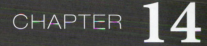
Eating and Weight

CHAPTER OUTLINE

- **Real-World Profile of Kirstie Alley**
- *The Digestive System*
- *Factors in Weight Maintenance*
- *Overeating and Obesity*
- *Dieting*
- *Eating Disorders*

QUESTIONS

This chapter focuses on six basic questions:

1. How does the digestive system function?
2. What factors are involved in weight maintenance?

☑ CHECK YOUR HEALTH RISKS

Regarding Eating and Controlling Your Weight

☐ 1. I feel comfortable with my present weight.

☐ 2. Although I don't eat much, I stay heavier than I would like.

☐ 3. I have lost 15 pounds or more over the past 2 years.

☐ 4. I have gained 15 pounds or more over the past 2 years.

☐ 5. I am more than 30 pounds overweight.

☐ 6. My weight has fluctuated about 5 or 10 pounds during the past 2 years, but I'm not concerned about it.

☐ 7. If I were thinner, I would be happier.

☐ 8. My waist is as big as or bigger than my hips.

☐ 9. I have been on at least 10 different diet programs in my life.

☐ 10. I have fasted, used laxatives, or used diet drugs to lose weight.

☐ 11. My family has been concerned that I am too thin, but I disagree.

☐ 12. A coach, instructor, or trainer has suggested that weighing less could improve my athletic performance.

☐ 13. I sometimes lose control over eating and eat far more than I planned.

☐ 14. I would like to have liposuction or gastric bypass surgery to lose weight.

☐ 15. I have vomited after eating as a way to control my weight.

☐ 16. Food is a danger that can be managed by careful thought and mental preparation in order not to eat too much.

Items 1 and 6 reflect a healthy attitude toward weight, but each of the other items represents a health risk from improper eating or unhealthy attitudes concerning eating. Unhealthy eating not only relates to the development of several diseases, but preoccupation with weight and frequent dieting can also be unhealthy.

Real-World Profile of
KIRSTIE ALLEY

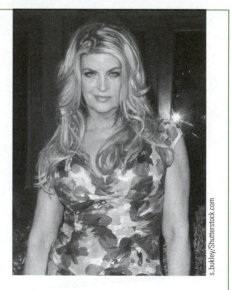

s_bukley/Shutterstock.com

Many celebrities struggle with losing weight, but Kirstie Alley's weight has become part of her celebrity. As a television and movie actress in the 1980s and 90s, she was thin, but by 2004, Kirstie Alley weighed over 200 pounds ("Gaining It Back," 2006). During her appearance on *The Oprah Winfrey Show*, she vowed to diet, and with the help of a commercial weight loss program, she succeeded. She showed off her slimmer body in a bikini on the same show in 2006. Like so many people who have succeeded in losing weight, she gained it back ("Kirstie Alley's Weight," 2009).

And then she began a program to lose weight again (James, 2010). During her stint on *Dancing With the Stars*, Alley lost weight rapidly. No mystery there; she was working out more than 5 hours a day and eating only 1,400 calories a day ("Only Eating," 2011). Her weight goal: to wear a size 2 dress (M. Brown, 2011).

How common are weight fluctuations such as those Kirstie Alley experienced? Are her strivings to be very thin typical or extreme? Are her drastic approaches to dieting common? Do these tactics pose health hazards? Do such extreme body images and dieting strategies signal the development of eating disorders? This chapter explores these questions and others concerning eating and weight.

This chapter examines in detail the four major problems of eating—overeating and dieting, anorexia nervosa, bulimia, and binge eating— each related to difficulties in weight maintenance. To put these in context, we first consider the organs and functions of the digestive system.

The Digestive System

The human body can digest a wide variety of plant and animal tissues, converting these foods into usable proteins, fats, carbohydrates, vitamins, and minerals. The digestive system takes in food, processes it into particles that can be absorbed, and excretes the undigested wastes. The particles that are absorbed through the digestive system are transported through the bloodstream so as to be available to all body cells. These molecules nourish the body by providing the energy for activity as well as the materials for body growth, maintenance, and repair.

The digestive tract is a modified tube, consisting of a number of specialized structures. Also included in the digestive system are several accessory structures connected to the digestive tract by ducts. These ducted glands produce substances that are essential for digestion, and the ducts provide a way for these substances to enter the digestive system. Figure 14.1 shows the digestive system.

In humans and other mammals, some digestion begins in the mouth. The teeth tear and grind food, mixing it with saliva. Several **salivary glands** furnish the moisture that allows the food to be tasted. Without such moisture, the taste buds on the tongue do not function. Saliva also contains an enzyme that digests starch, so some digestion actively begins before food particles leave the mouth.

Swallowing is a voluntary action, but once food is swallowed, its progress through the **pharynx** and **esophagus** is largely involuntary. **Peristalsis** propels food through the digestive system, beginning with the esophagus. Peristaltic movement is the rhythmic contraction and relaxation of the circular muscles of structures in the digestive system. In the stomach, rhythmic contractions mix the food with **gastric juices** secreted by the stomach and the glands that empty into the stomach. Little absorption of nutrients occurs in the stomach; only alcohol, aspirin, and some fat-soluble drugs are absorbed through the stomach lining. The major function of the stomach is to mix food particles

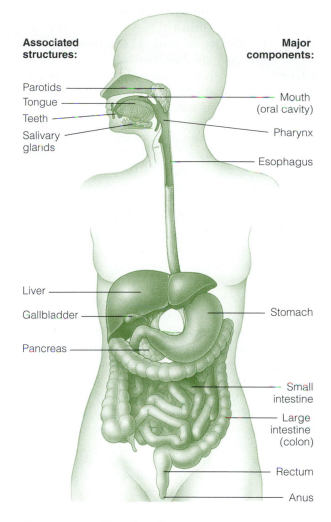

Associated structures:
- Parotids
- Tongue
- Teeth
- Salivary glands
- Liver
- Gallbladder
- Pancreas

Major components:
- Mouth (oral cavity)
- Pharynx
- Esophagus
- Stomach
- Small intestine
- Large intestine (colon)
- Rectum
- Anus

FIGURE 14.1 The digestive system.

Source: Introduction to microbiology (p. 556), by J. L. Ingraham & C. A. Ingraham. From INGRAHAM/INGRAHAM, Introduction to Microbiology, 1E. © 1995 Cengage Learning.

with gastric juices, preparing the mixture for absorption in the small intestine.

The mixture of food particles and gastric juices moves into the small intestine a little at a time. The high acidity of the gastric juices results in a very acidic mixture, and the small intestine cannot function in high acidity. To reduce the level of acidity, the pancreas secretes several acid-reducing enzymes into the small intestine. These **pancreatic juices** are also essential for digesting carbohydrates and fats.

The digestion of starch that begins in the mouth is completed in the small intestine. The upper third of the small intestine absorbs starch and other carbohydrates. Protein digestion, initiated in the stomach, is also completed when proteins are absorbed in the upper portion of the small intestine. Fats, however, enter the small intestine almost entirely undigested. **Bile salts** produced in the **liver** and stored in the **gall bladder** break down fat molecules into a form that is acted on by a pancreatic enzyme. Absorption of fats occurs in the middle third of the small intestine. The bile salts that aid the process are reabsorbed later in the lower third of the small intestine.

Large quantities of water pass through the small intestine. In addition to the water that people drink, digestive juices increase the fluid volume. Of all the water that passes into the small intestine, 90% is absorbed. This absorption process also causes vitamins and electrolytes to pass into the body at this point in digestion.

From the small intestine, digestion proceeds to the large intestine. As with other portions of the digestive system, movement through the large intestine occurs through peristalsis. However, the peristaltic movement in the large intestine is more sluggish and irregular than in the small intestine. Bacteria inhabit the large intestine and manufacture several vitamins. Although the large intestine has absorptive capabilities, it typically absorbs only water, a few minerals, and the vitamins manufactured by its bacteria.

Feces consist of the materials left after digestion has taken place. Feces are composed of undigested fiber, inorganic material, undigested nutrients, water, and bacteria. Peristalsis carries the feces through the large intestine, through the **rectum**, and finally through the **anus**, where they are eliminated.

In summary, the digestive system turns food into nutrients by a process that begins in the mouth with the breakdown of food into smaller particles. Digestive juices continue to act on food particles in the stomach, but digestion of most types of nutrients occurs in the small intestine. Digestion is completed with the elimination of the undigested residue. The digestive system is plagued by more diseases and disorders than any other body system. Many digestive disorders are not of active concern to health psychology, but several, such as obesity, anorexia nervosa, bulimia, and binge eating, have important behavioral components. In addition, maintaining a stable weight depends on behaviors—eating and activity.

Factors in Weight Maintenance

Stable weight occurs when the calories absorbed from food equal those expended for body metabolism plus physical activity. This balance is not a simple calculation but, rather, the result of a complex set of actions and interactions. Caloric content varies with foods; fat has more calories per volume than carbohydrates or proteins. The degree of absorption depends on how rapidly food passes through the digestive system and even the nutrient composition of the foods. Furthermore, metabolic rates can differ from person to person and from time to time. Activity level is another source of variability, with greater activity requiring greater caloric expenditures.

To obtain calories, people (and other animals) eat. Eating and weight balance have regulating components in the nervous system. A variety of hormones and neurotransmitters form a short-term and a long-term regulation system (Majdič, 2009). **Leptin**, a protein hormone discovered in 1994, is produced by white adipose tissue (fat) and acts on receptors in the central nervous system as part of a signaling system involved in the long-term regulation of weight. Low leptin levels signal low fat stores, prompting eating. High levels signal adequate fat stores and satiation. *Insulin* is a second hormone involved in weight maintenance. Produced by the pancreas, this hormone allows body cells to take in glucose for their use. (Deficiency in insulin production or use results in diabetes, which is covered in Chapter 11.) High insulin production leads to the intake of more glucose than cells can use, and the excess is converted into fat in the body. In the brain, insulin acts on the **hypothalamus**, sending signals of satiation and decreasing appetite.

The hormone **ghrelin**, a peptide hormone discovered in 1999, also plays a role in eating (Majdič, 2009). This hormone is produced by cells in the stomach wall, and its level rises before and falls after meals; thus, ghrelin seems to be involved in the short-term regulation of food intake by prompting eating. Ghrelin also acts in the hypothalamus to activate *neuropeptide Y*, which secretes *Agouti-related peptide*. This peptide stimulates appetite and decreases metabolism, thus affecting the weight balance equation in two ways.

In addition to the hormones that prompt eating, a variety of hormones are related to feelings of satiation and thus tend to decrease or terminate eating. The hormone **cholecystokinin** (**CCK**), a peptide hormone produced by the intestines, acts on the brain to produce feelings of satiation. CCK, *glucagon-like peptide 1*, and *peptide YY* are all produced in the intestines but act on the hypothalamus to signal satiation (Majdič, 2009). Thus, the picture of hormone and neurotransmitter action in relation to hunger and eating is very complex and not yet fully understood. One system appears to initiate eating, and one seems to produce satiation and thus decrease eating. Table 14.1 lists each set of hormones and shows where they are produced. Notice that many are produced in the hypothalamus, and all may act on different nuclei in the hypothalamus to form a complex mechanism for the short-term and long-term regulation of weight.

To understand the complexities of weight metabolism and weight maintenance, consider an extreme example: an experiment in which participants were systematically starved.

Experimental Starvation

More than 60 years ago, Ancel Keys and his colleagues (Keys, Brozek, Henschel, Mickelsen, & Taylor, 1950) began a study on the physical effects of human starvation. The research took place during World War II; the participants were conscientious objectors who volunteered to be part of the study as an alternative to military service. In most ways these volunteers were quite normal young men; their weights were normal, their IQs were in the normal to bright range, and they were emotionally stable.

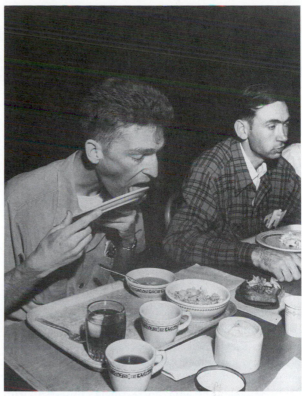

Experimental starvation produced an obsession with food and a variety of negative changes in the behavior of these volunteers.

For the first 3 months of the project, the 36 volunteers ate regularly to establish their normal caloric requirements. Next, the men received half their previous rations, with the goal of reducing their body weight

TABLE 14.1   Hormones Involved in Appetite and Satiation

Hormones That Increase Appetite		Hormones That Increase Satiation	
Hormone	**Produced in**	**Hormone**	**Produced in**
Ghrelin	Stomach	Leptin	Adipose tissue
Neuropeptide Y	Hypothalamus	Insulin	Pancreas
Orexins	Hypothalamus	Cholecystokinin (CCK)	Intestines
Agouti-related peptide	Hypothalamus	Glucagon-like peptide 1	Intestines
Melanin-concentrating hormone (MCH)	Hypothalamus	Peptide YY	Intestines

to 75% of previous levels. Although the researchers cut the participants' caloric intake in half, they were careful to give them adequate nutrients so that the men were never in any danger of actually starving. However, the men were hungry almost constantly.

At first the men lost weight rapidly, but the initial pace of weight loss did not last. To continue losing weight, the men had to consume even fewer calories, which led to considerable suffering. Nevertheless, most stayed with the project through the entire 6 months, and most met their goal of losing 25% of their body weight.

The behaviors that accompanied the semistarvation were quite surprising to Keys and his colleagues. The men were optimistic and cheerful initially, but these feelings soon vanished. The men became irritable, aggressive, and began to fight among themselves—behavior that was completely out of character. Although the men continued this bellicose behavior throughout the 6 months of the starvation phase, they also became apathetic and avoided physical activity as much as they could. They became neglectful of their dormitory, their own physical appearance, and their girlfriends.

The men became increasingly obsessed with thoughts of food. Mealtimes became the center of their lives; they tended to eat very slowly and to be very sensitive to the taste of their food. At the beginning of the period of caloric reduction, the researchers saw no need to place physical restrictions on the men to prevent them from cheating on their diets. But about 3 months into the starvation, the men felt that they would be tempted to cheat if they left the dormitory alone. As a result, they were allowed to go out only in pairs or in larger groups. These dedicated, polite, normal, stable young men had become abnormal and unpleasant under conditions of semistarvation.

Obsession with food and a continuing negative outlook also characterized the refeeding phase of the project. The plan for refeeding was for the men to regain the weight they had lost over a 3-month period. This phase was to have lasted 3 months, with food introduced at gradually increasing levels. The men objected so strongly that the pace of refeeding was accelerated. As a result, the men ate as much and as often as they could, some as many as five large meals a day. By the end of the refeeding period, most men had regained their pre-experimental weight; in fact, many were slightly heavier. About half were still preoccupied

with food, and for many, their prestarvation optimism and cheerfulness had not completely returned.

Experimental Overeating

A study of experimental starvation does not seem very attractive, but an experiment on overeating might sound appealing to many people. Ethan Allen Sims and his associates (Sims, 1974, 1976; Sims et al., 1973; Sims & Horton, 1968) found a group of people who should have been especially interested and appreciative—prisoners. Inmates at the Vermont State Prison volunteered to gain 20 to 30 pounds as part of an experiment on overeating. Sims's interest was analogous to Keys's—an understanding of the physical and psychological components of overeating. Special living arrangements were made for these prisoners, including plentiful and delicious food. In addition, the experiment included a restriction of physical activity to make weight gain easier.

Increased calories and decreased physical activity would seem to assure weight gain. Did these men gain weight? At first they gained fairly easily. But soon the rate of weight gain slowed, and the participants had to eat more and more to continue gaining. As with the men in the starvation study, these men needed about 3,500 calories to maintain their weight at normal levels, but many had to double that amount to continue gaining. Not all the men were able to attain their weight goals, regardless of how much they ate. One man did not reach his goal even though he ate more than 10,000 calories per day.

Were the overeating prisoners as miserable as the starving conscientious objectors? No, but they did find overeating unpleasant. Food became repulsive to them, despite the excellent quality and preparation. They had to force themselves to eat, and many considered dropping out of the study.

When the weight gain phase of the study was over, the prisoners cut down their food intake dramatically and lost weight. Not all lost as quickly as others, and two had some trouble returning to their original weight. An examination of these two men's medical backgrounds revealed some family history of obesity, although the men themselves had never been overweight. These results indicate that normal weight people have trouble increasing their weight substantially and that, even if they do, the increased weight is difficult to maintain.

IN SUMMARY

Weight maintenance depends largely on two factors: the number of calories absorbed through food intake and the number expended through body metabolism and physical activity. Underlying this balance is a complex set of hormones and neurotransmitters that have selective effects on various brain sites, including the hypothalamus. Weight gain occurs when more nutrients are present than are required for maintenance of body metabolism and physical activity. Weight loss occurs when insufficient nutrients are present to furnish the necessary energy for body metabolism and activity. An experiment in starvation showed that loss of too much weight leads to irritability, aggression, apathy, lack of interest in sex, and preoccupation with food. Another experiment in overeating showed that some people find gaining weight almost as difficult as losing it.

Overeating and Obesity

Overeating is not the sole cause of obesity, but it is an important part of the weight maintenance equation. As the studies on experimental starvation and overeating show, metabolic-level changes with food intake as well as with energy output alter the efficiency of nutrient use by the body. Thus, individual variations in body metabolism allow some people to burn calories faster than others. Two people who eat the same amount may have different weights.

Although many overweight people report that they eat less than others, these self-reports are not very accurate, and objective measurements usually indicate that overweight people eat more (Jeffery & Harnack, 2007; Pietiläinen et al., 2010). They are especially likely to eat food rich in fat, which has a higher caloric density than carbohydrates or protein. They may eat less food but more calories. Overweight individuals also have a tendency to be less physically active than leaner people, which contributes to overweight. These behaviors contribute to obesity and its related health consequences, but the underlying reasons for obesity and even its definition remain controversial.

What Is Obesity?

Answers to the question of what obesity is vary by personal and social standards. Should obesity be defined in

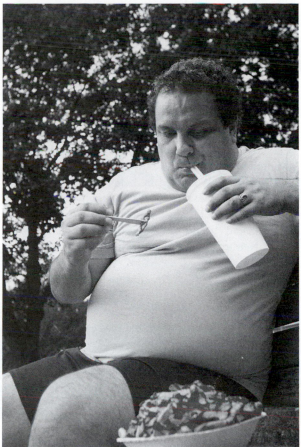

Peter Reali/Jupiter Images

The weight maintenance equation is complex, but overeating is a cause of obesity.

terms of health? Appearance? Body mass? Percentage of body fat? Weight charts? Total weight? No good definition of obesity would consider only body weight, because some individuals have a small skeletal frame, whereas others are larger, and some people's weight is in muscle, whereas others carry weight in fat. Muscle tissue and bone weigh more than fat, so some people can be heavier yet leaner, as athletes often are.

Determining percentage and distribution of body fat is not as easy as consulting a chart, and several different methods exist to assess body fat (Skybo & Ryan-Wenger, 2003). Many new technologies for imaging the body—computer tomography, ultrasound, magnetic resonance imaging, and PET scanning—can be applied to assessing fat content, but these methods have the drawbacks of being very expensive and relatively inaccessible. Simpler methods include the skinfold technique, which involves measuring the thickness of a pinch of skin, and bioelectrical impedance measurement, which involves sending a harmless level of electrical current through the body to measure levels of fat in various parts of the body. The bioelectric impedance measurement is more accurate than the skinfold technique.

Even the skinfold technique is not as easy as consulting a chart, which is the traditional method of assessing overweight and obesity. Height–weight charts were popular, but the **body mass index** (**BMI**) is an alternative approach. BMI is defined as body weight in kilograms (kg) divided by height in meters squared (m^2)—that is, BMI = kg/m^2. Although BMI does not consider a person's age, gender, or body build, this measurement began to gain popularity in the early 1990s. Neither weight charts nor BMI measures body

fat, but this index can provide a standard for measuring overweight and obesity (National Task Force on the Prevention and Treatment of Obesity, 2000). Overweight is usually defined as a BMI of 25 through 29.9 and obesity as a BMI of 30 or more. (A 5'10" man with a BMI of 30 would weigh 207 pounds, and a 5"4" woman with a BMI of 30 would weigh 174 pounds.) Table 14.2 shows a sample of BMI levels and their corresponding heights and weights.

Another measure that can be useful in assessing overweight is fat distribution, measured as the ratio of waist to hip size. People who have waists that approach the size of their hips tend to have fat distributed around their middles, whereas people who have large hips compared with their waists have lower hip-to-waist ratios.

TABLE 14.2   Body Mass Index Scores and Their Corresponding Heights and Weights

Body Mass Index (kg/m^2)							
17.5*	21	23	25	27	30	35	40**
Height in Inches (Weight in Pounds)							
60	90	107	118	128	138	153	179	204
61	93	111	122	132	143	158	185	211
62	96	115	126	136	147	164	191	218
63	99	118	130	141	152	169	197	225
64	102	122	134	145	157	174	202	232
65	105	126	138	150	162	180	210	240
66	109	130	142	155	167	186	216	247
67	112	134	146	159	172	191	223	255
68	115	138	151	164	177	197	230	262
69	118	142	155	169	182	203	236	270
70	122	146	160	174	188	207	243	278
71	125	150	165	179	193	215	250	286
72	129	154	169	184	199	221	258	294
73	132	159	174	189	204	227	265	302
74	136	163	179	194	210	233	272	311
75	140	168	184	200	216	240	279	319
76	144	172	189	205	221	246	287	328

*BMI of 17.5 after intentional starvation meets one *DSM-IV* definition of anorexia nervosa.
**BMI of 40 is considered morbid obesity by Bender, Trautner, Spraul, & Berger (1998).

Regardless of the definitions that researchers have used to study obesity, overweight is often defined in terms of social standards and fashion. These definitions usually have little to do with health and are subject to variations by culture and time. Numerous examples come from human history. During times when food supply was uncertain (the most frequent situation throughout history), carrying some supply of fat on the body was a type of insurance and thus often considered attractive (Nelson & Morrison, 2005). Fat could also be considered a mark of prosperity; fat advertised to the world that a person could afford an ample supply of food. Only in very recent history has this standard changed. Before 1920, thinness was considered unattractive, possibly due to its association with diseases or poverty.

Thinness is no longer considered unattractive. Indeed, today it is as highly desirable as plumpness was in previous centuries, especially for women. Early studies that examined changes in the body weight of *Playboy* centerfolds and Miss America candidates from 1959 to 1978 (Garner, Garfinkel, Schwartz, & Thompson, 1980), from 1979 to 1988 (Wiseman, Gray, Mosimann, & Ahrens, 1992), and another from 1922 to 1999 (Rubenstein & Caballero, 2000) found that weights for both groups had decreased relative to average weight of the general population. More recent analysis of centerfolds (Seifert, 2005; Sypeck et al., 2006) confirms this trend toward thinness over the past 50 years. These ideal bodies are so thin that 99% of centerfolds and 100% of Miss America winners were in the underweight range (Spitzer, Henderson, & Zivian, 1999).

This thin ideal for women's bodies has become so widely accepted that even normal weight women often consider themselves too heavy (Maynard, Serdula, Galuska, Gillespie, & Mokdad, 2006). The acceptance of thinness as attractive for women begins as early as 3 years old (Harriger, Calogero, Witherington, & Smith, 2010) and persists into adulthood (Brown & Slaughter, 2011). Clearly, obesity, like beauty, is in the eye of the beholder, and the ideal body has become thinner over the past 50 years.

Despite the emphasis on thinness, obesity has become epidemic, not only in the United States but also around the world. As Barry Popkin (2009) concluded, "The world is fat." In the United States, adult obesity increased by 50% from the early 1980s to the late 1990s (NCHS, 2011). Extreme obesity more than doubled during the 1990s. That increase has leveled, but no decline has occurred. Nor is the increase in obesity confined to adults or even to humans; other animals such as dogs, cats, and rats that live in close proximity to humans have also become fatter over the past several decades (Klimentidis, 2011).

Researchers have proposed several reasons for the dramatic increase in obesity over the past two decades, including an increase in consumption of fast food and sweetened sodas, growing portion sizes, and a decrease in physical activity. Not only people in the United States (Pereira et al., 2005) but also those in many other countries, including developing nations (Popkin, 2009), have begun eating more fast food and viewing more television and videos. Both behaviors are related to a larger body mass index and to weight gain. Indeed, adolescents whose schools are located within half a mile of a fast-food restaurant experience an increased likelihood of being overweight compared with those without a fast-food restaurant so close to their school (Davis & Carpenter, 2009). The consumption of sugar-sweetened sodas is another (possible) factor that studies have related to increased incidence of overweight (Bermudez & Gao, 2011; Bray, 2004; Must, Barrish, & Bandini, 2009). Large portion size also contributes to increasing obesity, and despite pleas by health authorities, fast-food restaurants continue to "supersize" meals (Young & Nestle, 2007), which tends to supersize diners. This trend affects the United States more than European and Asian countries, but obesity is a growing epidemic around the world (James, 2008).

If obesity is defined as having a BMI of 30 or higher, then 33% of U.S. adults are obese, and an additional 34% are overweight, defined as a BMI of 25.0 to 29.9 (NCHS, 2011). The rates of obesity are lower in children (10.4%) and adolescents (19%), but these rates indicate higher numbers than 20 years ago. Obesity and overweight occur in both genders, all ethnic groups, all geographic regions, and all educational levels. As Figure 14.2 shows, however, the rates of obesity and overweight vary by gender and ethnic background. Overweight and obesity rates are high in the United States and much lower in countries such as Japan (Kobayashi, 2007). However, many parts of the world have also experienced an increase in obesity, including Canada (Bélanger-Ducharme & Tremblay, 2005), Great Britain (Wardle & Johnson, 2002), Australia (Thorburn, 2005), Latin America (Fraser, 2005), Iran (Rashidi, Mohammadpour-Ahranjani, Vafa, & Karandish, 2005), and many countries in Europe (Berghöfer et al., 2008).

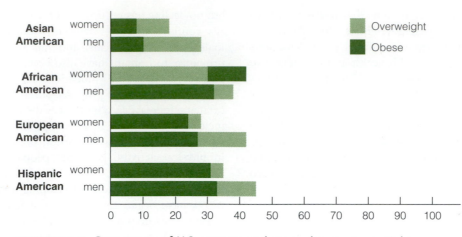

FIGURE 14.2 Percentage of U.S. women and men who are overweight and obese, by ethnic group.

Source: Data from *Statistical Abstract of the United States adults and national health interview survey,* 2009, 2010, by J.R Plei, B.W word and J.W lucas, National center for health statistics. *Vital health statistics, 10*(249) Table 31, p. 106.

Why Are Some People Obese?

Understanding the biology of eating and energy regulation is challenging, but explaining why that regulation fails to work for some people is even more difficult. Several models attempt to explain why some people are obese and others maintain a normal weight. These models, which should be able to explain both the development and the maintenance of obesity, include the setpoint model, genetic explanations, and the positive incentive model.

The Setpoint Model The setpoint model holds that weight is regulated around a **setpoint**, a type of internal thermostat. When fat levels rise above or fall below a certain level, physiological and psychological mechanisms are activated that encourage a return to setpoint. The discovery of leptin and the other hormones related to weight regulation is consistent with this view. Leptin is produced by body fat and acts as a signaling system to the hypothalamus in the brain. The findings from the study on experimental starvation and the studies on experimental overeating are also consistent with the concept of a setpoint, which predicts that deviations from normal weight in either direction are achieved only with difficulty. When fat levels fall below setpoint, the body takes action to preserve its fat stores. Part of that action includes slowing the metabolic process to require fewer calories, thus making the body more conservative in its energy expenditures. People on diets have difficulty in continuing to lose weight because their bodies fight against the depletion of fat stores. With conditions of prolonged and serious starvation, this slowed metabolism is expressed behaviorally as listlessness and apathy—both of which were exhibited by Keys's starving volunteers.

Increased hunger is the body's other corrective action when fat supplies fall below setpoint. Again, this mechanism seems to be consistent with the action of leptin and the results of the Keys et al. study on starvation. When fat stores fall, leptin levels decrease, which activates the hypothalamus in ways that result in hunger (Majdič, 2009). In Keys's study, the men became miserable as they dieted, and they stayed that way until they were back to their original weight. During the time they were below their normal weight (which would be below setpoint), they were obsessed with food. When they were allowed to eat, they preferred the high-calorie foods that tended to increase their fat stores most rapidly, a situation that is consistent with setpoint theory. They acted as though they were receiving messages from their bodies to eat. Results from a study of grocery shoppers (Paradis & Cabanac, 2008) were also consistent with this view. This research showed that people who had been involved in weight-loss diets chose higher calorie foods than those who had not been dieting.

The experiment on overeating also fits with setpoint theory. The prisoners who tried to gain more than their normal weight were fighting their natural setpoint and the increased amount of leptin produced by their added fat cells. This signal should have translated into something like "Stop eating," which seems to have happened—the prisoners found eating unpleasant.

Questions remain concerning the setpoint model, including why the setpoint should vary so much from person to person and why some people have a setpoint that is set at obese. One answer may be that the setpoint is at least partly established through a hereditary component.

Genetic Explanations of Obesity   One genetic explanation of obesity looks to prehistory to explain why people have a tendency to put on weight, hypothesizing that humans (and other animals) have evolved a "thrifty" metabolism that tends to store fat (Cummings & Schwartz, 2003). This tendency would be adaptive if food supplies were scarce, as they have been throughout most of history and prehistory. With the plentiful supply of food available to most people in high-income countries, this thrifty metabolism results in overweight and obesity. Indeed, some speculation holds that this availability makes obesity almost inevitable (Walker, Walker, & Adam, 2003). However, not all people are obese, and within any environment, some individuals are fatter than others. Some of that variation must be attributable to factors other than a general tendency to store fat.

Obesity tends to run in families, which suggests the possibility of a specific genetic basis. However, eating patterns are also shared in families, so researchers have examined twins and adopted children to disentangle genetic and environmental influences in weight. Results from early studies on adopted children (Stunkard et al., 1986) and identical twins reared together or apart (Stunkard, Harris, Pedersen, & McClean, 1990) suggested a role for heredity in weight. Adopted children's weights were more similar to their biological parents' than to their adoptive parents', and the weights of twins were highly correlated, even when the twins had not been raised together. Heritability also affects BMI (Schousboe et al., 2004) and fat distribution on the body (Fox et al., 2004).

These studies suggest that weight and fat distribution have strong genetic components, but no authorities claim that any single gene determines most human obesity (Cummings & Schwartz, 2003). Indeed, even researchers who claim a strong genetic influence for weight are focusing on the interaction among many genes and various environmental circumstances to understand weight regulation and obesity (Levin, 2010; Morrison, 2008; Rooney & Ozanne, 2011; Wells, 2011). Some combinations of genes may function in faulty ways that dysregulate the setpoint system and produce obesity. Another possibility emphasizes maternal overnutrition during late pregnancy and nursing, which may activate genes that produce permanent changes in metabolism. Other possibilities include combinations of many genes that respond to the food environment (such as availability of high-fat or sweetened food) and create obesity.

This emphasis on the food environment is well founded—obesity occurs in a specific context; a person cannot be obese without an adequate food supply. Although the genetic components of obesity may explain some of the variation in weight among people in a given environment, the increase in obesity that is occurring around the world has developed too rapidly to be the result of genes. Researchers must look beyond inheritance to attain a complete explanation of obesity. (See Would You Believe …? box for another suggestion of an environmental influence on the development of obesity.)

The Positive Incentive Model   The shortcomings of setpoint theory and genetics in explaining all factors related to eating and obesity led to the formulation of the *positive incentive model*. This model holds that the positive reinforcement of eating has important consequences for weight maintenance. This view suggests that people have several types of motivation to eat, including personal pleasure and social context as well as biological factors (Pinel, Assanand, & Lehman, 2000). The personal pleasure factors revolve around the pleasures from the type and taste of food. The social context of eating includes the cultural background of the person eating as well as the surroundings, the people present, and whether or not they are eating. Biological factors include the length of time since eating and blood glucose levels. In addition, some proponents of the positive incentive theory (Pinel et al., 2000) take an evolutionary view, contending that humans have an evolved tendency to eat in the presence of food. Scarcity of food has built animals that survived when they laid on fat, making eating and the selection of food an important evolved ability. Therefore, this model includes biological factors but holds

Would You BELIEVE...? You May Need a Nap Rather Than a Diet

Would you believe that sleep deprivation is related to obesity? It's not that being awake longer creates more opportunities for eating (which may be true) or that nighttime snacking may lead to obesity (which it may; Coles, Dixon, & O'Brien, 2007). Rather, sleep may be related to weight regulation, and missing sleep may produce problems in this system.

A suggestion of the importance of sleep for weight regulation came from the observation that sleep deprivation has become increasingly common for large numbers of people, and this trend has coincided with the growth in obesity. Researchers began to wonder: Is this relationship a coincidence or is there some underlying connection?

First, researchers attended to the basic question: Does inadequate sleep correlate with overweight? An examination of the sleep habits of a representative sample of the U.S. population (Wheaton et al., 2011) led to the conclusion that individuals who get less than 7 hours of sleep per night are more likely to be overweight or obese than people who sleep more. This relationship also occurs in obese children (Seegers et al., 2011). Research has also established that short sleep duration precedes weight gain (Lyytikäinen, Rahkonen, Lahelma, & Lallukka, 2011), which is a necessary link in establishing any causal relationship.

Next, researchers attempted to connect lack of sleep with hormonal mechanisms that might underlie the relationship between sleep deprivation and obesity. Reviews of that research (Knutson & van Cauter, 2008; van Cauter et al., 2007) led to the conclusion that the type of partial sleep deprivation that is so common is also capable of altering the regulation of the hormones involved in appetite and eating in ways that may cause weight gain and insulin resistance. Specifically, sleep deprivation increases ghrelin, which stimulates eating, and decreases leptin, which acts as a satiation signal (Knutson & van Cauter, 2008). Missing sleep may increase the risks for obesity and diabetes by altering the brain chemistry that underlies weight regulation. Thus, getting adequate sleep may be more beneficial than keeping you well rested—sleeping may protect against obesity.

that eating is a process involving self-regulation, with important individual, learned, and cultural components (Epstein, Leddy, Temple, & Faith, 2007; Finlayson, King, & Blundell, 2007).

The setpoint model ignores the factors of taste, learning, and social context in eating, and these factors are unquestionably important (Bessesen, 2011; Rozin, 2005; Stroebe, Papies, & Aarts, 2008). For each person in each instance, the act of choosing something to eat has a long history of personal experience and cultural learning. But a preferred food will not be equally appealing under all circumstances. For example, some foods—such as pickles and ice cream—do not seem to go together (at least for most people), even if both foods are individually tasty.

Social setting is important to eating, which is often a social activity. People tend to eat more in the presence of others, unless they believe that the others are judging them, and then they eat less (Vartanian, Herman, & Polivy, 2007), suggesting that social norms govern eating situations (Herman & Polivy, 2005). Culture provides an even wider context for eating, and various cultures have restrictions (and requirements) on what, when, and how much to eat. People tend to get hungry on a schedule that corresponds to mealtimes, but people in the United States are much more likely to eat cereal for breakfast than for dinner. In contrast, people in Spain do not eat cold cereal, and the lack of cultural tradition for this type of food made marketing it difficult in that country (Visser, 1999). These cultural and learned factors also affect the caloric value of chosen foods and how much a person eats, and these choices influence body weight. For example, when people choose "comfort foods," they often choose either food that carries personal nostalgic emotions or food that represents a personal indulgence (Locher, Yoels, Maurer, & Van Ells, 2005).

The positive incentive view predicts a variety of body weights, depending on food availability, individual experience with food, cultural encouragement to eat various foods, and the cultural ideal for body weight. Thus, the availability of an abundant food supply is necessary but not sufficient to produce obesity. People must overeat to become obese, and the quantity of food a person eats is related to how palatable the food is. Some tastes, such as sweet, are innately determined through the action of taste buds, and an overabundance of sweet food may be a factor in the dysregulaton of body weight (Swithers, Martin, Clark, Laboy, & Davidson, 2010). In high-income countries, a huge food industry promotes food products as desirable through massive advertising campaigns, and many of these foods are high in sugar and fat. This situation influences individual food choices that promote population-wide obesity (Brownell & Horgen, 2004). Indeed, even rats eat more when food cues are abundant in the environment (Polivy, Coelho, Hargreaves, Fleming, & Herman, 2007).

Another factor that promotes overeating is the availability of a variety of foods. Eating a very desirable food leads to a decreased evaluation of how pleasant that food is (Brondel et al., 2009); that is, people become satiated for any particular food. When food supplies are limited in variety (but not in quantity), this factor can lead to lower levels of food consumption, but a new taste can tempt someone who is full to eat more. Indeed, if eating a sufficient amount terminated a meal, dessert would not be so popular (Pinel, 2009).

Variety is important in boosting eating, even in rats. A large body of research (Ackroff et al., 2007; Raynor & Epstein, 2001; Sclafani, 2001) indicates that variety is important in the amount eaten, for rats and for humans. An early study (Sclafani & Springer, 1976) showed that a "supermarket" diet produced weight gains of 269% in laboratory rats. The diet consisted of a changing variety of foods chosen from the supermarket, including chocolate chip cookies, salami, cheese, bananas, marshmallows, chocolate, peanut butter, and sweetened condensed milk. The combination of high fat and high sugar plus the changing variety led to enormous weight gain.

Are humans very different? The availability of a wide variety of tasty food should produce widespread obesity, which is exactly the situation that exists in a number of countries today. This wide variety of foods allows people to always have some foods that furnish a new taste, and people in such situations never become satiated for all available foods.

However, fat may be more important than other ingredients in producing obesity. Not only is fat denser in calories, but some evidence indicates that fat intake is also capable of affecting the biology of weight regulation. One hypothesis (Niswender, Daws, Avison, & Galli, 2011) holds that ingestion of foods high in fat and sugar disrupts satiation signals and boosts appetite signals in the brain. Thus, eating a diet high in fat and sugar increases appetite rather than leading to satiation. Results from a twin study (Rissanen et al., 2002) support this contention. To control for genetics, this study examined twin pairs in which one twin was obese and the other was normal weight. This procedure assured that the weight difference was due to environmental rather than genetic factors. The results indicated that the obese twins not only ate a diet higher in fat than their leaner twins but also reported memories of preferences for such foods from adolescence and young adulthood.

Thus, the positive incentive theory of eating and weight maintenance takes into account factors that the setpoint model ignores, including individual food preferences, cultural influences on eating, cultural influences on body composition, and the relationship between food availability and obesity. Both models draw on biological factors and inheritance, and many advocates of the setpoint theory acknowledge that the factors highlighted by the positive incentive theory are important to weight regulation and contribute to obesity.

How Unhealthy Is Obesity?

Overweight and obesity are undesirable from a fashion point of view, but does overweight endanger health? These effects depend partly on the degree of overweight and the distribution of fat on the body. Being slightly overweight is not much of a health risk (McGee, 2005), but being obese places a person at an elevated risk for several types of health problems and premature death.

A U-shaped relationship has appeared between weight and poor health; that is, the very thinnest and the very heaviest people seem to be at greatest risk for all-cause mortality in Europe (Pischon et al., 2008) and in the United States (Flegal, Graubard, Williamson, & Gail, 2005). Low body weight is not as much of a risk as obesity, and some researchers (Pinel et al., 2000) have argued that low body weight can be healthier than normal weight, which may be attributable to the association between overweight and death from cardiovascular disease (Heir, Erikssen, & Sandvik, 2011).

Without any question, obesity is a mortality risk, but those who are overweight yet not obese may not experience much more risk than those in the normal weight range. For example, studies from the United States (Flegal et al., 2005) and the European Union (Banegas, López-García, Gutiérrez-Fisac, Guallar-Castillón, & Rodríguez-Artalejo, 2003) found little

TABLE 14.3   Categories of Obesity and Risks for All-Cause Mortality Based on Body Mass Index (BMI)

Degree of Obesity	BMI Range	Risk for Men	Relative Risk	Risk for Women	Relative Risk
Moderate	25 to 32	None	1.0	Very low	1.1
Obese	32 to 36	Low	1.3	Low	1.2
Gross	36 to 40	High	1.9	Low	1.3
Morbid	40>	Very high	3.1	Very high	2.3

Source: Based on Bender et al. (1998).

elevation in risk for people who were overweight but substantial risk for those who were obese. A summary of these levels of risk appears in Table 14.3.

Other studies show similar results: Obesity is associated not only with increased mortality but also with increased use of medical care (Bertakis & Azari, 2005) and increased chances for developing Type 2 diabetes, osteoarthritis, high blood pressure, heart disease, and stroke (NCHS, 2011). Obesity also raises the risks for gallbladder disease (Smelt, 2010); migraine headache (Peterlin, Rosso, Rapoport, & Scher, 2010); kidney stones (Taylor, Stampfer, & Curhan, 2005); and sleep apnea, respiratory problems, liver disease, osteoarthritis, reproductive problems in women, and colon cancer (National Task Force on the Prevention and Treatment of Obesity, 2000). A large-scale study in Europe found that mortality risk was lowest for women with a BMI of 24.3 and for men with a BMI of 25.3 (Pischon et al., 2008).

Both age and ethnicity complicate the interpretation of risk from obesity. For young and middle-aged adults, being obese is a risk for all-cause mortality and especially for death due to cardiovascular disease (McGee, 2005). Indeed, being overweight during childhood and adolescence predicts increased mortality in the years to come (Bjørge, Engeland, Tverdal, & Smith, 2008). After age 55, the relationship no longer exists (Lantz, Golberstein, House, & Morenoff, 2010).

Another weight-related factor associated with morbidity and mortality is weight distribution. People who accumulate excess weight around their abdomen are at greater risk than people who carry their excess weight on their hips and thighs, and the tendency for this distribution has a genetic component (Fox et al., 2004). A variety of studies have shown that patterns of body weight and the waist-to-hip ratio may be better predictors of all-cause mortality than the body mass index (Pischon et al., 2008). Excess abdominal fat raises the risk for Type 2 diabetes (Hu, 2003) and cardiovascular disease (Pi-Sunyer, 2004).

The dangers of "beer bellies" were noted more than 25 years ago (Hartz, Rupley, & Rimm, 1984), but more recently this pattern of fat distribution has been integrated into a pattern of risk factors called the *metabolic syndrome*, a collection of factors proposed to elevate the risk for cardiovascular disease and diabetes. In addition to excess abdominal fat, components of the metabolic syndrome include elevated blood pressure, insulin resistance, and problems with the levels of two components of cholesterol. A large waistline is the most visible symptom of this syndrome, and research has indicated that abdominal fat is positively related to the metabolic syndrome, but fat on the thighs has a negative relationship (Goodpaster et al., 2005).

In conclusion, obese people have heightened risks of developing certain health problems, especially diabetes, gallstones, and cardiovascular disease. Table 14.4 summarizes studies showing that obesity and fat distributed around the waist both relate to increased mortality rates, especially from heart disease.

IN SUMMARY

Obesity can be defined in terms of health or social standards, and the two are not always the same. Assessment of body fat requires complex technology for accurate measurement, so the body mass index is often used as the assessment for overweight and obesity. Social standards, however, have dictated a standard of thinness with a lower body weight than is ideal for health.

Obesity has been explained by the setpoint model, genetic factors, and the positive incentive model. Setpoint theory explains weight regulation

TABLE 14.4   The Relationship Between Weight and Disease or Death

Results	Sample	Authors
Effects of Obesity		
Obesity is a risk for all-cause mortality.	U.S. population	Flegal et al., 2005
Obesity and underweight are risks for all-cause mortality.	Adults from nine countries in Europe	Pischon et al., 2008
Obesity is a stronger risk than overweight, but both contribute to mortality.	Adults from 15 members of the European Union	Banegas et al., 2003
Obese adults sought health care more often than normal-weight adults.	Obese and normal-weight adults	Bertakis & Azari, 2005
Headaches are more common among obese, especially those with abdominal obesity.	Large sample of U.S. adults	Peterlin et al., 2010
Obesity is a risk for kidney stones.	Men, older women, younger women	Taylor et al., 2005
Obesity increases risk for all-cause mortality.	Young and middle-aged adults	McGee, 2005
Overweight did not increase mortality risk for those over age 55.	U.S adults	Lantz et al., 2010
Overweight during childhood and adolescence raises the risk for later mortality.	Overweight children and adolescents	Bjørge et al., 2008
Effects of Abdominal Fat		
Abdominal fat is strongly associated with all-cause mortality.	Adults from nine countries in Europe	Pischon et al., 2008
Central fat is related to Type 2 diabetes and all-cause mortality.	Women	Hu, 2003
Central fat is related to the development of cardiovascular disease.	Review of studies, including cross-cultural comparisons	Pi-Sunyer, 2004
Abdominal fat is related to the metabolic syndrome.	Older women and men	Goodpaster et al., 2005

in terms of biological control systems that are sensitive to body fat. This model hypothesizes that obesity is a defect in this control mechanism. Such a defect is the primary component of genetic models of obesity, which hypothesize that obesity occurs when a person inherits some configuration of defective genes that affect the neurochemicals that signal hunger or satiation. However, neither of these models takes learned and environmental factors of eating into account, but the positive incentive model does. This view holds that people (and other animals) gain weight when they have ready access to an abundant and varied supply of tasty food.

Dieting

Many people in the United States have some knowledge of the risks of obesity and even know about the risks of an unfavorable waist-to-hip ratio, but media portrayals of idealized thin bodies are even more influential in the motivation to diet (Wiseman, Sunday, & Becker, 2005). Despite the idealization of thinness, obesity in the United States rose sharply during the 1990s and has not decreased since (NCHS, 2011). Acceptance of the ideal body as thin, combined with the growing prevalence of overweight, produces a situation in which dieting and weight loss are the subjects of a great many people's concern. What are people doing to try to lose weight, and how well do these strategies work?

People are inundated with messages about diets—television, magazine, and newspapers are filled with advertisements for miracle diets that take off pounds almost effortlessly. Those diets may seem too good to be true, and they are. In September 2002, the U.S. Federal Trade Commission issued a report that described how widespread false and misleading diets have become ("Federal Trade Commission," 2002). Despite the customer testimonials and the before-and-after photos, these "miracle" diets do not work. U.S. Surgeon General Richard Carmona said, "There is no such thing as a miracle pill for weight loss. The surest and safest way to weight loss and healthier living is by combining healthful eating and exercising" ("Federal Trade Commission," 2002, p. 8). Despite this prudent advice, many people fail to make wise choices when they want to lose weight. For example, people may concentrate on cutting fat in their diet without attending to the amount of sugar and other sweeteners they consume (Bray, Nielsen, & Popkin, 2004), or they cut carbohydrates yet eat a high-fat diet.

Other unwise decisions abound in choice of diet. The trend toward dieting has become more severe in the past few decades. During the mid-1960s, only 10% of overweight adults were dieting (Wyden, 1965), but during subsequent years those percentages steadily increased; in 2009, 52% of high school girls and 28% of high school boys were trying to lose weight (Eaton et al., 2010). Adults, too, are increasingly likely to diet. A survey of adults (Kruger, Galuska, Serdula, & Jones, 2004) showed that almost 38% of women and 24% of men were trying to lose weight. However, many of these adolescent and adult dieters do not have sufficient excess weight to put them at risk for disease or death, and many take unwise approaches to losing weight.

Approaches to Losing Weight

To lose weight or keep from gaining weight, people have several choices. They can (1) reduce portion size, (2) restrict the types of food they eat, (3) increase their level of exercise, (4) rely on drastic medical procedures such as fasting, diet pills, or surgery, or (5) use a combination of these approaches. Regardless of the approach, *all diets that prompt weight loss do so through restriction of calories.*

Restricting Types of Food Maintaining a diet consisting of a variety of foods with smaller portions is a reasonable and healthy strategy. The Weight Watchers program emphasizes eating a healthy variety of foods. This program proved most effective in an evaluation of a variety of dieting strategies (Dansinger et al., 2005), producing the best combination of weight loss and low dropout rate of any of the programs in this study. However, a healthy, balanced diet is not the most common diet approach; many programs rely on restricting types of foods.

Common approaches to restricting types of food include restricting carbohydrates (such at the Atkins diet) or restricting fat (LEARN diet). Diets that follow these different approaches produce slight differences in terms of weight loss and effects on health risks (Gardner et al., 2007; Hession, Rolland, Kulkarni, Wise, & Broom, 2009). The low-fat approach is more successful in terms of weight loss, but overweight people who follow low-carbohydrate, high-fat diets can also be successful in losing weight. Despite warnings from nutritionists about the dangers of such diet plans, people who follow these diets have not experienced unfavorable changes in cholesterol levels or risks for cardiovascular disease (Gardner et al., 2007). In addition, these diets tend to produce lower dropout rates than low-fat diets (Hession et al., 2009). Neither type of diet produced an impressive weight loss—an average of 10 to 12 pounds.

Some diets are more extreme, restricting the dieter to a limited group of foods or even a single food. All-fruit diets, egg diets, cabbage soup diet, and even the ice cream diet fall into this category. Of course, such diets are nutritional disasters. They produce weight loss by restricting calories; dieters get tired of the monotony of one food and eat less than they would if they were eating a variety. "All the hard-boiled eggs you want" turns out to be not many!

Taking monotony a step further are the liquid diets, which exist in a variety of forms and under various brand names. Liquid diets have the advantage of being nutritionally more balanced than most restricted food diets. Still, liquid diets and their equivalent meals in the form of puddings or bars have the disadvantage of being monotonous and repetitive, and tend to be low in fiber. Like all other diets, these work by restricting calorie intake. Although current researchers may disagree on the advantages of low-fat or low-carbohydrate diets, they are likely to agree that diets high in fiber from fruits and vegetables are good choices (Schenker, 2001). However, even this approach can be successful. An intensive behavioral program using meal replacements (Anderson, Conley, & Nicholas, 2007) was successful for very overweight people, producing weight losses of 50 to 100 pounds, with better maintenance rates than most diet programs.

In conclusion, all food restriction strategies can be successful in producing weight loss, but many are bad approaches. Most of these diets fail to teach new eating habits that people can maintain over the long term. This problem was Kirstie Alley's dieting downfall; she has lost weight successfully several times but failed to maintain the loss. She knew how to diet to lose weight quickly, and she knew how to overeat. Her approach to weight loss did not include learning how to eat in moderation ("Kirstie Alley's Weight," 2009).

Behavior Modification Programs

Although dieting should be seen as a permanent modification in one's eating habits, such change is difficult. The behavior modification approach toward treating weight loss begins with the assumption that eating is a behavior that is subject to change. This application of behavioral theory was originated by Richard Stuart (1967), who reported a much higher success rate than that achieved through previous diet approaches. Most behavior modification programs focus on eating and exercise, helping overweight people to monitor and change their behavior. Clients in these programs often keep eating diaries to focus their awareness on the types of foods they eat and under what circumstances, as well as to provide data the therapist can use to devise a personal plan for changing unhealthy eating habits. The outcome of one weight loss trial (Hollis et al., 2008) indicated that dieters who kept a diary lost twice as much weight as those on the same program who did not. In addition, exercise goals are a typical component of behavior modification programs. The most common format for these programs is a group setting with weekly meetings that include instruction in nutrition and in self-monitoring to attain individual goals (Wing & Polley, 2001). Almost all weight control programs include some modification of eating, physical activity, or both, and these programs may be referred to as behavioral or behavior modification programs (Wadden, Crerand, & Brock, 2005).

Because weight loss is not a behavior, these behavioral programs tend to reinforce good eating habits rather than the number of pounds lost. In other words, the behaviors, not the consequences, are the targets for reward and change. People who are overweight to moderately obese may be fairly successful in

these types of programs (Moldovan & David, 2011). The goal is typically gradual weight loss and maintenance of that loss. The average amount of weight lost is about 20 pounds over 6 months, but dieters maintain only about 60% of that loss over a year (Wing & Polley, 2001). Thus, even moderate, gradual weight loss may be difficult to maintain.

Exercise   The importance of exercise in weight loss has become increasingly apparent (Wu, Gao, Chen, & van Dam, 2009). Exercise alone is not very effective for weight loss (Thorogood et al., 2011), but adding physical activity to a program to change eating is important. Because metabolic rate slows down when food intake decreases, physical activity can counteract this metabolic slowdown and thus may be an indispensable part of weight reduction programs. A large-scale survey of dieters ("Federal Trade Commission Weighs in on Losing Weight," 2002) found that 73% of successful dieters exercised at least three times a week, and a meta-analysis of successful components in a diet program (Wu et al., 2009) indicated that physical activity was such a component. Exercise can also change body composition, adding muscle while dieting decreases fat levels. (The role of exercise is discussed more fully in Chapter 15.)

Drastic Methods of Losing Weight   People sometimes take drastic measures to lose weight, and physicians sometimes recommend drastic measures for severely obese patients. Even with medical supervision, some weight reduction programs present risks, sometimes to the point of being life threatening.

One approach that has turned out to carry substantial risks is taking drugs to reduce appetite. In the 1950s and 1960s, amphetamines were widely prescribed as diet pills to increase the activity of the nervous system, speed up metabolism, and suppress appetite. Unfortunately, the effects are short term, and dependence may become a more serious problem than obesity. Increasing evidence of the dangers of amphetamines led to the development of other diet drugs, but the quest for a safe, effective drug that helps people lose weight has proven difficult. Currently available drugs include sibutramine (Meridia) and orlistat (Xenical), both of which offer the possibility of only modest weight loss (Czernichow et al., 2010; Osei-Assibey, Adi, Kryou, Kumar, & Matyka, 2011). The developing knowledge of hormones and neurochemicals related to weight regulation suggests that more effective drugs are possible, but that promise has not developed, so a growing number of obese people are turning to surgery as a way to manage their weight.

Several types of surgery can affect weight, but most current surgeries either restrict the size of the stomach by gastric banding (placing a band around the stomach) or gastric bypass (routing food around most of the stomach and part of the intestines) (Buchwald et al., 2004). People are candidates for these surgeries if their BMI is 35 or higher and if they have health problems that make weight loss imperative. These procedures are successful in promoting drastic weight loss and changing eating behaviors (Moldovan & David, 2011). These changes improve diabetes, hypertension, and other risk factors for cardiovascular disease. Like any surgery, these procedures carry some risks, and patients typically must be prepared to monitor their food intake and to take nutritional supplements for the rest of their lives (Tucker, Szomstein, & Rosenthal, 2007). Despite the risks and maintenance requirements, these surgeries increased dramatically from the 1990s to 2004 and then decreased slightly, but about 125,000 occur each year in the United States (Nguyen, Masoomi, et al., 2011).

Another surgical approach to weight loss is to remove adipose tissue through a fat-suctioning technique called liposuction. The technique produces a recontouring of the body rather than an overall weight loss (Sattler, 2005). This procedure is not useful in controlling the health complications of obesity; rather, it is a cosmetic procedure to change body shape, not a way to lose weight or affect health. Despite the discomfort and expense of the surgery, liposuction is the most common type of plastic surgery worldwide (Sattler, 2005). Like all surgery, it presents risks such as infection and reactions to anesthesia.

Drastic means of losing weight are poor solutions to obesity for most people. However, they are fairly common. High school girls reported using such drastic strategies for weight loss as fasting (14.5%), taking appetite suppressant drugs (6.3%), and using laxatives or purging (5.4%); a majority (52%) admitted chronic dieting (Eaton et al., 2010). Having a friend who uses these methods increases adolescent girls' risks for doing so (Eisenberg, Neumark-Sztainer, Story, & Perry, 2005), and being overweight raises the percentages of those who have used such methods to 40% for girls and 20% for boys (Neumark-Sztainer et al., 2007). All these drastic means of losing weight can be dangerous. In addition, all are difficult to maintain long enough to produce significant weight loss. Even when dieters succeed with these strategies, they usually regain the weight they have lost because these approaches do not enable them to learn how to make good diet choices for permanent weight loss. Indeed, keeping weight off is a major challenge, regardless of weight loss method.

Maintaining Weight Loss   In Chapters 12 and 13, we saw that about two thirds of the people who initially quit smoking or stop drinking will eventually relapse. For people who succeed in losing weight, maintaining that loss is comparably difficult. A systematic review of commercial weight loss programs (Tsai & Wadden, 2005) indicated that people who managed to lose weight on these programs (not all do) had a high probability of regaining 50% of the weight they lost within 1 to 2 years. However, this review evaluated highly selected dieters, including those who were extremely obese and those who sought professional help in losing weight. For those people, weight control is now considered to be a chronic illness, with continued professional assistance needed to maintain weight loss (Kubetin, 2001). Kirstie Alley provides an example of these findings: After losing weight on the Jenny Craig program, she regained all that she had lost, plus a bit, then sought another approach and lost again.

Effective formal weight reduction interventions typically include posttreatment programs to help dieters maintain weight loss. These programs are usually more successful than those that lack a posttreatment phase. For example, a comparison of two follow-up interventions in dieters who had completed a 6-month weight loss program (Svetkey et al., 2008) included three groups of dieters. One group received no follow-up, one received an intervention that involved brief personal contact on a monthly basis, and another consisted of an interactive, technology-based intervention. The personal follow-up was more effective, but both interventions produced dieters who weighed less than before they started the program. Thus, the follow-up need not be intensive or complex; simple procedures can be effective. For example, people who lost weight and weighed themselves daily were less likely to regain the lost weight than those who did not step on the scales so often (Wing et al., 2007).

A survey by *Consumer Reports* ("The Truth About Dieting," 2002) supplied information about a wide selection of dieters, both successful and unsuccessful. This survey included more than 32,000 dieters, 25%

of whom had lost at least 10% of their starting weight and kept it off for at least a year. This number confirmed that people have problems both with losing weight and with maintaining weight loss, but it also showed that some people are successful.

Most of the dieters in the *Consumer Reports* survey lost weight on their own rather than through a formal weight loss program. Consistent with the systematic review of commercial programs (Tsai & Wadden, 2005), more of the unsuccessful dieters (26%) than successful dieters (14%) tried a program such as Weight Watchers or Jenny Craig. Those who were successful tended to use a variety of approaches, including exercising and increasing physical activity, eating fewer fatty and sweet foods, increasing consumption of fruits and vegetables, and cutting down on portion size. Not surprisingly, those dieters who were successful in maintaining their weight loss rarely used any of the drastic means of losing weight reviewed in the prior section, except for surgery; individuals who undergo surgery to lose weight tend to lose large amounts of weight and maintain some of that weight loss (Douketis, Macie, Thabane, & Williamson, 2005). People who lose weight without surgery and keep it off tend to alter their eating and physical activity, forming new habits that they are able to maintain.

Childhood obesity has increased, even among children as young as preschool age, and has become a worldwide epidemic and thus of great concern (Spruijt-Metz, 2011). Interventions may include strategies for preventing the development of overweight, dietary programs, family interventions, physical activity programs, school-based programs, or some combination of these elements. Although dietary modification can result in reducing weight among overweight children (Collins, Warren, Neve, McCoy, & Stokes, 2007), adding a physical activity component boosts effectiveness (Safron, Cislak, Gaspar, & Luszczynska, 2011). A meta-analysis of family-based behavioral interventions (Young, Northern, Lister, Drummond, & O'Brien, 2007) and residential weight loss programs for children (Kelly & Kirschenbaum, 2011) indicated that both approaches can be effective in changing eating and physical activity habits.

Is Dieting a Good Choice?

Although dieting can produce weight loss, it may not be a good choice for everyone. Dieting has psychological costs, may not be effective in improving health, and

may be a signal of body dissatisfaction that is a risk for eating disorders. A group of dieters rated their overall experience as positive early in their diet (Jeffery, Kelly, Rothman, Sherwood, & Boutelle, 2004), but as the dieting continued, positive feelings decreased. Some dieters exhibit strong reactions, behaving very much like starving people: They are irritable, obsessed with food, finicky about taste, easily distractible, and hungry. These behavioral reactions make dieting foolish for those who are close to the best weight for their health. For those who are sufficiently overweight to endanger their health, losing weight may still be an unwise choice. Developing reasonable and healthy eating patterns is a far better choice than dieting. That is, dieting is not the same as eliminating overeating (Herman, van Strien, & Polivy, 2008). The former is not a good choice for many people, whereas the latter is a good choice for everyone.

Ironically, weight loss may be a health risk for some people and a health benefit for others. Involuntary weight loss is often associated with disease, so the association between unintentional weight loss and mortality is no surprise. Older people are more likely to lose weight due to illness, and a study that considered participants' age (Kuk & Ardern, 2009) indicated that younger people are at risk from overweight but that after age 65, overweight is no longer a predictor of mortality. However, when overweight and obese adults were assigned randomly to a weight loss program (Shea et al., 2010), those who lost weight did not experience any increase in mortality; indeed, their risk was lowered.

Thus, the benefits of weight loss may not apply equally to all people. Even modest weight loss can be important for individuals who are obese and who can maintain the loss. However, the risks of dieting may be greater than the risks of moderate, stable overweight (Gaesser, 2003). Obesity, however, is not healthy.

IN SUMMARY

The near obsession with thinness in our culture has led to a plethora of diets, many of which are neither safe nor permanently effective. Most diets will produce some initial weight loss in response to the restriction of caloric intake, but maintaining the reduced weight levels is a matter of permanent changes in basic eating habits and activity levels. Despite attempts to be thin, people in the United

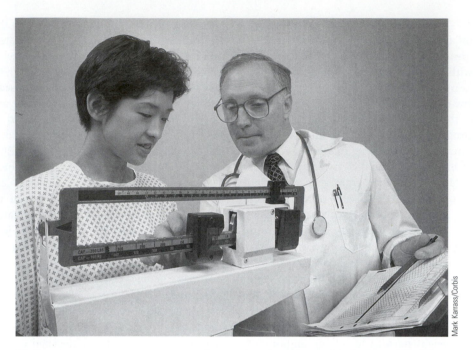

Mark Karrass/Corbis

Dieting is common, even among those who do not need to lose weight for health reasons.

States are now heavier than ever because they have increased the number of calories they consume and lowered their amount of physical activity.

Losing weight is easier than maintaining weight loss, but programs that include posttreatment and frequent follow-up can be successful in helping people maintain a healthy weight. Whether part of a formal program or a personal attempt, eating a variety of healthy foods and maintaining physical activity are more likely than drastic programs to result in long-term weight loss. Like programs for adults, programs for obese children and adolescents face similar challenges and include the same effective components—healthy food choices and physical activity.

Dieting is a good choice for some people but not for others. Obese people and those with a high waist-to-hip ratio should try to lose weight and keep it off. However, most people who diet for cosmetic reasons would be healthier (and happier) if they did not diet, and even people who are slightly overweight may not benefit from dieting.

Eating Disorders

The eating disorders that have received the most attention, both in the popular media and in the scientific literature, are anorexia nervosa and bulimia, but binge eating is also an eating disorder diagnosis. An **eating disorder** is a serious and habitual disturbance in eating behavior that produces unhealthy consequences. This definition of eating disorders excludes starvation resulting from the inability to find suitable food supplies and also unhealthy eating resulting from inadequate information about nutrition. Also excluded are disturbances in eating behavior such as pica, or the eating of nonnutritive substances such as plastic and wood, and the rumination disorder of infancy—that is, regurgitation of food without nausea or gastrointestinal illness. Neither of these disorders presents serious health problems to adults, and they are of relatively minor importance in health psychology.

The term *anorexia nervosa* literally means lack of appetite due to a nervous or psychological condition; *bulimia* means continuous, morbid hunger. Neither meaning, however, is quite accurate. **Anorexia nervosa** is an eating disorder that includes intentional starvation and a distorted body image. People with anorexia nervosa have not lost their appetite. Ordinarily, they are perpetually hungry, but they insist that they do not wish to eat.

Bulimia has come to mean more than continuous, morbid hunger. The chief identifying mark of this eating disorder is repeated bingeing and purging, the purge usually coming after eating huge quantities of food, typically high in calories and loaded with carbohydrates, fat, or both. Eating large quantities of food is critical to the definition of binge eating; people with this disorder binge but do not purge, resulting in overweight and obesity.

These three eating disorders obviously have much in common. Indeed, some authorities regard anorexia and bulimia as two dimensions of the same illness. Others see the three as separate but related disorders (Polivy & Herman, 2002). For example, binge eating is common to all three. In addition, the core components of all three include body dissatisfaction combined with preoccupation with food, weight, and body shape. The basis for body dissatisfaction is easy to understand: Overweight and obesity have become more common, yet the ideal body is thin. This combination has created a discontent that touches everyone in the culture. Children as young as early elementary school age express body dissatisfaction (Brown & Slaughter, 2011; Harriger et al., 2010), and discontent with body shape is so common among women that it is the norm (Grogan, 2007; Rodin, Silberstein, & Striegel-Moore, 1985). However, only a small percentage of people with body dissatisfaction develop eating disorders, indicating that other factors operate to produce these disorders (Tylka, 2004).

Janet Polivy and Peter Herman (2002, 2004) suggested that body dissatisfaction constitutes an essential precursor to the development of eating disorders, but those who develop eating problems must also come to see being thin as a solution to other problems in their lives. People who channel their distress into body concerns and focus on their bodies as a way to change their dissatisfaction have the cognitions that lead to eating disorders (Evans, 2003). Such cognitions include the feeling that being thin will lead to happiness.

Other risks for eating disorders include family and personality correlates such as a great deal of negative family interaction; a history of sexual abuse during childhood; low self-esteem; and high levels of negative mood, anxiety, and depression (Polivy & Herman,

2002). In addition, some genetic or neuroendocrine predisposition may contribute to the development of eating disorders; the neurotransmitter serotonin has been implicated (Kaye, 2008), and leptin exerts a variety of actions in the brain (Zupancic & Mahajan, 2011). Test of factors related to unhealthy weight control strategies (Liechty, 2010; Neumark-Sztainer, Wall, Story, & Perry, 2003) show that concern about body weight appears to be a primary factor in eating disorders.

Anorexia Nervosa

Despite the current focus on anorexia, neither the disorder nor the term is new. The first two documented cases of intentional self-starvation were reported by Richard Morton in 1689 (Sours, 1980). Morton wrote about an 18-year-old English girl who had died of the effects of anorexia some 25 years earlier and about an 18-year-old boy who had survived. Both had shown a remarkable indifference to starvation, and both had been described as sad and anxious. In London, Sir William Gull (1874) studied several cases of intentional self-starvation during the 1860s. He regarded the condition as a psychological disorder and coined the term *anorexia nervosa* to indicate loss of appetite due to "nervous" causes—that is, psychological factors.

During the 1940s and 1950s, psychiatrists who took a psychoanalytic view hypothesized that the ailment was a denial of femininity and a fear of motherhood. Other theorists suggested that it represented an attempt on the part of the young woman to reestablish unity with her mother. Unfortunately, none of these hypotheses proved fruitful in expanding the scientific understanding of anorexia nervosa. The past five decades have seen a shift away from this sort of speculation and a turn toward the view that anorexia involves a complex of sociocultural, family, and biological factors (Polivy & Herman, 2002). Recent emphasis has been on describing the disorder in terms of behaviors and their physiological effects, demographic correlates, and effective treatment procedures.

What Is Anorexia? Anorexia nervosa is an eating disorder characterized by intentional self-starvation or semistarvation, sometimes to the point of death. People with anorexia are extremely afraid of gaining weight and have a distorted body image, seeing themselves as being too heavy even though they are exceedingly thin. Research using brain imaging (Sachdev, Mondraty,

Wen, & Gulliford, 2008) has revealed that women who are anorexic process images of their own bodies differently than they do images of other women's bodies—even when the two bodies are the same weight.

The *Diagnostic and Statistical Manual of Mental Disorders* (4th edition, text revision [*DSM-IV-TR*]) of the American Psychiatric Association (APA, 2000) defines *anorexia nervosa* as intentional weight loss to a point that the person weighs less than 85% of the weight considered normal by the Metropolitan Life Insurance tables or has a body mass index of 17.5 or less, along with a fear of being fat, a distorted body image, and for women, **amenorrhea**, the cessation of menstrual periods for at least three cycles.

The *DSM-IV-TR* (APA, 2000) identifies two subtypes of anorexia: the restricting type and the binge–purge type. Anorexics with the restricting type eat almost nothing, losing weight by dieting, fasting, exercising, or a combination of these strategies. Anorexics with the binge–purge type may eat large quantities of food and use vomiting or laxatives to purge the food they have eaten. Alternatively, these anorexics may eat small amounts of food and purge. Research has confirmed that these two subtypes are distinct (Kaye, 2008). Purging is typical of bulimia, and binge eating occurs in binge eating disorder, but bulimics use purging to maintain a normal body weight. Anorexics purge to lose weight.

Anorexia is not confined to any demographic group, but young women are at higher risk than older women or men of any age. Typically, they are preoccupied with food, often like to cook for others, insist that others eat their food, but eat almost nothing themselves. They lose from 15% to 50% of their body weight, yet continue to see themselves as overweight. These young women tend to be ambitious, perfectionist, from high-achieving families, and unhappy with their bodies. Anorexics are preoccupied with body fat, which usually leads to a strenuous program of exercise—dancing, jogging, doing calisthenics, or playing tennis. Excessively active and energetic behavior continues until their weight loss reaches a level that produces fatigue and weakness, making further activity impossible.

After substantial weight loss has occurred, individual differences tend to disappear, and accounts of individuals with the disorder are remarkably similar. Interestingly, many of the characteristics match the sketch of starving conscientious objectors drawn by Keys et al. (1950). Thus, these characteristics are probably an effect of starvation and not its cause. As weight loss reaches more than 25% of one's previous normal weight, the person constantly feels chilled, grows a soft, downy covering of body hair, loses scalp hair, loses interest in sex, and develops an unusual preoccupation with food. As starvation nears a perilous level, the anorexic individual becomes more hostile toward family and friends who try to reverse the weight loss.

Many authorities, including Hilde Bruch (1973, 1978, 1982), have regarded anorexia nervosa as a means of gaining control. Bruch, who spent more than 40 years studying eating disorders and the effects of starvation, reported that prior to dieting, anorexics typically are troubled girls who feel incapable of changing their lives. These young women often see their parents as overdemanding and in absolute control of their life, yet they remain too compliant to rebel openly. They try to seize control of their life in the most personal manner possible: by changing the shape of their body. Short of force-feeding, no one can stop these young women from controlling their own body size and shape. Anorexics take great pleasure and pride in doing something that is difficult and often compare their superior willpower with that of others who are overweight or who shun exercise. Bruch (1978) reported that anorexics enjoy being hungry and eventually regard any food in the stomach as dirty or damaging.

Who Has Anorexia? Although anorexia is associated with Western culture, it appears in non-Western cultures around the world (Keel & Klump, 2003) and cuts across ethnic groups (Marques et al., 2011). This diagnosis was once more common among upper-middle-class and upper-class women of European ancestry in North America and Europe, but a recent assessment of many ethnic groups (Marques et al., 2011) showed that the prevalence of anorexia is similar in Hispanic American, Asian American, and African American women. Anorexia has become more common than it was 50 years ago (Keel & Klump, 2003), but anorexia nervosa is still a very rare disorder in the general population. The *DSM-IV-TR* (APA, 2000) estimated the lifetime prevalence of anorexia at 0.5% for women and one tenth of that for men. Other analyses (Hudson, Hiripi, Pope, & Kessler, 2007) yield higher (but still low) estimates—0.9% for women and 0.3% for men. However, among some groups the incidence rates are much higher. For example, 26% of young women who had competed in beauty pageants reported that they believed they had or had received a diagnosis of an eating disorder (Thompson & Hammond, 2003). The competitive, weight-conscious atmosphere of professional schools for dance and modeling prompt the development of anorexia, and 6.5% of dance students and 7% of modeling students met the diagnostic criteria for anorexia nervosa (Garner & Garfinkel, 1980). A survey of college students involved in theater, dance, cheerleading, and athletics (Robles, 2011) indicated that 12% had been treated for eating disorders. Female athletes who participate in sports that emphasize appearance, thin body type, or low body fat are especially at risk (Torstveit, Rosenvinge, & Sundgot-Borgen, 2008). Level of involvement in these activities may be more at risk; for example, more elite dancers experience more frequent and severe symptoms of eating disorders (Thomas, Keel, & Heatherton, 2005).

Individuals with anorexia often report family difficulties, but it is difficult to determine if the difficulties precede the onset of eating problems or are a result of them (Polivy & Herman, 2002). Family environment is important in several ways. Families with children who have eating disorders tend to include a lot of negative emotion and little emotional support. Family violence—either as an observer or a target—is

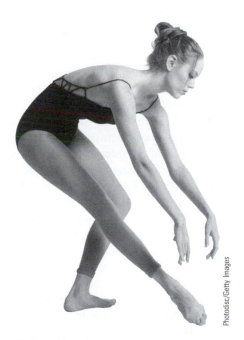

Eating disorders are more common among models, dancers, and athletes whose sports demand thinness.

a risk for eating disorders for both men and women (Bardy, 2008). In addition, a family member with an eating disorder raises the risk for others in the family (Tylka, 2004), but so does having friends with unhealthy weight control practices (Eisenberg et al., 2005) or joining a sorority (Basow, Foran, & Bookwala, 2007). Thus, disordered eating is affected by social context as well as family dynamics. In addition, physical or sexual abuse is a more common experience in the history of those who are anorexic than for individuals who eat normally (Rayworth, 2004).

Over the years, a large majority of those diagnosed as anorexic have been women, who have been the focus of research and treatment. Men make up about 10% of all anorexics (APA, 2000). This estimate—that 90% or more of all anorexics are women—has remained constant over a period of years, but it is based mostly on clinical impressions rather than on complete population data. Reviews of eating disorders in men (Jones & Morgan, 2010; Woodside, 2002) claim that more representative assessments of eating disorders reveal much higher numbers, with men constituting at least 20% of cases. Thus, this eating disorder may be more common among men than the clinical impressions suggest.

Male anorexics are quite similar to female anorexics in terms of social class and family configuration, symptoms, treatment, and prognosis, but they differ in terms of the factors that pushed them toward disordered eating (Ricciardelli, McCabe, Williams, & Thompson, 2007). In addition, some studies have found that sexual orientation is a factor that differs for male and female anorexics, with more male anorexics being gay (Boisvert & Harrell, 2009), but a comparison of symptoms and characteristics (Crisp et al., 2006) revealed many more similarities than differences.

Boys and young men may take drastic measures to achieve their ideal body, just as girls and young women do (Olivardia, Pope, & Phillips, 2000). The ideal body for boys is muscular, and escaping this indoctrination is as difficult as avoiding the thin body ideal is for girls (Mosley, 2009). However, both ideals share the abhorrence of fat. Thus, both women and men have concerns about body shape and size that may appear as disordered eating.

Treatment for Anorexia Treatment for anorexia suffers from an unfortunate dilemma: This disorder has the highest mortality rate of any psychiatric diagnosis, but no treatment has demonstrated a high degree of effectiveness (Cardi & Treasure, 2010). About 3% of all anorexics die from causes related to their disorder (Keel & Brown, 2010). Most die of cardiac arrhythmia, but suicide is also a frequent cause of death for those with the bingeing–purging type of anorexia (Foulon et al., 2007). Despite the very real possibility of death, anorexia nervosa remains one of the most difficult behavior disorders to treat. About 75% of anorexics recover (Keel & Brown, 2010). Of those who do not recover, some improve but struggle with eating-related body image problems, obsessive-compulsive disorder, or depression. Between 9% and 18% continue to exhibit symptoms of anorexia, and those who are treated on an inpatient basis fare more poorly than those who receive community-based treatment.

An initial complication for treatment is that most anorexics are focused on losing weight, resent suggestions that they are too thin, and resist any attempt to change their eating. That attitude appears on a number of websites hosted by individuals who are anorexic and promote it as a lifestyle alternative rather than a disorder (Davis, 2008). Readiness for change predicts more successful treatment (McHugh, 2007). Motivating anorexics to seek treatment is thus a major challenge that may be addressed by the application of motivational interviewing (Hogan & McReynolds, 2004). This technique is a directive intervention to change attitudes about problems and make people more willing to work toward change.

As starvation continues, anorexics eventually reach the point of fatigue, exhaustion, and possible physical collapse, and they are forced into treatment. This situation seems undesirable, but even those who have been subjected to involuntary treatment later agreed that this strategy was justified (Tan, Stewart, Fitzpatrick, & Hope, 2010). The immediate aim of almost any treatment program for advanced anorexia is medical stabilization of any physical dangers from starvation. Then, anorexics need to work toward restoration of normal weight, healthy eating, and improved body image. Recommendations concerning the methods of achieving these goals are not universally accepted, and systematic reviews have yet to reach firm conclusions concerning what treatments are most effective for people with anorexia (Bulik, Berkman, Brownley, Sedway, & Lohr, 2007; Fisher, Hetrick, & Rushford, 2010; Hay, 2004).

Since the mid-1970s, cognitive behavioral therapy has become increasingly popular as a treatment for anorexia nervosa, and it has shown some success in changing both cognitive distortions that accompany body image problems and eating behavior (Fairburn & Harrison, 2003). Cognitive behavioral therapists attack these irrational beliefs while maintaining a warm and accepting attitude toward patients. Anorexics are taught to discard the absolutist, all-or-nothing thinking pattern expressed in such self-statements as "If I gain one pound, I'll go on to gain a hundred." Addressing cognitive distortions may be more important than previously recognized—a developing body of research indicates that anorexics experience significant cognitive distortions that apply to the processing of food-related words (Nikendei et al., 2008). In addition, people with anorexia are more likely than others to believe that they cannot control their thoughts, and half reported that they used cognitive strategies to make themselves feel worse (Woolrich, Cooper, & Turner, 2008). The cognitive component of cognitive behavioral therapy has the potential to address these problems.

Cognitive behavioral therapy is not greatly more effective than other types of psychological and multimodal interventions such as the standard programs for anorexia, which consist of individual and group therapy plus supervised meals, meal planning, and nutrition education (Williamson, Thaw, & Varnado-Sullivan, 2001). Such programs are effective for some individuals with anorexia. Unfortunately, none of the treatments for anorexia show impressive success rates (Hay & de M. Claudino, 2010), and researchers are searching for improvements, especially in treating adults with anorexia.

For adolescents, the picture is somewhat more optimistic. An approach developed at the Maudsley Hospital in London emphasizes the role of family and family involvement in treatment for anorexia (Locke, le Grange, Agras, & Dare, 2001). Rather than treat parents as part of the problem, this approach accepts them as an essential part of the solution. Acknowledging that it is relatively easy to get anorexics to gain weight in the hospital, this approach focuses on helping them eat at home by equipping parents with strategies to get their children to eat. The value of including families in treatment of anorexia in adolescents has become well accepted (Cardi & Treasure, 2010).

Treatment of anorexia may also include antidepressant and antipsychotic drugs. A systematic review of the use of fluoxetine (Prozac) found insufficient evidence to recommend this treatment for anorexia (Claudino et al., 2006). Another systematic review (Court, Mulder, Hetrick, Purcell, & McGorry, 2008) failed to find evidence that antipsychotic drugs were an effective therapy for anorexia. Thus, the arsenal for treating this difficult disease remains understocked.

Relapse always remains a possibility. Even with intensive therapy that targets irrational eating patterns and distorted body image, some anorexics retain elements of these maladaptive thought processes. Some slip back to self-starvation, some attempt suicide, some become depressed, and some develop other eating disorders (Carter, Blackmore, Sutandar-Pinnock, & Woodside, 2004; Castellini et al, 2011). Follow-up care is often included in comprehensive programs, and cognitive behavioral therapy seems especially useful to prevent relapses (Pike, Timothy, Vitousek, Wilson, & Bauer, 2003).

Bulimia

Bulimia is often regarded as a companion disorder to anorexia nervosa, and some cases have been identified of individuals who have moved from one diagnosis to the other (Eddy et al., 2007). Unlike those with anorexia, who rely mostly on strict fasts to lose more and more weight, individuals with bulimia consume huge quantities of food in an uncontrolled manner (binge) and then purge, either by vomiting or by taking laxatives. The seemingly bizarre practice of binge eating followed by purging is not new. The ancient Romans sometimes indulged in very similar eating rituals. After they had feasted on great quantities of rich food, these Romans would retire to the vomitorium, empty their stomachs, and then return to eat some more (Friedländer, 1968). Unlike bulimia, this practice may not have been oriented toward weight control. Today, bulimia is defined as an eating disorder and affects millions of people.

What Is Bulimia?   As defined by the *Diagnostic and Statistical Manual of Mental Disorders* (*DSM-IV-TR*) of the American Psychiatric Association (APA, 2000), *bulimia nervos*a involves recurrent episodes of binge eating, a sense of lack of control over eating, and inappropriate, drastic measures to compensate for the binge. Some bulimics fast or exercise excessively, but most use self-induced vomiting or laxatives and maintain a relatively normal weight.

One factor that distinguishes bulimia from anorexia is lack of impulse control (Polivy & Herman, 2002), although this characteristic may apply to some people who are bulimic more strongly than to others (Myers, Wonderlich, et al., 2006). Bulimics often experience problems related to impulsivity, such as a history of alcohol or drug abuse, sexual promiscuity, suicide attempts, and stealing or shoplifting. This factor may be critical; a person may become bulimic rather than

anorexic if she or he cannot resist the impulse to eat, yet feels the body dissatisfaction that is common to both of these disorders.

Childhood experiences with sexual abuse, physical abuse, and posttraumatic stress are additional correlates of bulimia (Rayworth, 2004; Treur, Koperdák, Rózsa, & Füredi, 2005). In addition, recent involvement with sexual assault raises the risk (Fischer, Stojek, & Hartzell, 2010). A survey of a representative sample of bulimic women in the United States (Wonderlich, Wilsnack, Wilsnack, & Harris, 1996) revealed that nearly one fourth of all female victims of childhood sexual abuse displayed bulimic behaviors later on. These women tend to have more severe symptoms than others (Treur et al., 2005). A relationship also exists between bulimia and depression, but childhood sexual abuse is also related to depression, as are suicide attempts. Body image and eating disorders tend to precede the development of depression in adolescent girls (Blodgett Salafia & Gondoli, 2011; Kaye, 2008), which suggests a developmental sequence and may allow the establishment of a chain of causality for the development of bulimia.

Personality factors also differ in bulimics; those who binge and purge fall into different categories (Duncan et al., 2005; Wonderlich et al., 2005). One subgroup of bulimics exhibited more pathology than the other, including more concomitant mental disorders and stronger symptoms of bulimia, whereas another group showed less pathology and less severe symptoms of bulimia. However, depression and anxiety are part of the experience of bulimia.

Who Is Bulimic?   In at least one way, the population of bulimics is quite similar to that of anorexics. Both eating disorders occur far more often in women than in men, with women comprising about 90% to 95% of those diagnosed in both groups (APA, 2000). Bulimia occurs with equal prevalence in various social classes and ethnic groups in the United States (Franko et al., 2007).

How prevalent is bulimia? Is its incidence increasing or decreasing? Approximately 1% to 3% of American women and 0.2% of men meet the current diagnostic criteria for bulimia (APA, 2000), making this disorder much more common than anorexia. In a survey of high school students (Eaton et al., 2010), 5.4% of girls and 2.6% of boys said that they had vomited or used laxatives to lose or avoid gaining weight. These percentages reflect a high rate of these behaviors, which suggests a growing prevalence of bulimia. An analysis of the history of this disorder (Keel & Klump, 2003) indicated a substantial increase during the second half of the 20th century. Furthermore, bulimia is restricted to Western cultures and those cultures influenced by Western values, making this eating disorder a culture-bound syndrome.

Is Bulimia Harmful?

To many people, bingeing and purging may seem an acceptable means of controlling weight. For others, guilt is a nearly inevitable part of bulimia, and some mental health problems accompany this disorder. However, the question remains: Is bulimia harmful to physical health? Unlike anorexia nervosa, which has a mortality rate of 3% (Keel & Brown, 2010), bulimia is very seldom fatal (Steinhausen & Weber, 2010). Nevertheless, bulimia has serious detrimental consequences.

The combination of binge eating and purging is harmful in several ways. First, the intake of large quantities of sweets can result in **hypoglycemia**, or a deficiency of sugar in the blood. This may seem paradoxical because the typical binge eater consumes huge amounts of sugar, but the metabolism of sugar prompts insulin release, which drives down blood sugar levels. Low blood sugar results in dizziness, fatigue, depression, and cravings for more sugar, which may prompt another binge. Second, binge eaters seldom eat a balanced diet, and poor nutrition may lead to lethargy and depression. Third, binge eating is expensive. Bulimics can spend more than $100 a day on food and this expense can lead to other problems, such as financial difficulties or stealing. Also, binge eaters are preoccupied with food in an obsessive way, thinking and planning the next binge. This obsession may leave bulimics with limited time to attend to other activities (Polivy & Herman, 2002).

Purging also leads to several physical problems (Mehler, 2011). One of the most common consequences of frequent vomiting is damaged teeth; hydrochloric acid from the stomach erodes the enamel that protects the teeth. Many longtime bulimics need extensive dental work, and dentists are sometimes the first health care professionals to see evidence of bulimia. Hydrochloric acid may also lead to damage in the mouth and esophagus. Bleeding and tearing of the esophagus are not common among bulimics but are very dangerous. Some longtime sufferers report reverse peristalsis, an involuntary regurgitation of food, often after eating quite moderately. Other potential dangers of frequent purging include **anemia**, a reduction in the number of red blood cells; **electrolyte imbalance** caused by the loss of minerals such as sodium, potassium, magnesium, and calcium; and **alkalosis**, an abnormally high level of alkaline in the body tissues resulting from the loss of hydrochloric acid. These conditions may lead to weakness and fatigue. Purging through excessive use of laxatives and diuretics may lead to kidney damage, dehydration, and a spastic colon or the loss of voluntary control over excretory functions. In addition, ingredients in the substances used as laxatives may have toxic properties, adding to the dangers (Steffen, Mitchell, Roerig, & Lancaster, 2007). In summary, bulimia is not a harmless weight control strategy but a serious disorder with a multitude of potential dangers.

Treatment for Bulimia

In one important respect, the treatment of bulimia has a critical advantage over therapy programs for anorexia nervosa—those with bulimia are more likely to be motivated to change their eating behaviors. Unfortunately, this motivation does not guarantee that bulimics will seek therapy.

Cognitive behavioral therapy is recognized as the preferred treatment for bulimia (Cardi & Treasure, 2010). Cognitive behavioral therapists work toward changing both distorted cognitions, such as obsessive body concerns, and behaviors such as bingeing, vomiting, and laxative use. Specific techniques may include keeping a diary on the factors related to bingeing and on feelings after purging, monitoring caloric intake, eating slowly, eating regular meals, and clarifying distorted views of eating and weight control. A systematic review of treatments for bulimia (Shapiro et al., 2007) revealed that cognitive behavioral treatment is effective, including assessments at long-term follow-up.

Interpersonal psychotherapy has also been used successfully in treating bulimia (Tanofsky-Kraff & Wilfley, 2010) Interpersonal psychotherapy is a nonintrospective, short-term therapy that was originally applied to depression. It focuses on present interpersonal problems and not on eating, taking the approach that eating problems tend to appear in late adolescence when interpersonal issues present major developmental challenges. In this view, eating problems represent maladaptive attempts to cope. The success rate of interpersonal therapy is comparable to that of cognitive behavioral therapy, but it does not work as quickly. Some research (Constantino, Arnow, Blasey, & Agras, 2005) indicates that matching patient characteristics and expectations to therapy intervention improves the success of both cognitive behavioral and interpersonal therapy.

Although the antidepressant fluoxetine (Prozac) is not very effective in treating anorexia, the results for bulimia are more positive (Shapiro et al., 2007). Psychotherapy is a better choice for most patients than drugs alone, but the combination of drugs and psychotherapy may also be a good choice for some bulimic patients.

Therapy for bulimia is usually successful (Keel & Brown, 2010); about 70% of bulimics recover as a result of therapy, and others improve. However, between 11% and 14% do not respond positively to therapy, and these individuals experience continuing problems with bingeing and purging, which may continue for years.

Preventing bulimia would be more desirable than treatment, and some programs attempt to change the attitudes that put people at risk. These programs are aimed at young women with the risk factors of low self-esteem, poor body image, high acceptance of the thin body ideal, a strong need for perfection, a history of repeated dieting, and other dysfunctional eating behaviors or attitudes. Some programs are school based, whereas others target young women at high risk. One typical strategy is psychoeducational, which attempts to change the acceptance of the thin body ideal and boost self-esteem. Adding a weight control component oriented toward building healthy eating while controlling weight has resulted in better success (Stice, Presnell, Groesz, & Shaw, 2005; Stice, Trost, & Chase, 2003). Another successful strategy involves attempting to create dissonance by encouraging participants to critique the thin ideal (Stice, Rohde, Shaw, & Gau, 2011). Thus, programs that address the cognitive component of bulimia and offer a healthy way to manage body concerns may be more successful in averting this disorder.

Binge Eating Disorder

Many people eat too much at times, such as parties or holidays, but binge eating disorder is more than an occasional overindulgence. Binge eating consists of the same type of out-of-control eating that is symptomatic of bulimia, but without any form of purging. Although binge eating did not appear in *DSM-IV*, this category will be designated as a disorder in *DSM-V* (American Psychiatric Association, 2011). To be diagnosed with this disorder, people must exhibit frequent binge eating episodes (an average of at least once a week for at least 3 months) with feelings of a lack of control, and they must experience distress over this behavior.

Becoming Healthier

1. Develop your eating competence (Stotts et al., 2007) by getting good information about nutrition and using that information in deciding on a healthy diet.
2. Give up dieting, but also give up overeating.
3. Consult a chart that contains body mass index rather than a fashion magazine to determine what the correct weight is for you.
4. Be more concerned with eating a healthy diet than with your weight.
5. Concentrate less on food restriction and more on exercise as a way to change your body shape.
6. Do not skip meals as a way to lose weight, especially breakfast; people who eat breakfast are less likely to be overweight than those who skip it (Purslow et al., 2008).
7. Do not compare your body to those of models and actors or actresses. These images furnish unrealistic and unattainable body images that tend to make people unhappy with their own bodies.
8. Understand that losing weight will not solve all your problems.
9. If you lose weight, know when to stop. Listen to people who tell you that you have lost enough.
10. Do not hide how little you weigh from friends or family by wearing baggy clothing.
11. When you make dietary changes, find ways to keep eating a pleasurable activity. Feelings of deprivation and going without favorite foods can make you too miserable to care about eating correctly.
12. Do not use diet drugs, fast, or go on a very low-calorie diet to lose weight, even if you are very obese.
13. Do not vomit as a way to keep from gaining weight.
14. Learn how to see someone who is normal weight or slightly overweight as attractive. Look for such people in the news and in the media.

Who Are Binge Eaters? Eating large quantities of food would seem to be a risk for obesity, and it is (Stice, Presnell, & Spangler, 2002). Many individuals who are obese experience binge eating. An examination of women with eating disorders (Striegel-Moore et al., 2004) revealed that binge eaters had higher BMIs than women with other eating disorders and experienced an even greater degree of body dissatisfaction. Binge eating is common to bulimia and, to a lesser degree, to anorexia; thus, it is not surprising that individuals with any of these eating disorders exhibit similar self-esteem, body dissatisfaction, and weight concerns (Decaluwé & Braet, 2005; Grilo et al., 2008). Alcohol problems are also common to both bulimics and binge eaters (Krahn, Kurth, Gomberg, & Drewnowski, 2005). These symptoms are consistent with Kirstie Alley's behavior and weight battles; she experienced binges that led to her weight gains and once experienced a problem with cocaine abuse (Mock & Wang, 2011).

As with anorexics, binge eaters are more likely to be female than male, but binge eating is more common among men than anorexia or bulimia is (Hudson et al., 2007). The loss of control that characterizes binge eating even occurs among children younger than 12 years old (Tanofsky-Kraff, Marcus, Yanovski, & Yanovski, 2008) and among adolescents (Goldschmidt et al., 2008), representing a major factor in obesity for these age groups. In addition, all ethnic groups are represented, and binge eating occurs in non-Western societies at rates that are similar to those in the United States and Europe (Becker, Burwell, Navara, & Gilman, 2003). Binge eating is also more common than either anorexia or bulimia—the estimated prevalence is at least 2% of the population. As with other eating disorders, most people with symptoms are not diagnosed and thus do not receive treatment.

Like others with eating disorders, people who experience eating binges also tend to have other behavioral or psychiatric problems, which complicate the diagnosis of this disorder (Hilbert et al., 2011; Stunkard & Allison, 2003). Indeed, the presence of personality disorders is one criterion that distinguishes binge eaters from those who are obese but do not binge (van Hanswijck de Jonge, van Furth, Lacey, & Waller, 2003). Table 14.5 presents a comparison of anorexia, bulimia, and binge eating.

TABLE 14.5 Comparison of Anorexia, Bulimia, and Binge Eating

	Anorexia	**Bulimia**	**Binge Eating**
Body weight	<17.5 BMI	Normal	Overweight
Distorted body image	Yes	Yes	Yes
Percent affected			
Women	0.9%	1%–3%	3.5%
Men	0.3%	0.5%	2.0%
Vulnerability			
Gender	Women	Women	Women
Age	Adolescent & young adult	Adolescent & young adult	Adults
Ethnicity	European & European American	All	All
Prominent characteristics	Ambitious, perfectionist, anxiety disorders	Impulsive, sensation-seeking	Personality disorders
Alcohol or drug abuse problems	Not common	Common	Common
Obsessive thoughts	Body fat and control	Food and next binge	Food and next binge
Health risks	3% mortality	Hypoglycemia, anemia, electrolyte imbalance	Obesity
Treatment success	75%; relapse is a risk	80%; relapse is a risk	Good success for binges but weight loss is difficult

Treatment for Binge Eating   Treatments for binge eating face the challenge of changing an established eating pattern plus helping binge eaters lose weight. Cognitive behavioral therapy is effective in helping people control binge eating, but it is not as effective in promoting weight loss (Striegel-Moore et al., 2010; Yager, 2008). Nor are obese binge eaters good candidates for weight loss surgery; this drastic intervention does not help in managing binges (Yager, 2008).

Thus, researchers have searched for a component to add to therapy programs. One consideration was SSRI (selective serotonin reuptake inhibitor) antidepressant drugs, such as fluoxetine (Prozac), which has some use in relieving psychiatric problems. These drugs produce a significant decrease in binge eating (Leombruni et al., 2008) but do not prompt weight loss. Adding the weight loss drug orlistat produced a modest weight loss (Reas & Grilo, 2008); the weight loss drug sibutramine may be more effective (Yager, 2008). However, these results highlight the difficulties of addressing the two problem components that binge eaters encounter.

Perception of the problem also plays a role in treatment for binge eaters. Some people who experience binges seek treatment for the bingeing behavior, whereas others see their main problem as overweight. Those who focus on their binge eating tend to choose cognitive behavioral therapy; those who see their problem as weight are more likely to choose a therapy with that goal (Brody, Masheb, & Grilo, 2005). This type of tailoring is an advantage not only for binge eating but also for many therapies and problems.

IN SUMMARY

Some people begin a weight loss program that seemingly gets out of control and turns into an almost total fasting regimen. This eating disorder, called anorexia nervosa, is uncommon but most prevalent among young, high-achieving women who have high body dissatisfaction and believe that being thin will solve their problems. Anorexia is very difficult to treat successfully because people with this disorder continue to see themselves as too fat and thus resist attempts to change their eating habits. A type of family therapy and cognitive behavioral therapy are more effective than other approaches.

Bulimia is an eating disorder characterized by uncontrolled binge eating, usually accompanied by guilt and followed by vomiting or other purgative methods. In general terms, people with bulimia are more likely than others to be depressed and impulsive, which may lead to alcohol and other drug abuse and stealing. In addition, they are more likely to have been victims of childhood family or sexual abuse, to be dissatisfied with their bodies, and to use food as a coping strategy.

Treatment for bulimia has generally been more successful than treatment for anorexia, partly because of bulimics' greater motivation to change. The more successful programs for eating disorders are those that include cognitive behavioral techniques, which seek to change not only eating patterns but also the pathological concerns about weight and eating, and interpersonal therapy, which focuses on relationship issues. Antidepressant drugs may also be useful in treating bulimia.

Binge eating was not classified as a disorder in *DSM-IV* but will appear in *DSM-V*. Those who experience binges are often overweight or obese and share impulse control and other psychological problems common to those with bulimia. Women are more likely to be binge eaters, but more men have this than any other eating disorder. Treatment faces the problems of altering maladaptive eating patterns and body image problems as well as promoting weight loss. Cognitive behavioral therapy is effective with the former, but losing weight is a difficult problem for binge eaters, as we have seen that it is for others.

Answers

This chapter has addressed six basic questions:

1. How does the digestive system function?

The digestive system turns food into nutrients by breaking down food into particles that can be absorbed. The process of breaking down food begins in the mouth and continues in the stomach, but absorption of most nutrients occurs in the small intestine. A complex signaling system involves hormones produced in the body and brain and received by the hypothalamus and other brain structures to control eating and weight. Hormones such as ghrelin, neuropeptide Y, agouti-related peptide, and melanin-concentrating hormone increase appetite and feelings of hunger, whereas leptin, insulin, cholecystokinin, glucagon-like peptide 1, and peptide YY are involved in satiation.

2. What factors are involved in weight maintenance?

Weight maintenance depends largely on two factors: the number of calories absorbed through food intake and the number expended through body metabolism and physical activity. Experimental starvation has demonstrated that losing weight leads to irritability, aggression, apathy, lack of interest in sex, and preoccupation with food. Initial weight loss may be easy, but the slowing of metabolic rate makes drastic weight loss difficult. Experimental overeating has demonstrated that gaining weight can be almost as difficult and unpleasant as losing it.

3. What is obesity, and how does it affect health?

Obesity can be defined in terms of percent body fat, body mass index, or social standards, all of which yield different estimates for the prevalence of obesity. Over the past 25 years, obesity has become more common in countries around the world, but the ideal body has become thinner in many Western countries. The difficulty of either losing or gaining weight and the discovery of leptin, ghrelin, and other hormones involved in weight regulation are consistent with the notion of a natural setpoint for weight maintenance. Obesity seems to be a deviation from this regulation that has genetic components, but the recent rapid growth of obesity is not compatible with a genetic model. An alternative view holds that positive aspects of eating lead people to overeat when a variety of tasty foods are available, which is the situation in the United States and other high-income countries.

Obesity is associated with increased mortality, heart disease, Type 2 diabetes, and digestive tract diseases, and the very thinnest and the very heaviest people are at the greatest risk for death. Severe obesity and carrying excess weight around the waist rather than hips are both risks of death from several causes, especially heart disease.

4. Is dieting a good way to lose weight?

A cultural obsession with thinness has led to a plethora of diets, many of which are neither safe nor permanently effective. Changing from overeating to healthier eating patterns and incorporating exercise are wise choices for weight change, whereas liposuction, diet drugs, fasting, and very low-calorie diets are not.

5. What is anorexia nervosa, and how can it be treated?

Anorexia nervosa is an eating disorder characterized by self-starvation. This disorder is most prevalent among young, high-achieving women with body image problems, but anorexia is uncommon, affecting less than 1% of the population. Anorexics are very difficult to treat successfully because they continue to see themselves as too fat and thus lack the motivation to change their eating habits. Cognitive behavioral therapy and a specific type of family therapy are more effective than other approaches.

6. What is bulimia, and how does it differ from binge eating?

Bulimia is an eating disorder characterized by uncontrolled binge eating, usually accompanied by guilt and followed by vomiting or other purgative methods. Bulimia is more common than anorexia, affecting between 1% and 3% of the population. Their motivation to change eating patterns has made bulimics better therapy candidates than anorexics. Treatment for bulimia, especially cognitive behavioral therapy and interpersonal therapy, has generally been successful.

Binge eating is similar to bulimia in terms of binges, but binge eaters do not purge. Thus, they are often overweight or obese, whereas bulimics tend to be normal weight. Binge eating is also more common than bulimia, especially among men. The two disorders are similar in terms of impulsivity, history of family violence, and coexisting personality disorders. Binge eating is more difficult to treat because therapy must address both binge eating and weight problems.

Suggested Readings

Brownell, K. D., & Horgen, K. B. (2004). *Food fight: The inside story of the food industry, America's obesity crisis, and what we can do about it.* New York: McGraw-Hill. In this controversial book, Kelly Brownell and Katherine Horgen contend that obesity is the result not of a lack of willpower but of a "toxic food environment" created by the food industry.

Hurley, D. (2011, June). The hungry brain. *Discover*, *32*(5), 53–59. Hurley's readable story reviews research on the complexities of the physiology and neurochemistry of eating and obesity.

Polivy, J., & Herman, C. P. (2004). Sociocultural idealization of thin female body shapes: An introduction to the special issues on body image and eating disorders. *Journal of Social and Clinical Psychology*, 23, 1–6. These prominent researchers provide an interesting perspective on eating and eating disorders that summarizes the findings of articles from a special issue devoted to this topic.

Popkin, B. (2009). *The world is fat: The fads, trends, policies, and products that are fattening the human race*. New York: Avery/Penguin. Barry Popkin takes a worldwide view of eating and obesity, examining how obesity has become a more urgent problem than hunger.

CHAPTER 15

Exercising

CHAPTER OUTLINE

- **Real–World Profile of Tara Costa**
- *Types of Physical Activity*
- *Reasons for Exercising*
- *Physical Activity and Cardiovascular Health*
- *Other Health Benefits of Physical Activity*
- *Hazards of Physical Activity*
- *How Much Is Enough but Not Too Much?*
- *Improving Adherence to Physical Activity*

QUESTIONS

This chapter focuses on six basic questions:

1. What are the different types of physical activity?

2. Does physical activity benefit the cardiovascular system?

✔CHECK YOUR HEALTH RISKS

Regarding Exercise and Physical Activity

1. Whenever the urge to exercise comes over me, I sit down until the urge goes away.

2. My family history of heart disease means that I am going to have a heart attack whether I exercise or not.

3. When it comes to exercise, I subscribe to the motto "No pain, no gain."

4. I have changed jobs in order to have more time to train for competitive athletic events.

5. I use exercise along with diet as a means of controlling my weight.

6. People have advised me to start an exercise program, but I just never seem to have the time or energy.

7. One of the reasons I exercise is that I believe that a person can't be too thin and that exercise will help me continue to lose weight.

8. I may begin an exercise program when I'm older, but now I'm young and in good shape.

9. I'm too old and out of shape to begin exercising.

10. I'd probably have a heart attack if I started to jog or run.

11. I'd like to exercise, but I can't run, and walking isn't strenuous enough to be good exercise.

12. I try not to let injuries interfere with my regular exercise routine.

Except for item 5, each of these items represents a health risk from either too little or too much exercise. Count your checkmarks to evaluate your risks. As you read this chapter, you will learn that some of these items are riskier than others.

Real–World Profile of
TARA COSTA

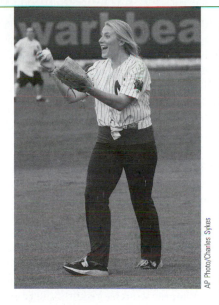

AP Photo/Charles Sykes

The Ironman Triathlon is one of the most grueling competitions in the world. Not only do competitors run a marathon—which, in itself is a feat—but they bicycle for 112 miles and swim for 2.4 miles *before* they run the marathon. Completing an Ironman Triathlon is a source of pride for even the most avid of fitness enthusiasts.

On October 8, 2011, Tara Costa completed her first Ironman Triathlon with a total time of 13 hours and 56 minutes. Why was the performance of this 26-year-old woman so impressive?

Three years earlier, Tara was not physically active and was severely obese, weighing in at 294 pounds. To get into shape, Tara took an extreme measure: She joined the cast of the 7th season of the American television show *The Biggest Loser*. Contestants on *The Biggest Loser* spend close to 6 hours a day in strenuous exercise, spurred on by a team of "in-your-face" fitness coaches, the pressure of being on national television, and the chance to win a huge cash prize.

These pressures would make nearly anyone committed to a fitness regimen. However, Tara impressed her audience by setting the show's record for winning the most physical challenges of any contestant ever on the show. In doing so, Tara inspired millions of viewers with her spirit and determination. After 8 months on *The Biggest Loser*, Tara lost over half of her body weight, with a combination of dietary change and a strenuous regimen of physical activity. This dramatic weight loss—as well as the intensity of Tara's fitness regimen—is extreme. Tara now seeks to maintain this state of fitness, for example, by competing in the New York City Marathon and the Ironman Triathlon.

I n becoming more physically active, Tara Costa likely reduced her risk for a number of health problems. However, her exercise regimen was grueling and her weight loss was extreme. While shows like *The Biggest Loser* pressure people toward dramatic weight losses, critics warn of the dangers of losing weight so quickly. Furthermore, many contestants on shows like *The Biggest Loser* risk falling back into old habits once the pressures and supports of the show go away.

In this chapter, we discuss the importance of physical activity in maintaining a healthy lifestyle, the benefits and risks of increasing physical activity, and provide examples of interventions that may help the rest of us—that is, people who are not stars on the *The Biggest Loser*—successfully initiate and maintain a program of physical activity.

Types of Physical Activity

Although exercise can include hundreds of different kinds of physical activities, physiologically there are only five types of exercise: isometric, isotonic, isokinetic, anaerobic, and aerobic. Each has different goals, different activities, and different advocates. Each can contribute to some aspect of fitness or health, but only aerobic exercise produces benefits for cardiorespiratory health.

Isometric exercise involves contracting muscles against an immovable object. Although the body does not move in isometric exercise, muscles push hard against each other or against an immovable object and thus produce increases in strength. Pushing hard against a solid wall is an example of isometric exercise. This type of physical activity can improve muscle strength, which can be especially important for older people in preserving independent living.

Isotonic exercise requires the contraction of muscles and the movement of joints. Weight lifting and many forms of calisthenics fit into this category. Programs based on isotonic exercise can improve muscle strength and muscle endurance if the program is sufficiently lengthy. Again, older people can profit from isotonic exercise, but many people in a weight-lifting program are bodybuilders interested in improving the appearance of their body rather than improving health.

Isokinetic exercise is similar to isotonic exercise, except that isokinetic exercise involves exerting effort to move muscles and joints against a variable amount

of resistance. This type of exercise requires specialized equipment that adjusts the amount of resistance according to the amount of force applied. People who suffer muscle injuries often receive prescriptions to perform isokinetic exercise as a way to restore muscle strength and endurance. Isokinetic exercise is an important adjunct in physical rehabilitation, helping injured people to regain strength and flexibility with more safety than other types of exercise.

Anaerobic exercises require short, intensive bursts of energy but no increased amount of oxygen use. This form of exercise includes short-distance running, some calisthenics, softball, and other exercises that require intense, short-term energy. Such exercises improve speed and endurance, but they may carry risks for people with coronary heart disease.

Aerobic exercise is any exercise that requires dramatically increased oxygen consumption over an extended period of time. Aerobic exercise includes jogging, walking at a brisk pace, cross-country skiing, dancing, rope skipping, swimming, cycling, and other activities that increase oxygen consumption.

The important characteristics of aerobic exercise are intensity and duration. Exercise must be intense enough to elevate the heart rate into a certain range, based on a person's age and maximum possible heart rate. This type of program requires elevated oxygen use and provides a workout for both the respiratory system, which furnishes the oxygen, and the coronary system, which pumps the blood. Of the various approaches to fitness, aerobic activity is superior to other types of exercise in developing cardiorespiratory health.

Current recommendations call for a person to engage in some aerobic exercise at least three times a week. However, any aerobic exercise is better than none.

Reasons for Exercising

People exercise for a variety of reasons, some that are consistent with good health and some that are not. Reasons for adhering to a physical activity program include physical fitness, weight control, cardiovascular health, increased longevity, protection against cancer, prevention of osteoporosis, control of diabetes, better cognitive functioning, and as a buffer against depression, anxiety, and stress. This chapter looks at evidence relating to each of these reasons as well as to the potential hazards of physical activity.

Physical Fitness

Does physical activity help people become physically fit? The effects of exercise on fitness depend both on the duration and intensity of the exercise and on the definition of fitness. To most exercise physiologists, fitness is a complex condition consisting of muscle strength, muscle endurance, flexibility, and cardiorespiratory (aerobic) fitness. Each of the five types of exercise can contribute to these four different aspects of fitness, but no one type fulfills all the requirements.

In addition, fitness has both organic and dynamic aspects. *Organic fitness* is the capacity for action and movement that is determined by inherent characteristics of the body. These organic factors include genetic endowment, age, and health limitations. *Dynamic fitness* arises through physical activity, whereas organic fitness does not. A person can have a good level of organic fitness and yet be "out of shape" and perform poorly. Another person may train and improve dynamic fitness but still be unable to win races because of relatively poor organic fitness. Athletes who want to be champions need to have been very selective about choosing their biological parents in order to have inherited a high level of organic fitness. Aspiring champions must train in order to gain the dynamic fitness necessary for optimal athletic performance. Michael Phelps, who broke records for swimming in the 2008 Olympics, had an excellent balance of organic and dynamic fitness—he inherited a body suited to swimming, but he needed to work hard to break records. The rest of this chapter deals almost exclusively with dynamic fitness and its components, because this type of fitness arises from exercise, whereas organic fitness does not.

Muscle Strength and Endurance

Two components of physical fitness are muscle strength and muscle endurance. Muscle strength is a measure of how strongly a muscle can contract. This type of fitness can come from isometric, isotonic, isokinetic, and to a lesser extent, anaerobic exercise. All these types of exercise have the capability to increase muscle strength because they involve contracting muscles.

Muscle endurance differs from muscle strength in that it requires continued performance. Some strength is necessary for muscle endurance, but the opposite is not true: A muscle may be strong but not have the endurance to continue its performance. Exercises that improve strength require greater exertion for limited repetitions; exercises that improve endurance require less exertion but more frequent repetition (Knuttgen, 2007). Both muscle strength and muscle endurance improve through similar types of exercises, including isometric, isotonic, and isokinetic.

Flexibility

Flexibility is the range-of-motion capacity of a joint. The types of exercises that develop muscle strength and muscle endurance generally do not improve flexibility. Moreover, flexibility is specific to each joint, so that exercises designed to develop flexibility are varied. In addition to being a component of fitness, flexibility also decreases the likelihood of injury in other types of physical activity, especially aerobic and anaerobic exercise.

Slow and sustained stretching exercises promote muscle flexibility. In contrast, fast, jerky, bouncing movements cause muscle soreness and injury. Flexibility training is typically not as intense as strength and endurance training. Yoga and tai chi provide the types of movements that increase flexibility.

Aerobic Fitness

Of all the types of physical activity, aerobic exercise contributes most to cardiorespiratory fitness. When people acquire aerobic fitness, they improve cardiorespiratory health in several ways. First, they increase the amount of oxygen available during strenuous exercise, and second, they increase the amount of blood pumped with each heartbeat. These changes result in a lowering of both resting heart rate and resting blood pressure and increase the efficiency of the cardiovascular system (Cooper, 2001). This type of exercise helps protect both men and women from heart disease and a variety of other diseases (Murphy, Nevill, Murtagh, & Holder, 2007).

Weight Control

Obesity continues to be a worldwide problem. Many people adopt a sedentary lifestyle, spending much of their time watching television, viewing videos, playing computer games, surfing the Internet, and talking on cell phones. There is a link between these two phenomena, as research shows that physical activity contributes to weight control.

Most experts see obesity as a long-term accumulation of excess body fat (Forbes, 2000; Hansen, Shriver, & Schoeller, 2005). Obesity can arise over time, when a person's dietary caloric intake exceeds his or her expenditure of energy through physical activity. However, the level of exercise needed for cardiovascular health is not necessarily the same as that needed for weight control.

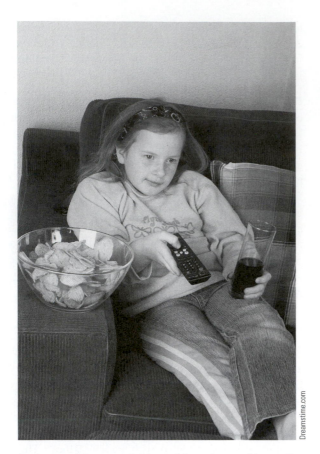

Dreamstime.com

Sedentary leisure activities add to the problem of childhood obesity.

For example, 15 minutes of walking or cycling to and from work can be enough to reduce both cardiovascular mortality and all-cause mortality (Barengo et al., 2004). However, the amount of exercise necessary to prompt weight loss is far greater. Some authorities (Hill & Wyatt, 2005; Jakicic & Otto, 2005) recommend that obese people need to spend at least 60 minutes a day engaged in moderate to heavy physical activity to bring about initial weight loss and to maintain that loss. Thus, longer and more intense physical activity is required for long-lasting weight control, which exceeds the amount of physical activity needed for cardiovascular health.

Exercise can also serve as a means for sculpting an ideal body shape. Unfortunately, exercise is limited as a method of spot reduction. Muscle and fat have little to do with one another, and a person can have both in the same part of the body. If people exercise during weight reduction, they build muscle tissue while losing fat, which may build a more attractive body shape. Spot reduction appears to be the result because fat tends to be lost from the places where it was most abundant. However, fat distribution is under strong genetic control, and people with large hips or thighs in relation to other body parts will have large hips or thighs after they lose weight. Despite some exercise promoters' claims, a particular calisthenic exercise will not reduce fat in a specific part of the body.

Inactive people who are concerned about weight and who have recently stopped smoking should strongly consider beginning a physical activity program. Steven Blair and Tim Church (2004) claimed that such an exercise program would be at least as effective as dieting in controlling weight and much better than dieting in changing the ratio of fat to muscle tissue. An early study supported this view. Investigators randomly assigned sedentary, obese men to one of three groups: dieters, runners, or controls (Wood et al., 1988). The dieters did not exercise, the runners did not diet, and the controls did neither. After a year, people in both the exercise group and the dieting group had lost about the same amount of weight, and both of these groups had lost more than people in the control group. However, some important differences emerged in comparing the dieters and the runners. Although both groups had lost an equal amount of weight, the dieters lost both fat and lean tissue, whereas the runners lost only fat tissue and retained more lean muscle tissue.

Exercise does not produce much weight loss through burning calories; for example, more than 30 minutes of tennis is required to work off the calories in two doughnuts. However, sitting and eating doughnuts is a risk for obesity in two ways—the sitting and the eating. Rather, most of the weight loss associated with exercise comes from elevation of the metabolic rate, the rate at which the body metabolizes calories. The resulting increase in the number of calories burned can produce changes in weight that exceed the number of calories spent in any activity.

IN SUMMARY

Five basic categories subsume all forms of physical activity: isometric, isotonic, isokinetic, anaerobic, and aerobic. Each of these five exercise types has advantages and disadvantages for improving physical fitness, but only aerobic exercise benefits cardiorespiratory health.

People have a variety of reasons for maintaining an exercise regimen, including physical fitness, aerobic health, and weight control. The various types of exercise can increase dynamic fitness, strengthen muscles, improve endurance, and increase flexibility. Aerobic fitness reduces death not only from cardiovascular disease but also from all causes.

One popular reason for remaining physically active is to control weight and achieve a sculpted body. Physical activity can help people lose weight, but its capacity for spot reduction is very limited. Overweight people can lose weight through moderate physical activity, highly active thin people can maintain lean body mass through proper diet, and people of moderate weight can increase lean body weight without an overall weight gain.

Physical Activity and Cardiovascular Health

Nowadays, most people recognize the health benefits of physical activity. This knowledge, however, did not exist until relatively recently. During the early years of the 20th century, physicians often advised patients with heart disease to avoid strenuous physical activity, based on the belief that too much physical activity could damage the heart and threaten a person's life. (Figure 9.7 in Chapter 9 paints a dramatic picture of the rise and fall of death rates from cardiovascular disease throughout the 20th century.) During the middle of the 20th century, some cardiologists rethought this advice and recommended aerobic exercise both as an adjunct to standard treatment and as a protection against heart disease. Later in this section, we describe the cardiovascular benefits of exercise, but first we look briefly at the history of studies that examined exercise and cardiovascular health.

Early Studies

Jeremy Morris and his colleagues (Morris, Heady, Raffle, Roberts, & Parks, 1953) made history with their observation of a link between physical activity and cardiovascular disease. This observation took place in England and involved London's famous double-decker buses. Morris and his colleagues discovered that physically active male conductors differed from the sedentary drivers in their incidence of heart disease. Ten years later, Harold Kahn (1963) investigated the relationship between physical activity and heart disease among postal workers in Washington, D.C. Kahn found lower coronary heart disease (CHD) death rates among the physically active men. These studies, of course, did not prove that physical activity decreased the risk of CHD, because the high- and low-activity workers may also have differed on the basis of body type, personality, or some other factor associated with a high or low risk of CHD.

Ralph Paffenbarger, a professor of epidemiology at Stanford University School of Medicine and the Harvard School of Public Health, built upon this earlier work with the publication of several landmark studies on the relationship between physical activity and CHD. The first studies followed a group of San Francisco longshoremen in 1951 and tracked CHD deaths over time (Paffenbarger, Gima, Laughlin, & Black, 1971; Paffenbarger, Laughlin, Gima, & Black, 1970). In general, they found that CHD death rates were much higher for workers with low versus high activity. In these studies, all workers in both the high- and low-activity groups had begun their employment with at least 5 years of strenuous cargo handling; thus, all workers were likely in good shape at the start of the study. Yet, physical activity level emerged as a significant predictor of subsequent risk for CHD death.

In the late 1970s, Paffenbarger and his associates (Paffenbarger, Wing, & Hyde, 1978) published a landmark epidemiological study based on extensive medical records of former Harvard University students, their weekly total energy expenditure, and a composite physical activity index that took into account all activity, both on and off the job. With this data, Paffenbarger and his colleagues divided the Harvard alumni into high- and low-activity groups. Of those men whose energy levels could be determined, about 60% expended fewer than 2,000 kcal per week and placed in the low-activity group; the 40% who expended more than 2,000 kcal made up the high-activity group. (Note that 2,000 kcal of energy is approximately that expended in 20 miles of jogging or its equivalent.) The results showed that the least active Harvard alumni had an increased risk of heart attack over their more physically active classmates, with 2,000 kcal per week as the breaking point. In addition, exercise benefited men who smoked, had a history of hypertension, or both. Beyond the 2,000 kcal per week expenditure, increased exercise paid no dividends in terms of

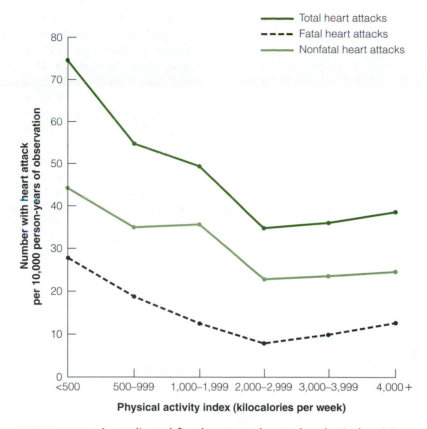

FIGURE 15.1   Age-adjusted first heart attack rates by physical activity index in a 6- to 10-year follow-up of male Harvard alumni.

Source: Adapted from "Physical activity as an index of heart attack risk in college alumni," by R. S. Paffenbarger, Jr., A. L. Wing, and R. T. Hyde, 1978, *American Journal of Epidemiology, 108,* p. 166. Copyright © 1978 by The Johns Hopkins University School of Hygiene and Public Health. Reprinted by permission of Oxford University Press.

reduced risk of fatal or nonfatal heart attacks. Figure 15.1 shows this relationship.

Later Studies

Dozens of more recent studies have examined the relationship between physical activity and cardiovascular mortality. A systematic review of these studies shows that physical activity confers a 35% reduction in risk of death due to cardiovascular causes (Nocon et al., 2008). The same review concludes that physical activity confers a 33% reduction in risk of death due to all causes. Furthermore, both men and women benefit from physical activity, but risk reductions may be larger for women than for men (Nocon et al., 2008).

Evidence also shows cardiovascular benefits among people in a variety of nations and different ethnic groups. For example, many Mexican Americans are at risk for obesity, high cholesterol, and other cardiovascular risk factors, which suggests that they can probably profit from a routine exercise program. A study of Mexican Americans in the San Antonio Heart Study (Rainwater et al., 2000) found that changes in physical activity over a 5-year period tended to mirror changes in cardiovascular disease (CVD) risk factors.

Thus, it is unmistakably clear that physical activity protects against CVD (Myers, 2000; Nocon et al., 2008; Schlicht, Kanning, & Bös, 2007). First, people who are already active receive some gains by increasing their level of activity, but the largest gains occur when people go from a sedentary lifestyle to an active one. Second, walking, especially for older people, confers protection against CVD (Murphy et al., 2007). Third, an inactive lifestyle is equal to diabetes, high cholesterol level,

smoking, and high blood pressure as a CVD risk factor. Fourth, physically fit men and women in all age groups can reduce their CVD risk through leisure-time activities. Fifth, exercise accumulated several years ago does not provide much current protection against all-cause mortality. Similarly, people who survive a heart attack and who include physical activity as part of their cardiac rehabilitation program decrease their all-cause mortality as well as their risk for a subsequent heart attack. However, those benefits disappear after 5 years if participants stop exercising. Thus, because previous physical activity loses its benefit after a few years, heart attack survivors should maintain their exercise program.

Exercise also offers protection against stroke. Researchers from the Nurses' Health Study (Hu et al., 2000) found that the most active women, compared with sedentary women, reduced their risk of death from ischemic stroke by about 34%, compared with sedentary women. Furthermore, there was a dose–response relationship between levels of physical activity and protection from ischemic stroke. Individuals who had a stroke were less physically active than others, including less physical activity in the week preceding their stroke (Krarup et al., 2007). Similarly, a meta-analysis (Wendel-Vos et al., 2004) found that high levels of occupational and leisure-time physical activity reduce the risk of both ischemic stroke and hemorrhagic stroke.

These and other reports on cardiovascular disease suggest that a lifestyle that includes at least some physical activity can help protect people against premature cardiovascular disease, including stroke. Even small amounts of activity can help, but more is better, at least to a point. (In a later section, we discuss how much is enough without being too much.)

Do Women and Men Benefit Equally?

All the early studies on the cardiovascular effects of exercise had one important limitation: They focused exclusively on men. To complete the picture of the health benefits of exercise, later researchers extended their investigations to women. Gender differences in degree of physical activity, leisure-time activity, and job-related activity might suggest differences between men and women in their level of protection against cardiovascular disease and all-cause mortality.

Do the benefits of physical activity extend to women as well as men? Paffenbarger and his associates (Oguma, Sesso, Paffenbarger, & Lee, 2002) looked at 37 prospective cohort studies and one retrospective study that dealt with the association between all-cause mortality and both physical activity and physical fitness in women. The results indicated that women can gain about as much as men from physical activity, a finding confirmed in a more recent review (Nocon et al., 2008). Inactive women were much more likely than active women to have died during the study period. An energy expenditure of about 1,000 kilocalories per week (equivalent to approximately 10 miles of jogging) is probably adequate to avoid premature death. (See Figure 15.1 for a relationship between level of kilocalories and first heart attack in men.)

In summary, both women and men can improve their cardiovascular health and live longer with light to moderate exercise. Physically active people can expect an average increase in longevity of about 2 years (Blair, Cheng, & Holder, 2001). A cynic might note that a person would need to jog a total of about 2 years between the ages of 20 and 80 to increase longevity by 2 years. Why live another 2 years if one must spend that time exercising? However, physical activity does more than simply add quantity to a person's life span; it adds *quality* to those years as well, by improving well-being, mental health, and cognitive functioning (as we will discuss later in this chapter).

Physical Activity and Cholesterol Levels

How does exercise protect against cardiovascular disease? Exercise increases high-density lipoprotein (HDL, or "good" cholesterol) while decreasing LDL ("bad" cholesterol; Hausenloy & Yellen, 2008). The combination of raising HDL and lowering LDL may leave total cholesterol the same, but the ratio of total cholesterol to HDL becomes more favorable, and the risk for heart disease decreases. Thus, physical activity can benefit cardiac patients in two ways: by lowering LDL and by raising HDL (Szapary, Bloedon, & Foster, 2003).

Moderate levels of exercise, with or without dietary changes, bring about a favorable ratio of total cholesterol to HDL. Reviews of studies from the Toronto symposium (Leon & Sanchez, 2001; Williams, 2001) generally found that moderate exercise, such as walking and

gardening, increases HDL and less frequently decreases both LDL and triglycerides. The combination of a low-fat diet and exercise is even more effective (Varady & Jones, 2005). Thus, moderate activity may lead to a more favorable ratio of total cholesterol to HDL, but prolonged strenuous physical activity does not seem to confer additional protection against heart disease; that is, there is inconsistent evidence for a dose–response relationship between levels of physical activity and death from heart disease (Leon & Sanchez, 2001).

If adults can improve their lipid numbers through moderate exercise, could children and adolescents also benefit from regular physical activity? Identifying the link between fitness and cardiovascular risk factors in children is difficult, as many children and adolescents who are sedentary are also overweight or obese. Despite this challenge, low fitness is related to high cholesterol levels and other cardiovascular risk factors for children in Europe (Andersen et al., 2008) and the United States (Eisenmann, Welk, Wickel, & Blair, 2007). Programs to improve these risk factors typically include both weight loss and exercise, yielding little research that evaluates only the influence of physical activity on cardiovascular risk factors (Kelley & Kelley, 2007).

In general, physically active children can profit from exercise, but probably not as much as adults (Tolfrey, 2004). However, children as young as 4 can profit from an enhanced exercise program (Sääkslahti et al., 2004). This research looked at 4- to 7-year-old children and found that both girls and boys with highly active play time had low levels of total cholesterol, high levels of HDL cholesterol, and a favorable ratio between total cholesterol and high-density lipoprotein cholesterol. A study of preadolescent and early adolescent children showed results similar to studies with adults; that is, exercise seems to lower LDL while raising HDL and leaving total cholesterol basically unchanged (Tolfrey, Jones, & Campbell, 2000). Regular aerobic exercise may protect against heart disease in both adults and children by increasing HDL and by improving the ratio of total cholesterol to HDL.

IN SUMMARY

Accumulating evidence suggests that physical activity reduces the incidence of coronary heart disease. Early research had many flaws and tended to include only men. However, more recent research confirms a strong association between a regimen of moderate physical activity and cardiovascular health, including heart disease and stroke. In addition, physical activity can raise HDL, thereby improving the ratio of total cholesterol to high-density lipoprotein. As a result, regular activity may add as much as 2 years to one's life while decreasing disability, especially in later years.

Other Health Benefits of Physical Activity

Although most people who exercise do so for physical fitness, weight control, or cardiovascular health, other benefits accrue to those who adopt a physical activity regimen, including protection against some kinds of cancer, prevention of bone density loss, control of diabetes, and improved psychological health.

Protection Against Cancer

Several reviews (Miles, 2007; Thune & Furberg, 2001) examine the connection between physical activity and various cancers. Of the hundreds of studies evaluated, most focused on cancers of the colon and rectum, breast, endometrium, prostate, and lung. Physical activity offers protection against each of these types of cancer, with the strongest evidence for colorectal and breast cancer. The protective effects for colorectal cancer seem as strong for women as for men (Wolin, Yan, Colditz, & Lee, 2009), and exercise appears to protect postmenopausal more than premenopausal women from breast cancer (Friedenreich & Cust, 2008). Furthermore, exercise may be more likely to protect non-Caucasian women against breast cancer better than Caucasian women (Friedenreich & Cust, 2008). Results from a meta-analysis (Tardon et al., 2005) are consistent with the systematic reviews, suggesting that moderate to high levels of physical activity reduce incidence of lung cancer in both women and men, but the relationship is stronger for women.

How does physical activity lower risk for cancer? Although the answer is unclear, physical activity may do so by influencing tumor initiation and growth (Rogers, Colbert, Greiner, Perkins, & Hursting, 2008). Furthermore, physical activity affects proinflammatory cytokines, which are involved in the development of both cardiovascular disease (Stewart et al., 2007) and

cancer. Thus, research has not only established the protective benefits of physical activity for cancer but also has begun to show how those benefits may occur.

Exercise may also be helpful for people with cancer. Cancer patients undergoing chemotherapy benefit from physical activity training by increasing strength, aerobic fitness, and weight (Quist et al., 2006). A systematic review (Speck, Courneya, Masse, Duval, & Schmitz, 2010) also indicates that exercise helps manage the fatigue that often accompanies cancer treatment. Thus, physical activity is effective in preventing several types of cancer and is helpful in managing some of the distressing side effects of cancer treatment.

Prevention of Bone Density Loss

Exercise also protects against **osteoporosis**, a disorder characterized by a reduction in bone density due to calcium loss that results in brittle bones. Physical activity can protect both men and women against loss of bone mineral density (BMD), especially those who were active during their youth. Bone minerals accrue during childhood and early adolescence, and activity during those years may be especially important for bone health (Hind & Burrows, 2007). For example, one comparison of retired athletes and a comparison group found that the former athletes retained more BMD and had fewer fractures at age 60 than those who had not been athletes.

Both men and women can benefit from high-impact exercise such as running and jumping. However, this type of exercise may leave people (especially older individuals) vulnerable to injuries. We discuss these and other injuries later in this chapter, but as the Would You Believe …? box explains, both older and young people benefit from exercise. An experimental study (Vainionpää, Korpelainen, Leppäluoto, & Jämsä, 2005) indicated that young, premenopausal women in the experimental (high-impact) group had significantly higher bone mineral density than young women in the control group. However, an intervention featuring walking (Palombaro, 2005) and another using tai chi (Wayne et al., 2007) did not demonstrate effectiveness as clearly as the program with higher-impact exercise (Zehnacker & Bemis-Dougherty, 2007).

Control of Diabetes

Because obesity is a factor in Type 2 diabetes and because exercise is an established means of controlling weight, it follows that physical activity may be a useful weapon in the control of diabetes. Systematic reviews of research on this topic confirm the benefits of exercise for improvement of insulin resistance (Plasqui & Westerterp, 2007), for prevention of Type 2 diabetes (Jeon, Lokken, Hu, & van Dam, 2007), and for the management of this condition (Kavookjian, Elswick, & Whetsel, 2007). Thus, the benefits of exercise for Type 2 diabetes are well established.

Does physical activity protect Type 1 diabetics? A meta-analysis of behavior change interventions (Conn et al., 2008) shows that exercise is an important component in managing Type 1 diabetes. Physically active adolescents with Type 1 diabetes exhibit lower cardiovascular risk factors than those who are less active (Herbst, Kordonouri, Schwab, Schmidt, & Holl, 2007). Although these studies reported a modest protective benefit for physical activity, they do not suggest that exercise is a panacea for the control of diabetes. Nevertheless, they do indicate that physical activity can be a useful component in the treatment of insulin-dependent diabetes and can offer some protection against the development of non-insulin-dependent diabetes.

Psychological Benefits of Physical Activity

As stated earlier, physical activity increases not only the quantity of life, but also its quality. The gains from regular physical activity extend to psychological benefits, including a defense against depression, a reduction of anxiety, a buffer against stress, and a contributor to better cognitive functioning. People who exercise list psychological reasons nearly as often as physiological ones when asked about the benefits they receive from exercise. Does the evidence support these claims?

In general, the link between physical activity and psychological functioning is less clearly established than the link between physical activity and physiological health. In addition, any evaluation of the therapeutic effects of exercise on psychological disorders must consider the problems raised by the placebo effect. For this reason, quality research is difficult, and some areas lack adequate research to evaluate the effects (Larun, Nordheim, Ekeland, Hagen, & Heian, 2006). Nevertheless, evidence suggests that a regular exercise regimen can decrease depression, reduce anxiety, buffer stress, and improve cognitive functioning.

Would You BELIEVE...? It's Never Too Late—or Too Early

Physical activity is a healthy habit, but would you believe that it's never too late in the life span to start exercising? Or too early?

Older adults benefit from being physically active in many ways. Cardiovascular benefits include lower blood pressure, improved symptoms of congestive heart failure, and decreased risk for cardiovascular disease (Karani, McLaughlin, & Cassel, 2001). In addition, physically active older adults have lower risk for diabetes, osteoporosis, osteoarthritis, and depression. All of these benefits result in lowered sickness and death among physically active older adults (Everett, Kinser, & Ramsey, 2007).

Despite these many benefits, 56% of Americans over age 75 are sedentary (USCB, 2011). People tend to become less active as they age, and they also reduce their exercising when they experience pain (Nied & Franklin, 2002). For example, arthritis causes knee and hip joint pain that makes older people less willing to exercise. Also, people who have had a stroke may experience balance or weakness problems that make them feel uneasy about even normal levels of activity. Older people are more likely than younger ones to fall, and resulting broken bones may make a permanent change in their mobility

and independence. Although all of these concerns have some foundation, the risks are manageable. Physical activity offers more benefits than risks for older people, even for those over age 85 and for those who are frail. They may need supervision for their exercise, but older adults benefit from physical activity. Exercise such as tai chi even helps quell fears and risks of falling (Sattin, Easley, Wolf, Chen, & Kutner, 2005; Zijlstra et al., 2007). Almost all older people can decrease health risks and gain mobility from exercising.

It's also never too early to begin an active lifestyle. Physical activity furnishes lifetime benefits, and even young children benefit. Very young children may not seem to be at any risk from inactivity, but they are. To maintain their goals of safety and convenience, parents and caregivers often confine infants in strollers, infant seats, or playpens that limit their movement (National Association for Sport and Physical Education, 2002). These experiences not only limit mobility during infancy but may also delay developmental goals such as crawling and walking. Lack of physical activity during toddlerhood can lead to a sedentary childhood. Inactive children may also lag in developing motor skills and join the

growing number of overweight and obese children in the United States (Floriani & Kennedy, 2008).

The National Association for Sport and Physical Education (NASPE, 2002) proposed guidelines for physical activity, beginning during infancy. For all children, NASPE emphasized supervision and safety. The recommendations for infants included allowing them to experience settings in which they can move while maintaining safety, and playing a variety of games such as peekaboo and hide-and-seek. NASPE recommended at least 30 minutes a day of structured physical activity for toddlers, and 60 minutes for preschool children. Scott Roberts (2002) went a step further, recommending workouts for children. He argued that the prohibitions against weight lifting and other types of strength training for children have no research basis. On the contrary, Roberts maintained that children experience the same benefits from this type of exercise as do adults, including protection against cardiovascular disease, hypertension, and obesity as well as improved strength, flexibility, and posture.

Remember, physical activity brings lifetime benefits, so it's never too early—or too late—to begin a lifetime exercise program.

Decreased Depression   The *Diagnostic and Statistical Manual of Mental Disorders* (4th edition, text revision [*DSM-IV-TR*]) of the American Psychiatric Association (APA, 2000) defines a major depressive episode as "a period of at least 2 weeks during which there is either depressed mood or the loss of interest or pleasure in nearly all activities" (p. 349). During a lifetime, as many as 25% of women and 12% of men may suffer from major

depression (APA, 2000). If physical activity can relieve major depression, then millions of people can benefit from a therapy that is easily available to nearly everyone.

People who exercise regularly are generally less depressed than sedentary people (Martinsen, 2008). When researchers compare groups of exercisers with groups of sedentary people on different measures of depression, they find that highly active people are usually less depressed. One possible explanation is that, rather than improve mood, exercising may be restricted to healthy people. Depressed people may simply be less motivated to exercise.

Experimental studies aim to determine the direction of causation. For example, one randomized controlled trial (Annesi, 2005) divided moderately depressed individuals into an experimental group that performed 10 weeks of moderate physical activity three times a week for 20 to 30 minutes and a control group that did not exercise. Clear differences emerged between the two groups, with those who exercised experiencing much lower levels of depression than participants in the control group. Furthermore, a similar research design (Dunn, Trivedi, Kampert, Clark, & Chambliss, 2005) found evidence for a dose–response relationship between physical activity and relief from depressive symptomatology.

Exercise is certainly more effective than no treatment and may be comparable to cognitive therapy (Donaghy, 2007) or antidepressant medication (Daley, 2008). The long-term effects of physical activity on depression, however, have not been substantiated. Nevertheless, an evaluation of the significance of exercise programs (Rethorst, Wipfli, & Landers, 2007) determined that such programs produced not only statistically significant differences but also clinically significant effects. In summarizing the effects of physical activity on depression, Rod Dishman (2003) emphasized the benefits. Dishman explained: "I am not proposing that exercise is a replacement for psychotherapy or drug therapy, but these findings about exercise are not trivial and suggest that physical activity may be an important addition or complement to standard treatment for mild depression" (p. 45).

Reduced Anxiety Many people report that they exercise to feel more relaxed and less anxious. Does exercise play a role in anxiety reduction? The answer may depend on the type of anxiety under study. **Trait anxiety** is a general personality characteristic or trait that manifests itself as a more or less constant feeling of dread or uneasiness. **State anxiety** is a temporary, affective condition that stems from a specific situation. Feelings of worry or concern over a final examination or a job interview are examples of state anxiety. Physiological changes such as increased perspiration and heart rate typically accompany this type of anxiety.

Research on the effects of physical activity on state anxiety suffers from many of the same methodological limitations as research on physical activity and depression; that is, only a few of the studies have had an adequate number of participants and have used random assignment to experimental and control groups (Dunn, Trivedi, & O'Neal, 2001). A meta-analysis of randomized controlled trials (Wipfli, Rethorst, & Landers, 2008) indicated that exercise is more effective than no treatment and has comparable or superior effects to other forms of therapy. Furthermore, physical activity is also effective in reducing anxiety symptoms among chronic illness patients (Herring, O'Connor, & Dishman, 2010).

How does physical activity reduce anxiety? One hypothesis is that exercise simply provides a change of pace—a chance to relax and forget one's troubles. In support of this change-of-pace hypothesis, exercise demonstrated no stronger therapeutic effect than meditation (Bahrke & Morgan, 1978). Studies show that other techniques to reduce anxiety, including biofeedback, transcendental meditation, "time-out" therapy, and even beer drinking in a pub atmosphere, can also be effective (Morgan, 1981). Each of these interventions provides a change of pace, and all are associated with reduced levels of state anxiety.

Another hypothesis involves changes in brain chemistry. Studies with rats (Greenwood et al., 2005) show that exercise changes the transport of the neurotransmitter serotonin, which is related to positive mood. Studies with humans (Broocks et al., 2003) also suggest that changes occur in the metabolism of this neurotransmitter after exercise. Thus, physical activity may reduce anxiety by providing a change of pace, by altering neurotransmitter activity, or through some combination of the two.

Buffer Against Stress Two questions arise in relation to exercise and stress: (1) can exercise enhance psychological well-being? (2) can it protect people against the harmful effects of stress? Research on the first question has generally produced an affirmative answer. For example, older adults who exercise more regularly report greater well-being as well as greater quality of life than older adults who do not (Paxton, Motl, Aylward, & Nigg, 2010). Furthermore, a meta-analysis (Netz, Wu, Becker, & Tenenbaum, 2005) finds that physical activity relates to psychological well-being, but longer exercise duration does not always lead to continuing increases in feelings of well-being. Thus, even moderate exercise can boost well-being.

Answers to the second question are more difficult because a direct causal link between stress and subsequent physical illness has not yet been established (see Chapter 6 on stress and disease). However, several studies suggest that physical activity helps people deal with stress. Fitness appears to act as a buffer for both physical and psychological stress (Ensel & Lin, 2004); individuals who are more fit experience less distress.

Why might fitness reduce feelings of stress? One pathway may involve cardiovascular responses to stress, as exercise moderates the increase in blood pressure that accompanies psychological stress (Hamer, Taylor, & Steptoe, 2006). A second pathway may involve immune responses, as the effect of stress on the release of

proinflammatory cytokines is moderated in fit individuals (Hamer & Steptoe, 2007). Thus, exercise acts to decrease stress, on both a psychological and a physiological level.

The duration of exercise required to produce positive effects is not extreme; as little as 10 minutes of moderately strenuous exercise is capable of elevating mood (Hansen, Stevens, & Coast, 2001). The results of the studies on stress buffering do not indicate a strong effect for exercise, but physical activity is a strategy that many people use to help them manage stress. Figure 15.2 shows some of the positive effects of exercise.

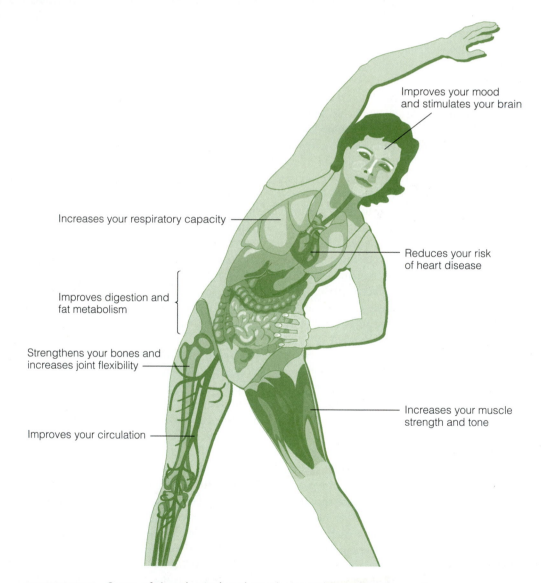

Improves your mood and stimulates your brain

Increases your respiratory capacity

Reduces your risk of heart disease

Improves digestion and fat metabolism

Strengthens your bones and increases joint flexibility

Improves your circulation

Increases your muscle strength and tone

FIGURE 15.2 Some of the physical and psychological benefits of exercise.

Source: An invitation to health (7th ed., p. 493), by D. Hales, 1997, Pacific Grove, CA: Brooks/Cole. Copyright © 1997 by Brooks/Cole Publishing Company. Reprinted by permission.

Better Cognitive Functioning   Physical activity may make you feel better, but can it also make you think better? Researchers are increasingly discovering a link between physical activity and cognitive functioning. Cognitive functioning includes diverse abilities such as the ability to focus attention, the speed of processing new information, and memory. Cognitive functioning also includes executive functioning, which refers to the ability to plan for and successfully pursue goals.

Aging often brings about a decline in cognitive functioning. Consequently, most research that focuses on the link between physical activity and cognitive functioning involves adults, particularly older adults. Indeed, a recent review of 29 exercise intervention studies (Smith, Blumenthal, et al., 2010) concludes that adults who participate in regular physical activity programs show greater attention, processing speed, memory, and executive functioning than adults who do not participate in physical activity programs. Moreover, physical activity appears to reduce some of the cognitive declines that occur with aging. For example, physical activity interventions show a stronger protective effect on memory among older adults than among younger adults, as well as among adults who are at greatest risk for Alzheimer's disease. Aerobic fitness training also contributes to increases in brain volume among older adults, but not younger adults (Colcombe et al., 2006).

One Australian study focused on older adults who reported memory problems that were indicative of risk for Alzheimer's disease (Lautenschlager et al., 2008). Through random assignment, some of these adults participated in a 6-month, home-based physical activity intervention; others adults did not. At an 18-month follow-up, the adults assigned to the intervention *improved* in their cognitive functioning. In contrast, those who did not receive the physical activity intervention showed no change in cognitive functioning.

Can physical activity also improve cognitive function in children? Recent research suggests it can. Children who are physically fit show better memory performance than those who are less fit, as well as greater volume of the hippocampus, a brain structure that plays an important role in memory (Chaddock et al., 2010). Intervention research also shows this link between physical activity and cognitive functioning. For example, a 3-month physical activity intervention program for overweight and sedentary children led to greater planning abilities as well as greater performance on a standardized math test (Davis et al., 2011).

Why does physical activity improve cognitive functioning? While the exact reason remains unknown, researchers speculate that these benefits may derive from increased cerebral blood flow or increased expression of brain-derived neurotrophic factor (BDNF), a protein that contributes the growth and differentiation of neurons in the brain (Brown, McMorris, et al., 2010; Smith, Blumenthal, et al., 2010).

IN SUMMARY

During the past 50 years, research supports the hypothesis that physical activity improves health and psychological functioning. Regular moderate physical activity can reduce the incidence of cardiovascular disease, including heart disease and stroke. Exercise improves both blood pressure and cholesterol profile, showing some ability to raise HDL. Physical activity also shows benefits for decreasing the risk for the development of diabetes and several types of cancer, including colon and breast cancer. Exercise can also promote bone growth in young people and slow the loss of bone minerals in older individuals. Moreover, physical activity shows psychological benefits. Indeed, exercise may be a useful intervention for depression. Benefits also appear for reducing anxiety, buffering stress, and improving cognitive functioning.

An earlier section of this chapter examined several reasons why people exercise. Table 15.1 lists some of these reasons, summarizes research evidence, and cites at least one study pertaining to each reason.

Hazards of Physical Activity

Although physical activity can enhance physical functioning, reduce anxiety, stress, and depression, and improve cognitive functioning, it also poses hazards to one's physical and psychological health. Some athletes overtrain to the point of staleness and, as a consequence, suffer from negative mood, fatigue, and depression (Tobar, 2005). In addition, some highly active people suffer from exercise-related injuries. For example, Tara Costa suffered a fractured tibia during her training for the Ironman Triathlon (Costa, 2010). Other people allow exercise to assume an almost addictive importance in their lives. In this section, we look at some of these potential hazards related to physical activity.

TABLE 15.1   Reasons for Exercising and Research Supporting These Reasons

Reasons for Exercising	Findings	Principal Source(s)
Weight control	Obesity can be reduced through exercise; 60 to 90 minutes a day may be necessary.	Hill & Wyatt, 2005; Jakicic & Otto, 2005
Weight control	Exercise is as effective as dieting; sculpting the perfect body won't work.	Blair & Church, 2004; Wood et al., 1988
Heart disease and aerobic fitness	Light to moderate exercise provides sufficient protection.	Barengo et al., 2004; Paffenbarger et al., 1978
	Both physical fitness and physical activity have a dose–response relationship with aerobic health.	Blair et al., 2001
	Walking confers benefits for older people.	Murphy et al., 2007
Stroke	Active women reduce risk of stroke.	Hu et al., 2000
	Inactive people are more likely to have strokes.	Krarup et al., 2007
	Physical activity can reduce two types of stroke.	Wendel-Vos et al., 2004
All-cause mortality	Nurses' Health Study reviewed 37 prospective cohort studies.	Oguma et al., 2002
Cholesterol level	Exercise increases HDL and decreases LDL.	Hausenloy & Yellen, 2008; Szapary et al., 2003
	Exercise reduces LDL and triglycerides.	Leon & Sanchez, 2001
	Low fitness is related to high cholesterol in children and adolescents.	Andersen et al., 2008; Eisenmann et al., 2007
	Exercise relates to low cholesterol in children.	Sääkslahti et al., 2004; Tolfrey, 2004; Tolfrey et al., 2000
Cancer	Meta-analyses show inverse relationship between exercise and cancer of various sites.	Miles, 2007; Thune & Furberg, 2001
	Exercise reduces risk for lung cancer, with a stronger relationship for women.	Tardon et al., 2005
	Exercise may protect against both tumor initiation and growth.	Rogers et al., 2008
	Physical activity helps people with cancer manage the effects of cancer treatment.	Quist et al., 2006; Speck et al., 2010
Bone density loss (osteoporosis)	Exercise helps build bone mass in children and adolescents.	Hind & Burrows, 2007
	Retired male athletes retain much of bone mineral density.	Nordström et al., 2005
	High-impact activity can delay loss of bone minerals in women.	Vainionpää et al., 2005
	Low-impact activities are not as effective as high-impact exercise.	Palombaro, 2005; Wayne et al., 2007; Zehnacker et al., 2007
Diabetes	Exercise improves insulin resistance.	Plasqui & Westerterp, 2007
	Exercise lowers risk for Type 2 diabetes.	Jeon et al., 2007
	Exercise can help in managing Type 2 diabetes.	Kavookjian et al., 2007

TABLE 15.1   Reasons for Exercising and Research Supporting These Reasons — *Continued*

Reasons for Exercising	Findings	Principal Source(s)
	Exercise is an important component in managing Type 1 diabetes.	Conn et al., 2008
	Exercise lowers risk for CVD in individuals with Type 1 diabetes.	Herbst et al., 2007
Decreased depression	Moderate exercise three times a week for 20 to 30 minutes reduces depression.	Annesi, 2005
	A dose–response relationship occurs with exercise and depression.	Dunn et al., 2005
	Exercise compares with cognitive therapy and antidepressant medication in effectiveness.	Daley, 2008; Donaghy, 2007
	Benefits of exercise are clinically significant.	Rethorst et al., 2007
Reduced anxiety	Moderate exercise can reduce state anxiety.	Dunn et al., 2001; Wipfli et al., 2008
	Physical activity is effective in reducing anxiety among chronic illness patients.	Herring et al., 2010
Buffer against stress	Exercise enhances mood, feelings of well-being, and quality of life.	Ensel & Lin, 2004; Hansen et al., 2001; Paxton et al., 2010
	Exercise increases well-being, but more is not always better.	Netz et al., 2005
	Exercise affects blood pressure and immune system response to stress.	Hamer et al., 2006; Hamer & Steptoe, 2007
Better cognitive functioning	Exercise is linked to greater attention, processing speed, memory, and executive functioning in adults.	Smith et al., 2010
	Aerobic fitness training is linked to increases in brain volume among older adults.	Colcombe et al., 2006
	6-month exercise program led to improved cognitive functioning.	Lautenschlager et al., 2008
	Children who exercise more show better memory, planning, and math performance.	Chaddock et al., 2010; Davis et al., 2011

Exercise Addiction

Some people become so involved with exercise that they ignore injuries to continue exercising or allow their exercise regimen to interfere with other parts of their lives such as work or family responsibilities. Others may think these people have an *exercise addiction*, but their behavior may not match the description of an addiction. In Chapter 13, we saw that addictions produce tolerance, dependence, and withdrawal symptoms.

William Morgan (1979) compared the process of excessive exercising to the development of other addictions. Initially, the tolerance for running is low, and it has many unpleasant side effects. But persistence eases the unpleasant aspects, and the pleasure of meeting goals becomes a powerful reinforcer. Like most social drinkers who have a casual, nonobsessive relationship with alcohol, most exercisers are able to incorporate physical activity into their lives without drastic changes in lifestyle. Other exercisers, however, cannot. Those who continue to increase their exercise must make changes in their lives to accommodate the time required, with consequences for other responsibilities and activities.

A high level of commitment to exercise is not the same as addiction (Terry, Szabo, & Griffiths, 2004). Some people's exercise habits reflect a high degree of commitment, whereas others fit the description of dependence, showing a strong emotional attachment to exercise (Ackard, Brehm, & Steffen, 2002) and exhibiting withdrawal symptoms such as depression and anxiety when prevented from exercising (Hausenblas & Symons Downs, 2002a, 2002b). Committed exercisers tend to have rational reasons for their exercise behavior such as extrinsic rewards, whereas addicted exercisers tend to use exercise as a way to manage negative emotions and problems in their lives (Warner & Griffiths, 2006). Some research opens up the possibility that exercise may be analogous to other types of addiction (Hamer & Karageorghis, 2007). This contention remains controversial, however, and some authorities prefer the term *obligatory exercise* or *exercise dependence* rather than exercise addiction.

Obligatory exercisers share several characteristics with people with eating disorders, especially anorexia. For example, they continue their chosen activity even when they are injured, continuing behavior that is harmful and even self-destructive. They also show a progressive self-absorption, with a great deal of concentration on internal experiences. In addition, many people who are anorexic experience a compulsion to exercise excessively (Klein et al., 2004). This observation prompted the proposal that teenage female anorexics and addicted male runners are analogous (Davis & Scott-Robertson, 2000); both show the need for mastery of the body, unusually high expectations of self, tolerance or denial of physical discomfort and pain, and a single-minded commitment to endurance. Other researchers (Ackard et al., 2002) found that obligatory exercisers exhibited body obsession, were more likely to have eating disorders, and showed symptoms of other psychological problems. The motivation for excessive exercise is a critical mediating factor that connects exercise to eating disorders (Cook & Hausenblas, 2008). For these individuals, the connection between exercising and eating disorders is a strong emotional attachment to exercise. These individuals experience injuries yet continue to exercise, neglect their personal relationships, and short-change their jobs to devote time to exercise. Perhaps

this fanaticism can be best expressed in the words of one obligatory runner:

> One day last spring I was having an exceptionally good run. I was running about 10 miles a day at that time and on this particular day I had decided to extend my workout. I was around the 14-mile point and I was preparing to cross a one-lane bridge when all of a sudden a large cement mixer turned the corner and began to cross the bridge. I never thought for a second about stopping and letting the truck pass. I simply continued and said to myself, "Come on you son-of-a-bitch and I'll split you right down the middle—there will be concrete all over the road!" The driver slammed on the brakes and swerved to the side as I sailed by. That was really scary afterward, but at the time I really felt good. I have felt equally strong and indestructible many times since, but never have taken on a cement truck again. (Morgan, 1979, pp. 63, 67)

Injuries From Physical Activity

Excluding head-to-head challenges with cement trucks, what are the chances of experiencing injuries from exercise? Many people with a regular exercise program accept minor injuries and soreness as an almost inevitable component of their program. However, irregular exercise produces even more injuries and more discomfort, with "weekend athletes" accounting for a disproportional number of injuries.

Musculoskeletal injuries are common, and the greater the frequency and intensity of exercise, the more likely it is that people will injure themselves (Powell, Paluch, & Blair, 2011). The Surgeon General's report (USDHHS, 1996) found that about half of runners had experienced an injury during the past year. This review also found, as expected, that the injury rate was lower for walkers than for joggers and that previous injury is a risk factor for subsequent injury. Physical activity is the source of 83% of all musculoskeletal injuries, and at least one fourth of exercisers must interrupt their regimen because of such injuries (Hootman et al., 2002). The decision to decrease exercise in response to injury is a wise one; "working through the pain" is an exercise myth that is associated with further injury.

Besides muscular and skeletal injuries, avid exercisers encounter a number of other health hazards. Heat, cold, dogs, and drivers can all be sources of danger. During exercise, body temperature rises. Both heat and cold present problems, some of which can be dangerous (Roberts, 2007). Fluid intake before, after, and even during exercise can protect against overheating by allowing cooling through sweating. However, conditions of extremely high air temperature, high humidity, and sunlight can combine to raise body temperature and prevent sweat from evaporating from the skin surface. If the body cannot cool itself, dangerous overheating may occur. Managing the risks for heat stress is a challenge for those who manage sports teams (Cleary, 2007).

Cold temperatures can also be dangerous for outdoor exercising (Roberts, 2007), but proper clothing can provide protection. Layered clothing for the body and gloves, hat, and even a face mask can protect against temperatures of 20°F and below (Pollock, Wilmore, & Fox, 1978). Temperatures below zero,

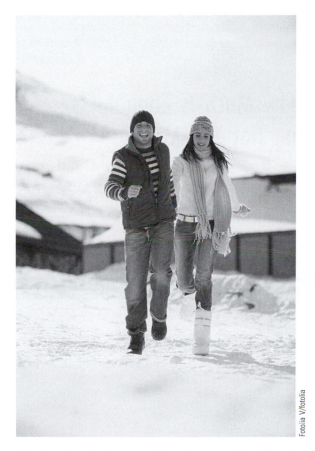

Fotolia V/fotolia

Wearing appropriate clothing decreases the risks of injury during exercise.

especially when combined with wind, can be dangerous even to people who are not exercising.

Death During Exercise

Many patients who have had a heart attack go into cardiac rehabilitation programs that include an exercise program, which generally includes close supervision. Although these coronary patients are at elevated risk during exercise, the cardiovascular benefit they gain from exercising ordinarily outweighs the risk (USDHHS, 1996). Nevertheless, individuals diagnosed with coronary heart disease should undertake exercise only with a physician's permission and under the supervision of specialists in cardiac rehabilitation.

What about people who have no known disease? Is it possible for a person who looks and feels well to die unexpectedly during exercise? Yes—but it is also possible to die unexpectedly while watching TV or sleeping. However, exercise increases the risk of such sudden death (Thompson et al., 2007). A 12-year follow-up analysis of male physicians (Albert et al., 2000) showed that sudden death was more than 16 times more likely during or immediately after vigorous physical exertion than during other times. However, the risk was very low for any specific episode of exercise—one death per 1.5 million episodes of exercise. This study also showed that the benefits of exercise outweighed the risks: Men who exercised regularly were less likely to die during exercise than those who were unaccustomed to exertion. Although the men in this follow-up study (Albert et al., 2000) did not identify themselves as having cardiovascular disease when the study began, either they were affected without their knowledge or developed this disease during the 12 years of the study. Indeed, most sudden deaths during exercise are the result of some type of heart disease, but people may be unaware of their risks.

Under most circumstances, exercise shows benefits for the cardiovascular system, but for those with CVD and for those who have exercised heavily for years of their lives (Raum, Rothenbacher, Ziegler, & Brenner, 2007), this pattern of physical activity is a risk. Even young people may be vulnerable to sudden cardiac death during exercise (Virmani, Burke, & Farb, 2001). In children, adolescents, and young adults, the cause of sudden cardiac death is most often congenital heart abnormalities or arrhythmias (abnormal heartbeat patterns). Among adults, about 60% of sudden cardiac deaths are due to blood clots that precipitate heart attacks, the typical case of the most frequent cause of death in the United States. Thus, most sudden deaths during exercise are those of individuals who had underlying cardiovascular problems, whether they knew it or not.

Reducing Exercise Injuries

Adequate caution can decrease the probability of injury. For people who have or are at risk for cardiovascular disease, supervised training is a wise precaution, especially when initiating an exercise program. Others, such as people who have been sedentary for a long time, may also benefit from supervision or training. With the guidance of a trainer, people will be less likely to attempt exercise that is inappropriate for their fitness level or to continue to exercise for too long as they start a program. In addition, an exercise professional will teach proper warm-up and stretching routines that are important in preventing injuries (Cooper, 2001).

Regardless of the level of fitness, the use of appropriate equipment decreases injuries. For example, proper running shoes are a necessity for running, jogging, or even exercise walking (Cooper, 2001). The correct type and amount of clothing are also important, either to allow for cooling or to retain heat. In addition to dressing properly for heat or cold, exercisers need to recognize the symptoms of heat stress. These include dizziness, weakness, nausea, muscle cramps, and headache. Each of these symptoms is a signal to stop exercising.

IN SUMMARY

Exercise has hazards as well as benefits. Potential hazards include exercise addiction—that is, a compulsive need to devote long periods of time to strenuous physical activity. Also, exercise may lead to injuries, the majority of which are musculoskeletal and relatively minor. Exercisers should avoid working out in extreme temperatures, and they should know how to avoid dogs, drivers, and darkness.

Death during exercise is a possibility. Those most vulnerable are individuals with cardiovascular disease, who are often older, but young people with heart abnormalities are also at risk. Nevertheless, people who exercise regularly are much less likely than sporadic exercisers to die of a heart attack during intense physical exertion. Exercise-related injuries can be reduced by appropriate preparation such as choosing the appropriate level of exercise, using appropriate equipment, and recognizing signs of trouble and reacting appropriately.

How Much Is Enough but Not Too Much?

How much physical activity is enough but not too much? Table 15.2 lists the current physical activity recommendations, by age group. In recent years, estimates have decreased for the amount of exercise that

TABLE 15.2 Current Physical Activity Recommendations

Age Group	Recommendation
Children and adolescents (aged 6–17)	1 hour of aerobic physical activity every day; most of this activity should be of moderate to vigorous intensity. Muscle-strengthening and bone-strengthening activity on at least 3 days per week.
Adults (aged 18–64)	2.5 hours of moderate-intensity aerobic activity per week, or 1.25 hours of vigorous-intensity aerobic activity per week. Muscle-strengthening activities on at least 2 days per week.
Older adults (aged 65 and older)	Same recommendations as for adults, or as much as abilities allow. Exercise that maintains or improves balance is recommended as well.

Source: Garber, C. E., Blissmer, B., Deschenes, M. R., Franklin, B. A., Lamonte, M. J., Lee, I-M., Nieman, D. C., & Swain, D. P. (2011). Quantity and quality of exercise for developing and maintaining cardiorespiratory, musculoskeletal, and neuromotor fitness in apparently healthy adults: Guidance for prescribing exercise. *Medicine & Science in Sports & Exercise, 43,* 1334–1359; U.S. Department of Health and Human Services (USDHHS). (2008). *Physical activity guidelines for Americans.* Retrieved February 20, 2012, from http://www.health.gov/PAGuidelines/factsheetprof.aspx

produces health benefits. In 2011, the American College of Sports Medicine revised its recommendations for the amount and type of activity for health benefits (Garber et al., 2011). These recommendations clarified earlier recommendations, taking new research into account. According to this official view, a healthy adult under age 65 should participate in 30 minutes of moderately vigorous activity five times a week or vigorous activity 20 minutes three times a week. In addition, people should engage in 8 to 10 strength training exercises for 12 repetitions at least twice a week. These experts described this level of exercise as adequate to protect against chronic disease, including cardiovascular disease.

The moderately vigorous activity recommendations reflect the evidence that less intense exercise produces health benefits and that vigorous exercise is not necessary. For example, a program of walking decreased cardiovascular risk factors in previously sedentary individuals (Murphy et al., 2007). Indeed, moderate exercise may be superior to more intense activity for some cardiovascular risk factors (Johnson, Slentz,

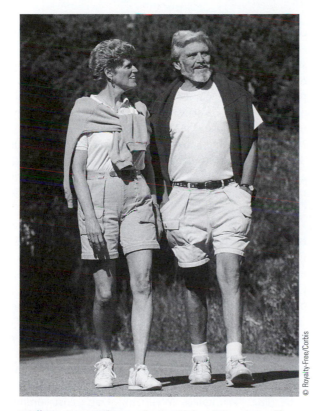

© Royalty-Free/Corbis

Walking is one form of physical activity that offers more advantages than hazards for most people.

et al., 2007). However, moderately vigorous activity three times a week will not prompt weight loss or maintain weight loss; those goals require more lengthy and more intense exercise (Garber et al., 2011). Therefore, how much is enough depends on the health goals.

Improving Adherence to Physical Activity

Adherence to nearly all medical and health regimens is a serious problem (see Chapter 4), and exercise is no exception. Only 33% of adults in the United States get regular physical activity at either a moderate or vigorous intensity (USBC, 2011); the percentage is similar in the European Union (Sjöström, Oja, Hagströmer, Smith, & Bauman, 2006). For individuals who participate in prescribed exercise regimens, the dropout rates closely parallel the relapse rates reported in smoking and alcohol cessation programs.

Everybody could use some extra motivation to get up off the couch and exercise. For some people, a membership at a health club, a personal trainer, or an opportunity to be a contestant on *The Biggest Loser* provides the motivation. Unfortunately, with so much of the population being sedentary, interventions are needed that do not require such costly face-to-face contact with a fitness professional. Thus, interventions that aim to improve physical activity often rely on other methods and channels, such as the computers and the Internet, telephone, mass media, and changes to the environment. In this section, we review some of these interventions and describe their effectiveness. As you will learn, one of the challenges in improving adherence to physical activity is maintaining the activity over time. Furthermore, you will learn that even some of the simplest interventions can have surprising effects.

Informational Interventions Informational interventions seek to raise public awareness of the importance of physical activity and its benefits, as well as highlight opportunities to engage in exercise. These informational interventions take a variety of forms, ranging from mass media campaigns to "point-of-decision" prompts.

Mass media campaigns use widespread media channels such as television and radio commercials, newspaper and magazine advertisements, billboards,

Becoming Healthier

1. If you don't exercise, make specific plans to start a program of regular physical activity, concentrating on choosing an activity that is convenient and that you feel capable of performing (and even enjoying).

2. If you are overweight and over 40, consult a physician before beginning.

3. Don't start too fast. Once you have determined that you are ready to begin an exercise program, start slowly. The first day you may feel as though you can run a mile. Don't give in to that temptation.

4. Exercising too vigorously on the first day will result in injuries or at least sore muscles. If you are stiff and sore the next day, you overdid it, and you won't feel like exercising.

5. If you are exercising for weight control, don't weigh yourself every day, and try not to become preoccupied with your weight or body shape.

6. If you are in the process of quitting smoking, use exercise as a way to prevent weight gain.

7. Social support helps. Enlist a friend to exercise with you, or join a team or group exercise program.

8. If you jog or cycle in a location unfamiliar to you, check out your surroundings before you begin. Dogs, ditches, and dangerous detours may be in your path.

9. Remember that in order to receive maximum health benefits from your exercise program, you must stick to it. Don't expect quick or dramatic results.

10. To acquire muscle tone as well as aerobic fitness, include a combination of types of exercise such as working out with weights or other isotonic exercise as well as aerobics.

and bus wraps to inform people about the importance of physical activity. A recent review of 18 mass media interventions—implemented in a variety of countries, including the United States, New Zealand, Australian, Canada, Columbia, and Brazil—finds that these mass media campaigns are generally successful at raising awareness, as measured by people's ability to recall information from the campaign (Leavy, Bull, Rosenberg, & Bauman, 2011).

Does this awareness translate into increases in physical activity? The evidence regarding this question is mixed. While some of these mass media campaigns led to greater levels of self-reported physical activity, other interventions did not. Furthermore, there is little evidence that any mass media campaign has effects on physical activity that persist long after a campaign ends (Leavy et al., 2011). Thus, the effectiveness of mass media campaigns on adoption of physical activity remains unclear.

Informational interventions can occur in simpler and less expensive forms, such as through "point-of-decision" prompts. When you need to get to a higher floor in a building, do you take the elevator or do you take the stairs? This is a choice that many people make on an everyday basis, and taking the stairs is an opportunity to inject physical activity into an otherwise sedentary day. Yet, most people choose the elevator. Dozens of studies show that signs placed near stairs—whether they be in the workplace, shopping malls, or subway exits—motivate people to make the physically active choice. In fact, reviews of research on these point-of-decision prompts show that they increase stair use by approximately 50% (Nocon, Müller-Riemenschneider, Nitzschke, & Willich, 2010; Soler et al., 2010). Furthermore, people who are obese are more likely than normal-weight individuals to respond to these signs by taking the stairs (Webb & Cheng, 2010).

These point-of-decision prompts may also be cost effective. One team of British researchers (Olander & Eves, 2011) compared the effects of two interventions aimed at increasing stair use on a university campus. One intervention, called "Workplace Wellbeing Day," placed research staff at an information booth in the center of campus at midday, where informational leaflets were handed out to over 1,000 people. The other intervention simply had point-of-decision signs strategically placed between the elevators and the stairs of several buildings. How much did these interventions cost? The "Workplace Wellbeing Day" cost almost $800 to implement and had no effect on stair use. In contrast, the point-of-decision signs cost merely $30 to implement and significantly increased stair use. Thus, informational interventions can work, particularly when people are exposed to the information at the point of decision (Wakefield, Loken, & Hornik, 2010). However, informational interventions seek to raise awareness or generate positive attitudes toward physical activity. These are only the first steps toward maintaining an activity regimen; changing behavior patterns is much more difficult.

Behavioral and Social Interventions Behavioral interventions attempt to teach people the skills necessary for adoption and maintenance of physical activity. Social interventions aim to create a social environment that makes adoption and maintenance of physical activity more successful. These types of interventions range from school-based physical education programs, to interventions designed to increase social support, to individually tailored health behavior change programs.

School-based physical education programs are often a mix of structured physical activity and education about the benefits of regular exercise. There is strong evidence that school-based physical activity programs increase the amount of time that students spend in moderate to vigorous physical activity, and this increased activity often leads to improvements in aerobic fitness (Kahn et al., 2002). However, these benefits are largely due to the physical activity incorporated directly into these programs, rather than the educational aspect. For example, classroom-based educational programs that focus on reducing sedentary behaviors—such as watching television and playing video games—do not reliably increase physical activity (Kahn et al., 2002). Furthermore, school-based physical education programs are less effective at increasing physical activity outside of school hours than they are at increasing physical activity during school hours (Cale & Harris, 2006). Thus, school-based physical education programs are moderately successful at increasing students' physical activity but do not appear to teach skills that enable students to increase physical activity on their own time.

Social support interventions focus on changing physical activity by building and maintaining social relationships that can facilitate behavior change. Examples of these interventions include developing a "buddy system," making a contract with another person to exercise for a specific period of time, or participating in a group exercise program. A systematic review of

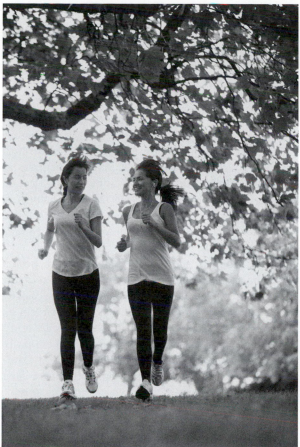

The "buddy system" can make physical activity easier and more enjoyable.

social support interventions (Kahn et al., 2002) concludes that they are effective. Social support interventions generally increase the amount of time spent in physical activity, increase the frequency of exercise, and lead to improvements in aerobic fitness and decreases in body fat. Thus, the power of social support is clear in the context of physical activity; enlisting the support of a friend, family member, or coworker can increase a person's likelihood of staying physically active.

Individually tailored health behavior change programs constitute a third form of behavioral intervention for physical activity. These typically involve information and activities that address goal setting, self-monitoring, reinforcement, development of self-efficacy, problem solving, and relapse prevention; in other words, many of the successful behavior change strategies described in Chapter 4. Individually tailored health behavior change programs are also generally successful, as they are associated with increases in time spent in physical activity and increases in aerobic fitness (Kahn et al., 2002).

However, individually tailored health behavior change programs can be expensive if delivered in person by a trained counselor. Therefore, many individually tailored programs are delivered via telephone, Internet, or computer. Interventions delivered through these channels generally yield significant increases in physical activity during the intervention period (Goode, Reeves, & Eakin, 2012; Hamel, Robbins, & Wilbur, 2010; Neville, O'Hara, & Milat, 2009) and can be as successful as face-to-face programs (Mehta & Sharma, 2012).

Unfortunately, individually tailored health behavior change programs suffer the problem that many interventions have: They are generally not successful at maintaining physical activity postintervention (Goode et al., 2012; Hamel et al., 2010; Neville et al., 2009). One phenomenon that contributes to the problem of relapse is the **abstinence violation effect** (Marlatt & Gordon, 1980). When people go 5 or 6 days without exercising, they tend to adopt the attitude "I'm out of shape now. It would take too much energy and pain to start over again." As with the smoker or the abuser of alcohol, this exerciser is allowing one lapse to turn into a full-blown relapse. Research with dropouts from an exercise program (Sears & Stanton, 2001) attempted to warn participants that they may be tempted to permanently quit exercising after a period of inactivity but that resuming exercise is a better choice than continued inactivity. The abstinence violation effect is an example of one of many psychological factors that influences adherence to physical activity recommendations. However, it would be shortsighted to believe that only psychological factors matter; the physical environment influences adherence as well.

Environmental Interventions Physical activity can be far easier and far more enjoyable if it takes place in a pleasing environment, such as a hike on a trail, a jog on a neighborhood sidewalk, or a stroll through a park. Thus, characteristics of a person's neighborhood can predict the likelihood of physical activity.

A large study of over 11,000 adults living in 11 different countries confirms the link between characteristics of neighborhood environments and physical activity (Sallis et al., 2009). People are more likely to

meet physical activity guidelines if their neighborhoods have sidewalks on most streets, plenty of shops, bicycle facilities, and free or low-cost recreational facilities. The importance of the neighborhood environment for physical activity among children is critical as well. Children who live in neighborhoods with access to playgrounds, parks, and recreational facilities tend to be more active and less obese (Veugelers, Sithole, Zhang, & Muhajarine, 2008). These associations may emerge for two reasons. First, easier access to recreational locations makes it easier to exercise. Second, people are more likely to be physically active when they see other people doing the same. For example, simply viewing people engaging in physical activity in and around one's neighborhood can motivate exercise (Kowal & Fortier, 2007).

Thus, one way to increase levels of physical activity is through enhancing access to places that encourage physical activity. These kinds of interventions may include providing access to fitness equipment in the workplace or in community centers, creating trails, or improving park amenities and facilities. Environmental interventions do work, in terms of increasing the physical activity and fitness of those working or living nearby (Kahn et al., 2002). However, these types of interventions can be quite expensive, and there is limited evidence available regarding their cost effectiveness. Regardless, it is important to recognize the key role that the physical environment plays in physical activity.

IN SUMMARY

In the United States and other industrialized countries, a sedentary lifestyle is more common than a physically active one; about 67% of adults fail to comply with recommendations for regular, vigorous exercise. Interventions for improving physical activity include: informational interventions, behavioral and social interventions, and environmental interventions. Informational interventions, such as mass media campaigns, have little effectiveness in changing behavior, unless "point-of-decision" prompts are used. Behavioral and social interventions are more successful in improving physical activity but do not have a good record of maintaining physical activity after the intervention concludes. Environmental interventions may be effective in changing behavior long-term, but the cost effectiveness of environmental interventions is not clear.

Answers

This chapter has addressed six basic questions:

1. What are the different types of physical activity?

All physical activity can be subsumed under one or more of five basic categories: isometric, isotonic, isokinetic, anaerobic, and aerobic. Each of these five exercise types has advantages and disadvantages for improving physical fitness. Most people who exercise do so for the benefits from one or another of these five types of physical activity, but no one type of exercise promotes all types of fitness.

2. Does physical activity benefit the cardiovascular system?

Most results on the health benefits of exercise have confirmed a positive relationship between regular physical activity and enhanced cardiovascular health, including weight control and a favorable cholesterol ratio. This research suggests that a regimen of moderate, brisk physical activity should be prescribed as one of several components in a program of coronary health.

3. What are some other health benefits of physical activity?

In addition to improving cardiovascular health, regular physical activity may protect against some kinds of cancer, especially colon and breast cancer; help prevent bone density loss, thus lowering one's risk of osteoporosis; prevent and control Type 2 diabetes and help manage Type 1 diabetes; and help people live longer.

Besides improving physical fitness and health, regular exercise can confer certain psychological benefits. Specifically, research has demonstrated that exercises can decrease depression, reduce anxiety, buffer against the harmful effects of stress, and improve cognitive functioning.

4. Can physical activity be hazardous?

Several hazards accompany both regular and occasional exercise. Some runners appear to be addicted to exercise, becoming obsessed with body image and fearful of being prevented from following their exercise regimen. Injuries are frequent among those who exercise regularly, especially if they train intensively. However, the most serious hazard is sudden death while exercising, which almost always occurs in people with cardiovascular disease. People who exercise regularly are much less likely than occasional exercisers to die of a heart attack during heavy physical exertion.

5. How much is enough but not too much?

The current pronouncement from the American College of Sports Medicine allowed for two routes to achieve acceptable levels of physical activity. One possibility is moderately vigorous exercise for 30 minutes five times per week, and the other involves intense exercise for 20 minutes three times a week. In addition, individuals should participate in strength training. Although the less intense program of physical activity is not sufficient to promote a high level of fitness, health benefits occur at lower levels of exercise. For cardiovascular health, almost any amount of exercise is better than no exercise.

6. What are effective interventions for improving physical activity?

More than 50% of adults in the United States are too sedentary for good health. One simple and effective intervention for improving physical activity is using "point-of-decision" prompts, which highlight opportunities for people to engage in exercise—such as using stairs instead of an elevator. Social and behavioral interventions are also effective in promoting adoption of physical activity; these interventions can be delivered in person, as well as through the computer, telephone, and Internet. However, the effects of social and behavioral interventions may not be maintained for long after the intervention concludes. One challenge in maintaining physical activity over time is the abstinence violation effect, when people give up on a regimen after a short setback.

Suggested Readings

Burfoot, A. (2005, August). Does running lower your risk of cancer? *Runner's World, 40*, 60–61. In this article, Amby Burfoot looks at some of the research on exercise and cancer and takes issue with Ken Cooper's statement that anyone who exercises more than the equivalent of 15 miles a week is running for something other than health. Burfoot considers the growing evidence that physical activity may protect against cancer as well as help people recover from cancer.

Powell, K. E., Paluch, A. E., & Blair, S. N. (2011). Physical activity for health: What kind? How much? How intense? On top of what? *Annual Review of Public Health*, *32*, 349–365. This excellent and up-to-date review chapter summarizes a number of key concepts important in understanding the relationship between physical activity and health, such as the intensity of activity, the dose–response relationship, and the importance of initiating even light-intensity activity to improve health.

Silver, J. K., & Morin, C. (Eds.). (2008). *Understanding fitness: How exercise fuels health and fights disease*. Westport, CT: Praeger Publishers/Greenwood Publishing Group. This book provides an explanation of the biological processes that occur when people exercise, including a review of the many diseases that exercise can help prevent.

CHAPTER 16

Future Challenges

CHAPTER OUTLINE

- **Real-World Profile of Dwayne and Robyn**
- *Challenges for Healthier People*
- *Outlook for Health Psychology*
- *Making Health Psychology Personal*

QUESTIONS

This chapter focuses on three basic questions:

1. What role does health psychology play in contributing to the goals of *Healthy People 2020*?

2. What is the outlook for the future of health psychology?

3. How can you use health psychology to cultivate a healthier lifestyle?

Real-World Profile of
DWAYNE AND ROBYN

Dwayne Brown* is a 21-year-old college junior who seldom thinks about his health—either his present or future health. Dwayne feels good, believes that his present lack of obvious illness is a sign that he is in good health, and assumes that he will always be free of disease and disability.

Dwayne has a number of habits that have consequences for his health. One of these is his diet, which consists mostly of fast-food burgers, with an occasional fried fish sandwich for variety. However, variety is not a high priority for Dwayne, who eats three meals a day, 6 days a week at the same fast-food restaurant. Breakfast usually consists of a biscuit, scrambled eggs, sausage, and a soft drink (because he doesn't like coffee). For lunch, he has a burger, fries, and another soft drink. Dinner is a repeat of lunch. He also snacks and often chooses ice cream and candy bars. Despite his "junk food" diet, Dwayne is not overweight.

Dwayne holds other attitudes, beliefs, and behaviors that present risks. He seldom exercises or wears seat belts and has few close friends. He believes that his future health is beyond his personal control—that genetics and fate are the underlying determinants of heart disease, cancer, and accidents. Thus, he has thought little about ways of maintaining his health or decreasing his chances of chronic illness or premature death. He does not see a physician regularly. When he feels ill, he takes over-the-counter medication, hoping that he will feel better.

However, Dwayne does some things right. He does not smoke cigarettes or drink alcohol and considers his life as low stress. His abstinence from drinking stems from his religious rather than health beliefs, and his avoidance of smoking comes from an incident during his adolescence when he smoked a cigarette and became sick. His score on the Social Readjustment Rating Scale (Holmes & Rahe, 1967; see Chapter 5) was as low as anyone's could be, including only one stressful life event—Christmas. Dwayne sees himself as a healthy person.

Robyn Green* is also a 21-year-old college junior, but her attitudes and behaviors concerning health differ a great deal from Dwayne's. Her differences include a basic attitude—that she has the primary responsibility for her health. Consistent with this attitude, Robyn has adopted a lifestyle that she believes will keep her healthy. Like Dwayne, she does not smoke; she took a puff from a cigarette when she was in fourth grade and coughed for a long time, which discouraged her from smoking. Her father was a smoker during her childhood and adolescence, but she and her mother convinced him to stop smoking in their home. To further avoid exposure to secondhand smoke, Robyn avoids enclosed places where people are smoking. Unlike Dwayne, Robyn drinks alcohol. Her drinking is moderate, and she does not binge drink. Her parents are also moderate drinkers, and Robyn's home was one in which alcohol was consumed but not abused.

Robyn's diet differs dramatically from Dwayne's diet. She seldom eats eggs, whole milk products, beef, or pork; she concentrates on eating lots of fruits and vegetables (yet is not vegetarian). She occasionally allows herself a dessert. Robyn is careful about choosing a low-fat diet because she is concerned about cholesterol. Her grandfather died of heart disease at age 63, and she believes that his smoking and high-fat, high-cholesterol diet hastened his death. Robyn also follows an exercise program, which she finds somewhat difficult to maintain with her school schedule. She takes an aerobic dance class 3 days a week; she walks 30 minutes a day on those days with no dance class. So far, she has been faithful in maintaining this workout schedule. Robyn sees herself as a healthy person.

*The names have been changed to protect these persons' privacy.

How do Dwayne's and Robyn's health habits and attitudes compare with yours? Dwayne is less knowledgeable and concerned with his health than most college students, whereas Robyn is more so. Both Dwayne and Robyn see themselves as healthy people; yet, you should know by now that Robyn is more likely to maintain her health, whereas Dwayne is likely to see his deteriorate if his habits persist. In this chapter, we will examine some health issues specific to college students and hope to convince you of health psychology's relevance to your life. But first, let's look at health care and the challenges facing not only health psychologists but also all health care providers in the United States and around the world.

Challenges for Healthier People

People in the United States, Canada, and other high-income countries are inundated with health information telling about the dangers of smoking, abusing alcohol, eating improperly, and not exercising regularly. As you learned in Chapters 3 and 4, knowledge does not always translate into action, and people have difficulty in adopting these healthy habits. Still, over the past 35 years U.S. residents have managed to make some healthy changes in their lifestyles, and these changes contribute to the declining mortality for heart disease, stroke, cancer, homicide, and unintentional injuries (USCB, 2011). However, unhealthy and risky behaviors still contribute to an increasing rate of obesity, diabetes, and lower respiratory disease.

What are the most current public health goals of the United States? *Healthy People 2020* (USDHHS, 2010a) is a report that establishes the United States' health objectives for the years 2010 through 2020. These objectives include 40 focus areas and nearly 600 specific goals, along with 12 leading indicators, which appear in Table 16.1. Notice that most of these indicators are major areas of concern to health psychologists. In addition, two overarching goals summarize the focus of the *Health People 2020* report: to

TABLE 16.1 Leading Health Indicators for Healthy People 2020

© Cengage Learning 2014

Nutrition, physical activity, and obesity

- Increase number of adults who meet physical activity guidelines
- Reduce number of children, adolescents, and adults who are obese
- Increase total vegetable intake in children, adolescents, and adults

Oral health

- Increase number of children and adults who use oral health services regularly

Tobacco use

- Reduce number of adults who are current cigarette smokers
- Reduce number of adolescents who smoked in past 30 days

Substance abuse

- Reduce number of adolescents who use alcohol or illicit drugs
- Reduce number of adults engaging in binge drinking

Reproductive and sexual health

- Increase number of sexually active females who receive reproductive health services
- Increase number of persons living with HIV who know their HIV status

Mental health

- Reduce suicides
- Reduce number of adolescents who experience major depressive episodes

(continued)

TABLE 16.1   Leading Health Indicators for Healthy People 2020 — *Continued*

Injury and violence

- Reduce fatal injuries
- Reduce homicides

Environmental quality

- Increase air quality
- Reduce number of children exposed to secondhand smoke

Access to health services

- Increase number of people with medical insurance
- Increase number of people with a usual primary care provider

Clinical preventive services

- Increase number of adults who receive colorectal cancer screenings
- Increase number of adults with hypertension whose blood pressure is under control
- Increase number of adult diabetics with good glycemic control
- Increase number of children who receive recommended vaccinations

Maternal, infant, and child health

- Reduce infant mortality
- Reduce number of preterm births

Social determinants of health

- Increase number of students who graduate with a high-school equivalency diploma

increase quality and years of healthy life, and to elimi- nate health disparities. Although these goals are ambi- tious and have presented challenges in the past (USDHHS, 2007), the United States has progressed toward or met many prior *Healthy People* goals (USDHHS, 2010a).

Increasing the Span of Healthy Life

The first goal—to increase the span of healthy life—is a bit different from increasing **life expectancy**. Rather than striving for longer lives, many people are now trying to increase their number of well-years. A **well-year** is "the equivalent of a year of completely well life, or a year of life free of dysfunction, symptoms, and health-related problems" (Kaplan & Bush, 1982, p. 64). A concept closely related to well-years is **health expectancy**, defined as the number of years a person can anticipate spending free from disability (Robine & Ritchie, 1991). For exam- ple, life expectancy in the United States is about 76 for men and 81 for women, but health expectancy is about

68 for men and 72 for women, leaving both men and women with a discrepancy of about 8 to 9 years of dis- ability (WHO, 2010). Japan boasts both the highest life expectancy (83) and the highest health expectancy (76) of any country; even in Japan, people can expect approx- imately 7 years of disability (WHO, 2010).

In the United States, years of life are increasing, but years of life without chronic illness are declining (USDHHS, 2007). U.S. residents are not benefiting from increases in healthy life expectancy as much as residents of many other countries (Mathers et al., 2004). Although people in the United States may expect 70 years of healthy life, this figure ranks 32nd in the world in terms of disability-free life expectancy. The United States trails most other industrialized countries because of high rates of smoking-related dis- ease, violence, and AIDS-related health problems. Although the decline in tobacco use in recent decades improves Americans' healthy life expectancy, these gains will likely be offset by the increasing rate of obe- sity in the United States (Stewart, Cutler, & Rosen,

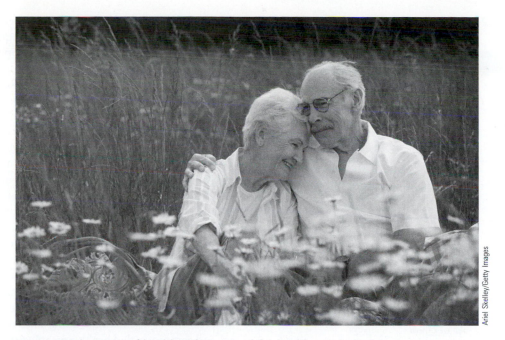

Increasing the span of healthy life is a goal for health psychologists.

2009). Table 16.2 shows the healthy life expectancy for a selection of countries with both high and low values. As other industrialized countries have health expectancy much greater than the United States, improvements should be possible in the United States.

What explains the difference between life expectancy and health expectancy? Economic factors play an important role. The differences between life expectancy and health expectancy are even larger when comparing the richest and poorest countries, or even the richest and poorest segments of the population within a country (Jagger et al., 2009; Mathers et al., 2004; McIntosh, Fines, Wilkins, & Wolfson, 2009). Wealthy people not only live longer but also have more years of healthy life.

The changing nature of disease also accounts for the difference between life expectancy and health expectancy. Diseases that kill people will influence life expectancy; diseases that compromise health will influence health expectancy. For example, circulatory disorders head both lists, but disorders producing restricted movement and respiratory disorders are responsible for producing lost health expectancy, whereas cancer and accidents are major sources of lost life expectancy. Depression also compromises health expectancy more so than it compromises life expectancy (Reynolds, Haley, & Kozlenko, 2008). Thus, interventions aimed at increasing life expectancy will not necessarily improve

health expectancy and quality of life. For this reason, experts recommend using a population's health expectancy as an indicator of overall population health (Steifel, Perla, & Zell, 2010).

Reducing Health Disparities

Healthy People 2020 defines a **health disparity** as "a particular type of health difference that is closely linked with social, economic, and/or environmental disadvantage" (USDHHS, 2008b). Disparities exist based on race and ethnicity, education, income, gender, sexual orientation, disability status, special health care needs, and geographic location. All of these disparities are important to understand and reduce; however, racial and ethnic disparities are the most documented health disparities in the United States. In the United States, ethnicity is not separable from social, economic, and educational factors that contribute to disease as well as to seeking and receiving medical care (Kawachi, Daniels, & Robinson, 2005). Being poor with a low educational level elevates risks for many diseases and provides a poorer prognosis for those who are ill. These disadvantages also apply to children in these socioeconomic groups (Wen, 2007). African Americans, Hispanic Americans, and Native Americans have lower average educational levels and incomes than European

Ariel Skelley/Getty Images

TABLE 16.2 Healthy Life Expectancy for Selected Nations, 2007

Country	Healthy Life Expectancy
Japan	76
San Marino	75
Switzerland	75
Sweden	74
Iceland	74
Australia	74
Italy	74
Canada	73
Germany	73
United Kingdom	72
USA	70
Costa Rica	69
Mexico	67
China	66
Colombia	66
Vietnam	64
Brazil	64
Russian Federation	60
India	56
Iraq	54
Haiti	54
Rwanda	43
Afghanistan	36
Sierra Leone	35

Source: Data from *World Health Statistics 2010*, by World Health Organization. Retrieved April 9, 2012, from www.who.int/gho

Americans and Asian Americans (USCB, 2011), and education relates to income. Thus, the racial and ethnic disparities are intertwined with income and education disparities, complicating our understanding of the underlying reasons for health disparities among people of different ethnic backgrounds.

Racial and Ethnic Disparities   African Americans, compared with European Americans, have a shorter life expectancy as well as a higher infant mortality rate, more homicide deaths, higher rates of cardiovascular disease, higher cancer mortality, and more tuberculosis and diabetes (USCB, 2011). They also experience lower health expectancy (USDHHS, 2007). Inadequate medical treatment may be a factor: African Americans receive poorer care than European Americans on nearly half of the quality measures of medical care (AHRQ, 2011). But even when equating for income (De Lew & Weinick, 2000) and access to medical care (Schneider, Zaslavsky, & Epstein, 2002), African Americans have poorer outcomes than European Americans. Part of the discrepancy may be due to limited **health literacy,** the ability to read and understand health information to make health-related decisions (Paasche-Orlow, Parker, Gazmararian, Nielsen-Bohlman, & Rudd, 2005; Rudd, 2007). Disparities in health literacy account for some ethnic health disparities, such as ethnic differences in vaccination (Bennett, Chen, Soroui, & White, 2009), HIV and diabetes management (Osborn, White, Cavanaugh, Rothman, & Wallston, 2009; Waldrop-Valverde et al., 2010), and medication use (Bailey et al., 2009). The Would You Believe …? box discusses the importance of health literacy and some ways that health psychologists can increase people's understanding of health information.

Discrimination may also be a factor contributing to inadequate medical treatment for African Americans (Brown et al., 2008; Smiles, 2002). For example, African Americans receive less aggressive treatment for symptoms of coronary heart disease, are less likely to be referred to a cardiologist than European Americans, are less likely to receive kidney dialysis, and are less likely to receive the most effective treatments for HIV infection (Institute of Medicine, 2002). Many physicians believe that race or ethnicity plays no role in the care they provide (Lillie-Blanton, Maddox, Rushing, & Mensah, 2004), but these results and the reports of African Americans (Brown et al., 2008) indicate otherwise.

Low economic status, lack of access to medical care, and poor health literacy affect Native Americans at least as strongly as African Americans (AHRQ, 2011; USDHHS, 2007). Native Americans have a shorter life expectancy, a higher mortality rate, higher infant mortality, and higher rates of infectious illness than European Americans (Hayes-Bautista et al., 2002). Many Native Americans receive medical care from the Indian Health Service, but that organization has a history of poor funding as well as mistreatment of Native American patients that has led to mistrust (Keltner, Kelley, & Smith, 2004). In addition, many Native Americans live in rural settings in which medical care services are limited. These circumstances contribute to decreased access to medical care, which is related to poor health,

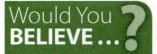

Would You BELIEVE...? Health Literacy Can Improve by "Thinking Outside the Box"

Sometimes, even the most well-intentioned health interventions may not work for one simple reason: People do not understand the information presented. This is a problem faced not merely by people with low levels of health literacy. It is a problem likely faced by you.

In the 1990s, several countries—including the United States, Canada, Mexico, and United Kingdom—passed laws requiring food manufacturers to post a "Nutrition Facts" box on food packaging. The governments' goal with this legislation was to help consumers make healthier and more informed food choices. In the United States, the "Nutrition Facts" box typically appears on the back of the product and reports information such as serving size, calories, fat, cholesterol, sodium, vitamins, and minerals.

If you are like most people, you probably do not pay much attention to—or even understand—the information presented in these boxes. People's use of nutrition information boxes declined from 1996 to 2006 (Todd & Variyam, 2008). Why? Despite the government's best efforts to design a box that would be easy to

read, many people find it difficult to interpret all the numerical information (Institute of Medicine [IOM], 2012). How much fat is too much fat? How big is a serving size? Is one snack food more or less healthy than another snack food? These are the kinds of questions that consumers need answers to, but current nutrition boxes effectively hide this information by tacking it to the back of a package and presenting it as a list of nearly indecipherable numbers.

Most experts think the cause of this problem is not people's lack of health literacy, but rather, problems with how we design the labels. For example, experts in health literacy know that images often convey information better than numbers do (Houts, Doak, Doak, & Loscalzo, 2006). Recently, a group of health psychologists, public health experts, marketers, and nutritionists convened to recommend broad changes to food nutrition labels (IOM, 2012). This group concluded that consumers should be able to make better food choices when nutrition information appears on the *front* of the package, and use symbols and images rather than

numbers to convey important information. Furthermore, the symbols should represent only the most essential nutrition information, such as calories, saturated and *trans* fats, sodium, and added sugars. An example of a front-of-package nutrition symbol system designed by the United Kingdom appears in this box. It uses standard traffic light colors to inform consumers that a product is high, medium, or low in a particular element. Which system is easier for you to understand: the current United States fact box or the redesigned UK symbols?

This is one example of how health psychologists can address literacy issues by rethinking how marketers and interventions present information. Another example of an innovative approach to addressing health literacy issues is the use of *telenovelas* to communicate health information to Latino populations. Telenovelas are short, dramatic "soap operas," immensely popular in Latino culture, that focus on romantic and middle class issues. Some health psychologists created "entertainment interventions" using the *telenovela* format to communicate to Spanish-speaking audiences about the importance of breast screening (Wilkin et al., 2007) and HIV testing (Olshefsky, Zive, Scolari, & Zuniga, 2007). Both interventions were deemed successful, largely because they presented health information in a format that the audience was famili[ar] with and could easily understand.

Thus, addressing dispariti[es] health literacy is a public health [chal]lenge and will require ext[ra] efforts to ensure that people [under]stand important informatio[n]. more "thinking outside of [the box]" efforts to address dispariti[es] literacy may be more su[ccessful].

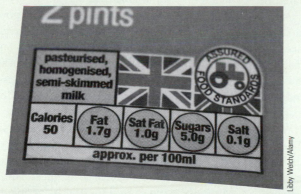

The UK Traffic Light system of nutrition labeling makes it easier for people to understand important health information.

Libby Welch/Alamy

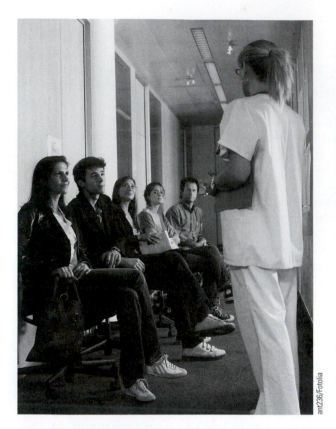

Many people in the United States face barriers in obtaining medical care.

Hispanic Americans are much more likely to develop diabetes, obesity, and hypertension than European Americans (USDHHS, 2000). Hispanic American young men are at sharply increased risk of violent death (Hayes-Bautista et al., 2002), which may be the reason for the overall lower life expectancy of Hispanic Americans. In other age groups, Hispanics fare about the same as or better than European Americans on some health and mortality measures. Hispanic Americans have a lower death rate than many other ethnic groups, including European Americans, for heart disease, stroke, and lung cancer (NCHS, 2011). These low death rates seem puzzling, given the high rates of smoking, obesity, and hypertension among Hispanic Americans. The poor health habits of Hispanic Americans, combined with their low disease prevalence, may reflect a transition in which immigrants adopt American lifestyles but have not yet had time to develop the chronic diseases typical of the United States (Borrell, 2005).

Asian Americans have lower infant mortality, longer life expectancy, fewer lung and breast cancer deaths, and lower cardiovascular death rates than other ethnic groups (NCHS, 2011). Like Hispanic Americans, Asian Americans come from a variety of ethnicities, including Chinese, Korean, Japanese, Vietnamese, and Cambodian. Many Asian cultures share values that promote good health, such as strong social and family ties, but other factors present barriers to good health. For example, Vietnamese and Cambodian cultures show a higher tolerance for family violence than European American culture (Weil & Lee, 2004). Overall, Asian Americans have the longest life expectancy and best health of any ethnic group in the United States.

Educational and Socioeconomic Disparities Low income has an obvious connection to lower standards of medical care. After adjusting for poverty, many of the health disadvantages of ethnicity disappear (Krieger, Chen, Waterman, Rehkopf, & Subramanian, 2005). One medical care disadvantage related to poverty is lack of insurance, which makes access to medical care more difficult in the United States. However, universal access to medical care does not completely remove the disparities among socioeconomic groups (Lasser, Himmelstein, & Woolhandler, 2006; Martikainen, Valkonen, & Martelin, 2001). Even in countries that have universal access to medical care, health disparities between poor and wealthy people persist, suggesting that factors other than access to medical care are involved in maintaining health.

but Native Americans who live in urban areas also experience poor health and limited access to medical care (Castor et al., 2006). Native Americans also exhibit many risky behaviors that influence their health, including high rates of smoking and alcohol abuse, poor diet, and behaviors that increase injuries and deaths from violence. Native Americans, then, are one of the groups poorly served by the current system of medical care and health education in the United States.

Many Hispanic Americans also experience low income and educational status. However, Hispanics in the United States include a variety of groups, and their health and longevity tend to vary with income and education. Cuban Americans generally have higher education and economic levels than Mexican Americans or Puerto Ricans, and Cuban Americans are more likely to have access to regular medical care and physician visits (LaVeist, Bowie, & Cooley-Quille, 2000). Cubans have better health, and Puerto Ricans tend to have poorer health, than other groups of Hispanics in the United States (Borrell, 2005).

Education and socioeconomic level are two factors that may influence health status—independent of access to medical care. Across ethnic groups and in countries around the world, people who have higher education and income also have better health and longevity than those with lower education and income (Crimmins & Saito, 2001; Mackenbach et al., 2008). As the Chapter 1 Would You Believe …? box detailed, people who attend college have many health advantages. Compared with those with a high school education or less, those who attend college live longer and healthier, with lower rates of infectious and chronic diseases and unintentional injuries (NCHS, 2011). These advantages should not be surprising, considering the low rate of smoking among those who attend or graduate from college compared with people with fewer than 12 years of education; smoking is a leading contributor to ill health and death.

In addition, people with low education and low socioeconomic status are more likely to have risky health habits, such as eating a high-fat diet and leading a sedentary life, than people with higher incomes and more education. Although improved access to medical care and decreased discrimination in medical care delivery will probably eliminate some of the health disparities among ethnic groups, changes in health-related behaviors and improved living conditions will also be necessary to achieve the goal of eliminating health disparities in the United States.

IN SUMMARY

People in the United States and other industrialized countries are becoming more health conscious, and both government policy and individual behavior reflect this concern. *Healthy People 2020* states two overarching goals for the U.S. population: (1) to increase the quality and years of healthy life and (2) to eliminate health disparities. The first goal includes increasing the number of well-years or health expectancy—that is, years free of dysfunction, disease symptoms, and health-related problems. The second goal—eliminating disparities in health care—is far from being met, in part because people at the upper socioeconomic level continue to make greater gains in health status than do those at the lower levels. Ethnicity remains a factor in health and medical care, not only in the United States but also in other countries. In the United

States, African Americans and Native Americans experience great disadvantages compared with Asian Americans and European Americans. Some Hispanics experience health advantages, and others disadvantages. The factors of education and income are intertwined with ethnicity, complicating understanding of the source of disparities in health.

Outlook for Health Psychology

Since the founding of health psychology more than 30 years ago, the field has blossomed, prompting a plethora of research and clinical applications to a variety of health-related behaviors and outcomes. That progress has touched many areas of health care, but social and economic forces will influence the future of the field.

Progress in Health Psychology

Until the 1970s, very few psychologists focused on physical health as an area of research (APA Task Force on Health Research, 1976). However, during the past 30 years, psychology research on health issues accelerated to the point that it has changed the field of psychology, making health-related issues common topics in psychology journals. Health psychologists are now frequent contributors to journals in medicine and health care.

Despite the growth of health psychology and its ability to contribute to health care, the field faces several challenges. One major challenge is acceptance by other health care practitioners, an acceptance that continues to grow. Like physicians and patients, health psychologists also face the most serious problem within medical care—namely, escalating costs. In an environment of limited resources, psychologists will need to justify the costs that their services add to health care (Thielke, Thompson, & Stuart, 2011; Tovian, 2004). Although the diagnostic and therapeutic techniques used by health psychologists have demonstrated effectiveness, these procedures also have financial costs. Health psychology must justify its costs by offering services that meet the needs of individuals and society while fitting within a troubled health care system (IOM, 2010).

Future Challenges for Health Care

Health and medical care in the United States face enormous challenges. The two goals of *Healthy People 2020*—to add years of healthy life and to eliminate disparities in providing health care—will be difficult to achieve. Adding years of healthy life to an aging population is a daunting task. As the population ages, chronic illnesses and chronic pain become more common.

In 1900, only 4% of the population was over 65; in 2006, more than 13% of U.S. citizens had reached that age (USCB, 2011). During this same period, life expectancy increased from 47 years to 78 years. Experts project that life expectancy in the United States will reach 80 years by the year 2020 (see Figure 16.1), with more than 19 million people, or 6.1% of the total population, over age 75.

As the population continues to age during the next few decades, psychology will play an important role in helping older people achieve and maintain healthy and productive lifestyles and adjust to the problems of chronic illness. As we have seen, health psychology plays an important role in preventing illness, promoting healthy aging, and helping people cope with pain. In old age, lifestyles can still be changed to help prevent illness, but health psychology's alliance with gerontology will more likely produce an emphasis on promoting and maintaining health, managing pain, and formulating health care policy.

The elimination of health disparities based on gender, ethnicity, age, income, educational level, and disability also will prove difficult, and increasing diversity will continue to challenge the health care system. As we discussed earlier in this chapter, many ethnic disparities trace back to economic, educational, and health literacy differences among ethnic groups (Lasser et al., 2006; USDHHS, 2007). The health disparity attributable to gender is not so easy to understand. Women receive poorer health care yet have longer life expectancies. This survival advantage was small in 1900, grew to more than 7 years during the 1970s, and has declined to about 5 years (USCB, 2011). Efforts to trace this gender difference to biology have been largely unsuccessful, but health-related behaviors, social support, and coping strategies favor women (Whitfield, Weidner, Clark, & Anderson, 2002). Importantly, the escalating costs of medical care in the United States will place limits on the extent that health care policies and interventions can successfully address disparities.

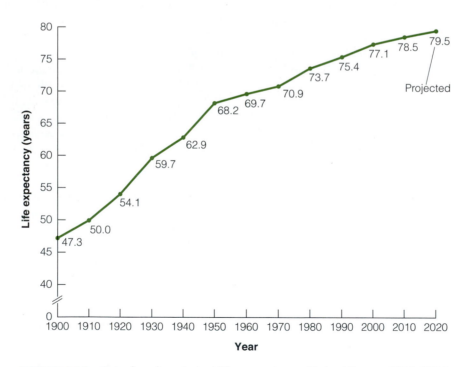

FIGURE 16.1 Actual and projected life expectancy, United States, 1900–2020.

Sources: Data from *Historical statistics of the United States: Colonial times to 1970* (p. 55), by U.S. Department of Commerce, Bureau of the Census, 1975, Washington, DC: U.S. Government Printing Office; *Statistical abstracts of the United States: 2001* (p. 73); *Statistical abstracts of the United States, 2012*, by U.S. Bureau of the Census, 2011, Washington, DC: U.S. Government Printing Office.

Controlling Health Care Costs The richest nation in the world is having trouble paying its medical bills. Health and medical care costs in the United States have escalated at a higher rate than inflation and other costs of living (Bodenheimer, 2005a; Mongan, Ferris, & Lee, 2008), leaving many people unable to afford medical care and others in the position of fearing that they will not be able to do so in the future.

A number of factors contribute to the high costs. These factors include the proliferation of expensive technology, a large proportion of physicians who are specialists, inefficient administration, inappropriate treatments, and a profit-oriented system that resists controls (IOM, 2010).

Figure 16.2 shows where health care dollars go. Hospitals receive 33% and physicians 22% of the dollars spent (USCB, 2011). Although physicians receive less of the health care dollar than hospitals, their fees contribute significantly to the high cost of health care (Bodenheimer, 2005c). Managed care curtailed physicians' fees during the late 1980s and early 1990s, but the backlash against managed care loosened these restrictions, and physicians' fees began to increase again in the late 1990s. The number of specialists adds to the cost of medical care, and the scarcity of primary care/family practitioners (and the lack of incentive for going into primary care) also plays a role (Sepulveda, Bodenheimer, & Grundy, 2008). Ironically, more physicians created competition, but rather than decreasing costs, this situation has contributed to higher costs (Weitz, 2010).

Administrative costs also contribute to the high health care costs in the United States (Bodenheimer, 2005a; Mongan et al., 2008). The complex system of insurance, private physicians, private and public hospitals, and government-supported medical programs such as Medicare produced different procedures, forms, payment plans, expenses allowed, maximum payments, and deductibles involved in payment for medical services. Thus, payment is a complex matter, which adds to people's frustration in dealing with the medical care system and creates possibilities for errors and fraud.

Health care reform is an urgent priority for the United States, but many conflicting interests have prevented widespread changes (Bodenheimer, 2005c; Mongan et al., 2008). During the 1980s, health maintenance organizations (HMOs) proliferated as a way to control costs (Weitz, 2010). Originally, HMOs were nonprofit organizations oriented toward preventive

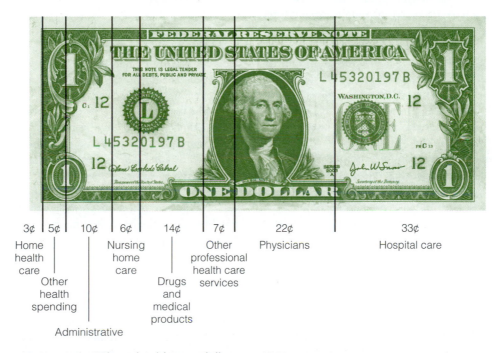

FIGURE 16.2 Where health care dollars go, 2011.

Source: Statistical abstract of the United States, 2011 (130th edition). Washington, DC: U.S. Government Printing Office. Retrieved June 1, 2011 from http://www.census.gov

care, but corporations entered the HMO market and profit became a motive. The growth of HMOs and the restriction of care received through these organizations contributed to slowing the medical care cost escalation. A backlash against the restrictions on care imposed by HMOs produced patients' rights movements, which have edged the system back toward high spending.

Can the United States provide quality medical care more efficiently? Other industrialized countries such as Canada, Japan, Australia, the countries of Western Europe, and Scandinavia share certain factors with the United States—aging populations with high rates of cardiovascular disease, cancer, and other chronic diseases—that pose similar challenges for their medical care systems (Bodenheimer, 2005b). Many of these countries do a better job of providing medical care to a larger percentage of their residents at lower cost than does the U.S. system. Their longer life expectancies and health expectancies are testimony to the effectiveness of their systems.

Germany, Canada, Japan, and Great Britain all face the problem of escalating medical care costs, and these nations also struggle to contain rising costs (Weitz, 2010). The history of medical care costs in these countries and the United States appears in Figure 16.3. These countries have managed to contain expenditures by controlling at least some of the factors that account for the rise in medical costs in the United States: Canada has a single-payer system, which minimizes administrative costs; Great Britain limits access to high-technology medicine; Germany imposes some limits on payments to physicians and limits hospitals' purchases of high-technology equipment. Japan has an insurance system as the United States does, but insurers do not compete with one another, as the government regulates the cost of services and fees. Japan, however, has lower rates of obesity than many other countries, which contributes to a healthier population.

All of the strategies for cost containment have drawbacks. For example, people have quicker access to medical procedures such as MRIs, mammograms, and knee replacement surgery in the United States than in Canada, but these procedures are significantly more expensive in the United States (Bodenheimer, 2005b). Time delays for some services may pose risks, but in other cases, patients in the United States are overtreated, and limiting access could minimally influence health outcomes (IOM, 2010) or may actually boost health and life expectancy (Emanuel & Fuchs,

2008; Research and Policy Committee, 2002). Canadians' longer life expectancy suggests that the delays they experience do not pose major threats (Lasser et al., 2006).

By devising systems in which all people have access to health care, Germany, Canada, Great Britain, and Japan have diminished competitive profit making, which remains a central feature of the U.S. system (Mahar, 2006). These four countries have different systems for paying for medical care, and all have experienced cost problems, but each has universal coverage, whereas a growing percentage of people in the United States have limited access to medical care. In 2010, U.S. President Barack Obama signed into law the Patient Protection and Affordable Care Act, which would require all Americans to maintain health insurance coverage, while also establishing a marketplace in which Americans choose from various health care insurance plans and coverage. Implementation of this reform plan has been challenged on a number of grounds, including its constitutionality. As of late 2012, the United States Supreme Court upheld the constitutionality of most of this law, and its provisions are gradually being enacted. Still, health care reform has been—and remains—an urgent issue in the United States (IOM, 2010).

The Importance of Prevention About 70% of the cost of medical care is spent on 10% of the population, whereas healthy people (about 50% of the population) account for about 3% of medical care expenditures (Bodenheimer & Fernandez, 2005). These statistics highlight the importance of maintaining and promoting health as a way to contain medical care costs. Thus, health psychologists can have a role in reducing medical care costs because unhealthy behaviors contribute to the chronic diseases that generate the majority of expenses, such as cardiovascular disease, cancer, diabetes, and chronic lower respiratory disease. Those with good health habits have lifetime medical costs of about *half* those for people with poor health habits. However, people who live longer have years to accrue medical costs, so even good health can be costly in the long run (van Baal et al., 2008). Promotion of good health habits is an important way to decrease the need for medical services in the short run.

Reducing the demand for medical services is another approach to controlling medical care costs (Fries, 1998), which may be a good strategy to move people toward self-care. The availability of a wide range

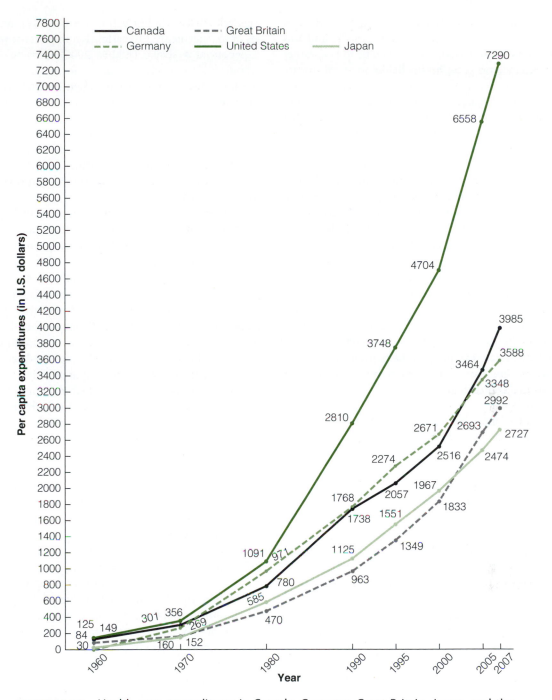

FIGURE 16.3 Health care expenditures in Canada, Germany, Great Britain, Japan, and the United States, 1960–2007.

Source: Health, United States, 2010, 2011, by National Center for Health Statistics, Hyattsville, MD: U.S. Government Printing Office, Table 121.

of medical technology has led to the widespread belief that modern medicine can cure any disease, and this belief fosters an overreliance on medicine to heal rather than a reliance on good health habits to avoid disease and on self-management for people with chronic conditions. As we discussed in Chapter 4, building feelings of personal efficacy for health—such as the beliefs that Robyn held—can help reduce the demand for medical services, and this approach has potential benefits for health in U.S. society. For example, encouraging individuals with chronic health problems to join self-help groups may reduce their need for intensive medical care (Humphreys & Moos, 2007). Additional research in this area may reveal that this approach can be a good strategy for containing medical care costs.

Controlling medical care costs will require substantial changes in the U.S. health care system. Insurance companies, hospitals, and physicians are all affected by health care reform and have all fought against changes (Mongan et al., 2008). As our examination of health care systems in other countries showed, no system can provide the best quality of medical care for low costs, but many countries do a better job than the United States.

Adapting to Changing Health Care Needs Chronic illnesses now are the leading cause of death and disability in the United States and other industrialized countries. Yet, the medical care system remains oriented toward providing acute care for sick people rather than providing services that will prevent, ameliorate, or manage chronic conditions. That is, the medical care system has not responded to meet the needs created by changed patterns of disease that occurred during the 20th century (Bodenheimer, 2005c). Controlling chronic illness can occur through two routes: management to control these disabling conditions and prevention to avoid them.

Management of chronic illness is a current need and will become even more important in the future. Cardiovascular disease, cancer, chronic lower respiratory disease, and diabetes account for nearly 70% of deaths in the United States (USCB, 2011). However, medical care for these and other chronic illnesses is plagued by undertreatment, overtreatment, and mistreatment. For example, overtreatment occurred with 30% of individuals attending a primary care clinic, who were diagnosed with asthma and prescribed inhaled corticosteroids despite a lack of evidence for symptoms of asthma (Lucas, Smeenk, Smeele, & van

Schayck, 2008). Undertreatment occurred in an analysis of management of hypertension in patients who had experienced a stroke (Elkins, 2006), 20% to 30% of whom did not receive treatment for diagnosed hypertension. Mistreatment occurs when health care providers make medical errors, which occurs with alarming frequency (HealthGrades, 2011). A system that provides more effective management of chronic illnesses will demand a shift from hospital- and physician-based care to a team approach that includes access to medical care and patient education to improve monitoring and self-care.

Self-care—rather than medical care—is a priority for prevention, which is a strategy that can reduce the need for medical services. In general, primary prevention offers more savings than secondary prevention. *Primary prevention* consists of immunizations and programs that encourage lifestyle changes; this type of prevention is usually a good bargain. Immunizations have some potential for harm but remain good choices unless the risk from side effects of the immunization is comparable to the risk of catching the disease. Programs that encourage people to quit smoking, eat properly, exercise, and moderate their drinking generally have low cost and little potential to do harm (Clark, 2008). In addition, some of these behaviors, such as smoking and inactivity, are risks for many health problems, and efforts oriented toward changing these behaviors can pay off by decreasing risks for several disorders. For example, a study of people who led a life that included the recommended exercise, body mass index, eating habits, and no history of smoking (Fraser & Shavlike, 2001) concluded that healthy lifestyle can add 10 years of life. Thus, primary prevention efforts pose few risks and offer many potential benefits.

Most prevention efforts target young and middle-aged adults who feel the need to change their behavior for health reasons. Such people are generally more responsive to prevention efforts than adolescents because adults generally recognize greater susceptibility to disease. Health habits begun later in life can add health years to life (Siegler, Bastian, Steffens, Bosworth, & Costa, 2002), but lifelong health habits should reap greater rewards. Thus, broadening prevention efforts to adolescents and young adults would be even more advantageous, but this group has been even more neglected in terms of lifestyle interventions (Williams, Holmbeck, & Greenley, 2002). Most of the health research and interventions for adolescents center on injury prevention and smoking deterrence, but adolescents build a foundation for a lifetime of health-related behaviors. Thus, primary prevention efforts tailored for people throughout the life span have the potential to improve health and life expectancy.

Secondary prevention consists of screening people at risk for developing a disease in order to find potential problems in their early and more treatable stages. However, such efforts can be costly because the number of people at risk may be much larger than the number who will develop the disease. Based on the economic considerations of cost–benefit analysis—that is, how much money is spent and how much is saved—secondary prevention may cost more than it saves.

However, neither hospitals' nor physicians' primary focus is on prevention services. Hospitals focus on acute care, and physicians' time is too expensive to focus on health education. Public health agencies, health educators, and health psychologists can provide health education in a more cost-effective manner than hospitals and physicians. Broadening the role of these entities in the health care system may provide better care as well as offer the potential for controlling medical care costs.

Will Health Psychology Continue to Grow?

The problems in the U.S. health care system influence people in clinical health psychology and behavioral medicine because these practitioners must work within that troubled system and demonstrate that the services they provide have value (IOM, 2010; Tovian, 2004). However, health psychologists are also working to reform the system. Their commitment to the biopsychosocial model has helped to promote this model as a more comprehensive view of health and to end the false dichotomy between mental and physical health (Suls & Rothman, 2004). Clinical health psychologists have firmly established their expertise as consultants, but health psychologists may become even more prominent as health care providers. Kaiser Permanente of Northern California designated psychologists as primary health care providers in its health maintenance facilities more than a decade ago (Bruns, 1998), and programs are currently in place for training health psychologists to be primary providers (McDaniel & le Roux, 2007). These psychologists typically become behavioral health or behavioral medicine specialists and serve as part of teams that implement an integrated care approach to health care services.

Psychologists are increasingly involved in team-based approaches to primary care (Nash, McKay, Vogel, & Masters, 2012), a trend that is likely to continue as long as the cost effectiveness of the psychologist's role can be demonstrated (Thielke et al, 2011).

Technological and medical advances create not only new opportunities to improve health, but also new issues for health psychology to address. One of the greatest scientific achievements of the last decade was the mapping of the human genome, which allowed researchers unprecedented opportunity to identify the genes that predispose people to various health conditions. As the genetic basis of health conditions becomes clearer, genetic tests will become increasingly available to the public. Health psychologists are ideally poised to help the health care system find ways to improve people's understanding of genetic risk information, to understand their emotional responses to test results, and to encourage high-risk individuals to maintain a healthy lifestyle (Saab et al., 2004). Other technological advances such as the Internet and smartphones allow for new methods of intervention, as these channels are being used to facilitate smoking cessation (Wetter et al., 2011), pain management (Rosser & Eccleston, 2011), and diabetes self-management (Arsand, Tatara, Ostengen, & Hartvigsen, 2010). Given their expertise in understanding health behavior, health literacy, and risk communication, psychologists will play an important role in designing and evaluating technology-based interventions for health behavior.

IN SUMMARY

Health psychology has made significant contributions to health care research and practice, but must meet a number of challenges to continue to grow. Several of these challenges relate to the troubled health care system in the United States. Medical care costs have risen in the United States more rapidly than in other industrialized countries, many of which manage to provide health care to a wider segment of their population and with a better outcome in terms of life expectancy and health expectancy. The United States needs to reform its inefficient medical care system so that a larger segment of the population can receive quality health care services.

The future of health care will demand better management of chronic illnesses and a greater emphasis on prevention. The aging population will increase the need for management of chronic conditions that are more common among older people. Prevention may be the key both to better health and to controlling medical care costs. Health psychology has a role to play in both the management and prevention of chronic illness, as reflected in the growth of the field of primary care psychology. Technological and medical advances such as genetic testing and smartphone technology present new opportunities for psychologists to contribute to the changing landscape of health care.

Making Health Psychology Personal

At the beginning of this chapter, we met Dwayne Brown and Robyn Green, two college students with varying attitudes toward health and differing health-related behaviors. You may see similarities and differences between Dwayne's and Robyn's behavior and your own. By contrasting their behavior with that of typical college students and analyzing their actions and attitudes, you may be able to understand your risks and form a plan to adopt health behaviors that will lead you to a healthier and longer life.

Understanding Your Risks

Like Dwayne and Robyn, more than 90% of college students rate their health as good, if not excellent (American College Health Association [ACHA], 2012). That perception is consistent with statistics on morbidity and mortality (USCB, 2011); young adults have a lower incidence of disease and death than older adults. The perception of good health may be beneficial, but that view may also create hazards by leading young adults (like Dwayne) to believe that their good health will continue, regardless of their behavior. This view is dangerously incorrect and may even increase the risks for the leading cause of death to this age group—unintentional injury (accidents). Indeed, both unintentional injury and intentional violence are leading causes of injury and death for people before age 45.

Injury and Violence   As the leading killers of young people, injuries and violence lead to more lost years of life than any other source. For example, each cancer-related death accounts for an average of 19 lost years of life, but each death due to unintentional injury steals an average of 33 years from a person's life expectancy (USCB, 2011). Sadly, most deaths among college students result from behaviors that contribute to either unintentional or intentional injuries.

Automobile crashes are by far the leading cause of fatal injuries among adolescents and young adults; they account for about two thirds of fatalities from unintentional injuries for young people 15 to 24 (USCB, 2011). Nearly half of these deaths are due to drinking and driving (Hingson, Heeren, Winter, & Wechsler, 2005). In the United States, young adults aged 21 to 24 lead all other age groups in a frightening statistic: fatalities due to drunk driving (USCB, 2011). In countries around the world, driving after drinking is an unfortunately common practice for college students, and countries with higher rates of this practice also have higher rates of traffic fatalities (Steptoe et al., 2004). The university environment appears to contribute to this dangerous behavior; college students are more likely than their nonstudent peers to drive after drinking (Hingson et al., 2005). College students are also more likely than their peers to use cell phones while driving, which is another behavior that sharply increases the risk of a crash (Cramer, Mayer, & Ryan, 2007). In the United States, the percentage of traffic fatalities due to such distracted driving nearly doubled from 2005 to 2009 (USCB, 2011).

Failure to use seat belts also contributes to the injury and death rate for automobile crashes; unrestrained drivers are 5 times more likely to be injured than those using restraints (Bustamante, Zhang, O'Connell, Rodriguez, & Borroto-Ponce, 2007). A substantial difference appears for male and female college students in driving-related risks. College men are less likely to use seat belts than college women (Henson, Carey, Carey, & Maisto, 2006). However, women are more likely to use cell phones while driving (Cramer et al., 2007).

College students are also victims (and perpetrators) of intentional violence, including assaults, robberies, rapes, and murders, but at a lower rate than nonstudents of comparable age (Carr, 2007). Crime rates in general have decreased in the United States, and that trend has also appeared on college campuses; only about one fourth of campus injuries are the result of intentional violence. However, many campus crimes go unreported, and people fail to report sexual and

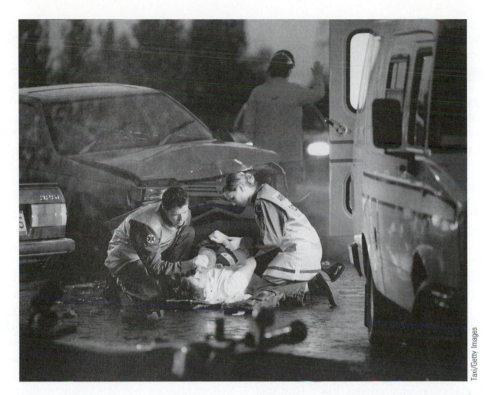

Automobile crashes are the leading cause of fatal injuries for adolescents and young adults in the United States.

partner violence more often than they report these acts of violence.

Two percent of college women and 1% of college men have been raped within the past school year (ACHA, 2012); nearly twice as many students report being the target of an attempted rape. These percentages are small but represent thousands of people per year. In addition, the percentage is cumulative; by the end of college life, the chance of a college woman experiencing a rape or attempted rape is more than 20% (Carr, 2007). Unwanted sexual touching and threats are much more common. Sexual victimization relates to a variety of health risks for women, including smoking, drug use, thoughts of suicide, and eating disorders (Gidycz, Orchowski, King, & Rich, 2008). Thus, sexual violence can initiate a cascade of health problems.

Dating violence is also a common experience during college, although emotionally abusive relationships are much more common (13% within the past year) than physically abusive ones (2% within the past year) (Carr, 2007). Women who are involved in physically abusive relationships are at increased risk for sexual violence and for victimization by a stalker, a form of victimization that is more common among college students than other groups. However, both women and men are perpetrators as well as victims of dating violence. A large, international study of dating violence (Straus, 2008) revealed that women are almost as likely as men to initiate dating violence. Couples in which one partner is more dominant than the other are at increased risk for violent behavior.

Suicide and suicide attempts are other forms of intentional violence that occur among college students. About 7% of college women and 6% of college men have seriously considered suicide within the past school year (ACHA, 2012); 1% had attempted suicide within that time span. Feelings of hopelessness and depression; involvement in an abusive relationship; and being lesbian, gay, or bisexual increase the risk for suicidal thoughts and suicide attempts (Carr, 2007). As Joetta Carr (2007) commented, "Some campus violence is a reflection of society's sexism, racism, and homophobia" (p. 311). Drinking, drug use, and mental health problems magnify the risks for all types of campus violence. However, college campuses are safer environments than most places, and students are safer on campus than in most communities.

Lifestyle Choices Although young adulthood presents hazards due to intentional and unintentional violence, it is also a time during which individuals adopt health-related behaviors that influence their health for decades. These health behaviors contribute to the risks for the leading causes of death during middle age and later. Dwayne and Robyn exhibit both risky and protective health behaviors, the most important of which is their status as nonsmokers. The choice to be a nonsmoker is typical of college students; a lower percentage of college students smoke than of those who have not attended college (Wetter et al., 2005). Indeed, education is currently the best predictor of smoking status. Thus, it may not be surprising that individuals with a college education live longer and experience better health than others.

Dwayne's abstention from alcohol and Robyn's social drinking are patterns that appear among college students, but many students choose less wisely and engage in binge drinking. Binge drinking represents the most dangerous pattern of drinking among young people. Such behavior can bring many health problems, and almost 4% of college students report that drinking interfered with their academic performance (ACHA, 2012). Even occasional binge drinking is risky because of its association with injury and violence. Over 40% of those between ages 18 and 25 engage in binge drinking (NCHS, 2011), and college students are more likely than others to do so.

College students often fail to eat a healthy diet. When students begin college, they often enter a new living situation in which they make dietary choices rather than eat at home. A study of college students in Greece (Papadaki, Hondros, Scott, & Kapsokefalou, 2007) found that students who moved away from home tended to change their diet to less healthy choices that included more sugar, alcohol, and fast food. Those who continued to live at home made few changes. Like Dwayne, few college students in the United States meet the guidelines for fruit and vegetable consumption (Adams & Colner, 2008). Like Robyn, those who do tend to adhere to other healthy behaviors, including using seat belts, engaging in physical activity, and sleeping well, along with decreased chances of smoking and driving after drinking.

College students are less likely than the general population to be overweight and more likely to engage in physical exercise; yet, significant percentages of students fall short of those health goals. One study of eating, weight, and physical activity among college students (Burke, Lofgren, Morrell, & Reilly, 2007) indicated that 33% of male and 22% of female college students were overweight; 11% and 7% were obese. A third of the women and 23% of the men accumulated less than 30 minutes of physical activity per day. As we would expect, these students had elevated cholesterol and blood pressure, laying the foundations for cardiovascular disease. Neither Dwayne nor Robyn is overweight, but Dwayne's diet and lack of exercise puts him at greater risk for high cholesterol and high blood pressure than Robyn, who does not want to repeat her grandfather's experience with heart disease.

College students also encounter stress, and Robyn's rating of her stress is more typical than Dwayne's rating, which was very low. Most college students report many more sources of stress, which is the most frequently named reason for academic problems (ACHA, 2012). Thus, stress is a major challenge for college students, but developing problem-focused strategies to manage stress is important (Largo-Wight, Peterson, & Chen, 2005). Indeed, college students can lead healthy lives during their college years by cultivating a healthy lifestyle, and these habits provide the basis for a longer life as well as a healthier one.

What Can You Do to Cultivate a Healthy Lifestyle?

Health psychologists and other health researchers generate a massive amount of information about health and health-related behaviors. Electronic media, including television and the Internet, inundate people with health information; some of this information may come from valid sources, but some may not. People are often confused by what they perceive as an overwhelming amount of information, which even seems contradictory at times (Kickbusch, 2008). Evaluating all the information and translating it into personal terms is a substantial task, which requires *health literacy*—the ability to read and understand health information to make health decisions. This ability is related, of course, to literacy in general but goes further to include an understanding and evaluation of scientific information related to health (White, Chen, & Atchison, 2008; Zaarcadoolas, Pleasant, & Greer, 2005).

Increase Your Health Literacy

Despite their educational level, college students do not necessarily have a high degree of health literacy. They actively seek health information but tend to consult friends and family rather than more expert sources (Baxter, Egbert, & Ho, 2008). To increase your health literacy, begin to evaluate health claims critically, considering the source of the claim (Chapter 2 presents useful tips for evaluating the trustworthiness of information on the Internet). Expertise matters, so listen to the experts. Health research has produced a large body of evidence that allows health researchers to make recommendations. The massive research findings from health psychology represent an authoritative source, with recommendations on smoking, drinking alcohol, eating a healthy diet, exercising, decreasing the risk of unintentional injury, and managing stress.

Adopt Good Health Behaviors—Now   One way to summarize the recommendations from health research is to work toward integrating the findings from the Alameda County study into your life. Recall from Chapter 2 that this study identified five behaviors that led to better health and lower mortality (Belloc, 1973; Berkman & Breslow, 1983): (1) refraining from smoking cigarettes, (2) engaging in regular physical exercise, (3) drinking alcohol in moderation or not at all, (4) maintaining a healthy weight, and (5) sleeping 7 to 8 hours per night.

Of these habits, avoiding tobacco is probably the most important health behavior you can adopt, as it is the health behavior most strongly linked to longevity (Ford, Bergmann, Boeing, Li, & Capewell, 2012; Ford, Zhao, Tsai, & Li, 2011). The damage from tobacco takes years to become apparent, but smoking cigarettes and exposure to secondhand smoke are both hazardous. The evidence is also overwhelming concerning the benefits of adopting an active lifestyle. For individuals of any age, physical activity boosts health and prevents disease and disability. These two health habits are more important for long-term health benefits than for immediate ones, but nonsmokers who exercise regularly experience short-term health advantages as well as longer life expectancies.

Moderating alcohol intake is also an important health behavior. Light drinkers are healthier than those who drink more, and probably than those who do not drink at all. However, these findings apply to older adults more strongly than to younger ones. For college students, light drinking can often turn into

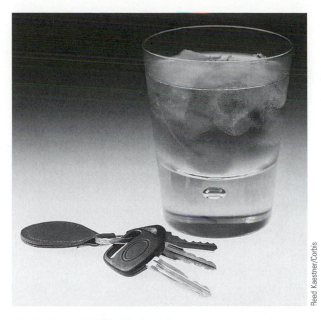

Reed Kaestner/Corbis

Alcohol is a significant contributor to motor vehicle crashes, and college students are more likely than others to binge drink.

binge drinking, which presents many serious risks to college students. Thus, good advice for college students is to work toward moderating drinking and avoiding the hazards of mixing alcohol and motor vehicles. Also, alcohol increases the risk of all types of violence, which is the leading cause of death for young adults. Avoiding heavy or binge drinking is the wise choice for college students.

Maintaining a healthy weight is important, but so are food choices. The foundation for cardiovascular disease begins during adolescence and young adulthood, and food choices are important. A high-fat diet is a component in this process. Even if you are able to maintain close to an ideal weight while eating a high-fat diet (as Dwayne was), this choice is a bad one. Strong evidence shows that a diet with lots of fruits and vegetables provides many health benefits. Choosing such a diet while balancing work, school, and personal demands is not an easy task but will lead to short-term benefits through weight maintenance and long-term advantages through decreasing the risks for cardiovascular disease, diabetes, and cancer. How much do these health habits matter? People who do not smoke, get adequate physical activity, moderate their alcohol consumption, and keep a healthy diet can benefit from an estimated *14 more years of life* than those who do not practice these four behaviors (Khaw et al., 2008)!

The fifth recommendation from the Alameda County study may be the most difficult for college students to follow: Get 7 to 8 hours of sleep a night. People who sleep more than 8 or less than 6 hours per night experience higher death rates than those who get 7 to 8 hours of sleep (Patel et al., 2004). Setting a priority on sleep may be difficult but will also pay off immediately in terms of energy, concentration, and perhaps even improved immune function (Motivala & Irwin, 2007).

A final recommendation from the Alameda County study emphasized the importance of social support (Camacho & Wiley, 1983; Wiley & Camacho, 1980). People with a social network are healthier than those with few social contacts. College students have many opportunities to form a social network of friends, which they may add to their families as sources of social support. Remember that social support provides one type of coping strategy, but it is wise to cultivate a range of such strategies, including problem-focused as well as emotion-focused strategies, and use them appropriately.

The combination of these health behaviors will extend your life and improve your health, not only in the future but also during your college years. We (Linda, Jess, and John) sincerely wish you a healthy and happy future.

IN SUMMARY

Improving the health of college students requires understanding the risks specific to this group and finding ways to diminish those risks, including changes in their health-related behaviors. Injuries from intentional and unintentional violence are major health threats to young adults, including college students. Vehicle crashes are the most common threat, but injuries and deaths occur as a result of assault, rape, partner violence, suicide, and homicide. Alcohol is a factor in all of those types of violence.

Health habits adopted during young adulthood lay the foundation for health or disease in later years. To make healthy choices, individuals need to develop their health literacy so that they can evaluate the health information that that they receive from others and from the media. A good guideline for cultivating a healthy lifestyle comes from the Alameda County study, which found that people are healthier and live longer if they (1) refrain from smoking cigarettes, (2) engage in physical activity regularly, (3) drink alcohol in moderation or not at all, (4) maintain a healthy weight, and (5) sleep 7 to 8 hours per night. In addition, developing a social support network enhances health.

Answers

This chapter has addressed three basic questions:

1. What role does health psychology play in contributing to the goals of *Healthy People 2020*?

Health psychology is one of several disciplines that have a role in helping the nation achieve the goals and objectives of *Healthy People 2020*. The two broad goals of this document are (1) increasing the span of healthy life and (2) eliminating health disparities among various ethnic groups. Health psychologists emphasize adding healthy years of life, not merely more years. They cooperate with other health professionals in understanding and reducing health discrepancies among different ethnic groups, but this goal has proven difficult to accomplish.

2. What is the outlook for the future of health psychology?

Health psychology faces challenges in the 21st century. Finding ways to control health care costs is a major goal for all health care providers. Health psychologists can contribute to that goal through their expertise in understanding and treating the chronic diseases that have become the leading causes of death in industrialized countries. Even more important, health psychologists have advocated for prevention, which has the potential to decrease the need for health care. Prevention through behavior change can help in controlling health care costs. To be included in future health care, health psychologists must continue to add to both the research and practice components of the field: Build a research base and develop more effective strategies for behavior change.

3. **How can you use health psychology to cultivate a healthier lifestyle?**

The habits that you adopt during young adulthood form a foundation for your health-related behavior throughout middle and older adulthood, so the choices you make now are important for your future health. Health psychology offers suggestions concerning how to cultivate healthy choices in terms of smoking, drinking and drug use, diet, exercise, and stress management. Increasing your health literacy and relying on research rather than information from the media or from friends provide a strategy for making good health choices.

Suggested Readings

Kickbusch, I. (2008). Health literacy: An essential skill for the twenty-first century. *Health Education, 108,* 101–104. This article examines the challenges to developing health literacy and emphasizes the importance of doing so in light of the ever-increasing complexity of health research.

Mongan, J. J., Ferris, T. G., & Lee, T. H. (2008). Options for slowing the growth of health care costs. *New England Journal of Medicine, 358,* 1509–1514. This recent article examines some possibilities for controlling health care costs without a drastic overhaul of the U.S. health care system.

Whitfield, K. E., Weidner, G., Clark, R., & Anderson, N. B. (2002). Sociodemographic diversity in behavioral medicine. *Journal of Consulting and Clinical Psychology, 70,* 463–481. Keith Whitfield and his colleagues provide a comprehensive review of ethnic, gender, and economic factors that affect health and life expectancy, analyzing the risks and protective factors associated with each demographic group.

Glossary

A-beta fibers Large sensory fibers involved in rapidly transmitting sensation and possibly in inhibiting the transmission of pain. (Chapter 7)

A-delta fibers Small sensory fibers that are involved in the experience of "fast" pain. (Chapter 7)

absolute risk A person's chances of developing a disease or disorder independent of any risk that other people may have for that disease or disorder. (Chapter 2)

abstinence violation effect Feelings of guilt and loss of control often experienced after a person lapses into an unhealthy habit after a period of abstinence. (Chapters 12, 15)

acceptance and commitment therapy A type of therapy that teaches people to notice and accept unwanted thoughts and feelings, while also committing to valued goals and activities. (Chapter 7)

acetylcholine One of the major neurotransmitters of the autonomic nervous system. (Chapter 5)

acquired immune deficiency syndrome (AIDS) An immune deficiency caused by viral infection and resulting in vulnerability to a wide range of bacterial, viral, and malignant diseases. (Chapter 6)

acrolein A yellowish or colorless, pungent liquid produced as a by-product of tobacco smoke; one of the aldehydes. (Chapter 12)

acupressure The application of pressure rather than needles to the points used in acupuncture. (Chapter 8)

acupuncture An ancient Chinese form of analgesia that consists of inserting needles into specific points on the skin and continuously stimulating the needles. (Chapter 8)

acute pain Short-term pain that results from tissue damage or other trauma. (Chapter 7)

addiction Dependence on a drug such that stopping its use results in withdrawal symptoms. (Chapter 13)

adherence A patient's ability and willingness to follow recommended health practices. (Chapter 4)

adrenal cortex The outer layer of the adrenal glands; secretes glucocorticoids. (Chapter 5)

adrenal glands Endocrine glands, located on top of each kidney, that secrete hormones and affect metabolism. (Chapter 5)

adrenal medulla The inner layer of the adrenal glands; secretes epinephrine and norepinephrine. (Chapter 5)

adrenocortical response The response of the adrenal cortex, prompted by ACTH, that results in the release of glucocorticoids, including cortisol. (Chapter 5)

adrenocorticotropic hormone (ACTH) A hormone produced by the anterior portion of the pituitary gland that acts on the adrenal gland and is involved in the stress response. (Chapter 5)

adrenomedullary response The response of the adrenal medulla, prompted by sympathetic nervous system activation, that results in the release of epinephrine. (Chapter 5)

aerobic exercise Exercise that requires an increased amount of oxygen consumption over an extended period of time. (Chapter 15)

afferent neurons Sensory neurons that relay information from the sense organs toward the brain. (Chapter 7)

agoraphobia An anxiety state characterized by fear about or avoidance of places or situations from which escape might be difficult. (Chapter 6)

alarm reaction The first stage of the general adaptation syndrome (GAS), in which the body's defenses are mobilized against a stressor. (Chapter 5)

alcohol dehydrogenase A liver enzyme that metabolizes alcohol into aldehyde. (Chapter 13)

aldehyde dehydrogenase An enzyme that converts aldehyde to acetic acid. (Chapter 13)

aldehydes A class of organic compounds obtained from alcohol by oxidation and also found in cigarette smoke; they cause mutations and are related to the development of cancer. (Chapter 12)

alkalosis An abnormally high level of alkaline in the body. (Chapter 14)

allergy An immune system response characterized by an abnormal reaction to a foreign substance. (Chapter 6)

allostasis The concept that different circumstances require different levels of physiological activation. (Chapter 5)

alternative medicine A group of diverse medical and health care systems, practices, and products that are not currently considered part of conventional medicine and are used as alternatives to conventional treatment. (Chapter 8)

amenorrhea Cessation of the menses. (Chapter 14)

amphetamines One type of stimulant drug. (Chapter 13)

anabolic steroids Steroid drugs that increase muscle bulk and decrease body fat but also have toxic effects. (Chapter 13)

anaerobic exercise Exercise that requires short, intensive bursts of energy but does not require an increased amount of oxygen use. (Chapter 15)

analgesic drugs Drugs that decrease the perception of pain. (Chapter 7)

anemia A low level of red blood cells, leading to generalized weakness and lack of vitality. (Chapter 14)

angina pectoris A disorder involving a restricted blood supply to the myocardium, which results in chest pain and restricted breathing. (Chapter 9)

anorexia nervosa An eating disorder characterized by intentional starvation, distorted body image, excessive amounts of energy, and an intense fear of gaining weight. (Chapter 14)

antibodies Protein substances produced in response to a specific invader or antigen, marking it for destruction and thus creating immunity to that invader. (Chapter 6)

antigens Substances that provoke the immune system to produce antibodies. (Chapter 6)

anus Opening through which feces are eliminated. (Chapter 14)

arteries Vessels carrying blood away from the heart. (Chapter 9)

arterioles Small branches of an artery. (Chapter 9)

arteriosclerosis A condition marked by loss of elasticity and hardening of arteries. (Chapter 9)

asthma A chronic disease that causes constriction of the bronchial tubes, preventing air from passing freely and causing wheezing and difficulty breathing during attacks. (Chapters 6, 11)

atheromatous plaques Deposits of cholesterol and other lipids, connective tissue, and muscle tissue. (Chapter 9)

atherosclerosis The formation of plaque within the arteries. (Chapter 9)

autoimmune diseases Disorders that occur as a result of the immune system's failure to differentiate between body cells and foreign cells, resulting in the body's attack and destruction of its own cells. (Chapter 6)

autonomic nervous system (ANS) The part of the peripheral nervous system that primarily serves internal organs. (Chapter 5)

aversion therapy A type of behavioral therapy, based on classical conditioning techniques, that uses some aversive stimulus to counter-condition the patient's response. (Chapter 13)

Ayurveda A system of medicine that originated in India more than 2,000 years ago; it emphasizes the attainment of health through balance and connection with all things in the universe. (Chapter 8)

B-cell A variety of lymphocyte that attacks invading microorganisms. (Chapter 6)

barbiturates Synthetic sedative drugs used medically to induce sleep. (Chapter 13)

behavior modification Shaping behavior by manipulating reinforcement in order to obtain a desired behavior. (Chapter 7)

behavioral medicine An interdisciplinary field concerned with developing and integrating behavioral and biomedical sciences. (Chapter 1)

behavioral willingness A person's motivation in a given situation to engage in a risky behavior, often as a reaction to social and situational pressures. (Chapter 4)

benign Limited in cell growth to a single tumor. (Chapter 10)

beta-carotene A form of vitamin A found in abundance in vegetables such as carrots and sweet potatoes. (Chapter 10)

bile salts Salts produced in the liver and stored in the gall bladder that aid in digestion of fats. (Chapter 14)

biofeedback The process of providing feedback information about the status of a biological system to that system. (Chapter 8)

biomedical model A perspective that considers disease to result from exposure to a specific disease-causing organism. (Chapter 1)

biopsychosocial model The approach to health that includes biological, psychological, and social influences. (Chapter 1)

body mass index (BMI) An estimate of obesity determined by body weight and height. (Chapter 14)

bronchitis Any inflammation of the bronchi. (Chapter 12)

bulimia An eating disorder characterized by periodic bingeing and purging, the latter usually taking the form of self-induced vomiting or laxative abuse. (Chapter 14)

C fibers Small-diameter nerve fibers that provide information concerning slow, diffuse, lingering pain. (Chapter 7)

cancer A group of diseases characterized by the presence of new cells that grow and spread beyond control. (Chapter 10)

capillaries Very small vessels that connect arteries and veins. (Chapter 9)

carcinogenic Cancer-inducing. (Chapter 10)

carcinoma Cancer of the epithelial tissues. (Chapter 10)

cardiac rehabilitation A complex of approaches designed to restore heart patients to cardiovascular health. (Chapter 9)

cardiologist A medical doctor who specializes in the diagnosis and treatment of heart disease. (Chapter 9)

cardiovascular disease (CVD) Disorders of the circulatory system, including coronary artery disease and stroke. (Chapter 9)

cardiovascular reactivity (CVR) An increase in blood pressure and heart rate as a reaction to frustration or harassment. (Chapter 9)

cardiovascular system The system of the body that includes the heart, arteries, and veins. (Chapter 9)

case–control study A retrospective epidemiological study in which people affected by a given disease (cases) are compared with others not affected (controls). (Chapter 2)

catecholamines A class of chemicals containing epinephrine and norepinephrine. (Chapter 5)

catharsis The spoken or written expression of strong negative emotion, which may result in improvement in physiological or psychological health. (Chapter 5)

central control trigger A nerve impulse that descends from the brain and influences the perception of pain (Chapter 7)

central nervous system (CNS) All the neurons within the brain and spinal cord. (Chapter 5)

cholecystokinin (CCK) A peptide hormone released by the intestines that may be involved in feelings of satiation after eating. (Chapter 14)

chronic disease A long-lasting disease that can be controlled but not cured. (Chapters 1, 11)

chronic pain Pain that endures beyond the time of normal healing; frequently experienced in the absence of detectable tissue damage. (Chapter 7)

chronic recurrent pain Alternating episodes of intense pain and no pain. (Chapter 7)

cirrhosis A liver disease resulting in the production of nonfunctional scar tissue. (Chapter 13)

clinical trial A research design that tests the effects of medical treatment. Many clinical trials are randomized controlled trials that allow researchers to determine whether a new treatment is or is not effective. (Chapter 2)

cluster headache A type of severe headache that occurs in daily clusters for 4 to 16 weeks. Symptoms are similar to migraine, but duration is much briefer. (Chapter 7)

cocaine A stimulant drug extracted from the coca plant. (Chapter 13)

cognitive behavioral therapy (CBT) A type of therapy that aims to develop beliefs, attitudes, thoughts, and skills to make positive changes in behavior. (Chapter 5)

cognitive therapy A type of therapy that aims to change attitudes and beliefs, assuming that behavior change will follow. (Chapter 7)

complementary medicine A group of diverse medical and health care systems, practices, and products that are not currently considered part of conventional medicine and are used in addition to conventional techniques. (Chapter 8)

conscientiousness A personality trait marked by a tendency to be planful and goal-oriented, to delay gratification, and to follow norms and rules. (Chapter 4)

continuum theory A theory that explains adherence with a single set of factors that should apply equally to all people. (Chapter 4)

control group In an experiment or clinical trial, the group of participants who do not receive an active treatment. The control group serves as a comparison to the experimental group. (Chapter 2)

coping Strategies that individuals use to manage the distressing problems and emotions in their lives. (Chapter 5)

coronary artery disease (CAD) A disorder of the myocardium arising from atherosclerosis and/or arteriosclerosis. (Chapter 9)

coronary heart disease (CHD) Any damage to the myocardium resulting from insufficient blood supply. (Chapter 9)

correlation coefficient Any positive or negative relationship between two variables. Correlational evidence cannot prove causation, but only that two variables vary together. (Chapter 2)

correlational studies Studies designed to yield information concerning the degree of relationship between two variables. (Chapter 2)

cortisol A type of glucocorticoid that provides a natural defense against inflammation and regulates carbohydrate metabolism. (Chapter 5)

cross-sectional study A type of research design in which subjects of different ages are studied at one point in time. (Chapter 2)

crowding A person's perception of discomfort in a high-density environment. (Chapter 5)

cytokines Chemical messengers secreted by cells in the immune system, forming a communication link between the nervous and immune systems. (Chapter 6)

daily hassles Everyday events that people experience as harmful, threatening, or annoying. (Chapter 5)

delirium tremens A condition induced by alcohol withdrawal and characterized by excessive trembling, sweating, anxiety, and hallucinations. (Chapter 13)

delta alcoholism A drinking pattern characterized by an inability to abstain from alcohol. (Chapter 13)

dependence A condition in which a drug becomes incorporated into the functioning of the body's cells so that it is needed for "normal" functioning. (Chapters 7, 13)

dependent variable In an experiment or clinical trial, the variable that represents the effect or outcome of interest. (Chapter 2)

diabetes mellitus A disorder caused by insulin deficiency. (Chapters 6, 11)

diaphragm The partition separating the cavity of the chest from that of the abdomen. (Chapter 12)

diastolic pressure A measure of blood pressure between contractions of the heart. (Chapter 9)

diathesis–stress model A theory of stress that suggests that some individuals are vulnerable to stress-related illnesses because they are genetically predisposed to those illnesses. (Chapter 6)

disulfiram A drug that causes an aversive reaction when taken with alcohol; used to treat alcoholism; Antabuse. (Chapter 13)

dopamine A neurotransmitter that is especially important in mediating the reward associated with taking psychoactive drugs. (Chapter 13)

dorsal horns The part of the spinal cord away from the stomach that receives sensory input and that may play an important role in the perception of pain. (Chapter 7)

dose–response relationship A direct, consistent relationship between an independent variable, such as a behavior, and a dependent variable, such as an illness. For example, the greater the number of cigarettes one smokes, the greater the likelihood of lung cancer. (Chapter 2)

double-blind design An experimental design in which neither the subjects nor those who dispense the treatment condition have knowledge of who receives the treatment and who receives the placebo. (Chapter 2)

eating disorder Any serious and habitual disturbance in eating behavior that produces unhealthy consequences. (Chapter 14)

efferent neurons Motor neurons that convey impulses away from the brain. (Chapter 7)

electrolyte imbalance A condition caused by loss of body minerals. (Chapter 14)

electromyograph (EMG) biofeedback Feedback that reflects activity of the skeletal muscles. (Chapter 8)

emotion-focused coping Coping strategies oriented toward managing the emotions that accompany the perception of stress. (Chapter 5)

emotional disclosure A therapeutic technique whereby people express their strong emotions by talking or writing about the events that precipitated them. (Chapter 5)

emphysema A chronic lung disease in which scar tissue and mucus obstruct the respiratory passages. (Chapter 12)

endocrine system The system of the body consisting of ductless glands. (Chapter 5)

endorphins Naturally occurring neurochemicals whose effects resemble those of the opiates. (Chapter 7)

environmental tobacco smoke (ETS) The smoke of spouses, parents, or coworkers to which nonsmokers are exposed; passive smoking. (Chapter 12)

epidemiology A branch of medicine that investigates the various factors that contribute either to positive health or to the frequency and distribution of a disease or disorder. (Chapter 2)

epinephrine A chemical manufactured by the adrenal medulla that accounts for much of the hormone production of the adrenal glands; sometimes called adrenaline. (Chapter 5)

esophagus The tube leading from the pharynx to the stomach. (Chapter 14)

essential hypertension Elevations of blood pressure that have no known cause. (Chapter 9)

ethanol The variety of alcohol used in beverages. (Chapter 13)

ex post facto design A scientific study in which the values of the independent variable are not manipulated, but selected by the experimenter after the groups have naturally divided themselves. (Chapter 2)

exhaustion stage The final stage of the general adaptation syndrome (GAS), in which the body's ability to resist a stressor has been depleted. (Chapter 5)

experimental group In an experiment or clinical trial, the group of participants who receive an active treatment. (Chapter 2)

feces Any materials left over after digestion. (Chapter 14)

fetal alcohol syndrome (FAS) A pattern of physical and psychological symptoms found in infants whose mothers drank heavily during pregnancy. (Chapter 13)

fibromyalgia A chronic pain condition characterized by tender points throughout the body; this condition produces symptoms of fatigue, headache, cognitive difficulties, anxiety, and sleep disturbances. (Chapter 7)

formaldehyde A colorless, pungent gas found in cigarette smoke; it causes irritation of the respiratory system and has been found to be carcinogenic; one of the aldehydes. (Chapter 12)

gall bladder A sac on the liver in which bile is stored. (Chapter 14)

gamma alcoholism A drinking pattern characterized by loss of control. (Chapter 13)

gastric juices Stomach secretions that aid in digestion. (Chapter 14)

gate control theory A theory of pain holding that structures in the spinal cord act as a gate for sensory input that is interpreted as pain. (Chapter 7)

general adaptation syndrome (GAS) The body's generalized attempt to defend itself against stress; consists of alarm reaction, resistance, and exhaustion. (Chapter 5)

ghrelin A peptide hormone produced primarily in the stomach, the level of which rises before and falls after meals. (Chapter 14)

glucagon A hormone secreted by the pancreas that stimulates the release of glucose, thus elevating blood sugar level. (Chapter 11)

granulocyte A type of lymphocyte that acts rapidly to kill invading organisms. (Chapter 6)

health disparity A difference in a health condition that exists between specific population groups. (Chapter 16)

health expectancy The period of life that a person spends free from disability. (Chapter 16)

health literacy The ability to read and understand health information to make health decisions. (Chapter 16)

health psychology A field of psychology that contributes to both behavioral medicine and behavioral health; the scientific study of behaviors that relate to health enhancement, disease prevention, and rehabilitation. (Chapter 1)

high-density lipoprotein (HDL) A form of lipoprotein that confers some protection against coronary artery disease. (Chapter 9)

hormones Chemical substances released into the blood and having effects on other parts of the body. (Chapter 5)

human immunodeficiency virus (HIV) A virus that attacks the human immune system, depleting the body's ability to fight infection; the infection that causes AIDS. (Chapter 11)

humoral immunity Immunity created through the process of exposure to antigens and production of antibodies in the bloodstream. (Chapter 6)

hydrocyanic acid A poisonous acid produced by treating a cyanide with an acid; one of the products of cigarette smoke. (Chapter 12)

hypertension Abnormally high blood pressure, with either a systolic reading in excess of 160 or a diastolic reading in excess of 105. (Chapter 9)

hypoglycemia Deficiency of sugar in the blood. (Chapter 14)

hypothalamus A small structure beneath the thalamus, involved in the control of eating, drinking, and emotional behavior. (Chapter 14)

illness behavior Those activities undertaken by people who feel ill and who wish to discover their state of health, as well as suitable remedies. Illness behavior precedes formal diagnosis. (Chapter 3)

immunity A response to foreign microorganisms that occurs with repeated exposure and results in resistance to a disease. (Chapter 6)

implementational intentions Detailed plans that link a specific situation with a goal that a person wants to achieve. (Chapter 4)

incidence A measure of the frequency of new cases of a disease or disorder during a specified period of time. (Chapter 2)

independent variable In an experiment or clinical trial, the variable that represents the presumed cause of an effect or outcome. (Chapter 2)

induction The process of being placed into a hypnotic state. (Chapter 8)

inflammation A general immune system response that works to restore damaged tissue. (Chapter 6)

insulin A hormone that enhances glucose intake to the cells. (Chapter 11)

integrative medicine The approach to treatment that attempts to integrate techniques from both conventional and alternative medicine. (Chapter 8)

interneurons Neurons that connect sensory neurons to motor neurons; association neurons. (Chapter 7)

ischemia Restriction of blood flow to tissue or organs; often used with reference to the heart. (Chapter 9)

islet cells The part of the pancreas that produces glucagon and insulin. (Chapter 11)

isokinetic exercise Exercise requiring exertion for lifting and additional effort for returning weight to the starting position. (Chapter 15)

isometric exercise Exercise performed by contracting muscles against an immovable object. (Chapter 15)

isotonic exercise Exercise that requires the contraction of muscles and the movement of joints, as in weight lifting. (Chapter 15)

Kaposi's sarcoma A malignancy characterized by multiple soft, dark blue or purple nodules on the skin, with hemorrhages. (Chapter 10)

laminae Layers of cell bodies. (Chapter 7)

lay referral network The network of family and friends from whom a person may first seek medical information and advice. (Chapter 3)

leptin A protein hormone produced by fat cells in the body that is related to eating and weight control. (Chapter 14)

leukemia Cancer originating in blood or blood-producing cells. (Chapter 10)

life events Major events in a person's life that require change or adaptation. (Chapter 5)

life expectancy The expected number of years of life that remain for a person of a given age. (Chapters 1, 16)

lipoproteins Substances in the blood consisting of lipid and protein. (Chapter 9)

liver The largest gland in the body; it aids digestion by producing bile, regulates organic components of the blood, and acts as a detoxifier of blood. (Chapter 14)

longitudinal study A type of research design in which one group of subjects is studied over a period of time. (Chapter 2)

low-density lipoprotein (LDL) A form of lipoprotein found to be positively related to coronary artery disease. (Chapter 9)

lymph Tissue fluid that has entered a lymphatic vessel. (Chapter 6)

lymph nodes Small nodules of lymphatic tissue spaced throughout the lymphatic system that help clean lymph of debris. (Chapter 6)

lymphatic system System that transports lymph through the body. (Chapter 6)

lymphocytes White blood cells found in lymph that are involved in the immune function. (Chapter 6)

lymphoma Cancer of the lymphoid tissues, including lymph nodes. (Chapter 10)

macrophage A type of lymphocyte that attacks invading organisms. (Chapter 6)

malignant Having the ability not only to grow but also to spread to other parts of the body. (Chapter 10)

medulla The structure of the hindbrain just above the spinal cord. (Chapter 7)

meta-analysis A statistical technique for combining results of several studies when these studies have similar definitions of variables. (Chapter 2)

metastasize To undergo metastasis, the spread of malignancy from one part of the body to another by way of the blood or lymph systems. (Chapter 10)

migraine headache Recurrent headache pain originally believed to be caused by constriction and dilation of the vascular arteries but now accepted as involving neurons in the brain stem. (Chapter 7)

model A set of related principles or hypotheses constructed to explain significant relationships among concepts or observations. (Chapter 2)

motivational interviewing A therapeutic approach that originated within substance abuse treatment that attempts to change a client's motivation and prepares the client to enact changes in behavior. (Chapter 4)

motivational phase In the health action process approach, the stage in which a person develops an intention to pursue a health-related goal. (Chapter 4)

myelin A fatty substance that acts as insulation for neurons. (Chapter 7)

myocardial infarction Heart attack. (Chapter 9)

myocardium The heart muscle. (Chapter 9)

natural killer (NK) cell A type of lymphocyte that attacks invading organisms. (Chapter 6)

negative reinforcement Removing an unpleasant or negatively valued stimulus from a situation, thereby strengthening the behavior that precedes this removal. (Chapter 4)

neoplastic Characterized by new, abnormal growth of cells. (Chapter 10)

neuroendocrine system Those endocrine glands that are controlled by and interact with the nervous system. (Chapter 5)

neurons Nerve cells. (Chapter 5)

neuroticism A personality trait marked by a tendency to experience negative emotional states. (Chapter 3)

neurotransmitters Chemicals that are released by neurons and that affect the activity of other neurons. (Chapter 5)

nitric oxide A colorless gas prepared by the action of nitric acid on copper and also produced in cigarette smoke; it affects oxygen metabolism and may be dangerous. (Chapter 12)

nocebo effect Adverse effect of a placebo. (Chapter 2)

nociceptors Sensory receptors in the skin and organs that are capable of responding to various types of stimulation that may cause tissue damage. (Chapter 7)

non-Hodgkin's lymphoma A malignancy characterized by rapidly growing tumors that are spread through the circulatory or lymphatic systems. (Chapter 10)

norepinephrine One of two major neurotransmitters of the autonomic nervous system. (Chapter 5)

oncologist A physician who specializes in the treatment of cancer. (Chapter 10)

opiates Drugs derived from the opium poppy, including codeine, morphine, and heroin. (Chapter 13)

optimistic bias The belief that other people, but not oneself, will develop a disease, have an accident, or experience other negative events. (Chapters 4, 9, 12)

osteoarthritis Progressive inflammation of the joints. (Chapter 7)

osteoporosis A disease characterized by a reduction in bone density, brittleness of bones, and a loss of calcium from the bones. (Chapter 15)

outcome expectations The beliefs that carrying out a specific behavior will lead to valued outcomes. (Chapter 4)

pancreas An endocrine gland, located below the stomach, that produces digestive juices and hormones. (Chapter 11)

pancreatic juices Acid-reducing enzymes secreted by the pancreas into the small intestine. (Chapter 14)

parasympathetic nervous system A division of the autonomic nervous system that promotes relaxation and functions under normal, nonstressful conditions. (Chapter 5)

passive smoking The exposure of nonsmokers to the smoke of spouses, parents, or coworkers; environmental tobacco smoke. (Chapter 12)

pathogen Any disease-causing organism. (Chapter 1)

periaqueductal gray An area of the midbrain that, when stimulated, decreases pain. (Chapter 7)

peripheral nervous system (PNS) The nerves that lie outside the brain and spinal cord. (Chapter 5)

peristalsis Contractions that propel food through the digestive tract. (Chapter 14)

personal control Confidence that people have in their ability to control the events that shape their lives. (Chapter 5)

phagocytosis The process of engulfing and killing foreign particles. (Chapter 6)

phantom limb pain The experience of chronic pain in an absent body part. (Chapter 7)

pharynx Part of the digestive tract between the mouth and the esophagus. (Chapter 14)

pituitary gland An endocrine gland that lies within the brain and whose secretions regulate many other glands. (Chapter 5)

placebo An inactive substance or condition that has the appearance of an active treatment and that may cause improvement or change because of people's belief in the placebo's efficacy. (Chapter 2)

plasma cells Cells, derived from B-cells, that secrete antibodies. (Chapter 6)

population density A physical condition in which a large population occupies a limited space. (Chapter 5)

positive reinforcement Adding a positively valued stimulus to a situation, thereby strengthening the behavior it follows. (Chapter 4)

positive reinforcer Any positively valued stimulus that, when added to a situation, strengthens the behavior it follows. (Chapter 7)

posttraumatic stress disorder (PTSD) An anxiety disorder caused by experience with an extremely traumatic event and characterized by recurrent and intrusive reexperiencing of the event. (Chapters 5, 6)

prechronic pain Pain that endures beyond the acute phase but has not yet become chronic. (Chapter 7)

prevalence The proportion of a population that has a disease or disorder at a specific point in time. (Chapter 2)

primary afferents Sensory neurons that convey impulses from the skin to the spinal cord. (Chapter 7)

primary appraisal One's initial appraisal of a potentially stressful event (Lazarus and Folkman). (Chapter 5)

problem-focused coping Coping strategies aimed at changing the source of the stress. (Chapter 5)

proinflammatory cytokine A chemical secreted by the immune system that promotes inflammation, and is associated with feelings of sickness, depression, and social withdrawal. (Chapter 6)

prospective studies Longitudinal studies that begin with a disease-free group of subjects and follow the occurrence of disease in that population or sample. (Chapter 2)

psychoneuroimmunology (PNI) A multidisciplinary field that focuses on the interactions among behavior, the nervous system, the endocrine system, and the immune system. (Chapter 6)

punishment The presentation of an aversive stimulus or the removal of a positive one. Punishment sometimes, but not always, weakens a response. (Chapter 4)

Raynaud's disease A vasoconstrictive disorder characterized by inadequate circulation in the extremities, especially the fingers or toes, resulting in pain. (Chapter 8)

reappraisal One's nearly constant reevaluation of stressful events (Lazarus and Folkman). (Chapter 5)

reciprocal determinism Bandura's model that includes environment, behavior, and person as mutually interacting factors. (Chapter 4)

rectum The end of the digestive tract leading to the anus. (Chapter 14)

relative risk The risk a person has for a particular disease compared with the risk of other people who do not have that person's condition or lifestyle. (Chapter 2)

reliability The extent to which a test or other measuring instrument yields consistent results. (Chapter 2)

resistance stage The second stage of the general adaptation syndrome (GAS), in which the body adapts to a stressor. (Chapter 5)

retrospective studies Longitudinal studies that look back at the history of a population or sample. (Chapter 2)

rheumatoid arthritis An autoimmune disorder characterized by a dull ache within or around a joint. (Chapters 6, 7)

risk factor Any characteristic or condition that occurs with greater frequency in people with a disease than it does in people free from that disease. (Chapter 2)

salivary glands Glands that furnish moisture that helps in tasting and digesting food. (Chapter 14)

sarcoma Cancer of the connective tissues. (Chapter 10)

secondary appraisal One's perceived ability to control or cope with harm, threat, or challenge (Lazarus and Folkman). (Chapter 5)

sedatives Drugs that induce relaxation and sometimes intoxication by lowering the activity of the brain, the neurons, the muscles, the heart, and even by slowing the metabolic rate. (Chapter 13)

selenium A trace element found in grain products and in meat from grain-fed animals. (Chapter 10)

self-efficacy The belief that one is capable of performing the behaviors that will produce desired outcomes in any particular situation. (Chapter 4)

self-selection A condition of an experimental investigation in which subjects are allowed, in some manner, to determine their own placement in either the experimental or the control group. (Chapter 2)

setpoint A hypothetical ratio of fat to lean tissue at which a person's weight will tend to stabilize. (Chapter 14)

sick role behavior Those activities undertaken by people who have been diagnosed as sick that are directed at getting well. (Chapter 3)

single-blind design A design in which the participants do not know if they are receiving the active or inactive treatment, but the providers are not blind to treatment conditions. (Chapter 2)

social contacts Number and kinds of people with whom one associates; members of one's social network. (Chapter 5)

social isolation The absence of specific role relationships. (Chapter 5)

social network The number and kinds of people with whom one associates; social contacts. (Chapter 5)

social support Both tangible and intangible support a person receives from other people. (Chapters 4, 5)

somatic nervous system The part of the PNS that serves the skin and voluntary muscles. (Chapter 5)

somatosensory cortex The part of the brain that receives and processes sensory input from the body. (Chapter 7)

somatosensory system The part of the nervous system that carries sensory information from the body to the brain. (Chapter 7)

spleen A large organ near the stomach that serves as a repository for lymphocytes and red blood cells. (Chapter 6)

spontaneous remission Disappearance of problem behavior or illness without treatment. (Chapter 13)

stage theory A theory that proposes that people pass through discrete stages as they attempt to change a health behavior. Stage theories propose that different factors become important at different times, depending on a person's stage. (Chapter 4)

state anxiety A temporary condition of dread or uneasiness stemming from a specific situation. (Chapter 15)

stroke Damage to the brain resulting from lack of oxygen; typically the result of cardiovascular disease. (Chapter 9)

subject variable A variable chosen (rather than manipulated) by a researcher to provide levels of comparison for groups of subjects. (Chapter 2)

substantia gelatinosa Two layers of the dorsal horns of the spinal cord. (Chapter 7)

sympathetic nervous system A division of the autonomic nervous system that mobilizes the body's resources in emergency, stressful, and emotional situations. (Chapter 5)

synaptic cleft The space between neurons. (Chapter 5)

syndrome A cluster of symptoms that characterize a particular condition. (Chapter 7)

synergistic effect The combined effect of two or more variables that exceeds the sum of their individual effects. (Chapter 10)

systolic pressure A measure of blood pressure generated by the heart's contraction. (Chapter 9)

T-cells The cells of the immune system that produce immunity. (Chapter 6)

tension headache Pain produced by sustained muscle contractions in the neck, shoulders, scalp, and face, as well as by activity in the central nervous system. (Chapter 7)

thalamus Structure in the forebrain that acts as a relay center for incoming sensory information and outgoing motor information. (Chapter 7)

theory A set of related assumptions from which testable hypotheses can be drawn. (Chapter 2)

thermal biofeedback Feedback concerning changes in skin temperature. (Chapter 8)

thermistor A temperature-sensitive resistor used in thermal biofeedback. (Chapter 8)

thymosin A hormone produced by the thymus. (Chapter 6)

thymus An organ located near the heart that secretes thymosin and thus processes and activates T-cells. (Chapter 6)

tolerance The need for increasing levels of a drug in order to produce a constant level of effect. (Chapters 7, 13)

tonsils Masses of lymphatic tissue located in the pharynx. (Chapter 6)

trait anxiety A personality characteristic that manifests itself as a more or less constant feeling of dread or uneasiness. (Chapter 15)

tranquilizers A type of sedative drug that reduces anxiety. (Chapter 13)

transcutaneous electrical nerve stimulation (TENS) Treatment for pain involving electrical stimulation of neurons from the surface of the skin. (Chapter 7)

triglycerides A group of molecules consisting of glycerol and three fatty acids; one of the components of serum lipids that has been implicated in the formation of atherosclerotic plaque. (Chapter 9)

urban press The many environmental stressors that affect city living, including noise, crowding, crime, and pollution. (Chapter 5)

vaccination A method of inducing immunity in which a weakened form of a virus or bacterium is introduced into the body. (Chapter 6)

validity Accuracy; the extent to which a test or other measuring instrument measures what it is supposed to measure. (Chapter 2)

veins Vessels that carry blood to the heart. (Chapter 9)

venules The smallest veins. (Chapter 9)

volitional phase In the health action process approach, the stage in which a person pursues a health-related goal. (Chapter 4)

well-year The equivalent of a year of complete wellness. (Chapter 16)

withdrawal Adverse physiological reactions exhibited when a drug-dependent person stops using that drug; the withdrawal symptoms are typically unpleasant and opposite to the drug's effects. (Chapter 13)

References

Abbott, R. B., Hui, K.-K., Hays, R. D., Li, M.-D., & Pan, T. (2007). A randomized controlled trial of tai chi for tension headaches. *Evidence Based Complementary and Alternative Medicine, 4*, 107–113.

Abi-Saleh, B., Iskandar, S. B., Elgharib, N., & Cohen, M. V. (2008). C-reactive protein: The harbinger of cardiovascular diseases. *Southern Medical Journal, 101*, 525–533.

Abnet, C. C. (2007). Carcinogenic food contaminants. *Cancer Investigation, 25*, 189–196.

Ackard, D. M., Brehm, B. J., & Steffen, J. J. (2002). Exercise and eating disorders in college-aged women: Profiling excessive exercisers. *Eating Disorders, 10*, 31–47.

Ackroff, L., Bonacchi, K., Magee, M., Yijn, Y.-M., Graves, J. V., & Sclafani, A. (2007). Obesity by choice revisited: Effects of food availability, flavor variety and nutrient composition on energy intake. *Physiology and Behavior, 92*, 468–478.

Adams, B., Aranda, M. P., Kemp, B., & Takagi, K. (2002). Ethnic and gender differences in distress among Anglo American, African American, Japanese American, and Mexican American spousal caregivers of persons with dementia. *Journal of Clinical Geropsychology, 8*, 279–301.

Adams, T. B., & Colner, W. (2008). The association of multiple risk factors with fruit and vegetable intake among a nationwide sample of college students. *Journal of American College Health, 56*, 455–461.

Adamson, J., Ben-Shlomo, Y., Chaturvedi, N., & Donovan, J. (2003). Ethnicity, socio-economic position and gender: Do they affect reported health-care seeking behavior? *Social Science and Medicine, 47*, 895–904.

Ader, R., & Cohen, N. (1975). Behaviorally conditioned immunosuppression. *Psychosomatic Medicine, 37*, 333–340.

Agardh, E., Allebeck, P., Hallqvist, J., Moradi, T., & Sidorchuk, A. (2011). Type 2 diabetes incidence and socio-economic position: A systematic review and meta-analysis. *International Journal of Epidemiology, 40*, 804–818.

Agboola, S., McNeill, A., Coleman, T., & Leonardi Bee, J. (2010). A systematic review of the effectiveness of smoking relapse prevention interventions for abstinent smokers. *Addiction, 105*(8), 1362–1380.

Agency for Healthcare Research and Quality (AHRQ). (2011). *2010 National healthcare disparities report* (AHRQ Publication No. 11-0005). Rockville, MD: U.S. Department of Health and Human Services.

Ai, A. L., Peterson, C., Tice, T. N., Bolling, S. F., & Koenig, H. G. (2004). Faith-based and secular pathways to hope and optimism subconstructs in middle-aged and older cardiac patients. *Journal of Health Psychology, 9*, 435–452.

Aiken, L. S. (2006). Angela Bryan: Award for distinguished scientific early career contributions to psychology. *American Psychologist, 61*, 802–804.

Aiken, L. S., West, S. G., Woodward, C. K., Reno, R. R., & Reynolds, K. D. (1994). Increasing screening mammography in asymptomatic women: Evaluation of a second-generation, theory-based program. *Health Psychology, 13*, 526–538.

Ajzen, I. (1985). From intentions to actions: A theory of planned behavior. In J. Kuhland & J. Beckman (Eds.), *Action-control: From cognitions to behavior* (pp. 11–39). Heidelberg, Germany: Springer.

Ajzen, I. (1991). The theory of planned behavior. *Organizational Behavior and Human Decision Processes, 50*, 179–211.

Alaejos, M. S., González, V., & Afonso, A. M. (2008). Exposure to heterocyclic aromatic amines from the consumption of cooked red meat and its effect on human cancer risk: A review. *Food Additives and Contaminants, 25*, 2–24.

Albert, C. M., Mittleman, M. A., Chae, C. U., Lee, I.-M., Hennekens, C. H., & Manson, J. E. (2000). Triggering of sudden death from cardiac causes by vigorous exertion. *New England Journal of Medicine, 343*, 1355–1361.

Aldana, S. G., Greenlaw, R., Salberg, A., Merrill, R. M., Hager, R., & Jorgensen, R. B. (2007). The effects of an intensive lifestyle modification program on carotid artery intima-media thickness: A randomized trial. *American Journal of Health Promotion, 21*, 510–516.

Aldridge, A. A., & Roesch, S. C. (2007). Coping and adjustment in children and cancer: A meta-analytic study. *Journal of Behavioral Medicine, 30*, 115–129.

Alexander, F. (1950). *Psychosomatic medicine*. New York: Norton.

Allen, K. (2003). Are pets a healthy pleasure? The influence of pets on blood pressure. *Current Directions in Psychological Science, 12*, 236–239.

Allen, K., Blascovich, J., & Mendes, W. B. (2002). Cardiovascular reactivity and the presence of pets, friends, and spouses: The truth about cats and dogs. *Psychosomatic Medicine, 64*, 727–739.

Alper, J. (1993). Ulcers as infectious diseases. *Science, 260*, 159–160.

Alzheimer's Organization. (2004). *Text of President Reagan's letter announcing his own Alzheimer's diagnosis, November 5, 1994.* Retrieved July 1, 2005, from http://www.alz.org/Media/news releases/ronaldreagan/reaganletter.asp

Amanzio, M., Corazzini, L. L., Vase, L., & Benedetti, F. (2009). A systematic review of adverse events in placebo groups of anti-migraine clinical trials. *Pain, 146*, 261–269.

Amato, P. R., & Hohmann-Marriott, B. (2007). A comparison of high- and low-distress marriages that end in divorce. *Journal of Marriage and Family, 69*, 621–638.

American Cancer Society. (2007). *Macrobiotic diet*. Retrieved May 5, 2008, from http://www.cancer.org/docroot/ETO/content/ETO_5_3X_Macrobiotic_Diet.asp

American Cancer Society. (2012). *Cancer facts and figures 2012*. Atlanta, GA: American Cancer Society.

American College Health Association (ACHA). (2012). *American College Health Association National College Health Assessment: Fall 2011 Reference Group Data Report*. Retrieved on April 10, 2012, from http://www.acha-ncha.org/docs/

American Lung Association. (2007). *Trends in asthma morbidity and mortality*. Retrieved August 3, 2008, from http://www.lungusa.org/site/c.dvLUK9OO0E/b.33347/

American Psychiatric Association. (2000). *Diagnostic and statistical manual of mental disorders* (4th ed., text revision). Washington, DC: Author.

American Psychiatric Association. (2011). *Proposed revisions: K 05 Binge Eating Disorder*. Retrieved August 12, 2011, from http://www.dsm5.org/ProposedRevisions/Pages/proposedrevision.aspx?rid=372#

American Psychological Association (APA). (2002). Ethical principles of psychologists and code of conduct. *American Psychologist, 57*, 1060–1073.

American Psychological Association (APA) Task Force on Health Research. (1976). Contributions of psychology to health research: Patterns, problems, and potentials. *American Psychologist*, 31, 263–274.

Amico, R., Harman, J. J., & Johnson, B. T. (2006). Efficacy of antiretroviral therapy adherence interventions: A research synthesis of trials, 1996 to 2004. *Journal of Acquired Immune Deficiency Syndromes*, 41, 285–297.

Anand, S. S., Islam, S., Rosengren, A., Franzosi, M. G., Steyn, K., Yusufali, A. H., et al. (2008). Risk factors for myocardial infarction in women and men: Insights from the INTERHEART study. *European Heart Journal*, 29, 932–940.

Andel, R., Crowe, M., Pedersen, N. L., Mortimer, J., Crimmins, E., Johansson, B., et al. (2005). Complexity of work and risk of Alzheimer's disease: A population-based study of Swedish twins. *Journal of Gerontology Series B: Psychological Sciences and Social Sciences*, 60B(5), 251–258.

Andersen, B. L., Yang, H.-C. Y., Farrar, W. B., Golden-Kreutz, D. M., Emery, C. F., Thornton, L. M., et al. (2008). Psychologic intervention improves survival for breast cancer patients: A randomized clinical trial. *Cancer*, 113, 3450–3458.

Andersen, L. B., Sardinha, L. B., Froberg, K., Riddoch, C. J., Page, A. S., & Anderssen, S. A. (2008). Fitness, fatness and clustering of cardiovascular risk factors in children from Denmark, Estonia and Portugal: The European Youth Heart Study. *International Journal of Pediatric Obesity*, 3(Suppl. 1), 58–66.

Anderson, J. L., Horne, B. D., Jones, H. U., Reyna, S. P., Carlquist, J. F., Bair, T. L., et al. (2004). Which features of the metabolic syndrome predict the prevalence and clinical outcomes of angiographic coronary artery disease? *Cardiology*, 101, 185–193.

Anderson, J. W., Conley, S. B., & Nicholas, A. S. (2007). One hundred pound weight losses with an intensive behavioral program: Changes in risk factors in 118 patients with long-term follow-up. *American Journal of Clinical Nutrition*, 86, 301–307.

Anderson, K. O., Green, C. R., & Payne, R. (2009). Racial and ethnic disparities in pain: Causes and consequences of unequal care. *The Journal of Pain*, 10, 1187–1204.

Anderson, K. O., Syrjala, K. L., & Cleeland, C. S. (2001). How to assess cancer pain. In D. C. Turk & R. Melzack (Eds.), *Handbook of pain assessment* (2nd ed., pp. 579–600). New York: Guilford Press.

Anderson, P. (2006). Global use of alcohol, drugs and tobacco. *Drug and Alcohol Review*, 25, 489–502.

Andersson, K., Melander, A., Svensson, C., Lind, O., & Nilsson, J. L. G. (2005). Repeat prescriptions: Refill adherence in relation to patient and prescriber characteristics, reimbursement level and type of medication. *European Journal of Public Health*, 15, 621–626.

Andrasik, F. (2001). Assessment of patients with headache. In D. C. Turk & R. Melzack (Eds.), *Handbook of pain assessment* (2nd ed., pp. 454–474). New York: Guilford Press.

Andrasik, F. (2003). Behavioral treatment approaches to chronic headache. *Neurological Science*, 24, S80–S85.

Andrews, J. A., Hampson, S. E., Barckley, M., Gerrard, M., & Gibbons, F. X. (2008). The effect of early cognitions on cigarette and alcohol use during adolescence. *Psychology of Addictive Behaviors*, 22, 96–106.

Aneshensel, C. S., Botticello, A. L., & Yamamoto–Mitani, N. (2004). When caregiving ends: The course of depressive symptoms after bereavement. *Journal of Health and Social Behavior*, 45, 422–440.

Anisman, H., Merali, Z., Poulter, M. O., & Hayley, S. (2005). Cytokines as a precipitant of depressive illness: Animal and human studies. *Current Pharmaceutical Design*, 11, 963–972.

Annesi, J. J. (2005). Changes in depressed mood associated with 10 weeks of moderate cardiovascular exercise in formerly sedentary adults. *Psychological Reports*, 96, 855–862.

Antall, G. F., & Kresevic, D. (2004). The use of guided imagery to manage pain in an elderly orthopaedic population. *Orthopaedic Nursing*, 23, 335–340.

Antoni, M. H., Baggett, L., Ironson, G., LaPerriere, A., August, S., Klimas, N., et al. (1991). Cognitive-behavioral stress management intervention buffers distress responses and immunologic changes following notification of HIV-1 seropositivity. *Journal of Consulting and Clinical Psychology*, 59, 906–915.

Antoni, M. H., Cruess, D. G., Cruess, S., Lutgendorf, S., Kumar, M., Ironson, G., et al. (2000). Cognitive-behavioral stress management intervention effects on anxiety, 24-hr urinary norepinephrine output, and T-cytotoxic/suppressor cells over time among symptomatic HIV-infected gay men. *Journal of Consulting and Clinical Psychology*, 68, 31–45.

Antoni, M. H., Ironson, G., & Scheiderman, N. (2007). *Cognitive-behavioral stress management workbook*. New York: Oxford University Press.

Antoni, M. H., Lechner, S., Diaz, A., Vargas, S., Holley, H., Phillips, K., et al. (2009). Cognitive behavioral stress management effects on psychosocial and physiological adaptation in women undergoing treatment for breast cancer. *Brain, Behavior, and Immunity*, 23, 580–591.

Antoni, M. H., & Lutgendorf, S. (2007). Psychosocial factors in disease progression in cancer. *Current Directions in Psychological Science*, 16, 42–46.

Apkarian, A. V., Bushnell, M. C., Treede, R.-D., & Zubieta, J.-K. (2005). Human brain mechanisms of pain perception and regulation in health and disease. *European Journal of Pain*, 9, 463–484.

Applebaum, A. J., Richardson, M. A., Brady, S. M., Brief, D. J., & Keane, T. M. (2009). Gender and other psychosocial factors as predictors of adherence to highly active antiretroviral therapy (HAART) in adults with comorbid HIV/AIDS, psychatric and substance-related disorder. *AIDS and Behavior*, 13, 60–65.

Arbisi, P. A., & Seime, R. J. (2006). Use of the MMPI-2 in medical settings. In J. N. Butcher (Ed.), *MMPI-2: A practitioner's guide* (pp. 273–299). Washington, DC: American Psychological Association.

Armeli, S., Tennen, H., Todd, M., Carney, A., Mohr, C., Affleck, G., et al. (2003). A daily process examination of the stress-response dampening effects of alcohol consumption. *Psychology of Addictive Behaviors*, 17, 266–276.

Armitage, C. J. (2004). Evidence that implementation intentions reduce dietary fat intake: A randomized trial. *Health Psychology*, 23, 319–323.

Armitage, C. J. (2009). Is there utility in the transtheoretical model? *British Journal of Health Psychology*, 14, 195–210.

Armitage, C. J., & Conner, M. (2000). Social cognition models and health behaviour: A structured review. *Psychology & Health*, 15, 173–189.

Armitage, C. J., Sheeran, P., Conner, M., & Arden, M. A. (2004). Stages of change or changes of stage? Predicting transitions in transtheoretical model stages in relation to healthy food choice. *Journal of Consulting and Clinical Psychology*, 72, 491–499.

Armor, D. J., Polich, J. M., & Stambul, H. B. (1976). *Alcoholism and treatment*. Santa Monica, CA: Rand.

Armour, B. S., Woollery, T., Malarcher, A., Pechacek, T. F., & Husten, C. (2005). Annual smoking-attributable mortality, years of potential life lost, and productivity losses—United States, 1997–2001. *Mortality and Morbidity Weekly Reports*, 54(25), 625–628.

Arnold, R., Ranchor, A. V., Sanderman, R., Kempen, G. I. J. M., Ormel, J., & Suurmeijer, T. P. B. M. (2004). The relative contribution of domains of quality of life to overall quality of life for different chronic diseases. *Quality of Life Research*, 13, 883–896.

Arntz, A., & Claassens, L. (2004). The meaning of pain influences its experienced intensity. *Pain*, 109, 20–25.

Aro, A. R., De Koning, H. J., Schreck, M., Henriksson, M., Anttila, A., & Pukkala, E. (2005). Psychological risk factors of incidence of breast cancer: A prospective cohort study in Finland. *Psychological Medicine*, 35, 1515–1521.

Arora, N. K., Rutten, L. J. F., Gustafson, D. H., Moser, R., & Hawkins, R. P. (2007). Perceived helpfulness and impact of social support provided by family, friends, and health care providers to women newly diagnosed with breast cancer. *Psycho-Oncology*, 16, 474–486.

Arsand, E., Tatara, N., Ostengen, G., & Hartvigsen, G. (2010). Mobile phone-based self-management tools for type 2 diabetes: The Few

Touch application. *Journal of Diabetes Science and Technology, 4,* 328–336.

"The art and science of natural products." (2010, May). *Complementary and alternative medicine: Focus on research and care.* Bethesda, MD: National Institutes of Health, National Center for Complementary and Alternative Medicine.

Arthur, C. M., Katkin, E. S., & Mezzacappa, E. S. (2004). Cardiovascular reactivity to mental arithmetic and cold pressor in African Americans, Caribbean Americans, and White Americans. *Annals of Behavioral Medicine, 27,* 31–37.

Ashton, W., Nanchahal, K., & Wood, D. (2001). Body mass index and metabolic risk factors for coronary heart disease in women. *European Health Journal, 22,* 46–55.

Aspden, P., Wolcott, J., Bootman, J. L., & Cronenwett, L. R. (Eds.). (2007). *Preventing medication errors: Quality chasm series.* Washington, DC: National Academies Press.

Associated Press. (2004). Clinton leaves hospital after surgery. *Associated Press Heart Health.* Retrieved June 16, 2005, from http://www.msnbc.msn.com/id/5906976/

Asthma Action America. (2004). *Children and asthma in America.* Retrieved July 7, 2005, from http://www.asthmainamerica.com/frequency.html

Astin, J. A. (1998). Why patients use alternative medicine. *Journal of the American Medical Association, 279,* 1548–1553.

Astin, J. A. (2004). Mind-body therapies for the management of pain. *Clinical Journal of Pain, 20,* 27–32.

Atkinson, N. L., Saperstein, S. L., & Pleis, J. (2009). Using the Internet for health-related activities: Findings from a national probability sample. *Journal of Medical Internet Research, 11,* e4.

Averbuch, M., & Katzper, M. (2000). A search for sex differences in response to analgesia. *Archives of Internal Medicine, 160,* 3424–3428.

Awad, G. H., Sagrestano, L. M., Kittleson, M. J., & Sarvela, P. D. (2004). Development of a measure of barriers to HIV testing among individuals at high risk. *AIDS Education and Prevention, 16,* 115–125.

Ayers, S. L., & Kronenfeld, J. J. (2011). Using zero-inflated models to explain chronic illness, pain, and complementary and alternative medicine use. *American Journal of Health Behavior, 35*(4), 447–457.

Back, S. E., Gentilin, S., & Brady, K. T. (2007). Cognitive-behavioral stress management for individuals with substance use disorders: A pilot study. *Journal of Nervous and Mental Disease, 195,* 662–668.

Baer, H. A. (2008). The growing legitimation of complementary medicine in Australia: Successes and dilemmas. *Australian Journal of Medical Herbalism, 20,* 5–11.

Baer, H. J., Glynn, R. J., Hu, F. B., Hankinson, S. E., Willett, W. C., Colditz, G. A., et al. (2011). Risk factors for mortality in the Nurses' Health Study: A competing risk analysis. *American Journal of Epidemiology, 173*(3), 319–329.

Bahrke, M. S., & Morgan, W. P. (1978). Anxiety reduction following exercise and meditation. *Cognitive Therapy and Research, 2,* 323–334.

Bailey, B. N., Delaney-Black, V., Covington, C. Y., Ager, J., Janisse, J., Hannigan, J. H., et al. (2004). Prenatal exposure to binge drinking and cognitive and behavioral outcomes at age 7 years. *American Journal of Obstetrics and Gynecology, 191,* 1037–1042.

Bailey, S. C., Pandit, A. U., Yin, S., Federman, A., Davis, T. C., Parker, R. M., & Wolf, M. S. (2009). Predictors of misunderstanding pediatric liquid medication instructions. *Family Medicine, 41,* 715–721.

Bailis, D. S., Segall, A., Mahon, M. J., Chipperfield, J. G., & Dunn, E. M. (2001). Perceived control in relation to socioeconomic and behavioral resources for health. *Social Science and Medicine, 52,* 1661–1676.

Baker, S. G., Lichtenstein, P., Kaprio, J., & Holm, N. (2005). Genetic susceptibility to prostate, breast, and colorectal cancer among Nordic twins. *Biometrics, 61,* 55–63.

Bala, M., Strzeszynski, L., & Cahill, K. (2008). Mass media interventions for smoking cessation in adults. *Cochrane Database of Systematic Reviews,* Cochrane Art. No.: CD004704, DOI: 10.1002/14651858. CD004704.pub2.

Baliki, M. N., Geha, P. Y., Apkarian, A. V., & Chialvo, D. R. (2008). Beyond feeling: Chronic pain hurts the brain, disrupting the default-mode network dynamics. *Journal of Neuroscience, 28,* 1398–1403.

Balkrishnan, R., & Jayawant, S. S. (2007). Medication adherence research in populations: Measurement issues and other challenges. *Clinical Therapeutics, 29,* 1180–1183.

Ball, D. (2008). Addiction science and its genetics. *Addiction, 103,* 360–367.

Banaji, M. R., & Steele, C. M. (1989). The social cognition of alcohol use. *Social Cognition, 7,* 137–151.

Bandura, A. (1986). *Social foundations of thought and action: A social cognitive theory.* Englewood Cliffs, NJ: Prentice-Hall.

Bandura, A. (1997). *Self-efficacy: The exercise of control.* New York: Freeman.

Bandura, A. (2001). Social cognitive theory: An agentic perspective. *Annual Review of Psychology, 52,* 1–26.

Banegas, J. R., López-García, E., Gutiérrez-Fisac, J. L., Guallar-Castillón, P., & Rodríguez-Artalejo, F. (2003). A simple estimate of mortality attributable to excess weight in the European Union. *European Journal of Clinical Nutrition, 57,* 201–208.

Bánóczy, J., & Squier, C. (2004). Smoking and disease. *European Journal of Dental Education, 8,* 7–10.

Bär, K.-J., Boettger, M. K., Schulz, S., Neubauer, R., Jochum, T., Voss, A., et al. (2008). Reduced cardio-respiratory coupling in acute alcohol withdrawal. *Drug & Alcohol Dependence, 98*(3), 210–217.

"Barack Obama Quits." (2011, Feb. 9). Barack Obama quits smoking after 30 years. *The Telegraph.* Retrieved June 2, 2011, from http://www.telegraph.co.uk/news/worldnews/barackobama/8314049/Barack-Obama-quits-smoking-after-30-years.html

Barber, J. (1996). A brief introduction to hypnotic analgesia. In J. Barber (Ed.), *Hypnosis and suggestion in the treatment of pain: A clinical guide* (pp. 3–32). New York: Norton.

Barber, T. X. (1984). Hypnosis, deep relaxation, and active relaxation: Data, theory, and clinical applications. In R. L. Woolfolk & P. M. Lehrer (Eds.), *Principles and practice of stress management.* New York: Guilford Press.

Barber, T. X. (2000). A deeper understanding of hypnosis: Its secrets, its nature, its essence. *American Journal of Clinical Hypnosis, 42,* 208–272.

Bardia, A., Tleyjeh, I. M., Cerhan, J. R., Sood, A. K., Limburg, P. J. Erwin, P. J., et al. (2008). Efficacy of antioxidant supplementation in reducing primary cancer incidence and mortality: Systematic review and meta-analysis. *Mayo Clinic Proceedings, 83,* 23–34.

Bardy, S. S. (2008). Lifetime family violence exposure is associated with current symptoms of eating disorders among both young men and women. *Journal of Traumatic Stress, 21,* 347–351.

Barengo, N. C., Hu, G., Lakka, T. A., Pekkarinen, H., Nissinen, A., & Tuomilehto, J. (2004). Low physical activity as predictor for total and cardiovascular disease mortality in middle-aged men and women in Finland. *European Heart Journal, 25,* 2204–2211.

Barlow, J. H., & Ellard, D. R. (2004). Psycho-educational interventions for children with chronic disease, parents and siblings: An overview of the research evidence base. *Child: Care, Health and Development, 30,* 637–645.

Barnes, P. J. (2008). Immunology of asthma and chronic obstructive pulmonary disease. *Nature Reviews Immunology, 8,* 183–192.

Barnes, P. M., Bloom, B., & Nahin, R. L. (2008). Complementary and alternative medicine use among adults and children, United States, 2007. *National Health Statistics Reports,* no. 12. Hyattsville, MD: National Center for Health Statistics.

Barnett, R. C., & Hyde, J. S. (2001). Women, men, work, and family: An expansionist theory. *American Psychologist, 56,* 781–796.

Barrett, S. P. (2010). The effects of nicotine, denicotinized tobacco, and nicotine-containing tobacco on cigarette craving, withdrawal, and self-administration in male and female smokers. *Behavioural Pharmacology, 21*(2), 144–152.

Barron, F., Hunter, A., Mayo, R., & Willoughby, D. (2004). Acculturation and adherence: Issues for health care providers working with clients of Mexican origin. *Journal of Transcultural Nursing, 15,* 331–337.

(ENRICHD) randomized trial. *Journal of the American Medical Association, 289,* 3106–3116.

Berkman, L. F., & Breslow, L. (1983). *Health and ways of living: The Alameda County Study.* New York: Oxford University Press.

Berkman, L. F., & Syme, S. L. (1979). Social networks, host resistance, and mortality: A nine-year follow-up study of Alameda County residents. *American Journal of Epidemiology, 109,* 186–204.

Berman, J. D., & Straus, S. E. (2004). Implementing a research agenda for complementary and alternative medicine. *Annual Review of Medicine, 55,* 239–254.

Bermudez, O. I., & Gao, X. (2011). Greater consumption of sweetened beverages and added sugars is associated with obesity among US young adults. *Annals of Nutrition & Metabolism, 57*(3/4), 211–218.

Bernards, S., Graham, K., Kuendig, H., Hettige, S., & Obot, I. (2009). 'I have no interest in drinking': A cross-national comparison of reasons why men and women abstain from alcohol use. *Addiction, 104*(10), 1658–1668.

Berne, R. M., & Levy, M. N. (2000). *Principles of physiology* (3rd ed.). St. Louis, MO: Mosby.

Bernstein, L., Henderson, B. E., Hanisch, R., Sullivan-Halley, J., & Ross, R. K. (1994). Physical exercise and reduced risk of breast cancer in young women. *Journal of the National Cancer Institute, 86,* 1403–1408.

Bertakis, K. D., & Azari, R. (2005). Obesity and the use of health care services. *Obesity Research, 13,* 372–379.

Bertram, L., & Tanzi, R. E. (2005). The genetic epidemiology of neurodegenerative disease. *Journal of Clinical Investigation, 115,* 1449–1457.

Bessesen, D. H. (2011). Regulation of body weight: What is the regulated parameter? *Physiology & Behavior, 104*(4), 599–607.

Bhat, V. M., Cole, J. W., Sorkin, J. D., Wozniak, M. A., Malarcher, A. M., Giles, W. H., et al. (2008). Dose-response relationship between cigarette smoking and risk of ischemic stroke in young women. *Stroke, 39,* 2439–2443.

Bhatt, S. P., Luqman-Arafath, T. K., & Guleria, R. (2007). Non-pharmacological management of hypertension. *Indian Journal of Medical Sciences, 61,* 616–624.

Bhogal, S., Zemek, R., & Ducharme, F. M. (2006). Written action plans for asthma in children. *Cochrane Database of Systematic Reviews,* Cochrane Art. No.: CD005306, DOI: 10.1002/14651858.CD005306.pub2.

Bianchini, K. J., Etherton, J. L., Greve, K. W., Heinly, M. T., & Meyers, J. E. (2008). Classification accuracy of MMPI-2 validity scales in the detection of pain-related malingering: A known-groups study. *Assessment, 15,* 435–449.

Bickel-Swenson, D. (2007). End-of-life training in U.S. medical schools: A systematic literature review. *Journal of Palliative Medicine, 10,* 229–235.

Bigal, M. E., & Lipton, R. B. (2008a). Concepts and mechanisms of migraine chronification. *Headache, 48,* 7–15.

Bigal, M. E., & Lipton, R. B. (2008b). The epidemiology and burden of headaches. In M. Levin (Ed.), *Comprehensive review of headache medicine* (pp. 39–59). New York: Oxford University Press.

Bigatti, S., & Cronan, T. A. (2002). A comparison of pain measures used with patients with fibromyalgia. *Journal of Nursing Measurement, 10,* 5–14.

Bird, S. T., Harvey, S. M., Beckman, L. J., & Johnson, C. H. (2000). Getting your partner to use condoms: Interviews with men and women at risk of HIV/STDs. *Journal of Sex Research, 38,* 233–240.

Biron, C., Brun, J., Ivers, H., & Cooper, C. L. (2006). At work but ill: Psychosocial work environment and well-being determinants of presenteeism propensity. *Journal of Public Mental Health, 5,* 26–37.

Birtane, M., Uzunca, K., Tastekin, N., & Tuna, H. (2007). The evaluation of quality of life in fibromyalgia syndrome: A comparison with rheumatoid arthritis by using SF-36 Health Survey. *Clinical Rheumatology, 26,* 679–684.

Bisson, J., & Andrew, M. (2007). Psychological treatment of post-traumatic stress disorder (PTSD). *Cochrane Database of Systematic Reviews,* Cochrane Art. No.: CD003388, DOI: 10.1002/14651858.CD003388.pub3.

Bjartveit, K. (2009). Health consequences of sustained smoking cessation. *Tobacco Control, 18*(3), 197–205.

Bjørge, T., Engeland, A., Tverdal, A., & Smith, G. D. (2008). Body mass index in adolescence in relation to cause-specific mortality: A follow-up to 230,000 Norwegian adolescents. *American Journal of Epidemiology, 168,* 30–37.

Black, E., Holst, C., Astrup, A., Toubro, S., Echwald, S., Pedersent, O., et al. (2005). Long-term influences of body-weight changes, independent of the attained weight, on risk of impaired glucose tolerance and Type 2 diabetes. *Diabetic Medicine, 22,* 1100–1205.

Black, P. H. (2003). The inflammatory response is an integral part of the stress response: Implications for atherosclerosis, insulin resistance, Type II diabetes and metabolic syndrome X. *Brain, Behavior and Immunity, 17,* 350–364.

Blackmore, E. R., Stansfeld, S. A., Weller, I., Munce, S., Zagorski, B. M., & Stewart, D. E. (2007). Major depressive episodes and work stress: Results from a national population survey. *American Journal of Public Health, 97,* 2088–2093.

Blair, S. N., Cheng, Y., & Holder, J. S. (2001). Is physical activity or physical fitness more important in defining health benefits? *Medicine and Science in Sports & Exercise, 33,* S379–S399.

Blair, S. N., & Church, T. (2004). The fitness, obesity, and health equation: Is physical activity the common denominator? *Journal of the American Medical Association, 292,* 1232–1234.

Blalock, J. E., & Smith, E. M. (2007). Conceptual development of the immune system as a sixth sense. *Brain, Behavior and Immunity, 21,* 23–33.

Blalock, S. J. (2007). Predictors of calcium intake patterns: A longitudinal analysis. *Health Psychology, 26,* 251–258.

Blanchard, C. M., Kupperman, J., Sparling, P. B., Nehl, E., Rhodes, R. E., Courneya, K. S., et al. (2009). Do ethnicity and gender matter when using the theory of planned behavior to understand fruit and vegetable consumption? *Appetite, 52,* 15–20.

Blanchard, E. B., & Andrasik, F. (1985). *Management of chronic headaches: A psychological approach.* New York: Pergamon Press.

Blanchard, E. B., Appelbaum, K. A., Radniz, C. L., Morrill, B., Michultka, D., Kirsch, C., et al. (1990). A controlled evaluation of thermal biofeedback and thermal biofeedback combined with cognitive therapy in the treatment of vascular headache. *Journal of Consulting and Clinical Psychology, 58,* 216–224.

Blanchard, J., & Lurie, N. (2004). R-E-S-P-E-C-T: Patient reports of disrespect in health care setting and its impact on care. *Journal of Family Practice, 53,* 721–730.

Blascovich, J., Spencer, S. J., Quinn, D., & Steele, C. (2001). African Americans and high blood pressure: The role of stereotype threat. *Psychological Science, 12,* 225–229.

Bleil, M. E., Gianaros, P. J., Jennings, J. R., Flory, J. D., & Manuck, S. B. (2008). Trait negative affect: Toward an integrated model of understanding psychological risk for impairment in cardiac autonomic function. *Psychosomatic Medicine, 70,* 328–337.

Blodgett Salafia, E. H., & Gondoli, D. M. (2011). A 4-year longitudinal investigation of the processes by which parents and peers ifluence the development of early adolescent girls' bulimic symptoms. *Journal of Early Adolescence, 31*(3), 390–414.

Bloomfield, K., Stockwell, T., Gmel, G., & Rehn, N. (2003). *International comparison of alcohol consumption.* National Institute of Alcoholism and Alcohol Abuse. Retrieved April 12, 2005, from http://www.niaaa.nih.gov/publications/arh27–1/95–109.htm

Bloor, M. (2005). Observations of shipboard illness behavior: Work discipline and the sick role in a residential work setting. *Qualitative Health Research, 15,* 766–777.

Bode, C., & Bode, J. C. (1997). Alcohol absorption, metabolism, and production in the gastrointestinal tract. *Alcohol Health & Research World, 21,* 82–83.

Bodenheimer, T. (2005a). High and rising health care costs: Part 1. Seeking an explanation. *Archives of Internal Medicine, 142,* 847–854.

Barth, J., Critchley, J., & Bengel, J. (2008). Psychosocial interventions for smoking cessation in patients with coronary heart disease. *Cochrane Database of Sytematic Reviews*, Cochrane Art. No.: CD006886, DOI: 10.1002/14651858.CD006886.

Barton-Donovan, K., & Blanchard, E. B. (2005). Psychosocial aspects of chronic daily headache. *Journal of Headache and Pain*, 6, 30–39.

Baseman, J. G., & Koutsky, L. A. (2005). The epidemiology of human papillomavirus infections. *Journal of Clinical Virology*, 32, 16–24.

Basow, S. A., Foran, K. A., & Bookwala, J. (2007). Body objectification, social pressure, and disordered eating behavior in college women: The role of sorority membership. *Psychology of Women Quarterly*, 31(4), 394–400.

Bassman, L. E., & Uellendahl, G. (2003). Complementary/alternative medicine: Ethical, professional, and practical challenges for psychologists. *Professional Psychology: Research and Practice*, 34, 264–270.

Batty, G. D., Kivimaki, M., Gray, L., Smith, G. D., Marmot, M. G., & Shipley, M. J. (2008). Cigarette smoking and site-specific cancer mortality: Testing uncertain associations using extended follow-up of the original Whitehall study. *Annals of Oncology*, 19, 996–1002.

Batty, G. D., Shipley, M. J., Mortensen, L. H., Boyle, S. H., Barefoot, J., Grønbæk, M., et al. (2008). IQ in late adolescence/early adulthood, risk factors in middle age and later all-cause mortality in men: The Vietnam Experience Study. *Journal of Epidemiology and Community Health*, 62, 522–531.

Baum, A., Perry, N. W., Jr., & Tarbell, S. (2004). The development of psychology as a health science. In R. G. Frank, A. Baum, & J. L. Wallander (Eds.), *Handbook of clinical health psychology* (Vol. 3, pp. 9–28). Washington, DC: American Psychological Association.

Baumann, L. J., Cameron, L. D., Zimmerman, R. S., & Leventhal, H. (1989). Illness representations and matching labels with symptoms. *Health Psychology*, 8, 449–469.

Baumann, P., Schild, C., Hume, R. F., & Sokol, R. J. (2006). Alcohol abuse—A persistent preventable risk for congenital anomalies. *International Journal of Gynecology and Obstetrics*, 95, 66–72.

Baxter, L., Egbert, N., & Ho, E. (2008). Everyday health communication experiences of college students. *Journal of American College Health*, 56, 427–436.

Beacham, G. (2011, November 7). Magic Johnson still beating HIV 20 years later. *Houston Chronicle*. Retrieved March 24, 2012, from http://www.chron.com/sports/article/Magic-Johnson-still-beating-HIV-20-years-later-2257066.php

Beaglehole, R., Bonita, R., & Kjellström, T. (1993). *Basic epidemiology*. Geneva: World Health Organization.

Beck, A. T. (1976). *Cognitive therapy and the emotional disorders*. New York: International Universities Press.

Beck, A. T., Ward, C. H., Mendelson, M., Mock, J., & Erbaugh, J. (1961). An inventory for measuring depression. *Archives of General Psychiatry*, 4, 561–571.

Becker, A. E., Burwell, R. A., Navara, K., & Gilman, S. E. (2003). Binge eating and binge eating disorder in a small-scale, indigenous society: The view from Fiji. *International Journal of Eating Disorders*, 34, 423–431.

Becker, M. H., & Rosenstock, I. M. (1984). Compliance with medical advice. In A. Steptoe & A. Mathews (Eds.), *Health care and human behavior* (pp. 135–152). London: Academic Press.

Bédard, M., Kuzik, R., Chambers, L., Molloy, D. W., Dubois, S., & Lever, J. A. (2005). Understanding burden differences between men and women caregivers: The contribution of care-recipient problem behaviors. *International Psychogeriatrics*, 17, 99–118.

Beecher, H. K. (1946). Pain of men wounded in battle. *Annals of Surgery*, 123, 96–105.

Beecher, H. K. (1955). The powerful placebo. *Journal of the American Medical Association*, 149, 1602–1607.

Beecher, H. K. (1956). Relationship of significance of wound to pain experience. *Journal of the American Medical Association*, 161, 1609–1613.

Beecher, H. K. (1957). The measurement of pain. *Pharmacological Review*, 9, 59–209.

Beetz, A., Kotrschal, K., Turner, D. C., Hediger, K., Uvnäs-Moberg, K., Julius, H. (2011). The effect of a real dog, toy dog, and friendly person on insecurely attached children during a stressful task: An exploratory study. *Anthrozoos: A Multidisciplinary Journal of The Interactions of People & Animals*, 24, 349–368.

Beilin, L., & Huang, R.-C. (2008). Childhood obesity, hypertension, the metabolic syndrome and adult cardiovascular disease. *Clinical and Experimental Pharmacology and Physiology*, 35, 409–411.

Bekke-Hansen, S., Trockel, M., Burg, M. M., & Taylor, C. B. (2012). Depressive symptom dimensions and cardiac prognosis following myocardial infarction: Results from the ENRICHD clinical trial. *Psychological Medicine*, 42, 51–60.

Bélanger-Ducharme, F., & Tremblay, A. (2005). Prevalence of obesity in Canada. *Obesity Reviews*, 6, 183–186.

Bélanger-Gravel, A., Godin, G., & Amireault, S. (2011). A meta-analytic review of the effect of implementation intentions on physical activity. *Health Psychology Review*, DOI: 10.1080/17437199.2011.560095.

Belar, C. D. (1997). Clinical health psychology: A specialty for the 21st century. *Health Psychology*, 16, 411–416.

Belar, C. D. (2008). Clinical health psychology: A health care specialty in professional psychology. *Professional Psychology: Research and Practice*, 39, 229–233.

Bell, R. A., Kravitz, R. L., Thom, D., Krupat, E., & Azari, R. (2001). Unsaid but not forgotten: Physician-patient relationship. *Archives of Internal Medicine*, 161, 1977–1983.

Bell, R. A., Kravitz, R. L., Thom, D., Krupat, E., & Azari, R. (2002). Unmet expectations for care and the patient-physician relationship. *Journal of General Internal Medicine*, 17, 817–824.

Belloc, N. (1973). Relationship of health practices and mortality. *Preventive Medicine*, 2, 67–81.

Benaim, C., Froger, J., Cazottes, C., Gueben, D., Porte, M., Desnuelle, C., et al. (2007). Use of the Faces Pain Scale by left and right hemispheric stroke patients. *Pain*, 128, 52–58.

Bendapudi, N. M., Berry, L. L., Frey, K. A., Parish, J. T., & Rayburn, W. L. (2006). Patients' perspectives on ideal physician behaviors. *Mayo Clinic Proceedings*, 81, 338–344.

Bender, R., Trautner, C., Spraul, M., & Berger, M. (1998). Assessment of excess mortality in obesity. *American Journal of Epidemiology*, 147, 42–48.

Benedetti, F. (2006). Placebo analgesia. *Neurological Sciences*, 27(Suppl. 2), S100–S102.

Benight, C. C., Ruzek, J. I., & Waldrep, E. (2008). Internet interventions for traumatic stress: A review and theoretically based example. *Journal of Traumatic Stress*, 21, 513–520.

Bennett, G. G., Merritt, M. M., Sollers, J. J., III, Edwards, C. L., Whitfield, K. E., Brandon, D. T., et al. (2004). Stress, coping, and health outcomes among African-Americans: A review of the John Henryism hypothesis. *Psychology and Health*, 19, 369–383.

Bennett, I. M., Chen, J., Soroui, J. S., & White, S. (2009). The contribution of health literacy to disparities in self-rated health status and preventive health behaviors in older adults. *Annals of Family Medicine*, 7, 204–211.

Benyamini, Y., Leventhal, E. A., & Leventhal, H. (2000). Gender differences in processing information for making self-assessments of health. *Psychosomatic Medicine*, 62, 354–364.

Berghöfer, A., Pischon, T., Reinhold, T., Apovian, C. M., Sharma, A. M., & Willich, S. N. (2008). Obesity prevalence from a European perspective: A systematic review. *BMC Public Health*, 8, 200–209.

Bergmark, K. H., & Kuendig, H. (2008). Pleasures of drinking: A cross-cultural perspective. *Journal of Ethnicity and Substance Abuse*, 7(2), 131–153.

Berkman, L. F., Blumenthal, J., Burg, M., Carney, R. M., Catellier, D., Cowan, M. J., et al. (2003). Effects of treating depression and low perceived social support on clinical events after myocardial infarction: The Enhancing Recovery in Coronary Heart Disease Patients

Bodenheimer, T. (2005b). High and rising health care costs: Part 2. Technologic innovation. *Archives of Internal Medicine, 142,* 932–937.

Bodenheimer, T. (2005c). High and rising health care costs: Part 3. The role of health care providers. *Archives of Internal Medicine, 142,* 996–1002.

Bodenheimer, T., & Fernandez, A. (2005). High and rising health care costs: Part 4. Can costs be controlled while preserving quality? *Archives of Internal Medicine, 143,* 26–31.

Bodhi, B. (2011). What does mindfulness really mean? A canonical perspective. *Contemporary Buddhism, 12*(1), 19–39.

Boffetta, P. (2004). Epidemiology of environmental and occupational cancer. *Oncogene, 23,* 6392–6403.

Bogart, L. M., & Delahanty, D. L. (2004). Psychosocial models. In T. J. Boll, R. G. Frank, A. Baum, & J. L. Wallander (Eds.), *Handbook of clinical health psychology: Vol. 3. Models and perspectives in health psychology* (pp. 201–248). Washington, DC: American Psychological Association.

Bogg, T., & Roberts, B. W. (2004). Conscientiousness and health-related behaviors: A meta-analysis of the leading behavioral contributors to mortality. *Psychological Bulletin, 130,* 887–919.

Boice, J. D., Jr., Bigbee, W. L., Mumma, M. T., & Blot, W. J. (2003). Cancer mortality in counties near two former nuclear materials processing facilities in Pennsylvania, 1950–1995. *Health Physics, 85,* 691–700.

Boisvert, J. A., & Harrell, W. A. (2009). Homosexuality as a risk factor for eating disorder symptomatology in men. *Journal of Men's Studies, 17*(3), 210–225.

Bolger, N., Zuckerman, A., & Kessler, R. C. (2000). Invisible support and adjustment to stress. *Journal of Personality and Social Psychology, 79,* 953–961.

Bolognesi, M., Nigg, C. R., Massarini, M., & Lippke, S. (2006). Reducing obesity indicators through brief physical activity counseling (PACE) in Italian primary care settings. *Annals of Behavioral Medicine, 31,* 179–185.

Bonica, J. J. (1990). Definitions and taxonomy of pain. In J. J. Bonica (Ed.), *The management of pain* (2nd ed., pp. 18–27). Malvern, PA: Lea & Febiger.

Bonilla, K. (2007, June 29). Diabetes, pregnancy and Halle Berry. *MyDiabetesCentral.com.* Retrieved June 29, 2008, from http://www.healthcentral.com/diabetes/c/5868/13828/halle-berry/

Borrell, L. N. (2005). Racial identity among Hispanics: Implications for health and well-being. *American Journal of Public Health, 95,* 379–381.

Bos, V., Kunst, A. E., Garssen, J., & Mackenbach, J. P. (2005). Socioeconomic inequalities in mortality within ethnic groups in the Netherlands, 1995–2000. *Journal of Epidemiology and Community Health, 59,* 329–335.

Bosch-Capblanch, S., Abba, K., Prictor, M., & Garner, P. (2007). Contracts between patients and healthcare practitioners for improving patients' adherence to treatment, prevention and health promotion activities. *Cochrane Database of Systematic Reviews,* Cochrane Art. No.: CD004808, DOI: 10.1002/14651858.CD004808.pub3.

Bottonari, K. A., Roberts, J. W., Ciesla, J. A., & Hewitt, R. G. (2005). Life stress and adherence to antiretroviral therapy among HIV-positive individuals: A preliminary investigation. *AIDS Patient Care and STDs, 19,* 719–727.

Bottos, S., & Dewey, D. (2004). Perfectionists' appraisal of daily hassles and chronic headache. *Headache, 44,* 772–779.

Botvin, G. J., & Griffin, K. W. (2004). Life skills training: Empirical findings and future directions. *Journal of Primary Prevention, 25,* 211–232.

Boudreaux, E. D., & O'Hea, E. L. (2004). Patient satisfaction in the emergency department: A review of the literature and implications for practice. *The Journal of Emergency Medicine, 26,* 13–26.

Bowers, S. L., Bilbo, S. D., Dhabhar, F. S., & Nelson, R. J. (2008). Stressor-specific alterations in corticosterone and immune responses in mice. *Brain, Behavior, and Immunity, 22,* 105–113.

Boyd, D. B. (2007). Integrative oncology: The last ten years—A personal retrospective. *Alternative Therapies in Health and Medicine, 13,* 56–64.

Brace, M. J., Smith, M. S., McCauley, E., & Sherry, D. D. (2000). Family reinforcement of illness behavior: A comparison of adolescents with chronic fatigue syndrome, juvenile arthritis, and healthy controls. *Journal of Developmental and Behavioral Pediatrics, 21,* 332–339.

Bramlett, M. D., & Blumberg, S. J. (2008). Prevalence of children with special health care needs in metropolitan and micropolitan statistical areas in the United States. *Maternal and Child Health Journal, 12,* 488–498.

Brantley, P. J., Bodenlos, J., Cowles, M., Whitehead, D., Ancona, M., & Jones, G. (2007). Development and validation of the Weekly Stress Inventory—Short Form. *Journal of Psychopathology and Behavioral Assessment, 29,* 54–59.

Brantley, P. J., Jones, G. N., Boudreaux, E., & Gatz, S. L. (1997). The Weekly Stress Inventory. In C. P. Zalaaquett (Ed.), *Evaluating stress: A book of resources* (pp. 405–420). Lanham, MD: Scarecrow Press.

Bray, G. A. (2004). The epidemic of obesity and changes in food intake: The fluoride hypothesis. *Physiology and Behavior, 82,* 115–121.

Bray, G. A., Nielsen, S. J., & Popkin, B. M. (2004). Consumption of high-fructose corn syrup in beverages may play a role in the epidemic of obesity. *American Journal of Clinical Nutrition, 79,* 537–543.

Brecher, E. M. (1972). *Licit and illicit drugs.* Boston, MA: Little, Brown.

Breibart, W., & Payne, D. (2001). Psychiatric aspects of pain management in patients with advanced cancer. In H. Chochinov & W. Breibart (Eds.), *Handbook of psychiatry in palliative medicine* (pp. 131–199). New York: Oxford University Press.

Breslin, M. J., & Lewis, C. A. (2008). Theoretical models of the nature of prayer and health: A review. *Mental Health, Religion & Culture, 11*(1), 9–21.

Breuer, B., Fleishman, S. B., Cruciani, R. A., & Portenoy, R. K. (2011). Medical oncologists' attitudes and practice in cancer pain management: A national survey. *Journal of Clinical Oncology, 29,* 4769–4775.

Breuer, J., & Freud, S. (1955). *Studies on hysteria.* In J. Strachey (Ed. and Trans.), *The standard edition of the complete psychological works of Sigmund Freud* (Vol. 2). London: Hogarth Press. (Original work published 1895)

Bricker, J. B., Petersen, A. V., Andersen, M. R., Rajan, K. B., Leroux, B. G., & Sarason, I. G. (2006). Childhood friends who smoke: Do they influence adolescents to make smoking transitions? *Addictive Behaviors, 31,* 889–900.

Brinn, M. P., Carson, K. V., Esterman, A. J., Chang, A. B., & Smith, B. J. (2010). Mass media interventions for preventing smoking in your people. *Cochrane Database of Systematic Reviews,* Cochrane Art No.: CD001006.

Briones, T. L. (2007). Psychoneuroimmunology and related mechanisms in understanding health disparities in vulnerable populations. *Annual Review of Nursing Research, 25,* 219–256.

Broadbent, E., Kahokeher, A., Booth, R. J., Thomas, J., Windsor, J. A., Buchanan, C. M., et al. (2012). A brief relaxation intervention reduces stress and improves surgical wound healing response: A randomized trial. *Brain, Behavior, and Immunity, 26,* 212–217.

Brody, M. L., Masheb, R. M., & Grilo, C. M. (2005). Treatment preferences of patients with binge eating disorder. *International Journal of Eating Disorders, 37,* 352–356.

Brondel, L., Van Wymelbeke, V., Pineau, N., Jiang, T., Hanus, C., & Rigaud, D. (2009). Variety enhances food intake in humans: Role of sensory-specific satiety. *Physiology & Behavior, 97*(1), 44–51.

Broocks, A., Meyer, T., Opitz, M., Bartmann, U., Hillmer-Vogel, U., George, A., et al. (2003). 5-HT-1A responsivity in patients with panic disorder before and after treatment with aerobic exercise, clomipramine or placebo. *European Neuropsychopharmacology, 13,* 153–164.

Brooks, V. L., Haywood, J. R., & Johnson, A. K. (2005). Translation of salt retention to central activation of the sympathetic nervous system in hypertension. *Clinical and Experimental Pharmacology and Physiology, 32,* 426–432.

Brown, A. D., McMorris, C. A., Longman, R. S., Leigh, R., Hill, M. D., Friedenreich, C. M., et al. (2010). Effects of cardiorespiratory fitness and cerebral blood flow on cognitive outcomes in older women. *Neurobiology of Aging, 31,* 2047–2057

Brown, B. (1970). Recognition of aspects of consciousness through association with EEG alpha activity represented by a light signal. *Psychophysics, 6,* 442–446.

Brown, D. (2011, March 2). In Charlie Sheen rants, mental-health and drug experts see lessons for others. *The Denver Post.* Retrieved June 19, 2011, from http://www.denverpost.com/recommended/ci_17515950

Brown, D. R., Hernández, A., Saint-Jean, G., Evans, S., Tafari, I., Brewster, L. G., et al. (2008). A participatory action research pilot study on urban health disparities using rapid assessment response and evaluation. *American Journal of Public Health, 98,* 28–38.

Brown, F. L., & Slaughter, V. (2011). Normal body, beautiful body: Discrepant perceptions reveal a pervasive 'thin ideal' from childhood to adulthood. *Body Image, 8*(2), 119–125.

Brown, I., Sheeran, P., & Reuber, M. (2009). Enhancing antiepileptic drug adherence: A randomized controlled trial. *Epilepsy & Behavior, 16,* 634–639.

Brown, M. (2011, April 21). Kirstie Alley weight loss goal is crazy talk. *The Stir Healthy Living.* Retrieved July 17, 2011, from http://thestir.cafemom.com/healthy_living/119292/kirstie_alley_weight_loss_goal

Brownell, K. D., & Horgen, K. B. (2004). *Food fight: The inside story of the food industry, America's obesity crisis, and what we can do about it.* New York: McGraw-Hill.

Bruch, H. (1973). *Eating disorders. Obesity, anorexia nervosa and the person within.* New York: Basic Books.

Bruch, H. (1978). *The golden cage: The enigma of anorexia nervosa.* Cambridge, MA: Harvard University Press.

Bruch, H. (1982). Anorexia nervosa: Therapy and theory. *American Journal of Psychiatry, 139,* 1531–1538.

Brugts, J. J., Yetgin, T., Hoeks, S. E., Gotto, A. M., Shepherd, J., Westendorp, R. G. J., et al. (2009). The benefits of statins in people without established cardiovascular disease but with cardiovascular risk factors: Meta-analysis of randomized controlled trials. *British Medical Journal, 338,* 2376.

Brumback, T., Cao, D., & King, A. (2007). Effects of alcohol on psychomotor performance and perceived impairment in heavy binge social drinkers. *Drug and Alcohol Dependence, 91,* 10–17.

Brummett, B. H., Barefoot, J. C., Siegler, I. C., Clapp-Channing, N. E., Lytle, B. L., Bosworth, H. B., et al. (2001). Characteristics of socially isolated patients with coronary artery disease who are at elevated risk for mortality. *Psychosomatic Medicine, 63,* 267–272.

Bruns, D. (1998). Psychologists as primary care providers: A paradigm shift. *Health Psychologist, 20*(4), 19.

Bryan, A., Fisher, J. D., & Fisher, W. A. (2002). Tests of the mediational role of preparatory safer sexual behavior in the context of the theory of planned behavior. *Health Psychology, 21,* 71–80.

Buchert, R., Thomasius, R., Wilke, F., Petersen, K., Nebeling, B., Obrocki, J., et al. (2004). A voxel-based PET investigation of the long-term effects of "Ecstasy" consumption on brain serotonin transporters. *American Journal of Psychiatry, 161*(7), 1181–1189.

Buchwald, H., Avidor, Y., Braunwald, E., Jensen, M. D., Pories, W., Fahrbach, K., et al. (2004). Bariatric surgery: A systematic review and meta-analysis. *Journal of the American Medical Association, 292,* 1724–1737.

Buchwald, H., Estok, R., Fahrbach, K., Banel, D., Jensen, M. D., Pories, W. J., et al. (2009). Weight and Type 2 diabetes after bariatric surgery: Systematic review and meta-analysis. *The American Journal of Medicine, 122,* 248–256.

Buddie, A. M. (2004). Alternatives to twelve-step programs. *Journal of Forensic Psychology Practice, 4,* 61–70.

Buffington, A. L. H., Hanlon, C. A., & McKeown, M. J. (2005). Acute and persistent pain modulation of attention-related anterior cingulate fMRI activations. *Pain, 113,* 172–184.

Bulik, C. M., Berkman, N. D., Brownley, K. A., Sedway, J. A., & Lohr, K. N. (2007). Anorexia nervosa treatment: A systematic review of randomized controlled trials. *International Journal of Eating Disorders, 40,* 310–320.

Burckhardt, C. S., & Jones, K. D. (2003a). Adult measures of pain: Short-Form McGill Pain Questionnaire (SF-MPQ). *Arthritis & Rheumatism: Arthritis Care & Research, 49*(S5), S98–S99.

Burckhardt, C. S., & Jones, K. D. (2003b). Adult measures of pain: Short-Visual Analog Scale (VAS). *Arthritis & Rheumatism: Arthritis Care & Research, 49*(S5), S100–S101.

Burgess, D. J., Ding, Y., Hargreaves, M., van Ryn, M., & Phelan, S. (2008). The association between perceived discrimination and underutilization of needed medical and mental health care in a multi-ethnic community sample. *Journal of Health Care for the Poor and Underserved, 19,* 1049–1089.

Burke, A., & Upchurch, D. M. (2006). Patterns of acupuncture use: Highlights from the National Health Interview Survey. *American Acupuncturist, 37,* 30–31.

Burke, A., Upchurch, D. M., Dye, C., & Chyu, L. (2006). Acupuncture use in the United States: Findings from the National Health Interview Survey. *Journal of Alternative and Complementary Medicine, 12,* 639–648.

Burke, J. D., Lofgren, I. E., Morrell, J. S., & Reilly, R. A. (2007). Health indicators, body mass index and food selection practices in college age students. *FASEB Journal, 21,* A1063.

Burkert, S., Knoll, N., Scholz, U., Roigas, J., & Gralla, O. (2012). Self-regulation following prostatectomy: Phase-specific self-efficacy beliefs for pelvic-floor exercise. *British Journal of Health Psychology, 17,* 273–293.

Bussey-Smith, K. L., & Rossen, R. D. (2007). A systematic review of randomized control trials evaluating the effectiveness of interactive computerized asthma patient education programs. *Annals of Allergy, Asthma and Immunology, 98,* 507–516.

Bustamante, M. X., Zhang, G., O'Connell, E., Rodriguez, D., & Borroto-Ponce, R. (2007). Motor vehicle crashes and injury among high school and college aged drivers. Miami–Dade County, FL 20005. *Annals of Epidemiology, 17,* 742.

Cahill, K., Lancaster, T., & Green, N. (2010). Stage-based interventions for smoking cessation. *Cochrane Database of Systematic Reviews, 11.* DOI: 10.1002/14651858.CD004492.pub4.

Cahill, K., Stead, L. F., & Lancaster, T. (2011). Nicotine receptor partial agonists for smoking cessation. *Cochrane Database of Systematic Reviews 2011,* Issue 2, Cochrane Art. No.: CD006103, DOI: 10.1002/14651858.CD006103.pub5.

Cahill, S. P., & Foa, E. B. (2007). PTSD: Treatment efficacy and future directions. *Psychiatric Times, 24,* 32–34.

Cale, L., & Harris, J. (2006). Interventions to promote young people's physical activity: Issues, implications and recommendations for practice. *Health Education Journal, 65,* 320–337.

Calhoun, J. B. (1956). A comparative study of the social behavior of two inbred strains of house mice. *Ecological Monogram, 26,* 81.

Calhoun, J. B. (1962, February). Population density and social pathology. *Scientific American, 206,* 139–148.

Calipel, S., Lucaspolomeni, M.-M., Wodey, E., & Ecoffey, C. (2005). Premedication in children: Hypnosis versus midazolam. *Pediatric Anesthesia, 15,* 275–281.

Callaway, E. (2011, September 16). Clues emerge to explain first successful HIV vaccine trial. *Nature.* DOI: 10.1038/news.2011.541.

Callister, L. C. (2003). Cultural influences on pain perceptions and behavior. *Home Health Care Management & Practice, 15,* 207–211.

Camacho, T. C., & Wiley, J. A. (1983). Health practices, social networks, and change in physical health. In L. F. Berkman & L. Breslow (Eds.), *Health and ways of living: The Alameda County Study* (pp. 176–209). New York: Oxford University Press.

Camelley, K. B., Wortman, C. B., Bolger, N., & Burke, C. T. (2006). The time course of brief reactions to spousal loss: Evidence from a national probability sample. *Journal of Personality and Social Psychology, 91,* 476–492.

Cameron, L. D., Booth, R. J., Schlatter, M., Ziginskas, D., & Harman, J. E. (2007). Changes in emotion regulation and psychological adjustment following use of a group psychosocial support program for women recently diagnosed with breast cancer. *Psycho-Oncology, 16*, 171–180.

Cameron, L. D., Leventhal, E. A., & Leventhal, H. (1995). Seeking medical care in response to symptoms and life stress. *Psychosomatic Medicine, 57*, 37–47.

Cameron, L. D., Petrie, K. J., Ellis, C., Buick, D., & Weinman, J. A. (2005). Symptom experiences, symptom attributions, and causal attributions in patients following first-time myocardial infarction. *International Journal of Behavioral Medicine, 12*, 30–38.

Camí, J., & Farré, M. (2003). Drug addiction. *New England Journal of Medicine, 349*, 975–986.

Campbell, J. M., & Oei, T. P. (2010). A cognitive model for the intergenerational tranference of alcohol use behavior. *Addictive Behaviors, 35*(2), 73–83.

Cancian, F. M., & Oliker, S. J. (2000). *Caring and gender.* Thousand Oaks, CA: Pine Forge Press.

Cannon, W. (1932). *The wisdom of the body.* New York: Norton.

Cardi, V., & Treasure, J. (2010). Treatments in eating disorders: Towards future directions. *Minerva Psichiatrica, 51*(3), 191–206.

Carmody, J., & Baer, R. A. (2008). Relationships between mindfulness practice and level of mindfulness, medical and psychological symptoms and well-being in a mindfulness-based stress reduction program. *Journal of Behavioral Medicine, 31*, 23–33.

Carpenter, C. J. (2010). A meta-analysis of the effectiveness of health belief model variables in predicting behavior. *Health Communication, 25*, 661–669.

Carr, D. (2003). A "good death" for whom? Quality of spouse's death and psychological distress among older widowed persons. *Journal of Health and Social Behavior, 44*, 215–232.

Carr, J. L. (2007). Campus violence white paper. *Journal of American College Health, 55*, 304–319.

Carrillo, J. E., Carrillo, V. A., Perez, H. R., Salas-Lopez, D., Natale-Pereira, A., & Byron, A. T. (2011). Defining and targeting health care access barriers. *Journal of Health Care for the Poor and Underserved, 22*, 562–575.

Carter, J. C., Blackmore, E., Sutandar-Pinnock, K., & Woodside, D. B. (2004). Relapse in anorexia nervosa: A survival analysis. *Psychological Medicine, 34*, 671–679.

Carver, C. S., Smith, R. G., Antoni, M. H., Petronis, V. M., Weiss, S., & Derhagopian, R. P. (2005). Optimistic personality and psychosocial well-being during treatment predict psychosocial well-being among long-term survivors of breast cancer. *Health Psychology, 24*, 508–516.

Caspi, A., Harrington, H., Moffitt, T. E., Milne, B. J., & Poulton, R. (2006). Socially isolated children 20 years later. *Archives of Pediatric Adolescent Medicine, 160*, 805–811.

Caspi, A., Sugden, K., Moffitt, T. E., Taylor, A., Craig, I. W., Harrington, H., et al. (2003). Influence of life stress on depression: Moderation by a polymorphism in the 5-HTT gene. *Science, 301*, 386–389.

Castellini, G., Lo Sauro, C., Mannucci, E., Ravaldi, C., Rotella, C. M., Faravelli, C., et al. (2011). Diagnostic crossover and outcome predictors in eating disorders to DSM-IV and DSM-V proposed criteria:
6-year follow-up study. *Psychosomatic Medicine, 73*(3), 270–279.

Castor, M. L., Smyser, M. S., Taualii, M. M., Park, A. N., Lawson, S. A., & Forquera, R. A. (2006). A nationwide population-based study identifying health disparities between American Indians/Alaska Natives and the general populations living in select urban counties. *American Journal of Public Health, 96*, 1478–1484.

Castro, C. M., Wilson, C., Wang, F., & Schillinger, D. (2007). Babel babble: Physicians' use of unclarified medical jargon with patients. *American Journal of Health Behavior, 31*, S85–S95.

Celebrity central: Lindsay Lohan. (2011). *People.* Retrieved November 17, 2011, from http://www.people.com/people/lindsay_lohan

Celentano, D. D., Valleroy, L. A., Sifakis, F., MacKellar, D. A., Hylton, J., Thiede, H., et al. (2006). Associations between substance use and sexual risk among very young men who have sex with men. *Sexually Transmitted Diseases, 33*, 265–271.

Centers for Disease Control and Prevention (CDC). (1992). 1993 revised classification system for HIV infection and expanded surveillance case definition for AIDS among adolescents and adults. *Morbidity and Mortality Weekly Report, 41*, No. RR-17.

Centers for Disease Control and Prevention (CDC). (1994). Reasons for tobacco use and symptoms of nicotine withdrawal among adolescent and young adult tobacco users—United States, 1993. *Morbidity and Mortality Weekly Report, 43*, 745–750.

Centers for Disease Control and Prevention (CDC). (2008). *HIV/AIDS surveillance report, 2006* (Vol. 18). Atlanta, GA: U.S. Department of Health and Human Services, Centers for Disease Control and Prevention. Retrieved August 3, 2008, from http://www.cdc.gov/hiv/topics/surveillance/resources/reports/

Centers for Disease Control and Prevention (CDC). (2009). *Chronic diseases—The power to prevent, the call to control: At a glance, 2009.* Atlanta, GA: U.S. Department of Health and Human Services, Centers for Disease Control and Prevention. Retrieved March 20, 2012, from http://www.cdc.gov/chronicdisease/resources/publications/aag/pdf/chronic.pdf

Centers for Disease Control and Prevention (CDC). (2010a). *HIV among gay, bisexual and other men who have sex with men (MSM).* Atlanta, GA: U.S. Department of Health and Human Services, Centers for Disease Control and Prevention. Retrieved March 20, 2012, from http://www.cdc.gov/hiv/topics/msm/pdf/msm.pdf

Centers for Disease Control and Prevention (CDC). (2010b). Vital signs: Current cigarette smoking among adults ≥18 years—United States, 2009. *Morbidity and Mortality Weekly Report, 59*(35), 1135–1140.

Centers for Disease Control and Prevention (CDC). (2011a). *HIV among African Americans.* Atlanta, GA: U.S. Department of Health and Human Services, Centers for Disease Control and Prevention. Retrieved March 20, 2012, from http://www.cdc.gov/hiv/topics/aa/PDF/aa.pdf

Centers for Disease Control and Prevention (CDC). (2011b). *HIV among youth.* Retrieved on March 20, 2012, from http://www.cdc.gov/hiv/youth/pdf/youth.pdf

Centers for Disease Control and Prevention (CDC). (2011c). *National diabetes fact sheet, 2011.* Atlanta, GA: U.S. Department of Health and Human Services, Centers for Disease Control and Prevention. Retrieved March 20, 2012, from http://www.cdc.gov/diabetes/pubs/pdf/ndfs_2011.pdf

Centers for Disease Control and Prevention (CDC). (2011d). *Safe on the outs.* Retrieved April 18, 2012, from http://www.cdc.gov/hiv/topics/research/prs/resources/factsheets/safe-on-the-outs.htm

Centers for Disease Control and Prevention (CDC) and NCHS. (2010a). *Health, United States, 2010. Chartbook, special feature on death and dying.* Hyattsville, MD: Author.

Centers for Disease Control and Prevention (CDC) and NCHS (CDC/NCHS). (2010b). *National Health Interview Survey, 2010.*

Central Intelligence Agency (CIA). (2012). *World factbook, 2012.* Washington, DC: Author.

Cepeda, M. S., Berlin, J. A., Gao, Y., Wiegand, F., & Wada, D. R. (2012). Placebo response changes depending on the neuropathic pain syndrome: Results of a systematic review and meta-analysis. *Pain Medicine, 13*, 575–595.

Ceylan-Isik, A. F., McBride, S. M., & Ren, J. (2010). Sex difference in alcoholism: Who is at a greater risk for development of alcoholic complication? *Life Sciences, 87*(5/6), 133–138.

Cha, E. S., Doswell, W. M., Kim, K. H., Charron-Prochownik, D., & Patrick, T. E. (2007). Evaluating the Theory of Planned Behavior to explain intention to engage in premarital sex amongst Korean college students: A questionnaire survey. *International Journal of Nursing Studies, 44*, 1147–1157.

Chaddock, L., Erickson, K. I., Prakash, R. S., Kim, J. S., Voss, M. W., VanPatter, M., et al. (2010). A neuroimaging investigation of the association between aerobic fitness, hippocampal volume, and memory performance in preadolescent children. *Brain Research, 1358*, 172–183.

Chakrabarty, S., & Zoorob, R. (2007). Fibromyalgia. *American Family Physician, 76*, 247–254.

Chandrashekara, S., Jayashree, K., Veeranna, H. B., Vadiraj, H. S., Ramesh, M. N., Shobha, A., et al. (2007). Effects of anxiety on TNF-a levels during psychological stress. *Journal of Psychosomatic Research, 63*, 65–69.

Chang, L., Ernst, T., Speck, O., Patel, H., DeSilva, M., Leonido-Yee, M., et al. (2002). Perfusion MRI and computerized cognitive test abnormalities in abstinent methamphetamine users. *Psychiatry Research: Neuroimaging Section, 114*, 65–79.

Chapman, C. R., Nakamura, Y., & Flores, L. Y. (1999). Chronic pain and consciousness: A constructivist perspective. In R. J. Gatchel & D. C. Turk (Eds.), *Psychosocial factors in pain: Critical perspectives* (pp. 35–55). New York: Guilford Press.

Chapman, R. H., Petrilla, A. A., Benner, J. S., Schwartz, J. S., & Tang, S. S. K. (2008). Predictors of adherence to concomitant antihypertensive and lipid-lowering medications in older adults: A retrospective, cohort Study. *Drugs & Aging, 25*, 885–892.

Charlee, C., Goldsmith, L. J., Chambers, L., & Haynes, R. B. (1996). Provider-patient communication among elderly and nonelderly patients in Canadian hospitals: A national survey. *Health Communication, 8*, 281–302.

Charles, S. T., Gatz, M., Kato, K., & Pedersen, N. L. (2008). Physical health 25 years later: The predictive ability of neuroticism. *Health Psychology, 27*, 369–378.

"Charlie Sheen." (2011, February 14). Charlie Sheen. *Famous and celebrity drug addicts.* Retrieved June 19, 2011, from http://www.famouscelebritydrugaddicts.com/charlie-sheen.htm

Chassin, L., Presson, C. C., Rose, J., & Sherman, S. J. (2007). What is addiction? Age-related differences in the meaning of addiction. *Drug and Alcohol Dependence, 87*, 30–38.

Chaturvedi, A. K., Engels, E. A., Anderson, W. F., & Gillison, M. L. (2008). Incidence trends for human papillomavirus-related and -unrelated oral squamous cell carcinomas in the United States. *Journal of Clinical Oncology, 26*, 612–619.

Chaturvedi, A. K., Engels, E. A., Pfeiffer, R. M., Hernandez, B. Y., Xiao, W., Kim, E., et al. (2011). Human papillomavirus and rising oropharyngeal cancer incidence in the United States. *Journal of Clinical Oncology, 29*, 4294–4301.

Chei, C. L., Iso, H., Yamagishi, K., Inoue, M., & Tsugane, S. (2008). Body mass index and weight change since 20 years of age and risk of coronary heart disease among Japanese: The Japan Public Health Center–Based Study. *International Journal of Obesity, 32*, 144–151.

Chen, E., Cohen, S., & Miller, G. E. (2010). How low socioeconomic status affects 2-year hormonal trajectories in children. *Psychological Science, 21*(1), 31–37.

Chen, E., & Miller, G. E. (2007). Stress and inflammation in exacerbations of asthma. *Brain, Behavior and Immunity, 21*, 993–999.

Chen, E., Strunk, R. C., Bacharier, L. B., Chan, M., & Miller, G. E. (2010). Socioeconomic status associated with exhaled nitric oxide responses to acute stress in children with asthma. *Brain, Behavior and Immunity, 24*, 444–450.

Chen, H. Y., Shi, Y., Ng, C. S., Chan, S. M., Yung, K. K., Lam, Z., et al. (2007). Auricular acupuncture treatment for insomnia: A systematic review. *Journal of Alternative and Complementary Medicine, 13*, 669–676.

Chen, J. Y., Fox, S. A., Cantrell, C. H., Stockdale, S. E., & Kagawa-Singer, M. (2007). Health disparities and prevention: Racial/ethnic barriers to flu vaccinations. *Journal of Community Health, 32*, 5–20.

Cheng, B. M. T., Lauder, I. J., Chu-Pak, L., & Kumana, C. R. (2004). Meta-analysis of large randomized controlled trials to evaluate the impact of statins on cardiovascular outcomes. *British Journal of Clinical Pharmacology, 57*, 640–651.

Cheng, T. Y. L., & Boey, K. W. (2002). The effectiveness of a cardiac rehabilitation program on self-efficacy and exercise. *Clinical Nursing Research, 11*, 10–19.

Cherkin, D. C., Sherman, K. J., Kahn, J., Wellman, R., Cook, A. J., Johnson, E., et al. (2011). A comparison of the effects of 2 types of massage and usual care on chronic low-back pain: A randomized, controlled trial. *Annals of Internal Medicine, 155*(1), 1–9.

Chia, L. R., Schlenk, E. A., & Dunbar-Jacob, J. (2006). Effect of personal and cultural beliefs on medication adherence in the elderly. *Drugs and Aging, 23*, 191–202.

Chida, T., Hamer, M., & Steptoe, A. (2008). A bidirectional relationship between psychosocial factors and atopic disorders: A systematic review and meta-analysis. *Psychosomatic Medicine, 70*, 102–116.

Chida, Y., & Hamer, M. (2008). An association of adverse psychosocial factors with diabetes mellitus: A meta-analytic review of longitudinal cohort studies. *Diabetologia, 51*, 2168–2178.

Chida, Y., & Mao, X. (2009). Does psychosocial stress predict symptomatic herpes simplex virus recurrence? A meta-analytic investigation on prospective studies. *Brain, Behavior, and Immunity, 23*, 917–925.

Chida, Y., & Steptoe, A. (2008). Positive psychological well-being and mortality: A quantitative review of prospective observational studies. *Psychosomatic Medicine, 70*, 741–756.

Chida, Y., & Steptoe, A. (2009). The association of anger and hostility with future coronary heart disease: A meta-analytic review of prospective evidence. *Journal of the American College of Cardiology, 53*, 936–946.

Chida, Y., & Vedhara, K. (2009). Adverse psychological factors predict poorer prognosis in HIV disease: A meta-analytic review of prospective investigations. *Brain, Behavior, and Immunity, 23*, 434–445.

Chiesa, A., & Serretti, A. (2010). A systematic review of neurobiological and clinical features of mindfulness meditations. *Psychological Medicine, 40*(8), 1239–1252.

Chinn, S., Jarvis, D., Melotti, R., Luczynska, C., Ackermann-Liebrich, U., Antó, J. M., et al. (2005). Smoking cessation, lung function, and weight gain: A follow-up study. *Lancet, 365*, 1629–1635.

Cholesterol Treatment Trialists' (CTT) Collaboration, Baigent, C., Blackwell, L., Emberson, J., Holland, L. E., Reith, C., et al. (2010). Efficacy and safety of more intensive lowering of LDL cholesterol: A meta-analysis of data from 170,000 participants in 26 randomised trials. *The Lancet, 376*, 1670–1681.

Chong, C. S., Tsunaka, M., Tsang, H. W., Chan, E. P., & Cheung, W. M. (2011). Effects of yoga on stress management in healthy adults: A systematic review. *Alternative Therapies in Health & Medicine, 17*(1), 32–38.

Chou, F., Holzemer, W. L., Portillo, C. J., & Slaughter, R. (2004). Self-care strategies and sources of information for HIV/AIDS symptom management. *Nursing Research, 53*, 332–339.

Chou, R., Qaseem, A., Snow, V., Casey, D., Cross, J. T., Jr., Shekelle, P., et al. (2007). Diagnosis and treatment of low back pain: A joint clinical practice guideline from the American College of Physicians and the American Pain Society. *Annals of Internal Medicine, 147*, 478–491, W118–W120.

Chow, C. K., Islam, S., Bautista, L., Rumboldt, Z., Yusufali, A., Xie, C., et al. (2011). Parental history and myocardial infarction risk across the world. *Journal of the American College of Cardiology, 57*, 619–627.

Christenfeld, N., Glynn, L. M., Phillips, D. P., & Shrira, I. (1999). Exposure to New York City as a risk factor for heart attack mortality. *Psychosomatic Medicine, 61*, 740–743.

Chumbler, N. R., Grimm, J. W., Cody, M., & Beck, C. (2003). Gender, kinship and caregiver burden: The case of community-dwelling memory impaired seniors. *International Journal of Geriatric Psychiatry, 18*, 722–732.

Chung, M. L., Moser, D. K., Lennie, T. A., Worrall-Carter, L., Bentley, B., Trupp, R., et al. (2006). Gender differences in adherence to the sodium-restricted diet in patients with heart failure. *Journal of Cardiac Failure, 12*, 628–634.

Cibulka, N. J. (2006). HIV infection. *American Journal of Nursing, 106*, 59.

Ciesla, J. A., & Roberts, J. E. (2007). Rumination, negative cognition, and their interactive effects on depressed mood. *Emotion, 7*, 555–565.

Cintron, A., & Morrison, R. S. (2006). Pain and ethnicity in the United States: A systematic review. *Journal of Palliative Medicine, 9,* 1454–1473.

Clague, J., Cinciripini, P., Blalock, J., Wu, X., & Hudmon, K. S. (2010). The D2 dopamine receptor gene and nicotine dependence among bladder cancer patients and controls. *Behavior Genetics, 40*(1), 49–58.

Clark, A. D. (2008). The new frontier of wellness. *Benefits Quarterly, 24,* 23–28.

Clark, A. M., Whelan, H. K., Barbour, R., & MacIntyre, P. D. (2005). A realist study of the mechanisms of cardiac rehabilitation. *Journal of Advanced Nursing, 52,* 362–371.

Clark, L., Jones, K., & Pennington, K. (2004). Pain assessment practices with nursing home residents. *Western Journal of Nursing Research, 26,* 733–750.

Clark, M. M., Decker, P. A., Offord, K. P., Patten, C. A., Vickers, K. S., Croghan, I. T., et al. (2004). Weight concerns among male smokers. *Addictive Behaviors, 29,* 1637–1641.

Clark, P. A. (2006). The need for new guidelines for AIDS testing and counseling: An ethical analysis. *Internet Journal of Infectious Diseases, 5*(2), 8.

Clark, R. (2003). Self-reported racism and social support predict blood pressure reactivity in Blacks. *Annals of Behavioral Medicine, 25,* 127–136.

Clark-Grill, M. (2007). Questionable gate-keeping: Scientific evidence for complementary and alternative medicines (CAM): Response to Malcolm Parker. *Journal of Bioethical Inquiry, 4,* 21–28.

Claudino, A. M., Hay, P., Lima, M. S., Bacaltchuk, J., Schmidt, U., & Treasure, J. (2006). Antidepressants for anorexia nervosa. *Cochrane Database of Systematic Reviews,* Cochrane Art. No.: CD004365, DOI: 10.1002/14651858.CD004365.pub2.

Claxton, A. J., Cramer, J., & Pierce, C. (2001). A systematic review of the association between dose regimens and medication compliance. *Clinical Therapeutics, 23,* 1296–1310.

Claydon, L. S., Chesterton, L. S., Barlas, P., & Sim, J. (2011). Dose-specific effects of transcutaneous electrical nerve stimulation (TENS) on experimental pain: A systematic review. *Clinical Journal of Pain, 27,* 635–647.

Cleary, M. (2007). Predisposing risk factors on susceptibility to exertional heat illness: Clinical decision-making considerations. *Journal of Sport Rehabilitation, 16,* 204–214.

Cleland, J. A., Palmer, J. A., & Venzke, J.W. (2005). Ethnic differences in pain perception. *Physical Therapy Reviews, 10,* 113–122.

Clever, S. L., Jin, L., Levinson, W., & Meltzer, D. O. (2008). Does doctor-patient communication affect patient satisfaction with hospital care? Results of an analysis with a novel instrumental variable. *Health Services Research, 43,* 1505–1519.

Clinton, W. J. (2005, September 25). I was a heart attack waiting to happen. *Parade Magazine,* 4–5.

Coe, C. L., & Laudenslager, M. L. (2007). Psychosocial influences on immunity, including effects on immune maturation and senescence. *Brain, Behavior and Immunity, 21,* 1000–1008.

Coffman, J. M., Cabana, M. D., Halpin, H. A., & Yelin, E. H. (2008). Effects of asthma education on children's use of acute care services: A meta-analysis. *Pediatrics, 121,* 575–586.

Cohen, S. (2005). Keynote presentation at the eighth International Congress of Behavioral Medicine. *International Journal of Behavioral Medicine, 12*(3), 123–131.

Cohen, S., Alper, C. M., Doyle, W. J., Treanor, J. J., & Turner, R. B. (2006). Positive emotional style predicts resistance to illness after experimental exposure to rhinovirus or influenza A virus. *Psychosomatic Medicine, 68,* 809–815.

Cohen, S., Doyle, W. J., Alper, C. M., Janicki-Deverts, D., & Turner, R. B. (2009). Sleep habits and susceptibility to the common cold. *Archives of Internal Medicine, 169,* 62–67.

Cohen, S., Doyle, W. J., Skoner, D. P., Rabin, B. S., & Gwaltney, J. M., Jr. (1997). Social ties and susceptibility to the common cold. *Journal of the American Medical Association, 277,* 1940–1944.

Cohen, S., Doyle, W. J., Turner, R., Alper, C. M., & Skoner, D. P. (2003). Sociability and susceptibility to the common cold. *Psychological Science, 14,* 389–395.

Cohen, S., Frank, E., Doyle, W. J., Skoner, D. P., Rabin, B. S., & Gwaltney, J. M., Jr. (1998). Types of stressors that increase susceptibility to the common cold in healthy adults. *Health Psychology, 17,* 214–223.

Cohen, S., Kamarck, T., & Mermelstein, R. (1983). A global measure of perceived stress. *Journal of Health and Social Behavior, 24,* 385–396.

Cohen, S., Tyrrell, D. A. J., & Smith, A. P. (1991). Psychological stress and susceptibility to the common cold. *New England Journal of Medicine, 325,* 606–612.

Cohen, S., Tyrrell, D. A. J., & Smith, A. P. (1993). Negative life events, perceived stress, negative affect, and susceptibility to the common cold. *Journal of Personality and Social Psychology, 64,* 131–140.

Cohn, L., Elias, J. A., & Chupp, G. L. (2004). Asthma: Mechanisms of disease persistence and progression. *Annual Review of Immunology, 22,* 789–818.

Colcombe, S. J., Erickson, K. I., Scalf, P. E., Kim, J. S., Prakash, R., McAuley, E., et al. (2006). Aerobic exercise training increases brain volume in aging humans. *The Journals of Gerontology: Series A, 61,* 1166–1170.

Colditz, G. A., Willett, W. C., Hunter, D. J., Stampfer, M. J., Manson, J. E., Hennekens, C. H., et al. (1993). Family history, age, and risk of breast cancer. *Journal of the American Medical Association, 270,* 338–343.

Cole, S. W., Naliboff, B. D., Kemeny, M. E., Griswold, M. P., Fahey, J. L., & Zack, J. A. (2001). Impaired response to HAART in HIV-infected individuals with high autonomic nervous system activity. *Proceedings of the National Academy of Sciences of the United States of America, 98,* 12695–12700.

Coles, S. L., Dixon, J. B., & O'Brien, P. E. (2007). Night eating syndrome and nocturnal snacking: Association with obesity, binge eating and psychological distress. *International Journal of Obesity, 31,* 1722–1730.

Colilla, S. A. (2010). An epidemiologic review of smokeless tobacco health effects and harm reduction potential. *Regulatory Toxicology & Pharmacology, 56*(2), 197–211.

Collins, C. E., Warren, J. M., Neve, M., McCoy, P., & Stokes, B. (2007). Review of interventions in the management of overweight and obese children which include a dietary component. *International Journal of Evidence-Based Healthcare, 5,* 2–53.

Collins, M. A. (2008). Protective mechanisms against neuroinflammatory proteins induced by preconditioning braincultures with moderate ethanol concentrations. *Neurotoxicity Research, 13,* 130.

Collins, R. L., Orlando, M., & Klein, D. J. (2005). Isolating the nexus of substance use, violence and sexual risk for HIV infection among young adults in the United States. *AIDS and Behavior, 9,* 73–87.

Colloca, L., Lopiano, L., Lanotte, M., & Benedetti, F. (2004). Overt versus covert treatment for pain, anxiety, and Parkinson's disease. *The Lancet: Neurology, 3,* 679–684.

Committee on the Use of Complementary and Alternative Medicine by the American Public, Institute of Medicine. (2005). *Complementary and alternative medicine in the United States.* Washington, DC: National Academic Press.

Cona, C. (2010). Integrative oncology combines conventional, CAM therapies. *HemOnc Today, 11*(14), 1, 10–12.

Conger, J. (1956). Reinforcement theory and the dynamics of alcoholism. *Quarterly Journal of Studies on Alcohol, 17,* 296–305.

Conn, V. S., Hafdahl, A. R., LeMaster, J. W., Ruppar, T. M., Cochran, J. E., & Nielsen, P. J. (2008). Meta-analysis of health behavior change interventions in Type 1 diabetes. *American Journal of Health Behavior, 32,* 315–392.

Constantino, M. J., Arnow, B. A., Blasey, C., & Agras, W. S. (2005). The association between patient characteristics and the therapeutic alliance in cognitive-behavioral and interpersonal therapy for bulimia nervosa. *Journal of Consulting and Clinical Psychology, 73,* 203–211.

Cook, A. J., Roberts, D. A., Henderson, M. D., Van Winkle, L. C., Chastain, D. C., & Hamill-Ruth, R. J. (2004). Electronic pain questionnaires: A randomized, crossover comparison with paper questionnaires for chronic pain assessment. *Pain, 110,* 310–317.

Cook, B. J., & Hausenblas, H. A. (2008). The role of exercise dependence for the relationship between exercise behavior and eating pathology: Mediator or moderator? *Journal of Health Psychology, 13,* 495–502.

Coon, D. W., & Evans, B. (2009). Empirically based treatments for family caregiver distress: What works and where do we go from here? *Geriatric Nursing, 30,* 426–436.

Cooper, B. (2001, March). Long may you run. *Runner's World, 36*(3), 64–67.

Corasaniti, M. T., Amantea, D., Russo, R., & Bagetta, G. (2006). The crucial role of plasticity in pain and cell death. *Cell Death and Differentiation, 13,* 534–536.

Cornford, C. S., & Cornford, H. M. (1999). 'I'm only here because of my family': A study of lay referral networks. *The British Journal of General Practice, 49,* 617–620.

Costa, L. C. M., Maher, C. G., McAuley, J. H., & Costa, L. O. P. (2009). Systematic review of cross-cultural adaptations of McGill Pain Questionnaire reveals a paucity of clinimetric testing. *Journal of Clinical Epidemiology, 62,* 934–943.

Costa, T. (2010, September 30). Setbacks—we all have them. *Tara's blog.* Retrieved from www.taracosta.com/?m=201009.

Costanza, M. E., Luckmann, R., White, M. J., Rosal, M. C., LaPelle, N., & Cranos, C. (2009). Moving mammogram-reluctant women to screening: A pilot study. *Annals of Behavioral Medicine, 37,* 343–349.

Cottington, E. M., & House, J. S. (1987). Occupational stress and health: A multivariate relationship. In A. Baum & J. E. Singer (Eds.), *Handbook of psychology and health: Vol. 5. Stress* (pp. 41–62). Hillsdale, NJ: Erlbaum.

Couper, J. W. (2007). The effects of prostate cancer on intimate relationships. *Journal of Men's Health and Gender, 4,* 226–232.

Court, A., Mulder, C., Hetrick, S. E., Purcell, R., & McGorry, P. D. (2008). What is the scientific evidence for the use of antipsychotic medication in anorexia nervosa? *Eating Disorders: The Journal of Treatment and Prevention, 16,* 217–223.

Courtney, A. U., McCarter, D. F., & Pollart, S. M. (2005). Childhood asthma: Treatment update. *American Family Physician, 71,* 1959–1968.

Cousins, N. (1979). *Anatomy of an illness as perceived by the patient: Reflections on healing and regeneration.* New York: Norton.

Coussons-Read, M. E., Okun, M. L., & Nettles, C. D. (2007). Psychosocial stress increases inflammatory markers and alters cytokine production across pregnancy. *Brain, Behavior and Immunity, 21,* 343–350.

Covington, E. C. (2000). The biological basis of pain. *International Review of Psychiatry, 12,* 128–147.

Coyne, J. C., Stefanek, M., & Palmer, S. C. (2007). Psychotherapy and survival in cancer: The conflict between hope and evidence. *Psychological Bulletin, 133,* 367–394.

Coyne, J. C., & Tennen, H. (2010). Positive psychology in cancer care: Bad science, exaggerated claims, and unproven medicine. *Annals of Behavioral Medicine, 39,* 16–26.

Craciun, C., Schüz, N., Lippke, S., & Schwarzer, R. (2012). Facilitating sunscreen use in women by a theory-based online intervention: A randomized controlled trial. *Journal of Health Psychology, 17,* 207. DOI: 10.1177/1359105311414955.

Craig, A. D. (2003). Pain mechanisms: Labeled lines versus convergence in central processing. *Annual Review of Neuroscience, 26,* 1–30.

Cramer, J. A. (2004). A systematic review of adherence with medications for diabetes. *Diabetes Care, 27,* 1218–1224.

Cramer, S., Mayer, J., & Ryan, S. (2007). College students use cell phones while driving more frequently than found in government study. *Journal of American College Health, 56,* 181–184.

Crandall, C. S., Preisler, J. J., & Aussprung, J. (1992). Measuring life event stress in the lives of college students: The Undergraduate Stress Questionnaire (USQ). *Journal of Behavioral Medicine, 15,* 627–662.

Crepaz, N., Passin, W. F., Herbst, J. H., Rama, S. M., Malow, R. M., Purcell, D. W., et al. (2008). Meta-analysis of cognitive-behavioral interventions on HIV-positive persons' mental health and immune functioning. *Health Psychology, 27,* 4–14.

Crimmins, E. M., Ki Kim, J., Alley, D. E., Karlamangla, A., & Seeman, T. (2007). Hispanic paradox in biological risk profiles. *American Journal of Public Health, 97,* 1305–1310.

Crimmins, E. M., & Saito, Y. (2001). Trends in healthy life expectancy in the United States, 1970–1990: Gender, racial, and educational differences. *Social Science and Medicine, 52,* 1629–1642.

Crisp, A., Gowers, S., Joughin, N., McClelland, L., Rooney, B., Nielsen, S., et al. (2006). Anorexia nervosa in males: Similarities and differences to anorexia nervosa in females. *European Eating Disorders Review, 14*(3), 163–167.

Crispo, A., Brennan, P., Jockel, K.-H., Schaffrath-Rosario, A., Wichman, H.-E., Nyberg, F., et al. (2004). The cumulative risk of lung cancer among current, ex- and never-smokers in European men. *British Journal of Cancer, 91,* 1280–1286.

Critchley, J. A., & Capewell, S. (2003). Mortality risk reduction associated with smoking cessation in patients with coronary heart disease: A systematic review. *Journal of the American Medical Association, 290,* 86–97.

Croft, P., Blyth, F. M., & van der Windt, D. (2010). The global occurrence of chronic pain: An introduction. In P. Croft, F. M. Blyth, & D. van der Windt (Eds.), *Chronic pain epidemiology: From Aetiology to public health* (pp. 9–18). New York: Oxford University Press.

Crowell, T. L., & Emmers-Sommer, T. M. (2001). "If I knew then what I know now": Seropositive individuals' perceptions of partner trust, safety and risk prior to HIV infection. *Communication Studies, 52,* 302–323.

Cruess, D. G., Petitto, J. M., Leserman, J., Douglas, S. D., Gettes, D. R., Ten Have, T. R., et al. (2003). Depression and HIV infection: Impact on immune function and disease progression. *CNS Spectrums, 8,* 52–58.

Cummings, D. E., & Schwartz, M. W. (2003). Genetics and pathophysiology of human obesity. *Annual Review of Medicine, 54,* 453–471.

Cunningham, J. A., Blomqvist, J., Koski-Jännes, A., & Cordingley, J. (2005). Maturing out of drinking problems: Perceptions of natural history as a function of severity. *Addiction Research & Theory, 13,* 79–84.

Cutrona, C. E., Russell, D. W., Brown, P. A., Clark, L. A., Hessling, R. M., & Gardner, K. A. (2005). Neighborhood context, personality, and stressful life events as predictors of depression among African American women. *Journal of Abnormal Psychology, 114,* 3–15.

Cutting Edge Information. (2004). *Pharmaceutical patient compliance and disease management.* Retrieved July 18, 2004, from http://www.pharmadiseasemanagement.com/metrics.htm

Czernichow, S., Lee, C. M. Y., Barzi, F., Greenfield, J. R., Baur, L. A., Chalmers, J., et al. (2010). Efficacy of weight loss drugs on obesity and cardiovascular risk factors in obese adolescents: A meta-analysis of randomized controlled trials. *Obesity Reviews, 11*(2), 150–158.

Czerniecki, J. M., & Ehde, D. M. (2003). Chronic pain after lower extremity amputation. *Critical Reviews in Physical and Rehabilitation Medicine, 15,* 309–332.

Dagenais, S., Caro, J., & Haldeman, S. (2008). A systematic review of low back pain cost of illness studies in the United States and internationally. *Spine Journal, 8,* 8–20.

Dalal, H. M., Zawada, A., Jolly, K., Moxham, T., & Taylor, R. S. (2010). Home based versus centre based cardiac rehabilitation: Cochrane systematic review and meta-analysis. *British Medical Journal, 340,* b5631.

Daley, A. (2008). Exercise and depression: A review of reviews. *Journal of Clinical Psychology in Medical Settings, 15,* 140–147.

D'Amico, D., Grazzi, L., Usai, S., Raggi, A., Leonardi, M., & Bussone, G. (2011). Disability in chronic daily headache: State of the art and future directions. *Neurological Sciences, 32,* 71–76.

Damjanovic, A. K., Yang, Y., Glaser, R., Kiecolt-Glaser, J. K., Huy, N., Laskowski, B., et al. (2007). Accelerated telomere erosion is associated with a declining immune function of caregivers of Alzheimer's disease patients. *Journal of Immunology, 179,* 4249–4254.

Damschroder, L. J., Zikmund-Fisher, B. J., & Ubel, P. A. (2005). The impact of considering adaptation in health state valuation. *Social Science and Medicine, 61*, 267–277.

Danaei, G., Ding, E. L., Mozffarian, D., Taylor, B., Rehm, J., Murray, C. J. L., et al. (2009). The preventable causes of death in the United States: Comparative risk assessment of dietary, lifestyle, and metabolic risk factors. *PLoS Medicine, 6*(4), 1–23.

Danaei, G., Vander Hoorn, S., Lopez, A. D., Murray, C. J. L., & Ezzati, M. (2005). Causes of cancer in the world: Comparative risk assessment of nine behavioural and environmental risk factors. *Lancet, 366*, 1784–1793.

Daniels, M. C., Goldberg, J., Jacobsen, C., & Welty, T. K. (2006). Is psychological distress a risk factor for the incidence of diabetes among American Indians? The Strong Heart Study. *Journal of Applied Gerontology, 25*(S1), 60S–72S.

Dansinger, M. L., Gleason, J. A., Griffith, J. L., Selker, H. P., & Schaefer, E. J. (2005). Comparison of the Atkins, Ornish, Weight Watchers, and Zone diets for weight loss and heart disease risk reduction: A randomized trial. *Journal of the American Medical Association, 293*, 43–53.

Dantzer, R., O'Connor, J. C., Freund, G. C., Johnson, R. W., & Kelley, K. W. (2008). From inflammation to sickness and depression: When the immune system subjugates the brain. *Nature Reviews Neuroscience, 9*, 46–57.

D'Arcy, Y. (2005). Conquering pain: Have you tried these new techniques? *Nursing, 35*(3), 36–42.

Datta, S. D., Koutsky, L. A., Ratelle, S., Unger, E. R., Shlay, J., McClain, T., et al. (2008). Human papillomavirus infection and cervical cytology in women screened for cervical cancer in the United States, 2003–2005. *Annals of Internal Medicine, 148*, 493–501.

"David Beckham's biggest secret revealed as star admits he has asthma." (2009, November 25). David Beckham's biggest secret revealed as star admits he has asthma. *Daily Mail*. Retrieved April 19, 2012, from http://www.dailymail.co.uk/tvshowbiz/article-1230404/

Davidson, K., MacGregor, M. W., Stuhr, J., Dixon, K., & MacLean, D. (2000). Constructive anger verbal behavior predicts blood pressure in a population-based sample. *Health Psychology, 19*, 55–64.

Davidson, K. W., & Mostofsky, E. (2010). Anger expression and risk of coronary heart disease: Evidence from the Nova Scotia Health Survey. *American Heart Journal, 159*, 199–206.

Davies, D. L. (1962). Normal drinking in recovered alcohol addicts. *Quarterly Journal of Studies on Alcohol, 24*, 321–332.

Davis, B., & Carpenter, C. (2009). Proximity of fast-food restaurants to schools and adolescent obesity. *American Journal of Public Health, 99*(3), 505–510.

Davis, C., & Scott-Robertson, L. (2000). A psychological comparison of females with anorexia nervosa and competitive male bodybuilders: Body shape ideals in the extreme. *Eating Behaviors, 1*, 33–46.

Davis, C. L., Tomporowski, P. D., McDowell, J. E., Austin, B. P., Miller, P. H., Yanasak, N. E., et al. (2011). Exercise improves executive function and achievement and alters brain activation in overweight children: A randomized, controlled trial. *Health Psychology, 30*, 91–98.

Davis, J. (2008). Pro-anorexia sites—A patient's perspective. *Child and Adolescent Mental Health, 13*, 97.

Davis, K. D. (2000). Studies of pain using functional magnetic resonance imaging. In K. L. Casey & M. C. Bushnell (Eds.), *Pain imaging: Progress in pain research and management* (pp. 195–210). Seattle, WA: IASP Press.

Davis, M. C., Zautra, A. J., Younger, J., Motivala, S. J., Attrep, J., & Irwin, M. R. (2008). Chronic stress and regulation of cellular markers of inflammation in rheumatoid arthritis: Implications for fatigue. *Brain, Behavior and Immunity, 22*, 24–32.

Dawson, D. A., Grant, B. F., Stinson, F. S., Chou, P. S., Huang, B., & Ruan, W. J. (2005). Recovery from DSM-IV alcohol dependence: United States, 2001–2002. *Addiction, 100*, 281–292.

Deandrea, S., Montanari, M., Moja, L., & Apolone, G. (2008). Prevalence of undertreatment in cancer pain: A review of published literature. *Annals of Oncology, 19*, 1985–1991.

De Andrés, J., & Van Buyten, J.-P. (2006). Neural modulation by stimulation. *Pain Practice, 6*, 39–45.

DeBar, L. L., Stevens, V. J., Perrin, N., Wu, P., Pearson, J., Yarborough, B. J., et al. (2012). A primary care-based, multicomponent lifestyle intervention for overweight adolescent females. *Pediatrics, 129*, e611–e620.

De Benedittis, G. (2003). Understanding the multidimensional mechanisms of hypnotic analgesia. *Contemporary Hypnosis, 20*, 59–80.

de Bloom, J., Geurts, S. A. E., Taris, T. W., Sonnentag, S., de Weerth, C., & Kompier, M. A. J. (2010). Effects of vacation from work on health and well-being: Lots of fun, quickly gone. *Work & Stress, 2*, 196–216.

de Bloom, J., Kompier, M., Geurts, S., de Weerth, C., Taris, T., & Sonnentag, S. (2009). Do we recover from vacation? Meta-analysis of vacation effects on health and well-being. *Journal of Occupational Health, 51*, 13–25.

de Brouwer, S. J. M., Kraaimaat, F. W., Sweep, F. C. G. J., Creemers, M. C. W., Radstake, T. R. D. J., Laarhoven, A. I. M., et al. (2010). Experimental stress in inflammatory rheumatic diseases: A review of psychophysiological stress responses. *Arthritis Research & Therapy, 12*, R89.

Decaluwé, V., & Braet, C. (2005). The cognitive behavioural model for eating disorders: A direct evaluation in children and adolescents with obesity. *Eating Behaviors, 6*, 211–220.

De Civita, M., & Dobkin, P. L. (2005). Pediatric adherence: Conceptual and methodological considerations. *Children's Health Care, 34*, 19–34.

Dehle, C., Larsen, D., & Landers, J. E. (2001). Social support in marriage. *American Journal of Family Therapy, 29*, 307–324.

de Leeuw, R., Schmidt, J. E., & Carlson, C. R. (2005). Traumatic stressors and post-traumatic stress disorder symptoms in headache patients. *Headache, 45*, 1365–1374.

DeLeo, J. A. (2006). Basic science of pain. *Journal of Bone and Joint Surgery, 88*(Suppl. 2), 58–62.

De Lew, N., & Weinick, R. M. (2000). An overview: Eliminating racial, ethnic, and SES disparities in health care. *Health Care Financing Review, 21*(4), 1–7.

DeLongis, A., Folkman, S., & Lazarus, R. S. (1988). The impact of daily stress on health and mood: Psychological and social resources as mediators. *Journal of Personality and Social Psychology, 54*, 486–495.

Delvaux, T., & Nostlinger, C. (2007). Reproductive choice for women and men living with HIV: Contraception, abortion and fertility. *Reproductive Health Matters, 15*(S29), 46–66.

De Marzo, A. M., Platz, E. A., Sutcliffe, S., Xu, J., Grönberg, H., Drake, C. G., et al. (2007). Inflammation in prostate carcinogenesis. *Nature Reviews Cancer, 7*, 256–269.

Dembroski, T. M., MacDougall, J. M., Williams, R. B., Haney, T. L., & Blumenthal, J. A. (1985). Components of Type A, hostility, and anger-in: Relationship to angiographic findings. *Psychosomatic Medicine, 47*, 219–233.

Deniz, O., Aygül, R., Koçak, N., Orhan, A., & Kaya, M. D. (2004). Precipitating factors of migraine attacks in patients with migraine with and without aura. *Pain Clinic, 16*, 451–456.

Dennis, J., Krewski, D., Côté, F.-S., Fafard, E., Little, J., & Ghadirian, P. (2011). Breast cancer risk in relation to alcohol consumption and BRCA gene mutations: A case-only study of gene-environment interaction. *The Breast Journal, 17*, 477–484.

Dennis, L. K., Vanbeek, M. J., Freeman, L. E. B., Smith, B. J., Dawson, D. V., & Coughlin, J. A. (2008). Sunburns and risk of cutaneous melanoma: Does age matter? A comprehensive meta-analysis. *Annals of Epidemiology, 18*, 614–627.

de Oliveira, C., Watt, W., & Hamer, M. (2010). Toothbrushing, inflammation, and risk of cardiovascular disease: Results from Scottish Health Survey. *British Medical Journal, 340*, c2451.

Derogatis, L. R. (1977). *Manual for the Symptom Checklist-90, Revised.* Baltimore, MD: Johns Hopkins University School of Medicine.

de Vet, E., de Nooijer, J., Oenema, A., de Vries, N. K., & Brug, J. (2008). Predictors of stage transitions in the Precaution Adoption Process Model. *American Journal of Health Promotion, 22*, 282–290.

DeVoe, J. E., Baez, A., Angier, H., Krois, L., Edlund, C., & Carney, P. A. (2007). Insurance + access ≠ health care: Typology of barriers to health care access for low-income families. *Annals of Family Medicine, 5,* 511–518.

DeVries, A. C., Glasper, E. R., & Detillion, C. E. (2003). Social modulation of stress responses. *Physiology and Behavior, 79,* 399–407.

DeWall, C. N., MacDonald, G., Webster, G. D., Masten, C. L., Baumeister, R. F., Powell, C., et al. (2010). Acetaminophen reduces social pain: Behavioral and neural evidence. *Psychological Science, 21,* 931–937.

Dewaraja, R., & Kawamura, N. (2006). Trauma intensity and posttraumatic stress: Implications of the tsunami experience in Sri Lanka for the management of future disasters. *International Congress Series, 1287,* 69–73.

Dhanani, N. M., Caruso, T. J., & Carinci, A. J. (2011). Complementary and alternative medicine for pain: An evidence-based review. *Current Pain & Headache Reports, 15*(1), 39–46.

Dickerson, F., Bennett, M., Dixon, L., Burke, E., Vaughan, C., Delahanty, J., et al. (2011). Smoking cessation in persons with serious mental illnesses: The experience of successful quitters. *Psychiatric Rehabilitation Journal, 34*(4), 311–316.

Dickerson, S. S., & Kemeny, M. E. (2004). Acute stressors and cortisol responses: A theoretical integration and synthesis of laboratory research. *Psychological Bulletin, 130,* 355–391.

Dietz, P. M., England, L. J., Shapiro-Mendoza, C. K., Tong, V. T., Farr, S. L., & Callaghan, W. M. (2010). Infant morbidity and mortality attributable to prenatal smoking in the U.S. *American Journal of Preventive Medicine, 39*(1), 45–52.

DiIorio, C., McCarty, F., Resnicow, K., Holstad, M. M., Soet, J., Yeager, K., et al. (2008). Using motivational interviewing to promote adherence to antiretroviral medications: A randomized controlled study. *AIDS Care, 20,* 273–283.

Dillard, J., with Hirchman, L. A. (2002). *The chronic pain solution.* New York: Bantam.

DiMatteo, M. R. (2004a). Social support and patient adherence to medical treatment: A meta-analysis. *Health Psychology, 23,* 207–218.

DiMatteo, M. R. (2004b). Variations in patients' adherence to medical recommendations: A quantitative review of 50 years of research. *Medical Care, 42,* 200–209.

DiMatteo, M. R., & DiNicola, D. D. (1982). *Achieving patient compliance: The psychology of the medical practitioner's role.* New York: Pergamon Press.

DiMatteo, M. R., Giordani, P. J., Lepper, H. S., & Croghan, T. W. (2002). Patient adherence and medical treatment outcomes: A meta-analysis. *Medical Care, 40,* 794–811.

DiMatteo, M. R., Haskard, K. B., & Williams, S. L. (2007). Health beliefs, disease severity, and patients adherence: A meta-analysis. *Medical Care, 45,* 521–528.

DiMatteo, M. R., Lepper, H. S., & Croghan, T. W. (2000). Meta-analysis of the effects of anxiety and depression on patient adherence. *Archives of Internal Medicine, 160,* 2101–2107.

Dimsdale, J. E., Eckenrode, J., Haggerty, R. J., Kaplan, B. H., Cohen, F., & Dornbusch, S. (1979). The role of social supports in medical care. *Social Psychiatry, 14,* 175–180.

Dingwall, G. (2005). *Alcohol and crime.* Cullompton, UK: Willan Publishing.

DiNicola, D. D., & DiMatteo, M. R. (1984). Practitioners, patients, and compliance with medical regimens: A social psychological perspective. In A. Baum, S. E. Taylor, & J. E. Singer (Eds.), *Handbook of psychology and health: Vol. 4. Social psychological aspects of health* (pp. 55–84). Hillsdale, NJ: Erlbaum.

di Sarsina, R. (2007). The social demand for a medicine focused on the person: The contribution of CAM to healthcare and health genesis. *Evidence-Based Complementary and Alternative Medicine, 4*(Suppl. 1), 45–51.

Dishman, R. K. (2003). The impact of behavior on quality of life. *Quality of Life Research, 12*(Suppl. 1), 43–49.

Distefan, J. M., Pierce, J. P., & Gilpin, E. A. (2004). Do favorite movie stars influence adolescent smoking initiation? *American Journal of Public Health, 94,* 239–244.

Dittmann, M. (2005). Publicizing diabetes' behavioral impact. *Monitor on Psychology, 36*(7), 35–36.

Dixon, L., Medoff, D. R., Wohlheiter, K., DiCelmente, C., Goldberg, R., Kreyenbuhl, J., et al. (2007). Correlates of severity of smoking among persons with severe mental illness. *American Journal of Addictions, 16*(2), 101–110.

Dobbins, M., DeCorby, K., Manske, S., & Goldblatt, E. (2008). Effective practices for school-based tobacco use prevention. *Preventive Medicine, 46,* 289–297.

Dobson, R. (2005). High cholesterol may increase risk of testicular cancer. *British Medical Journal, 330,* 1042.

Doevendans, P. A., Van der Smagt, J., Loh, P., De Jonge, N., & Touw, D. J. (2003). Prognostic implications of genetics in cardiovascular disease. *Current Pharmacogenomics, 1,* 217–228.

Donaghy, M. E. (2007). Exercise can seriously improve your mental health: Fact or fiction? *Advanced in Physiology, 9*(2), 76–88.

Donohue, K. F., Curtin, J. J., Patrick, C. J., & Lang, A. R. (2007). Intoxication level and emotional response. *Emotion, 7,* 103–112.

Dorenlot, P., Harboun, M., Bige, V., Henrard, J.-C., & Ankri, J. (2005). Major depression as a risk factor for early institutionalization of dementia patients living in the community. *International Journal of Geriatric Psychiatry, 20,* 471–478.

Dorn, J. M., Genco, R. J., Grossi, S. G., Falkner, K. L., Hovey, K. M., Iacoviello, L., et al. (2010). Periodontal disease and recurrent cardiovascular events in survivors of myocardial infarction (MI): The Western New York Acute MI Study. *Journal of Periodontology, 81,* 502–511.

Dorr, N., Brosschot, J. F., Sollers, J. J., & Thayer, J. F. (2007). Damned if you do, damned if you don't: The differential effect of expression and inhibition of anger on cardiovascular recovery in Black and White males. *International Journal of Psychophysiology, 66,* 125–134.

Doty, H. E., & Weech-Maldonado, R. (2003). Racial/ethnic disparities in adult preventive dental care use. *Journal of Health Care for the Poor and Underserved, 14,* 516–534.

Dougall, A. L., & Baum, A. (2001). Stress, health, and illness. In A. Baum, T. A. Revenson, & J. E. Singer (Eds.), *Handbook of health psychology* (pp. 321–337). Mahwah, NJ: Erlbaum.

Douketis, J. D., Macie, C., Thabane, L., & Williamson, D. F. (2005). Systematic review of long-term weight loss studies in obese adults: Clinical significance and applicability to clinical practice. *International Journal of Obesity, 29,* 1153–1167.

Dovidio, J. F., Penner, L. A., Albrecht, T. L., Norton, W. E., Gaertner, S. L., & Shelton, J. N. (2008). Disparities and distrust: The implications of psychological processes for understanding racial disparities in health and health care. *Social Science and Medicine, 67,* 478–486.

Dresler, C. M., Leon, M. E., Straif, K., Baan, R., & Secretan, B. (2006). Reversal of risk upon quitting smoking. *Lancet, 368,* 348–349.

D'Souza, G., & Dempsey, A. (2011). The role of HPV in head and neck cancer and review of the HPV vaccine. *Preventive Medicine, 53,* S5–S11.

Du, X. L., Meyer, T. E., & Franzini, L. (2007). Meta-analysis of racial disparities in survival in association with socioeconomic status among men and women with color cancer. *Cancer, 109,* 2161–2170.

Duangdao, K. M., & Roesch, S. C. (2008). Coping with diabetes in adulthood: A meta-analysis. *Journal of Behavioral Medicine, 31,* 291–300.

Dunbar, H. F. (1943). *Psychosomatic diagnosis.* New York: Hoeber.

Duncan, A. E., Neuman, R. J., Kramer, J., Kuperman, S., Hesselbrock, V., Reich, T., et al. (2005). Are there subgroups of bulimia nervosa based comorbid psychiatric disorders? *International Journal of Eating Disorders, 37,* 19–25.

Dunkel-Schetter, C. (2011). Psychological science on pregnancy: Stress processes, biopsychosocial models, and emerging research issues. *Annual Review of Psychology, 62,* 531–58.

Dunn, A. L., Trivedi, M. H., Kampert, J. B., Clark, C. G., & Chambliss, H. O. (2005). Exercise treatment for depression: Efficacy and dose response. *American Journal of Preventive Medicine, 28,* 1–8.

Dunn, A. L., Trivedi, M. H., & O'Neal, H. A. (2001). Physical activity dose-response effects on outcomes of depression and anxiety. *Medicine and Science in Sports and Exercise, 33,* S587–S597.

Dunton, G. F., Liao, Y., Intille, S. S., Spruijt-Metz, D., & Pentz, M. (2011). Investigating children's physical activity and sedentary behavior using ecological momentary assessment with mobile phones. *Pediatric Obesity, 19,* 1205–1212.

Durkheim, E. (1967). *The elementary forms of religious life* (J. W. Swain, Trans.). New York: Free Press. (Original work published 1912)

Dusseldrop, E., van Elderen, T., Maes, S., Meulman, J., & Kraaj, V. (1999). A meta-analysis of psychoeducational programs for coronary heart disease patients. *Health Psychology, 18,* 506–519.

Dutra, L., Stathopoulou, G., Basden, S. L., Leyro, T. M., Powers, M. B., & Otto, M. W. (2008). A meta-analytic review of psychosocial interventions for substance use disorders. *American Journal of Psychiatry, 165,* 179–187.

Dwan, K., Altman, D. G., Arnaiz, J. A., Bloom, J., Chan, A.-W., Cronin, E., et al. (2008). Systematic review of the empirical evidence of study publication bias and outcome reporting bias. *PLoS ONE, 3,* e3081.

Eaker, E. D., Sullivan, L. M., Kelly-Hayes, M., D'Agostino, R. B., Sr., & Benjamin, E. J. (2007). Marital status, marital strain, and risk of coronary heart disease or total mortality: The Framingham Offspring Study. *Psychosomatic Medicine, 69,* 509–513.

Eaton, D. K., Kann, L., Kinchen, S., Shanklin, S., Ross, J., Hawkins, J., et al. (2010). Youth risk behavior surveillance—United States, 2009. *Morbidity and Mortality Weekly Reports Surveillance Summaries, 59*(SS-5), 1–142.

Ebrecht, M., Hextall, J., Kirtley, L.-G., Taylor, A., Dyson, M., & Weinman, J. (2004). Perceived stress and cortisol levels predict speed of wound healing in healthy male adults. *Psychoneuroendocrinology, 29,* 798–809.

Eckhardt, C. I., & Crane, C. (2008). Effects of alcohol intoxication and aggressivity on aggressive verbalizations during anger arousal. *Aggressive Behavior, 34,* 428–436.

Eddy, K. T., Dorer, D. J., Franko, D. L., Tahilani, K., Thompson-Brenner, H., & Herzog, D. B. (2007). Should bulimia nervosa be subtyped by history of anorexia nervosa? A longitudinal validation. *International Journal of Eating Disorders, 40*(S3), S67–S71.

Edwards, A. G. K., Hulbert-Williams, N., & Neal, R. D. (2008). Psychological interventions for women with metastatic breast cancer. *Cochrane Database of Systematic Reviews,* Cochrane Art. No.: CD004253. DOI: 10.1002/14651858.CD004253.pub3.

Edwards, C. L., Fillingim, R. B., & Keefe, F. (2001). Race, ethnicity and pain. *Pain, 94,* 133–137.

Edwards, G. (1977). The alcohol dependence syndrome: Usefulness of an idea. In G. Edwards & M. Grant (Eds.), *Alcoholism: New knowledge and new responses.* London: Croom Helm.

Edwards, G. (2000). *Alcohol: The world's favorite drug.* New York: Thomas Dunne Books.

Edwards, G., & Gross, M. M. (1976). Alcohol dependence: Provisional description of a clinical syndrome. *British Medical Journal, 1,* 1058–1061.

Edwards, G., Gross, M. M., Keller, M., Moser, J., & Room, R. (1977). *Alcohol-related disabilities* (WHO Offset Pub. No. 32). Geneva: World Health Organization.

Edwards, L. M., & Romero, A. J. (2008). Coping with discrimination among Mexican descent adolescents. *Hispanic Journal of Behavioral Sciences, 30,* 24–39.

Ege, M. J., Mayer, M., Normand, A.-C., Genuneit, J., Cookson, W. O. C. M., Braun-Fahrlander, C., et al. (2011). Exposure to environmental microorganisms and childhood asthma. *The New England Journal of Medicine, 364,* 701–709.

Eggert, J., Theobald, H., & Engfeldt, P. (2004). Effects of alcohol consumption on female fertility during an 18-year period. *Fertility and Sterility, 81,* 379–383.

Ehrlich, G. E. (2003). Low back pain. *Bulletin of the World Health Organization, 81,* 671–676.

Eisenberg, M. E., Neumark-Sztainer, D., Story, M., & Perry, C. (2005). The role of social norms and friends' influences on unhealthy weight-control behaviors among adolescent girls. *Social Science and Medicine, 60,* 1165–1173.

Eisenberger, N. I., Gable, S. L., & Lieberman, M. D. (2007). Functional magnetic resonance imaging responses relate to differences in real-world social experience. *Emotion, 7,* 745–754.

Eisenberger, N. I., Inagaki, T. K., Mashal, N. M., & Irwin, M. R. (2010). Inflammation and social experience: An inflammatory challenge induces feelings of social disconnection in addition to depressed mood. *Brain, Behavior, and Immunity, 24,* 558–563.

Eisenberger, N. I., & Lieberman, M. D. (2004). Why rejection hurts: A common neural alarm system for physical and social pain. *Trends in Cognitive Sciences, 8,* 294–300.

Eisenberger, N. I., Lieberman, M. D., & Williams, K. D. (2003). Does rejection hurt? An fMRI study of social exclusion. *Science, 302,* 290–292.

Eisenmann, J. C., Welk, G. J., Wickel, E. E., & Blair, S. N. (2007). Combined influence of cardiorespiratory fitness and body mass index on cardiovascular disease risk factors among 8–18 year old youth: The Aerobics Center Longitudinal Study. *International Journal of Pediatric Obesity, 2*(2), 66–72.

Ekelund, U., Brage, S., Franks, P. W., Hennings, S., Emms, S., & Wareham, N. J. (2005). Physical activity energy expenditure predicts progression toward the metabolic syndrome independently of aerobic fitness in middle-aged healthy Caucasians. *Diabetes Care, 28,* 1195–1200.

Elbel, B., Gyamfi, J., & Kersh, R. (2011). Child and adolescent fast-food choice and the influence of calorie labeling: A natural experiment. *International Journal of Obesity, 35,* 493–500.

Elkins, J. S. (2006). Management of blood pressure in patients with cerebrovascular disease. *Johns Hopkins Advanced Studies in Medicine, 6*(8), 363–369, 349–350.

Eller, N. H., Netterstrøm, B., & Hansen, Å. M. (2006). Psychosocial factors at home and at work and levels of salivary cortisol. *Biological Psychology, 73,* 280–287.

Elliott, J. O., Seals, B. F., & Jacobson, M. P. (2007). Use of the precaution adoption process model to examine predictors of osteoprotective behavior in epilepsy. *Seizure, 16,* 424–437.

Elliott, R. A. (2006). Poor adherence to anti-inflammatory medication in asthma: Reasons, challenges, and strategies for improved disease management. *Disease Management and Health Outcomes, 14,* 223–233.

Ellis, A. (1962). *Reason and emotion in psychotherapy.* New York: Stuart.

Ellis, D. A., Podolski, C.-L., Frey, M., Naar-King, S., Wang, B., & Moltz, K. (2007). The role of parental monitoring in adolescent health outcomes: Impact on regimen adherence in youth with Type 1 diabetes. *Journal of Pediatric Psychology, 32,* 907–917.

Ellis, L. (2004). Thief of time. *InteliHealth.* Retrieved July 1, 2005, from http://www.intelihealth.com/IH/ihtIH/WSIHW000/8303/24299.html

Emanuel, A. S., McCully, S. N., Gallagher, K. M., & Updegraff, J. A. (2012). Theory of planned behavior explains gender difference in fruit and vegetable consumption. *Appetite.* DOI: 10.1016/j.appet.2012.08.007.

Emanuel, E. J., & Fuchs, V. R. (2008). The perfect storm of overutilization. *Journal of the American Medical Association, 299,* 2789–2791.

Emanuel, L., Bennett, K., & Richardson, V. E. (2007). The dying role. *Journal of Palliative Medicine, 10,* 159–168.

Empana, J.-P., Jouven, X., Lemaitre, R., Sotoodehnia, N., Rea, T., Raghunathan, T., et al. (2008). Marital status and risk of out-of-hospital sudden cardiac arrest in the population. *European Journal of Preventive Cardiology, 15,* 577–582.

Endresen, G. K. M. (2007). Fibromyalgia: A rheumatologic diagnosis? *Rheumatology International, 27,* 999–1004.

Engler, M. B., & Engler, M. M. (2006). The emerging role of flavonoid-rich cocoa and chocolate in cardiovascular health and disease. *Nutrition Reviews, 64,* 109–118.

Ensel, W. M., & Lin, N. (2004). Physical fitness and the stress process. *Journal of Community Psychology, 32,* 81–101.

Enstrom, J. E., & Kabat, G. C. (2006). Environmental tobacco smoke and coronary heart disease mortality in the United States—A meta-analysis and critique. *Inhalation Toxicology, 18*(3), 199–210.

Ephraim, P. L., Wegener, S. T., MacKenzie, E. J., Dillingham, T. R., & Pezzin, L. E. (2005). Phantom pain, residual limb pain, and back pain in amputees: Results of a national survey. *Archives of Physical Medicine and Rehabilitation, 86,* 1910–1919.

Epstein, L. H., Leddy, J. J., Temple, J. L., & Faith, M. S. (2007). Food reinforcement and eating: A multilevel analysis. *Psychological Bulletin, 133,* 884–906.

Ernster, V. L., Grady, D., Müke, R., Black, D., Selby, J., & Kerlikowske, K. (1995). Facial wrinkling in men and women by smoking status. *American Journal of Public Health, 85,* 78–82.

Ertekin-Taner, N. (2007). Genetics of Alzheimer's disease: A centennial review. *Neurologic Clinics, 25,* 611–667.

European Vertebral Osteoporosis Study Group. (2004). Variation in back pain between countries: The example of Britain and Germany. *Spine, 29,* 1017–1021.

Evans, D., & Norman, P. (2009). Illness representations, coping and psychological adjustment to Parkinson's disease. *Psychology & Health, 24,* 1181–1197.

Evans, G. W., & Stecker, R. (2004). Motivational consequences of environmental stress. *Journal of Environmental Psychology, 24,* 143–165.

Evans, M. A., Shaw, A. R. G., Sharp, D. J., Thompson, E. A., Falk, S., Turton, P., et al. (2007). Men with cancer: Is their use of complementary and alternative medicine a response to needs unmet by conventional care? *European Journal of Cancer Care, 16,* 517–525.

Evans, P. C. (2003). "If only I were thin like her, maybe I could be happy like her": The self-implications of associating a thin female ideal with life success. *Psychology of Women Quarterly, 27,* 209–214.

Everett, M. D., Kinser, A. M., & Ramsey, M. W. (2007). Training for old age: Production functions for the aerobic exercise inputs. *Medicine and Science in Sports and Exercise, 39,* 2226–2233.

Evers, A., Klusmann, V., Ziegelmann, J. P., Schwarzer, R., & Heuser, I. (2011). Long-term adherence to a physical activity intervention: The role of telephone-assisted vs. self-administered coping plans and strategy use. *Psychology & Health.* DOI: 10.1080/08870446.2011.582114.

Everson, S. A., Lynch, J. W., Kaplan, G. A., Lakka, T. A., Sivenius, J., & Salonen, J. T. (2001). Stress-induced blood pressure reactivity and incident stroke in middle-aged men. *Stroke, 32,* 1263–1270.

Ezekiel, J. E., & Miller, F. G. (2001). The ethics of placebo-controlled trials: A middle ground. *New England Journal of Medicine, 345,* 915–920.

Ezzo, J., Streitberger, K., & Schneider, A. (2006). Cochrane systematic reviews examine p6 acupuncture-point stimulation for nausea and vomiting. *Journal of Complementary and Alternative Medicine, 12,* 489–495.

Faden, R. R. (1987). Ethical issues in government sponsored public health campaigns. *Health Education Quarterly, 14,* 27–37.

Fairburn, C. G., & Harrison, P. J. (2003). Eating disorders. *Lancet, 361,* 407–416.

Fairhurst, M., Wiech, K., Dunckley, P., & Tracey, I. (2007). Anticipatory brainstem activity predicts neural processing of pain in humans. *Pain, 128,* 101–110.

Falagas, M. E., Zarkadoulia, E. A., Pliatsika, P. A., & Panos, G. (2008). Socioeconomic status (SES) as a determinant of adherence to treatment in HIV infected patients: A systematic review of the literature. *Retrovirology, 5,* 13.

Fang, C. V., & Myers, H. F. (2001). The effects of racial stressors and hostility on cardiovascular reactivity in African American and Caucasian men. *Health Psychology, 20,* 64–70.

Farley, J. J., Rodrigue, J. R., Sandrik, L. L., Tepper, V. J., Marhefka, S. L., & Sleasman, J. W. (2004). Clinical assessment of medication adherence among HIV-infected children: Examination of the Treatment Interview Protocol (TIP). *AIDS Care, 16,* 323–337.

Farrell, S. P., Hains, A. A., Davies, W. H., Smith, P., & Parton, E. (2004). The impact of cognitive distortions, stress, and adherence on metabolic control in youths with Type 1 diabetes. *Journal of Adolescent Health, 34,* 461–467.

Favier, I., Haan, J., & Ferrari, M. D. (2005). Chronic cluster headache: A review. *Journal of Headache and Pain, 6,* 3–9.

Federal Trade Commission weighs in on losing weight. (2002). *FDA Consumer, 36,* 8.

Feist, J., & Feist, G. J. (2006). *Theories of personality* (6th ed.). Boston, MA: McGraw-Hill.

Feldman, P. J., Cohen, S., Gwaltney, J. M., Jr., Doyle, W. J., & Skoner, D. P. (1999). The impact of personality on the reporting of unfounded symptoms and illness. *Journal of Personality and Social Psychology, 77,* 370–378.

Feldt, K. (2007). Pain measurement: Present concern and future directions. *Pain Medicine, 8,* 541–543.

Felson, R. B., & Staff, J. (2010). The effects of alcohol intoxication on violent versus other offending. *Criminal Justice and Behavior, 37*(12), 1343–1360.

Ferguson, J., Bauld, L., Chesterman, J., & Judge, K. (2005). The English smoking treatment services: One-year outcomes. *Addiction, 100*(Suppl. 2), 59–69.

Ferguson, J. K., Willemsen, E. W., & Castañeto, M. V. (2010). Centering prayer as a healing response to everyday stress: A psychological spiritual process. *Pastoral Psychology, 59*(3), 305–329.

Ferlay, J., Parkin, D. M., & Steliarova-Foucher, E. (2010). Estimates of cancer incidence and mortality in Europe in 2008. *European Journal of Cancer, 46,* 765–781.

Fernandez, E., & Sheffield, J. (1996). Relative contributions of life events versus daily hassles to the frequency and intensity of headaches. *Headache, 36,* 595–602.

Fernandez, R., Griffiths, R., Everett, B., Davidson, P., Salamonson, Y., & Andrew, S. (2007). Effectiveness of brief structured interventions on risk factor modification for patients with coronary heart disease: A systematic review. *International Journal of Evidence-Based Healthcare, 5,* 370–405.

Ferri, M., Amato, L., & Davoli, M. (2006). Alcoholics Anonymous and other 12-step programmes for alcohol dependence. *Cochrane Database of Systematic Reviews,* Cochrane Art. No.: CD005032, DOI: 10.1002/14651858.CD005032.pub2.

Fichtenberg, C. M., & Glantz, S. A. (2002). Effect of smoke-free workplaces on smoking behaviour: *Systematic Review, 325,* 188–195.

Fichter, M., Quadflieg, N., & Fischer, U. (2011). Severity of alcohol-related problems and mortality: Results from a 20-year prospective epidemiological community study. *European Archives of Psychiatry & Clinical Neuroscience, 261*(4), 293–302.

Fidler, J. A., West, R., van Jaarsveld, C. H. M., Jarvis, M. J., & Wardle, J. (2008). Smoking status of step-parents as a risk factor for smoking in adolescence. *Addiction, 103*(3), 496–501.

Fifield, J., Mcquillan, J., Armeli, S., Tennen, H., Reisine, S., & Affleck, G. (2004). Chronic strain, daily work stress and pain among workers with rheumatoid arthritis: Does job stress make a bad day worse? *Work and Stress, 18,* 275–291.

Fillingim, R. B., King, C. D., Ribeiro-Dasilva, M. C., Rahim-Williams, B., & Riley, J. L. (2009). Sex, gender, and pain: A review of recent clinical and experimental findings. *The Journal of Pain, 10,* 447–485.

Finkelstein, A., Taubman, S., Wright, B., Bernstein, M., Gruber, J., Newhouse, J. P., et al. (2011). *The Oregon Health Insurance Experiment: Evidence from the first year* (NBER Working Paper No. 17190). Washington, DC: National Bureau of Economic Research.

Finlayson, G., King, N., & Blundell, J. E. (2007). Liking vs. wanting food: Importance for human appetite control and weight regulation. *Neuroscience and Biobehavioral Reviews, 31,* 987–1002.

Finley, J. W., Davis, C. D., & Feng, Y. (2000). Selenium from high selenium broccoli protects rats from colon cancer. *Journal of Nutrition, 130,* 2384–2389.

Finniss, D. G., & Benedetti, F. (2005). The neural matrix of pain processing and placebo analgesia: Implications for clinical practice. *Headache Currents, 2*(6), 132–138.

Firenzuoli, F., & Gori, L. (2007). Herbal medicine today: Clinical and research issues. *Evidence Based Complementary and Alternative Medicine, 4*(Suppl. 1), 37–40.

Fischer, S., Stojek, M., & Hartzell, E. (2010). Effects of multiple forms of childhood abuse and adult sexual assault on current eating disorder symptoms. *Eating Behaviors, 11*(3), 190–192.

Fishbain, D. A., Cole, B., Lewis, J., Rosomoff, H. L., & Rosomoff, R. S. (2008). What percentage of chronic nonmalignant pain patients exposed to chronic opioid analgesic therapy develop abuse/addiction and/or aberrant drug-related behaviors? A structured evidence-based review. *Pain Medicine, 9*, 444–459.

Fisher, C. A., Hetrick, S. E., & Rushford, N. (2010). Family therapy for anorexia nervosa. *Cochrane Database of Systematic Reviews 2010*, Issue 4, Cochrane Art. No.: CD004780, DOI: 10.1002/14651858. CD004780.pub2.

Fitzpatrick, A. L., Kuller, L. H., Ives, D. G., Lopez, O. L., Jagust, W., Breitner, J. C. S., et al. (2004). Incidence and prevalence of dementia in the Cardiovascular Health Study. *Journal of the American Geriatrics Society, 52*, 195–204.

Fjorback, L. O., Arendt, M., Ørnbøl, E., Fink, P., & Walach, H. (2011). Mindfulness-based stress reduction and mindfulness-based cognitive therapy—A systematic review of randomized controlled trials. *Acta Psychiatrica Scandinavica, 124*(2), 102–119.

Flay, B. R. (2009). The promise of long-term effectiveness of school-based smoking prevention programs: A critical review of reviews. *Tobacco Induced Diseases, 5*(7), 1–12.

Flegal, K. M., Carroll, M. D., Kit, B. K., & Ogden, C. L. (2012). Prevalence of obesity and trends in the distribution of body mass index among US adults, 1999–2010. *Journal of the American Medical Association, 307*, 491–497.

Flegal, K. M., Graubard, B. I., Williamson, D. F., & Gail, M. H. (2005). Excess deaths associated with underweight, overweight, and obesity. *Journal of the American Medical Association, 293*, 1861–1867.

Fleshner, M., & Laudenslager, M. L. (2004). Psychoneuroimmunology: Then and now. *Behavioral and Cognitive Neuroscience Reviews, 3*, 114–130.

Flor, H. (2001). Psychophysiological assessment of the patient with chronic pain. In D. C. Turk & R. Melzack (Eds.), *Handbook of pain assessment* (2nd ed., pp. 70–96). New York: Guilford Press.

Flor, H., Nikolajsen, L., & Staehelin Jensen, T. (2006). Phantom limb pain: A case of maladaptive CNS plasticity? *Nature Reviews Neuroscience, 7*, 873–881.

Flores, G. (2006). Language barriers to health care in the United States. *New England Journal of Medicine, 355*, 229–231.

Floriani, V., & Kennedy, C. (2008). Promotion of physical activity in children. *Current Opinion in Pediatrics, 20*, 90–95.

Flynn, B. S., Worden, J. K., Bunn, J. Y., Solomon, L. J., Ashikaga, T., Connolly, S. W., et al. (2010). Mass media interventions to reduce youth smoking prevalence. *American Journal of Preventive Medicine, 39*(1), 53–62.

Folkman, S., & Lazarus, R. S. (1980). An analysis of coping in a middle-aged community sample. *Journal of Health and Social Behavior, 21*, 219–239.

Folkman, S., & Moskowitz, J. T. (2000). Positive affect and the other side of coping. *American Psychologist, 55*, 647–654.

Folkman, S., & Moskowitz, J. T. (2004). Coping: Pitfalls and promise. *Annual Review of Psychology, 55*, 745–774.

Foltz, V., St. Pierre, Y., Rozenberg, S., Rossignol, M., Bourgeois, P., Joseph, L., et al. (2005). Use of complementary and alternative therapies by patients with self-reported chronic back pain: A nationwide survey in Canada. *Joint Bone Spine, 72*, 571–577.

Foran, H., & O'Leary, K. (2008). Problem drinking, jealousy, and anger control: Variables predicting physical aggression against a partner. *Journal of Family Violence, 23*, 141–148.

Forbes, G. B. (2000). Body fat content influences the body composition response to nutrition and exercise. *Annals of the New York Academic of Sciences, 904*, 359–368.

Ford, E. S., Ajani, U. A., Croft, J. B., Critchley, J. A., Labarthe, D. R., Kottke, T. E., et al. (2007). Explaining the decrease in U. S. deaths from coronary disease, 1980–2000. *New England Journal of Medicine, 356*, 2388–2398.

Ford, E. S., Bergmann, M. M., Boeing, H., Li, C., & Capewell, S. (2012). Healthy lifestyle behaviors and all-cause mortality among adults in the United States. *Preventive Medicine, 55*, 23–27.

Ford, E. S., Zhao, G., Tsai, J., & Li, C. (2011). Low-risk lifestyle behaviors and all-cause mortality: Findings from the National Health and Nutrition Examination Survey III Mortality Study. *American Journal of Public Health, 101*, 1922–1929.

Fordyce, W. E. (1974). Pain viewed as learned behavior. In J. J. Bonica (Ed.), *Advances in neurology* (Vol. 4; pp. 415–422). New York: Raven Press.

Fordyce, W. E. (1976). *Behavioral methods for chronic pain and illness*. St. Louis, MO: Mosby.

Forlenza, J. J., & Baum, A. (2004). Psychoneuroimmunology. In R. G. Frank, A. Baum, & J. L. Wallander (Eds.), *Handbook of clinical health psychology* (Vol. 3, pp. 81–114). Washington, DC: American Psychological Association.

Foroud, T., Edenberg, H. J., & Crabbe, J. C. (2010). Genetic research: Who is at risk for alcoholism? *Alcohol Research & Health, 33*(1/2), 64–75.

Fortmann, A., Gallo, L. C., & Philis-Tsimkas, A. (2011). Glycemic control among Latinos with Type 2 diabetes: The role of social-environmental support resources. *Health Psychology, 30*, 251–258.

Foulon, C., Guelfi, J. D., Kipman, A., Adès, J., Romo, L., Houdeyer, K., et al. (2007). Switching to the bingeing/purging subtype of anorexia nervosa is frequently associated with suicidal attempts. *European Psychiatry, 22*, 513–519.

Fournier, J. C., DeRubeis, R. J., Hollon, S. D., Dimidjian, S., Amsterdam, J. D., Shelton, R. C., et al. (2010). Antidepressant drug effects and depression severity: A patient-level meta-analysis. *Journal of the American Medical Association, 303*, 47–53.

Fournier, M., de Ridder, D., & Bensing, J. (2002). Optimism and adaptation to chronic disease: The role of optimism in relation to self-care options for Type 1 diabetes mellitus, rheumatoid arthritis and multiple sclerosis. *British Journal of Health Psychology, 7*, 409–432.

Fox, C. S., Heard-Costa, N. L., Wilson, P. W. F., Levy, D., D'Agostino, R. B., Sr., & Atwood, L. D. (2004). Genome-wide linkage to chromosome 6 for waist circumference in the Framingham Heart Study. *Diabetes, 53*, 1399–1402.

Frank, E., Ratanawongsa, N., & Carrera, J. (2010). American medical students' beliefs in the effectiveness of alternative medicine. *International Journal of Collaborative Research on Internal Medicine & Public Health, 2*(9), 292–305.

Franklin, V. L., Waller, A., Pagliari, C., & Greene, S. A. (2006). A randomized controlled trial of Sweet Talk, a text-messaging system to support young people with diabetes. *Diabetic Medicine, 23*, 1332–1338.

Franko, D. L., Becker, A. E., Thomas, J. J., & Herzog, D. B. (2007). Cross-ethnic differences in eating disorder symptoms and related distress. *International Journal of Eating Disorders, 40*, 156–164

Franks, H. M., & Roesch, S. C. (2006). Appraisals and coping in people living with cancer: A meta-analysis. *Psycho-Oncology, 15*, 1027–1037.

Fraser, B. (2005). Latin America's urbanisation is boosting obesity. *Lancet, 365*, 1995–1996.

Fraser, G. E., & Shavlik, D. J. (2001). Ten years of life: Is it a matter of choice? *Archives of Internal Medicine, 161*, 1645–1652.

Frattaroli, J. (2006). Experimental disclosure and its moderators: A meta-analysis. *Psychological Bulletin, 132*, 823–865.

Frattaroli, J., Thomas, M., & Lyubomirsky, S. (2011). Opening up in the classroom: Effects of expressive writing on graduate school entrance exam performance. *Emotion, 11*, 691–696.

Frattaroli, J., Weidner, G., Merritt-Worden, T. A., Frenda, S., & Ornish, D. (2008). Angina pectoris and atherosclerotic risk factors in the Multisite Cardiac Lifestyle Intervention Program. *American Journal of Cardiology, 101,* 911–918.

Freedman, D. H. (2011). The triumph of new-age medicine. *The Atlantic, 308*(1), 90–100.

Freedman, D. S., Khan, L. K., Dietz, W. H., Srinivasan, S. R., & Berenson, G. S. (2001). Relationship of childhood obesity to coronary heart disease risk factors in adulthood: The Bogalusa Heart Study. *Pediatrics, 108,* 712–718.

Freedman, L. S., Kipnis, V., Schatzkin, A., & Potischman, N. (2008). Methods of epidemiology: Evaluating the fat-breast cancer hypothesis—Comparing dietary instruments and other developments. *Cancer Journals, 14*(2), 69–74.

Friedenreich, C. M., & Cust, A. E. (2008). Physical activity and breast cancer risk: Impact of timing, type and dose of activity and population subgroup effects. *British Journal of Sports Medicine, 42,* 636–647.

Friedländer, L. (1968). *Roman life and manners under the early empire.* New York: Barnes & Noble.

Friedman, M., & Rosenman, R. H. (1974). *Type A behavior and your heart.* New York: Knopf.

Friedmann, E., & Thomas, S. A. (1995). Pet ownership, social support, and one-year survival after acute myocardial infarction in the Cardiac Arrhythmia Suppression Trial (CAST). *The American Journal of Cardiology, 76,* 1213–1217.

Friedson, E. (1961). *Patients' views of medical practice.* New York: Russell Sage.

Fries, J. F. (1998). Reducing the need and demand for medical services. *Psychosomatic Medicine, 60,* 140–142.

Frisina, P. G., Borod, J. C., & Lepore, S. J. (2004). A meta-analysis of the effects of written emotional disclosure on the health outcomes of clinical populations. *Journal of Nervous and Mental Disease, 192,* 629–634.

Frone, M. R. (2008). Are work stressors related to employee substance use? The importance of temporal context assessment of alcohol and illicit drug use. *Journal of Applied Psychology, 93,* 199–206.

Froom, P., Kristal-Boneh, E., Melamed, S., Gofer, D., Benbassat, J., & Ribak, J. (1999). Smoking cessation and body mass index of occupationally active men: The Israeli CORDIS Study. *American Journal of Public Health, 89,* 718–722.

Fuertes, J. N., Mislowack, A., Bennett, J., Paul, L., Gilbert, T. C., Fontan, G., et al. (2007). The physician-patient working alliance. *Patient Education and Counseling, 66,* 29–36.

Fujino, Y., Tamakoshi, A., Iso, H., Inaba, Y., Kubo, T., Ide, R., et al. (2005). A nationwide cohort study of educational background and major causes of death among the elderly population in Japan. *Preventive Medicine, 40,* 444–451.

Fulkerson, J. A., & French, S. A. (2003). Cigarette smoking for weight loss or control among adolescents: Gender and racial/ethnic differences. *Journal of Adolescent Health, 32,* 306–313.

Fumal, A., & Schoenen, J. (2008). Tension-type headache: Current research and clinical management. *Lancet Neurology, 7,* 70–83.

Fung, T. T., Chiuve, S. E., McCullough, M. L., Rexrode, K. M., Logroscino, G., & Hu, F. B. (2008). Adherence to a DASH-style diet and risk of coronary heart disease and stroke in women. *Archives of Internal Medicine, 168,* 713–720.

Furberg, H., YunJung, K., Dackor, J., Boerwinkle, E., Franceschini, N., Ardissinio, D., et al. (2010). Genome-wide meta-analyses identify multiple loci associated with smoking behavior. *Nature Genetics, 42*(5), 441–447.

Furlan, A. D., Imamura, M., Dryden, T., & Irvin, E. (2008). Massage for low-back pain. *Cochrane Database of Systematic Reviews 2008,* Issue 4, Cochrane Art. No.: CD001929, DOI: 10.1002/14651858.CD001929.pub2.

Furnham, A. (2007). Are modern health worries, personality and attitudes to science associated with the use of complementary and alternative medicine? *British Journal of Health Psychology, 12,* 229–243.

Gaab, J., Sonderegger, L., Scherrer, S., & Ehlert, U. (2007). Psychoneuroendocrine effects of cognitive-behavioral stress management in a naturalistic setting—A randomized controlled trial. *Psychoneuroendocrinology, 31,* 428–438.

Gabriel, R., Ferrando, L., Cortón, E. S., Mingote, C., García-Camba, E., Liria, A. F., et al. (2007). Psychopathological consequences after a terrorist attack: An epidemiological study among victims, the general population, and police officers. *European Psychiatry, 22,* 339–346.

Gaesser, G. A. (2003). Weight, weight loss, and health: A closer look at the evidence. *Healthy Weight Journal, 17,* 8–11.

Gagliese, L., Weizblit, N., Ellis, W., & Chan, V. W. S. (2005). The measurement of postoperative pain: A comparison of intensity scales in younger and older surgical patients. *Pain, 117,* 412–420.

"Gaining it back." (2006, November 6). *Oprah Follow-Ups.* Retrieved July 17, 2011, from http://www.oprah.com/oprahshow/Oprah-Follow-Ups

Galdas, P. M., Cheater, F., & Marshall, P. (2005). Men and health help-seeking behavior: Literature review. *Journal of Advanced Nursing, 49,* 616–623.

Gallagher, B. (2003). Tai chi chuan and qigong. *Topics in Geriatric Rehabilitation, 19,* 172–182.

Gallagher-Thompson, D., & Coon, D. W. (2007). Evidence-based psychological treatments for distress in family caregivers of older adults. *Psychology and Aging, 22,* 37–51.

Galland, L. (2006). Patient-centered care: Antecedents, triggers, and mediators. *Alternative Therapies, 12,* 62–70.

Gallegos-Macias, A. R., Macias, S. R., Kaufman, E., Skipper, B., & Kalishman, N. (2003). Relationship between glycemic control, ethnicity and socioeconomic status in Hispanic and white non-Hispanic youths with Type 1 diabetes mellitus. *Pediatric Diabetes, 4,* 19–23.

Galloway, G. P., Coyle, J. R., Guillén, J. E., Flower, K., & Mendelson, J. E. (2011). A simple, novel method for assessing medication adherence: Capsule photographs taken with cellular telephones. *Journal of Addiction Medicine, 5,* 170–174.

Gambrill, S. (2008, April). Magic Johnson—Celebrity spokesperson for minority patient recruitment? *Clinical Trials Today.* Retrieved June 30, 2008, from http://www.clinicaltrialstoday.com/2008/04/magic-johnsonce.html

Gan, T. J., Gordon, D. B., Bolge, S. C., & Allen, J. G. (2007). Patient-controlled analgesia: Patient and nurse satisfaction with intravenous delivery systems and expected satisfaction with transdermal delivery systems. *Current Medical Research and Opinion, 23,* 2507–2516.

Gandini, S., Botteri, E., Iodice, S., Boniol, M., Lowenfels, A. B., Maisonneuve, P., et al. (2008). Tobacco smoking and cancer: A meta-analysis. *International Journal of Cancer, 122,* 155–164.

Gans, J. A., & McPhillips, T. (2003). Medication compliance-adherence-persistence. *Medication Compliance-Adherence-Persistence (CAP) Digest, 1,* 1–32.

Gao, L., Weck, M. N., Stegmaier, C., Rothenbacher, D., Brenner, H. (2010). Alcohol consumption, serum gamma-glutamyltransferase, and Helicobacter pylori infection in a population-based study among 9733 adults. *Annals of Epidemiology, 20*(2), 122–128.

Garavello, W., Negri, E., Talamini, R., Levi, F., Zambon, P., Dal Maso, L., et al. (2005). Family history of cancer, its combination with smoking and drinking, and risk of squamous cell carcinoma of the esophagus. *Cancer Epidemiology, Biomarkers, and Prevention, 14,* 1390–1393.

Garber, C. E., Blissmer, B., Deschenes, M. R., Franklin, B. A., Lamonte, M. J., Lee, I.-M., et al. (2011). Quantity and quality of exercise for developing and maintaining cardiorespiratory, musculoskeletal, and neuromotor fitness in apparently healthy adults: Guidance for prescribing exercise. *Medicine & Science in Sports & Exercise, 43,* 1334–1359.

Garber, M. C. (2004). The concordance of self-report with other measures of medication adherence: A summary of the literature. *Medical Care, 42,* 649–652.

García, J., Simón, M. A., Durán, M., Canceller, J., & Aneiros, F. J. (2006). Differential efficacy of a cognitive-behavioral intervention versus pharmacological treatment in the management of fibromyalgic syndrome. *Psychology, Health and Medicine, 11,* 498–506.

Garcia, K., & Mann, T. (2003). From "I wish" to "I will": Social-cognitive predictors of behavioral intentions. *Journal of Health Psychology, 8*, 347–360.

Gardner, C. D., Kiazand, A., Alhassan, S., Kim, S., Stafford, R. S., Balise, R. R., et al. (2007). Comparison of the Atkins, Zone, Ornish, and LEARN diets for change in weight and related risk factors among overweight premenopausal women: The A to Z weight loss study: A randomized trial. *Journal of the American Medical Association, 297*, 969–977.

Garner, D. M., & Garfinkel, P. E. (1980). Social-cultural factors in the development of anorexia nervosa. *Psychological Medicine, 10*, 647–656.

Garner, D. M., Garfinkel, P. E., Schwartz, D., & Thompson, M. (1980). Cultural expectations of thinness in women. *Psychological Reports, 47*, 483–491.

Garofalo, R., Herrick, A., Mustanski, B. S., & Donenberg, G. R. (2007). Tip of the iceberg: Young men who have sex with men, the Internet, and HIV risk. *American Journal of Public Health, 97*, 1113–1117.

Garssen, B. (2004). Psychological factors and cancer development. Evidence after 30 years of research. *Clinical Psychology Review, 24*, 115–338.

Gatchel, R. J. (2005). The biopsychosocial approach to pain assessment and management. In R. J. Gatchel (Ed.), *Clinical essentials of pain management* (pp. 23–46). Washington, DC: American Psychological Association.

Gatchel, R. J., & Epker, J. (1999). Psychosocial predictors of chronic pain and response to treatment. In R. J. Gatchel & D. C. Turk (Eds.), *Psychosocial factors in pain: Critical perspectives* (pp. 412–434). New York: Guilford Press.

Geary, D. C., & Flinn, M. V. (2002). Sex differences in behavioral and hormonal response to social threat: Commentary on Taylor et al. (2000). *Psychological Review, 109*, 745–750.

Geisser, M. E., Ranavaya, M., Haig, A. J., Roth, R. S., Zucker, R., Ambroz, C., et al. (2005). A meta-analytic review of surface electromyography among persons with low back pain and normal, healthy controls. *Journal of Pain, 6*, 711–726.

Gelhaar, T., Seiffge-Krenke, I., Borge, A., Cicognani, E., Cunha, M., Loncaric, D., et al. (2007). Adolescent coping with everyday stressors: A seven-nation study of youth from central, eastern, southern, and northern Europe. *European Journal of Developmental Psychology, 4*, 129–156.

Gellad, W. F., Haas, J. S., & Safran, D. G. (2007). Race/ethnicity and nonadherence to prescription medications among seniors: Results of a national study. *Journal of General Internal Medicine, 22*, 1572–1578.

Gemmell, L., & DiClemente, C. C. (2009). Styles of physician advice about smoking cessation in college students. *Journal of American College Health, 58*(2), 113–119.

George, S., Rogers, R. D., & Duka, T. K. (2005). The acute effect of alcohol on decision making in social drinkers. *Psychopharmacology, 182*, 160–169.

Georges, J., Jansen, S., Jackson, J., Meyrieux, A., Sadowska, A., & Selmes, M. (2008). Alzheimer's disease in real life—The dementia carer's survey. *International Journal of Geriatric Psychiatry, 23*, 546–553.

Gibbons, F. X., Gerrard, M., Blanton, H., & Russell, D. W. (1998). Reasoned action and social reaction: Willingness and intention as independent predictors of health risk. *Journal of Personality and Social Psychology, 74*, 1164–1180.

Gidycz, C. A., Orchowski, L. M., King, C. R., & Rich, C. L. (2008). Sexual victimization and health-risk behaviors: A prospective analysis of college women. *Journal of Interpersonal Violence, 23*, 744–763.

Gielen, A. C., McKenzie, L. B., McDonald, E. M., Shields, W. C., Wang, M.-C., Cheng, Y.-J., et al. (2007). Using a computer kiosk to promote child safety: Results of a randomized, controlled trial in an urban pediatric emergency department. *Pediatrics, 120*, 330–339.

Gielkens-Sijstermans, C. M., Mommers, M. A., Hoogenveen, R. T., Feenstra, T. L., de Vreede, J., Bovens, F. M., et al. (2010). Reduction of smoking in Dutch adolescents over the past decade and its health gains: A repeated cross-sectional study. *European Journal of Public Health, 20*(2), 146–150.

Gilbert, M. T. P., Rambaut, A., Wlasiuk, G., Spira, T. J., Pitchenik, A. E., & Worobey, M. (2007). The emergence of HIV/AIDS in the Americas and beyond. *Proceedings of the National Academy of Sciences of the United States of America, 104*, 18566–18570.

Gildea, K. M., Schneider, T. R., & Shebilske, W. L. (2007). Appraisals and training performance on a complex laboratory task. *Human Factors, 49*, 745–758.

Gillies, C. L., Abrams, K. R., Lambert, P. C., Cooper, N. J., Sutton, A. J., & Hsu, R. T. (2007). Pharmacological and lifestyle interventions to prevent or delay Type 2 diabetes in people with impaired glucose tolerance: Systematic review and meta-analysis. *British Medical Journal, 334*, 299–302.

Gilpin, E. A., White, M. M., Messer, K., & Pierce, J. P. (2007). Receptivity to tobacco advertising and promotions among young adolescents as a predictor of established smoking in young adulthood. *American Journal of Public Health, 97*, 1489–1495.

Ginsberg, J., Mohebbi, M. H., Patel, R. S., Brammer, L., Smolinski, M. S., & Brilliant, L. (2009). Detecting influenza epidemics using search engine query data. *Nature, 457*, 1012–1014.

Glaser, R. (2005). Stress-associated immune dysregulation and its importance for human health: A personal history of psychoneuroimmunology. *Brain, Behavior and Immunity, 19*, 3–11.

Glassman, A. H., Bigger, T., & Gaffney, M. (2009). Psychiatric characteristics associated with long-term mortality among 361 patients having an acute coronary syndrome and major depression. *Archives of General Psychiatry, 66*, 1022–1029.

Glueckauf, R. L., Ketterson, T. U., Loomis, J. S., & Dages, P. (2004). Online support and education for dementia caregivers: Overview, utilization, and initial program evaluation. *Telemedicine Journal and e-Health, 10*(2), n.p.

Glynn, L. M., Dunkel Schetter, C., Hobel, C. J., & Sandman, C. (2008). Pattern of perceived stress and anxiety in pregnancy predicts preterm birth. *Health Psychology, 27*, 43–51.

Godfrey, J. R. (2004). Toward optimal health: The experts discuss therapeutic humor. *Journal of Women's Health, 13*, 474–479.

Goffaux, P., Redmond, W. J., Rainville, P., & Marchand, S. (2007). Descending analgesia: When the spine echoes what the brain expects. *Pain, 130*, 137–143.

Gold, D. R., & Wright, R. (2005). Population disparities in asthma. *Annual Review of Public Health, 26*, 89–113.

Goldman, R. (2007, November 6). Halle Berry says she cured herself of Type 1 diabetes, but doctors say that's impossible. *ABC News on Call.* Retrieved June 28, 2008, from http://abcnews.go.com/Health/DiabetesResource/Story?id=3822870&page=1

Goldring, M. B., & Goldring, S. R. (2007). Osteoarthritis. *Journal of Cellular Physiology, 213*, 626–634.

Goldschmidt, A. B., Jones, M., Manwaring, J. L., Luce, K. H., Osborne, M. I., Cunning, D., et al. (2008). The clinical significance of loss of control over eating in overweight adolescents. *International Journal of Eating Disorders, 41*, 153–158.

Goldsmith, C. (2004). Fetal alcohol syndrome: A preventable tragedy. *Access, 18*(5), 34–38.

Goldstein, A. (1976). Opioid peptides (endorphins) in pituitary and brain. *Science, 193*, 1081–1086.

Goldston, K., & Baillie, A. J. (2008). Depression and coronary heart disease: A review of the epidemiological evidence, explanatory mechanisms and management approaches. *Clinical Psychology Review, 28*, 289–307.

Gonçalves, R. B., Coletta, R. D., Silvério, K. G., Benevides, L., Casati, M. Z., da Silva, J. S., et al. (2011). Impact of smoking on inflammation: Overview of molecular mechanisms. *Inflammation Research, 60*(5), 409–424.

Gonder-Frederick, L. A., Cox, D. J., & Ritterband, L. M. (2002). Diabetes and behavioral medicine: The second decade. *Journal of Consulting and Clinical Psychology, 70*, 611–625.

Gonzalez, J. S., Penedo, F. J., Antoni, M. H., Durán, R. E., Fernandez, M. I., McPherson-Baker, S., et al. (2004). Social support, positive states of mind, and HIV treatment adherence in men and women living with HIV/AIDS. *Health Psychology*, 23, 413–418.

Gonzalez, J. S., Peyrot, M., McCarl, L. A., Collins, E. M., Serpa, L., Mimiaga, M. J., et al. (2008). Depression and diabetes treatment nonadherence: A meta-analysis. *Diabetes Care*, 31, 2398–2403.

Gonzalez, R., Nolen-Hoeksema, S., & Treynor, W. (2003). Rumination reconsidered: A psychometric analysis. *Cognitive Therapy and Research*, 27, 247–259.

Goode, A. D., Reeves, M. M., & Eakin, E. G. (2012). Telephone-delivered interventions for physical activity and dietary behavior change: An updated systematic review. *American Journal of Preventive Medicine*, 42, 81–88.

Goodpaster, B. H., Krishnaswami, S., Harris, T. B., Katsiaras, A., Kritchevsky, S. B., Simonsick, E. M., et al. (2005). Obesity, regional body fat distribution, and the metabolic syndrome in older men and women. *Archives of Internal Medicine*, 165, 777–783.

Goodwin, D. G. (1976). *Is alcoholism hereditary?* New York: Oxford University Press.

Goodwin, R. D., & Friedman, H. S. (2006). Health status and the five-factor personality traits in a nationally representative sample. *Journal of Health Psychology*, 11, 643–654.

Gottfredson, L. S., & Deary, I. J. (2004). Intelligence predicts health and longevity, but why? *Current Directions in Psychological Science*, 13, 1–4.

Gouzoulis-Mayfrank, E., & Daumann, J. (2006). The confounding problem of polydrug use in recreational ecstacy/MDMA users: A brief overview. *Journal of Psychopharmacology*, 20, 188–193.

Grafton, K. V., Foster, N. E., & Wright, C. C. (2005). Test- retest reliability of the Short-Form McGill Pain Questionnaire: Assessment of intraclass correlation coefficients and limits of agreement in patients with osteoarthritis. *Clinical Journal of Pain*, 21, 73–82.

Graham, J. E., Christian, L. M., & Kiecolt-Glaser, J. K. (2006). Marriage, health, and immune function. In S. R. H. Beach, M. Z. Wamboldt, N. J. Kaslow, R. E. Heyman, M. B. First, L. G. Underwood, et al. (Eds.), *Relational processes and DSM-V: Neuroscience, assessment, prevention, and treatment* (pp. 61–76). Washington, DC: American Psychiatric Association.

Graham, J. E., Glaser, R., Loving, T. J., Malarkey, W. B., Stowell, J. R., & Kiecolt-Glaser, J. K. (2009). Cognitive word use during marital conflict and increases in proinflammatory cytokines. *Health Psychology*, 28, 621–630.

Graham, K., Bernards, S., Wilsnack, S. C., & Gmel, G. (2011). Alcohol may not cause partner violence but it seems to make it worse: A cross national comparison of the relationship between alcohol and severity of partner violence. *Journal of Interpersonal Violence*, 26(8), 1503–1523.

Graig, E. (1993). Stress as a consequence of the urban physical environment. In L. Goldberger & S. Breznitz (Eds.), *Handbook of stress: Theoretical and clinical aspects* (2nd ed., pp. 316–332). New York: Free Press.

Grant, B. F., Hasin, D. S., Chou, S. P., Stinson, F. S., & Dawson, D. A. (2004). Nicotine dependence and psychiatric disorders in the United States. *Archives of General Psychiatry*, 61, 1107–1115.

Grant, J. A., Courtemanche, J., Duerden, E. G., Duncan, G. H., & Rainville, P. (2010). Cortical thickness and pain sensitivity in Zen Meditators. *Emotion*, 10(1), 43–53.

Greenwood, B. N., Foley, T. E., Day, H. E. W., Burhans, D., Brooks, L., Campeau, S., et al. (2005). Wheel running alters serotonin (5-HT) transporter, 5-HT1A, 5-HT1B, and alpha1b-adrenergic receptor mRNA in the rat raphe nuclei. *Biological Psychiatry*, 57, 559–568.

Griffin, J. A., Umstattd, M. R., & Usdan, S. L. (2010). Alcohol use and high-risk sexual behavior among collegiate women: A review of research on alcohol myopia theory. *Journal of American College Health*, 58(6), 523–532.

Griffing, S., Lewis, C. S., Chu, M., Sage, R. E., Madry, L., & Primm, B. J. (2006). Exposure to interpersonal violence as a predictor of PTSD symptomatology in domestic violence survivors. *Journal of Interpersonal Violence*, 21, 936–954.

Grilo, C. M., Hrabosky, J. I., White, M. A., Allison, K. C., Stunkard, A. J., & Masheb, R. M. (2008). Overvaluation of shape and weight in binge eating disorder and overweight controls: Refinement of a diagnostic construct. *Journal of Abnormal Psychology*, 117, 414–419.

Grogan, S. (2007). *Body image: Understanding body dissatisfaction in men, women, and children* (rev. ed.). New York: Routledge.

Grossman, P., Niemann, L., Schmidt, S., & Walach, H. (2004). Mindfulness-based stress reduction and health benefits: A meta-analysis. *Journal of Psychosomatic Research*, 57, 35–43.

Grover, S. A., Gray-Donald, K., Joseph, L., Abrahamowicz, M., & Coupal, L. (1994). Life expectancy following dietary modification or smoking cessation. *Archives of Internal Medicine*, 154, 1697–1704.

Grundy, S. M. (2007). Cardiovascular and metabolic risk factors: How can we improve outcomes in the high-risk patient? *American Journal of Medicine*, 120(Suppl. 1), S3–S8.

Grundy, S. M., Cleeman, J. I., Bairey Merz, C. N., Brewer, B., Jr., Clark, L. T., Hunninghake, D. B., et al. (2004). Implications of recent clinical trials for the National Cholesterol Education Program Adult Treatment Panel III guidelines. *Circulation*, 110, 227–239.

Grzywacz, J. G., Almeida, D. M., Neupert, S. D., & Ettner, S. L. (2004). Socioeconomic status and health: A micro-level analysis of exposure and vulnerability to daily stressors. *Journal of Health and Social Behavior*, 45, 1–16.

Guck, T. P., Kavan, M. G., Elsasser, G. N., & Barone, E. J. (2001). Assessment and treatment of depression following myocardial infarction. *American Family Physician*, 64, 641–656.

Guevara, J. P., Wolf, F. M., Grum, C. M., & Clark, N. M. (2003). Effects of educational interventions for self management of asthma in children and adolescents: Systematic review and meta-analysis. *British Medical Journal*, 326, 1308–1309.

Guillot, J., Kilpatrick, M., Hebert, E., & Hollander, D. (2004). Applying the transtheoretical model to exercise adherence in clinical settings. *American Journal of Health Studies*, 19, 1–10.

Gull, W. W. (1874). Anorexia nervosa (apepsia hysterica, anorexia hysterica). *Transactions of the Clinical Society of London*, 7, 22–28. [Reprinted in R. M. Kaufman & M. Heiman (Eds.), *Evolution of psychosomatic concepts: Anorexia nervosa, a paradigm*. New York: International University Press, 1964.]

Guo, Q., Johnson, C. A., Unger, J. B., Lee, L., Xie, B., Chou, C.-P., et al. (2007). Utility of the theory of reasoned action and theory of planned behavior for predicting Chinese adolescent smoking. *Addictive Behaviors*, 32, 1066–1081.

Guo, X., Zhou, B., Nishimura, T., Teramukai, S., & Fukushima, M. (2008). Clinical effect of qigong practice on essential hypertension: A meta-analysis of randomized controlled trials. *Journal of Alternative and Complementary Medicine*, 14, 27–37.

Gustafson, E. M., Meadows-Oliver, M., & Banasiak, N. C. (2008). Asthma in childhood. In T. P. Gullotta & G. M. Blau (Eds.), *Handbook of childhood behavioral issues: Evidence-based approaches to prevention and treatment* (pp. 167–186). New York: Routledge/Taylor & Francis.

Gustavsson, P., Jakobsson, R., Nyberg, F., Pershagen, G., Järup, L., & Schéele, P. (2000). Occupational exposure and lung cancer risk: A population-based case-referent study in Sweden. *American Journal of Epidemiology*, 152, 32–40.

Ha, M., Mabuchi, K., Sigurdson, A. J., Freedman, D. M., Linet, M. S., & Doody, M. M. (2007). Smoking cigarettes before first childbirth and risk of breast cancer. *American Journal of Epidemiology*, 166, 55–61.

Haak, T., & Scott, B. (2008). The effect of qigong on fibromyaliga (FMS): A controlled randomized study. *Disability and Rehabilitation*, 30, 625–633.

Haan, M. N., & Wallace, R. (2004). Can dementia be prevented? Brain aging in a population-base. *Annual Review of Public Health*, 25, 1–24.

Haas, M., Spegman, A., Peterson, D., Aickin, M., & Vavrek, D. (2010). Dose response and efficacy of spinal manipulation for chronic cervicogenic headache: A pilot randomized controlled trial. *Spine Journal*, 10(2), 117–128.

Hagedoorn, M., Kujer, R. G., Buuk, B. P., DeJong, G. M., Wobbes, T., & Sanderman, R. (2000). Marital satisfaction in patients with cancer: Does support from intimate partners benefit those who need it the most? *Health Psychology, 19,* 274–282.

Hagger, M. S., Chatzisarantis, N. L., & Biddle, S. J. H. (2002). A meta-analytic review of the theories of reasoned action and planned behavior in physical activity: Predictive validity and the contribution of additional variables. *Journal of Sport and Exercise Psychology, 24,* 3–28.

Hagger, M. S., & Orbell, S. (2003). A meta-analytic review of the common-sense model of illness representations. *Psychology & Health, 18,* 141–184.

Hagimoto, A., Nakamura, M., Morita, T., Masui, S., & Oshima, A. (2010). Smoking cessation patterns and predictors of quitting smoking among the Japanese general population: A 1-year follow-up study. *Addiction, 105*(1), 164–173.

Haimanot, R. T. (2002). Burden of headache in Africa. *Journal of Headache & Pain, 4,* 47–54.

Halberstadt, A. L., & Geyer, M. A. (2011). Multiple receptors contribute to the behavioral effects of indoleamine hallucinogens. *Neuropharmacology, 61*(3), 364–381.

Hale, C. J., Hannum, J. W., & Espelage, D. L. (2005). Social support and physical health: The importance of belonging. *Journal of American College Health, 53,* 276–284.

Hale, S., Grogan, S., & Willott, S. (2007). Patterns of self-referral in men with symptoms of prostate disease. *British Journal of Health Psychology, 12,* 403–419.

Hall, C. B., Verghese, J., Sliwinski, M., Chen, Z., Katz, M., Derby, C., et al. (2005). Dementia incidence may increase more slowly after age 90: Results from the Bronx Aging Study. *Neurology, 65,* 882–886.

Hall, J. A., Blanch-Hartigan, D., & Roter, D. L. (2011). Patients' satisfaction with male versus female physicians: A meta-analysis. *Medical Care, 49,* 611–617.

Hall, M. A., & Schneider, C. E. (2008). Patients as consumers: Courts, contracts, and the new medical marketplace. *Michigan Law Review, 106,* 643–689.

Halpern, P., Moskovich, J., Avrahami, B., Bentur, Y., Soffer, D., & Peleg, K. (2011). Morbidity associated with MDMA (ecstacy) abuse: A survey of emergency department admissions. *Human & Experimental Toxicology, 30*(4), 259–266.

Hamel, L. M., Robbins, L. B., & Wilbur, J. (2011). Computer- and web-based interventions to increase preadolescent and adolescent physical activity: A systematic review. *Journal of Advanced Nursing, 67,* 251–268.

Hamer, M., & Karageorghis, C. (2007). Psychobiological mechanisms of exercise dependence. *Sports Medicine, 37,* 477–485.

Hamer, M., & Steptoe, A. (2007). Association between physical fitness, parasympathetic control, and proinflammatory responses to mental stress. *Psychosomatic Medicine, 69,* 660–666.

Hamer, M., Taylor, A., & Steptoe, A. (2006). The effect of acute aerobic exercise on stress related blood pressure responses: A systematic review and meta-analysis. *Biological Psychology, 71,* 183–190.

Hammond, D. (2005). Smoking behaviour among young adults: Beyond youth prevention. *Tobacco Control, 14,* 181–185.

Hanewinkel, R., & Sargent, J. D. (2007). Exposure to smoking in popular contemporary movies and youth smoking in Germany. *American Journal of Preventive Medicine, 32,* 466–473.

Hanley, M. A., Jensen, M. P., Smith, D. G., Ehde, D. M., Edwards, W. T., & Robinson, L. R. (2007). Preamputation pain and acute pain predict chronic pain after lower extremity amputation. *Journal of Pain, 8,* 102–109.

Hansen, C. J., Stevens, L. C., & Coast, J. R. (2001). Exercise duration and mood state: How much is enough to feel better? *Health Psychology, 20,* 267–275.

Hansen, K., Shriver, T., & Schoeller, D. (2005). The effects of exercise on the storage and oxidation of dietary fat. *Sports Medicine, 35,* 363–373.

Hansen, P. E., Floderus, B., Frederiksen, K., & Johansen, C. B. (2005). Personality traits, health behavior, and risk for cancer: A prospective study of a Swedish twin cohort. *Cancer, 103,* 1082–1091.

Hanson-Turton, T., Ryan, S., Miller, K., Counts, M., & Nash, D. B. (2007). Convenient care clinics: The future of accessible health care. *Disease Management, 10*(2), 61–73.

Hanvik, L. J. (1951). MMPI profiles in patients with low back pain. *Journal of Consulting and Clinical Psychology, 15,* 350–353.

Harakeh, Z., Engels, R. C. M. E., Monshouwer, K., & Hanssen, P. F. (2010). Adolescent's weight concerns and the onset of smoking. *Substance Use & Misuse, 45*(12), 1847–1860.

Harburg, E., Julius, M., Kaciroti, N., Gleiberman, L., & Schork, M. A. (2003). Expressive/suppressive anger-coping responses, gender, and types of mortality: A 17-year follow-up (Tecumseh, Michigan, 1971–1988). *Psychosomatic Medicine, 65,* 588–597.

Harder, B. (2004). Asthma counterattack. *Science News, 166,* 344–345.

Harper, C., & Matsumoto, I. (2005). Ethanol and brain damage. *Current Opinion in Pharmacology, 5,* 73–78.

Harriger, J., Calogero, R., Witherington, D., & Smith, J. (2010). Body size stereotyping and internalization of the thin ideal in preschool girls. *Sex Roles, 63*(9/10), 609–620.

Harrington, A. (2008). *The cure within: A history of mind-body medicine.* New York: Norton.

Harrington, J., Noble, L. M., & Newman, S. P. (2004). Improving patients' communication with doctors: A systematic review of intervention studies. *Patient Education and Counseling, 52,* 7–16.

Harris, M. I. (2001). Racial and ethnic differences in health care access and health outcomes for adults with Type 2 diabetes. *Diabetes Care, 24,* 454–459.

Harrison, B. J., Olver, J. S., Norman, T. R., & Nathan, P. J. (2002). Effects of serotonin and catecholamine depletion on interleukin-6 activation and mood in human volunteers. *Human Psychopharmacology: Clinical and Experimental, 17,* 293–297.

Harter, J. K., & Stone, A. A. (2012). Engaging and disengaging work conditions, momentary experiences and cortisol response. *Motivation and Emotion, 36*(2), 104–113.

Hartz, A., Kent, S., James, P., Xu, Y., Kelly, M., & Daly, J. (2006). Factors that influence improvement for patients with poorly controlled Type 2 diabetes. *Diabetes Research and Clinical Practice, 74,* 227–232.

Hartz, A. J., Rupley, D. C., & Rimm, A. A. (1984). The association of girth measurements with disease in 32,856 women. *American Journal of Epidemiology, 119,* 71–80.

Hasin, D. S., Keyes, K. M., Hatzenbuehler, M. L., Aharonovich, E. A., & Alderson, D. (2007). Alcohol consumption and posttraumatic stress after exposure to terrorism: Effects of proximity, loss, and psychiatric history. *American Journal of Public Health, 97,* 2268–2275.

Hatfield, J., & Job, R. F. S. (2001). Optimism bias about environmental degradation: The role of the range of impact of precautions. *Journal of Environmental Psychology, 21,* 17–30.

Hausenblas, H. A., & Symons Downs, D. (2002a). Exercise dependence: A systematic review. *Psychology of Sport and Exercise, 3,* 89–123.

Hausenblas, H. A., & Symons Downs, D. (2002b). Relationship among sex, imagery, and exercise dependence symptoms. *Psychology of Addictive Behaviors, 16,* 169–172.

Hausenloy, D. J., & Yellon, D. M. (2008). Targeting residual cardiovascular risk: Raising high-density lipoprotein cholesterol levels. *Heart, 94,* 706–714.

Hawkley, L. C., & Cacioppo, J. T. (2003). Loneliness and pathways to disease. *Brain, Behavior and Immunity, 17,* 98–105.

Hawkley, L. C., & Cacioppo, J. T. (2007). Aging and loneliness: Downhill quickly? *Current Directions in Psychological Science, 16,* 187–191.

Hay, P. (2004). Australian and New Zealand clinical practice guidelines for the treatment of anorexia nervosa. *Australian and New Zealand Journal of Psychiatry, 38,* 659–670.

Hay, P. J., & de M. Claudino, A. (2010). Evidence-based treatment for eating disorders. In W. S. Agras (Ed.), *The Oxford handbook of eating disorders* (pp. 452–479). New York: Oxford University Press.

Hayes, S., Bulow, C., Clarke, R., Vega, E., Vega-Perez, E., Ellison, L., et al. (2000). Incidence of low back pain in women who are pregnant. *Physical Therapy, 80,* 34.

Hayes-Bautista, D. E., Hsu, P., Hayes-Bautista, M., Iniguez, D., Chamberlin, C. L., Rico, C., et al. (2002). An anomaly within the Latino epidemiological paradox: The Latino adolescent male mortality peak. *Archives of Pediatrics and Adolescent Medicine, 156,* 480–484.

Haynes, R. B. (1976). Strategies for improving compliance: A methodologic analysis and review. In D. L. Sackett & R. B. Haynes (Eds.), *Compliance with therapeutic regimens* (pp. 69–82). Baltimore, MD: Johns Hopkins University Press.

Haynes, R. B. (1979). Introduction. In R. B. Haynes, D. W. Taylor, & D. L. Sackett (Eds.), *Compliance in health care* (pp. 1–7). Baltimore, MD: Johns Hopkins University Press.

Haynes, R. B. (2001). Improving patient adherence: State of the art, with a special focus on medication taking for cardiovascular disorders. In L. E. Burke & I. S. Ockene (Eds.), *Compliance in healthcare and research* (pp. 3–21). Armonk, NY: Futura.

Haynes, R. B., Ackloo, E., Sahota, N., McDonald, H. P., & Yao, X. (2008). Interventions for enhancing medication adherence. *Cochrane Database of Systematic Reviews,* Cochrane Art. No.: CD000011, DOI: 10.1002/14651858.CD000011.pub3.

Haynes, R. B., McDonald, H. P., & Garg, A. X. (2002). Helping patients follow prescribed treatment: Clinical applications. *Journal of the American Medical Association, 288,* 2880–2883.

He, D. (2005). An introduction to Chinese medical qi gong. *New England Journal of Traditional Chinese Medicine, 4,* 42–44.

HealthGrades. (2011). *Eighth annual patient safety in American hospitals study.* Retrieved November 2, 2011, from http://www.healthgrades.com

Hearn, W. L., Flynn, D. D., Hime, G. W., Rose, S., Cofino, J. C., Mantero-Atienza, E., et al. (1991). Cocaethylene: A unique cocaine metabolite displays high affinity for the dopamine transporter. *Journal of Neurochemistry, 56,* 698–701.

Heather, N. (2006). Controlled drinking, harm reduction and their roles in the response to alcohol-related problems. *Addiction Research and Theory, 14,* 7–18.

Heckman, C. J., Egleston, B. L., & Hofmann, M. T. (2010). Efficacy of motivational interviewing for smoking cessation: A systematic review and meta-analysis. *Tobacco Control: An International Journal, 19*(5), 410–416.

Heijmans, M., Rijken, M., Foets, M., de Ridder, D., Schreurs, K., & Bensing, J. (2004). The stress of being chronically ill: From disease-specific to task-specific aspects. *Journal of Behavioral Medicine, 27,* 255–271.

Heimer, R. (2008). Community coverage and HIV prevention: Assessing metrics for estimating HIV incidence through syringe exchange. *International Journal of Drug Policy, 19*(Suppl. 1), S65–S73.

Heinrich, K. M., Lee, R. E., Regan, G. R., Reese-Smith, J. Y., Howard, H. H., Haddock, C. K., et al. (2008). How does the built environment relate to body mass index and obesity prevalence among public housing residents? *American Journal of Health Promotion, 22,* 187–194.

Heir, T., Erikssen, J., & Sandvik, L. (2011). Overweight as predictor of long-term mortality among healthy, middle-aged men: A prospective cohort study. *Preventive Medicine, 52*(3/4), 223–226.

Held, C., Iqbal, R., Lear, S. A., Rosengren, A., Islam, S., Mathew, J., et al. (2012). Physical activity levels, ownership of goods promoting sedentary behavior and risk of myocardial infarction: Results of the INTERHEART study. *European Heart Journal, 33,* 452–466.

Helgeson, V. S. (2003). Cognitive adaptation, psychological adjustment, and disease progression among angioplasty patients: 4 years later. *Health Psychology, 22,* 30–38.

Helgeson, V. S., Cohen, S., Schulz, R., & Yasko, J. (2000). Group support interventions for women with breast cancer: Who benefits from what? *Health Psychology, 19,* 107–114.

Helgeson, V. S., Reynolds, K. A., Tomich, P. L. (2006). A meta-analytic review of benefit finding and growth. *Journal of Consulting and Clinical Psychology, 74,* 797–816.

Helgeson, V. S., Snyder, P., & Seltman, H. (2004). Psychological and physical adjustment of breast cancer over 4 years: Identifying distinct trajectories of change. *Health Psychology, 23,* 3–15.

Helweg-Larsen, M., & Nielsen, G. (2009). Smoking cross-culturally: Risk perceptions among young adults in Denmark and the United States. *Psychology and Health, 24,* 81–93.

Hembree, E. A., & Foa, E. B. (2003). Interventions for trauma-related emotional disturbances in adult victims of crime. *Journal of Traumatic Stress, 16,* 187–199.

Hemminki, K., Försti, A., & Bermejo, J. L. (2006). Gene-environment interactions in cancer. *Annals of the New York Academy of Science, 1076,* 137–148.

Henderson, L. A., Gandevia, S. C., & Macefield, V. G. (2008). Gender differences in brain activity evoked by muscle and cutaneous pain: A retrospective study of singe-trial fMRI data. *NeuroImage, 39,* 1867–1876.

Hendriks, H. F. J. (2007). Moderate alcohol consumption and insulin sensitivity: Observations and possible mechanisms. *Annals of Epidemiology, 17*(5 Suppl.), S40–S42.

Heneghan, C. J., Glasziou, P., & Perera, R. (2007). Reminder packaging for improving adherence to self-administered long-term medications. *Cochrane Database of Systematic Reviews,* Cochrane Art. No.: CD005025, DOI: 10.1002/14651858.CD005025.pub2.

Henke-Gendo, C., & Schulz, T. F. (2004). Transmission and disease association of Kaposi's sarcoma–associated herpes virus: Recent developments. *Current Opinion in Infectious Diseases, 17,* 53–57.

Henley, S. J., Thun, M. J., Chao, A., & Calle, E. E. (2004). Association between exclusive pipe smoking and mortality from cancer and other diseases. *Journal of the National Cancer Institute, 96,* 853–861.

Henriksen, L., Schleicher, N. C., Feighery, E. C., & Fortmann, S. P. (2010). A longitudinal study of exposure to retail cigarette advertising and smoking initiation. *Pediatrics, 126*(2), 232–238.

Henschke, N., Ostelo, R. W. J. G., van Tulder, M. W., Vlaeyen, J. W. S., Morley, S., Assendelft, W. J. J., et al. (2010). Behavioural treatment for chronic low-back pain. *Cochrane Database of Systematic Reviews,* Cochrane Art. No.: CD002014, DOI: 10.1002/14651858.CD002014. pub3.

Henson, J. M., Carey, M. P., Carey, K. B., & Maisto, S. A. (2006). Associations among health behaviors and time perspective in young adults: Model testing with boot-strapping replication. *Journal of Behavioral Medicine, 29,* 127–137.

Herbst, A., Kordonouri, O., Schwab, K. O., Schmidt, F., & Holl, R. W. (2007). Impact of physical activity on cardiovascular risk factors in children with Type 1 diabetes. *Diabetes Care, 30,* 2098–2100.

Herd, N., Borland, R., & Hyland, A. (2009). Predictors of smoking relapse by duration of abstinence: Findings from the International Tobacco Control (ITC) Four Country Survey. *Addiction, 104*(12), 2088–2099.

Herman, C. P., & Polivy, J. (2005). Normative influences on food intake. *Physiology and Behavior, 86,* 762–772.

Herman, C. P., van Strien, T., & Polivy, J. (2008). Undereating or eliminating overeating? *American Psychologist, 63,* 202–203.

Hernán, M. A., Jick, S. S., Logroscino, G., Olek, M. J., Ascherio, A., & Jick, H. (2005). Cigarette smoking and the progression of multiple sclerosis. *Brain, 128*(Pt. 6), 1461–1465.

Herring, M. P., O'Connor, P. J., & Dishman, R. K. (2010). The effect of exercise training on anxiety symptoms among patients: A systematic review. *Archives of Internal Medicine, 170,* 321–331.

Herrmann, S., McKinnon, E., John, M., Hyland, N., Martinez, O. P., Cain, A., et al. (2008). Evidence-based, multifactorial approach to addressing non-adherence to antiretroviral therapy and improving standards of care. *Internal Medicine Journal, 38,* 8–15.

Herzog, T. (2008). Analyzing the transtheoretical model using the framework of Weinstein, Rothman, and Sutton (1998). The example of smoking cessation. *Health Psychology, 27,* 548–556.

Hession, M., Rolland, C., Kulkarni, U., Wise, A., & Broom, J. (2009). Systematic review of randomized controlled trials of low-carbohydrate vs. low fat/low calorie diets in the management of obesity and its comorbidities. *Obesity Reviews, 10*(1), 36–50.

Hester, R. K., Delaney, H. D., & Campbell, W. (2011). ModerateDrinking. com and moderation management: Outcomes of a randomized clinical trial with non-dependent problems drinkers. *Journal of Consulting & Clinical Psychology, 79*(2), 215–224.

Hilbert, A., Pike, K. M., Wilfley, D. E., Fairburn, C. G., Dohm, F.-A., & Striegel-Moore, R. H. (2011). Clarifying boundaries of binge eating disorder and psychiatric comorbidity: A latent structure analysis. *Behaviour Research & Therapy, 49*(3), 202–211.

Hilgard, E. R. (1978). Hypnosis and pain. In R. A. Sternbach (Ed.), *The psychology of pain* (p. 219). New York: Raven Press.

Hilgard, E. R., & Hilgard, J. R. (1994). *Hypnosis in the relief of pain* (rev. ed.). Los Altos, CA: Kaufmann.

Hill, J. O., & Wyatt, H. R. (2005). Role of physical activity in preventing and treating obesity. *Journal of Applied Physiology, 99*, 765–770.

Hill, P. L., & Roberts, B. W. (2011). The role of adherence in the relationship between conscientiousness and perceived health. *Health Psychology, 30*, 797–804.

Himmelstein, D. U., Thorne, D., Warren, E., & Woolhandler, S. (2009). Medical bankruptcy in the United States, 2007: Results of a national study. *The American Journal of Medicine, 122*, 741–746.

Hind, K., & Burrows, M. (2007). Weight-bearing exercise and bone mineral accrual in children and adolescents: A review of controlled trials. *Bone, 40*, 14–27.

Hingson, R., Heeren, T., Winter, M., & Wechsler, H. (2005). Magnitude of alcohol-related mortality and morbidity among U.S. college students ages 18–24: Changes from 1998 to 2001. *Annual Review of Public Health, 26*, 259–279.

Hochbaum, G. (1958). *Public participation in medical screening programs* (DHEW Publication No. 572, Public Health Service). Washington, DC: U.S. Government Printing Office.

Hodgins, D. (2005). Can patients with alcohol use disorders return to social drinking? Yes, so what should we do about it? *Canadian Journal of Psychiatry, 50*(5), 264–265.

Hoey, L. M., Ieropoli, S. C., White, V. M., & Jefford, M. (2008). Systematic review of peer-support programs for people with cancer. *Patient Education and Counseling, 70*, 315–337.

Hoeymans, N., van Lindert, H., & Westert, G. P. (2005). The health status of the Dutch population as assessed by the EQ-6D. *Quality of Life Research, 14*, 655–643.

Hoffman, B. M., Papas, R. K., Chatkoff, D. K., & Kerns, R. D. (2007). Meta-analysis of psychological interventions for chronic low back pain. *Health Psychology, 26*, 1–9.

Hogan, B. E., & Linden, W. (2004). Anger responses styles and blood pressure: At least don't ruminate about it! *Annals of Behavioral Medicine, 27*, 38–49.

Hogan, E. M., & McReynolds, C. J. (2004). An overview of anorexia nervosa, bulimia nervosa, and binge eating disorders: Implications for rehabilitation professionals. *Journal of Applied Rehabilitation Counseling, 35*(4), 26–34.

Hogan, N. S., & Schmidt, L. A. (2002). Testing the grief to personal growth model using structural equation modeling. *Death Studies, 26*, 615–634.

Holahan, C. J., Schutte, K. K., Brennan, P. L., Holahan, C. K., Moos, B. S., & Moos, R. H. (2010). Late-life alcohol consumption and 20-year mortality. *Alcoholism: Clinical & Experimental Reserch, 34*(11), 1061–1071.

Holden, C. (2003, September 8). Party drug paper pulled. *Science Now*, 1–2.

Holick, M. F. (2004). Sunlight and vitamin D for bone health and prevention of autoimmune disease, cancers, and cardiovascular disease. *American Journal of Clinical Nutrition, 80*(Suppl. 6), S1678–S1688.

Hollis, J. F., Gullion, C. M., Stevens, V. J., Brantley, P. J., Appel, L. J., Ard, J. D., et al. (2008). Weight loss during the intensive intervention phase of the weight-loss maintenance trial. *American Journal of Preventive Medicine, 35*, 118–126.

Holman, E. A., Silver, R. C., Poulin, M., Andersen, J., Gil-Rivas, V., & McIntosh, D. N. (2008). Terrorism, acute stress, and cardiovascular health: A 3-year national study following the September 11th attacks. *Archives of General Psychiatry, 65*, 73–80.

Holmes, T. H., & Rahe, R. H. (1967). The Social Readjustment Rating Scale. *Journal of Psychosomatic Research, 11*, 213–218.

Holsti, L., & Grunau, R. E. (2007). Initial validation of the Behavioral Indicators of Infant Pain (BIIP). *Pain, 132*, 264–272.

Holt-Lunstad, J., Birmingham, W., & Jones, B. Q. (2008). Is there something unique about marriage? The relative impact of marital status, relationship quality, and network social support on ambulatory blood pressure and mental health. *Annals of Behavioral Medicine, 35*, 239–244.

Holtzman, D., Bland, S. D., Lansky, A., & Mack, K. A. (2001). HIV-related behaviors and perceptions among adults in 25 states: 1997 Behavioral Risk Factor Surveillance System. *American Journal of Public Health, 91*, 1882–1888.

Hölzel, B. K., Carmody, J., Vangel, M., Congleton, C., Yerramsetti, S. M., Gard, T., et al. (2011). Mindfulness practice leads to increases in regional brain gray matter density. *Psychiatry Research: Neuroimaging, 191*(1), 36–43.

Hootman, J. M., Macera, C. A., Ainsworth, B. E., Addy, C. L., Martin, M., & Blair, S. N. (2002). Epidemiology of musculoskeletal injuries among sedentary and physically active adults. *Medicine and Science in Sports and Exercise, 34*, 838–844.

Horne, R., Buick, D., Fisher, M., Leake, H., Cooper, V., & Weinman, J. (2004). Doubts about necessity and concerns about adverse effects: Identifying the types of beliefs that are associated with non-adherence to HAART. *International Journal of STD and AIDS, 15*, 38–44.

Horowitz, S. (2010). Health benefits of meditation: What the newest research shows. *Alternative and Complementary Therapies, 16*(4), 223–228.

Houts, P. S., Doak, C. C., Doak, L. G., & Loscalzo, M. J. (2006). The role of pictures in improving health communication: A review of research on attention, comprehension, recall, and adherence. *Patient Education and Counseling, 61*, 173–190.

Howe, G. W., Levy, M. L., & Caplan, R. D. (2004). Job loss and depressive symptoms in couples: Common stressors, stress transmission, or relationship disruption? *Journal of Family Psychology, 18*, 639–650.

Hróbjartsson, A., & Gøtzsche, P. C. (2001). An analysis of clinical trials comparing placebo with no treatment. *New England Journal of Medicine, 344*, 1594–1602.

Hróbjartsson, A., & Gøtzsche, P. C. (2004). Is the placebo powerless? Update of a systematic review with 52 new randomized trials comparing placebo with no treatment. *Journal of Internal Medicine, 256*, 91–100.

Hróbjartsson, A., & Gøtzsche, P. C. (2010). Placebo interventions for all clinical conditions. *The Cochrane Database of Systematic Reviews*, Cochrane Art. No.: CD003974, DOI: 10.1002/14651858.CD003974.pub3.

Hsiao, A.-F., Ryan, G. W., Hays, R. D., Coulter, I. D., Andersen, R. M., & Wenger, N. S. (2006). Variations in provider conceptions of integrative medicine. *Social Science and Medicine, 62*, 2973–2987.

Hsiao, A.-F., Wong, M. D., Goldstein, M. S., Becerra, L. S., Cheng, E. M., & Wenger, N. S. (2006). Complementary and alternative medicine use among Asian-American subgroups: Prevalence, predictors, and lack of relationship to acculturation and access to conventional health care. *Journal of Alternative and Complementary Medicine, 12*, 1003–1010.

Hsu, C., BlueSpruce, J., Sherman, K., & Cherkin, D. (2010). Unanticipated benefits of CAM therapies for back pain: An exploration of patient experiences. *Journal of Alternative & Complementary Medicine, 16*(2), 157–163.

Hu, B., Li, W., Wang, X., Liu, L., Teo, K., & Yusuf, S. (2012). Marital status, education, and risk of acute myocardial infarction in mainland China: The INTERHEART study. *Journal of Epidemiology, 22*, 123–129.

Hu, F. B. (2003). Overweight and obesity in women: Health risks and consequences. *Journal of Women's Health, 12*, 163–172.

Hu, F. B., Stampfer, M. J., Colditz, G. A., Ascherio, A., Rexrode, K. M., Willett, W. C., et al. (2000). Physical activity and risk of stroke in women. *Journal of the American Medical Association, 283,* 7961–7967.

Huang, J.-Q., Sridhar, S., & Hunt, R. H. (2002). Role of *Helicobacter pylori* infection and non-steroidal anti-inflammatory drugs in peptic-ulcer disease: A meta-analysis. *Lancet, 359,* 14–21.

Hudson, J. I., Hiripi, E., Pope, H. G., Jr., & Kessler, R. C. (2007). The prevalence and correlates of eating disorders in the National Comorbidity Survey replication. *Biological Psychiatry, 61,* 348–358.

Huebner, D. M., & Davis, M. C. (2007). Perceived antigay discrimination and physical health outcomes. *Health Psychology, 26,* 627–634.

Huebner, R. B., & Kantor, L. W. (2011). Advances in alcoholism treatment. *Alcohol Research & Health, 33*(4), 295–299.

Hufford, D. J. (2003). Evaluating complementary and alternative medicine: The limits of science and of scientists. *Journal of Law, Medicine and Ethics, 31,* 198–212.

Hughes, J. (1975). Isolation of an endogenous compound from the brain with pharmacological properties similar to morphine. *Brain Research, 88,* 295–308.

Hughes, J. (2003). Motivating and helping smokers to stop smoking. *Journal of General Internal Medicine, 18,* 1053–1057.

Hughes, J., Gulliver, S. B., Fenwick, J. W., Valliere, W. A., Cruser, K., Pepper, S., et al. (1992). Smoking cessation among self-quitters. *Health Psychology, 11,* 331–334.

Hughes, J. R. (2009). How confident should we be that smoking cessation treatments work? *Addiction, 104*(10), 1637–1640.

Hulme, C., Wright, J., Crocker, T., Oluboyede, Y., & House, A. (2010). Non-pharmacological approaches for dementia that informal carers might try or access: A systematic review. *International Journal of Geriatric Psychiatry, 25,* 756–763.

Humane Society of the United States. (2011). *U.S. pet ownership statistics.* Retrieved August 31, 2012, from http://www.humanesociety.org/issues/pet_overpopulation/facts/pet_ownership_statistics.html

Humphrey, L. L., Fu, R., Buckley, D. I., Freeman, M., & Helfand, M. J. (2008). Periodontal disease and coronary heart disease incidence: A systematic review and meta-analysis. *Journal of General Internal Medicine, 23,* 2079–2020.

Humphreys, K., & Moos, R. H. (2007). Encouraging posttreatment self-help group involvement to reduce demand for continuing care services: Two-year clinical and utilization outcomes. *Alcoholism: Clinical and Experimental Research, 31,* 64–68.

Hunt, W. A., Barnett, L. W., & Branch, L. G. (1971). Relapse rates in addiction programs. *Journal of Clinical Psychology, 27,* 455–456.

Huq, F. (2007). Molecular modeling analysis of the metabolism of cocaine. *Journal of Pharmacology and Toxicology, 2,* 114–130.

Hurley, S. F., & Matthews, J. P. (2007). The quit benefits model: A Markov model for assessing the health benefits and health care cost savings of quitting smoking. *Cost Effectiveness & Resource Allocation, 5,* 2–20.

Hutchinson, A. B., Branson, B. M., Kim, A., & Farnham, P. G. (2006). A meta-analysis of the effectiveness of alternative HIV counseling and testing methods to increase knowledge of HIV status. *AIDS, 20,* 1597–1604.

Huth, M. M., Broome, M. E., & Good, M. (2004). Imagery reduces children's post-operative pain, *Pain, 110,* 439–448.

Huxley, R., Ansary-Moghaddam, A., de González, A. B., Barzi, F., & Woodward, M. (2005). Type-II diabetes and pancreatic cancer: A meta-analysis of 36 studies. *British Journal of Cancer, 92,* 2076–2083.

Huxley, R. R., & Neil, H. A. W. (2003). The relation between dietary flavonol intake and coronary heart disease mortality: A meta-analysis of prospective cohort studies. *Journal of Clinical Nutrition, 57,* 904–908.

Hvidtfeldt, U. A., Tolstrup, J. S., Jakobsen, M. U., Heitmann, B. L., Grønbaek, M., O'Reilly, E., et al. (2010). Alcohol intake and risk of coronary heart disease in younger, middle-aged, and older adults. *Circulation, 121*(14), 1589–1597.

Iagnocco, A., Perella, C., Naredo, E., Meenagh, G., Ceccarelli, F., Tripodo, E., et al. (2008). Etanercept in the treatment of rheumatoid arthritis: Clinical follow-up over one year by ultrasonography. *Clinical Rheumatology, 27,* 491–496.

Iannotti, R. J., Schneider, S., Nansel, T. R., Haynie, D. L., Plotnick, L. P., Clark, L. M., et al. (2006). Self-efficacy, outcome expectations, and diabetes self-management in adolescents with Type 1 diabetes. *Journal of Developmental and Behavioral Pediatrics, 27,* 98–105.

Ickovics, J. R., Milan, S., Boland, R., Schoenbaum, E., Schuman, P., Vlahov, D. (2006). Psychological resources protect health: 5-year survival and immune function among HIV-infected women from four US cities. *AIDS, 20,* 1851–1860.

Iglesias, S. L., Azzara, S., Squillace, M., Jeifetz, M., Lores Arnais, M. R., Desimone, M. F., et al. (2005). A study on the effectiveness of a stress management programme for college students. *Pharmacy Education, 5,* 27–31.

Ijadunola, K. T., Abiona, T. C., Odu, O. O., & Ijadunola, M. Y. (2007). College students in Nigeria underestimate their risk of contacting HIV/AIDS infection. *European Journal of Contraception and Reproductive Health Care, 12,* 131–137.

Ilies, R., Schwind, K. M., Wagner, D. T., Johnson, M. D., DeRue, D. S., & Ilgen, D. R. (2007). When can employees have a family life? The effects of daily workload and affect on work-family conflict and social behaviors at home. *Journal of Applied Psychology, 92,* 1368–1379.

Imes, R. S., Bylund, C. L., Sabee, C. M., Routsong, T. R., & Sanford, A. A. (2008). Patients' reasons for refraining from discussing Internet health information with their healthcare providers. *Health Communication, 23,* 538–547.

Ingersoll, K. S., & Cohen, J. (2008). The impact of medication regimen factors on adherence to chronic treatment: A review of the literature. *Journal of Behavioral Medicine, 31,* 213–224.

Ingraham, B. A., Bragdon, B., & Nohe, A. (2008). Molecular basis for the potential of vitamin D to prevent cancer. *Current Medical Research and Opinion, 24,* 139–149.

Innes, K. E., & Vincent, H. K. (2007). The influence of yoga-based programs on risk profiles in adults with Type 2 diabetes mellitus: A systematic review. *Evidence Based Complementary and Alternative Medicine, 4,* 469–486.

Institute of Medicine (IOM). (2002). *Unequal treatment: Confronting racial and ethnic disparities in health care.* Washington, DC: Author.

Institute of Medicine (IOM) (2010). *Value in health care: Accounting for cost, quality, safety, outcomes, and innovations: Workshop summary.* Washington, DC: Author.

Institute of Medicine (IOM). (2011). *Relieving pain in America: A blueprint for transforming prevention, care, education, and research.* Washington, DC: Author.

Institute of Medicine (IOM). (2012). *Front-of-package nutrition rating systems and symbols: Promoting healthier choices.* Washington, DC: Author.

International Agency for Research on Cancer Working Group on artificial ultraviolet (UV) light and skin cancer (IARC). (2007). The association of use of sunbeds with cutaneous malignant melanoma and other skin cancers: A systematic review. *International Journal of Cancer, 120,* 1116–1122.

International Association for the Study of Pain (IASP), Subcommittee on Taxonomy. (1979). Pain terms: A list with definitions and notes on usage. *Pain, 6,* 249–252.

Iqbal, R., Anand, S., Ounpuu, S., Islam, S., Zhang, X., Rangarajan, S., et al. (2008). Dietary patterns and the risk of acute myocardial infarction in 52 countries: Results of the INTERHEART study. *Circulation, 118,* 1929–1937.

Iribarren, C., Darbinian, J. A., Lo, J. C., Fireman, B. H., & Go, A. S. (2006). Value of the sagittal abdominal diameter in coronary heart disease risk assessment: Cohort study in a large, multiethnic population. *American Journal of Epidemiology, 164,* 1150–1159.

Iribarren, C., Sidney, S., Bild, D. E., Liu, K., Markovitz, J. H., Roseman, J. M., et al. (2000). Association of hostility with coronary artery calcification in young adults. *Journal of the American Medical Association, 283,* 2546–2551.

Ironson, G., Weiss, S., Lydston, D., Ishii, M., Jones, D., Asthana, D., et al. (2005). The impact of improved self-efficacy on HIV viral load and distress in culturally diverse women living with AIDS: The SMART/EST women's project. *AIDS Care, 17*, 222–236.

Irwin, D. E., Milsom, I., Kopp, Z., Abrams, P., & EPIC Study Group. (2008). Symptom bother and health care-seeking behavior among individuals with overactive bladder. *European Urology, 53*, 1029–1039.

Irwin, M. R. (2008). Human psychoneuroimmunology: 20 years of discovery. *Brain, Behavior and Immunity, 22*, 129–139.

Irwin, M. R., Pike, J. L., Cole, J. C., & Oxman, M. N. (2003). Effects of a behavioral intervention, tai chi chih, on varicella-zoster virus specific immunity and health functioning in older adults. *Psychosomatic Medicine, 65*, 824–830.

Isaacson, W. (2011). *Steve Jobs.* New York: Simon & Schuster.

Islam, T., Gauderman, W. J., Berhane, K., McConnell, R., Avol, E., Peters, J. M., et al. (2007). Relationship between air pollution, lung function and asthma in adolescents. *Thorax, 62*, 957–963.

Iso, H., Rexrode, K. M., Stampfer, M. J., Manson, J. E., Colditz, G. A., Speizer, F. E., et al. (2001). Intake of fish and omega-3 fatty acids and risk of stroke in women. *Journal of the American Medical Association, 285*, 304–312.

Ito, T., Takenaka, K., Tomita, T., & Agari, I. (2006). Comparison of ruminative responses with negative rumination as a vulnerability factor for depression. *Psychological Reports, 99*, 763–772.

Ivanovski, B., & Malhi, G. S. (2007). The psychological and neurophysiological concomitants of mindfulness forms of meditation. *Acta Neuropsychiatrica, 19*(2), 76–91.

Iwamoto, D. K., Cheng, A., Lee, C. S., Takamatsu, S., & Gordon, D. (2011). "Man-ing" up and getting drunk: The role of masculine norms, alcohol intoxication and alcohol-related problems among college men. *Addictive Behaviors, 36*(9), 906–911.

Jackson, G. (2004). Treatment of erectile dysfunction in patients with cardiovascular disease: Guide to drug selection. *Drugs, 64*, 1533–1545.

Jackson, K. M., Sher, K. J., Gotham, H. J., & Wood, P. K. (2001). Transitioning into and out of large-effect drinking in young adulthood. *Journal of Abnormal Psychology, 110*, 378–391.

Jacobs, G. D. (2001). Clinical applications of the relaxation response and mind-body interventions. *Journal of Alternative and Complementary Medicine, 7*(Suppl. 1), 93–101.

Jacobson, E. (1938). *Progressive relaxation: A physiological and clinical investigation of muscle states and their significance in psychology and medical practice* (2nd ed.). Chicago, IL: University of Chicago Press.

Jager, R. D., Mieler, W. F., & Miller, J. W. (2008). Age-related macular degeneration. *New England Journal of Medicine, 358*, 2606–2617.

Jagger, C., Gillies, C., Moscone, F., Cambois, E., Van Oyen, H., Nusselder, W., et al. (2009). Inequalities in healthy life years in the 25 countries of the European Union in 2005: A cross-national meta-regression analysis. *The Lancet, 372*, 2124–2131.

Jahnke, R., Larkey, L., Rogers, C., & Etnier, J. (2010). A comprehensive review of health benefits of qigong and tai chi. *American Journal of Health Promotion, 24*(6), e1–e25.

Jakicic, J. M., & Otto, A. D. (2005). Physical activity considerations for the treatment and prevention of obesity. *American Journal of Clinical Nutrition, 82*(Suppl. 1), 226S–229S.

James, A. (2010, March 19). Kirstie Alley: Industry called me fat at 114 pounds. *HuffPost Celebrity.* Retrieved July 18, 2011, from http://www.popeater.com/2010/03/19/kirstie-alleys-big-life/

James, W. P. T. (2008). The epidemiology of obesity: The size of the problem. *Journal of Internal Medicine, 263*, 336–352.

Janssen, R. S., Onorato, I. M., Valdiserri, R. O., Durham, T. M., Nichols, W. P., Seiler, E. M., et al. (2003). Advancing HIV prevention: New strategies for a changing epidemic—United States, 2003. *Morbidity and Mortality Weekly Report, 52*, 329–332.

Janssen, S. A. (2002). Negative affect and sensitization to pain. *Scandinavian Journal of Psychology, 43*, 131–137.

Jay, S. M., Elliott, C. H., Woody, P. D., & Siegel, S. (1991). An investigation of cognitive-behavior therapy combined with oral valium for children undergoing painful medical procedures. *Health Psychology, 10*, 317–322.

Jeffery, R. W., & Harnack, L. J. (2007). Evidence implicating eating as a primary driver for the obesity epidemic. *Diabetes, 56*, 2673–2676.

Jeffery, R. W., Kelly, K. M., Rothman, A. J., Sherwood, N. E., & Boutelle, K. N. (2004). The weight loss experience: A descriptive analysis. *Annals of Behavioral Medicine, 27*, 100–106.

Jellinek, E. M. (1960). *The disease concept of alcoholism.* New Haven, CT: College and University Press.

Jenkins, S., & Armstrong, L. (2001). *It's not about the bike: My journey back to life.* New York: Penguin Books.

Jenks, R. A., & Higgs, S. (2007). Associations between dieting and smoking-related behaviors in young women. *Drug and Alcohol Dependence, 88*, 291–299.

Jensen, M. P., & Karoly, P. (2001). Self-report scales and procedures for assessing pain in adults. In D. C. Turk & R. Melzack (Eds.), *Handbook of pain assessment* (2nd ed., pp. 15–34). New York: Guilford Press.

Jeon, C. Y., Lokken, R. P., Hu, F. B., & van Dam, R. M. (2007). Physical activity of moderate intensity and risk of Type 2 diabetes: A systematic review. *Diabetes Care, 30*, 744–752.

Jha, A. P., Krompinger, J., & Baime, M. J. (2007). Mindfulness training modifies subsystems of attention. *Cognitive, Affective and Behavioral Neuroscience, 7*, 109–119.

John, U., Meyer, C., Rumpf, H.-J., Hapke, U., & Schumann, A. (2006). Predictors of increased body mass index following cessation of smoking. *American Journal of Addictions, 15*, 192–197.

Johnson, A., Sandford, J., & Tyndall, J. (2007). Written and verbal information versus verbal information only for patients being discharged from acute hospital settings to home. *Cochrane Database of Systematic Reviews*, Cochrane Art. No.: CD003716, DOI: 10.1002/14651858.CD003716.

Johnson, J. L., Eaton, D. K., Pederson, L. L., & Lowry, R. (2009). Associations of trying to lose weight, weight control behaviors, and current cigarette use among US high school students. *Journal of School Health, 79*(8), 355–360.

Johnson, J. L., Slentz, C. A., Houmard, J. A., Samsa, G. P., Duscha, B. D., Aiken, L. B., et al. (2007). Exercise training amount and intensity effects on metabolic syndrome (from Studies of a Targeted Risk Reduction Intervention through Defined Exercise). *American Journal of Cardiology, 100*, 1759–1766.

Johnson, L. W., & Weinstock, R. S. (2006). The metabolic syndrome: Concepts and controversy. *Mayo Clinic Proceedings, 81*, 1615–1621.

Johnson, M. I. (2006). The clinical effectiveness of acupuncture for pain relief—You can be certain of uncertainty. *Acupuncture in Medicine, 24*, 71–79.

Johnson, S. S., Driskell, M.-M., Johnson, J. L., Dyment, S. J., Prochaska, J. O., Prochaska, J. M., et al. (2006). Transtheoretical model intervention for adherence to lipid-lowering drugs. *Disease Management, 9*, 102–114.

Johnston, L. D., O'Malley, P. M., Bachman, J. G., & Schulenberg, J. E. (2007). *Monitoring the Future: National survey results on drug use, 1975–2006: Vol. 2. College students and adults ages 19–45* (NIH Publication No. 07-6206). Bethesda, MD: National Institute on Drug Abuse.

Johnston, L. D., O'Malley, P. M., Bachman, J. G., & Schulenberg, J. E. (2011). *Monitoring the Future national survey results on drug use, 1975–2010. Volume I: Secondary school students.* Ann Arbor, MI: Institute for Social Research, The University of Michigan.

Jolliffe, C. D., & Nicholas, M. K. (2004). Verbally reinforcing pain reports: An experimental test of the operant model of chronic pain. *Pain, 107*, 167–175.

Jones, D. W., Chambless, L. E., Folsom, A. R., Heiss, G., Hutchinson, R. G., Sharrett, A. R., et al. (2002). Risk factors for coronary heart disease in African Americans: The Atherosclerosis Risk in Communities Study, 1987–1997. *Archives of Internal Medicine, 162*, 2565–2571.

Jones, W. R., & Morgan, J. F. (2010). Eating disorders in men: A review of the literature. *Journal of Public Mental Health, 9*(2), 23–31.

Jorgensen, R. S., & Kolodziej, M. E. (2007). Suppressed anger, evaluative threat, and cardiovascular reactivity: A tripartite profile approach. *International Journal of Psychophysiology, 66*, 102–108.

Juliano, L. M., & Griffiths, R. R. (2004). A critical review of caffeine withdrawal: Empirical validation of symptoms and signs, incidence, severity, and associated features. *Psychopharmacology, 176*, 1–29.

Julien, R. M., Advokat, C., & Comaty, J. E. (2010). *A primer of drug action* (12th ed.). New York: Worth.

Juster, R. P., McEwen, B. S., & Lupien, S. J. (2010). Allostatic load biomarkers of chronic stress and impact on health and cognition. *Neuroscience & Biobehavioral Reviews, 35*, 2–16.

Ju Wang, & Li, Ming D. (2010). Common and unique biological pathways associated with smoking initiation/progression, nicotine dependence, and smoking cessation. *Neuropsychopharmacology, 35*(3), 702–719.

Kabat-Zinn, J. (1993). Mindfulness meditation: Health benefits of an ancient Buddhist practice. In D. Goleman & J. Gurin (Eds.), *Mind/body medicine: How to use your mind for better health* (pp. 259–275). Yonkers, NY: Consumer Reports Books.

Kahende, J. W., Woollery, T. A., & Lee, C.-W. (2007). Assessing medical expenditures on 4 smoking-related diseases, 1996–2001. *American Journal of Health Behavior, 31*, 602–611.

Kahn, E. B., Ramsey, L. T., Brownson, R. C., Heath, G. W., Howze, E. H., Powell, K. E., et al. (2002). The effectiveness of interventions to increase physical activity: A systematic review. *American Journal of Preventive Medicine, 22*, 73–107.

Kahn, H. A. (1963). The relationship of reported coronary heart disease mortality to physical activity of work. *American Journal of Public Health, 53*, 1058–1067.

Kaholokula, J. K., Saito, E., Mau, M. K., Latimer, R., & Seto, T. B. (2008). Pacific Islanders' perspectives on heart failure management. *Patient Education and Counseling, 70*, 281–291.

Kalant, H. (2004). Adverse effects of cannabis on health: An update of the literature since 1996. *Progress in Neuro-Psychopharmacology and Biological Psychiatry, 28*, 849–863.

Kalichman, S. C., Eaton, L., Cain, D., Cherry, C., Fuhrel, A., Kaufman, M., et al. (2007). Changes in HIV treatment beliefs and sexual risk behaviors among gay and bisexual men, 1997–2005. *Health Psychology, 26*, 650–656.

Kamarck, T. W., Muldoon, M. F., Shiffman, S. S., & Sutton-Tyrrell, K. (2007). Experiences of demand and control during daily life are predictors of carotid atherosclerotic progression among healthy men. *Health Psychology, 26*, 324–332.

Kambouropoulos, N. (2003). The validity of the tension-reduction hypothesis in alcohol cue-reactivity research. *Australian Journal of Psychology, 55*(S1), 6.

Kamer, A. R., Craig, R. G., Dasanayke, A. P., Brys, M., Glodzik-Sobanska, L., & de Leon, M. J. (2008). Inflammation and Alzheimer's disease: Possible role of periodontal diseases. *Alzheimer's and Dementia, 4*, 242–250.

Kamiya, J. (1969). Operant control of the EEG alpha rhythm and some of its reported effects on consciousness. In C. Tart (Ed.), *Altered states of consciousness* (pp. 519–529). New York: Wiley.

Kaner, E. F. S., Beyer, F., Dickinson, H. O., Pienaar, E., Campbell, F., Schlesinger, C., et al. (2007). Effectiveness of brief alcohol interventions in primary care populations. *Cochrane Database of Systematic Reviews*, Cochrane Art. No.: CD004148, DOI: 10.1002/14651858.CD004148.pub3.

Kanner, A. D., Coyne, J. C., Schaefer, C., & Lazarus, R. S. (1981). Comparison of two modes of stress measurement: Daily hassles and uplifts versus major life events. *Journal of Behavioral Medicine, 4*, 1–39.

Ka'opua, L. S. I., & Mueller, C. W. (2004). Treatment adherence among Native Hawaiians living with HIV. *Social Work, 49*, 55–62.

Kaplan, R. M., & Bush, J. W. (1982). Health-related quality of life measurement for evaluation research and policy analysis. *Health Psychology, 1*, 61–80.

Kaptchuk, T., Eisenberg, D., & Komaroff, A. (2002). Pondering the placebo effect. *Newsweek, 140*(23), 71, 73.

Kaptchuk, T. J., Friedlander, E., Kelley, J. M., Sanchez, M. N., Kokkotou, E., Singer, J. P., et al. (2010). Placebos without deception: A randomized controlled trial in irritable bowel syndrome. *PLoS ONE, 5*, e15591.

Karam, E., Kypri, K., & Salamoun, M. (2007). Alcohol use among college students: An international perspective. *Current Opinion in Psychiatry, 20*, 213–221.

Karani, R., McLaughlin, M. A., & Cassel, C. K. (2001). Exercise in the healthy older adult. *American Journal of Geriatric Cardiology, 10*, 269–273.

Karavidas, M. K., Tsai, P.-S., Yucha, C., McGrady, A., & Lehrer, P. M. (2006). Thermal biofeedback for primary Raynaud's phenomenon: A review of the literature. *Applied Psychophysiology and Biofeedback, 31*, 203–216.

Karl, A., Mühlnickel, W., Kurth, R., & Flor, H. (2004). Neuroelectric source imaging of steady-state movement-related cortical potentials in human upper extremity amputees with and without phantom limb pain. *Pain, 110*, 90–102.

Karlamangla, A. S., Singer, B. H., Williams, D. R., Schwartz, J. E., Matthews, K. A., Kiefe, C. I., et al. (2005). Impact of socioeconomic status on longitudinal accumulation of cardiovascular risk in young adults: The CARDIA Study (USA). *Social Science and Medicine, 60*, 999–1015.

Karoly, P., & Ruehlman, L. S. (2007). Psychosocial aspects of pain-related life task interference: An exploratory analysis in a general population sample. *Pain Medicine, 8*, 563–572.

Karp, A., Andel, R., Parker, M., Wang, H.-X., Winblad, B., & Fratiglioni, L. (2009). Mentally stimulating activities at work during midlife and dementia risk after 75: Follow-up study from the Kungsholmen project. *The American Journal of Geriatric Psychiatry, 17*, 227–236.

Karvinen, K. H., Courneya, K. S., Plotnikoff, R. C., Spence, J. C., Venner, P. M., & North, S. (2009). A prospective study of the determinants of exercise in bladder cancer survivors using the Theory of Planned Behavior. *Supportive Care in Cancer, 17*, 171–179.

Kasl, S. V., & Cobb, S. (1966a). Health behavior, illness behavior, and sick role behavior: I. Health and illness behavior. *Archives of Environmental Health, 12*, 246–266.

Kasl, S. V., & Cobb, S. (1966b). Health behavior, illness behavior, and sick role behavior: II. Sick role behavior. *Archives of Environmental Health, 12*, 531–541.

Kato, M., Noda, M., Inoue, M., Kadowaki, T., & Tsugane, S. (2009). Psychological factors, coffee and risk of diabetes mellitus among middle-aged Japanese: A population-based prospective study in the JPHC study cohort. *Endocrine Journal, 56*, 459–468.

Katon, W. J., Russo, J. E., Heckbert, S. R., Lin, E. H. B., Ciechanowski, P., Ludman, E., et al. (2010). The relationship between changes in depression symptoms and changes in health risk behaviors in patients with diabetes. *International Journal of Geriatric Psychiatry, 25*, 466–475.

Kaufmann, R. B., Babb, S., O'Halloran, A., Asman, K., Bishop, E., Tynan, M., et al. (2010). Vital signs: Nonsmokers' exposure to secondhand smoke—United States, 1999–2008. *Morbidity and Mortality Weekly Report, 59*(35), 1141–1146.

Kaur, S., Cohen, A., Dolor, R., Coffman, C. J., & Bastian, L. A. (2004). The impact of environmental tobacco smoke on women's risk of dying from heart disease: A meta-analysis. *Journal of Women's Health, 13*, 888–897.

Kavookjian, J., Elswick, B. M., & Whetsel, T. (2007). Interventions for being active among individuals with diabetes: A systematic review of the literature. *Diabetes Educator, 33*, 962–988.

Kawachi, I., Daniels, N., & Robinson, D. E. (2005). Health disparities by race and class: Why both matter. *Health Affairs, 24*, 343–352.

Kaye, W. (2008). Neurobiology of anorexia and bulimia nervosa. *Physiology and Behavior, 94*, 121–135.

Keefe, F. J. (1982). Behavioral assessment and treatment of chronic pain: Current status and future directions. *Journal of Consulting and Clinical Psychology, 50*, 896–911.

Keefe, F. J., & Smith, S. J. (2002). The assessment of pain behavior: Implications for applied psychophysiology and future research directions. *Applied Psychophysiology and Biofeedback, 27*, 117–127.

Keefe, F. J., Smith, S. J., Buffington, A. L. H., Gibson, J., Studts, J. L., & Caldwell, D. S. (2002). Recent advances and future directions in the biopsychosocial assessment and treatment of arthritis. *Journal of Consulting and Clinical Psychology, 70*, 640–655.

Keel, P. K., & Brown, T. A. (2010). Update on course and outcome in eating disorders. *International Journal of Eating Disorders, 43*(3), 195–204.

Keel, P. K., & Klump, K. L. (2003). Are eating disorders culture-bound syndromes? Implications for conceptualizing their etiology. *Psychological Bulletin, 129*, 747–769.

Keith, V., Kronenfeld, J., Rivers, P., & Liang, S. (2005). Assessing the effects of race and ethnicity on use of complementary and alternative therapies in the USA. *Ethnicity and Health, 10*, 19–32.

Keller, A., Hayden, J., Bombardier, C., & van Tulder, M. (2007). Effect sizes of non-surgical treatments of non-specific low-back pain. *European Spine Journal, 16*, 1776–1788.

Kelley, G. A., & Kelley, K. S. (2007). Aerobic exercise and lipids and lipoproteins in children and adolescents: A meta-analysis of randomized controlled trials. *Atherosclerosis, 191*, 447–453.

Kelley, K. W., Bluthé, R.-M., Dantzer, R., Zhou, J.-H., Shen, W.-H., Johnson, R. W., et al. (2003). Cytokine-induced sickness behavior. *Brain, Behavior and Immunity, 17*(S1), 112–118.

Kelly, J. A., & Kalichman, S. C. (2002). Behavioral research in HIV/AIDS primary and secondary prevention: Recent advances and future directions. *Journal of Consulting and Clinical Psychology, 70*, 626–639.

Kelly, J. F., Stout, R. L., Magill, M., & Tonigan, J. S. (2011). The role of Alcoholics Anonymous in mobilizing adaptive social network changes: A prospective lagged mediational analysis. *Drug & Alcohol Dependence, 114*(2/3), 119–126.

Kelly, K. P., & Kirschenbaum, D. S. (2011). Immersion treatment of childhood and adolescent obesity: The first review of a promising intervention. *Obesity Reviews, 12*(1), 37–49.

Keltner, B., Kelley, F. J., & Smith, D. (2004). Leadership to reduce health disparities. *Nursing Administration Quarterly, 28*, 181–190.

Kemeny, M. E. (2003). The psychobiology of stress. *Current Directions in Psychological Science, 12*, 124–129.

Kemeny, M. E., & Schedlowski, M. (2007). Understanding the interaction between psychosocial stress and immune-related diseases: A stepwise progression. *Brain, Behavior and Immunity, 21*, 1009–1018.

Kendler, K. S., Gatz, M., Gardner, C. O., & Pedersen, N. L. (2007). Clinical indices of familial depression in the Swedish Twin Registry. *Acta Psychiatrica Scandinavica, 115*, 214–220.

Kendzor, D. E., Businelle, M. S., Costello, T. J., Castro, Y., Reitzel, L. R., Cofta-Woerpel, L. M., et al. (2010). Financial strain and smoking cessation among racially/ethnically diverse smokers. *American Journal of Public Health, 100*(4), 702–706.

Kennedy, D. P., Tucker, J. S., Pollard, M. S., Go, M.-H., & Green, H. D. (2011). Adolescent romantic relationships and change in smoking status. *Addictive Behaviors, 36*(4), 320–326.

Keogh, E., Bond, F. W., & Flaxman, P. E. (2006). Improving academic performance and mental health through a stress management intervention: Outcomes and mediators of change. *Behaviour Research and Therapy, 44*, 339–357.

Kerns, R. D., Turk, D. C., & Rudy, T. E. (1985). The West Haven–Yale Multidimensional Pain Inventory. *Pain, 23*, 345–356.

Kerse, N., Buetow, S., Mainous, A. G., III, Young, G., Coster, G., & Arroll, A. (2004). Physician-patient relationship and medication compliance: A primary care investigation. *Annals of Family Medicine, 2*, 455–461.

Kertesz, L. (2003). The numbers behind the news. *Healthplan, 44*(5), 10–14, *16*, 18.

Kesmodel, U., Wisborg, K., Olsen, S. F., Henriksen, T. B., & Secher, N. J. (2002). Moderate alcohol intake during pregnancy and the risk of stillbirth and death in the first year of life. *American Journal of Epidemiology, 155*, 305–312.

Kessler, R. C., Berglund, P., Delmer, O., Jin, R., Merikangas, K. R., & Walters, E. E. (2005). Lifetime prevalence and age-of-onset distributions of DSM-IV disorders in the National Comorbidity Survey Replication. *Archives of General Psychiatry, 62*, 593–602.

Keys, A., Brozek, J., Henschel, A., Mickelsen, O., & Taylor, H. L. (1950). *The biology of human starvation* (2 Vols.). Minneapolis, MN: University of Minnesota Press.

Khan, C. M., Stephens, M. A. P., Franks, M. M., Rook, K. S., & Salem, J. K. (2012). Influences of spousal support and control on diabetes management through physical activity. *Health Psychology.* DOI: 10.1037/a0028609.

Kharbanda, R., & MacAllister, R. J. (2005). The atherosclerosis time-line and the role of the endothelium. *Current Medicinal Chemistry—Immunology, Endocrine, and Metabolic Agents, 5*, 47–52.

Khaw, K.-T., Wareham, N., Bingham, S., Luben, R., Welch, A., & Day, N. (2004). Association of hemoglobin A1c with cardiovascular disease and mortality in adults: The European Prospective Investigation Into Cancer in Norfolk. *Annals of Internal Medicine, 141*, 413–420.

Khaw, K.-T., Wareham, N., Bingham, S., Welch, A., Luben, R., & Day, N. (2008). Combined impact of health behaviours and mortality in men and women: The EPIC-Norfolk prospective population study. *PLoS Med, 5*, e12. DOI: 10.1371/journal.pmed.0050012.

Kickbusch, I. (2008). Health literacy: An essential skill for the twenty-first century. *Health Education, 108*, 101–104.

Kiecolt-Glaser, J. K. (1999). Stress, personal relationships, and immune function: Health implications. *Brain, Behavior and Immunity, 13*, 61–72.

Kiecolt-Glaser, J. K., Malarkey, W. B., Cacioppo, J. T., & Glaser, R. (1994). Stressful personal relationships: Immune and endocrine function. In R. Glaser & J. K. Kiecolt-Glaser (Eds.), *Handbook of human stress and immunity* (pp. 321–339). San Diego, CA: Academic Press.

Kiecolt-Glaser, J. K., Marucha, P. T., Malarkey, W. B., Mercado, A. M., & Glaser, R. (1995). Slowing of wound healing by psychological stress. *Lancet, 346*, 1194–1196.

Kiecolt-Glaser, J. K., McGuire, L., Robles, T. F., & Glaser, R. (2002). Emotions, morbidity, and mortality: New perspectives from psychoneuroimmunology. *Annual Review of Psychology, 53*, 83–108.

Kiecolt-Glaser, J. K., & Newton, T. L. (2001). Marriage and health: His and hers. *Psychological Bulletin, 127*, 472–503.

Kim, D., Kawachi, I., Hoorn, S. V., Ezzati, M. (2008). Is inequality at the heart of it? Cross-country associations of income inequality with cardiovascular diseases and risk factors. *Social Science and Medicine, 66*, 1719–1732.

Kim, H., Neubert, J. K., Rowan, J. S., Brahim, J. S., Iadarola, M. J., & Dionne, R. A. (2004). Comparison of experimental and acute clinical pain responses in humans as pain phenotypes. *Journal of Pain, 5*, 377–384.

Kim, H. S., Sherman, D. K., & Taylor, S. E. (2008). Culture and social support. *American Psychologist, 63*, 518–526.

Kim, Y., Myung, S.-K., Jeon, Y.-J., Lee, E.-H., Park, C.-H., Seo, H. G., et al. (2011). Effectiveness of pharmacologic therapy for smoking cessation in adolescent smokers: Meta-analysis of randomized controlled trials. *American Journal of Health-System Pharmacy, 68*(3), 219–226.

Kimball, C. P. (1981). *The biopsychosocial approach to the patient.* Baltimore, MD: Williams & Wilkins.

King, D., & Pace, L. (2005, April). Sports, steroids, and scandals. *Information Today, 22*, 25–27.

King, J., & Henry, E. (2004, September 4). Bill Clinton awaits heart surgery next week. *CNN Washington Bureau.* Retrieved June 16, 2005, from http://www.cnn.com/2004/ALLPOLITICS/09/03/clinton.tests/

King, L., Saules, K. K., & Irish, J. (2007). Weight concerns and cognitive style: Which carries more "weight" in the prediction of smoking among college women? *Nicotine and Tobacco Research, 9*, 535–543.

King, T. K., Matacin, M., White, K. S., & Marcus, B. H. (2005). A prospective examination of body image and smoking cessation in women. *Body Image, 2*, 19–28.

Kirschbaum, C., Tietze, A., Skoluda, N., & Dettenborn, L. (2009). Hair as a retrospective calendar of cortisol production: Increased cortisol incorporation into hair in the third trimester of pregnancy. *Psychoneuroendocrinology, 34*, 32–37.

"Kirstie Alley's weight." (2009, April 30). Kirstie Alley's weight struggle. *Oprah Winfrey Show*. Retrieved July 17, 2011, from http://www.oprah.com/entertainment/Kirstie-Alleys-Weight-Battle

Kivlinghan, K. T., Granger, D. A., & Booth, A. (2005). Gender differences in testosterone and cortisol response to competition. *Psychoneuroendocrinology, 30*, 58–71.

Kiyohara, C., & Ohno, Y. (2010). Sex differences in lung cancer susceptibility: A review. *Gender Medicine, 7*(5), 381–401.

Klatsky, A. L. (2010). Alcohol and cardiovascular health. *Physiology & Behavior, 100*(1), 76–81.

Klatsky, A. L., & Udaltsova, N. (2007). Alcohol drinking and total mortality risk. *Annals of Epidemiology, 17*(S5), S63–S67.

Klein, D. A., Bennett, A. S., Schebendach, J., Foltin, R. W., Devlin, M. J., & Walsh, B. T. (2004). Exercise "addiction" in anorexia nervosa: Model development and pilot study. *CNS Spectrums, 9*, 531–537.

Klein, H., Elifson, K. W., & Sterk, C. E. (2003). "At risk" women who think that they have no chance of getting HIV: Self-assessed perceived risks. *Women and Health, 38*, 47–63.

Klimentidis, Y. C. (2011). Canaries in the coal mine: A cross-species analysis of the plurality of obesity epidemics. *Proceedings of the Royal Society B: Biological Sciences, 278*(1712), 1626–1632.

Klonoff, E. A., & Landrine, H. (2000). Is skin color a marker for racial discrimination? Explaining the skin color–hypertension relationship. *Journal of Behavioral Medicine, 23*, 329–338.

Kluger, R. (1996). *Ashes to ashes: America's hundred-year cigarette war, the public health and the unabashed triumph of Philip Morris*. New York: Knopf.

Knafl, K. A., & Deatrick, J. A. (2002). The challenge of normalization for families of children with chronic conditions. *Pediatric Nursing, 28*, 49–54.

Knight, S. J., & Emanuel, L. (2007). Processes of adjustment to end-of-life losses: A reintegration model. *Journal of Palliative Medicine, 10*, 1190–1198.

Knutson, K. L., & van Cauter, E. (2008). Associations between sleep loss and increased risk of obesity and diabetes. *Annals of the New York Academy of Sciences, 1129*(Suppl. 1), 287–304.

Knuttgen, H. G. (2007). Strength training and aerobic exercise: Comparison and contrast. *Journal of Strength and Conditioning, 21*, 973–978.

Ko, N.-Y., & Muecke, M. (2005). Reproductive decision-making among HIV-positive couples in Taiwan. *Journal of Nursing Scholarship, 37*, 41–47.

Kobayashi, F. (2007). Assessing body types, diet, exercise, and sedentary behavior of American and Japanese college students. *Nutrition & Food Science, 37*(5), 329–337.

Kochanek, K. D., Xu, J., Murphy, S. L., Miniño, A. M., & Kung, H.-C. (2011). Deaths: Preliminary data for 2009. *National Vital Statistics Reports, 59*(4), 1–68.

Kofman, O. (2002). The role of prenatal stress in the etiology of developmental behavioural disorders. *Neuroscience and Biobehavioral Reviews, 26*, 457–470.

Kohn, L. T., Corrigan, J. M., & Donaldson, M. (Eds.). (1999). *To err is human: Building a safer health system*. Washington, DC: Institute of Medicine.

Köhnke, M. D. (2008). Approach to the genetics of alcoholism: A review based on pathophysiology. *Biochemical Pharmacology, 75*, 160–177.

Koopmans, G. T., & Lamers, L. M. (2007). Gender and health care utilization: The role of mental distress and help-seeking propensity. *Social Science & Medicine, 64*, 1216–1230.

Kop, W. J. (2003). The integration of cardiovascular behavioral medicine and psychoneuroimmunology: New developments based on converging research fields. *Brain, Behavior, and Immunity, 17*, 233–237.

Kop, W. J., Stein, P. K., Tracy, R. P., Barzilay, J. I., Schulz, R., & Gottdiener, J. S. (2010). Autonomic nervous system dysfunction and inflammation contribute to the increased cardiovascular mortality risk associated with depression. *Psychosomatic Medicine, 72*, 626–635.

Kopnisky, K. L., Stoff, D. M., & Rausch, D. M. (2004). Workshop report: The effects of psychological variables on the progression of HIV-1 disease. *Brain, Behavior and Immunity, 18*, 246–261.

Kosok, A. (2006). The moderation management programme in 2004: What type of drinker seeks controlled drinking? *International Journal of Drug Policy, 17*, 295–303.

Koss, M. P. (1990). The women's mental health research agenda: Violence against women. *American Psychologist, 45*, 374–380.

Koss, M. P., Bailey, J. A., Yuan, N. P., Herrara, V. M., & Lichter, E. L. (2003). Depression and PTSD in survivors of male violence: Research and training initiatives to facilitate recovery. *Psychology of Women Quarterly, 27*, 130–142.

Kottow, M. H. (2007). Should research ethics triumph over clinical ethics? *Journal of Evaluation in Clinical Practice, 13*, 695–698.

Koval, J. J., Pederson, L. L., Zhang, X., Mowery, P., & McKenna, M. (2008). Can young adult smoking status be predicted from concern about body weight and self-reported BMI among adolescents? Results from a ten-year cohort study. *Nicotine & Tobacco Research, 10*(9), 1449–1455.

Kowal, J., & Fortier, M. S. (2007). Physical activity behavior change in middle-aged and older women: The role of barriers and of environmental characteristics. *Journal of Behavioral Medicine, 30*, 233–242.

Kozlowski, L. T., Wilkinson, A., Skinner, W., Kent, C., Franklin, T., & Pope, M. (1989). Comparing tobacco cigarette dependence with other drug dependences. *Journal of the American Medical Association, 261*, 898–901.

Krahn, D. D., Kurth, C. L., Gomberg, E., & Drewnowski, A. (2005). Pathological dieting and alcohol use in college women—A continuum of behaviors. *Eating Behaviors, 6*, 43–52.

Krantz, D. S., & McCeney, K. T. (2002). Effects of psychological and social factors on organic disease: A critical assessment of research on coronary heart disease. *Annual Review of Psychology, 53*, 341–369.

Krantz, G., Forsman, M., & Lundberg, U. (2004). Consistency in physiological stress responses and electromyographic activity during induced stress exposure in women and men. *Integrative Physiological and Behavioral Science, 39*, 105–118.

Krarup, L.-H., Truelsen, T., Pedersen, A., Kerke, H., Lindahl, M., Hansen, L., et al. (2007). Level of physical activity in the week preceding an ischemic stroke. *Cerebrovascular Disease, 24*, 296–300.

Krewski, D., Lubin, J. H., Zielinski, J. M., Alavanja, M., Catalan, V. S., Field, R. W., et al. (2006). A combined analysis of North American case-control studies of residential radon and lung cancer. *Journal of Toxicology and Environmental Health, 69*, 533–597.

Krieger, N., Chen, J. T., Waterman, P. D., Rehkopf, D. H., & Subramanian, S. V. (2005). Painting a truer picture of US socioeconomic and racial/ethnic health inequalities: The public health disparities geocoding project. *American Journal of Public Health, 95*, 312–323.

Krisanaprakornkit, T., Krisanaprakornkit, W., Piyavhatkul, N., & Laopaiboon, M. (2006). Meditation therapy for anxiety disorders. *Cochrane Database of Systematic Reviews*, Cochrane Art. No.: CD004998, DOI: 10.1002/14651858.CD004998.pub2.

Krishna, S., & Boren, S. A. (2008). Diabetes self-management care via cell phone: A systematic review. *Journal of Diabetes, Science and Technology, 2*, 509–517.

Krishnan-Sarin, S., O'Malley, S., & Krysta, J. H. (2008). Treatment implications. *Alcohol Research & Health, 31*(4), 400–407.

Kröner-Herwig, B. (2009). Chronic pain syndromes and their teratment by psychological interventions. *Current Opinion in Psychiatry, 22*(2), 200–204.

Kronish, I. M., Rieckmann, N., Halm, E. A., Shimbo, D., Vorchheimer, D., Haas, D. C., et al. (2006). Persistent depression affects adherence to secondary prevention behaviors after acute coronary syndromes. *Journal of General Internal Medicine, 21*, 1178–1183.

Kruger, J., Galuska, D. A., Serdula, M. K., & Jones, D. A. (2004). Attempting to lose weight: Specific practices among U.S. adults. *American Journal of Preventive Medicine, 26*, 402–406.

Kubetin, S. K. (2001). Weight-loss maintenance requires long-term management. *Family Practice News, 31*(4), 6–7.

Kübler-Ross, E. (1969). *On death and dying.* New York: Macmillan.

Kuhnel, J., & Sonnentag, S. (2011). How long do you benefit from vacation? A closer look at the fade-out of vacation effects. *Journal of Organizational Behavior, 32,* 125–143.

Kuk, J. L., & Ardern, C. I. (2009). Influence of age on the association between various measures of obesity and all-cause mortality. *Journal of the American Geriatrics Society, 57*(11), 2007–2084.

Kung, H. C., Hoyert, D. L., Xu, J. Q., & Murphy, S. L. (2008). Deaths: Final data for 2005. *National Vital Statistics Reports, 56*(10), 1–66.

Kuntsche, S., Plant, M. L., Plant, M. A., Miller, P., & Gabriel, G. (2008). Spreading or concentrating drinking occasions—Who is most at risk? *European Addiction Research, 14*(2), 71–81.

Kurland, H. (2000). *History of t'ai chi chu'an.* Retrieved May 16, 2008, from http://www.dotaichi.com/Articles/HistoryofTaiChi.htm

Kyngäs, H. (2004). Support network of adolescents with chronic disease: Adolescents' perspective. *Nursing and Health Sciences, 6,* 287–293.

Laaksonen, M., Talala, K., Martelin, T., Rahkonen, O., Roos, E., Helakorpi, S., et al. (2008). Health behaviours as explanations for educational level differences in cardiovascular and all-cause mortality: A follow-up of 60,000 men and women over 23 years. *European Journal of Public Health, 18,* 38–43.

Laatikainen, T., Critchley, J., Vartiainen, E., Salomaa, V., Ketonen, M., & Capewell, S. (2005). Explaining the decline in coronary heart disease mortality in Finland between 1982 and 1997. *American Journal of Epidemiology, 162,* 764–773.

Lafferty, W. E., Tyree, P. T., Devlin, S. M., Andersen, M. R., & Diehr, P. K. (2008). Complementary and alternative medicine provider use and expenditures by cancer treatment phase. *American Journal of Managed Care, 14,* 326–334.

Lai, D. T. C., Cahill, K., Qin, Y., & Tang, J. L. (2010). Motivational interviewing for smoking cessation. *Cochrane Database of Systematic Reviews 2010,* Cochrane Art. No.: CD006936, DOI: 10.1002/14651858.CD006936.pub2.

Laitinen, M. H., Ngandu, T., Rovio, S., Helkala, E.-L., Uusitalo, U., Viitanen, M., et al. (2006). Fat intake at midlife and risk of dementia and Alzheimer's disease: A population-based study. *Dementia and Geriatric Cognitive Disorders, 22,* 99–107.

Lake, J. (2009). Complementary, alternative, and integrative Rx: Safety issues. *Psychiatric Times, 26*(7), 22–29.

Lamptey, P. R. (2002). Reducing heterosexual transmission of HIV in poor countries. *British Medical Journal, 324,* 207–211.

Landolt, A. S., & Milling, L. S. (2011). The efficacy of hypnosis as an intervention for labor and delivery pain: A comprehensive methodological review. *Clinical Psychology Review, 31*(6), 1022–1031.

Landrine, H., & Klonoff, E. A. (1996). The Schedule of Racist Events: A measure of racial discrimination and a study of its negative physical and mental health consequences. *Journal of Black Psychology, 22,* 144–168.

Lang, E. V., Benotsch, E. G., Fick, L. J., Lutgendorf, S., Berbaum, M. L., Berbaum, K. S., et al. (2000). Adjunctive non-pharmacological analgesia for invasive medical procedures: A randomised trial. *Lancet, 355,* 1486–1490.

Lang, F. R., Baltes, P. B., & Wagner, G. G. (2007). Desired lifetime and end-of-life desires across adulthood from 20 to 90: A dual-source information model. *Journals of Gerontology Series B: Psychological Sciences and Social Sciences, 62B,* 268–276.

Langa, K. M., Foster, N. L., & Larson, E. B. (2004). Mixed dementia: Emerging concepts and therapeutic implications. *Journal of the American Medical Association, 292,* 2901–2908.

Lange, T., Dimitrov, S., & Born, J. (2011). Effects of sleep and circadian rhythm on the human immune system. *Annals of the New York Academy of Sciences, 1193,* 48–59.

Langer, E. J., & Rodin, J. (1976). The effects of choice and enhanced personal responsibility for the aged: A field experiment in an institutional setting. *Journal of Personality and Social Psychology, 34,* 191–198.

Langhorne, P., Coupar, F., & Pollock, A. (2009). Motor recovery after stroke: A systematic review. *Lancet Neurology, 8*(8), 741–754.

Lantz, P. M., Golberstein, E., House, J. S., & Morenoff, J. (2010). Socioeconomic and behavioral risk factors for mortality in a national 19-year prospective study of U.S. adults. *Social Science & Medicine, 70*(10), 1558–1566.

López-Moreno, J. A., González-Cuevas, G., Moreno, G., & Navarro, M. (2008). The pharmacology of the endocannabinoid system: Functional structural interactions with other neurotransmitter systems and their repercussions in behavioral addiction. *Addiction Biology, 13,* 160–187.

Largo-Wight, E., Peterson, P. M., & Chen, W. W. (2005). Perceived problem solving, stress, and health among college students. *American Journal of Health Behavior, 29,* 360–370.

Larun, L., Nordheim, L. V., Ekeland, E., Hagen, K. B., & Heian, F. (2006). Exercise in prevention and treatment of anxiety and depression among children and young people. *Cochrane Database of Systematic Reviews,* Cochrane Art. No.: CD004691, DOI: 10.1002/14651858.CD004691.pub2.

Lash, S. J., Stephens, R. S., Burden, J. L., Grambow, S. C., DeMarce, J. M., Jones, M. E., et al. (2007). Contracting, prompting, and reinforcing substance use disorder continuing care: A randomized clinical trial. *Psychology of Addictive Behaviors, 21,* 387–397.

Lasser, K. E., Himmelstein, D. U., & Woolhandler, S. (2006). Access to care, health status, and health disparities in the United States and Canada: Results of a cross-national population-based survey. *American Journal of Public Health, 96,* 1300–1307.

Laucht, M., Becker, K., Frank, J., Schmidt, M. H., Esser, G., Treutlein, J., et al. (2008). Genetic variation in dopamine pathways differentially associated with smoking progression in adolescence. *Journal of the American Academy of Child and Adolescent Psychiatry, 47,* 673–681.

Lauerman, J. (2011, January 18). Jobs's cancer combined with transplant carries complications. *Bloomberg.* Retrieved April 20, 2012, from http://www.bloomberg.com/news/2011-01-17/jobs-s-liver-transplant-complicated-by-cancer-carries-risks-doctors-say.html

Laurent, M. R., & Vickers, T. J. (2009). Seeking health information online: Does Wikipedia matter? *Journal of the American Medical Informatics Association, 16,* 471–479.

Lautenschlager, N. T., Cox, K. L., Flicker, L., Foster, J. K., van Bockxmeer, F. M., Xiao, J., et al. (2008). Effect of physical activity on cognitive function in older adults at risk for Alzheimer Disease. *Journal of the American Medical Association, 300,* 1027–1037.

LaVeist, T. A., Bowie, J. V., & Cooley-Quille, M. (2000). Minority health status in adulthood: The middle years of life. *Health Care Financing Review, 21*(4), 9–21.

Lawler, P. R., Filion, K. B., & Eisenberg, M. J. (2011). Efficacy of exercise-based cardiac rehabilitation post-myocardial infarction: A systematic review and meta-analysis of randomized controlled trials. *American Heart Journal, 162,* 571–584.

Lawrence, D., Mitrou, F., Sawyer, M. G., & Zubrick, S. R. (2010). Smoking status, mental disorders and emotional and behavioural problems in young people: Child and adolescent component of the National Survey of Mental Health and Wellbeing. *Australian & New Zealand Journal of Psychiatry, 44*(9), 805–814.

Lazarou, J., Pomeranz, B. H., & Corey, P. N. (1998). Incidence of adverse drug reactions in hospitalized patients: A meta-analysis of prospective studies. *Journal of the American Medical Association, 278,* 1200–1205.

Lazarus, R. S. (1984). Puzzles in the study of daily hassles. *Journal of Behavioral Medicine, 7,* 375–389.

Lazarus, R. S. (1993). From psychological stress to the emotions: A history of changing outlooks. *Annual Review of Psychology, 44,* 1–21.

Lazarus, R. S. (2000). Toward better research on stress and coping. *American Psychologist, 55,* 665–673.

Lazarus, R. S., & Cohen, J. (1977). Environmental stress. In I. Altman & J. Wohlwill (Eds.), *Human behavior and environment: Advances in theory and research* (Vol. 2, pp. 89–127). New York: Plenum Press.

Lazarus, R. S., & DeLongis, A. (1983). Psychological stress and coping in aging. *American Psychologist, 38,* 245–254.

Lazarus, R. S., DeLongis, A., Folkman, S., & Gruen, R. (1985). Stress and adaptational outcomes. *American Psychologist, 40,* 770–779.

Lazarus, R. S., & Folkman, S. (1984). *Stress, appraisal, and coping.* New York: Springer.

Lazovich, D., Vogel, R. I., Berwick, M., Weinstock, M. A., Anderson, K. E., & Warshaw, E. M. (2010). Indoor tanning and risk of melanoma: A case-control study in a highly exposed population. *Cancer Epidemiology, Biomarkers, and Prevention, 19,* 1557–1568.

Leape, L. L., & Berwick, D. M. (2005). Five years after *To Err Is Human*: What have we learned? *Journal of the American Medical Association, 293,* 2384–2390.

Leavy, J. E., Bull, F. C., Rosenberg, M., & Bauman, A. (2011). Physical activity mass media campaigns and their evaluation: A systematic review of the literature 2003–2010. *Health Education Research, 26,* 1060–1085.

Lebovits, A. (2007). Cognitive-behavioral approaches to chronic pain. *Primary Psychiatry, 14*(9), 48–50, 51–54.

Lee, H. S., Engstrom, M., & Petersen, S. R. (2011). Harm reduction in 12 steps: Complementary, oppositional, or something in-between? *Substance Use & Misuse, 46*(9), 1151–1161.

Lee, L. M., Karon, J. M., Selik, R., Neal, J. J., & Fleming, P. L. (2001). Survival after AIDS diagnosis in adolescents and adults during the treatment era, United States, 1984–1997. *Journal of the American Medical Association, 285,* 1308–1315.

Lee, M. S., Kim, M. K., & Ryu, H. (2005). Qi-training (qigong) enhanced immune functions: What is the underlying mechanism? *International Journal of Neuroscience, 115,* 1099–1104.

Lee, M. S., Pittler, M. H., & Ernst, E. (2007a). External qigong for pain conditions: A systematic review of randomized clinical trials. *Journal of Pain, 8,* 827–831.

Lee, M. S., Pittler, M. H., & Ernst, E. (2007b). Tai chi for rheumatoid arthritis: Systematic review. *Rheumatology, 46*(11), 1648–1651.

Lee, P. N., & Forey, B. A. (2006). Environmental tobacco smoke exposure and risk of stroke in nonsmokers: A review with meta-analysis. *Journal of Stroke & Cerebrovascular Diseases, 15*(5), 190–201.

Lee, P. R., Lee, D. R., Lee, P., & Arch, M. (2010). 2010: U.S. drug and alcohol policy, looking back and moving forward. *Journal of Psychoactive Drugs, 42*(2), 99–114.

Leeuw, M., Goossens, M. E. J. B., Linton, S. J., Crombez, G., Boersma, K., & Vlaeyen, J. W. S. (2007). The fear-avoidance model of musculoskeletal pain: Current state of scientific evidence. *Journal of Behavioral Medicine, 30,* 77–94.

Lemstra, M., Nannapaneni, U., Neudorf, C., Warren, L., Kershaw, T., & Scott, C. (2010). A systematic review of school-based marijuana and alcohol prevention programs targeting adolescents aged 10–15. *Addiction Research & Theory, 18*(1), 84–96.

Lenssinck, M.-L. B., Damen, L., Verhagen, A. P., Berger, M. Y., Passchier, J., & Koes, B. W. (2004). The effectiveness of physiotherapy and manipulation in patients with tension-type headache: A systematic review. *Pain, 112,* 381–388.

Leo, R. J., & Ligot, J. S. A., Jr. (2007). A systematic review of randomized controlled trials of acupuncture in the treatment of depression. *Journal of Affective Disorders, 97,* 13–22.

Leombruni, P., Pierò, A., Lavagnino, L., Brustolin, A., Campisi, S., & Fassino, S. (2008). A randomized, double-blind trial comparing sertraline and fluoxetine 6-month treatment in obese patients with binge eating disorder. *Progress in Neuro-Psychopharmacology & Biological Psychiatry, 32*(6), 1599–1605.

Leon, A. S., & Sanchez, O. A. (2001). Response of blood lipids to exercise training alone or combined with dietary intervention. *Medicine and Science in Sports and Exercise, 33,* S502–S515.

Lepore, S. J., Fernandez-Berrocal, P., Ragan, J., & Ramos, N. (2004). It's not that bad: Social challenges to emotional disclosure enhance adjustment to stress. *Anxiety, Stress and Coping, 17,* 341–361.

Lepore, S. J., Revenson, T. A., Weinberger, S. L., Weston, P., Frisina, P. G., Robertson, R., et al. (2006). Effects of social stressors on cardiovascular reactivity in black and white women. *Annals of Behavioral Medicine, 31,* 120–127.

Leserman, J., Ironson, G., O'Cleirigh, C., Fordiani, J. M., & Balbin, E. (2008). Stressful life events and adherence in HIV. *AIDS Patient Care and STDs, 22,* 403–411.

Lestideau, O. T., & Lavallee, L. F. (2007). Structured writing about current stressors: The benefits of developing plans. *Psychology and Health, 22,* 659–676.

Leung, D. P., Chan, C. K., Tsang, H. W., Tsang, W. W., & Jones, A. Y. (2011). Tai chi as an intervention to improve balance and reduce falls in older adults: A systematic and meta-analytic review. *Alternative Therapies in Health & Medicine, 17*(1), 40–48.

Levenson, J. L., & Schneider, R. K. (2007). Infectious diseases. In J. L. Levenson (Ed.), *Essentials of psychosomatic medicine* (pp. 181–204). Washington, DC: American Psychiatric Publishing.

Levenson, R. W., Sher, K. J., Grossman, L. M., Newman, J., & Newlin, D. B. (1980). Alcohol and stress response dampening: Pharmacological effects, expectancy, and tension reduction. *Journal of Abnormal Psychology, 89,* 528–538.

Levenstein, S. (2000). The very model of a modern etiology: A biopsychosocial view of peptic ulcer. *Psychosomatic Medicine, 62,* 176–185.

Leventhal, H., & Avis, N. (1976). Pleasure, addiction, and habit: Factors in verbal report or factors in smoking behavior? *Journal of Abnormal Psychology, 85,* 478–488.

Leventhal, H., Breland, J. Y., Mora, P. A., & Leventhal, E. A. (2010). Lay representations of illness and treatment: A framework for action. In A. Steptoe (Ed.), *Handbook of behavioral medicine: Methods and application* (pp. 137–154). New York: Springer.

Leventhal, H., Leventhal, E. A., & Cameron, L. (2001). Representations, procedures, and affect in illness self-regulation: A perceptual-cognitive model. In A. Baum, T. A. Revenson, & J. E. Singer (Eds.), *Handbook of health psychology* (pp. 19–47). Mahwah, NJ: Erlbaum.

Levi, L. (1974). Psychosocial stress and disease: A conceptual model. In E. K. E. Gunderson & R. H. Rahe (Eds.), *Life stress and illness* (pp. 8–33). Springfield, IL: Thomas.

Levin, B. E. (2010). Interaction of perinatal and pre-pubertal factors with genetic predisposition in the development of neural pathways involved in the regulation of energy homeostasis. *Brain Research, 1350,* 10–17.

Levin, T., & Kissane, D. W. (2006). Psychooncology—The state of its development in 2006. *European Journal of Psychiatry, 20,* 183–197.

Levy, D., & Brink, S. (2005). *A change of heart: How the people of Framingham, Massachusetts, helped unravel the mysteries of cardiovascular disease.* New York: Knopf.

Lewis, E. T., Combs, A., & Trafton, J. A. (2010). Reasons for under-use of prescribed opioid medications by patients in pain. *Pain Medicine, 11,* 861–871.

Lewis, M., & Johnson, M. I. (2006). The clinical effectiveness of therapeutic massage for muscoloskeletal pain: A systematic review. *Physiotherapy, 92,* 146–158.

Li, G., Zhan, P., Wang, J., Gregg, E. W., Yang, W., Gong, Q., et al. (2008). The long-term effect of lifestyle interventions to prevent diabetes in the China Da Qing Diabetes Prevention Study: A 20-year follow-up study. *The Lancet, 371,* 1783–1789.

Li, Q.-Z., Li, P., Garcia, G. E., Johnson, R. J., & Feng, L. (2005). Genomic profiling of neutrophil transcripts in Asian qigong practitioners: A pilot study in gene regulation by mind-body interaction. *Journal of Alternative and Complementary Medicine, 11,* 29–39.

Liang, X., Wang, Q., Yang, X., Cao, J., Chen, J., Mo, X., et al. (2011). Effect of mobile phone intervention for diabetes on glycaemic control: A meta-analysis. *Diabetic Medicine, 28,* 455–463.

Lichtenstein, B. (2005). Domestic violence, sexual ownership, and HIV risk in women in the American deep south. *Social Science and Medicine, 60,* 701–715.

Lieberman, M. A., & Goldstein, B. A. (2006). Not all negative emotions are equal: The role of emotional expression in online support groups for women with breast cancer. *Psycho-Oncology, 15,* 160–168.

Liechty, J. M. (2010). Body image disortion and three types of weight loss behaviors among nonoverweight girls in the United States. *Journal of Adolescent Health*, *47*(2), 176–182.

Ligier, S., & Sternberg, E. M. (2001). The neuroendocrine system and rheumatoid arthritis: Focus on the hypothalamo-pituitary-adrenal axis. In R. Ader, D. L. Felten, & N. Cohen (Eds.), *Psychoneuroimmunology* (3rd ed., Vol. 2, pp. 449–469). San Diego, CA: Academic Press.

Lillie-Blanton, M., Maddox, T. M., Rushing, O., & Mensah, G. A. (2004). Disparities in cardiac care: Rising to the challenge of *Healthy People 2010*. *Journal of the American College of Cardiology*, *44*, 503–508.

Lin, Y., Furze, G., Spilsbury, K., & Lewin, R. J. (2009). Misconceived and maladaptive beliefs about heart disease: A comparison between Taiwan and Britain. *Journal of Clinical Nursing*, *18*, 46–55.

Lincoln, K. D., Chatters, L. M., & Taylor, R. J. (2003). Psychological distress among Black and White Americans: Differential effects of social support, negative interaction and personal control. *Journal of Health and Social Behavior*, *44*, 390–407.

Linde, K., Berner, M. M., & Kriston, L. (2008). St. John's wort for major depression. *Cochrane Database of Systematic Reviews, 2008*, Issue 4. Cochrane, Art. No.: CD000448, DOI: 10.1002/14651858.CD000448.pub3.

Linde, K., Witt, C. M., Streng, A., Weidenhammer, W., Wagenfeil, S., Brinkhaus, B., et al. (2007). The impact of patient expectations on outcomes in four randomized controlled trials of acupuncture in patients with chronic pain. *Pain*, *128*, 264–271.

Linden, W. (2000). Psychological treatments in cardiac rehabilitation: Review of rationales and outcomes. *Journal of Psychosomatic Research*, *48*, 443–454.

Lindsay, J., Sykes, E., McDowell, I., Verreault, R., & Laurin, D. (2004). More than epidemiology of Alzheimer's disease: Contributions of the Canadian Study of Health and Aging. *Canadian Journal of Psychiatry*, *49*, 83–91.

Lindstrom, H. A., Fritsch, T., Petot, G., Smyth, K. A., Chen, C. H., Debanne, S. M., et al. (2005). The relationship between television viewing in midlife and the development of Alzheimer's disease in a case-control study. *Brain and Cognition*, *58*, 157–165.

Lints-Martindale, A. C., Hadjistavropoulos, T., Barber, B., & Gibson, S. J. (2007). A psychophysical investigation of the Facial Action Coding System as an index of pain variability among older adults with and without Alzheimer's disease. *Pain Medicine*, *8*, 678–689.

Lippke, S., Schwarzer, R., Ziegelmann, J. P., Scholz, U., & Schuz, B. (2010). Testing stage-specific effects of a stage-matched intervention: A randomized controlled trial targeting physical exercise and its predictors. *Health Education & Behavior*, *37*, 533–546.

Lippke, S., Ziegelmann, J., & Schwarzer, R. (2004). Initiation and maintenance of physical exercise: Stage-specific effects of a planning intervention. *Research in Sports Medicine: An International Journal*, *12*, 221–240.

Lipton, R. B., Bigal, M. E., Diamond, M., Freitag, F., Reed, M. L., & Stewart, W. F. (2007). Migraine prevalence, disease burden, and the need for preventive therapy. *Neurology*, *68*, 343–349.

Litz, B. T., Williams, L., Wang, J., Bryant, R., & Engel, C. C. (2004). A therapist-assisted Internet self-help program for traumatic stress. *Professional Psychology: Research and Practice*, *35*, 628–634.

Liu, H., Golin, C. E., Miller, L. G., Hays, R. D., Beck, C. K., Sanandji, S., et al. (2001). A comparison study of multiple measures of adherence to HIV protease inhibitors. *Annals of Internal Medicine*, *134*, 968–977.

Livermore, M. M., & Powers, R. S. (2006). Unfulfilled plans and financial stress: Unwed mothers and unemployment. *Journal of Human Behavior in the Social Environment*, *13*, 1–17.

Livneh, H., & Antonak, R. F. (2005). Psychosocial adaptation to chronic illness and disability: A primer for counselors. *Journal of Counseling and Development*, *83*, 12–20.

Livneh, H., Lott, S. M., & Antonak, R. F. (2004). Patterns of psychosocial adaptation to chronic illness and disability: A cluster analytic approach, *Psychology, Health and Medicine*, *9*, 411–430.

Ljungberg, J. K., & Neely, G. (2007). Stress, subjective experience and cognitive performance during exposure to noise and vibration. *Journal of Environmental Psychology*, *27*, 44–54.

Lloyd-Williams, M., Dogra, N., & Petersen, S. (2004). First year medical students' attitudes toward patients with life-limiting illness: Does age make a difference? *Palliative Medicine*, *18*, 137–138.

Lobo, A., Dufouil, C., Marcos, G., Quetglas, B., Saz, P., & Guallar, E. (2010). Is there an association between low-to-moderate alcohol consumption and risk of cognitive decline? *American Journal of Epidemiology*, *172*(6), 708–716.

Locher, J. L., Yoels, W. C., Maurer, D., & Van Ells, J. (2005). Comfort foods: An exploratory journey into the social and emotional significance of food. *Food and Foodways: History and Culture of Human Nourishment*, *13*, 273–297.

Lock, K., Pomerleau, J., Causer, L., Altmann, D. R., & McKee, M. (2005). The global burden of disease attributable to low consumption of fruit and vegetables: Implications for the global strategy on diet. *Bulletin of the World Health Organization*, *83*, 100–108.

Locke, J., le Grange, D., Agras, W. S., & Dare, C. (2001). *Treatment manual for anorexia nervosa: A family-based approach*. New York: Guilford Press.

Loftus, M. (1995). The other side of fame. *Psychology Today*, *28*(3), 48–53, 70, 72, 74, 76, 78, 80–81.

Logan, D. E., & Rose, J. B. (2004). Gender differences in post-operative pain and patient controlled analgesia use among adolescent surgical patients. *Pain*, *109*, 481–487.

Loggia, M. L., Juneau, M., & Bushnell, M. C. (2011). Autonomic responses to heat pain: Heart rate, skin conductance, and their relation to verbal ratings and stimulus intensity. *Pain*, *152*, 592–598.

Lohaus, A., & Klein-Hessling, J. (2003). Relaxation in children: Effects of extended and intensified training. *Psychology and Health*, *18*, 237–249.

Lopez, C., Antoni, M., Penedo, F., Weiss, D., Cruess, S., Segotas, M., et al. (2011). A pilot study of cognitive behavioral stress management effects on stress, quality of life, and symptoms in persons with chronic fatigue syndrome. *Journal of Psychosomatic Research*, *70*, 328–334.

Lotufo, P. A., Gaziano, J. M., Chae, C. U., Ajani, U. A., Moreno-John, G., Buring, J. E., et al. (2001). Diabetes and all-cause and coronary heart disease mortality among US male physicians. *Archives of Internal Medicine*, *161*, 242–247.

Low, C. A., Stanton, A. L., Bower, J. E., & Gyllenhammer, L. (2010). A randomized controlled trial of emotionally expressive writing for women with metastatic breast cancer. *Health Psychology*, *29*, 460–466.

Lowes, L., Gregory, J. W., & Lyne, P. (2005). Newly diagnosed childhood diabetes: A psychosocial transition for parents? *Journal of Advanced Nursing*, *50*, 253–261.

Lowman, C., Hunt, W. A., Litten, R. Z., & Drummond, D. C. (2000). Research perspectives on alcohol craving: An overview. *Addiction*, *95*(Suppl. 2), 45–54.

Lu, Q., & Stanton, A. L. (2010). How benefits of expressive writing vary as a function of writing instructions, ethnicity and ambivalence over emotional expression. *Psychology & Health*, *25*, 669–684.

Lucas, A. E. M., Smeenk, F. W. J. M., Smeele, I. J., van Schayck, C. P. (2008). Overtreatment with inhaled corticosteroids and diagnostic problems in primary care patients, an exploratory study. *Family Practice*, *25*, 86–91.

Ludwig, D. S., & Ebbeling, C. B. (2001). Type 2 diabetes mellitus in children: Primary care and public health considerations. *Journal of the American Medical Association*, *286*, 1427–1430.

Lundahl, B., & Burke, B. L. (2009). The effectiveness and applicability of motivational interviewing: A practice-friendly review of four meta-analyses. *Journal of Clinical Psychology*, *65*, 1232–1245.

Lundahl, B. W., Kunz, C., Brownell, C., Tollefson, D., & Burke, B. L. (2010). A meta-analysis of motivational interviewing: Twenty-five years of empirical studies. *Research on Social Work Practice*, *20*(2), 137–160.

Luo, X. (2004). Estimates and patterns of direct health care expenditures among individuals with back pain in the United States. *Spine, 29*, 79–86.

Lustman, P. J., & Clouse, R. E. (2005). Depression in diabetic patients: The relationship between mood and glycemic control. *Journal of Diabetes and Its Complications, 19*, 113–122.

Luthar, S. S., & Latendresse, S. J. (2005). Children of the affluent: Challenges to well-being. *Current Directions in Psychological Science, 14*, 49–53.

Lutz, R. W., Silbret, M., & Olshan, W. (1983). Treatment outcome and compliance with therapeutic regimens: Long-term follow-up of a multidisciplinary pain program. *Pain, 17*, 301–308.

Lycett, D., Munafò, M., Johnstone, E., Murphy, M., & Aveyard, P. (2011). Associations between weight change over 8 years and baseline body mass index in a cohort of continuing and quitting smokers. *Addiction, 106*(1), 188–196.

Lynch, H. T., Deters, C. A., Snyder, C. L., Lynch, J. F., Villeneuve, P., Silberstein, J., et al. (2005). BRCA1 and pancreatic cancer: Pedigree findings and their causal relationships. *Cancer Genetics and Cytogenetics, 158*, 119–125.

Lyvers, M., Cholakians, E., Puorro, M., & Sundram, S. (2011). Alcohol intoxication and self-reported risky sexual behaviour intentions with highly attractive strangers in naturalistic settings. *Journal of Substance Use, 16*(2), 99–108.

Lyytikäinen, P., Rahkonen, O., Lahelma, E., & Lallukka, T. (2011). Association of sleep duration with weight and weight gain: A prospective follow-up study. *Journal of Sleep Research, 20*(2), 298–302.

MacDonald, G., & Leary, M. R. (2005). Why does social exclusion hurt? The relationship between social and physical pain. *Psychological Bulletin, 131*, 202–223.

MacDougall, J. M., Dembroski, T. M., Dimsdale, J. E., & Hackett, T. P. (1985). Components of Type A, hostility, and anger-in: Further relationships to angiographic findings. *Health Psychology, 4*, 137–142.

Macedo, A., Baños, J.-E., & Farré, M. (2008). Placebo response in the prophylaxis of migraine: A meta-analysis. *European Journal of Pain, 12*, 68–75.

Maciejewski, P. K., Zhang, B., Block, S. D., & Prigerson, H. G. (2007). An empirical examination of the stage theory of grief. *Journal of the American Medical Association, 297*, 716–723.

Mackay, J., & Mensah, G. (2004). *The atlas of heart disease and stroke*. Geneva: World Health Organization and Centers for Disease Control and Prevention.

MacKellar, D. A., Valleroy, L. A., Secura, G. M., Behel, S., Bingham, T., Celentano, D. D., et al. (2007). Perceptions of lifetime risk and actual risk for acquiring HIV among young men who have sex with men. *AIDS and Behavior, 11*, 263–270.

Mackenbach, J. P., Stirbu, I., Roskam, J.-A. R. Schaap, M. M., Menvielle, G., Leinsalu, M., et al. (2008). Socioeconomic inequalities in health in 22 European countries. *New England Journal of Medicine, 358*, 2468–2481.

Macrodimitris, S. D., & Endler, N. S. (2001). Coping, control, and adjustment in Type 2 diabetes. *Health Psychology, 20*, 208–216.

Maenthaisong, R., Chaiyakunapruk, N., Niruntraporn, S., & Kongkaew, C. (2007). The efficacy of aloe vera used for burn wound healing: A systematic review. *Burns, 33*, 713–718.

Magura, S. (2007). The relationship between substance user treatment and 12-step fellowships: Current knowledge and research questions. *Substance Use and Misuse, 42*, 343–360.

Mahar, M. (2006). *Money-driven medicine: The real reason health care costs so much*. New York: HarperCollins.

Maier, S. F. (2003). Bi-directional immune-brain communication: Implications for understanding stress, pain, and cognition. *Brain, Behavior and Immunity, 17*, 269–285.

Maier, S. F., & Watkins, L. R. (2003). Immune-to-central nervous system communication and its role in modulating pain and cognition: Implications for cancer and cancer treatment. *Brain, Behavior and Immunity, 17*, 125–131.

Maizels, M., & McCarberg, B. (2005). Antidepressants and antiepileptic drugs for chronic non-cancer pain. *American Family Physician, 71*, 483–490.

Majdič, G. (2009). Integrative role of brain and hypothalamus in the control of energy balance. *Acta Chimica Slovenica, 56*(2), 289–296.

Major, B., & O'Brien, L. T. (2005). The psychology of stigma. *Annual Review of Psychology, 56*, 393–421.

Malecka-Tendera, E., & Mazur, A. (2006). Childhood obesity: A pandemic of the twenty-first century. *International Journal of Obesity, 30*(Suppl. 2), S1–S3.

Manchikanti, L., Vallejo, R., Manchikanti, K. N., Benyamin, R. M., Datta, S., & Christo, P. J. (2011). Effectiveness of long-term opioid therapy for chronic non-cancer pain. *Pain Physician, 14*, E133–E156.

Mancini, A. D., Bonanno, G. A., & Clark, A. E. (2011). Stepping off the hedonic treadmill: Individual differences in response to major life events. *Journal of Individual Differences, 32*, 144–152.

Mancini, A. D., Griffin, P., & Bonanno, G. A. (2012). Recent trends in the treatment of prolonged grief. *Current Opinion in Psychiatry, 25*, 46–51.

Mandayam, S. (2004). Epidemiology of alcoholic liver disease. *Seminars in Liver Disease, 24*, 217–232.

Mangels, A. R., Messina, V., & Melina, V. (2003). Vegetarian diets. *Journal of the American Dietetic Association, 103*, 748–765.

Manheimer, E., White, A., Berman, B., Forys, K., & Ernst, E. (2005). Meta-analysis: Acupuncture for low back pain. *Annals of Internal Medicine, 142*, 651–663.

Manimala, M. R., Blount, R. L., & Cohen, L. L. (2000). The effects of parental reassurance versus distraction on child distress and coping during immunizations. *Children's Health Care, 29*, 161–177.

Mann, D. M., Ponieman, D., Leventhal, H., & Halm, E. (2009). Predictors of adherence to diabetes medications: The role of disease and medication beliefs. *Journal of Behavioral Medicine, 32*, 278–284.

Mann, D. M., Woodward, M., Muntner, P., Falzon, L., & Kronish, I. (2010). Predictors of nonadherence to statins: A systematic review and meta-analysis. *The Annals of Pharmacotherapy, 44*, 1410–1421.

Mann, K. (2004). Pharmacotherapy of alcohol dependence: A review of the clinical data. *CNS Drugs, 18*, 485–504.

Mann, K., & Hermann, D. (2010). Individualised treatment in alcohol-dependent patients. *European Archives of Psychiatry & Clinical Neuroscience, 260*, 116–120.

Manna, A., Raffone, A., Perrucci, M. G., Nardo, D., Ferretti, A., Tartaro, A., et al. (2010). Neural correlates of focused attention and cognitive monitoring in meditation. *Brain Research Bulletin, 82*(1/2), 46–56.

Mannan, H. R., Stevenson, C. E., Peeters, A., Walls, H. L., & McNeil, J. J. (2011). Age at quitting smoking as a predictor of risk of cardiovascular disease incidence independent of smoking status, time since quitting and pack-years. *BMC Research Notes, 4*(1), 39–47.

Manne, S. L., & Andrykowski, M. A. (2006). Are psychological interventions effective and accepted by cancer patients? II. Using empirically supported therapy guidelines to decide. *Annals of Behavioral Medicine, 32*, 98–103.

Manni, L., Albanesi, M., Guaragna, M., Barbaro Paparo, S., & Aloe, L. (2010). Neurotrophins and acupuncture. *Autonomic Neuroscience: Basic & Clinical, 157*(1/2), 9–17.

Manor, O., Eisenbach, Z., Friedlander, Y., & Kark, J. D. (2004). Educational differentials in mortality from cardiovascular disease among men and women: The Israel Longitudinal Mortality Study. *Annals of Epidemiology, 14*, 453–460.

Mantell, J. E., Stein, Z. A., & Susser, I. (2008). Women in the time of AIDS: Barriers, bargains, and benefits. *AIDS Education and Prevention, 20*, 91–106.

Mao, J. J., Palmer, C. S., Healy, K. E., Desai, K., & Amsterdam, J. (2011). Complementary and alternative medicine use among cancer survivors: A population-based study. *Journal of Cancer Survivorship: Research and Practice, 5*(1), 8–17.

Marcus, D. A. (2001). Gender differences in treatment-seeking chronic headache sufferers. *Headache, 41*, 698–703.

Margolis, R. D., & Zweben, J. E. (2011). *Treating patients with alcohol and other drug problems: An integrated approach* (2nd ed.). Washington, DC: American Psychological Association.

Mariotto, A. B., Yabroff, K. R., Shao, Y., Feuer, E. J., & Brown, M. L. (2011). Projections of the cost of cancer care in the United States: 2010–2020. *Journal of the National Cancer Institute, 103*, 117–128.

Markovitz, J. H., Matthews, K. A., Whooley, M., Lewis, C. E., & Greenlund, K. J. (2004). Increases in job strain are associated with incident hypertension in the CARDIA study. *Annals of Behavioral Medicine, 28*, 4–9.

Marlatt, G. A., Demming, B., & Reid, J. (1973). Loss of control drinking in alcoholics: An experimental analogue. *Journal of Abnormal Psychology, 81*, 233–241.

Marlatt, G. A., & Gordon, J. R. (1980). Determinants of relapse: Implication for the maintenance of behavior change. In P. O. Davidson & S. M. Davidson (Eds.), *Behavioral medicine: Changing health lifestyles* (pp. 410–452). New York: Brunner/Mazel.

Marlatt, G. A., & Rohsenow, D. J. (1980). Cognitive processes in alcohol use: Expectancy and the balanced placebo design. In N. Mello (Ed.), *Advances in substance abuse: Behavioral and biological research* (pp. 159–199). Greenwich, CT: JAI Press.

Marlowe, N. (1998). Stressful events, appraisal, coping and recurrent headache. *Journal of Clinical Psychology, 54*, 247–256.

Marques, L., Alegria, M., Becker, A. E., Chen, C.-N., Fang, A., Chosak, A., et al. (2011). Comparative prevalence, correlates of impairment, and service utilization for eating disorders across US ethnic groups: Implications for reducing ethnic disparities in health care access for eating disorders. *International Journal of Eating Disorders, 44*(5), 412–420.

Marquié, L., Raufaste, E., Lauque, D., Mariné, C., Ecoiffier, M., & Sorum, P. (2003). Pain rating by patients and physicians: Evidence of systematic miscalibration. *Pain, 102*, 289–296.

Marsland, A. L., Bachen, E. A., Cohen, S., & Manuck, S. B. (2001). Stress, immunity, and susceptibility to infectious disease. In A. Baum, T. A. Revenson, & J. E. Singer (Eds.), *Handbook of health psychology* (pp. 683–695). Mahwah, NJ: Erlbaum.

Marsland, A. L., Bachen, E. A., Cohen, S., Rabin, B., & Manuck, S. B. (2002). Stress, immune reactivity and susceptibility to infectious disease. *Physiology and Behavior, 77*, 711–716.

Martikainen, P., Valkonen, T., & Martelin, T. (2001). Change in male and female life expectancy by social class: Decomposition by age and cause of death in Finland 1971–95. *Journal of Epidemiology and Community Health, 55*, 494–499.

Martin, C. S., Fillmore, M. T., Chung, T., Easdon, C. M., & Miczek, K. A. (2006). Multidisciplinary perspectives on impaired control over substance use. *Alcoholism: Clinical and Experimental Research, 30*, 265–271.

Martin, P. D., & Brantley, P. J. (2004). Stress, coping, and social support in health and behavior. In J. M. Raczynsky & L. C. Leviton (Eds.), *Handbook of clinical health psychology* (Vol. 2, pp. 233–267). Washington, DC: American Psychological Association.

Martin, P. R., Forsyth, M. R., & Reece, J. (2007). Cognitive-behavioral therapy versus temporal pulse amplitude biofeedback training for recurrent headache. *Behavior Therapy, 38*, 350–363.

Martin, P. R., & Petry, N. M. (2005). Are non-substance- related addictions really addictions? *American Journal on Addictions, 14*, 1–3.

Martin, R., & Lemos, K. (2002). From heart attacks to melanoma: Do common sense models of somatization influence symptoms interpretation for female victims? *Health Psychology, 21*, 25–32.

Martin, R., & Leventhal, H. (2004). Symptom perception and health care–seeking behavior. In J. M. Raczynski & L. C. Leviton (Eds.), *Handbook of clinical health psychology* (Vol. 2, pp. 299–328). Washington, DC: American Psychological Association.

"Martin Sheen." (2008, May 27). Martin Sheen opens up about drug use. *Associated Press.* Retrieved June 26, 2011, from http://www.military.com/entertainment/movies/movie-news/martin-sheen-opens-up-about-drug-use

Martindale, D. (2001, May 26). Needlework: Whether it's controlling the flow of vital energy or releasing painkilling chemicals, acupuncture seems plausible enough. But does it really work? *New Scientist, 170*, 42–45.

Martinez, F. D. (2001). The coming-of-age of the hygiene hypothesis. *Respiratory Research, 2*, 129–132.

Martins, I. J., Hone, E., Foster, J. K., Sünram-Lea, S. I., Gnjec, A., Fuller, S. J., et al. (2006). Apolipoprotein E, cholesterol metabolism, diabetes, and the convergence of risk factors for Alzheimer's disease and cardiovascular disease. *Molecular Psychiatry, 11*, 721–736.

Martins, R. K., & McNeil, D. W. (2009). Review of motivational interviewing in promoting health behaviors. *Clinical Psychology Review, 29*, 283–293.

Martinsen, E. W. (2005). Exercise and depression. *International Journal of Sport and Exercise Psychology, 3*(Special Issue), 469–483.

Martire, L. M., Lustig, A. P., Schulz, R., Miller, G. E., & Helgeson, V. S. (2004). Is it beneficial to involve a family member? A meta-analysis of psychosocial intervention for chronic illness. *Health Psychology, 23*, 599–611.

Martire, L. M., & Schulz, R. (2007). Involving family in psychosocial interventions for chronic illness. *Current Directions in Psychological Science, 16*, 90–94.

Martire, L. M., Schulz, R., Helgeson, V. S., Small, B. J., & Saghafi, E. M. (2010). Review and meta-analysis of couple-oriented interventions for chronic illness. *Annals of Behavioral Medicine, 40*, 325–342.

Mason, J. W. (1971). A reevaluation of the concept of "non-specificity" in stress theory. *Journal of Psychiatric Research, 8*, 323–333.

Mason, J. W. (1975). A historical view of the stress field. *Journal of Human Stress, 1* (Pt. 2), 22–36.

Mason, P. (2005). Deconstructing endogenous pain modulation. *Journal of Neurophysiology, 94*, 1659–1663.

Masters, K. S., & Spielmans, G. I. (2007). Prayer and health: Review, meta-analysis, and research agenda. *Journal of Behavioral Medicine, 30*, 329–338.

Masters, K. S., Spielmans, G. I., & Goodson, J. T. (2005, August). *Meta-analytic review of distant intercessory prayer studies.* Paper presented at the 113th convention of the American Psychological Association, Washington, DC.

Masur, F. T., III. (1981). Adherence to health care regimens. In C. K. Prokop & L. A. Bradley (Eds.), *Medical psychology: Contributions to behavioral medicine* (pp. 441–470). New York: Academic Press.

Matarazzo, J. D. (1987). Postdoctoral education and training of service providers in health psychology. In G. C. Stone, S. M. Weiss, J. D. Matarazzo, N. E. Miller, J. Rodin, C. D. Belar, et al. (Eds.), *Health psychology: A discipline and a profession* (pp. 371–388). Chicago, IL: University of Chicago Press.

Matarazzo, J. D. (1994). Health and behavior: The coming together of science and practice in psychology and medicine after a century of benign neglect. *Journal of Clinical Psychology in Medical Settings, 1*, 7–39.

Mathers, M. I., Salomon, J. A., Tandon, A., Chatterji, S., Ustün, B., & Murray, C. J. L. (2004). Global patterns of healthy life expectancy in the year 2002. *BMC Public Health, 4*, record 66. Retrieved August 9, 2005, from http://www.biomedcentral.com/1471-2458/4/66

Matthews, A. M., Wilson, V. B., & Mitchell, S. H. (2011). The role of antipsychotics in smoking and smoking cessation. *CNS Drugs, 25*(4), 299–315.

Matthews, K. (2005). Former president to have scar tissue removed. *Associated Press.* Retrieved June 16, 2005, from http://www.greatdreams.com/political/clinton-heart.htm

Matthews, K. A. (2005). Psychological perspectives on the development of heart disease. *American Psychologist, 60*, 783–796.

Matthews, K. A., & Gallo, L. C. (2011). Psychological perspectives on pathways linking socioeconomic status and physical health. *Annual Review of Psychology, 62*, 501–530.

Matthews, K. A., Gallo, L. C., & Taylor, S. E. (2010). Are psychosocial factors mediators of socioeconomic status and health connections? A progress report and blueprint for the future. *Annals of the New York Academy of Sciences, 1186,* 146–173.

Matthews, K. A., Kuller, L. H., Chang, Y., & Edmundowicz, D. (2007). Premenopausal risk factors for coronary and aortic calcification: A 20-year follow-up in the healthy women study. *Preventive Medicine, 45,* 302–308.

Matthies, E., Hoeger, R., & Guski, R. (2000). Living on polluted soil: Determinants of stress symptoms. *Environment and Behavior, 32,* 270–286.

Matud, M. P. (2004). Gender differences in stress and coping styles. *Personality and Individual Differences, 37,* 1401–1415.

Mausbach, B. T., Coon, D. W., Depp, C., Rabinowitz, Y. G., Wilson-Arias, E., Kraemer, H. C., et al. (2004). Ethnicity and time to institutionalization of dementia patients: A comparison of Latina and Caucasian female family caregivers. *Journal of the American Geriatrics Society, 52,* 1077–1084.

Mausbach, B. T., Semple, S. J., Strathdee, S. A., & Patterson, T. L. (2009). Predictors of safer sex intentions and protected sex among heterosexual HIV-negative methamphetamine users: An expanded model of the Theory of Planned Behavior. *AIDS Care, 21,* 17–24.

Mayeaux, R. (2003). Epidemiology of neurogeneration. *Annual Review of Neuroscience, 26,* 81–104.

Mayfield, D. (1976). Alcoholism, alcohol intoxication, and assaultive behavior. *Diseases of the Nervous System, 37,* 228–291.

Maynard, L. M., Serdula, M. K., Galuska, D. A., Gillespie, C., & Mokdad, A. H. (2006). Secular trends in desired weight of adults. *International Journal of Obesity, 30,* 1375–1381.

Mayo Clinic Staff. (2008). *Vegetarian diet: How to get the best nutrition.* Retrieved May 5, 2008, from http://www.mayoclinic.com/print/vegetarian-diet/HQ01596/METHOD=print

Mayo-Smith, M. F., Beecher, L. H., Fischer, T. L., Gorelick, D. A., Guillaunce, J. L., Hill, A., et al. (2004). Management of alcohol withdrawal delirium: An evidence-based practice guideline. *Archives of Internal Medicine, 164,* 1405–1412.

Maziak, W. (2011). The global epidemic of waterpipe smoking. *Addictive Behaviors, 36*(1/2), 1–5.

McCaffrey, A. M., Eisenberg, D. M., Legedza, A. T. R., Davis, R. B., & Phillips, R. S. (2004). Prayer for health concerns: Results of a national survey on prevalence and patterns of use. *Archives of Internal Medicine, 164,* 858–862.

McCallie, M. S., Blum, C. M., & Hood, C. J. (2006). Progressive muscle relaxation. *Journal of Human Behavior in the Social Environment, 13,* 51–66.

McClave, A. K., McKnight-Eily, L. R., Davis, S. P., & Dube, S. R. (2010). Smoking characteristics of adults with selected lifetime mental illnesses: Results from the 2007 National Health Interview Survey. *American Journal of Public Health, 100*(12), 2464–2472.

McColl, K. E. L., Watabe, H., & Derakhshan, M. H. (2007). Sporadic gastric cancer: A complex interaction of genetic and environmental risk factors. *American Journal of Gastroenterology, 102,* 1893–1895.

McCracken, L. M., Eccleston, C., & Bell, L. (2005). Clinical assessment of behavioral coping responses: Preliminary results from a brief inventory. *European Journal of Pain, 9,* 69–78.

McCrae, R. R., & Costa, P. T., Jr. (2003). *Personality in adulthood: A five-factor theory perspective* (2nd ed.). New York: Guilford Press.

McCullough, M. L., Patel, A. V., Kushi, L. H., Patel, R., Willett, W. C., Doyle, C., et al. (2011). Following cancer prevention guidelines reduces risk of cancer, cardiovascular disease, and all-cause mortality. *Cancer Epidemiology, Biomarkers & Prevention, 20,* 1089. DOI: 10.1158/1055-9965.EPI-10-1173.

McDaniel, S. H., Belar, C. D., Schroeder, C., Hargrove, D. S., & Freeman, E. L. (2002). A training curriculum for professional psychologists in primary care. *Professional Psychology: Research and Practice, 33,* 65–72.

McDaniel, S. H., & le Roux, P. (2007). An overview of primary care family psychology. *Journal of Clinical Psychology in Medical Settings, 14,* 23–32.

McEachan, R. R. C., Conner, M., Taylor, N. J., & Lawton, R. J. (2011). Prospective prediction of health-related behaviours with the Theory of Planned Behaviour: A meta-analysis. *Health Psychology Review, 5,* 97–144.

McEwen, A., West, R., & McRobbie, H. (2008). Motives for smoking and their correlates in clients attending Stop Smoking treatment services. *Nicotine and Tobacco Research, 10,* 843–850.

McEwen, B. S. (2005). Stressed or stressed out: What is the difference? *Journal of Psychiatry and Neuroscience, 30,* 315–318.

McEwen, B. S., & Gianaros, P. J. (2010). Central role of the brain in stress and adaptation: Links to socioeconomic status, health, and disease. *Annals of the New York Academy of Sciences, 1186,* 190–222.

McGee, D. L. (2005). Body mass index and mortality: A meta-analysis based on person-level data from twenty-six observational studies. *Annals of Epidemiology, 15,* 87–97.

McGregor, B. A., & Antoni, M. H. (2009). Psychological intervention and health outcomes among women treated for breast cancer: A review of stress pathways and biological mediators. *Brain, Behavior, and Immunity, 23,* 159–166.

McGuire, B. E., & Shores, E. A. (2001). Simulated pain on the Symptom Checklist 90–Revised. *Journal of Clinical Psychology, 57,* 1589–1596.

McHugh, M. D. (2007). Readiness for change and short-term outcomes of female adolescents in residential treatment for anorexia nervosa. *International Journal of Eating Disorders, 40,* 602–612.

McIntosh, C. N., Fines, P., Wilkins, R., & Wolfson, M. C. (2009). Income disparities in health-adjusted life expectancy for Canadian adults, 1991 to 2001. *Health Reports, 20,* 55–64.

McKay, D., & Schare, M. L. (1999). The effects of alcohol and alcohol expectancies on subjective reports and physiological reactivity: A meta-analysis. *Addictive Behaviors, 24,* 633–647.

McKay, J. R., & Hiller-Sturmhöfel, S. (2010). Treating alcoholism as a chronic disease: Approaches to long-term continuing care. *Alcohol Research & Health, 33*(4), 356–370.

McKechnie, R., Macleod, R., & Keeling, S. (2007). Facing uncertainty: The lived experience of palliative care. *Palliative and Supportive Care, 5,* 367–376.

McKee, S. A., Sinha, R., Weinberger, A. H., Sofuoglu, M., Harrison, E. L. R., Lavery, M., et al. (2011). Stress decreases the ability to resist smoking and potentiates smoking intensity and reward. *Journal of Psychopharmacology, 25*(4), 490–502.

McLean, S., Skirboll, L. R., & Pert, C. B. (1985). Comparison of substance P and enkephalin distribution in rat brain: An overview using radio-immunocytochemistry. *Neuroscience, 14,* 837–852.

McLellan, A. T., Lewis, D. C., O'Brien, C. P., & Kleber, H. D. (2000). Drug dependence, a chronic medical illness: Implications for treatment, insurance, and outcomes. *Journal of the American Medical Association, 284,* 1689–1695.

McNally, R. J. (2003). Progress and controversy in the study of post-traumatic stress disorder. *Annual Review of Psychology, 54,* 229–252.

McRae, C., Cherin, E., Tamazaki, T. G., Diem, G., Vo, A. H., Russell, D., et al. (2004). Effects of perceived treatment on quality of life and medical outcomes in a double-blind placebo surgery trial. *Archives of General Psychiatry, 61,* 412–420.

McWilliams, J. M. (2009). Health consequences of uninsurance among adults in the United States: Recent evidence and implications. *The Milbank Quarterly, 87,* 443–494.

McWilliams, L. A., Goodwin, R. D., & Cox, B. J. (2004). Depression and anxiety associated with three pain conditions: Results from a nationally representative sample. *Pain, 111,* 77–83.

Mechanic, D. (1978). *Medical sociology* (2nd ed.). New York: Free Press.

Mehler, P. S. (2011). Medical complications of bulimia nervosa and their treatments. *International Journal of Eating Disorders, 44*(2), 95–104.

Mehta, P., & Sharma, M. (2012). Internet and cell phone based physical activity interventions in adults. *Archives of Exercise in Health and Disease, 2,* 108–113.

Meichenbaum, D. (2007). Stress inoculation training: A preventative and treatment approach. In P. M. Lehrer, R. L. Woolfolk, & W. E. Sime

(Eds.), *Principles and practices of stress management* (3rd ed., pp. 497–517). New York: Guilford Press.

Meichenbaum, D., & Cameron, R. (1983). Stress inoculation training: Toward a general paradigm for training coping skills. In D. Meichenbaum & M. E. Jaremko (Eds.), *Stress reduction and prevention* (pp. 115–154). New York: Plenum Press.

Meichenbaum, D., & Turk, D. C. (1976). The cognitive-behavioral management of anxiety, anger and pain. In P. O. Davidson (Ed.), *The behavioral management of anxiety, depression, and pain* (pp. 1–34). New York: Brunner/Mazel.

Melamed, B. G., Kaplan, B., & Fogel, J. (2001). Childhood health issues across the life span. In A. Baum, T. A. Revenson, & J. E. Singer (Eds.), *Handbook of health psychology* (pp. 449–457). Mahwah, NJ: Erlbaum.

Melzack, R. (1973). *The puzzle of pain*. New York: Basic Books.

Melzack, R. (1975). The McGill Pain Questionnaire: Major properties and scoring methods. *Pain, 1,* 277–299.

Melzack, R. (1987). The short-form McGill Pain Questionnaire. *Pain, 30,* 191–197.

Melzack, R. (1992, April). Phantom limbs. *Scientific American, 266,* 120–126.

Melzack, R. (1993). Pain: Past, present and future. *Canadian Journal of Experimental Psychology, 47,* 615–629.

Melzack, R. (2005). Evolution of the neuromatrix theory of pain. *Pain Practice, 5,* 85–94.

Melzack, R. (2008). The future of pain. *Nature Reviews Drug Discovery, 7,* 629.

Melzack, R., & Katz, J. (2001). The McGill Pain Questionnaire: Appraisal and current status. In D. C. Turk & R. Melzack (Eds.), *Handbook of pain assessment* (2nd ed., pp. 35–52). New York: Guilford Press.

Melzack, R., & Wall, P. D. (1965). Pain mechanisms: A new theory. *Science, 150,* 971–979.

Melzack, R., & Wall, P. D. (1982). *The challenge of pain*. New York: Basic Books.

Melzack, R., & Wall, P. D. (1988). *The challenge of pain* (rev. ed.). London: Penguin.

Mercken, L., Candel, M., Willems, P., & de Vries, H. (2007). Disentangling social selection and social influence effects on adolescent smoking: The importance of reciprocity in friendships. *Addiction, 102,* 1483–1492.

Merritt, M. M., Bennett, G. G., Williams, R. B., Sollers, J. J., III, & Thayer, J. F. (2004). Low educational attainment, John Henryism, and cardiovascular reactivity to and recovery from personally relevant stress. *Psychosomatic Medicine, 66,* 49–55.

Michael, K. C., Torres, A., & Seemann, E. A. (2007). Adolescents' health habits, coping styles and self-concept are predicted by exposure to interparental conflict. *Journal of Divorce and Remarriage, 48,* 155–174.

Michaud, D. S. (2007). Chronic inflammation and bladder cancer. *Urologic Oncology, 25,* 260–268.

"Michelle Obama." (2011, Feb. 8). Michelle Obama: President quit smoking. *HuffPost Politics.* Retrieved June 4, 2011, from http://www.huffingtonpost.com/2011/02/08/michelle-obama-president-_n_820340.html

Michie, S., O'Connor, D., Bath, J., Giles, M., & Earll, L. (2005). Cardiac rehabilitation: The psychological changes that predict health outcome and healthy behaviour. *Psychology, Health and Medicine, 10,* 88–95.

Milam, J. E. (2004). Posttraumatic growth among HIV/AIDS patients. *Journal of Applied Social Psychology, 34,* 2353–2376.

Miles, L. (2007). Physical activity and the prevention of cancer: A review of recent findings. *Nutrition Bulletin, 32,* 250–282.

Miligi, L., Costantini, A. S., Veraldi, A., Benvenuti, A., & Vineis, P. (2006). Cancer and pesticides. *Annals of the New York Academy of Sciences, 1076,* 366–377.

Miller, D. B., & Townsend, A. (2005). Urban hassles as chronic stressors and adolescent mental health: The Urban Hassles Index. *Brief Treatment and Crisis Intervention, 5,* 85–94.

Miller, F. G., & Wager, T. (2004). Painful deception. *Science, 304,* 1109–1111.

Miller, G. E., & Blackwell, E. (2006). Turning up the heat: Inflammation as a mechanism linking chronic stress, depression, and heart disease. *Current Directions in Psychological Science, 15,* 269–272.

Miller, G. E., & Cohen, S. (2001). Psychological interventions and the immune system: A meta-analytic review and critique. *Health Psychology, 20,* 47–63.

Miller, L. G., Liu, H., Hays, R. D., Golin, C. E., Beck, C. K., Asch, S. M., et al. (2002). How well do clinicians estimate patients' adherence to combination antiretroviral therapy? *Journal of General Internal Medicine, 17,* 1–11.

Miller, M., Hemenway, D., & Rimm, E. (2000). Cigarettes and suicide: A prospective study of 50,000 men. *American Journal of Public Health, 90,* 768–773.

Miller, N. E. (1969). Learning of visceral and glandular responses. *Science, 163,* 434–445.

Miller, V. A., & Drotar, D. (2003). Discrepancies between mother and adolescent perceptions of diabetes-related decision-making autonomy and their relationship to diabetes-related conflict and adherence to treatment. *Journal of Pediatric Psychology, 28,* 265–274.

Miller, W. R., & Rollnick, S. (2002). *Motivational interviewing: Preparing people for change* (2nd ed.). New York: Guilford Press.

Miller, W. R., Walters, S. T., & Bennett, M. E. (2001). How effective is alcoholism treatment in the United States? *Journal of Studies on Alcohol, 62,* 211–220.

Miller, W. R., Wilbourne, P. L., & Hettema, J. E. (2003). What works? A summary of alcohol treatment outcome research. In R. K. Hester & W. R. Miller (Eds.), *Handbook of alcoholism treatment approaches: Effective alternatives* (3rd ed., pp. 13–63). Boston: Allyn and Bacon.

Milling, L. S., Kirsch, I., Allen, G. J., & Reutenauer, E. L. (2005). The effects of hypnotic and nonhypnotic imaginative suggestion on pain. *Annals of Behavioral Medicine, 29,* 116–127.

Milling, L. S., Levine, M. R., & Meunier, S. A. (2003). Hypnotic enhancement of cognitive-behavioral interventions for pain: An analogue treatment study. *Health Psychology, 22,* 406–413.

Mills, N., Allen, J., & Morgan, S. C. (2000). Does tai chi/qi gong help patients with multiple sclerosis? *Journal of Bodywork and Movement Therapies, 4,* 39–48.

Miniño, A. M., Murphy, S. L., Xu, J., & Kochanek, K. D. (2011 December, 7). Deaths: Final data for 2008. *National Vital Statistics Reports, 59*(10).

Mitchell, M., Johnston, L., & Keppell, M. (2004). Preparing children and their families for hospitalization: A review of the literature. *Paediatric and Child Health Nursing, 7*(2), 5–15.

Mitchell, W. (2001). Neurological and developmental effects of HIV and AIDS in children and adolescents. *Mental Retardation and Developmental Disabilities Research Reviews, 7,* 211–216.

Miyazaki, T., Ishikawa, T., Iimori, H., Miki, A., Wenner, M., Fukunishi, I., et al. (2003). Relationship between perceived social support and immune function. *Stress and Health, 19,* 3–7.

Moak, Z. B., & Agrawal, A. (2010). The association between perceived interpersonal social support and physical and mental health: results from the national epidemiological survey on alcohol and related conditions. *Journal of Public Health, 32,* 191–201.

Mochly-Rosen, D., & Zakhari, S. (2010). Focus on: The cardiovascular system: What did we learn from the French (paradox)? *Alcohol Research & Health, 33*(1/2), 76–88.

Mock, J., & Wang, J. (2011, March 29). Celebrity central: Kirstie Alley biography. *People.* Retrieved August 13, 2011, from http://www.people.com/people/kirstie_alley/biography

Moen, P., & Yu, Y. (2000). Effective work/life strategies: Working couples, work conditions, gender, and life quality. *Social Problems, 47,* 291–326.

Moerman, D. (2003). Doctors and patients: The role of clinicians in the placebo effect. *Advances, 19*(1), 14–22.

Moerman, D. (2011). Examining a powerful healing effect through a cultural lens, and finding meaning. *The Journal of Mind-Body Regulation, 1,* 63–72.

Moerman, D., & Jonas, W. B. (2002). Deconstructing the placebo effect and finding the meaning response. *Annals of Internal Medicine, 136,* 471–476.

Moldovan, A. R., & David, D. (2011). Effect of obesity treatments on eating behavior: Psychosocial interventions versus surgical interventions: A systematic review. *Eating Behaviors, 12*(3), 161–167.

Molimard, M., & Le Gros, V. (2008). Impact of patient-related factors on asthma control. *Journal of Asthma, 45,* 109–113.

Molloy, G. J., Perkins-Porras, L., Bhattacharyya, M. R., Strike, P. C., & Steptoe, A. (2008). Practical support predicts medication adherence and attendance at cardiac rehabilitation following acute coronary syndrome. *Journal of Psychosomatic Research, 65,* 581–586.

Molloy, G. J., Perkins-Porras, L., Strike, P. C., & Steptoe, A. (2008). Social networks and partner stress as predictors of adherence to medication, rehabilitation attendance, and quality of life following acute coronary syndrome. *Health Psychology, 27,* 52–58.

Monahan, J. L., & Lannutti, P. J. (2000). Alcohol as social lubricant. *Human Communication Research, 26,* 175–202.

Mongan, J. J., Ferris, T. G., & Lee, T. H. (2008). Options for slowing the growth of health care costs. *New England Journal of Medicine, 358,* 1509–1514.

Monroe, S. M. (2008). Modern approaches to conceptualizing and measuring human life stress. *Annual Review of Clinical Psychology, 4,* 33–52.

Monroe, S. M., & Harkness, K. L. (2005). Life stress, the "kindling" hypothesis, and the recurrence of depression: Considerations from a life stress perspective. *Psychological Review, 112,* 417–445.

Montgomery, G. H., DuHamel, K. N., & Redd, W. H. (2000). A meta-analysis of hypnotically induced analgesia: How effective is hypnosis? *International Journal of Clinical and Experimental Hypnosis, 48,* 138–153.

Montgomery, G. H., Erblich, J., DiLorenzo, T., & Bovbjerg, D. H. (2003). Family and friends with disease: Their impact on perceived risk. *Preventive Medicine, 37,* 242–249.

Moore, J. (2004). The puzzling origins of AIDS. *American Scientist, 92,* 540–547.

Moore, L. L., Visioni, A. J., Qureshi, M. M., Bradlee, M. L., Ellison, R. C., & D'Agostino, R. (2005). Weight loss in overweight adults and the long-term risk of hypertension: The Framingham Study. *Archives of Internal Medicine, 165,* 1298–1303.

Moore, S., Sikora, P., Grunberg, L., & Greenberg, E. (2007). Expanding the tension-reduction model of work stess and alcohol use: Comparison of managerial and non-managerial men and women. *Journal of Management Studies, 44,* 261–283.

Moos, R. H., & Schaefer, J. A. (1984). The crisis of physical illness: An overview and conceptual analysis. In R. H. Moos (Ed.), *Coping with physical illness: Vol. 2. New perspectives* (pp. 3–25). New York: Plenum Press.

Moran, W. R. (2002, January 31). Jackie Joyner-Kersee races against asthma. *USA Today Health.* Retrieved July 7, 2005, from http://www.usatoday.com/news/health/spotlight/2002/01/31/spotlight-kersee.htm

Morgan, W. P. (1979, February). Negative addiction in runners. *The Physician and Sportsmedicine, 7,* 56–63, 67–70.

Morgan, W. P. (1981). Psychological benefits of physical activity. In F. J. Nagle & H. J. Montoye (Eds.), *Exercise in health and disease* (pp. 299–314). Springfield, IL: Thomas.

Morillo, L. E., Alarcon, F., Aranaga, N., Aulet, S., Chapman, E., Conterno, L., et al. (2005). Prevalence of migraine in Latin America. *Headache, 45,* 106–117.

Morley, S., de C. Williams, A. C., & Black, S. (2002). A confirmatory factor analysis of the Beck Depression Inventory in chronic pain. *Pain, 99,* 289–298.

Morris, J. C., Storandt, M., Miller, J. P., McKeel, D. W., Price, J. L., Rubin, E. H., et al. (2001). Mild cognitive impairment represents early-stage Alzheimer disease. *Archives of Neurology, 58,* 397–405.

Morris, J. N., Heady, J. A., Raffle, P. A. B., Roberts, C. G., & Parks, J. W. (1953). Coronary heart disease and physical activity of work. *Lancet, 2,* 1053–1057, 1111–1120.

Morrison, C. D. (2008). Leptin resistance and the response to positive energy balance. *Physiology and Behavior, 94,* 660–663.

Moseley, J. B., O'Malley, K. P., Petersen, N. J., Menke, T. J., Brody, B. A., Kuykendall, D. H., et al. (2002). A controlled trial of arthroscopic surgery for osteoarthritis of the knee. *New England Journal of Medicine, 347,* 81–88.

Moskowitz, J. T. (2003). Positive affect predicts lower risk of AIDS mortality. *Psychosomatic Medicine, 65,* 620–626.

Moskowitz, J. T., Hult, J. R., Bussolari, C., & Acree, M. (2009). What works in coping with HIV? A meta-analysis with implications for coping with serious illness. *Psychological Bulletin, 135,* 121–141.

Moskowitz, J. T., & Wrubel, J. (2005). Coping with HIV as a chronic illness: A longitudinal analysis of illness appraisals. *Psychology and Health, 20,* 509–531.

Mosley, P. E. (2009). Bigorexia: Bodybuilding and muscle dysmorphia. *European Eating Disorders Review, 17*(3), 191–198.

Motivala, S. J., & Irwin, M. R. (2007). Sleep and immunity: Cytokine pathways linking sleep and health outcomes. *Current Directions in Psychological Science, 16,* 21–25.

Mottillo, S., Filion, K. B., Genest, J., Joseph, L., Pilote, L., Poirier, P., et al. (2010). The metabolic syndrome and cardiovascular risk: A systematic review and meta-analysis. *Journal of the American College of Cardiology, 56,* 1113–1132.

Moussavi, S., Shatterji, S., Verdes, E., Tandon, A., Patel, V., & Ustun, B. (2007). Depression, chronic diseases, and decrements in health: Results from the World Health Surveys. *The Lancet, 370,* 851–858.

Moyer, C. A., Rounds, J., & Hannum, J. W. (2004). Meta-analysis of massage therapy research. *Psychological Bulletin, 130,* 3–18.

Mozaffarian, D., Longstreth, W. T., Lemaitre, R. N., Manolio, T. A., Kuller, L. H., Burke, G. L., et al. (2005). Fish consumption and stroke risk in elderly individuals: The Cardiovascular Health Study. *Archives of Internal Medicine, 165,* 200–206.

Mukamal, K. J., Chen, C. M., Rao, S. R., & Breslow, R. A. (2010). Alcohol consumption and cardiovascular mortality among U.S. adults, 1987 to 2002. *Journal of the American College of Cardiology, 55*(13), 1328–1335.

Mulvaney, C., Kendrick, D., Towner, E., Brussoni, M., Hayes, M., Powell, J., et al. (2009). Fatal and non-fatal fire injuries in England 1995–2004: Time trends and inequalities by age, sex and area of deprivation. *Journal of Public Health, 31*(1), 154–161.

Murgraff, V., White, D., & Phillips, K. (1996). Moderating binge drinking: It is possible to change behavior if you plan it in advance? *Alcohol and Alcoholism, 31,* 577–582.

Murphy, J. K., Stoney, C. M., Alpert, B. S., & Walker, S. S. (1995). Gender and ethnicity in children's cardiovascular reactivity: 7 years of study. *Health Psychology, 14,* 48–55.

Murphy, M. H., Nevill, A. M., Murtagh, E. M., & Holder, R. L. (2007). The effect of walking on fitness, fatness and resting blood pressure: A meta-analysis of randomized, controlled trials. *Preventive Medicine, 44,* 377–385.

Murray, E., Lo, B., Pollack, L., Donelan, K., Catania, J. White, M., et al. (2003). The impact of health information on the internet on the physician-patient relationship. *Archives of Internal Medicine, 163,* 1727–1734.

Murray, J. A. (2001). Loss as a universal concept: A review of the literature to identify common aspects of loss in diverse situations. *Journal of Loss and Trauma, 6,* 219–231.

Murtaugh, M. A. (2004). Meat consumption and the risk of colon and rectal cancers. *Clinical Nutrition, 13,* 61–64.

Murthy, P., Kudlur, S., George, S., & Mathew, G. (2009). A clinical overview of fetal alcohol syndrome. *Addictive Disorders & Their Treatment, 8*(1), 1–12.

Must, A., Barish, E. E., & Bandini, L. G. (2009). Modifiable risk factors in relation to changes in BMI and fatness: What have we learned from prospective studies of school-aged children? *International Journal of Obesity, 33*(7), 705–715.

Mustard, T. R., & Harris, A. V. E. (1989). Problems in understanding prescription labels. *Perceptual and Motor Skills, 69,* 291–299.

Muthen, B. O., & Muthen, L. K. (2000). The development of heavy drinking and alcohol-related problems from ages 18 to 37 in a U.S. national sample. *Journal of Studies on Alcohol, 61,* 290–300.

Mutti, S., Hammond, D., Borland, R., Cummings, M. K., O'Connor, R. J., & Fong, G. T. (2011). Beyond light and mild: Cigarette brand descriptors and perceptions of risk in the International Tobacco Control (ITC) Four Country Survey. *Addiction, 106*(6), 1166–1175.

Myers, J. (2000). Physical activity and cardiovascular disease. *IDEA Health and Fitness Source, 18,* 38–45.

Myers, T. C., Wonderlich, S. A., Crosby, R., Mitchell, J. E., Steffen, K. J., Smyth, J., et al. (2006). Is multi-impulsive bulimia a distinct type of bulimia nervosa: Psychopathology and EMA findings. *International Journal of Eating Disorders, 39,* 655–661.

Myung, S.-K., McDonnell, D. D., Kazinets, G., Seo, H. G., & Moskowitz, J. M. (2009). Effects of web- and computer-based smoking cessation programs. *Archives of Internal Medicine, 169*(10). 929–937.

Nahin, R. L., Barnes, P. M., Stussman, B. J., & Bloom, B. (2009). Costs of complementary and alternative medicine (CAM) and frequency of visits to CAM practitioners: United States, 2007. *National Health Statistics Reports, 18,* 1–16.

Napadow, V., Kettner, N., Liu, J., Li, M., Kwong, K. K., Vangel, M., et al. (2007). Hypothalamus and amygdala response to acupuncture stimuli in carpal tunnel syndrome. *Pain, 130,* 254–266.

Naparstek, B. (2007). Guided imagery: A best practice for pregnancy and childbirth. *Journal of Childbirth Education, 22,* 4–8.

Nash, J. M., McKay, K. M., Vogel, M. E., & Masters, K. S. (2012). Functional roles and foundational characteristics of psychologists in integrated primary care. *Journal of Clinical Psychology in Medical Settings.* DOI: 10.1007/s10880-011-9290-z.

Nash, J. M., Park, E. R., Walker, B. B., Gordon, N., & Nicholson, R. A. (2004). Cognitive-behavioral group treatment for disabling headache. *Pain Medicine, 5,* 178–186.

Nash, J. M., & Thebarge, R. W. (2006). Understanding psychological stress, its biological processes, and impact on primary headache. *Headache, 46,* 1377–1386.

Nassiri, M. (2005). The effects of regular relaxation on perceived stress in a group of London primary education teachers. *European Journal of Clinical Hypnosis, 6,* 21–29.

National Association for Sport and Physical Education (NASPE). (2002). *Guidelines for infants and toddlers.* Retrieved August 5, 2002, from www.aahperd.org/naspe/template.cfm?template=toddlers.html

National Center for Complementary and Alternative Medicine (NCCAM). (2005/2009). *Ayurvedic medicine: An introduction.* (NCCAM Publication No. D287). Revised July, 2009. Retrieved August 20, 2011, from http://nccam.nih.gov/health/ayurveda/introduction.htm

National Center for Complementary and Alternative Medicine (NCCAM). (2006/2009). *Reiki: An introduction* (NCCAM Publication No. D315). Retrieved August 22, 2011, from http://nccam.nih.gov/health/reiki/introduction.htm

National Center for Complementary and Alternative Medicine (NCCAM). (2006/2010a). *Massage therapy: An introduction* (NCCAM Publication No. D327). Revised August, 2010. Retrieved August 21, 2011, from http://nccam.nih.gov/health/massage/massageintroduction.htm

National Center for Complementary and Alternative Medicine (NCCAM). (2006/2010b). *Meditation: An introduction* (NCCAM Publication No. D308). Revised June, 2010. Retrieved August 21, 2011, from http://nccam.nih.gov/health/meditation/overview.htm

National Center for Complementary and Alternative Medicine (NCCAM). (2006/2010c). *Tai chi: An introduction* (NCCAM Publication No. D322). Revised August, 2010. Retrieved August 22, 2011, from http://nccam.nih.gov/health/taichi/introduction.htm

National Center for Complementary and Alternative Medicine (NCCAM). (2007/2010). *Chiropractic: An introduction* (NCCAM Publication No. D403). Revised October 2010. Retrieved August 20, 2011, from http://nccam.nih.gov/health/chiropractic/introduction.htm

National Center for Complementary and Alternative Medicine (NCCAM). (2007/2011). *Acupuncture: An introduction.* Bethesda, MD: Author. Revised August, 2011. Retrieved September 11, 2011, from http://nccam.nih.gov/health/acupuncture/introduction.htm

National Center for Complementary and Alternative Medicine (NCCAM). (2008). *Yoga for health: An introduction* (NCCAM Publication No. D412). Retrieved August 21, 2011, from http://nccam.nih.gov/health/yoga/introduction.htm

National Center for Complementary and Alternative Medicine (NCCAM). (2008/2011). *What is complementary and alternative medicine?* (NCCAM Publication No. D347). Revised July, 2011. Retrieved August 21, 2011, from http://nccam.nih.gov/health/whatiscam/

National Center for Health Statistics (NCHS). (2011). *Health, United States, 2010.* Hyattsville, MD: U.S. Government Printing Office.

National Task Force on the Prevention and Treatment of Obesity. (2000). Overweight, obesity, and health risk. *Archives of Internal Medicine, 160,* 898–904.

Nausheen, B., Gidron, Y., Peveler, R., & Moss-Morris, R. (2009). Social support and cancer progression: A systematic review. *Journal of Psychosomatic Research, 67,* 403–415.

Naylor, R. T., & Marshall, J. (2007). Autogenic training: A key component in holistic medical practice. *Journal of Holistic Healthcare, 4,* 14–19.

Nelson, H. D., Nevitt, M. C., Scott, J. C., Stone, K. L., & Cummings, S. R. (1994). Smoking, alcohol, and neuromuscular and physical functioning of older women. *Journal of the American Medical Association, 272,* 1825–1831.

Nelson, L. D., & Morrison, E. L. (2005). The symptoms of resource scarcity: Judgments of food and finances influence preferences for potential partners. *Psychological Science, 16,* 167–173.

Nemeroff, C. J. (1995). Magical thinking about illness virulence: Conceptions of germs from "safe" versus "dangerous" others. *Health Psychology, 14,* 147–151.

Nes, L. S., & Segerstrom, S. C. (2006). Dispositional optimism and coping: A meta-analytic review. *Personality and Social Psychology Review, 10,* 235–251.

Nestoriuc, Y., & Martin, A. (2007). Efficacy of biofeedback for migraine: A meta-analysis. *Pain, 128,* 111–127.

Netz, Y., Wu, M.-J., Becker, B. J., & Tenenbaum, G. (2005). Physical activity and psychological well-being in advanced age: A meta-analysis of intervention studies. *Psychology and Aging, 20,* 272–284.

Neumark-Sztainer, D. R., Wall, M. M., Haines, J. I., Story, M. T., Sherwood, N. E., & van den Berg, P. A. (2007). Shared risk and protective factors for overweight and disordered eating in adolescents. *American Journal of Preventive Medicine, 33,* 359–369.

Neumark-Sztainer, D. R., Wall, M. M., Story, M., & Perry, C. L. (2003). Correlates of unhealthy weight-control behaviors among adolescents: Implications for prevention programs. *Health Psychology, 22,* 88–98.

Neville, L. M., O'Hara, B., & Milat, A. J. (2009). Computer-tailored dietary behavior change interventions: A systematic review. *Health Education Research, 24,* 699–720.

Ng, B. H. P., & Tsang, H. W. H. (2009). Psychophysiological outcomes of health qigong for chronic conditions: A systematic review. *Psychophysiology, 46*(2), 257–269.

Ng, J. Y. Y., & Tam, S. F. (2000). Effects of exercise-based cardiac rehabilitation on mobility and self-esteem after cardiac surgery. *Perceptual and Motor Skills, 91,* 107–114.

Ng, M. K. C. (2007). New perspectives on Mars and Venus: Unravelling the role of androgens in gender differences in cardiovascular biology and disease. *Heart, Lung and Circulation, 16,* 185–192.

Nguyen, L. T., Davis, R. B., Kaptchuk, T. J., & Phillips, R. S. (2011). Use of complementary and alternative medicine and self-rated health status: Results of a national survey. *Journal of General Internal Medicine, 26*(4), 399–404.

Nguyen, N. T., Masoomi, H., Magno, C. P., Nguyen, X.-M. T., Laugenour, K., & Lane, J. (2011). Trends in use of bariatric surgery, 2003–2008. *Journal of the American College of Surgeons, 213*(2), 261–266.

Nicassio, P. M., Meyerowitz, B. E., & Kerns, R. D. (2004). The future of health psychology interventions. *Health Psychology, 23*, 132–137.

Nicoll, R. A., & Alger, B. E. (2004, December). The brain's own marijuana. *Scientific American, 291*, 68–75.

Nied, R. J., & Franklin, B. (2002). Promoting and prescribing exercise for the elderly. *American Family Physician, 65*, 419–426, 427–428.

Nielsen, T. S., & Hansen, K. B. (2007). Do green areas affect health? Results from a Danish survey of the use of green areas and health indicators. *Health and Place, 13*, 839–850.

Nieva, G., Ortega, L. L., Mondon, S., Ballbé, M., & Gual, A. (2011). Simultaneous versus delayed treatment of tobacco dependence in alcohol-dependent outpatients. *European Addiction Research, 17*(1), 1–9.

Nikendei, C., Weisbrod, M., Schild, S., Bender, S., Walther, S., & Herzog, W. (2008). Anorexia nervosa: Selective processing of food-related word and pictoral stimuli in recognition and free recall tests. *International Journal of Eating Disorders, 41*, 439–447.

Niswender, K. D., Daws, L. C., Avison, M. J., & Galli, A. (2011). Insulin regulation of monoamine signaling: Pathway to obesity. *Neuropsychopharmacology, 36*(1), 359–360.

Nivison, M. E., & Endresen, I. M. (1993). An analysis of relationships among environmental noise, annoyance and sensitivity to noise, and the consequences for health and sleep. *Journal of Behavior Medicine, 16*, 257–276.

Nocon, M., Hiemann, T., Müller-Riemenschneider, F., Thalau, F., Roll, S., & Willich, S. N. (2008). Association of physical activity with all-cause and cardiovascular mortality: A systematic review and meta-analysis. *European Journal of Cardiovascular Prevention & Rehabilitation, 15*, 239–246.

Nocon, M., Müller-Riemenschneider, F., Nitzschke, K., & Willich, S. N. (2010). Review article: Increasing physical activity with point-of-choice prompts – A systematic review. *Scandinavian Journal of Public Health, 38*, 633–638.

Nordström, A., Karlsson, C., Nyquist, F., Olsson, T., Nordström, P., & Karlsson, M. (2005). Bone loss and fracture risk after reduced physical activity. *Journal of Bone and Mineral Research, 20*, 202–207.

Nori Janosz, K. E., Koenig Berris, K. A., Leff, C., Miller, W. M., Yanez, J., Myers, S., et al. (2008). Clinical resolution of Type 2 diabetes with reduction in body mass index using meal replacement based weight loss. *Vascular Disease Prevention, 5*, 17–23.

Norris, F. H., Byrne, C. M., Diaz, E., & Kaniasty, K. (2001). *The range, magnitude, and duration of effects of natural and human-caused disasters: A review of the empirical literature.* Boston, MA: National Center for PTSD.

Nouwen, A., Winkley, K., Twisk, J., Lloyd, C. E., Peyrot, M., Ismail, K., et al. (2010). Type 2 diabetes mellitus as a risk factor for the onset of depression: A systematic review and meta-analysis. *Diabetologia, 53*, 2480–2486.

Novack, D. H., Cameron, O., Epel, E., Ader, R., Waldstein, S. R., Levenstein, S., et al. (2007). Psychosomatic medicine: The scientific foundation of the biopsychosocial model. *Academic Psychiatry, 31*, 388–401.

Novins, D. K., Beals, J., Moore, L. A., Spicer, P., & Manson, S. M. (2004). Use of biomedical services and traditional healing options among American Indians: Sociodemographic correlates, spirituality, and ethnic identity. *Medical Care, 42*, 670–679.

Nunez-Smith, M., Wolf, E., Huang, H. M., Chen, P., Lee, L., Emanuel, E., et al. (2010). Media exposure and tobacco, illicit drugs, and alcohol use among children and adolescents: A systematic review. *Substance Abuse, 31*(3), 174–192.

"Obama Admits." (2008, June 10). Obama admits smoking cigarettes in last few months. *ABC News.* Retrieved June 2, 2011, from http://blogs.abcnews.com/politicalradar/2008/06/obama-admits-sm.html

O'Brien, C. W., & Moorey, S. (2010). Outlook and adaptation in advanced cancer: A systematic review. *Psycho-Oncology, 19*, 1239–1249.

O'Carroll, R. E., Dryden, J., Hamilton-Barclay, T., & Ferguson, E. (2011). Anticipated regret and organ donor registration: A pilot study. *Health Psychology, 30*, 661–664.

O'Cleirigh, C., Ironson, G., Weiss, A., & Costa, P. T., Jr. (2007). Conscientiousness predicts disease progression (CD4 number and viral load) in people living with HIV. *Health Psychology, 26*, 473–480.

O'Connor, D. B., & Shimizu, M. (2002). Sense of personal control, stress and coping style: A cross-cultural study. *Stress and Health: Journal of the International Society for the Investigation of Stress, 18*, 173–183.

O'Connor, D. W., Ames. D., Gardner, B., & King, M. (2009). Psychosocial treatments of behavior symptoms in dementia: A systematic review of reports meeting quality standards. *International Psychogeriatrics, 21*, 225–240.

O'Connor, R. J., McNeill, A., Borland, R., Hammond, D., King, B., Boudreau, C., et al. (2007). Smokers' beliefs about the relative safety of other tobacco products: Findings from the ITC collaboration. *Nicotine and Tobacco Research, 9*, 1033–1042.

Ogden, C. L., Carroll, M. D., Kit, B. K., & Flegal, K. M. (2012). Prevalence of obesity and trends in body mass index among US children and adolescents, 1999–2010. *Journal of the American Medical Association, 307*, 483–490.

Ogden, J. (2003). Some problems with social cognition models: A pragmatic and conceptual analysis. *Health Psychology, 22*, 424–428.

Ogedegbe, G., Schoenthaler, A., & Fernandez, S. (2007). Appointment-keeping behavior is not related to medication adherence in hypertensive African Americans. *Journal of General Internal Medicine, 22*, 1176–1179.

Oguma, Y., Sesso, H. D., Paffenbarger, R. S., Jr., & Lee, I.-M. (2002). Physical activity and all cause mortality in women: A review of the evidence. *British Journal of Sports Medicine, 36*, 162–172.

Oh, K., Hu, F. B., Manson, J. E., Stampfer, M. J., & Willett, W. C. (2005). Dietary fat intake and risk of coronary heart disease in women: 20 years of follow-up of the Nurses' Health Study. *American Journal of Epidemiology, 161*, 672–679.

Oh, Y.-M., Kim, Y. S., Yoo, S. H., Kim, S. K., & Kim, D. S. (2004). Association between stress and asthma symptoms: A population-based study. *Respirology, 9*, 363–368.

O'Hare, P. (2007). Merseyside, the first harm reduction conferences, and the early history of harm reduction. *International Journal of Drug Policy, 18*, 141–144.

Okuda, M., & Nakazawa, T. (2004). *Helicobacter pylori* infection in childhood. *Journal of Gastroenterology, 39*, 809–810.

Olander, E. K., & Eves, F. F. (2011). Effectiveness and cost of two stair-climbing interventions—Less is more. *American Journal of Health Promotion, 25*, 231–236.

Oldenburg, R. A., Meijers-Heijboer, H., Cornelisse, C. J., & Devilee, P. (2007). Genetic susceptibility for breast cancer: How many more genes to be found? *Critical Reviews in Oncology/Hematology, 63*, 125–149.

O'Leary, C. M., Nassar, N., Zubrick, S. R., Kurinczuk, J. J., Stanley, F., & Bower, C. (2010). Evidence of a complex association between dose, pattern and timing of prenatal alcohol exposure and child behaviour problems. *Addiction, 105*(1), 74–86.

Olesen, J. (1988). Classification and diagnostic criteria for headache disorders, cranial neuralgias, and facial pain: Headache Classification Committee of the International Headache Society [Special issue]. *Cephalalgia, 8*(Suppl. 7), 1–96.

Olivardia, R., Pope, H. G., & Phillips, K. A. (2000). *The Adonis complex: The secret crisis of male body obsession.* New York: Free Press.

O'Loughlin, J., Karp, I., Koulis, T., Paradis, G., & DiFranza, J. (2009). Determinants of first puff and daily cigarette smoking in adolescents. *American Journal of Epidemiology, 170*(5), 585–597.

Olsen, R., & Sutton, J. (1998). More hassle, more alone: Adolescents with diabetes and the role of formal and informal support. *Child Care, Health and Development, 24*, 31–39.

Olshefsky, A. M., Zive, M. M., Scolari, R., & Zuniga, M. (2007). Promoting HIV risk awareness and testing in Latinos living on the U.S.-Mexico Border: The Tu No Me Conoces Social Marketing Campaign. *AIDS Education & Prevention, 19,* 422–435.

Olver, I. N., Taylor, A. E., & Whitford, H. S. (2005). Relationships between patients' pre-treatment expectations of toxicities and post chemotherapy experiences. *Psycho-Oncology, 14,* 25–33.

Oman, R. F., & King, A. C. (2000). The effect of life events and exercise program on the adoption and maintenance of exercise behavior. *Health Psychology, 19,* 605–612.

Ondeck, D. M. (2003). Impact of culture on pain. *Home Health Care Management and Practice, 15,* 255–257.

"Only Eating." (2011, May 10). Kirstie Alley: I'm only eating 1,400 calories a day. *Us Magazine.* Retrieved July 17, 2011, from http://www.usmagazine.com/healthylifestyle/news/kirstie-alley-im-only-eating-1400-calories-a-day-2011105

Operario, D., Adler, N. E., & Williams, D. R. (2004). Subjective social status: Reliability and predictive utility for global health. *Psychology and Health, 19,* 237–246.

Orbell, S., Hodgkins, S., & Sheeran, P. (1997). Implementation intentions and the theory of planned behavior. *Personality and Social Psychology Bulletin, 23,* 945–554.

Orford, J., Krishnan, M., Balaam, M., Everitt, M., & van der Graaf, K. (2004). University student drinking: The role of motivational and social factors. *Drugs: Education, Prevention and Policy, 11,* 407–421.

Organisation for Economic Co-operation and Development (OECD). (2008). *OECD health data 2008: Statistics and indicators for 30 countries.* Paris: Organisation for Economic Co-operation and Development.

Ornish, D., Brown, S. E., Scherwitz, L. W., Billings, J. H., Armstrong, W. T., Ports, T., et al. (1990). Can lifestyle changes reverse coronary heart disease? The Lifestyle Heart Trial. *Lancet, 336,* 129–133.

Ornish, D., Scherwitz, L. W., Billings, J. H., Gould, L., Merritt, T. A., Sparler, S., et al. (1998). Intensive lifestyle changes for reversal of coronary heart disease. *Journal of the American Medical Association, 280,* 2001–2007.

Ortner, C. N. M., MacDonald, T. K., & Olmstead, M. C. (2003). Alcohol intoxication reduces impulsivity in the delay-discounting paradigm. *Alcohol & Alcoholism, 38,* 151–156.

Osborn, C. Y., White, R. O., Cavanaugh, K., Rothman, R. L., & Wallston, K. A. (2009). Diabetes numeracy: An overlooked factor in understanding racial disparities in glycemic control. *Diabetes Care, 32,* 1614–1619.

Osborn, J. W. (2005). Hypothesis: Set-points and long-term control of arterial pressure: A theoretical argument for a long-term arterial pressure control system in the brain rather than the kidney. *Clinical and Experimental Pharmacology and Physiology, 32,* 384–393.

Osborn, R. L., Demoncada, A. C., & Feuerstein, M. (2006). Psychosocial interventions for depression, anxiety, and quality of life in cancer survivors: Meta-analyses. *International Journal of Psychiatry in Medicine, 36,* 13–34.

Osei-Assibey, G., Adi, Y., Kyrou, I., Kumar, S., & Matyka, K. (2011). Pharmacotherapy for overweight/obesity in ethnic minorities and White Caucasians: A systematic review and meta-analysis. *Diabetes, Obesity & Metabolism, 13*(5), 385–393.

Øystein, K. (2008). A broader perspective on education and mortality: Are we influenced by other people's education? *Social Science and Medicine, 66,* 620–636.

Ozer, E. J. (2005). The impact of violence on urban adolescents: Longitudinal effects of perceived school connection and family support. *Journal of Adolescent Research, 20,* 167–192.

Ozer, E. J., Best, S, R., Lipsey, T. L., & Weiss, D. S. (2003). Predictors of posttraumatic stress disorder and symptoms in adults: A meta-analysis. *Psychological Bulletin, 129,* 52–73.

Paasche-Orlow, M. K., Parker, R. M., Gazmararian, J. A., Nielsen-Bohlman, L. T., & Rudd, R. R. (2005). The prevalence of limited health literacy. *Journal of General Internal Medicine, 20,* 175–184.

Pabst, A., Baumeister, S. E., & Kraus, L. (2010). Alcohol-expectancy dimensions and alcohol consumption at different ages in the general population. *Journal of Studies on Alcohol & Drugs, 71*(1), 46–53.

Pace, T. W. W., & Heim, C. M. (2011). A short review on the psycho-neuroimmunology of posttraumatic stress disorder: From risk factors to medical comorbidities. *Brain, Behavior, and Immunity, 25,* 6–13.

Paffenbarger, R. S., Jr., Gima, A. S., Laughlin, M. E., & Black, R. A. (1971). Characteristics of longshoremen related to fatal coronary heart disease and stroke. *American Journal of Public Health, 61,* 1362–1370.

Paffenbarger, R. S., Jr., Laughlin, M. E., Gima, A. S., & Black, R. A. (1970). Work activity of longshoremen as related to death from coronary heart disease and stroke. *New England Journal of Medicine, 282,* 1109–1114.

Paffenbarger, R. S., Jr., Wing, A. L., & Hyde, R. T. (1978). Physical activity as an index of heart attack risk in college alumni. *American Journal of Epidemiology, 108,* 161–175.

Palm, J. (2004). The nature of and responsibility of alcohol and drug problems: Views among treatment staff. *Addiction Research and Theory, 12,* 413–431.

Palombaro, K. M. (2005). Effects of walking-only interventions on bone mineral density at various skeletal sites: A meta-analysis. *Journal of Geriatric Physical Therapy, 28*(3), 102–107.

Pambianco, G., Costacou, T., & Orchard, T. (2007). The determination of cardiovascular risk factor profiles in Type 1 diabetes. *Diabetes, 56*(Suppl. 1), A176–A177.

Panagiotidis, P., Papadopoulou, M., Diakogiannis, I., Iacovides, A., & Kaprinis, G. (2008). Young people and binge drinking. *Annals of General Psychiatry, 7*(Suppl. 1), 1.

Papadaki, A., Hondros, G., Scott, J. A., & Kapsokefalou, M. (2007). Eating habits of university students living at, or away from home in Greece. *Appetite, 49,* 169–176.

Papadopoulos, A., Guida, F., Cénée, S., Cyr, D., Schmaus, A., Radoï, L., et al. (2011). Cigarette smoking and lung cancer in women: Results of the French ICARE case-control study. *Lung Cancer, 74,* 369–377.

Papas, R. K., Belar, C. D., & Rozensky, R. H. (2004). The practice of clinical health psychology: Professional issues. In R. G. Frank, A. Baum, & J. L. Wallander (Eds.), *Handbook of clinical health psychology* (Vol. 3, pp. 293–319). Washington, DC: American Psychological Association.

Paradis, S., & Cabanac, M. (2008). Dieting and food choice in grocery shopping. *Physiology & Behavior, 93*(4/5), 1030–1032.

Parchman, M. L., Noel, P. H., & Lee, S. (2005). Primary care attributes, health care system hassles, and chronic illness. *Medical Care, 43,* 1123–1129.

Park, J. (2005). Use of alternative health care. *Health Reports, 16*(2), 39–42.

Parker, C. S., Zhen, C., Price, M., Gross, R., Metlay, J. P., Christie, J. D., et al. (2007). Adherence to warfarin assessed by electronic pill caps, clinician assessment, and patient reports: Results from the IN-RANGE study. *Journal of General Internal Medicine, 22,* 1254–1259.

Parker, R. M., Schaller, J., & Hansmann, S. (2003). Catastrophe, chaos, and complexity models and psychosocial adjustment to disability. *Rehabilitation Counseling Bulletin, 46,* 234–241.

Parrott, D. J., & Zeichner, A. (2002). Effects of alcohol and trait anger on physical aggression in men. *Journal of Studies on Alcohol, 63,* 196–204.

Parschau, L., Richert, J., Koring, M., Ernsting, A., Lippke, S., & Schwarzer, R. (2012). Changes in social-cognitive variables are associated with stage transitions in physical activity. *Health Education Research, 27,* 129–140.

Pascoe, E. A., & Richman, L. S. (2009). Perceived discrimination and health: A meta-analytic review. *Psychological Bulletin, 135,* 531–554.

Patel, S. R., Ayas, N. T., Malhotra, M. R., White, D. P., Schemhammer, E. S., Speizer, F. E., et al. (2004). A prospective study of sleep duration and mortality risk in women. *Sleep, 27,* 440–444.

Patra, J., Taylor, B., Irving, H., Roerecke, M., Baliunas, D., Mohapatra, S., et al. (2010). Alcohol consumption and the risk of morbidity and mortality for different stroke types—A systematic review and meta-analysis. *BMC Public Health, 10,* 258–269.

Patterson, D. R. (2010). *Clinical hypnosis for pain control.* Washington, DC: American Psychological Association.

Patterson, D. R., & Jensen, M. P. (2003). Hypnosis and clinical pain. *Psychological Bulletin, 129,* 495–521.

Paull, T. T., Cortez, D., Bowers, B., Elledge, S. J., & Gellert, M. (2001). Direct DNA binding by BRCA 1. *Proceedings of the National Academy of Sciences of the United States of America, 98,* 6086–6091.

Paulozzi, L., Baldwin, G., Franklin, G., Kerlikowske, R. G., Jones, C. M., Ghiya, N., et al. (2012). CDC grand rounds: Prescription drug overdoses—a U.S. epidemic. *Morbidity and Mortality Weekly Report, 61,* 10–13.

Pauly, M. V., & Pagán, J. A. (2007). Spillovers and vulnerability: The case of community uninsurance. *Health Affairs, 26,* 1304–1314.

Paun, O., Farran, C. J., Perraud, S., & Loukissa, D. A. (2004). Successful caregiving of persons with Alzheimer's disease. *Alzheimer's Care Quarterly, 5,* 241–251.

Pavlik, V. N., Doody, R. S., Massman, P. J., & Chan, W. (2006). Influence of premorbid IQ and education on progression of Alzheimer's disease. *Dementia and Geriatric Cognitive Disorders, 22,* 367–377.

Pavlin, D. J., Sullivan, M. J. L., Freund, P. R., & Roesen, K. (2005). Catastrophizing: A risk factor for postsurgical pain. *Clinical Journal of Pain, 21,* 83–90.

Paxton, R. J., Motl, R. W., Aylward, A., & Nigg, C. R. (2010). Physical activity and quality of life: The complementary influence of self-efficacy for physical activity and mental health difficulties. *International Journal of Behavioral Medicine, 17,* 255–263.

Paynter, J., & Edwards, R. (2009). The impact of tobacco promotion at the point of sale: A systematic review. *Nicotine & Tobacco Research, 11*(1), 25–35.

Peay, M. Y., & Peay, E. R. (1998). The evaluation of medical symptoms by patients and doctors. *Journal of Behavioral Medicine, 21,* 57–81.

Pedersen, A. F., Zachariae, R., & Bovbjerg, D. H. (2009). Psychological stress and antibody response to influenze vaccination: A meta-analysis. *Brain, Behavior, and Immunity, 23,* 427–433.

Peele, S. (2002, August 1). Harm reduction in clinical practice. *Counselor: The Magazine for Addiction Professionals,* 28–32.

Peele, S. (2007). Addiction as disease: Policy, epidemiology, and treatment consequences of a bad idea. In J. E. Henningfield, P. B. Santora, & W. K. Bickel (Eds.), Addiction treatment: Science and policy for the twenty-first century (pp. 153–164). Baltimore, MD: Johns Hopkins University Press.

Peila, R., Rodriguez, B. L., & Launer, L. J. (2002). Type 2 diabetes, APOE gene, and the risk for dementia and related pathologies. *Diabetes, 51,* 1256–1262.

Pelletier, K. R. (2002). Mind as healer, mind as slayer: Mind-body medicine comes of age. *Advances in Mind-Body Medicine, 18,* 4–15.

Pence, L. B., Thorn, B. E., Jensen, M. P., & Romano, J. M. (2008). Examination of perceived spouse responses to patient well and pain behavior in patients with headache. *The Clinical Journal of Pain, 24,* 654–661.

Penley, J. A., Tomaka, J., & Wiebe, J. S. (2002). The association of coping to physical and psychological health outcomes: A meta-analytic review. *Journal of Behavioral Medicine, 25,* 551–603.

Pennebaker, J. W., Barger, S. D., & Tiebout, J. (1989). Disclosure of traumas and health among Holocaust survivors. *Psychosomatic Medicine, 51,* 577–589.

Pennebaker, J. W., Colder, M., & Sharp, L. K. (1990). Accelerating the coping process. *Journal of Personality and Social Psychology, 58,* 528–537.

Penza-Clyve, S. M., Mansell, C., & McQuaid, E. L. (2004). Why don't children take their asthma medications? A qualitative analysis of children's perspectives on adherence. *Journal of Asthma, 41,* 189–197.

Penzien, D. B., Rains, J. C., & Andrasik, F. (2002). Behavioral management of recurrent headache: Three decades of experience and empiricism. *Applied Psychophysiology and Biofeedback, 27,* 163–181.

Pereira, M. A., Kartashov, A. I., Ebbeling, C. B., Van Horn, L., Slattery, M. L., Jacobs, D. R., Jr., et al. (2005). Fast-food habits, weight gain, and insulin resistance (the CARDIA study): 15-year prospective analysis. *Lancet, 365,* 36–42.

Peres, M. F. P., Mercante, J. P. P., Tanuri, F. C., & Nunes, M. (2006). Chronic migraine prevention with topiramate. *Journal of Headache and Pain, 7,* 185–187.

Peretti-Watel, P., Constance, J., Guilbert, P., Gautier, A., Beck, F., & Moatti, J.-P. (2007). Smoking too few cigarettes to be at risk? Smokers' perceptions of risk and risk denial, a French survey. *Tobacco Control, 16,* 351–356.

Permutt, M. A., Wasson, J., & Cox, N. (2005). Genetic epidemiology of diabetes. *Journal of Clinical Investigation, 115,* 1431–1439.

Perram, S. W. (2006). The results of 47 clinical studies examined in a 30-year period. *American Chiropractor, 28,* 42–44.

Pert, C. B., & Snyder, S. H. (1973). Opiate receptor: Demonstration in nervous tissue. *Science, 179,* 1011–1014.

Peterlin, B. L., Rosso, A. L., Rapoport, A. M., & Scher, A. I. (2010). Obesity and migraine: The effect of age, gender and adipose tissue distribution. *Headache, 50*(1), 52–62.

Petrie, K. J., Perry, K., Broadbent, E., & Weinman, J. (2012). A text message programme designed to modify patients' illness and treatment beliefs improves self-reported adherence to asthma preventer medication. *British Journal of Health Psychology, 17,* 74–84.

Petticrew, M., Bell, R., & Hunter, D. (2002). Influence of psychological coping on survival and recurrence in people with cancer: A systematic review. *British Medical Journal, 325,* 1066.

Pettman, E. (2007). A history of manipulative therapy. *Journal of Manual and Manipulative Therapy, 15,* 165–174.

Pew Internet. (2012). *Highlights of the Pew Internet Project's research related to health and health care.* Retrieved March 28, 2012, from http://www.pewinternet.org/Commentary/2011/November/Pew-Internet-Health.aspx

Phillips, J. G., & Ogeil, R. P. (2007). Alcohol consumption and computer blackjack. *Journal of General Psychology, 134,* 333–353.

Phillips, K. M., Antoni, M. H., Carver, C. S., Lechner, S. C., Penedo, F. J., McCullough, M. E., et al. (2011). Stress management skills and reductions in serum cortisol across the year after survey for non-metastatic breast cancer. *Cognitive Therapy & Research, 35,* 595–600.

Phipps, E., Braitman, L. E., Stites, S., & Leighton, J. C. (2008). Quality of life and symptom attribution in long-term colon cancer survivors. *Journal of Evaluation in Clinical Practice, 14,* 254–258.

Pho, L., Grossman, D., & Leachman, S. A. (2006). Melanoma genetics: A review of genetic factors and clinical phenotypes in familial melanoma. *Current Opinion in Oncology, 18,* 173–179.

Picavet, H. S. J. (2010). Musculoskeletal pain complaints from a sex and gender perspective. In P. Croft, F. M. Blyth, & D. van der Windt (Eds.), *Chronic pain epidemiology: From Aetiology to Public Health* (pp. 119–126). New York: Oxford University Press.

Pickup, J. C., & Renard, E. (2008). Long-acting insulin analogs versus insulin pump therapy for the treatment of Type 1 and Type 2 diabetes. *Diabetes Care, 31*(S2), S140–S145.

Pierce, J. P. (2005). Influence of movie stars on the initiation of adolescent smoking. *Pediatric Dentistry, 27,* 149.

Pierce, J. P., Distefan, J. M., Kaplan, R. M., & Gilpin, E. A. (2005). The role of curiosity in smoking initiation. *Addictive Behaviors, 30,* 685–696.

Pietiläinen, K. H., Korkeila, M., Bogl, L. H., Westerterp, K. R., Yki-Järvinen, H., Kaprio, J., et al. (2010). Inaccuracies in food and physical activity diaries of obese subjects: Complementary evidence from doubly labeled water and co-twin assessments. *International Journal of Obesity, 34*(3), 437–445.

Piette, J. D., Heisler, M., Horne, R., & Caleb Alexander, G. (2006). A conceptually based approach to understanding chronically ill patients' responses to medication cost pressures. *Social Science and Medicine, 62,* 846–857.

Pike, K. M., Timothy, B., Vitousek, K., Wilson, G. T., & Bauer, J. (2003). Cognitive behavior therapy in posthospitalization treatment of anorexia nervosa. *American Journal of Psychiatry, 160,* 2046–2049.

Pilote, L., Dasgupta, K., Guru, V., Humphries, K. H., McGrath, J., Norris, C., et al. (2007). A comprehensive view of sex-specific issues related to cardiovascular disease. *Canadian Medical Association Journal, 176*(6), S1–S44.

Pimlott-Kubiak, S., & Cortina, L. M. (2003). Gender, victimization, and outcomes: Reconceptualizing risk. *Journal of Consulting and Clinical Psychology, 71,* 528–539.

Pinel, J. P. J. (2009). *Biopsychology* (7th ed.). Boston, MA: Allyn and Bacon.

Pinel, J. P. J., Assanand, S., & Lehman, D. R. (2000). Hunger, eating, and ill health. *American Psychologist, 55,* 1105–1116.

Pingitore, D., Scheffler, R., Haley, M., Seniell, T., & Schwalm, D. (2001). Professional psychology in a new era: Practice-based evidence from California. *Professional Psychology, Research and Practice, 32,* 585–596.

Piotrowski, C. (1998). Assessment of pain: A survey of practicing clinicians. *Perceptual and Motor Skills, 86,* 181–182.

Piotrowski, C. (2007). Review of the psychological literature on assessment instruments used with pain patients. *North American Journal of Psychology, 9,* 303–306.

Pischon, T., Boeing, H., Hoffmann, K., Bergmann, M., Schulze, M. B., Overvad, K., et al. (2008). General and abdominal adiposity and risk of death in Europe. *New England Journal of Medicine, 359*(20), 2105–2120.

Pisinger, C., & Godtfredsen, N. S. (2007). Is there a health benefit of reduced tobacco consumption? A systematic review. *Nicotine and Tobacco Research, 9,* 631–646.

Pisinger, C., & Jorgensen, T. (2007). Weight concerns and smoking in a general population: The Inter99 study. *Preventive Medicine, 44,* 283–289.

Pi-Sunyer, F. X. (2004). The epidemiology of central fat distribution in relation to disease. *Nutrition Reviews, 62,* 120–126.

Plasqui, G., & Westerterp, K. R. (2007). Physical activity and insulin resistance. *Current Nutrition and Food Science, 3,* 157–160.

Pole, N., Best, S. R., Metzler, T., & Marmar, C. R. (2005). Why are Hispanics at greater risk for PTSD? *Cultural Diversity and Mental Health, 11,* 144–161.

Polgar, S., & Ng, J. (2005). Ethics, methodology and the use of placebo controls in surgical trials. *Brain Research Bulletin, 67,* 290–297.

Polich, J. M., Armor, D. J., & Braiker, H. B. (1980). *The course of alcoholism: Four years after treatment.* Santa Monica, CA: Rand.

Polivy, J., Coelho, J., Hargreaves, D., Fleming, A., & Herman, C. P. (2007). The effects of external cues on eating and body weight: Another look at obese humans and rats. *Appetite, 49,* 321.

Polivy, J., & Herman, C. P. (2002). Causes of eating disorders. *Annual Review of Psychology, 53,* 187–214.

Polivy, J., & Herman, C. P. (2004). Sociocultural idealization of thin female body shapes: An introduction to the special issues on body image and eating disorders. *Journal of Social and Clinical Psychology, 23,* 1–6.

Pollack, M., Chastek, B., Willaism, S. A., & Moran, J. (2010). Impact of treatment complexity on adherence and glycemic control: An analysis of oral antidiabetic agents. *Journal of Clinical Outcomes Management, 17,* 257–265.

Pollock, M. L., Wilmore, J. H., & Fox, S. M., III. (1978). *Health and fitness through physical activity.* New York: Wiley.

Pomerleau, O. F., & Kardia, S. L. R. (1999). Introduction to the features section: Genetic research on smoking. *Health Psychology, 18,* 3–6.

Pool, G. J., Schwegler, A. F., Theodore, B. R., & Fuchs, P. N. (2007). Role of gender norms and group identification on hypothetical and experimental pain tolerance. *Pain, 129,* 122–129.

Poole, H., Branwell, R., & Murphy, P. (2006). Factor structure of the Beck Depression Inventory-II in patients with chronic pain. *Clinical Journal of Pain, 22,* 790–798.

Pope, C., Mechoulam, R., & Parsons, L. (2010). Endocannabinoid signaling in neurotoxicity and neuroprotection. *NeuroToxicology, 31*(5), 562–571.

Pope, S. K., Shue, V. M., & Beck, C. (2003). Will a healthy lifestyle help prevent Alzheimer's disease? *Annual Review of Public Health, 24,* 111–132.

Popham, R. E. (1978). The social history of the tavern. In Y. Israel, F. B. Glaser, H. Kalant, R. E. Popham, W. Schmidt, & R. G. Smart (Eds.), *Research advances in alcohol and drug problems* (Vol. 2, pp. 225–302). New York: Plenum Press.

Popkin, B. (2009). *The world is fat: The fads, trends, policies, and products that are fattening the human race.* New York: Avery/Penguin.

Porter, J., & Jick, H. (1980). Addiction rate in patients treated with narcotics. *New England Journal of Medicine, 302,* 123.

Poss, J. E. (2000). Developing a new model for cross-cultural research: Synthesizing the health belief model and the theory of reasoned action. *Advances in Nursing Science, 23,* 1–15.

Possemato, K., Ouimette, P., & Geller, P. A. (2010). Internet-based expressive writing for kidney transplant recipients: Effects on posttraumatic stress and quality of life. *Traumatology, 16,* 49–54.

Poston, W. S. C., Taylor, J. E., Hoffman, K. M., Peterson, A. L., Lando, H. A., Shelton, S., et al. (2008). Smoking and deployment: Perspectives of junior enlisted U.S. Air Force and U.S. Army personnel and their supervisors. *Military Medicine, 173,* 441–447.

Pouchot, J., Le Parc, J.-M., Queffelec, L., Sichère, P., & Flinois, A. (2007). Perceptions in 7700 patients with rheumatoid arthritis compared to their families and physicians. *Joint Bone Spine, 74,* 622–626.

Pouletty, P. (2002). Opinion: Drug addictions: Towards socially accepted and medically treatable diseases. *Nature Reviews Drug Discovery, 1,* 731–736.

Powell, J., Inglis, N., Ronnie, J., & Large, S. (2011). The characteristics and motivations of online health information seekers: Cross-sectional survey and qualitative interview study. *Journal of Medical Internet Research, 13,* e20.

Powell, K. E., Paluch, A. E., & Blair, S. N. (2011). Physical activity for health: What kind? How much? How intense? On top of what? *Annual Review of Public Health, 32,* 349–365.

"Practical Nurse." (2008). Hereditary breast cancer risk overestimated. *Practical Nurse, 35*(9), 9.

Prapavessis, H., Cameron, L., Baldi, J. C., Robinson, S., Borries, K., Harper, T., et al. (2007). The effects of exercise and nicotine replacement therapy on smoking rates in women. *Addictive Behaviors, 32,* 1416–1432.

Prejean, J., Song, R., Hernandez, A., Zieball, R., Green, T., Walker, F., et al. (2011). Estimated HIV incidence in the United States, 2006–2009. *PLoS ONE, 6,* e17502. DOI: 10.1371/journal.pone.0017502.

Pressman, S. D., & Cohen, S. (2005). Does positive affect influence health? *Psychological Bulletin, 131,* 925–971.

Prestwich, A., Perugini, M., & Hurling, R. (2009). Can the effects of implementation intentions on exercise be enhanced using text messages? *Psychology and Health, 24,* 677–687.

Price, D. D., Finniss, D. G., & Benedetti, F. (2008). A comprehensive review of the placebo effect: Recent advances and current thought. *Annual Review of Psychology, 59,* 565–590

Prince, M. (2004). Care arrangements for people with dementia in developing countries. *International Journal of Geriatric Psychiatry, 19,* 170–177.

Prochaska, J. J., Spring, B., & Nigg, C. R. (2008). Multiple health behavior change research: An introduction and overview. *Preventive Medicine, 46,* 181–188.

Prochaska, J. O., DiClemente, C. C., & Norcross, J. C. (1992). In search of how people change: Applications to addictive behaviors. *American Psychologist, 47,* 1102–1114.

Prochaska, J. O., Norcross, J. C., & DiClemente, C. C. (1994). *Changing for good.* New York: Avon Books.

Psaty, B. M., Anderson, M., Kronmal, R. A., Tracy, R. P., Orchard, T., Fried, L. P., et al. (2004). The association between lipid levels and the risks of incident myocardial infarction, stroke, and total mortality: The Cardiovascular Health Study. *Journal of the American Geriatrics Society, 52,* 1639–1647.

Purslow, L. R., Sandhu, M. S., Forouhi, N., Young, E. H., Luben, R. N., Welch, A. A., et al. (2008). Energy intake at breakfast and weight change: Prospective study of 6,764 middle-aged men and women. *American Journal of Epidemiology, 167,* 188.

Puska, P. (2002). Nutrition and global prevention on non-communicable diseases. *Asia Pacific Journal of Clinical Nutrition, 11*(Suppl. 9), S755–S758.

Puska, P., Vartiainen, E., Tuomilehto, J., Salomaa, V., & Nissinen, A. (1998). Changes in premature death in Finland: Successful long-term prevention of cardiovascular diseases. *Bulletin of the World Health Organization, 76,* 419–425.

Qiu, C., Kivipelto, M., & von Strauss, E. (2011). Epidemiology of Alzheimer's disease: Occurrence, determinants, and strategies toward intervention. *Dialogues in Clinical Neuroscience, 11,* 111–128.

Quartana, P. J., Laubmeier, K. K., & Zakowski, S. G. (2006). Psychological adjustment following diagnosis and treatment of cancer: An examination of the moderating role of positive and negative emotional expressivity. *Journal of Behavioral Medicine, 29,* 487–498.

Quinn, J. F., Bodenhamer-Davis, E., & Koch, D. S. (2004). Ideology and the stagnation of AODA treatment modalities in America. *Deviant Behavior, 25,* 109–131.

Quinn, J. R. (2005). Delay in seeking care for symptoms of acute myocardial infarction: Applying a theoretical model. *Research in Nursing and Health, 28,* 283–294.

Quist, M., Rorth, M., Zacho, M., Andersen, C., Moeller, T., Midtgaard, J., et al. (2006). High-intensity resistance and cardiovascular training improve physical capacity in cancer patients undergoing chemotherapy. *Scandinavian Journal of Medicine and Science in Sports, 16,* 349–357.

Qureshi, A. A., Laden, F., Colditz, G. A., & Hunter, D. J. (2008). Geographic variation and risk of skin cancer in US women. *Archives of Internal Medicine, 168,* 501–507.

Rabin, C., Leventhal, H., & Goodin, S. (2004). Conceptualization of disease timeline predicts posttreatment distress in breast cancer patients. *Health Psychology, 23,* 407–412.

Rahim-Williams, F. B., Riley, J. L., III, Herrera, D., Campbell, C. M., Hastie, B. A., & Fillingim, R. B. (2007). Ethnic identity predicts experimental pain sensitivity in African Americans and Hispanics. *Pain, 129,* 177–184.

Rainville, P., & Price, D. D. (2003). Hypnosis phenomenology and the neurobiology of consciousness. *International Journal of Clinical and Experimental Hypnosis, 51*(Special Issue, Pt. 1), 105–129.

Rainwater, D. L., Mitchell, B. D., Gomuzzie, A. G., Vandeberg, J. L., Stein, M. P., & MacCluer, J. W. (2000). Associations among 5-year changes in weight, physical activity, and cardiovascular disease risk factors in Mexican Americans. *American Journal of Epidemiology, 152,* 974–982.

Rami, B., Popow, C., Horn, W., Waldhoer, T., & Schober, E. (2006). Telemedical support to improve glycemic control in adolescents with Type 1 diabetes mellitus. *European Journal of Pediatrics, 165,* 701–705.

Ramsay, S., Ebrahim, S., Whincup, P., Papacosta, O., Morris, R., Lennon, L., et al. (2008). Social engagement and the risk of cardiovascular disease mortality: Results of a prospective population-based study of older men. *Annals of Epidemiology, 18,* 476–483.

"RAND Corporation." (2011). RAND Corporation, Palmer Center for Chiropractic Research and Samueli Institute receive $7.4 million grand from Congressionally Directed Medical Research program; award is the largest in the history of the chiropractic profession. *American Chiropractor, 33*(3), 8.

Rapoff, M. A. (2003). Pediatric measures of pain: The Pain Behavior Observation Method, Pain Coping Questionnaire (PCQ), and Pediatric Pain Questionnaire (PPQ). *Arthritis and Rheumatism: Arthritis Care and Research, 49*(S5), S90–S91.

Rashidi, A., Mohammadpour-Ahranjani, B., Vafa, M. R., & Karandish, M. (2005). Prevalence of obesity in Iran. *Obesity Reviews, 6,* 191–192.

Rasmussen, H. N., Scheier, M. F., & Greenhouse, J. B. (2009). Optimism and physical health: A meta-analytic review. *Annals of Behavioral Medicine, 37,* 239–256.

Raum, E., Rothenbacher, D., Ziegler, H., & Brenner, H. (2007). Heavy physical activity: Risk or protective factor for cardiovascular disease? A life course perspective. *Annals of Epidemiology, 17,* 417–424.

Raynor, H. A., & Epstein, L. H. (2001). Dietary variety: Energy regulation and obesity. *Psychological Bulletin, 127,* 325–341.

Rayworth, B. B. (2004). Childhood abuse and risk of eating disorders in women. *Epidemiology, 15,* 271–278.

Read, J. P., Wood, M. D., & Capone, J. C. (2005). A prospective investigation of relations between social influences and alcohol involvement during the transition into college. *Journal of Studies on Alcohol, 66,* 23–34.

Reader, D. M. (2007). Medical nutrition therapy and lifestyle interventions. *Diabetes Care, 30*(Suppl. 2), S188–S193.

Reagan, N. (2000). *I love you Ronnie: The letters of Ronald Reagan to Nancy Reagan.* New York: Random House.

Reas, D. L., & Grilo, C. M. (2008). Review and meta-analysis of pharmacotherapy for binge-eating disorder. *Obesity, 16*(9), 2024–2038.

Reas, D. L., Nygård, J. F., & Sørensen, T. (2009). Do quitters have anything to lose? Changes in body mass index for daily, never, and former smokers over an 11-year period (1990–2001). *Scandinavian Journal of Public Health, 37*(7), 774–777.

Reed, G. M., & Scheldeman, L. (2004). News. *European Psychologist, 9,* 184–187.

Regoeczi, W. C. (2003). When context matters: A multilevel analysis of household and neighbourhood crowding on aggression and withdrawal. *Journal of Environmental Psychology, 23,* 457–470.

Rehm, J., Baliunas, D., Borges, G. L. G., Graham, K., Irving, H., Kehoe, T., et al. (2010). The relation between different dimensions of alcohol consumption and burden of disease: An overview. *Addiction, 105*(5), 817–843.

Rehm, J., Patra, J., & Taylor, B. (2007). Harm, benefits, and net effects on mortality of moderate drinking of alcohol among adults in Canada in 2002. *Annals of Epidemiology, 17*(5S), S81–S86.

Reich, A., Müller, G., Gelbrich, G., Deutscher, K., Gödicke, R., & Kiess, W. (2003). Obesity and blood pressure—Results from the examination of 2365 schoolchildren in Germany. *International Journal of Obesity, 27,* 1459–1464.

Reiche, E. M. V., Nunes, S. O. V., & Morimoto, H. K. (2004). Stress, depression, the immune system, and cancer. *Lancet Oncology, 5,* 617–625.

Reid, C. M., Gooberman-Hill, R., & Hanks, G. W. (2008). Opioid analgesics for cancer pain: Symptom control for the living or comfort for the dying? A qualitative study to investigate the factors influencing the decision to accept morphine for pain caused by cancer. *Annals of Oncology, 19,* 44.

Reilly, T., & Woo, G. (2004). Social support and maintenance of safer sex practices among people living with HIV/AIDS. *Health and Social Work, 29,* 97–105.

Reitz, C., Tang, M. X., Manly, J., Schupf, N., Mayeaux, R., & Luchsinger, J. A. (2008). Plasma lipid levels in the elderly are not associated with the risk of mild cognitive impairment. *Dementia and Geriatric Cognitive Disorders, 25,* 232–237.

Rentz, C., Krikorian, R., & Keys, M. (2005). Grief and mourning from the perspective of the person with a dementing illness: Beginning the dialogue. *Omega: Journal of Death and Dying, 50,* 165–179.

Renz, H., Blümer, N., Virna, S., Sel, S., & Garn, H. (2006). The immunological basis of the hygiene hypothesis. *Chemical Immunology and Allergy, 91,* 30–48.

Research and Policy Committee. (2002). *A new vision for healthcare: A leadership role for business.* New York: Committee for Economic Development.

Resnicow, K., Jackson, A., Wang, T., Aniridya, K. D., McCarty, F., Dudley, W. N., et al. (2001). A motivational interviewing intervention to increase fruit and vegetable intake through Black churches: Results of the Eat for Life trial. *American Journal of Public Health, 91,* 1686–1693.

Rethorst, C. D., Wipfli, B. M., & Landers, D. M. (2007). The effect of exercise on depression: Examining clinical significance. *Journal of Sport and Exercise Psychology, 29*(Suppl.), S198.

Reuben, A. (2008). Alcohol and the liver. *Current Opinion in Gastroenterology, 24,* 328–338.

Reuter, T., Ziegelmann, J. P., Wiedemann, A. U., Lippke, S., Schüz, B., & Aiken, L. S. (2010). Planning bridges the intention–behaviour gap: Age makes a difference and strategy use explains why. *Psychology & Health, 25,* 873–887.

Reynolds, S. L., Haley, W., & Kozlenko, N. (2008). The impact of depressive symptoms and chronic diseases on active life expectancy in older Americans. *American Journal of Geriatric Psychology, 16,* 425–432.

Rhee, Y., Taitel, M. S., Walker, D. R., & Lau, D. T. (2007). Narcotic drug use among patients with lower back pain in employer health plans: A retrospective analysis of risk factors and health care services. *Clinical Therapeutics, 29*(Suppl. 1), 2603–2612.

Riazi, A., Pickup, J., & Bradley, C. (2004). Daily stress and glycaemic control in Type 1 diabetes: Individual differences in magnitude, direction, and timing of stress-reactivity. *Diabetes Research and Clinical Practice, 66,* 237–244.

Ricciardelli, L. A., McCabe, M. P., Williams, R. J., & Thompson, J. K. (2007). The role of ethnicity and culture in body image and disordered eating among males. *Clinical Psychology Review, 27,* 582–606.

Rice, D. P., & Fineman, N. (2004). Economic implications of increased longevity in the United States. *Annual Review of Public Health, 25,* 457–473.

Richardson, J., Smith, J. E., McCall, G., Richardson, A., Pilkington, K., & Kirsch, I. (2007). Hypnosis for nausea and vomiting in cancer chemotherapy: A systematic review of the research evidence. *European Journal of Cancer Care, 16,* 402–412.

Richardson, K. M., & Rothstein, H. R. (2008). Effects of occupational stress management intervention programs: A meta-analysis. *Journal of Occupational Health Psychology, 13,* 69–93.

Richman, J. A., Cloninger, L., & Rospenda, K. M. (2008). Macrolevel stressors, terrorism, and mental health outcomes: Broadening the stress paradigm. *American Journal of Public Health, 98,* 323–329.

Rietveld, S., & Koomen, J. M. (2002). A complex system perspective on medication compliance: Information for healthcare providers. *Disease Management and Health Outcomes, 10,* 621–630.

Riley, J. L., III, Wade, J. B., Myers, C. D., Sheffield, D., Papas, R. K., & Price, D. D. (2002). Racial/ethnic differences in the experience of chronic pain. *Pain, 100,* 291–298.

Rimm, E. B., & Moats, C. (2007). Alcohol and coronary heart disease: Drinking patterns and mediators of effect. *Annals of Epidemiology, 17*(S5), S3–S7.

Ringen, P. A., Andreas, M. I., Birkenaes, A. B., Engh, J. A., Faerden, A., Vaskinn, A., et al. (2008). The level of illicit drug use is related to symptoms and premorbid functioning in severe mental illness. *Acta Psychiatrica Scandinavica, 118*(4), 297–304.

Ringström, G., Abrahamsson, H., Strid, H., & Simrén, M. (2007). Why do subjects with irritable bowel syndrome seek health care for their symptoms? *Scandinavian Journal of Gastroenterology, 42,* 1194–1203.

Rise, J., Sheeran, P., & Hukkelberg, S. (2010). The role of self-identity in the Theory of Planned Behavior: A meta-analysis. *Journal of Applied Social Psychology, 40,* 1085–1105.

Rissanen, A., Hakala, P., Lissner, L., Mattlar, C.-E., Koskenvuo, M., & Rönnemaa, T. (2002). Acquired preference especially for dietary fat and obesity: A study of weight-discordant monozygotic twin pairs. *International Journal of Obesity and Related Metabolic Disorders, 26,* 973–977.

Ritter, A., & Cameron, J. (2006). A review of the efficacy and effectiveness of harm reduction strategies for alcohol, tobacco and illicit drugs. *Drug and Alcohol Review, 25,* 611–624.

Rivis, A., Sheeran, P., & Armitage, C. J. (2009). Expanding the affective and normative components of the Theory of Planned Behavior: A meta-analysis of anticipated affect and moral norms. *Journal of Applied Social Psychology, 39,* 2985–3019.

Roberts, B. A., Fuhrer, R., Marmot, M., & Richards, M. (2011). Does retirement influence cognitive performance? The Whitehall II Study. *Journal of Epidemiology & Community Health, 65,* 958–963.

Roberts, L., Ahmed, I., Hall, S., & Davison, A. (2009). Intercessory prayer for the alleviation of ill health. *Cochrane Database of Systematic Reviews 2009,* Issue 2, Cochrane Art. No.: CD000368, DOI: 10.1002/14651858.CD000368.pub3.

Roberts, S. O. (2002). A strong start: Strength and resistance training guidelines for children and adolescents. *American Fitness, 20*(1), 34–38.

Roberts, W. O. (2007). Heat and cold: What does the environment do to marathon injury? *Sports Medicine, 37,* 400–403.

Robine, J.-M., & Ritchie, K. (1991). Healthy life expectancy: Evaluation of global indicator of change in population health. *British Medical Journal, 302,* 457–460.

Robins, L. N. (1995). The natural history of substance use as a guide to setting drug policy. *American Journal of Public Health, 85,* 12–13.

Robinson, L., Clare, L., & Evans, K. (2005). Making sense of dementia and adjusting to loss: Psychological reactions to a diagnosis of dementia in couples. *Aging and Mental Health, 9,* 337–347.

Robinson, M. E., Gagnon, C. M., Dannecker, E. A., Brown, J. L., Jump, R. L., & Price, D. D. (2003). Sex differences in common pain events: Expectations and anchors. *Journal of Pain, 4,* 40–45.

Robinson-Whelen, S., Tada, Y., MacCallum, R. C., McGuire, L., & Kiecolt-Glaser, J. K. (2001). Long-term caregiving: What happens when it ends? *Journal of Abnormal Psychology, 110,* 573–584.

Robles, D. S. (2011). The thin is in: Am I thin enough? Perfectionism and self-esteem in anorexia. *International Journal of Research & Review, 6*(1), 65–73.

Robles, T. F., Glaser, R., & Kiecolt-Glaser, J. K. (2005). Out of balance: A new look at chronic stress, depression, and immunity. *Current Directions in Psychological Science, 14,* 111–115.

Röder, C. H., Michal, M., Overbeck, G., van de Ven, V. G., & Linden, D. E. J. (2007). Pain response in depersonalization: A functional imaging study using hypnosis in health subjects. *Psychotherapy and Psychosomatics, 76,* 115–121.

Rodgers, W. M., Hall, C. R., Blanchard, C. M., McAuley, E., & Munroe, K. J. (2002). Task and scheduling self-efficacy as predictors of exercise behaviour. *Psychology & Health, 27,* 405–416.

Rodgers, W. M., & Sullivan, M. J. L. (2001). Task, coping and scheduling self-efficacy in relation to frequency of physical activity. *Journal of Applied Social Psychology, 31,* 741–753.

Rodin, J., & Langer, E. J. (1977). Long-term effects of a control-relevant intervention with the institutionalized aged. *Journal of Personality and Social Psychology, 35,* 897–902.

Rodin, J., Silberstein, L., & Striegel-Moore, R. (1985). Women and weight: A normative discontent. In T. B. Sonderegger (Ed.), *Psychology and gender* (pp. 267–307). Lincoln: University of Nebraska Press.

Rodriguez, J., Jiang, R., Johnson, W. C., MacKenzie, B. A., Smith, L. J., & Barr, R. G. (2010). The association of pipe and cigar use with cotinine levels, lung function, and airflow obstruction. *Annals of Internal Medicine, 152*(4), 201–210.

Rodu, B., & Cole, P. (2007). Declining mortality from smoking in the United States. *Nicotine and Tobacco Research, 9,* 781–784.

Roe, S., & Becker, J. (2005). Drug prevention with vulnerable young people: A review. *Drugs: Education, Prevention and Policy, 12,* 85–99.

Roelofs, J., Boissevain, M. D., Peters, M. L., de Jong, J. R., & Vlaeyen, J. W. S. (2002). Psychological treatments for chronic low back pain: Past, present, and beyond. *Pain Reviews, 9,* 29–40.

Roesch, S. L., Adams, L., Hines, A., Palmores, A., Vyas, P., Tran, C., et al. (2005). Coping with prostate cancer: A meta-analytic review. *Journal of Behavioral Medicine, 28,* 281–293.

Roger, V. L., Go, A. S., Lloyd-Jones, D. M., Benjamin, E. J., Berry, J. D., Borden, W. B., et al. (2012). Heart disease and stroke statistics—2012 update: A report from the American Heart Association. *Circulation*, *125*, e2–e220.

Rogers, C. J., Colbert, L. H., Greiner, J. W., Perkins, S. N., & Hursting, S. D. (2008). Physical activity and cancer prevention: Pathways and targets for intervention. *Sports Medicine*, *38*, 271–296.

Rollings, G. (2011, January 1). I smiled as I cut off my arm. I was grateful to be free. *The Sun*. Retrieved on February 4, 2012, from http://www.thesun.co.uk/sol/homepage/showbiz/film/3326119/I-smiled-as-I-cut-off-my-arm-I-was-just-grateful-to-be-free.html

Rollins, S. Z., & Garrison, M. E. B. (2002). The Family Daily Hassles Inventory: A preliminary investigation of reliability and validity. *Family and Consumer Sciences Research Journal*, *31*, 135–154.

Rollman, G. B. (1998). Culture and pain. In S. S. Kazarian & D. R. Evans (Eds.), *Cultural clinical psychology: Theory, research, and practice* (pp. 267–286). New York: Oxford University Press.

Ronan, G. F., Dreer, L. W., Dollard, K. M., & Ronan, D. W. (2004). Violent couples: Coping and communication skills. *Journal of Family Violence*, *19*, 131–137.

Room, R., & Day, N. (1974). Alcohol and mortality. In M. Keller (Ed.), *Second special report to the U.S. Congress: Alcohol and health* (pp. 79–92). Washington, DC: U.S. Government Printing Office.

Rooney, K., & Ozanne, S. E. (2011). Maternal over-nutrition and offspring obesity predisposition: Targets for preventative interventions. *International Journal of Obesity*, *35*(7), 883–890.

Rosal, M. C., Olendzki, B., Reed, G. W., Gumieniak, O., Scavron, J., & Ockene, I. (2005). Diabetes self-management among low-income Spanish-speaking patients: A pilot study. *Annals of Behavioral Medicine*, *29*, 225–235.

Rosario, M., Salzinger, S., Feldman, R. S., & Ng-Mak, D. S. (2008). The roles of social support and coping. *American Journal of Community Psychology*, *41*, 43–62.

Rose, J. P., Geers, A. L., Rasinski, H. M., & Fowler, S. L. (2011). Choice and placebo expectation effects in the context of pain analgesia. *Journal of Behavioral Medicine*. DOI:10.1007/s10865-011-9374-0.

Rosen, C. S. (2000). Is the sequencing of change processes by stage consistent across health problems? A meta-analysis. *Health Psychology*, *19*, 593–604.

Rosenberg, E., Leanza, Y., & Seller, R. (2007). Doctor-patient communication in primary care with an interpreter: Physician perceptions of professional and family interpreters. *Patient Education and Counseling*, *67*, 286–292.

Rosenberg, H., & Melville, J. (2005). Controlled drinking and controlled drug use as outcome goals in British treatment services. *Addiction Research and Theory*, *13*, 85–92.

Rosenberg, N. L., Grigsby, J., Dreisbach, J., Busenbark, D., & Grigsby, P. (2002). Neuropsychologic impairment and MRI abnormalities associated with chronic solvent abuse. *Journal of Toxicology: Clinical Toxicology*, *40*, 21–34.

Rosenberg, S. D., Lu, W., Mueser, K. T., Jankowski, M. K., & Cournos, F. (2007). Correlates of adverse childhood events among adults with schizophrenia spectrum disorders. *Psychiatric Services*, *58*, 245–253.

Rosenblatt, K. A., Wicklund, K. G., & Stanford, J. L. (2000). Sexual factors and the risk of prostate cancer. *American Journal of Epidemiology*, *152*, 1152–1158.

Rosengren, A., Hawken, S., Ounpuu, S., Sliwa, K., Zubaid, M., Almahmeed, W. A., et al. (2004). Association of psychosocial risk factors with risk of acute myocardial infarction in 11119 cases and 13648 controls from 52 countries (the INTERHEART study): Case-control study. *Lancet*, *364*, 953–962.

Rosengren, A., Subramanian, S. V., Islam, S., Chow, C. K., Avezum, A., Kazmi, K., et al. (2009). Education and risk for acute myocardial infarction in 52 high, middle and low-income countries: INTERHEART case-control study. *Heart*, *95*, 2014–2022.

Rosenman, R. H., Brand, R. J., Jenkins, C. D., Friedman, M., Straus, R., & Wurm, M. (1975). Coronary heart disease in the Western Collaborative Group Study: Final follow-up of 8 1/2 years. *Journal of the American Medical Association*, *233*, 872–877.

Rosier, E. M., Iadarola, M. J., & Coghill, R. C. (2002). Reproducibility of pain measurement and pain perception. *Pain*, *98*, 205–216.

Rosland, A., Kieffer, E., Israel, B., Cofield, M., Palmisano, G., Sinco, B., et al. (2008). When is social support important? The association of family support and professional support with specific diabetes self-management behaviors. *Journal of General Internal Medicine*, *23*, 1992–1999.

Rösner, S., Hackl-Herrwerth, A., Leucht, S., Vecchi, S., Srisurapanont, M., & Soyka, M. (2010). Opioid antagonists for alcohol dependence. *Cochrane Database of Systematic Reviews 2010*, *12*, Cochrane Art. No.: CD001867, DOI: 10.1002/14651858.CD001867.pub3.

Ross, M. J., & Berger, R. S. (1996). Effects of stress inoculation training on athletes' postsurgical pain and rehabilitation after orthopedic injury. *Journal of Consulting and Clinical Psychology*, *64*, 406–410.

Rosser, B. A., & Eccleston, C. (2011). Smartphone applications for pain management. *Journal of Telemedicine and Telecare*, *17*, 308–312.

Rössler, W., Lauber, C., Angst, J., Haker, H., Gamma, A., Eich, D., et al. (2007). The use of complementary and alternative medicine in the general population: Results from a longitudinal community study. *Psychological Medicine*, *37*, 73–84.

Rossow, I., Grøholt, B., & Wichstrøm, L. (2005). Intoxicants and suicidal behaviour among adolescents: Changes in levels and associations from 1992 to 2002. *Addiction*, *100*, 79–88.

Roter, D. L., & Hall, J. A. (2004). Physician gender and patient-centered communication: A critical review of empirical research. *Annual Review of Public Health*, *25*, 497–519.

Roth, M., & Kobayashi, K. (2008). The use of complementary and alternative medicine among Chinese Canadians: Results from a national survey. *Journal of Immigrant & Minority Health*, *10*(6), 517–528.

Rotskoff, L. (2002). *Love on the rocks: Men, women, and alcohol in post–World War II America*. Chapel Hill: University of North Carolina Press.

Rotter, J. B. (1966). Generalized expectancies for internal versus external control of reinforcement. *Psychological Monographs*, *80*(Whole No. 609).

Rozanski, A., Blumenthal, J. A., Davidson, K. W., Saab, P. G., & Kubzansky, L. (2005). The epidemiology, pathophysiology, and management of psychosocial risk factors in cardiac practice: The emerging field of behavioral cardiology. *Journal of the American College of Cardiology*, *45*, 637–651.

Rozin, P. (2005). The meaning of food in our lives: A cross-cultural perspective on eating and well-being. *Journal of Nutrition Education and Behavior*, *37*(Suppl. 2), S107–S112.

Rubak, S., Sanboek, A., Lauritzen, T., & Christensen, B. (2005). Motivational interviewing: A systematic review and meta-analysis. *British Journal of General Practice*, *55*, 305–312.

Rubenstein, S., & Caballero, B. (2000). Is Miss America an undernourished role model? *Journal of the American Medical Association*, *283*, 1569.

Rubinstein, S. M., van Middelkoop, M., Assendelft, W. J., de Boer, M. R., & van Tulder, M. W. (2011). Spinal manipulative therapy for chronic low-back pain. *Cochrane Database of Systematic Reviews, 2011*, Issue 2, Cochrane Art. No.: CD008112, DOI: 10.1002/14651858.CD008112.pub2.

Rudd, R. E. (2007). Health literacy skills of U.S. adults. *American Journal of Health Behavior*, *31*, S8–S18.

Rutledge, P. C., Park, A., & Sher, K. J. (2008). 21st birthday drinking: Extremely extreme. *Journal of Consulting and Clinical Psychology*, *76*, 511–516.

Rutten, G. (2005). Diabetes patient education: Time for a new era. *Diabetic Medicine*, *22*, 671–673.

Ryan, C. J., & Zerwic, J. J. (2003). Perceptions of symptoms of myocardial infarction related to health care seeking behaviors in the elderly. *Journal of Cardiovascular Nursing*, *18*, 184–196.

Sääkslahti, A., Numminen, P., Varstala, V., Helenius, H., Tammi, A., Viikari, J., et al. (2004). Physical activity as a preventive measure for coronary heart disease risk factors in early childhood. *Scandinavian Journal of Medicine and Science in Sports*, *14*, 143–149.

Sabia, S., Marmot, M., Dufouil, C., & Singh-Manoux, A. (2008). Smoking history and cognitive function in middle age from the Whitehall II study. *Archives of Internal Medicine, 168,* 1165–1173.

Sacco, R. L., Benson, R. T., Kargman, D. E., Boden-Albala, B., Tuck, C., Lin, I.-F., et al. (2001). High-density lipoprotein cholesterol and ischemic stroke in the elderly: The Northern Manhattan Stroke Study. *Journal of the American Medical Association, 285,* 2729–2735.

Sachdev, P., Mondraty, N., Wen, W., & Gulliford, K. (2008). Brains of anorexia nervosa patients process self-images differently from non-self-images: An fMRI study. *Neuropsychologia, 46,* 2161–2168.

Sackett, D. L., & Snow, J. C. (1979). The magnitude of compliance and noncompliance. In R. B. Haynes, D. W. Taylor, & D. L. Sackett (Eds.), *Compliance in health care* (pp. 11–22). Baltimore, MD: Johns Hopkins University Press.

Safron, M., Cislak, A., Gaspar, T., & Luszczynska, A. (2011). Behaviors and body weight change: A systematic umbrella review. *Behavioral Medicine, 37*(1), 15–25.

Sallis, J. F., Bowles, H. R., Bauman, A., Ainsworth, B. E., Bull, F. C., Craig, C. L., et al. (2009). Neighborhood environments and physical activity among adults in 11 countries. *American Journal of Preventive Medicine, 36,* 484–490.

Samuelson, M., Carmody, J., Kabat-Zinn, J., & Bratt, M. A. (2007). Mindfulness-based stress reduction in Massachusetts correctional facilities. *Prison Journal, 87,* 254–268.

Sánchez del Rio, M., & Alvarez Linera, J. (2004). Functional neuroimaging of headaches. *Lancet Neurology, 3,* 645–651.

Sánchez-Johnsen, L. A. P., Carpentier, M. R., & King, A. C. (2011). Race and sex associations to weight concerns among urban African American and Caucasian smokers. *Addictive Behaviors, 36*(1/2), 14–17.

Sancier, K. M., & Holman, D. (2004). Commentary: Multifaceted health benefits of medical Qigong. *Journal of Alternative and Complementary Medicine, 10,* 163–165.

Sanders, S. (2005). Is the glass half empty or half full? Reflections on strain and gain in caregivers of individuals with Alzheimer's disease. *Social Work in Health Care, 40*(3), 57–73.

Sanders, S. H. (2006). Behavioral conceptualization and treatment for chronic pain. *Behavior Analyst Today, 7,* 253–261.

Sapolsky, R. M. (1997, November). On the role of upholstery in cardiovascular physiology. *Discover Magazine.* Retrieved March 9, 2012, from http://discovermagazine.com/1997/nov/ontheroleofuphol1260

Sapolsky, R. M. (1998). *Why zebras don't get ulcers: An updated guide to stress, stress-related diseases, and coping.* New York: Freeman.

Sapolsky, R. M. (2004). Social status and health in humans and other animals. *Annual Review of Anthropology, 33,* 393–418.

Sattin, R. W., Easley, K. A., Wolf, S. L., Chen, Y., & Kutner, M. H. (2005). Reduction in fear of falling through intense tai chi exercise training in older, transitionally frail adults. *Journal of the American Geriatrics Society, 53,* 1168–1178.

Sattler, G. (2005). Advances in liposuction and fat transfer. *Dermatology Nursing, 17,* 133–139.

Saunders, T., Driskell, J. E., Johnston, J. H., & Sales, E. (1996). The effects of stress inoculation training on anxiety and performance. *Journal of Occupational Health Psychology, 1,* 170–186.

Savage, E., Farrell, D., McManus, V., & Grey, M. (2010). The science of intervention development for type 1 diabetes in childhood: Systematic review. *Journal of Advanced Nursing, 66,* 2604–2619.

Sayette, M. A., Kirchner, T. R., Moreland, R. L., Levine, J. M., & Travis, T. (2004). Effects of alcohol on risk-seeking behavior: A group-level analysis. *Psychology of Addictive Behaviors, 18,* 190–193.

Scarpa, A., Haden, S. C., & Hurley, J. (2006). Community violence victimization and symptoms of posttraumatic stress disorder: The moderating effects of coping and social support. *Journal of Interpersonal Violence, 21,* 446–469.

Scarscelli, D. (2006). Drug addiction between deviance and normality: A study of spontaneous and assisted remission. *Contemporary Drug Problems, 33,* 237–274.

Schaap, M. M., Kunst, A. E., Leinsalu, M., Regidor, E., Ekholm, O., Dzurova, D., et al. (2008). Effect of nationwide tobacco control policies on smoking cessation in high and low educated groups in 18 European countries. *Tobacco Control, 17*(4), 248–255.

Schaap, M. M., van Agt, H. M. E., & Kunst, A. E. (2008). Identification of socioeconomic groups at increased risk for smoking in European countries: Looking beyond educational level. *Nicotine & Tobacco Research, 10*(2), 359–369.

Schachter, S. (1980). Urinary pH and the psychology of nicotine addiction. In P. O. Davidson & S. M. Davidson (Eds.), *Behavioral medicine: Changing health lifestyles* (pp. 70–93). New York: Brunner/Mazel.

Schachter, S. (1982). Recidivism and self-cure of smoking and obesity. *American Psychologist, 37,* 436–444.

Schaffer, M., Jeglic, E. L., & Stanley, B. (2008). The relationship between suicidal behavior, ideation, and binge drinking among college students. *Archives of Suicide Research, 12,* 124–132.

Schaller, M., Miller, G. E., Gervais, W. M., Yager, S., & Chen, E. (2010). Mere visual perception of other people's disease symptoms facilitates a more aggressive immune response. *Psychological Science, 21,* 649–652.

Schell, L. M., & Denham, M. (2003). Environmental pollution in urban environments and human biology. *Annual Review of Anthropology, 32,* 111–134.

Schenker, S. (2001, September). The truth about fad diets. *Student BMJ,* 318–319.

Schindler, L., Kerrigan, D., & Kelly, J. (2002). *Understanding the immune system.* Retrieved January 29, 2002, from newscenter.cancer.gov/sciencebehind/immune

Schlenger, W. E., Caddell, J. M., Ebert, L., Jordan, B. K., Rourke, K. M., Wilson, D., et al. (2002). Psychological reactions to terrorist attacks: Findings from the National Study of Americans' Reactions to September 11. *Journal of the American Medical Association, 288,* 581–588.

Schlicht, W., Kanning, M., & Bös, K. (2007). Psychosocial interventions to influence physical inactivity as a risk factor: Theoretical models and practical evidence. In J. Dordan, B. Bardé, & A. M. Zeiher (Eds.), *Contributions toward evidence-based psychocardiology: A systematic review of the literature* (pp. 107–123). Washington, DC: American Psychological Association.

Schmaltz, H. N., Southern, D., Ghali, W. A., Jelinski, S. F., Parsons, G. A., King, K., et al. (2007). Living alone, patient sex and mortality after acute myocardial infarction. *Journal of General Internal Medicine, 22,* 572–578.

Schneider, E. C., Zaslavsky, A. M., & Epstein, A. M. (2002). Racial disparities in the quality of care for enrollees in Medicare managed care. *Journal of the American Medical Association, 287,* 1288–1294.

Schneiderman, N., Saab, P. G., Carney, R. M., Raczynski, J. M., Cowan, M. J., Berkman, L. F., et al. (2004). Psychosocial treatment within sex by ethnicity subgroups in the Enhancing Recovery in Coronary Heart Disease clinical trial. *Psychosomatic Medicine, 66,* 475–483.

Schnittker, J. (2004). Education and the changing shape of the income gradient in health. *Journal of Health and Social Behavior, 45,* 286–305.

Schnittker, J. (2007). Working more and feeling better: Women's health, employment, and family life. *American Sociological Review, 72,* 221–238.

Schoenbaum, M. (1997). Do smokers understand the mortality effects of smoking? Evidence from the Health Retirement Survey. *American Journal of Public Health, 87,* 755–759.

Schousboe, K., Visscher, P. M., Erbas, B., Kyvik, K. O., Hopper, J. L., Henriksen, J. E., et al. (2004). Twin study of genetic and environmental influences on adult body size, shape, and composition. *International Journal of Obesity, 28,* 39–48.

Schroeder, K., Fahey, T., & Ebrahim, S. (2007). Interventions for improving adherence to treatment in patients with high blood pressure in ambulatory settings. *Cochrane Database of Systematic

Reviews, Cochrane Art. No.: CD004804, DOI: 10.1002/14651858. CD004804.

Schroeder, K. E. E. (2004). Coping competence as predictor and moderator of depression among chronic disease patients. *Journal of Behavioral Medicine, 27*, 123–145.

Schroevers, M., Ranchor, A. V., & Sanderman, R. (2006). Adjustment to cancer in the 8 years following diagnosis: A longitudinal study comparing cancer survivors with healthy individuals. *Social Science and Medicine, 63*, 598–610.

Schuckit, M. A. (2000). Keep it simple. *Journal of Studies on Alcohol, 61*, 781–782.

Schulz, K. F., Altman, D. G., Moher, D., and the CONSORT Group. (2010). CONSORT 2010 statement: Updated guidelines for reporting parallel group randomized trials. *Annals of Internal Medicine, 152*(11), 726–732.

Schulz, R., & Aderman, D. (1974). Clinical research and the stages of dying. *Omega: Journal of Death and Dying, 5*, 137–143.

Schulze, A., & Mons, U. (2006). The evolution of educational inequalities in smoking: A changing relationship and a cross-over effect among German birth cohorts of 1921–70. *Addiction, 101*, 1051–1056.

Schüz, B., Sniehotta, F. F., & Schwarzer, R. (2007). Stage-specific effects of an action control intervention on dental flossing. *Health Education Research, 22*, 332–341.

Schieman, S., Milkie, M. A., & Glavin, P. (2009). When work interferes with life: Work-nonwork interference and the influence of work-related demands and resources. *American Sociological Review, 74*, 966–988.

Schwartz, B. S., Stewart, W. F., Simon, D., & Lipton, R. B. (1998). Epidemiology of tension-type headache. *Journal of the American Medical Association, 279*, 381–383.

Schwartz, G. E., & Weiss, S. M. (1978). Behavioral medicine revisited: An amended definition. *Journal of Behavioral Medicine, 1*, 249–251.

Schwarzer, R. (2008). Modeling health behavior change: How to predict and modify the adoption and maintenance of health behaviors. *Applied Psychology: An International Review, 57*, 1–29.

Schwarzer, R., Luszczynska, A., Ziegelmann, J. P., Scholz, U., & Lippke, S. (2008). Social-cognitive predictors of physical exercise adherence: Three longitudinal studies in rehabilitation. *Health Psychology, 27*(S1), S54–S63.

Schwarzer, R., & Renner, B. (2000). Social-cognitive predictors of health behavior: Action self-efficacy and coping self-efficacy. *Health Psychology, 19*, 487–495.

Sclafani, A. (2001). Psychobiology of food preferences. *International Journal of Obesity, 25*(Suppl. 5), S13–S16.

Sclafani, A., & Springer, D. (1976). Dietary obesity in adult rats: Similarities to hypothalamic and human obesity. *Physiology and Behavior, 17*, 461–471.

Scott, D. J., Stohler, C. S., Egnatuk, C. M., Wang, H., Koeppe, R. A., & Zubieta, J.-K. (2008). Placebo and nocebo effects are defined by opposite opioid and dopaminergic responses. *Archives of General Psychiatry, 65*, 220–231.

Scott-Sheldon, L. A., Kalichman, S. C., Carey, M. P., & Fielder, R. L. (2008). Stress management interventions for HIV+ adults: A meta-analysis of randomized controlled trials, 1989 to 2006. *Health Psychology, 27*, 129–139.

Scully, J. A., Tosi, H., & Banning, K. (2000). Life events checklists: Revisiting the Social Readjustment Rating Scale after 30 years. *Educational and Psychological Measurement, 60*, 864–876.

Searle, A., & Bennett, P. (2001). Psychological factors and inflammatory bowel disease: A review of a decade of literature. *Psychology and Health Medicine, 6*, 121–135.

Searle, A., Norman, P., Thompson, R., & Vedhara, K. (2007). A prospective examination of illness beliefs and coping in patients with Type 2 diabetes. *British Journal of Health Psychology, 12*, 621–638.

Sears, S. R., & Stanton, A. L. (2001). Expectancy-value constructs and expectancy violation as predictors of exercise adherence in previously sedentary women. *Health Psychology, 20*, 326–333.

Sebre, S., Sprugevica, I., Novotni, A., Bonevski, D., Pakalniskiene, V., Popescu, D., et al. (2004). Cross-cultural comparisons of child-reported emotional and physical abuse: Rates, risk factors and psychosocial symptoms. *Child Abuse and Neglect, 28*, 113–127.

Secker-Walker, R. H., Flynn, B. S., Solomon, L. J., Skelly, J. M., Dorwaldt, A. L., & Ashikaga, T. (2000). Helping women quit smoking: Results of a community intervention program. *American Journal of Public Health, 90*, 940–946.

Seegers, V., Petit, D., Falissard, B., Vitaro, F., Trembley, R. E., Montplaisir, J., et al. (2011). Short sleep duration and body mass index: A prospective longitudinal study in preadolescence. *American Journal of Epidemiology, 173*(6), 621–629.

Segall, A. (1997). Sick role concepts and health behavior. In D. S. Gochman (Ed.), *Handbook of health behavior research: Vol.1. Personal and social determinants* (pp. 289–301). New York: Plenum Press.

Segerstrom, S. C. (2005). Optimism and immunity: Do positive thoughts always lead to positive effects? *Brain, Behavior, and Immunity, 19*, 195–200.

Segerstrom, S. C. (2007). Stress, energy, and immunity: An ecological view. *Current Directions in Psychological Science, 16*, 326–330.

Segerstrom, S. C., & Miller, G. E. (2004). Psychological stress and the human immune system: A meta-analytic study of 30 years of inquiry. *Psychological Bulletin, 130*, 601–630.

Seifert, T. (2005). Anthropomorphic characteristics of centerfold models: Trends toward slender figures over time. *Journal of Eating Disorders, 37*, 271–274.

Selkoe, D. J. (2007). Developing preventive therapies for chronic diseases: Lessons learned from Alzheimer's disease. *Nutrition Reviews, 65*(S12), S239–S243.

Selye, H. (1956). *The stress of life.* New York: McGraw-Hill.

Selye, H. (1976). *Stress in health and disease.* Reading, MA: Butterworths.

Selye, H. (1982). History and present status of the stress concept. In L. Goldberger & S. Breznitz (Eds.), *Handbook of stress: Theoretical and clinical aspects* (pp. 7–17). New York: Free Press.

Seow, D., & Gauthier, S. (2007). Pharmacotherapy of Alzheimer disease. *Canadian Journal of Psychiatry, 52*, 620–629.

Sepa, A., Wahlberg, J., Vaarala, O., Frodi, A., & Ludvigsson, J. (2005). Psychological stress may induce diabetes-related autoimmunity in infancy. *Diabetes Care, 28*, 290–295.

Sephton, S. E., Dhabhar, F. S., Keuroghlian, A. S., Giese-Davis, J., McEwen, B. S., Ionan, A. C., et al. (2009). Depression, cortisol, and suppressed cell-mediated immunity in metastatic breast cancer. *Brain, Behavior, and Immunity, 23*, 1148–1155.

Sepulveda, M.-J., Bodenheimer, T., & Grundy, P. (2008). Primary care: Can it solve employers' health care dilemma? *Health Affairs, 27*, 151–158.

Severson, H. H., Forrester, K. K., & Biglan, A. (2007). Use of smokeless tobacco is a risk factor for cigarette smoking. *Nicotine and Tobacco Research, 9*, 1331–1337.

Shai, I., Spence, J. D., Schwarzfuchs, D., Henkin, Y., Parraga, G., Rudich, A., et al. (2010). Dietary intervention to reverse carotid atherosclerosis. *Circulation, 121*, 1200–1208.

Shannon, S., Weil, A., & Kaplan, B. J. (2011). Medical decision making in integrative medicine: Safety, efficacy, and patient preference. *Alternative & Complementary Therapies, 17*(2), 84–91.

Shapiro, D., Cook, I. A., Davydov, D. M., Ottaviani, C., Leuchter, A. F., & Abrams, M. (2007). Yoga is a complementary treatment of depression: Effects of traits and moods on treatment outcome. *Evidence-Based Complementary and Alternative Medicine, 4*, 493–502.

Shapiro, J. R., Berkman, N. D., Brownley, K. A., Sedway, J. A., Lohr, K. N., & Bulik, C. M. (2007). Bulimia nervosa treatment: A systematic review of randomized controlled trials. *International Journal of Eating Disorders, 40*(4), 321–336.

Sharpe, L., Sensky, T., Timberlake, N., Ryan, B., Brewin, C. R., & Allard, S. (2001). A blind, randomized controlled trial of cognitive-behavioral intervention for patients with recent onset rheumatoid arthritis: Preventing psychological and physical mobility. *Pain, 89*, 275–283.

Shea, M. K., Houston, D. K., Nichlas, B. J., Messier, S. P., Davis, C. C., Miller, M. E., et al. (2010). The effect of randomization to weight loss on total mortality in older overweight and obese adults: The ADAPT study. *Journals of Gerontology Series A: Biological Sciences & Medical Sciences, 65A*(5), 519–525.

Sheehy, R., & Horan, J. J. (2004). Effects of stress inoculation training for 1st-year law students. *International Journal of Stress Management, 11*, 41–55.

Sheeran, P. (2002). Intention-behavior relations: A conceptual and empirical review. *European Review of Social Psychology, 12*, 1–36.

Sheeran, P., & Orbell, S. (1999). Implementation intentions and repeated behaviour: Augmenting the predictive validity of the theory of planned behaviour. *European Journal of Social Psychology, 29*, 349–369.

Sheeran, P., & Orbell, S. (2000). Using implementation intentions to increase attendance for cervical cancer screening. *Health Psychology, 19*, 283–289.

Sheese, B. E., Brown, E. L., & Graziano, W. G. (2004). Emotional expression in cyberspace: Searching for moderators of the Pennebaker disclosure effect via e-mail. *Health Psychology, 23*, 457–464.

Shell, E. R. (2000, May). Does civilization cause asthma? *Atlantic Monthly, 285*, 90–92, 94, 96–98, 100.

Shen, B.-J., Avivi, Y. E., Todaro, J. F., Spiro, A., Laurenceau, J.-P., Ward, K. D., et al. (2008). Anxiety characteristics independently and prospectively predict myocardial infarction in men: The unique contribution of anxiety among psychologic factors. *Journal of the American College of Cardiology, 51*, 113–119.

Shen, B.-J., Stroud, L. R., & Niaura, R. (2004). Ethnic differences in cardiovascular responses to laboratory stress: A comparison between Asian and White Americans. *International Journal of Behavioral Medicine, 11*, 181–186.

Shen, Z., Chen, J., Sun, S., Yu, B., Chen, Z., Yang, J., et al. (2003). Psychosocial factors and immunity of patients with generalized anxiety disorder. *Chinese Mental Health Journal, 17*, 397–400.

Sheps, D. S. (2007). Psychological stress and myocardial ischemia: Understanding the link and implications. *Psychosomatic Medicine, 69*, 491–492.

Sher, K. J. (1987). Stress response dampening. In H. T. Blane & K. E. Leonard (Eds.), *Psychological theories of drinking and alcoholism* (pp. 227–271). New York: Guilford Press.

Sher, K. J., & Levenson, R. W. (1982). Risk for alcoholism and individual differences in the stress-response-dampening effect of alcohol. *Journal of Abnormal Psychology, 91*, 350–367.

Sherman, D. K., Updegraff, J. A., & Mann, T. L. (2008). Improving oral health behavior: A social psychological approach. *Journal of the American Dental Association, 139*, 1382–1387.

Sherman, K. J., Cherkin, D. C., Hawkes, R. J., Miglioretti, D. L., & Deyo, R. A. (2009). Randomized trial of therapeutic massage for chronic neck pain. *Clinical Journal of Pain, 25*(3), 233–238.

Shernoff, M. (2006). Condomless sex: Gay men, barebacking, and harm reduction. *Social Work, 51*, 106–113.

Sherwood, L. (2001). *Human physiology: From cells to systems* (4th ed.). Pacific Grove, CA: Brooks/Cole.

Shi, L., Liu, J., Fonseca, V., Walker, P., Kalsekar, A., & Pawaskar, M. (2010). Correlation between adherence rates measured by MEMS and self-reported questionnaires: A meta-analysis. *Health and Quality of Life Outcomes, 8*, 99.

Shi, S., & Klotz, U. (2008). Clinical use and pharmacological properties of selective COX-2 inhibitors. *European Journal of Clinical Pharmacology, 64*, 233–252.

Shiffman, S., Balabanis, M. H., Paty, J. A., Engberg, J., Gwaltney, C. J., Liu, K. S., et al. (2000). Dynamic effects of self-efficacy on smoking lapse and relapse. *Health Psychology, 19*, 315–323.

Shiffman, S., Brockwell, S. E., Pillitteri, J. L., & Gitchell, J. G. (2008). Use of smoking-cessation treatments in the United States. *American Journal of Preventive Medicine, 34*, 102–111.

Shimabukuro, J., Awata, S., & Matsuoka, H. (2005). Behavioral and psychological symptoms of dementia characteristics of mild Alzheimer patients. *Psychiatry and Clinical Neurosciences, 59*, 274–279.

Shinnick, P. (2006). Qigong: Where did it come from? Where does it fit in science? What are the advances? *Journal of Alternative and Complementary Medicine, 12*, 351–353.

Shmueli, A., Igudin, I., & Shuval, J. (2011). Change and stability: Use of complementary and alternative medicine in Israel: 1993, 2000 and 2007. *European Journal of Public Health, 21*(2), 254–259.

Siegel, M., & Biener, L. (2000). The impact of an antismoking media campaign on progression to established smoking: Results of a longitudinal youth study. *American Journal of Public Health, 90*, 380–386.

Siegel, M., & Skeer, M. (2003). Exposure to secondhand smoke and excess lung cancer mortality risk among workers in the "5 B's": Bars, bowling alleys, billiard halls, betting establishments, and bingo parlours. *Tobacco Control, 12*, 333–338.

Siegel, R., Naishadham, D., & Jemal, A. (2012). Cancer statistics, 2012. *CA: A Cancer Journal for Clinicians, 62*, 10–29.

Siegler, B. (2003, August 6–12). Actress Halle Berry battles diabetes. *Miami Times, 80*(48), 4B.

Siegler, I. C., Bastian, L. A., Steffens, D. C., Bosworth, H. B., & Costa, P. T. (2002). Behavioral medicine and aging. *Journal of Consulting and Clinical Psychology, 70*, 843–851.

Siegman, A. W. (1994). From Type A to hostility to anger: Reflections on the history of coronary-prone behavior. In A. W. Siegman & T. W. Smith (Eds.), *Anger, hostility, and the heart* (pp. 1–21). Hillsdale, NJ: Erlbaum.

Siemiatycki, J., Richardson, L., Straif, K., Latreille, B., Lakhani, R., Campbell, S., et al. (2004). Listing occupational carcinogens. *Environmental Health Perspectives, 112*, 1447–1459.

Sifri, R., Rosenthal, M., Hyslop, T., Andrel, J., Wender, R., Vernon, S. W., et al. (2010). Factors associated with colorectal cancer screening decision stage. *Preventive Medicine, 51*, 329–331.

Sigmon, S. T., Stanton, A. L., & Snyder, C. R. (1995). Gender differences in coping: A further test of socialization and role constraint theories. *Sex Roles, 33*, 565–587.

Silberstein, S. D. (2004). Migraine pathophysiology and its clinical implications. *Cephalalgia, 24*(Suppl. 2), 2–7.

Silverman, S. M. (2008). Lindsay Lohan opens up about recent troubles. *People*. Retrieved March 6, 2008, from http://www.people.com/people/article/0,20181019,00.html

Simoni, J. M., Frick, P. A., & Huang, B. (2006). A longitudinal evaluation of a social support model of medication adherence among HIV-positive men and women an antiretroviral therapy. *Health Psychology, 25*, 74–81.

Simoni, J. M., Pearson, C. R., Pantalone, D. W., Marks, G., & Crepaz, N. (2006). Efficacy of interventions in improving highly active antiretroviral therapy adherence and HIV-1 RNA viral load: A meta-analytic review of randomized controlled trials. *Journal of Acquired Immune Deficiency Syndromes, 43*, S23–S35.

Simonsick, E. M., Guralnik, J. M., Volpato, S., Balfour, J., & Fried, L. P. (2005). Just get out the door! Importance of walking outside the home for maintaining mobility: Findings from the Women's Health and Aging Study. *Journal of the American Geriatrics Society, 53*, 198–203.

Simpson, S. H., Eurich, D. T., Majundar, S. R., Padwal, R. S., Tsuyuki, R. T., Varney, J., et al. (2006). A meta-analysis of the association between adherence to drug therapy and mortality. *British Medical Journal, 333*, 15–18.

Sims, E. A. H. (1974). Studies in human hyperphagia. In G. Bray & J. Bethune (Eds.), *Treatment and management of obesity*. New York: Harper & Row.

Sims, E. A. H. (1976). Experimental obesity, dietary-induced thermogenesis, and their clinical implications. *Clinics in Endocrinology and Metabolism, 5*, 377–395.

Sims, E. A. H., Danforth, E., Jr., Horton, E. S., Bray, G. A., Glennon, J. A., & Salans, L. B. (1973). Endocrine and metabolic effects of experimental obesity in man. *Recent Progress in Hormonal Research, 29*, 457–496.

Sims, E. A. H., & Horton, E. S. (1968). Endocrine and metabolic adaptation to obesity and starvation. *American Journal of Clinical Nutrition, 21*, 1455–1470.

Singletary, K. W., & Gapstur, S. M. (2001). Alcohol and breast cancer: Review of epidemiologic and experimental evidence and potential mechanisms. *Journal of the American Medical Association, 286,* 2143–2151.

Sitzer, D. I., Twamley, E. W., & Jeste, D. V. (2006). Cognitive training in Alzheimer's disease: A meta-analysis of the literature. *Acta Psychiatrica Scandinavica, 114,* 75–90.

Sjöström, M., Oja, P., Hagströmer, M., Smith, B. J., & Bauman, A. (2006). Health-enhancing physical activity across European Union countries: The Eurobarometer study. *Journal of Public Health, 14,* 291–300.

Skinner, B. F. (1953). *Science and human behavior.* New York: Macmillan.

Skinner, T. C., Hampson, S. E., & Fife-Schaw, C. (2002). Personality, personal model beliefs, and self-care in adolescents and young adults with Type 1 diabetes. *Health Psychology, 21,* 61–70.

Skybo, T., & Ryan-Wenger, N. (2003). Measures of overweight status in school-age children. *Journal of School Nursing, 19,* 172–180.

Slater, J., & Depue, R. A. (1981). The contribution of environmental events and social support to serious suicide attempts in primary depressive disorder. *Journal of Abnormal Psychology, 90,* 275–285.

Slomkowski, C., Rende, R., Novak, S., Lloyd-Richardson, E., & Niaura, R. (2005). Sibling effects on smoking in adolescence: Evidence for social influence from a genetically informative design. *Addiction, 100,* 430–438.

Slugg, R. M., Meyer, R. A., & Campbell, J. N. (2000). Response of cutaneous A- and C-fiber nociceptors in the monkey to controlled-force stimuli. *Journal of Neurophysiology, 83,* 2179–2191.

Small, B. J., Rosnick, C. B., Fratiglioni, L., & Bäckman, L. (2004). Apolipoprotein ε and cognitive performance: A meta-analysis. *Psychology and Aging, 19,* 592–600.

Smedslund, G., & Ringdal, G. I. (2004). Meta-analysis of the effects of psychosocial interventions on survival time in cancer patents. *Journal of Psychosomatic Research, 57,* 123–131.

Smeets, R. J., Severens, J. L., Beelen, S., Vlaeyen, J. W., & Knottnerus, J. A. (2009). More is not always better: Cost-effectiveness analysis of combined, single behavioral and single physical rehabilitation programs for chronic low back pain. *European Journal of Pain, 13,* 71–81.

Smelt, A. H. M. (2010). Triglycerides and gallstone formation. *Clinica Chimica Acta, 411*(21/22), 1625–1631.

Smetana, G. W. (2000). The diagnostic value of historical features in primary headache syndromes: A comprehensive review. *Archives of Internal Medicine, 160,* 2729–2740.

Smiles, R. V. (2002). Race matters in health care: Experts say eliminating racial and ethnic health disparities is the civil rights issue of our day. *Black Issues in Higher Education, 19*(7), 22–29.

Smith, C. A., Hay, P. P., & MacPherson, H. (2010). Acupuncture for depression. *Cochrane Database of Systematic Reviews, 2010,* Issue 1, Cochrane Art. No.: CD004046, DOI: 10.1002/14651858.CD004046.pub3.

Smith, D. A., Ness, E. M., Herbert, R., Schechter, C. B., Phillips, R. A., Diamond, J. A., et al. (2005). Abdominal diameter index: A more powerful anthropometric measure for prevalent coronary heart disease risk in adult males. *Diabetes, Obesity and Metabolism, 7,* 370–380.

Smith, D. P., & Bradshaw B. S. (2006). Rethinking the Hispanic paradox: Death rates and life expectancy for US non-Hispanic white and Hispanic populations. *American Journal of Public Health, 96,* 1686–1692.

Smith, J. E., Richardson, J., Hoffman, C., & Pilkington, K. (2005). Mindfulness-based stress reduction as supportive therapy in cancer care: Systematic review. *Journal of Advanced Nursing, 52,* 315–327.

Smith, K. M., & Sahyoun, N. R. (2005). Fish consumption: Recommendations versus advisories, can they be reconciled? *Nutrition Reviews, 63,* 39–46.

Smith, L. A., Roman, A., Dollard, M. F., Winefield, A. H., & Siegrist, J. (2005). Effort-reward imbalance at work: The effects of work stress on anger and cardiovascular disease symptoms in a community

sample. *Stress and Health: Journal of the International Society for the Investigation of Stress, 21,* 113–128.

Smith, P. J., Blumenthal, J. A., Hoffman, B. M., Cooper, H., Strauman, T. A., Welsh-Bohmer, K., et al. (2010). Aerobic exercise and neurocognitive performance: A meta-analytic review of randomized controlled trials. *Psychosomatic Medicine, 72,* 239–252.

Smith, T. W., & Ruiz, J. M. (2002). Psychosocial influences on the development and course of coronary heart disease: Current status and implications for research and practice. *Journal of Consulting and Clinical Psychology, 70,* 548–568.

Smyth, J. M., Stone, A. A., Hurewitz, A., & Kaell, A. (1999). Effects of writing about stressful experiences on symptom reduction in patients with asthma or rheumatoid arthritis: A randomized trial. *Journal of the American Medical Association, 281,* 1304–1309.

Sniehotta, F. F., Scholz, U., & Schwarzer, R. (2005). Bridging the intention-behaviour gap: Planning, self-efficacy, and action control in the adoption and maintenance of physical exercise. *Psychology & Health, 20,* 143–160.

Snyder, S. H. (1977, March). Opiate receptors and internal opiates. *Scientific American, 236,* 44–56.

Sobel, B. E., & Schneider, D. J. (2005). Cardiovascular complications in diabetes mellitus. *Current Opinion in Pharmacology, 5,* 143–148.

Sobell, L. C., Cunningham, J. A., & Sobell, M. B. (1996). Recovery from alcohol problems with and without treatment: Prevalence in two population surveys. *American Journal of Public Health, 86,* 966–972.

Sola-Vera, J., Sáez, J., Laveda, R., Girona, E., García-Sepulcre, M. F., Cuesta, A., et al. (2008). Factors associated with non-attendance at outpatient endoscopy. *Scandinavian Journal of Gastroenterology, 43,* 202–206.

Soler, R. E., Leeks, K. D., Buchanan, L. R., Brownson, R. C., Heath, G. W., Hopkins, D. H., et al. (2010). Point-of-decision prompts to increase stair use: A systematic review update. *American Journal of Preventive Medicine, 38,* S292–S300.

Song, M.-Y., John, M., & Dobs, A. S. (2007). Clinicians' attitudes and usage of complementary and alternative integrative medicine: A survey at the Johns Hopkins Medical Institute. *Journal of Alternative and Complementary Medicine, 13,* 305–306.

Song, Z., Foo, M.-D., Uy, M. A., & Sun, S. (2011). Unraveling the daily stress crossover between unemployed individuals and their employed spouses. *Journal of Applied Psychology, 96,* 151–168.

Sont, W. N., Zielinski, J. M., Ashmore, J. P., Jiang, H., Krewski, D., Fair, M. E., et al. (2001). First analysis of cancer incidence and occupational radiation exposure based on the National Dose Registry of Canada. *American Journal of Epidemiology, 153,* 309–318.

Soole, D. W., Mazerolle, L., & Rombouts, S. (2008). School-based drug prevention programs: A review of what works. *Australian & New Zealand Journal of Criminology, 41*(2), 259–286.

Sours, J. A. (1980). *Starving to death in a sea of objects: The anorexia nervosa syndrome.* New York: Aronson.

Speck, R. M., Courneya, K. S., Masse, L. C., Duval, S., & Schmitz, K. H. (2010). An update of controlled physical activity trials in cancer survivors: A systematic review and meta-analysis. *Journal of Cancer Survivorship, 4,* 87–100.

Spiegel, D. (2004). Commentary on "Meta-analysis of the effects of psychosocial interventions on survival time and mortality in cancer patients" by Geir Smedslund and Gerd Inter Ringdal. *Journal of Psychosomatic Research, 57,* 133–135.

Spiegel, D., Bloom, J. R., Kraemer, H. C., & Gottheil, E. (1989). Effect of psychosocial treatment on survival of patients with metastatic breast cancer. *Lancet, ii,* 888–891.

Spiegel, D., & Giese-Davis, J. (2003). Depression and cancer: Mechanisms and disease progression. *Biological Psychiatry, 54,* 269–282.

Spierings, E. L. H., Ranke, A. H., & Honkoop, P. C. (2001). Precipitating and aggravating factors of migraine versus tension-type headache. *Headache, 41,* 554–558.

Spitzer, B. L., Henderson, K. A., & Zivian, M. T. (1999). Gender differences in population versus media body size: A comparison over four decades. *Sex Roles, 40,* 545–566.

Springer, J. F., Sale, E., Kasim, R., Winter, W., Sambrano, S., & Chipungu, S. (2004). Effectiveness of culturally specific approaches to substance abuse prevention: Findings for CSAP's national cross-site evaluation of high risk youth programs. *Journal of Ethnic and Cultural Diversity in Social Work, 13*, 1–23.

Spruijt-Metz, D. (2011). Etiology, treatment, and prevention of obesity in childhood and adolescence: A decade in review. *Journal of Research on Adolescence, 21*(1), 129–152.

Sri Vengadesh, G., Sistla, S. C., & Smile, S. R. (2005). Postoperative pain relief following abdominal operations: A prospective randomised study of comparison of patient controlled analgesia with conventional parental opioids. *Indian Journal of Surgery, 67*, 34–37.

Stacey, P. S., & Sullivan, K. A. (2004). Preliminary investigation of thiamine and alcohol intake in clinical and healthy samples. *Psychological Reports, 94*, 845–848.

Staessen, J. A., Wang, J., Bianchi, G., & Birkenhager, W. H. (2003). Essential hypertension. *Lancet, 361*, 1629–1641.

Stallworth, J., & Lennon, J. L. (2003). An interview with Dr. Lester Breslow. *American Journal of Public Health, 93*, 1803–1805.

Stamler, J., Elliott, P., Dennis, B., Dyer, A. R., Kesteloot, H., Liu, K., et al. (2003). INTERMAP: Background, aims, design, methods, and descriptive statistics (nondietary). *Journal of Human Hypertension, 17*, 591–608.

Stamler, J., Stamler, R., Neaton, J. D., Wentworth, D., Daviglus, M. L., Garside, D., et al. (1999). Low risk-factor profile and long-term cardiovascular and noncardiovascular mortality and life expectancy: Findings for 5 large cohorts of young adult and middle-aged men and women. *Journal of the American Medical Association, 282*, 2012–2018.

Stampfer, M. J., Hu, F. B., Manson, J. E., Rimm, E. B., & Willett, W. C. (2000). Primary prevention of coronary heart disease in women through diet and lifestyle. *New England Journal of Medicine, 343*, 16–22.

Standridge, J. B., Zylstra, R. G., & Adams, S. M. (2004). Alcohol consumption: An overview of benefits and risks. *Southern Medical Journal, 97*, 664–672.

Stanner, S. A., Hughes, J., Kelly, C. N. M., & Buttriss, J. (2004). A review of the epidemiological evidence for the "antioxidant hypothesis." *Public Health Nutrition, 7*, 407–422.

Stanton, A. L., Revenson, T. A., & Tennen, H. (2007). Health psychology: Psychological adjustment to chronic disease. *Annual Review of Psychology, 58*, 565–592.

Stanton, J. M., Balzer, W. K., Smith, P. C., Parra, L. F., & Ironson, G. (2001). A general measure of work stress: The Stress in General scale. *Educational and Psychological Measurement, 61*, 866–887.

Starkstein, S. E., Jorge, R., Mizrahi, R., Adrian, J., & Robinson, R. G. (2007). Insight and danger in Alzheimer's disease. *European Journal of Neurology, 14*, 455–460.

Stason, W., Neff, R., Miettinen, O., & Jick, H. (1976). Alcohol consumption and nonfatal myocardial infarction. *American Journal of Epidemiology, 104*, 603–608.

Staton, L. J., Panda, M., Chen, I., Genao, I., Kurz, J., Pasanen, M., et al. (2007). When race matters: Disagreement in pain perception between patients and their physicians in primary care. *Journal of the National Medical Association, 99*, 532–537.

Stayner, L., Bena, J., Sasco, A. J., Smith, R., Steenland, K., Kreuzer, M., et al. (2007). Lung cancer risk and workplace exposure to environmental tobacco smoke. *American Journal of Public Health, 97*(3), 545–551.

Stead, L. F., Bergson, G., & Lancaster, T. (2008). Physician advice for smoking cessation. *Cochrane Database of Systematic Reviews*, Cochrane Art. No.: CD000165, DOI: 10.1002/14651858.CD000165.pub2.

Stead, L. F., Perera, R., Bullen, C., Mant, D., & Lancaster, T. (2008). Nicotine replacement therapy for smoking cessation. *Cochrane Database of Systematic Reviews*, Cochrane Art. No.: CD000146, DOI: 10.1002/14651858.CD000146.pub3.

Steele, C. M., & Josephs, R. A. (1990). Alcohol myopia: Its prized and dangerous effects. *American Psychologist, 45*, 921–933.

Steffen, K. J., Mitchell, J. E., Roerig, J. L., & Lancaster, K. L. (2007). The eating disorders medicine cabinet revisited: A clinician's guide to ipecac and laxatives. *International Journal of Eating Disorders, 40*, 360–368.

Steifel, M. C., Perla, R. J., & Zell, B. L. (2010). A health bottom line: Healthy life expectancy as an outcome measure for health improvement efforts. *The Milbank Quarterly, 88*, 30–53.

Stein, M. B., Schork, N. J., & Gelernter, J. (2008). Gene-by-environment (serotonin transporter and childhood maltreatment) interaction for anxiety sensitivity, an intermediate phenotype for anxiety disorders. *Neuropsychopharmacology, 33*, 312–319.

Steinbrook, R. (2004). The AIDS epidemic in 2004. *New England Journal of Medicine, 351*, 115–117.

Steinhausen, H. C., & Weber, S. (2010). The outcome of bulimia nervosa: Findings from one-quarter century of research. *American Journal of Psychiatry, 166*(12), 1331–1341.

Stelfox, H. T., Gandhi, T. K., Orav, E. J., & Gustafson, M. L. (2005). The relation of patient satisfaction with complaints against physicians and malpractice lawsuits. *The American Journal of Medicine, 118*, 1126–1133.

Steptoe, A., Hamer, M., & Chida, Y. (2007). The effects of acute psychological stress on circulating inflammatory factors in humans: A review and meta-analysis. *Brain, Behavior and Immunity, 21*, 901–912.

Steptoe, A., Wardle, J., Bages, N., Sallis, J. F., Sanabria-Ferrand, P.-A., & Sanchez, M. (2004). Drinking and driving in university students: An international study of 23 countries. *Psychology and Health, 19*, 527–540.

Stetter, F., & Kupper, S. (2002). Autogenic training: A meta-analysis of clinical outcome studies. *Applied Psychophysiology and Biofeedback, 27*, 45–98.

Stevenson, R. J., Hodgson, D., Oaten, M. J., Barouei, J., & Case, T. I. (2011). The effect of disgust on oral immune function. *Psychophysiology, 48*, 900–907.

Stewart, J. C., Janicki, D. L., & Kamarck, T. W. (2006). Cardiovascular reactivity to and recovery from psychological challenge as predictors of 3-year change in blood pressure. *Health Psychology, 25*, 111–118.

Stewart, K. L. (2004). Pharmacological and behavioral treatments for migraine headaches: A meta-analytic review. *Dissertation Abstracts International: Section B, 65*(3-B), 1535.

Stewart, L. K., Flynn, M. G., Campbell, W. W., Craig, B. A., Robinson, J. P., Timmerman, K. L., et al. (2007). The influence of exercise training on inflammatory cytokines and C-reactive protein. *Medicine and Science in Sports and Exercise, 39*, 1714–1719.

Stewart, S. T., Cutler, D. M., & Rosen, A. B. (2009). Forecasting the effects of obesity and smoking on U.S. life expectancy. *The New England Journal of Medicine, 361*, 2252–2260.

Stewart-Knox, B. J., Sittlington, J., Rugkåsa, J., Harrisson, S., Treacy, M., & Abaunza, P. S. (2005). Smoking and peer groups: Results from a longitudinal qualitative study of young people in Northern Ireland. *British Journal of Social Psychology, 44*, 397–414.

Stewart-Williams, S. (2004). The placebo puzzle: Putting together the pieces. *Health Psychology, 23*, 198–206.

Stice, E., Presnell, K., Groesz, L., & Shaw, H. (2005). Effects of a weight maintenance diet on bulimic symptoms in adolescent girls: An experimental test of the dietary restraint theory. *Health Psychology, 24*, 402–412.

Stice, E., Presnell, K., & Spangler, D. (2002). Risk factors for binge eating onset in adolescent girls: A 2-year prospective investigation. *Health Psychology, 21*, 131–138.

Stice, E., Rohde, P., Shaw, H., & Gau, J. (2011). Disorder prevention program for female high school students: Long-term effects. *Journal of Consulting & Clinical Psychology, 79*(4), 500–508.

Stice, E., Trost, A., & Chase, A. (2003). Healthy weight control and dissonance-based eating disorder prevention programs: Results from a controlled trial. *International Journal of Eating Disorders, 33*, 10–21.

Stickney, S. R., Black, D. R. (2008). Physical self-perception, body dysmorphic disorder, and smoking behavior. *American Journal of Health Behavior, 32*, 295–304.

Stojanovich, L., & Marisavljevich, D. (2008). Stress as a trigger of autoimmune disease. *Autoimmunity Review, 7*, 209–213.

Stokols, D. (1972). On the distinction between density and crowding: Some implications for future research. *Psychological Review, 79*, 275–277.

Stone, A. A., Krueger, A. B., Steptoe, A., & Harter, J. K. (2010). The socioeconomic gradient in daily colds and influenza, headaches, and pain. *Archives of Internal Medicine, 170*, 570–572.

Stone, A. A., Reed, B. R., & Neale, J. M. (1987). Changes in daily event frequency precedes episodes of physical symptoms. *Journal of Human Stress, 13*, 70–74.

Stone, G. C. (1987). The scope of health psychology. In G. C. Stone, S. M. Weiss, J. D. Matarazzo, N. E. Miller, J. Rodin, C. D. Belar, et al. (Eds.), *Health psychology: A discipline and a profession* (pp. 27–40). Chicago: University of Chicago Press.

Storr, C. L., Lalongo, N. S., Anthony, J. C., & Breslau, N. (2007). Childhood antecedents of exposure to traumatic events and posttraumatic stress disorder. *American Journal of Psychiatry, 164*, 119–125.

Strachan, E., Saracino, M., Selke, S., Magaret, A., Buchwald, D., & Wald, A. (2011). The effects of daily distress and personality on genital HSV shedding and lesions in a randomized, double-blind, placebo-controlled, crossover trial of acyclovir in HSV-2 seropositive women. *Brain, Behavior, and Immunity, 25*, 1475–1481.

Strasser, A. A., Lerman, C., Sanborn, P. M., Pickworth, W. B., & Feldman, E. A. (2007). New lower nicotine cigarettes can produce compensatory smoking and increased carbon monoxide exposure. *Drug and Alcohol Dependence, 86*, 294–300.

Straus, M. A. (2008). Dominance and symmetry in partner violence by male and female university students in 32 nations. *Children and Youth Services Review, 30*, 252–275.

Strazdins, L., & Broom, D. H. (2007). The mental health costs and benefits of giving social support. *International Journal of Stress Management, 14*, 370–385.

Streltzer, J. (1997). Pain. In W.-S. Tseng & J. Streltzer (Eds.), *Culture and psychopathology: A guide to clinical assessment* (pp. 87–100). New York: Brunner/Mazel.

Streppel, M. T., Boshuizen, H. C., Ocké, M. C., Kok, F. J., & Kromhout, D. (2007). Mortality and life expectancy in relation to long-term cigarette, cigar and pipe smoking: The Zutphen study. *Tobacco Control, 16*, 107–113.

Striegel-Moore, R. H., DeBar, L., Perrin, N., Lynch, F., Kraemer, H. C., Wilson, G. T., et al. (2010). Cognitive behavioral guided self-help for the treatment of recurrent binge eating. *Journal of Consulting & Clinical Psychology, 78*, 312–321.

Striegel-Moore, R. H., Franko, D. L., Thompson, D., Barton, B., Schreiber, G. B., & Daniels, S. R. (2004). Changes in weight and body image over time in women with eating disorders. *International Journal of Eating Disorders, 36*, 315–327.

Strine, T. W., Mokdad, A. H., Balluz, L. S., Berry, J. T., & Gonzalez, O. (2008). Impact of depression and anxiety on quality of life, health behaviors, and asthma control among adults in the United States with asthma, 2006. *Journal of Asthma, 45*, 123–133.

Stroebe, W., Papies, E. K., & Aarts, H. (2008). From homeostatic to hedonic theories of eating: Self-regulatory failure in food-rich environments. *Applied Psychology: An International Review, 57*, 172–193.

Strong, C. A. (1895). The psychology of pain. *Psychological Review, 2*, 329–347.

Strong, D. R., Cameron, A., Feuer, S., Cohn, A., Abrantes, A. M., & Brown, R. A. (2010). Single versus recurrent depression history: Differentiating risk factors among current US smokers. *Drug & Alcohol Dependence, 109*(1–3), 90–95.

Stotts, J., Lohse, B., Patterson, J., Horacek, T., White, A., & Greene, G. (2007). Eating competence in college students nominates a non-dieting approach to weight management. *FASEB Journal, 21*, A301.

Stroebe, W. (2008). *Dieting, overweight, and obesity: Self-regulation in a food-rich environment.* Washington, DC: American Psychological Association.

Stroud, C. B., Davila, J., Hammen, C., & Vrshek-Schallhorn, S. (2011). Severe and nonsevere events in first onsets versus recurrences of depression: Evidence for stress sensitization. *Journal of Abnormal Psychology, 120*, 142–154.

Stroud, C. B., Davila, J., & Moyer, A. (2008). The relationship between stress and depression in first onsets versus recurrences: A meta-analytic review. *Journal of Abnormal Psychology, 117*, 206–213.

Stuart, R. B. (1967). Behavioral control of overeating. *Behavior Research and Therapy, 5*, 357–365.

Stunkard, A. J., & Allison, K. C. (2003). Binge eating disorder: Disorder or marker? *International Journal of Eating disorders, 34*(Suppl. 1), S107–S116.

Stunkard, A. J., Harris, J. R., Pedersen, N. L., & McClean, G. E. (1990). The body-mass index of twins who have been reared apart. *New England Journal of Medicine, 322*, 1483–1487.

Stunkard, A. J., Sørensen, T. I. A., Hanis, C., Teasdale, T. W., Chakraborty, R., Schull, W. J., et al. (1986). An adoption study of human obesity. *New England Journal of Medicine, 314*, 193, 198.

Stürmer, T., Hasselbach, P., & Amelang, M. (2006). Personality, lifestyle, and risk of cardiovascular disease and cancer: Follow-up of population based cohort. *British Medical Journal, 332*, 1359.

Su, D., Li, L., & Pagán, J. A. (2008). Acculturation and the use of complementary and alternative medicine. *Social Science and Medicine, 66*, 439–453.

Suarez, E. C., Saab, P. G., Llabre, M. M., Kuhn, C. M., & Zimmerman, E. (2004). Ethnicity, gender, and age effects on adrenoceptors and physiological responses to emotional stress. *Psychophysiology, 41*, 450–460.

Substance Abuse and Mental Health Services Administration (SAMHSA). (2010). *Results from the 2009 National Survey on Drug Use and Health: Vol. 1. Summary of national findings* (Office of Applied Studies NSDUH Series H-38A, DHHS Publication No. SMA 10-4586 Findings). Rockville, MD: National Clearinghouse for Alcohol and Drug Information.

Sufka, K. J., & Price, D. D. (2002). Gate control theory reconsidered. *Brain & Mind, 3*, 277–290.

Suls, J., & Bunde, J. (2005). Anger, anxiety, and depression as risk factors for cardiovascular disease: The problems and implications of overlapping affective dispositions. *Psychological Bulletin, 131*, 260–300.

Suls, J., Martin, R., & Leventhal, H. (1997). Social comparison, lay referral, and the decision to seek medical care. In B. P. Buunk & F. X. Gibbons (Eds.), *Health, coping and well-being: Perspectives from social comparison theory* (pp. 195–226). Mahwah, NJ: Lawrence Erlbaum Associates.

Suls, J., & Rothman, A. (2004). Evolution of the biopsychosocial model: Prospects and challenges for health psychology. *Health Psychology, 23*, 119–125.

Sundblad, G. M. B., Saartok, T., & Engström, L.-M. T. (2007). Prevalence and co-occurrence of self-rated pain and perceived health in schoolchildren: Age and gender differences. *European Journal of Pain, 11*, 171–180.

Surwit, R. S., Van Tilburg, M. A. L., Zucker, N., McCaskill, C. C., Parekh, P., Feinglos, M. N., et al. (2002). Stress management improves long-term glycemic control in Type 2 diabetes. *Diabetes Care, 25*, 30–34.

Susser, M. (1991). What is a cause and how do we know one? A grammar for pragmatic epidemiology. *American Journal of Epidemiology, 133*, 635–648.

Sutton, S., McVey, D., & Glanz, A. (1999). A comparative test of the theory of reasoned action and the theory of planned behavior in the prediction of condom use intentions in a national sample of English young people. *Health Psychology, 18*, 72–81.

Svansdottir, H. B., & Snaedal, J. (2006). Music therapy in moderate and severe dementia of Alzheimer's type: A case-control study. *International Psychogeriatrics, 18*, 613–621.

Svetkey, L. P., Stevens, V. J., Brantley, P. J., Appel, L. J., Hollis, J. F., Loria, C. M., et al. (2008). Comparison of strategies for sustaining weight loss. *Journal of the American Medical Association, 299,* 1139–1148.

Swaim, R. C., Perrine, N. E., & Aloise-Young, P. A. (2007). Gender differences in a comparison of two tested etiological models of cigarette smoking among elementary school students. *Journal of Applied Social Psychology, 37,* 1681–1696.

Sweeney, C. T., Fant, R. V., Fagerstrom, K. O., McGovern, F., & Henningfield, J. E. (2001). Combination nicotine replacement therapy for smoking cessation rationale, efficacy and tolerability. *CNS Drugs, 15,* 453–467.

Swinburn, B. A., Sacks, G., Hall, K. D., McPherson, K., Finegood, D. T., Moodie, M. L., et al. (2011). The global obesity pandemic: Shaped by global drivers and local environments. *The Lancet, 378,* 804–814.

Swithers, S. E., Martin, A. A., Clark, K. M., Laboy, A. F., & Davidson, T. L. (2010). Body weight gain in rats consuming sweetened liquids. Effects of caffeine and diet composition. *Appetite, 55*(3), 528–533.

Sypeck, M. F., Gray, J. J., Etu, S. F., Ahrens, A. H., Mosimann, J. E., & Wiseman, C. V. (2006). Cultural representations of thinness in women, redux: Playboy magazine's depiction of beauty from 1979 to 1999. *Body Image, 3,* 229–235.

Szapary, P. O., Bloedon, L. T., & Foster, B. D. (2003). Physical activity and its effects on lipids. *Current Cardiology Reports, 5,* 488–492.

Szekely, C. A., Breitner, J. C., Fitzpatrick, A. L., Rea, T. D., Psaty, B. M., Kuller, L. H., et al. (2008). NSAID use and dementia risk in the Cardiovascular Health Study: Role of APOE and NSAID type. *Neurology, 70,* 17–24.

Tacker, D. H., & Okorodudu, A. O. (2004). Evidence for injurious effect of cocaethylene in human microvascular endothelial cells. *Clinica Chimica Acta, 345,* 69–76.

Takkouche, B., Regueira, C., & Gestal-Otero, J. J. (2001). A cohort study of stress and the common cold. *Epidemiology, 12,* 345–349.

Talbot, M. (2000, January 9). The placebo prescription. *New York Times Magazine,* 34–39, 44, 58–60.

Tamres, L. K., Janicki, D., & Helgeson, V. S. (2002). Sex differences in coping behavior: A meta-analytic review and an examination of relative coping. *Personality and Social Psychology Review, 6,* 2–30.

Tan, J. O. A., Stewart, A., Fitzpatrick, R., & Hope, T. (2010). Attitudes of patients with anorexia nervosa to compulsory treatment and coercion. *International Journal of Law & Psychiatry, 33*(1), 13–19.

Tang, B. M. P., Eslick, G. D., Nowson, C., Smith, C., & Bensoussan, A. (2007). Use of calcium or calcium in combination with vitamin D supplementation to prevent fractures and bone loss in people aged 50 years and older: A meta-analysis. *Lancet, 370,* 657–666.

Tanofsky-Kraff, M., Marcus, M. D., Yanovski, S. Z., & Yanovski, J. A. (2008). Loss of control eating disorder in children age 12 years and younger: Proposed research criteria. *Eating Behaviors, 9,* 360–365.

Tanofsky-Kraff, M., & Wilfley, D. E. (2010). Interpersonal psychotherapy for the treatment of eating disorders. In W. S. Agras (Ed.), *The Oxford handbook of eating disorders* (pp. 348–372). New York: Oxford University Press.

Tardon, A., Lee, W. J., Delgaldo-Rodrigues, M., Dosemeci, M., Albanes, D., Hoover, R., et al. (2005). Leisure-time physical activity and lung cancer: A meta-analysis. *Cancer Causes and Control, 16,* 389–397.

Tashman, L. S., Tenenbaum, G., & Eklund, R. (2010). The effect of perceived stress on the relationship between perfectionism and burnout in coaches. *Anxiety, Stress & Coping, 23,* 195–212.

Tate, J. J., & Milner, C. E. (2010). Real-time kinematic, temporospatial, and kinetic biofeedback during gait retraining in patients: A systematic review. *Physical Therapy, 90*(8), 1123–1134.

Taylor, D. H., Jr., Hasselblad, V., Henley, S. J., Thun, M. J., & Sloan, F. A. (2002). Benefits of smoking cessation for longevity. *American Journal of Public Health, 92,* 990–996.

Taylor, E. N., Stampfer, M. J., & Curhan, G. C. (2005). Obesity, weight gain, and the risk of kidney stones. *Journal of the American Medical Association, 293,* 455–462.

Taylor, R., Najafi, F., & Dobson, A. (2007). Meta-analysis of studies of passive smoking and lung cancer: Effects of study type and continent. *International Journal of Epidemiology, 36*(5), 1048.

Taylor, S. E. (2002). *The tending instinct: How nurturing is essential to who we are and how we live.* New York: Times Books, Henry Holt and Company.

Taylor, S. E. (2006). Tend and befriend: Biobehavioral bases of affiliation under stress. *Current Directions in Psychological Science, 15,* 273–277.

Taylor, S. E., Gonzaga, G., Klein, L. C., Hu, P., Greendale, G. A., & Seeman, T. E. (2006). Relation of oxytocin to psychological and biological stress responses in women. *Psychosomatic Medicine, 68,* 238–245.

Taylor, S. E., Klein, L. C., Lewis, B. P., Gruenewald, T. L., Gurung, R. A. R., & Updegraff, J. A. (2000). Biobehavioral responses to stress in females: Tend-and-befriend, not fight-or-flight. *Psychological Review, 107,* 411–429.

Taylor, S. E., Saphire-Bernstein, S., & Seeman, T. E. (2010). Are plasma oxytocin in women and plasma vasopressin in men biomarkers of distressed pair-bond relationships? *Psychological Science, 21,* 3–7.

Taylor, G. H., Wilson, S. L., & Sharp, J. (2011). Medical, psychological, and sociodemographic factors associated with adherence to cardiac rehabilitation programs: A systematic review. *Journal of Cardiovascular Nursing, 26,* 202–209.

Taylor-Piliae, R. E., Haskell, W. L., Waters, C. M., & Froelicher, E. S. (2006). Change in perceived psychosocial status following a 12-week Tai Chi exercise programme. *Journal of Advanced Nursing, 54,* 313–329.

Tedeschi, R. G., & Calhoun, L. G. (2006). Time of change? The spiritual challenges of bereavement and loss. *Omega: Journal of Death and Dying, 53,* 105–116.

Tedeschi, R. G., & Calhoun, L. G. (2008). Beyond the concept of recovery: Growth and the experience of loss. *Death Studies, 32,* 27–39.

Templeton, D. (2008, April 15). Bill Clinton's heart troubles hard to detect, experts say. *Pittsburg Post-Gazette.* Retrieved June 1, 2008, from http://www.post-gazette.com/pg/08106/873418-114.stm

Teo, K. K., Ounpuu, S., Hawken, S., Pandey, M. R., Valentin, V., Hunt, D., et al. (2006). Tobacco use and risk of myocardial infarction in 52 countries in the INTERHEART study: A case-control study. *The Lancet, 368,* 19–25.

Terry, A., Szabo, A., & Griffiths, M. D. (2004). The Exercise Addiction Inventory: A new brief screening tool. *Addiction Research and Theory, 12,* 489–499.

Testa, M., Vazile-Tamsen, C., & Livingston, J. A. (2004). The role of victim and perpetrator intoxication on sexual assault outcomes. *Journal of Studies on Alcohol, 65,* 320–329.

Theberge, N. (2008). The integration of chiropractors into healthcare teams: A case study from sport medicine. *Sociology of Health and Illness, 30,* 19–34.

Theis, K. A., Helmick, C. G., & Hootman, J. M. (2007). Arthritis burden and impact are greater among U.S. women than men: Intervention opportunities. *Journal of Women's Health, 16,* 441–453.

Thielke, S., Thompson, A., & Stuart, R. (2011). Health psychology in primary care: Recent research and future directions. *Psychological Research and Behavior Management, 4,* 59–68.

Thomas, J. J., Keel, P. K., & Heatherton, T. E. (2005). Disordered eating attitudes and behaviors in ballet students: Examination of environmental and individual risk factors. *International Journal of Eating Disorders, 38,* 263–268.

Thomas, W., White, C. M., Mah, J., Geisser, M. S., Church, T. R., & Mandel, J. S. (1995). Longitudinal compliance with annual screening for fecal occult blood. *American Journal of Epidemiology, 142,* 176–182.

Thompson, O. M., Yaroch, A. L., Moser, R. P., Finney Rutten, L. J., Petrelli, J. M., Smith-Warner, S. A., et al. (2011). Knowledge of and adherence to fruit and vegetable recommendations and intakes: Results of the 2003 Health Information National Trends Survey. *Journal of Health Communication: International Perspectives, 16,* 328–340.

Thompson, P. D. (2001, January). Exercise rehabilitation for cardiac patients: A beneficial but underused therapy. *The Physician and Sportsmedicine, 29,* 69–75.

Thompson, P. D., Franklin, B. A., Balady, G. J., Blair, S. N., Corrado, D., Domenico, E., III, et al. (2007). Exercise and acute cardiovascular events: Placing the risks into perspective. *Medicine and Science in Sports and Exercise, 39,* 886–897.

Thompson, S. H., & Hammond, K. (2003). Beauty is as beauty does: Body image and self-esteem of pageant contestants. *Eating and Weight Disorders, 8,* 231–237.

Thorburn, A. W. (2005). Prevalence of obesity in Australia. *Obesity Reviews, 6,* 187–189.

Thorn, B. E., & Kuhajda, M. C. (2006). Group cognitive therapy for chronic pain. *Journal of Clinical Psychology, 62,* 1355–1366.

Thorn, B. E., Pence, L. B., Ward, L. C., Kilgo, G., Clements, K. L., Cross, T. H., et al. (2007). A randomized clinical trial of targeted cognitive behavioral treatment to reduce catastrophizing in chronic headache sufferers. *Journal of Pain, 8,* 938–949.

Thorogood, A., Mottillo, S., Shimony, A., Filion, K. B., Joseph, L., Genest, J., et al. (2011). Isolated aerobic exercise and weight loss: A systematic review and meta-analysis of randomized controlled trials. *American Journal of Medicine, 124*(8), 747–755.

Thun, M. J., Day-Lally, C. A., Calle, E. E., Flanders, W. D., & Heath, C. W., Jr. (1995). Excess mortality among cigarette smokers: Changes in a 20-year interval. *American Journal of Public Health, 85,* 1223–1230.

Thune, I., Brenn, T., Lund, E., & Gaard, M. (1997). Physical activity and the risk of breast cancer. *New England Journal of Medicine, 336,* 1269–1275.

Thune, I., & Furberg, A. S. (2001). Physical activity and cancer risk: Dose-response and cancer, all sites and site-specific. *Medicine and Science in Sports and Exercise, 33,* S530–S550.

Thuné-Boyle, I. C. V., Myers, L. B., & Newman, S. P. (2006). The role of illness beliefs, treatment beliefs, and perceived severity of symptoms in explaining distress in cancer patients during chemotherapy treatment. *Behavioral Medicine, 32,* 19–29.

Thygesen, L. C., Johansen, C., Keiding, N., Giovannucci, E., & Grønbæk, M. (2008). Effects of sample attrition in a longitudinal study of the association between alcohol intake and all-cause mortality. *Addiction, 103,* 1149–1159.

Tice, D. M., Bratslavsky, E., & Baumeister, R. F. (2001). Emotional distress regulation takes precedence over impulse control: If you feel bad, do it! *Journal of Personality and Social Psychology, 80,* 53–67.

Tilburt, J. C., Emanuel, E. J., Kaptchuk, T. J., Curlin, F. A., & Miller, F. G. (2008). Prescribing "placebo treatments": Results of national survey of US internists and rheumatologists. *British Medical Journal, 337,* a1938. DOI: 10.1136/bmj.a1938

Tobar, D. A. (2005). Overtraining and staleness: The importance of psychological monitoring. *International Journal of Sport and Exercise Psychology, 3,* 455–468.

Todd, J. E., & Variyam, J. N. (2008). *The decline in consumer use of food nutrition labels, 1995–2006.* Washigton, DC: U.S. Department of Agriculture.

Tolfrey, K. (2004). Lipid-lipoproteins in children: An exercise dose-response study. *Medicine and Science in Sports and Exercise, 36,* 418–427.

Tolfrey, K., Jones, A. M., & Campbell, I. G. (2000). The effect of aerobic exercise training on the lipid-lipoprotein profile of children and adolescents. *Sports Medicine, 29,* 99–112.

Tolstrup, J. S., Nordestgaard, B. G., Rasmussen, S., Tybjærg-Hansen, A., & Grønbæk, M. (2008). Alcoholism and alcohol drinking habits predicted from alcohol dehydrogenase genes. *Pharmacogenomics Journal, 8,* 220–227.

Tomar, S. L., & Hatsukami, D. K. (2007). Perceived risk of harm from cigarettes or smokeless tobacco among U.S. high school seniors. *Nicotine and Tobacco Research, 9,* 1191–1196.

Tomfohr, L. M., Martin, T. M., & Miller, G. E. (2008). Symptoms of depression and impaired endothelial function in healthy adolescent women. *Journal of Behavioral Medicine, 31,* 137–143.

Torchalla, I., Okoli, C. T. C., Hemsing, N., & Greaves, L. (2011). Gender differences in smoking behaviour and cessation. *Journal of Smoking Cessation, 6*(1), 9–16.

Torian, L., Chen, M., Rhodes, P., & Hall, H. R. (2011). HIV surveillance—United States, 1981–2008. *Morbidity and Mortality Weekly Report, 60*(21), 689–693.

Torpy, J. M. (2006). Eating fish: Health benefits and risks. *Journal of the American Medical Association, 296,* 1926.

Torstveit, M. K., Rosenvinge, J. H., & Sundgot-Borgen, J. (2008). Prevalence of eating disorders and the predictive power of risk models in female elite athletes: A controlled study. *Scandinavian Journal of Medicine and Science in Sports, 18,* 108–118.

Tousignant-Laflamme, Y., Rainville, P., & Marchand, S. (2005). Establishing a link between heart rate and pain in healthy subjects: A gender effect. *Journal of Pain, 6,* 341–347.

Tovian, S. M. (2004). Health services and health care economics: The health psychology marketplace. *Health Psychology, 23,* 138–141.

Tractenberg, R. E., Singer, C. M., & Kaye, J. A. (2005). Symptoms of sleep disturbance in persons with Alzheimer's disease and normal elderly. *Journal of Sleep Research, 14,* 177–185.

Travis, L. (2001). Training for interdisciplinary healthcare. *Health Psychologist, 23*(1), 4–5.

Treiber, F. A., Davis, H., Musante, L., Raunikar, R. A., Strong. W. G., McCaffrey, F., et al. (1993). Ethnicity, gender, family history of myocardial infarction, and menodynamic responses to laboratory stressors in children. *Health Psychology, 12,* 6–15.

Treur, T., Koperdák, M., Rózsa, S., & Füredi, J. (2005). The impact of physical and sexual abuse on body image in eating disorders. *European Eating Disorders Review, 13,* 106–111.

Troxel, W. M., Matthews, K. A., Bromberger, J. T., & Sutton-Tyrrell, K. (2003). Chronic stress burden, discrimination, and subclinical carotid artery disease in African American and Caucasian women. *Health Psychology, 22,* 300–309.

The truth about dieting. (2002, June). *Consumer Reports, 67*(6), 26–31.

Tsai, A. G., & Wadden, T. A. (2005). Systematic review: An evaluation of major commercial weight loss programs in the United States. *Annals of Internal Medicine, 142,* 56–66.

Tsao, J. C. I (2007). Effectiveness of massage therapy for chronic, nonmalignant pain: A review. *Evidence-Based Complementary and Alternative Medicine, 4,* 165–179.

Tsao, J. C. I., & Zeltzer, L. K. (2005). Complementary and alternative medicine approaches for pediatric pain: A review of the state-of-the-science. *Evidence-Based Complementary and Alternative Medicine, 2,* 149–159.

Tsiotra, P. C., & Tsigos, C. (2006). Stress, the endoplasmic reticulum, and insulin resistance. In G. P. Chrousos & C. Tsigos (Eds.), *Stress, obesity, and metabolic syndrome* (pp. 63–76). New York: Annals of the New York Academy of Sciences.

Tsoi, D. T., Porwal, M., & Webster, A. C. (2010). Interventions for smoking cessation and reduction in individuals with schizophrenia. *Cochrane Database of Systematic Reviews 2010, 6,* Cochrane Art. No.: CD007253, DOI:10.1002/14651858.CD007253.pub2.

Tucker, J. A., Phillips, M. M., Murphy, J. G., & Raczynski, J. M. (2004). Behavioral epidemiology and health psychology. In R. G. Frank, A. Baum, & J. L. Wallander (Eds.), *Handbook of clinical health psychology* (Vol. 3, pp. 435–464). Washington, DC: American Psychological Association.

Tucker, J. S., Orlando, M., & Ellickson, P. L. (2003). Patterns and correlates of binge drinking trajectories from early adolescence to young adulthood. *Health Psychology, 22,* 79–87.

Tucker, O. N., Szomstein, S., & Rosenthal, R. J. (2007). Nutritional consequences of weight loss surgery. *Medical Clinics of North America, 91,* 499–513.

Turk, D. C. (1978). Cognitive behavioral techniques in the management of pain. In J. P. Foreyt & D. P. Rathjen (Eds.), *Cognitive behavior therapy* (pp. 199–232). New York: Plenum Press.

Turk, D. C. (2001). Physiological and psychological bases of pain. In A. Baum, T. A. Revenson, & J. E. Singer (Eds.), *Handbook of health psychology* (pp. 117–131). Mahwah, NJ: Erlbaum.

Turk, D. C., & McCarberg, B. (2005). Non-pharmacological treatments for chronic pain: A disease management context. *Disease Management and Health Outcomes, 13*, 19–30.

Turk, D. C., & Melzack, R. (2001). The measurement of pain and the assessment of people experiencing pain. In D. C. Turk & R. Melzack (Eds.), *Handbook of pain assessment* (2nd ed., pp. 3–11). New York: Guilford Press.

Turk, D. C., Swanson, K. S., & Gatchel, R. J. (2008). Predicting opioid misuse by chronic pain patients: A systematic review and literature synthesis. *Clinical Journal of Pain, 24*, 497–508.

Turner, J., & Kelly, B. (2000). Emotional dimensions of chronic disease. *Western Journal of Medicine, 172*, 124–128.

Turner, J. A., Deyo, R. A., Loeser, J. D., Von Korff, M., & Fordyce, W. E. (1994). The importance of placebo effects in pain treatment and research. *Journal of the American Medical Association, 271*, 1609–1614.

Turner, R. J., & Avison, W. R. (2003). Status variations in stress exposure: Implications for the interpretation of research on race, socioeconomic status, and gender. *Journal of Health and Social Behavior, 44*, 488–505.

Turner, R. J., & Wheaton, B. (1995). Checklist measurement of stressful life events. In S. Cohen, R. C. Kessler, & L. U. Gordon (Eds.), *Measuring stress: A guide for health and social scientists* (pp. 29–58). New York: Oxford University Press.

Turpin, R. S., Simmons, J. B., Lew, J. F., Alexander, C. M., Dupee, M. A., Kavanagh, P., et al. (2004). Improving treatment regimen adherence in coronary heart disease by targeting patient types. *Disease Management and Health Outcomes, 12*, 377–383.

Twenge, J. M., Liqing, Z., & Im, C. (2004). It's beyond my control: A cross-temporal meta-analysis of increasing externality in locus of control, 1960–2002. *Personality and Social Psychology Review, 8*, 308–319.

Twicken, D. (2011). An introduction to medical qi gong. *Acupuncture Today, 12*(2), 20.

Tylka, T. L. (2004). The relation between body dissatisfaction and eating disorder symptomatology: An analysis of moderating variables. *Journal of Counseling Psychology, 51*, 178–191.

UCLA Cousins Center for Psychoneuroimmunology. (2011). *About us.* Retrieved September 6, 2011, from http://www.semel.ucla.edu/cousins/about

Ullman, D. (2010). A review of a historical summit on integrative medicine. *Evidence-Based Complementary & Alternative Medicine (eCAM), 7*(4), 511–514.

Ulrich, C. (2002). High stress and low income: The environment of poverty. *Human Ecology, 30*(4), 16–18.

UNAIDS. (2007). *AIDS epidemic update, 2007.* Geneva, Switzerland: Joint United Nations Programme on HIV/AIDS.

UNAIDS (2010). *Report on the global AIDS epidemic, 2010.* Geneva, Switzerland: World Health Organization.

Unger-Saldaña, K., & Infante-Castañeda, C. B. (2011). Breast cancer delay: A grounded model of help-seeking behavior. *Social Science and Medicine, 72*, 1096–1104.

Updegraff, J. A., Silver, R. C., & Holman, E. A. (2008). Searching for and finding meaning in a collective trauma: Results from a national longitudinal study of the 9/11 terrorist attacks. *Journal of Personality and Social Psychology, 95*, 709–722.

Updegraff, J. A., & Taylor, S. E. (2000). From vulnerability to growth: Positive and negative effects of stressful life events. In J. Harvey & E. Miller (Eds.), *Loss and Trauma: General and Close Relationship Perspectives* (pp. 3–28). Philadelphia, PA: Brunner-Routledge.

Updegraff, J. A., Taylor, S. E., Kemeny, M. E., & Wyatt, G. E. (2000). Positive and negative effects of HIV infection in women with low socioeconomic resources. *Personality and Social Psychology Bulletin, 28*, 382–394.

Urizar, G. G., & Muñoz, R. F. (2011). Impact of a prenatal cognitive-behavioral stress management intervention on salivary cortisol levels in low-income mothers and their infants. *Psychoneuroimmunology, 36*, 1480–1494.

U.S. Census Bureau (USCB). (2011). *Statistical abstract of the United States: 2012* (131st ed.). Washington, DC: U.S. Government Printing Office. Retrieved September 28, 2012, from http://www.census.gov/compendia/statab/

U.S. Department of Health and Human Services (USDHHS). (1990). *The health benefits of smoking cessation: A report of the Surgeon General* (DHHS Publication No. CDC 90-8416). Washington, DC: U.S. Government Printing Office.

U.S. Department of Health and Human Services (USDHHS). (1995). *Healthy People 2000 review, 1994* (DHHS Publication No. PHS 95-1256-1). Washington, DC: U.S. Government Printing Office.

U.S. Department of Health and Human Services (USDHHS). (1996). *Physical activity and health: A report of the Surgeon General.* Atlanta, GA: Centers for Disease Control and Prevention.

U.S. Department of Health and Human Services (USDHHS). (2000). *Healthy People 2010: Understanding and improving health* (2nd ed.). Washington, DC: U.S. Government Printing Office.

U.S. Department of Health and Human Services (USDHHS). (2003). *The seventh report of the Joint National Committee on Prevention, Detection, Evaluation and Treatment of High Blood Pressure* (NIH Publication No. 03-5233). Washington, DC: Author.

U.S. Department of Health and Human Services (USDHHS). (2004). *The health consequences of smoking: A report of the Surgeon General.* Atlanta, GA: Author.

U.S. Department of Health and Human Services (USDHHS). (2007). *Healthy people 2010 midcourse review.* Retrieved August 5, 2008, from http://www.healthypeople.gov/Data/midcourse/

U.S. Department of Health and Human Services (USDHHS). (2008a). *Physical activity guidelines for Americans.* Retrieved February 20, 2012, from http://www.health.gov/PAGuidelines/factsheetprof.aspx

U.S. Department of Health and Human Services (USDHHS). (2008b). *The Secretary's Advisory Committee on National Health Promotion and Disease Prevention Objectives for 2020. Phase I report: Recommendations for the framework and format of Healthy People 2020. Section IV. Advisory Committee findings and recommendations.* Retrieved April 12, 2012, http://www.healthypeople.gov/2020/about/advisory/PhaseI.pdf

U.S. Department of Health and Human Services (USDHHS). (2010a). *Healthy People 2020.* Washington, DC: U.S. Government Printing Office. Retrieved April 20, 2012, from http://www.healthypeople.gov/2020/

U.S. Department of Health and Human Services (USDHHS). (2010b). *HHS announces the nation's new health promotion and disease prevention agenda* (press release). Retrieved April 10, 2012, from http://www.hhs.gov/news/press/2010pres/12/20101202a.html

U.S. Department of Health and Human Services (USDHHS). (2010c). *How tobacco smoke causes disease: The biology and behavioral basis for smoking-attributable disease: A report of the Surgeon General.* Atlanta, GA: Centers for Disease Control and Prevention.

U.S. Department of Health and Human Services (USDHHS). (2010d). *A report of the Surgeon General: How tobacco smoke causes disease: What it means to you.* Retrieved February 27, 2012, from http://www.cdc.gov/tobacco/data_statistics/sgr/2010/consumer_booklet/pdfs/consumer.pdf

U.S. Public Health Service (USPHS). (1964). *Smoking and health: Public Health Service report of the Advisory Committee to the Surgeon General of the Public Health Service* (PHS Publication No. 1103). Washington, DC: U.S. Government Printing Office.

Vainionpää, A., Korpelainen, R., Leppäluoto, J., & Jämsä, T. (2005). Effects of high-impact exercise on bone mineral density: A randomized controlled trial in premenopausal women. *Osteoporosis International, 16*, 191–197.

van Baal, P. H. M., Polder, J. J., de Wit, G. A., Hoogenveen, R. T., Feenstra, T. L., Bohuizen, H. C., et al. (2008). Lifetime medical costs of obesity: Prevention no cure for increasing health expenditure. *PLoS Medicine, 5*(2), 242–249.

van Cauter, E., Holmbäck, U., Knutson, K., Leproult, R., Miller, A., Nedeltcheva, A., et al. (2007). Impact of sleep and sleep loss on neuroendocrine and metabolic function. *Hormone Research, 67*(Suppl. 1), 2–9.

Van der Does, A. J., & Van Dyck, R. (1989). Does hypnosis contribute to the care of burn patients? Review of evidence. *General Hospital Psychiatry, 11,* 119–124.

van Dillen, S. M. E., de Vries, S., Groenewegen, P. P., & Spreeuwenberg, P. (2011). Greenspace in urban neighborhoods and residents' health: Adding quality to quantity. *Journal of Epidemiology & Community Health.* DOI:10.1136/jech.2009.104695.

van Hanswijck de Jonge, P., van Furth, E. F., Lacey, J. H., & Waller, G. (2003). The prevalence of DSM-IV personality pathology among individuals with bulimia nervosa, binge eating disorder and obesity. *Psychological Medicine, 33,* 1311–1317.

van Reekum, R., Binns, M., Clarke, D., Chayer, C., Conn, D., & Herrmann, N. (2005). Is late-life depression a predictor of Alzheimer's disease? Results from a historical cohort study. *International Journal of Geriatric Psychiatry, 20,* 80–82.

van Ryn, M., & Burke, J. (2000). The effect of patient race and socioeconomic status on physicians' perception of patients. *Social Science and Medicine, 50,* 813–828.

van Zundert, J., & van Kleef, M. (2005). Low back pain: From algorithm to cost-effectiveness? *Pain Practice, 5,* 179–189.

Varady, K. A., & Jones, P. J. H. (2005). Combination diet and exercise interventions for the treatment of dyslipidemia: An effective preliminary strategy to lower cholesterol levels? *Journal of Nutrition, 135,* 1829–1835.

Vartanian, L. R., Herman, C. P., & Polivy, J. (2007). Consumption stereotypes and impression management: How you are what you eat. *Appetite, 48*(3), 265–277.

Veehof, M. M., Oskam, M.-J., Schreurs, K. M. G., & Bohlmeijer, E. T. (2010). Acceptance-based interventions for the treatment of chronic pain: A systematic review and meta-analysis. *Pain, 152,* 533–542.

Veldtman, G. R., Matley, S. L., Kendall, L., Quirk, J., Gibbs, J. L., Parsons, J. M., et al. (2001). Illness understanding in children and adolescents with heart disease. *Western Journal of Medicine, 174,* 171–173.

Velicer, W. F., & Prochaska, J. O. (2008). Stages and non-stage theories of behavior and behavior change: A comment on Schwarzer. *Applied Psychology: An International Review, 57,* 75–83.

Velligan, D. I., Wang, M., Diamond, P., Glahn, D. C., Castillo, D., Bendle, S., et al. (2007). Relationships among subjective and objective measures of adherence to oral antipsychotic medications. *Psychiatric Services, 58,* 1187–1192.

Vemuri, P., Gunter, J. L., Senjem, M. L., Whitwell, J. L., Kantarci, K., Knopman, D. S., et al. (2008). Alzheimer's disease diagnosis in individual subjects using structural MR images: Validation studies. *NeuroImage, 39,* 1186–1197.

Venn, A., & Britton, J. (2007). Exposure to secondhand smoke and biomarkers of cardiovascular disease risk in never-smoking adults. *Circulation, 115,* 900–995.

Verbeeten, K. C., Elks, C. E., Daneman, D., & Ong, K. K. (2011). Association between childhood obesity and subsequent Type 1 diabetes: A systematic review and meta-analysis. *Diabetic Medicine, 28,* 10–18.

Verhagen, A. P., Damen, L., Berger, M. Y., Passchier, J., & Koes, B. W. (2009). Behavioral treatments of chronic tension-type headache in adults: Are they beneficial? *CNS Neuroscience & Therapeutics, 15*(2), 183–205.

Verkaik, R., Van Weert, J. C. M., & Francke, A. L. (2005). The effects of psychosocial methods on depressed, aggressive and apathetic behaviors of people with dementia: A systematic review. *International Journal of Geriatric Psychiatry, 20,* 301–314.

Verma, K. B., & Khan, M. I. (2007). Social inhibition, negative affectivity and depression in cancer patients with Type D personality. *Social Science International, 23,* 114–122.

Vermeire, E., Hearnshaw, H., Van Royen, P., & Denekens, J. (2001). Patient adherence to treatment: Three decades of research. A comprehensive review. *Journal of Clinical Pharmacy and Therapeutics, 26,* 331–342.

Verplanken, B., & Faes, S. (1999). Good intentions, bad habits, and effects of forming implementation intentions on healthy eating. *European Journal of Social Psychology, 29,* 591–604.

Veugelers, P., Sithole, F., Zhang, S., Muhajarine, N. (2008). Neighborhood characteristics in relation to diet, physical activity and overweight of Canadian children. *International Journal of Pediatric Obesity, 3,* 152–159.

Victor, T. W., Hu, X., Campbell, J. C., Buse, D. C., & Lipton, R. B. (2010). Migraine prevalence by age and sex in the United States: A life-span study. *Cephalalgia, 30,* 1065–1072.

Villalba, D., Ham, L. S., & Rose, S. (2011). Alcohol intoxication and memory for events: A snapshot of alcohol myopia in a real-world drinking scenario. *Memory, 19*(2), 202–210.

Viner, R. M., & Taylor, B. (2007). Adult outcomes of binge drinking in adolescence: Findings from a UK national birth cohort. *Journal of Epidemiology and Community Health, 61*(10), 902–907.

Virmani, R., Burke, A. P., & Farb, A. (2001). Sudden cardiac death. *Cardiovascular Pathology, 10,* 211–218.

Visser, M. (1999). Food and culture: Interconnections. *Social Research, 66,* 117–132.

Vitória, P. D., Salgueiro, M. F., Silva, S. A., & De Vries, H. (2009). The impact of social influence on adolescent intention to smoke: Combining types and referents of influence. *British Journal of Health Psychology, 14*(4), 681–699.

Vlachopoulos, C., Rokkas, K., Ioakeimidis, N., & Stefanadis, C. (2007). Inflammation, metabolic syndrome, erectile dysfunction, and coronary artery disease: Common links. *European Urology, 52,* 1590–1600.

Voas, R. B., Roman, T. E., Tippetts, A. S., & Durr-Holden, C. D. M. (2006). Drinking status and fatal crashes: Which drinkers contribute most to the problem? *Journal of Studies on Alcohol, 67,* 722–729.

von Baeyer, C. L., & Spagrud, L. J. (2007). Systematic review of observational (behavioral) measures of pain for children and adolescents aged 3 to 18 years. *Pain, 127,* 140–150.

von Hertzen, L. C., & Haahtela, T. (2004). Asthma and atopy—The price of affluence? *Allergy, 59,* 124–137.

Von Korff, M., Barlow, W., Cherkin, D., & Deyo, R. A. (1994). Effects of practice style in managing back pain. *Annals of Internal Medicine, 121,* 187–195.

Waber, R. L., Shiv, B., Carmon, Z., & Ariely, D. (2008). Commercial features of placebo and therapeutic efficacy. *Journal of the American Medical Association, 299,* 1016–1017.

Wachholtz, A., & Sambamoorthi, U. (2011). National trends in prayer use as a coping mechanism for health concerns: Changes from 2002 to 2007. *Psychology of Religion and Spirituality, 3*(2), 67–77.

Wadden, T. A., Crerand, C. E., & Brock, J. (2005). Behavioral treatment of obesity. *Psychiatric Clinics of North America, 28,* 151–170.

Wager, T. D., Rilling, J. K., Smith, E. E., Sololik, A., Casey, K. L., Davidson, R. J., et al. (2004). Placebo-induced changes in fMRI in the anticipation and experience of pain. *Science, 303,* 1162–1167.

Wahlberg, A. (2007). A quackery with a difference—New medical pluralism and the problem of 'dangerous practitioners' in the United Kingdom. *Social Science & Medicine, 65*(11), 2307–2316.

Waite-Jones, J. M., & Madill, A. (2008a). Amplified ambivalence: Having a sibling with juvenile idiopathic arthritis. *Psychology and Health, 23,* 477–492.

Waite-Jones, J. M., & Madill, A. (2008b). Concealed concern: Fathers' experiences of having a child with juvenile idiopathic arthritis. *Psychology and Health, 23,* 585–601.

Wakefield, M., Loken, B., & Hornik, R. (2010). Use of mass media campaigns to change health behaviour. *The Lancet, 376,* 1261–1271.

Walach, H., & Jonas, W. B. (2004). Placebo research: The evidence base for harnessing self-healing capacities. *Journal of Alternative and Complementary Medicine, 10*(S1), S103–S112.

Walcher, T., Haenle, M. M., Mason, R. A., Koenig, W., Imhof, A., & Kratzer, W. (2010). The effect of alcohol, tobacco and caffeine consumption and vegetarian diet on gallstone prevalence. *European Journal of Gastroenterology & Hepatology, 22*(11), 1345–1351.

Wald, H. S., Dube, C. E., & Anthony, D. C. (2007). Untangling the Web—The impact of Internet use on health care and the physician-patient relationship. *Patient Education and Counseling, 68,* 218–224.

Waldrop-Valverde, D., Osborn, C. Y., Rodriguez, A., Rothman, R. L., Kumar, M., & Jones, D. L. (2010). Numeracy skills explain racial differences in HIV medication management. *AIDS & Behavior, 14,* 799–806.

Walen, H. R., & Lachman, M. E. (2000). Social support and strain from partner, family, and friends: Costs and benefits for men and women in adulthood. *Journal of Social and Personal Relationships, 17,* 5–30.

Walker, A. R. P., Walker, B. F., & Adam, F. (2003). Nutrition, diet, physical activity, smoking, and longevity: From primitive hunter-gatherer to present passive consumer—How far can we go? *Nutrition, 19,* 169–173.

Walker, E. A., Mertz, C. K., Kalten, M. R., & Flynn, J. (2003). Risk perception for developing diabetes. *Diabetes Care, 26,* 2543–2548.

Wall, P. (2000). *Pain: The science of suffering.* New York: Columbia University Press.

Waltenbaugh, A. W., & Zagummy, M. J. (2004). Optimistic bias and perceived control among cigarette smokers. *Journal of Alcohol and Drug Education, 47,* 20–33.

Walter, H., Gutierrez, K., Ramskogler, K., Hertling, I., Dvorak, A., & Lesch, O. M. (2003). Gender-specific differences in alcoholism: Implications for treatment. *Archives of Women's Mental Health, 6,* 253–258.

Wamala, S. P., Mittleman, M. A., Horsten, M., Schenck-Gustafsson, K., & Orth-Gomér, K. (2000). Job stress and the occupational gradient in coronary heart disease risk in women: The Stockholm Female Coronary Risk study. *Social Science and Medicine, 51,* 481–489.

Wang, C., Bannuru, R., Ramel, J., Kupelnick, B., Scott, T., & Schmid, C. H. (2010). Tai chi on psychological well-being: Systematic review and meta-analysis. *BMC Complementary & Alternative Medicine, 10, 23.* DOI:10.1186/1472-6882-10-23.

Wang, C., Schmid, C. H., Rones, R., Kalish, R., Yinh, J., Goldenberg, D. L., et al. (2010). A randomized trial of tai chi for fibromyalgia. *New England Journal of Medicine, 363*(8), 743–754.

Wang, H.-W., Mittleman, M. A., & Orth-Gomér, K. (2005). Influence of social support on progression of coronary artery disease in women. *Social Science and Medicine, 60,* 599–607.

Wang, H.-X., Leineweber, C., Kirkeeide, R., Svane, B., Schenck-Gustafsson, K., Theorell, T., et al. (2007). Psychosocial stress and atherosclerosis: Family and work stress accelerate progression of coronary disease in women. The Stockholm Female Coronary Angiography Study. *Journal of Internal Medicine, 261,* 245–254.

Wang, J. L., Lesage, A., Schmitz, N., & Drapeau, A. (2008). The relationship between work stress and mental disorders in men and women: Findings from a population-based study. *Journal of Epidemiology and Community Health, 62,* 42–47.

Wang, S.-W., Shih, J. H., Hu, A. W., Louie, J. Y., & Lau, A. S. (2010). Cultural differences in daily support experiences. *Cultural Diversity and Ethnic Minority Psychology, 16,* 413–420.

Wang, Y. (2004). Diet, physical activity, childhood obesity and risk of cardiovascular disease. *International Congress Series, 1262,* 176–179.

Wansink, B., & Payne, C. R. (2008). Eating behavior and obesity at Chinese buffets. *Obesity, 16,* 1957–1960.

Warburton, D. E. R., Nicol, C. W., & Bredin, S. S. D. (2006). Health benefits of physical activity: The evidence. *Canadian Medical Association Journal, 174,* 801–809.

Wardle, J., & Johnson, F. (2002). Weight and dieting: Examining levels of weight concern in British adults. *International Journal of Obesity, 26,* 1144–1149.

Warner, R., & Griffiths, M. D. (2006). A qualitative thematic analysis of exercise addiction: An exploratory study. *International Journal of Mental Health and Addiction, 4,* 13–26.

Warren, C. W., Jones, N. R., Peruga, A., Chauvin, J., Baptiste, J.-P., de Silva, V. C., et al. (2008). Global youth tobacco surveillance, 2000–2007. *Morbidity and Mortality Weekly Reports, 57*(SS-1), 1–27.

Watanabe, T., Higuchi, K., Tanigawa, T., Tominaga, K., Fujiwara, Y., & Arakawa, T. (2002). Mechanisms of peptic ulcer recurrence: Role of inflammation. *Inflammopharmacology, 10,* 291–302.

Watkins, L. R., Hutchinson, M. R., Ledeboer, A., Wieseler-Frank, J., Milligan, E. D., & Maier, S. F. (2007). Glia as the "bad guys": Implications for improving clinical pain control and the clinical utility of opioids. *Brain, Behavior and Immunity, 21,* 131–146.

Watkins, L. R., & Maier, S. F. (2003). When good pain turns bad. *Current Directions in Psychological Science, 12,* 232–236.

Watkins, L. R., & Maier, S. F. (2005). Immune regulation of central nervous system function: From sickness responses to pathological pain. *Journal of Internal Medicine, 257,* 139–155.

Waye, K. P., Bengtsson, J., Rylander, R., Hucklebridge, F., Evans, P., & Clow, A. (2002). Low frequency noise enhances cortisol among noise sensitive subjects during work performance. *Life Sciences, 70,* 745–758.

Wayne, P. M., Kiel, D. P., Krebs, D. E., Davis, R. B., Savetsky-German, J., Connelly, M., et al. (2007). The effects of tai chi on bone mineral density in postmenopausal women: A systematic review. *Archives of Physical Medicine and Rehabilitation, 88,* 673–680.

Webb, O. J., & Cheng, T.-F. (2010). An informational stair climbing intervention with greater effects in overweight pedestrians. *Health Education Research, 25,* 936–944.

Webb, T. L., Joseph, J., Yardley, L., & Michie, S. (2010). Using the Internet to promote health behavior change: A systematic review and meta-analysis of the impact of theretical basis, use of behavior change techniques, and mode of delivery on efficacy. *Journal of Medical Internet Research, 12,* e4.

Weems, C. F., Watts, S. E., Marsee, M. A., Taylor, L. K., Costa, N. M., Cannon, M. F., et al. (2007). The psychological impact of Hurricane Katrina: Contextual differences in psychological symptoms, social support, and discrimination. *Behavior Research and Therapy, 45,* 2295–2306.

Weidner, G. (2000). Why do men get more heart disease than women? An international perspective. *Journal of American College Health, 48,* 291–296.

Weidner, G., & Cain, V. S. (2003). The gender gap in heart disease: Lessons from Eastern Europe. *American Journal of Public Health, 93,* 768–770.

Weil, C. M., Wade, S. L., Bauman, L. J., Lynn, H., Mitchell, H., & Lavigne, J. (1999). The relationship between psychosocial factors and asthma morbidity in inner-city children with asthma. *Pediatrics, 104,* 1274–1280.

Weil, J. M., & Lee, H. H. (2004). Cultural considerations in understanding family violence among Asian American Pacific islander families. *Journal of Community Health Nursing, 21,* 217–227.

Weinberger, A. H., Krishnan-Sarin, S., Mazure, C. M., & McKee, S. A. (2008). Relationship of perceived risks of smoking cessation to symptoms of withdrawal, craving, and depression during short-term smoking abstinence. *Addictive Behaviors, 33,* 960–963.

Weiner, H., & Shapiro, A. P. (2001). *Helicobacter pylori,* immune function, and gastric lesions. In R. Ader, D. L. Felten, & N. Cohen (Eds.), *Psychoneuroimmunology* (3rd ed., Vol. 2, pp. 671–686). San Diego, CA: Academic Press.

Weiner, M. F., Hynan, L. S., Bret, M. E., & White, C., III. (2005). Early behavioral symptoms and course of Alzheimer's disease. *Acta Psychiatrica Scandinavica, 111,* 367–371.

Weingart, S. N., Pagovich, O., Sands, D. Z., Li, J. M., Aronson, M. D., Davis, R. B., et al. (2006). Patient-reported service quality on a medicine unit. *International Journal for Quality in Health Care, 18,* 95–101.

Weinstein, N. D. (1980). Unrealistic optimism about future life events. *Journal of Personality and Social Psychology, 39,* 806–820.

Weinstein, N. D. (1984). Why it won't happen to me: Perceptions of risk factors and susceptibility. *Health Psychology, 3,* 431–457.

Weinstein, N. D. (1988). The precaution adoption process. *Health Psychology, 7,* 355–386.

Weinstein, N. D. (2000). Perceived probability, perceived severity, and health-protective behavior. *Health Psychology, 19,* 65–74.

Weinstein, N. D. (2001). Smokers' recognition of their vulnerability to harm. In P. Slovic (Ed.), *Smoking: Risk, perception and policy* (pp. 81–96). Thousand Oaks, CA: Sage.

Weinstein, N. D., Lyon, J. E., Sandman, P. M., & Cuite, C. L. (2003). Experimental evidence for stages of health behavior change: The precaution adoption process model applied to home radon testing. In P. Salovey & A. J. Rothman (Eds.), *Social psychology of health* (pp. 249–260). New York: Psychology Press.

Weinstein, N. D., Sandman, P. M., & Blalock, S. J. (2008). The precaution adoption process model. In K. Glanz, B. K. Rimer, & F. M. Lewis (Eds.), *Health behavior and health education: Theory, research, and practice* (pp. 123–147). San Francisco, CA: Jossey-Bass.

Weir, H. K., Thun, M. J., Hankey, B. F., Ries, L. A. G., Howe, H. L., Wingo, P. A., et al. (2003). Annual report to the nation on the status of cancer, 1975–2000, featuring the uses of surveillance data for cancer prevention and control. *Journal of the National Cancer Institute, 95,* 1276–1299.

Weiss, J. W., Cen, S., Schuster, D. V., Unger, J. B., Johnson, C. A., Mouttapa, M., et al. (2006). Longitudinal effects of pro-tobacco and anti-tobacco messages on adolescent smoking susceptibility. *Nicotine and Tobacco Research, 8,* 455–465.

Weiss, R. (1999, November 30). Medical errors blamed for many deaths; as many as 98,000 a year in US linked to mistakes. *Washington Post,* p. A1.

Weitz, R. (2010). *The sociology of health, illness, and health care: A critical approach* (5th ed.). Belmont, CA: Wadsworth.

Wells, J. C. K. (2011). An evolutionary perspective on the trans-generational basis of obesity. *Annals of Human Biology, 38*(4), 400–409.

Wells, R. E., Phillips. R. S., Schachter, S. C., & McCarthy, E. P. (2010). Complementary and alternative medicine use among U.S. adults with common neurological conditions. *Journal of Neurology, 257,* 1822–1831.

Wen, C., Tsai, S. P., Cheng, T. Y., Chan, H., T., Chung, W. S. I., & Chen, C. J. (2005). Excess injury mortality among smokers: A neglected tobacco hazard. *Tobacco Control, 14*(Suppl. 1), 28–32.

Wen, M. (2007). Racial and ethnic differences in general health status and limiting health conditions among American children: Parental reports in the 1999 National Survey of America's Families. *Ethnicity and Health, 12,* 401–422.

Wendel-Vos, G. C., Schuit, A. J., Feskens, E. J., Boshuizen, H. C., Verschuren, W. M., Saris, W. H., et al. (2004). Physical activity and stroke: A meta-analysis of observational data. *International Journal of Epidemiology, 33,* 787–798.

Wenzel, S. E. (2006). Asthma: Defining of the persistent adult phenotypes. *Lancet, 368,* 804–813.

West, S. L., & O'Neal, K. K. (2004). Project D.A.R.E. outcome effectiveness revisited. *American Journal of Public Health, 94,* 1027–1029.

Wetter, D. W., Cofta-Gunn, L., Fouladi, R. T., Irvin, J. E., Daza, P., Mazas, C., et al. (2005). Understanding the association among education, employment characteristics, and smoking. *Addictive Behaviors, 30,* 905–914.

Wetter, D. W., McClure, J. B., Cofta-Woerpel, L., Costello, T. J., Reitzel, L. R., Businelle, M. S., et al. (2011). A randomized clinical trial of a palmtop computer-delivered treatment for smoking relapse prevention among women. *Psychology of Addictive Behaviors, 25,* 365–371.

Whang, W., Kubzansky, L. D., Kawachi, I., Rexrode, K. M., Kroenke, C. H., Glynn, R. J., et al. (2009). Depression and risk of sudden cardiac death and coronary heart disease in women: Results from the Nurses' Health Study. *Journal of the American College of Cardiology, 53,* 950–958.

Wheaton, A. G., Perry, G. S., Chapman, D. P., McKnight-Eily, L. R., Presley-Cantrell, L. R., & Croft, J. B. (2011). Relationship between body mass index and perceived insufficient sleep among U.S. adults: An analysis of 2008 BRFSS data. *BMC Public Health, 11*(1), 295–302.

White, S., Chen, J., & Atchison, R. (2008). Relationship of preventive health practices and health literacy: A national study. *American Journal of Health Behavior, 32,* 227–242.

White, W. L. (2004). Addiction recovery mutual aid groups: An enduring international phenomenon. *Addiction, 99,* 532–538.

Whitfield, K. E., Weidner, G., Clark, R., & Anderson, N. B. (2002). Sociodemographic diversity in behavioral medicine. *Journal of Consulting and Clinical Psychology, 70,* 463–481.

Wider, B., & Boddy, K. (2009). Conducting systematic reviews of complementary and alternative medicine: Common pitfalls. *Evaluation & the Health Professions, 32*(4), 417–430.

Wilbert-Lampen, U., Leistner, D., Greven, S., Pohl, T., Sper, S., Völker, C., et al. (2008). Cardiovascular events during World Cup Soccer. *New England Journal of Medicine, 358,* 475–483.

Wilbert-Lampen, U., Nickel, T., Leistner, D., Guthlin, D., Matis, T., Volker, C., et al. (2010). Modified serum profiles of inflammatory and vasoconstrictive factors in patients with emotional stress-induced acute coronary syndrome during World Cup Soccer 2006. *Journal of the American College of Cardiology, 55,* 637–642.

Wiley, J. A., & Camacho, T. C. (1980). Life-style and future health: Evidence from the Alameda County Study. *Preventive Medicine, 9,* 1–21.

Wilkin, H. A., Valente, T. W., Murphy, S., Cody, M. J., Huang, G., & Beck, V. (2007). Does entertainment education work with Latinos in the United States? Identification and the effects of a telenovela breast cancer storyline. *Health Communication, 21,* 223–233.

Williams, L. J., Jacka, F. N., Pasco, J. A., Dodd, S., & Berk, M. (2006). Depression and pain: An overview. *Acta Neuropsychiatrica, 18,* 79–87.

Williams, M. T., & Hord, H. G. (2005). The role of dietary factors in cancer prevention: Beyond fruits and vegetables. *Nutrition in Clinical Practice, 20,* 451–459.

Williams, P. G., Holmbeck, G. N., & Greenley, R. N. (2002). Adolescent health psychology. *Journal of Consulting and Clinical Psychology, 70,* 828–842.

Williams, P. T. (2001). Health effects resulting from exercise versus those from body fat loss. *Medicine and Science in Sports and Exercise, 33,* S611–S621.

Williams, R. B., Jr. (1989). *The trusting heart: Great news about Type A behavior.* New York: Times Books.

Williams, R. B., Barefoot, J. C., Califf, R. M., Haney, T. L., Saunders, W. B., Pryor, D. B., et al. (1992). Prognostic importance of social and economic resources among medically treated patients with angiographically documented coronary artery disease. *Journal of the American Medical Association, 267,* 520–524.

Williamson, D. A., Thaw, J. M., & Varnado-Sullivan, P. J. (2001). Cost-effectiveness analysis of a hospital-based cognitive-behavioral treatment program for eating disorders. *Behavior Therapy, 32,* 459–470.

Wills, T. A. (1998). Social support. In E. A. Blechman & K. D. Brownell (Eds.), *Behavioral medicine and women: A comprehensive handbook* (pp. 118–128). New York: Guilford Press.

Wills, T. A., Sargent, J. D., Stoolmiller, M., Gibbons, F. X., & Gerrard, M. (2008). Movie smoking exposure and smoking onset: A longitudinal study of meditation processes in a representative sample of U.S. adolescents. *Psychology of Addictive Behaviors, 22,* 269–277.

Wills-Karp, M. (2004). Interleukin-13 in asthma pathogenesis. *Immunological Reviews, 202,* 175–190.

Wilson, B., & McSherry, W. (2006). A study of nurses' inferences of patients' physical pain. *Journal of Clinical Nursing, 15,* 459–468.

Wilz, G., Schinkothe, D., & Soellner, R. (2011). Goal attainment and treatment compliance in a cognitive-behavioral telephone intervention for family caregivers of persons with dementia. *GeroPsych: The Journal of Gerontopsychology and Geriatric Psychiatry, 24,* 115–125.

Wimberly, S. R., Carver, C. S., Laurenceau, J.-P., Harris, S. D., & Antoni, M. H. (2005). Perceived partner reactions to diagnosis and treatment of breast cancer: Impact on psychosocial and psychosexual adjustment. *Journal of Consulting and Clinical Psychology, 73,* 300–311.

Wing, R. R., Gorin, A. A., Raynor, H. A., Tate, D. F., Fava, J. L., & Machan, J. (2007). "STOP Regain": Are there negative effects of daily weighing? *Journal of Consulting and Clinical Psychology, 75*, 652–656.

Wing, R. R., & Polley, B. A. (2001). Obesity. In A. Baum, T. A. Revenson, & J. E. Singer (Eds.), *Handbook of health psychology* (pp. 263–279). Mahwah, NJ: Erlbaum.

Wingard, D. L., Berkman, L. F., & Brand, R. J, (1982). A multivariate analysis of health-related practices: A nine-year mortality follow-up of the Alameda County study. *American Journal of Epidemiology, 116*, 765–775.

Winterling, J., Glimelius, B., & Nordin, K. (2008). The importance of expectations on the recovery period after cancer treatment. *Psycho-Oncology, 17*, 190–198.

Wipfli, B. M., Rethorst, C. D., & Landers, D. M. (2008). The anxiolytic effects of exercise: A meta-analysis of randomized trials and dose-response analysis. *Journal of Sport and Exercise Psychology, 30*, 392–410.

Wise, J. (2000). Largest-ever study shows reduction in cardiovascular mortality. *Bulletin of the World Health Organization, 78*, 562.

Wiseman, C. V., Gray, J. J., Mosimann, J. E., & Ahrens, A. H. (1992). Cultural expectations of thinness in women: An update. *International Journal of Eating Disorders, 11*, 85–89.

Wiseman, C. V., Sunday, S. R., & Becker, A. E. (2005). Impact of the media on adolescent body image. *Child and Adolescent Psychiatric Clinics of North America, 14*, 453–471.

Witkiewitz, K., & Marlatt, G. A. (2010). Behavioral therapy across the spectrum. *Alcohol Research & Health, 33*(4), 313–319.

Witt, C. M., Brinkhaus, B., Reinhold, T., & Willich, S. N. (2006). Efficacy, effectiveness, safety and costs of acupuncture for chronic pain—Results of a large research initiative. *Acupuncture in Medicine, 24*(S33), 33–39.

Wolff, N. J., Darlington, A.-S. E., Hunfeld, J. A. M., Verhulst, F. C., Jaddoe, V. W. V., Moll, H. A., et al. (2009). The association of parent behaviors, chronic pain, and psychological problems with venipuncture distress in infants: The Generation R Study. *Health Psychology, 28*, 605–613.

Wolfgang, M. E. (1957). Victim precipitated criminal homicide. *Journal of Criminal Law and Criminology, 48*, 1–11.

Wolin, K. Y., Yan, Y., Colditz, G. A., & Lee, I.-M. (2009). Physical activity and colon cancer prevention: A meta-analysis. *British Journal of Cancer, 100*, 611–616.

Wonderlich, S. A., Crosby, R. D., Joiner, T., Peterson, C. B., Bardone-Cone, A., Klein, M., et al. (2005). Personality subtyping and bulimia nervosa: Psychopathological and genetic correlates. *Psychological Medicine, 35*, 649–657.

Wonderlich, S. A., Wilsnack, R. W., Wilsnack, S. C., & Harris, T. R. (1996). Childhood sexual abuse and bulimic behavior in a nationally representative sample. *American Journal of Public Health, 86*, 1082–1086.

Wood, P. D., Stefanick, M. L., Dreon, D. M., Frey-Hewitt, B., Garay, S. C., Williams, P. T., et al. (1988). Changes in plasma lipids and lipoproteins in overweight men during weight loss through dieting compared with exercise. *New England Journal of Medicine, 319*, 1173–1179.

Woodhouse, A. (2005). Phantom limb sensation. *Clinical and Experimental Pharmacology and Physiology, 32*, 132–134.

Woodside, D. B. (2002). Eating disorders in men: An overview. *Healthy Weight Journal, 16*(4), 52–55.

Woodward, H. I., Mytton, O. T., Lemer, C., Yardley, I. E., Ellis, B. M., Rutter, P. D., et al. (2010). What have we learned about interventions to reduce medical errors? *Annual Review of Public Health, 31*, 479–497.

Woolrich, R. A., Cooper, M. J., & Turner, H. M. (2008). Metacognition in patients with anorexia nervosa, dieting and non-dieting women: A preliminary study. *European Eating Disorders Review, 16*, 11–20.

World Cancer Research Fund/American Institute for Cancer Research (WCRF/AICR). (2007). *Food, nutrition, physical activity, and the prevention of cancer: A global perspective*. Washington, DC: AICR.

World Health Organization (WHO). (2008a). *The WHO report on the global tobacco epidemic, 2008*. Geneva, Switzerland: Author.

World Health Organization (WHO). (2008b). *World health 2008*. Geneva, Switzerland: WHO Press.

World Health Organization (WHO). (2009). *WHO report on the global tobacco epidemic, 2009: Implementing smoke-free environments*. Geneva, Switzerland: Author.

World Health Organization (WHO). (2010). *World Health Statistics 2010*. Retrieved April 9, 2012, from www.who.int/gho

World Medical Association. (2004). *Declartion of Helsinki: Ethical principles for medical research involving human subjects*. Retrieved February 7, 2008, from http://www.wma.net/e/policy/b3.htm

Writing Group for the Women's Health Initiative Investigators. (2002). Risks and benefits of estrogen plus progestin in healthy postmenopausal women: Principal results from the Women's Health Initiative randomized controlled trial. *Journal of the American Medical Association, 288*, 321–333.

Wu, J.-R., Moser, D. K., Chung, M. L., & Lennie, T. A. (2008). Objectively measured, but not self-reported, medication adherence independently predicts event-free survival in patients with heart failure. *Journal of Cardiac Failure, 14*, 203–210.

Wu, T., Gao, X., Chen, M., & van Dam, R. M. (2009). Long-term effectiveness of diet-plus-exercise interventions vs. diet-only interventions for weight loss: A meta-analysis. *Obesity Reviews, 10*(3), 313–323.

Wyden, P. (1965). *The overweight society*. New York: Morrow.

Xin, L., Miller, Y. D., & Brown, W. J. (2007). A qualitative review of the role of qigong in the management of diabetes. *Journal of Alternative and Complementary Medicine, 13*, 427–434.

Xue, C. C. L., Zhang, A. L., Greenwood, K. M., Lin, V., & Story, D. F. (2010). Traditional Chinese medicine: An update on clinical evidence. *Journal of Alternative & Complementary Medicine, 16*(3), 301–312.

Xue, C. C. L., Zhang, A. L., Lin, V., Da Costa, C., & Story, D. F. (2007). Complementary and alternative medicine use in Australia: A national population-based survey. *Journal of Alternative and Complementary Medicine, 13*, 643–650.

Xutian, S., Zhange, J., & Louise, W. (2009). New exploration and understanding of traditional Chinese medicine. *American Journal of Chinese Medicine, 37*(3), 411–426.

Yager, J. (2008). Binge eating disorder: The search for better treatments. *American Journal of Psychiatry, 165*, 4–6.

Yamashita, H., & Tsukayama, H. (2008). Safety of acupuncture practice in Japan: Patient reactions, therapist negligence and error reduction strategies. *Evidence-Based Complementary & Alternative Medicine (eCAM), 5*(4), 391–398.

Yan, L. L., Liu, K., Daviglus, M. L., Colangelo, L. A., Kiefe, C. I., Sidney, S., et al. (2006). Education, 15-year risk factor progression, and coronary artery calcium in young adulthood and early middle age. *Journal of the American Medical Association, 295*, 1793–1800.

Yan, L. L., Liu, K., Matthews, K. A., Daviglus, M. L., Freguson, T. F., & Kiefe, C. I. (2003). Psychosocial factors and risk of hypertension. *Journal of the American Medical Association, 290*, 2138–2148.

Yang, Y., Verkuilen, J., Rosengren, K. S., Mariani, R. A., Reed, M., Grubisich, S. A., et al. (2007). Effects of a taiji and qigong intervention on the antibody response to influenza vaccine in older adults. *American Journal of Chinese Medicine, 35*, 597–607.

Yano, E., Wang, Z.-M., Wang, X.-R., Wang, M.-Z., & Lan, Y.-J. (2001). Cancer mortality among workers exposed to amphibole-free chrysotile, asbestos. *American Journal of Epidemiology, 154*, 538–543.

Ye, X., Gross, C. R., Schommer, J., Cline, R., & St. Peter, W. L. (2007). Association between copayment and adherence to statin treatment initiated after coronary heart disease hospitalization: A longitudinal, retrospective, cohort study. *Clinical Therapeutics, 29*, 2748–2757.

Yi, H.-Y., Chen, C. M., & Williams, G. D. (2006). *Trends in alcohol-related fatal traffic crashes, United States, 1982–2004* (Alcohol Epidemiologic Data System, Surveillance Report No. 76). Arlington, VA: National Institute of Alcohol Abuse and Alcoholism.

Ylvén, R., Björck-Åkesson, E., & Granlund, M. (2006). Literature review of positive functioning in families with children with a disability. *Journal of Policy and Practice in Intellectual Disabilities, 3*, 253–270.

Yong, H.-H., Borland, R., Hyland, A., & Siahpush, M. (2008). How does a failed quit attempt among regular smokers affect their cigarette consumption? Findings from the International Tobacco Control Four-Country Survey (ITC-4). *Nicotine and Tobacco Research, 10*, 897–905.

Yoshino, A., Okamoto, Y., Onoda, K., Yoshimura, S., Kunisato, Y., Demoto, Y., et al. (2010). Sadness enhances the experience of pain via neural activation of the anterior cingulate cortex and amygdala: An fMRI study. *NeuroImage, 50*, 1194–1201.

Young, K. A., Gobrogge, K. L., & Wang, Z. (2011). The role of mesocorticolimbic dopamine in regulating interactions between drugs of abuse and social behavior. *Neuroscience & Biobehavioral Reviews, 35*(3), 498–515.

Young, K. M., Northern, J. J., Lister, K. M., Drummond, J. A., & O'Brien, W. H. (2007). A meta-analysis of family-behavioral weight-loss treatments for children. *Clinical Psychology Reviews, 27*, 240–249.

Young, L. R., & Nestle, M. (2007). Portion sizes and obesity: Responses of fast-food companies. *Journal of Public Health Policy, 28*(2), 238–248.

Yu, Z., Nissinen, A., Vartiainen, E., Song, G., Guo, Z., Zheng, G., et al. (2000). Associations between socioeconomic status and cardiovascular risk factors in an urban population in China. *Bulletin of the World Health Organization, 78*, 1296–1305.

Yuhas, N., McGowan, B., Fontaine, T., Czech, J., & Gambrell-Jones, J. (2006). Psychosocial interventions for disruptive symptoms of dementia. *Journal of Psychosocial Nursing and Mental Health Services, 44*, 34–42.

Yusuf, S., Hawken, S., Ôunpuu, S., Bautista, L., Franzosi, M. G., Commerford, P., et al. (2005). Obesity and the risk of myocardial infarction in 2700 participants from 52 countries: A case-control study. *Lancet, 366*, 1640–1649.

Yusuf, S., Hawken, S., Ôunpuu, S., Dans, T., Avezum, A., Lanas, F., et al. (2004). Effect of potentially modifiable risk factors associated with myocardial infarction in 52 countries (the INTERHEART study): Case-control study. *Lancet, 364*, 937–952.

Zaarcadoolas, C., Pleasant, A., & Greer, D. S. (2005). Understanding health literacy: An expanded model. *Health Promotion International, 20*, 195–203.

Zack, M., Poulos, C. X., Aramakis, V. B., Khamba, B. K., & MacLeod, C. M. (2007). Effects of drink-stress sequence and gender on alcohol stress response dampening in high and low anxiety sensitive drinkers. *Alcoholism: Clinical and Experimental Research, 31*, 411–422.

Zautra, A. J. (2003). *Emotions, stress, and health.* New York: Oxford University Press.

Zehnacker, C. H., & Bemis-Dougherty, A. (2007). Effect of weighted exercises on bone mineral density in post menopausal women: A systematic review. *Journal of Geriatric Physical Therapy, 30*, 79–88.

Zelenko, M., Lock, J., Kraemer, H. C., & Steiner, H. (2000). Perinatal complications and child abuse in a poverty sample. *Child Abuse and Neglect, 24*, 939–950.

Zhan, C., & Miller, M. R. (2003). Excess length of stay, charges, and mortality attributable to medical injuries during hospitalization. *Journal of the American Medical Association, 290*, 1868–1874.

Zhang, B., Ferrence, R., Cohen, J., Bondy, S., Ashley, M. J., Rehm, J., et al. (2005). Smoking cessation and lung cancer mortality in a cohort of middle-aged Canadian women. *Annals of Epidemiology, 15*, 302–309.

Zhou, E. S., Penedo, F. J., Lewis, J. E., Rasheed, M., Traeger, L., Lechner, S., et al. (2010). Perceived stress mediates the effects of social support on health-related quality of life among men treated for localized prostate cancer. *Journal of Psychosomatic Research, 69*, 587–590.

Zijlstra, G. A., Rixt, H., Jolanda, C. M., van Rossum, E., van Eijk, J. T., Yardley, L., et al. (2007). Interventions to reduce fear of falling in community-living older people: A systematic review. *Journal of American Geriatrics Society, 55*, 603–615.

Zimmerman, M. (1983). Methodological issues in the assessment of life events: A review of issues and research. *Clinical Psychology Review, 3*, 339–370.

Zimmerman, T., Heinrichs, N., & Baucom, D. H. (2007). "Does one size fit all?" Moderators in psychosocial interventions for breast cancer patients: A meta-analysis. *Annals of Behavioral Medicine, 34*, 225–239.

Zinberg, N. E. (1984). *Drug, set, and setting: The basis for controlled intoxicant use.* New Haven, CT: Yale University Press.

Zolnierek, K. B., & DiMatteo, M. R. (2009). Physician communication and patient adherence: A meta-analysis. *Medical Care, 47*, 826–834.

Zorrilla, E. P., Luborsky, L., McKay, J. R., Rosenthal, R., Houldin, A., Tax, A., et al. (2001). The relationship of depression and stressors to immunological assays: A meta-analytic review. *Brain, Behavior and Immunity, 15*, 199–226.

Zubin, J., & Spring, B. (1977). Vulnerability: A new view of schizophrenia. *Journal of Abnormal Psychology, 86*, 103–127.

Zupancic, M. L., & Mahajan, A. (2011). Leptin as a neuroactive agent. *Psychosomatic Medicine, 73*(5), 407–414.

Zvolensky, M. J., Jenkins, E. F., Johnson, K. A., & Goodwin, R. D. (2011). Personality disorders and cigarette smoking among adults in the United States. *Journal of Psychiatric Research, 45*(6), 835–841.

Zyazema, N. Z. (1984). Toward better patient drug compliance and comprehension: A challenge to medical and pharmaceutical services in Zimbabwe. *Social Science and Medicine, 18*, 551–554.

Zywiak, W. H., Stout, R. L., Longabaugh, R., Dyck, I., Connors, G. J., & Maisto, S. A. (2006). Relapse-onset factors in Project MATCH: The relapse questionnaire. *Journal of Substance Abuse Treatment, 315*, 341–345.

Name Index

A

Aarts, H., 352
Abaunza, P. S., 292
Abba, K., 84
Abbott, R. B., 190, 193
Abiona, T. C., 275
Abi-Saleh, B., 205, 216
Abnet, C. C., 242, 244
Abrahamowicz, M., 306
Abrahamsson, H., 44, 46, 48, 49
Abrams, K. R., 266
Abrams, M., 189, 190
Abrams, P., 46
Abrantes, A. M., 298
Ackard, D. M., 388
Ackermann-Liebrich, U., 305
Ackloo, E., 62, 84
Ackroff, L., 353
Acree, M., 111, 276
Adam, F., 351
Adams, B., 112
Adams, L., 249
Adams, S. M., 317, 318
Adams, T. B., 414
Adamson, J., 45
Addy, C. L., 388
Ader, R., 127
Aderman, D., 278
Adès, J., 364
Adi, Y., 357
Adler, N. E., 7
Adrian, J., 259
Advokat, C., 164, 332
Affleck, G., 138, 325
Afonso, A. M., 242
Agardh, E., 263
Agari, I., 139
Agboola, S., 304
Ager, J., 318
Agras, W. S., 364, 366
Agrawal, A., 109
Aharonovich, E. A., 102
Ahmed, I., 183
Ahrens, A. H., 349
Ai, A. L., 183
Aickin, M., 191, 193
Aiken, L. B., 391
Aiken, L. S., 2, 69, 79
Ainsworth, B. E., 388, 394
Ajani, U. A., 210, 211
Ajzen, I., 68, 71, 72, 74
Alaejos, M. S., 242
Alavanja, M., 238
Albanes, D., 380, 386
Albanesi, M., 191
Albert, C. M., 389
Albrecht, T. L., 67
Aldana, S. G., 228
Alderson, D., 102
Aldridge, A. A., 249
Alexander, C. M., 83

Alexander, F., 9, 13
Alger, B. E., 335
Alhassan, S., 179
Allard, S., 168, 169
Allebeck, P., 263
Allen, G. J., 184
Allen, J., 195, 196
Allen, J. G., 165
Allen, K., 110, 220
Alley, D. E., 6
Allison, K. C., 368
Almahmeed, W. A., 135, 221
Almeida, D. M., 7, 104
Aloe, L., 191
Aloise-Young, P. A., 74
Alper, C. M., 10
Alper, J., 137
Alpert, B. S., 136
Altman, D. G., 29
Altmann, D. R., 218, 242
Alvarez Linera, J., 161
Amantea, D., 160, 161, 162
Amanzio, M., 21
Amato, L., 329
Amato, P. R., 103
Ambroz, C., 159
Amelang, M., 247
Amico, R., 277
Amireault, S., 81
Amsterdam, J., 20, 187
Anand, S., 214, 218
Ancona, M., 100
Andel, R., 259
Andersen, B. L., 250
Andersen, C., 381
Andersen, J., 102
Andersen, L. B., 380, 386
Andersen, M. R., 198, 292
Andersen, R. M., 198
Anderson, J. L., 216
Anderson, J. W., 357
Anderson, K. E., 246
Anderson, K. O., 153, 162
Anderson, M., 215
Anderson, N. B., 406
Anderson, P., 312, 314, 316
Anderson, W. F., 247
Anderssen, S. A., 380, 386
Andersson, K., 65
Andrasik, F., 112, 133, 167
Andreas, M. I., 337
Andrel, J., 78
Andrew, M., 115
Andrew, S., 229
Andrews, J. A., 80
Andrykowski, M. A., 250
Aneiros, F. J., 168, 169
Aneshensel, C. S., 261, 278
Angier, H., 51
Angst, J., 185
Aniridya, K. D., 224

Anisman, H., 140
Ankri, J., 140
Annesi, J. J., 383, 387
Ansary-Moghaddam, A., 264
Antall, G. F., 190, 193
Anthony, D. C., 50
Anthony, J. C., 131
Antó, J. M., 305
Antonak, R. F., 109, 255, 256, 278
Antoni, M. H., 66, 114, 115, 130, 248, 249, 250, 251, 277
Anttila, A., 247
Apkarian, A. V., 148, 162
Apolone, G., 162
Apovian, C. M., 349
Appel, L. J., 357, 358
Appelbaum, K. A., 191, 193
Applebaum, A. J., 64
Arakawa, T., 137
Aramakis, V. B., 325
Aranda, M. P., 112
Arbisi, P. A., 158
Arch, M., 323
Ard, J. D., 357
Arden, M. A., 76
Ardern, C. I., 359
Ardissinio, D., 292
Arendt, M., 189, 190
Ariely, D., 21
Armeli, S., 138, 325
Armitage, C. J., 69, 74, 76, 79, 81
Armor, D. J., 330
Armour, B. S., 33
Armstrong, L., 41–42
Arnaiz, J. A., 29
Arnold, R., 255
Arnow, B. A., 366
Arntz, A., 152
Aro, A. R., 247
Aronson, M. D., 54
Arora, N. K., 249
Arroll, A., 52
Arsand, E., 411
Arthur, C. M., 137
Ascherio, A., 264, 297, 379, 386
Ashikaga, T., 293, 303
Ashley, M. J., 306
Ashmore, J. P., 238
Ashton, W., 218
Asman, K., 299
Aspden, P., 54
Assanand, S., 351, 353
Assendelft, W. J., 167, 191, 193
Asthana, D., 71
Astin, J. A., 167, 168, 169, 187
Astrup, A., 264
Atchison, R., 414
Atkinson, N. L., 49
Attrep, J., 138
Atwood, L. D., 351, 354
August, S., 277

Austin, B. P., 385, 387
Averbuch, M., 154
Aveyard, P., 306
Avezum, A., 135, 212, 214, 215, 217, 219
Avidor, Y., 358
Avis, N., 294
Avison, M. J., 353
Avison, W. R., 101
Avivi, Y. E., 221
Avol, E., 268
Avrahami, B., 332
Awad, G. H., 275
Awata, S., 259
Ayers, S. L., 185, 187, 190
Aygül, R., 133
Aylward, A., 383, 387
Azari, R., 52, 53, 354, 355
Azzara, S., 113, 114

B

Baan, R., 306
Babb, S., 299
Bacaltchuk, J., 364
Bacharier, L. B., 138
Bachen, E. A., 132, 133–134
Bachman, J. G., 7, 290
Back, S. E., 115
Bäckman, L., 258
Baer, H. A., 185, 189, 190
Baer, H. J., 320
Baer, R. A., 189, 190
Baez, A., 51
Bages, N., 412
Bagetta, G., 160, 161, 162
Baggett, L., 277
Bahrke, M. S., 383
Bailey, B. N., 318
Bailey, J. A., 103
Bailey, S. C., 402
Bailis, D. S., 48
Baillie, A. J., 221, 227
Baime, M. J., 180
Bair, T. L., 216
Bairey Merz, C. N., 215
Baker, S. G., 238
Bala, M., 303
Balaam, M., 326
Balabanis, M. H., 70
Balady, G. J., 389
Balbin, E., 65
Baldi, J. C., 306
Balfour, J., 219
Baliki, M. N., 162
Balise, R. R., 179
Baliunas, D., 318, 319, 320
Balkrishnan, R., 61
Ball, D., 322
Ballbé, M., 304
Balluz, L. S., 268
Baltes, P. B., 277
Balzer, W. K., 100
Banaji, M. R., 326
Banasiak, N. C., 138
Bandini, L. G., 349
Bandura, A., 68, 69–70, 168
Banegas, J. R., 353, 355
Banel, D., 264

Banning, K., 101
Bannuru, R., 189, 190
Bánóczy, J., 297
Baños, J.-E., 20
Baptiste, J.-P., 300
Bär, K.-J., 317
Barbaro Paparo, S., 191
Barber, B., 159
Barber, J., 184
Barber, T. X., 184
Barbour, R., 228
Barckley, M., 80
Bardia, A., 243, 244
Bardone-Cone, A., 365
Bardy, S. S., 363
Barefoot, J., 7
Barefoot, J. C., 220
Barengo, N. C., 376, 386
Barger, S. D., 115, 116, 117
Barish, E. E., 349
Barlas, P., 166
Barlow, J. H., 256
Barlow, W., 165
Barnes, P. J., 267
Barnes, P. M., 174, 175, 176, 177, 178,
    179, 180, 182, 184, 185, 186, 187,
    195, 197
Barnett, L. W., 304, 330, 338
Barnett, R. C., 106
Barone, E. J., 140, 228
Barouei, J., 128
Barr, R. G., 298
Barrett, S. P., 294
Barron, F., 67
Barth, J., 303
Bartmann, U., 383
Barton, B., 368
Barton-Donovan, K., 133
Barzi, F., 264, 357
Barzilay, J. I., 217
Basden, S. L., 337
Baseman, J. G., 246
Basow, S. A., 363
Bassman, L. E., 112
Bastian, L. A., 218, 410
Bath, J., 228
Batty, G. D., 7, 239
Baucom, D. H., 250
Bauer, J., 365
Bauld, L., 303
Baum, A., 15, 17, 128, 129, 130
Bauman, A., 391, 392, 394
Bauman, L. J., 138
Baumann, L. J., 47
Baumann, P., 318
Baumeister, R. F., 141, 148
Baumeister, S. E., 325
Baur, L. A., 357
Bautista, L., 214, 218
Baxter, L., 415
Beacham, G., 269, 270
Beaglehole, R., 27
Beals, J., 67
Becerra, L. S., 186
Beck, A. T., 158, 168
Beck, C., 258, 261
Beck, V., 407
Becker, A. E., 355, 365, 368
Becker, B. J., 383, 387
Becker, J., 338

Becker, K., 292
Becker, M. H., 68, 69
Beckham, D., 266
Beckman, L. J., 274
Bédard, M., 261
Beecher, H. K., 20, 151
Beelen, S., 167, 169
Beetz, A., 110
Beilin, L., 224
Bekke-Hansen, S., 221
Bélanger-Ducharme, F., 349
Bélanger-Gravel, A., 81
Belar, C. D., 9, 13, 15, 17
Bell, L., 168
Bell, R., 249
Bell, R. A., 52, 53
Belloc, N., 31, 415
Bemis-Dougherty, A., 381, 386
Bena, J., 299
Benaim, C., 157
Benbassat, J., 306
Bendapudi, N. M., 52
Bender, R., 348, 354
Bendle, S., 61
Benedetti, F., 21, 22
Benevides, L., 297
Bengel, J., 303
Bengtsson, J., 103
Benight, C. C., 115
Benjamin, E. J., 209, 220
Benner, J. S., 65
Bennett, A. S., 388
Bennett, G. G., 136, 222
Bennett, I. M., 402
Bennett, J., 52
Bennett, K., 278
Bennett, M., 298
Bennett, M. E., 330
Bennett, P., 100
Benotsch, E. G., 192, 194
Ben-Shlomo, Y., 45
Bensing, J., 255, 256
Benson, R. T., 215
Bensoussan, A., 195
Bentley, B., 65
Bentur, Y., 332
Benvenuti, A., 238
Benyamini, Y., 44
Berbaum, K. S., 192, 194
Berbaum, M. L., 192, 194
Berenson, G. S., 25
Berger, M., 348, 354
Berger, M. Y., 191, 192, 193, 194
Berger, R. S., 168, 169
Berghöfer, A., 349
Berglund, P., 141
Bergmann, M., 353, 354, 415
Bergmark, K. H., 326
Bergson, G., 303
Berhane, K., 268
Berk, M., 153
Berkman, L. F., 31, 108, 228, 415
Berkman, N. D., 364, 366, 367
Berlin, J. A., 20
Berman, B., 191, 193
Berman, J. D., 174, 188
Bermejo, J. L., 238
Bermudez, O. I., 349
Bernards, S., 319, 326
Berne, R. M., 210

Berner, M. M., 189
Bernstein, L., 245
Bernstein, M., 51
Berry, J. D., 209
Berry, J. T., 268
Berry, L. L., 52
Bertakis, K. D., 354, 355
Bertram, L., 258
Berwick, D. M., 54
Berwick, M., 246
Bessesen, D. H., 352
Best, S. R., 141
Beyer, F., 329
Bhat, V. M., 34
Bhatt, S. P., 225
Bhattacharyya, M. R., 67
Bhogal, S., 269
Bianchi, G., 209
Bianchini, K. J., 158
Bickel-Swenson, D., 158
Biddle, S. J. H., 73
Biener, L., 301
Bigal, M. E., 161
Bigatti, S., 157
Bigbee, W. L., 238
Bige, V., 140
Bigger, T., 228
Biglan, A., 300
Bilbo, S. D., 130
Bild, D. E., 221
Bingham, S., 216, 416
Binns, M., 259
Bird, S. T., 274
Birkenaes, A. B., 337
Birkenhager, W. H., 209
Birmingham, W., 220
Biron, C., 48
Birtane, M., 162
Bishop, E., 299
Bisson, J., 115
Bjartveit, K., 306
Björck-Åkesson, E., 257
Bjørge, T., 354, 355
Black, D., 297
Black, D. R., 295
Black, E., 264
Black, P. H., 137
Black, R. A., 377
Black, S., 158
Blackmore, E., 365
Blackmore, E. R., 140
Blackwell, E., 216
Blair, S. N., 376, 379, 380, 386, 388, 389
Blalock, J., 292
Blalock, J. E., 127
Blalock, S. J., 77, 78
Blanchard, C. M., 72, 74, 79
Blanchard, E. B., 112, 133, 191, 193
Blanchard, J., 52, 53, 67
Blanch-Hartigan, D., 52
Bland, S. D., 275
Blanton, H., 80, 81
Blascovich, J., 110, 215
Blasey, C., 366
Bleil, M. E., 223
Blissmer, B., 390, 391
Block, S. D., 279
Blodgett Salafia, E. H., 365
Bloedon, L. T., 379, 386
Blomqvist, J., 328

Bloom, B., 174, 175, 176, 177, 178, 179, 180,
    182, 184, 185, 186, 187, 195, 197
Bloom, J., 29
Bloom, J. R., 250
Bloomfield, K., 316
Bloor, M., 48
Blot, W. J., 238
Blount, R. L., 56
BlueSpruce, J., 192
Blum, C. M., 113, 114, 167
Blumberg, S. J., 254
Blumenthal, J. A., 222, 227, 228, 385
Blümer, N., 267
Blundell, J. E., 352
Bluthé, R.-M., 127
Blyth, F. M., 153, 160
Boddy, K., 188
Bode, C., 316
Bode, J. C., 316
Boden-Albala, B., 215
Bodenhamer-Davis, E., 325
Bodenheimer, T., 407, 408, 410
Bodenlos, J., 100
Bodhi, B., 180
Boeing, H., 353, 354, 415
Boersma, K., 153, 154, 161, 162, 168
Boerwinkle, E., 292
Boettger, M. K., 317
Boey, K. W., 229
Boffetta, P., 238
Bogart, L. M., 76
Bogg, T., 66
Bohlmeijer, E. T., 169
Bohuizen, H. C., 408
Boice, J. D., Jr., 238
Boissevain, M. D., 167, 169, 192, 194
Boisvert, J. A., 363
Boland, R., 277
Bolge, S. C., 165
Bolger, N., 256, 279
Bolling, S. F., 183
Bolognesi, M., 26
Bombardier, C., 191, 193
Bonacchi, K., 353
Bonanno, G. A., 279
Bond, F. W., 115
Bondy, S., 306
Bonevski, D., 103
Bonica, J. J., 152
Bonilla, K., 264
Boniol, M., 239
Bonita, R., 27
Bookwala, J., 363
Booth, A., 95
Booth, R. J., 113, 114, 250
Bootman, J. L., 54
Borden, W. B., 209
Boren, S. A., 265
Borge, A., 112
Borges, G. L. G., 318, 319, 320
Borland, R., 304
Born, J., 141
Borod, J. C., 116, 117
Borrell, L. N., 404
Borries, K., 306
Borroto-Ponce, R., 412
Bös, K., 378
Bos, V., 219
Bosch-Capblanch, S., 84
Boshuizen, H. C., 298, 379, 386

Bosworth, H. B., 220, 410
Botteri, E., 239
Botticello, A. L., 261, 278
Bottonari, K. A., 65
Bottos, S., 133
Botvin, G. J., 338
Boudreaux, E., 54, 100
Bourgeois, P., 185
Boutelle, K. N., 359
Bovbjerg, D. H., 134, 265
Bovens, F. M., 306
Bower, J. E., 116, 117
Bowers, B., 238
Bowers, S. L., 130
Bowie, J. V., 404
Bowles, H. R., 394
Boyd, D. B., 198, 243
Boyle, S. H., 7
Brace, M. J., 256, 257
Bradley, C., 137
Bradshaw B. S., 6
Brady, K. T., 115
Brady, S. M., 64
Braet, C., 368
Bragdon, B., 246
Brage, S., 219
Brahim, J. S., 154
Braiker, H. B., 330
Bramlett, M. D., 254
Brammer, L., 49
Branch, L. G., 304, 330, 338
Brand, R. J., 31, 221
Brandon, D. T., 136
Branson, B. M., 276
Brantley, P. J., 44, 100, 109, 357, 358
Branwell, R., 158
Bratslavsky, E., 141
Bratt, M. A., 194, 196
Braun-Fahrlander, C., 267
Braunwald, E., 358
Bray, G. A., 346, 349, 356
Brecher, E. M., 287
Bredin, S. S. D., 218
Brehm, B. J., 388
Breibart, W., 168
Breitner, J. C., 257, 258
Breland, J. Y., 46
Brenn, T., 245
Brennan, P., 33, 320, 321
Brenner, H., 321, 389
Breslau, N., 131
Breslin, M. J., 183
Breslow, L., 31, 415
Breslow, R. A., 320
Bret, M. E., 259, 260
Breuer, B., 165
Breuer, J., 116
Brewer, B., Jr., 215
Brewin, C. R., 168, 169
Brewster, L. G., 402
Bricker, J. B., 292
Brief, D. J., 64
Brilliant, L., 49
Brink, S., 33, 211, 212, 218
Brinkhaus, B., 188, 191, 193
Brinn, M. P., 301
Briones, T. L., 122
Britton, J., 299
Broadbent, E., 113, 114, 269
Brock, J., 357

Brockwell, S. E., 301, 304
Brody, M. L., 369
Bromberger, J. T., 105
Brondel, L., 353
Broocks, A., 383
Brooks, L., 383
Brooks, V. L., 218
Broom, D. H., 109
Broom, J., 356
Broome, M. E., 190, 193
Brosschot, J. F., 223
Brown, A. D., 385
Brown, P. A., 140
Brown, B., 183
Brown, D., 311
Brown, D. R., 402
Brown, E. L., 117
Brown, F. L., 349, 361
Brown, I., 81
Brown, J. L., 153
Brown, M., 342
Brown, M. L., 162
Brown, R. A., 298
Brown, T. A., 364, 366, 367
Brown, W. J., 194, 196
Brownell, C., 329
Brownell, K. D., 353, 370
Brownley, K. A., 364, 366, 367
Brownson, R. C., 392, 393–394
Brozek, J., 345, 362
Bruch, H., 362
Brug, J., 78
Brugts, J. J., 226
Brumback, T., 320
Brummett, B. H., 220
Brun, J., 48
Bruns, D., 411
Brustolin, A., 369
Bryan, A., 74
Bryant, R., 114, 115
Brys, M., 258
Buchanan, C. M., 113, 114
Buchanan, L. R., 392
Buchert, R., 335
Buchwald, D., 134
Buchwald, H., 264, 358
Buckley, D. I., 217
Buddie, A. M., 329
Buetow, S., 52
Buffington, A. L. H., 148, 162
Buick, D., 47, 135
Bulik, C. M., 364, 366, 367
Bull, F. C., 392, 394
Bullen, C., 302, 303
Bulow, C., 162
Bunde, J., 141, 221, 223
Bunn, J. Y., 293
Burckhardt, C. S., 157, 158
Burden, J. L., 73
Burg, M., 221, 228
Burgess, D. J., 45
Burhans, D., 383
Buring, J. E., 264
Burke, A., 186, 197
Burke, A. P., 389
Burke, B. L., 83, 329
Burke, C. T., 279
Burke, E., 298
Burke, J., 67
Burke, J. D., 414
Burkert, S., 79
Burrows, M., 381, 386
Burwell, R. A., 368

Buse, D. C., 161
Busenbark, D., 332
Bush, J. W., 400
Bushnell, M. C., 148, 160
Businelle, M. S., 290, 411
Bussey-Smith, K. L., 269
Bussolari, C., 111, 276
Bussone, G., 133
Bustamante, M. X., 412
Buttriss, J., 218
Buuk, B. P., 249
Bylund, C. L., 50
Byron, A. T., 50

C

Caballero, B., 349
Cabana, M. D., 269
Cabanac, M., 350
Cacioppo, J. T., 129, 141, 220
Caddell, J. M., 102
Cahill, K., 76, 83, 302, 303
Cahill, S. P., 114, 115
Cain, A., 64, 65
Cain, D., 273
Cain, V. S., 212, 214
Caldwell, D. S., 162
Cale, L., 393
Caleb Alexander, G., 64, 66
Calhoun, J. B., 104
Calhoun, L. G., 279
Califf, R. M., 220
Calipel, S., 192, 194
Callaghan, W. M., 297
Callaway, E., 270
Calle, E. E., 296, 298
Callister, L. C., 153
Calogero, R., 349, 361
Camacho, T. C., 31, 416
Cambois, E., 401
Camelley, K. B., 279
Cameron, A., 298
Cameron, J., 338
Cameron, L. D., 44, 46, 47, 135, 250, 306
Cameron, R., 114
Camí, J., 330
Campbell, C. M., 153
Campbell, F., 329
Campbell, I. G., 380, 386
Campbell, J. C., 161
Campbell, J. M., 326
Campbell, J. N., 146
Campbell, S., 238
Campbell, W., 330, 380
Campeau, S., 383
Campisi, S., 369
Canceller, J., 168, 169
Cancian, F. M., 261
Candel, M., 292
Cannon, M. F., 101
Cannon, W., 94
Cantrell, C. H., 194, 196
Cao, D., 320
Capewell, S., 212, 306, 415
Caplan, R. D., 103
Capone, J. C., 326
Cardi, V., 363, 364, 366
Carey, K. B., 412
Carey, M. P., 277, 412
Carinci, A. J., 191
Carlquist, J. F., 216
Carlson, C. R., 133

Carmody, J., 180, 189, 190, 194, 196
Carmon, Z., 21
Carney, A., 325
Carney, P. A., 51
Carney, R. M., 228
Caro, J., 162
Carpenter, C., 69, 349
Carpentier, M. R., 295, 296
Carr, D., 277
Carr, J. L., 412, 413
Carrera, J., 197, 198
Carrillo, J. E., 50
Carrillo, V. A., 50
Carroll, M. D., 24
Carson, K. V., 301
Carter, J. C., 365
Caruso, T. J., 191
Carver, C. S., 248, 249
Casati, M. Z., 297
Case, T. I., 128
Casey, D., 162
Casey, K. L., 21
Caspi, A., 140, 220
Cassel, C. K., 382
Castañeto, M. V., 183
Castellini, G., 365
Castillo, D., 61
Castor, M. L., 404
Castro, C. M., 52
Castro, Y., 290
Catalan, V. S., 238
Catellier, D., 228
Causer, L., 218, 242
Cavanaugh, K., 402
Cazottes, C., 157
Ceccarelli, F., 166
Celentano, D. D., 273, 275
Cen, S., 293, 300
Cepeda, M. S., 20
Cerhan, J. R., 243, 244
Ceylan-Isik, A. F., 316
Cha, E. S., 72
Chaddock, L., 385, 387
Chae, C. U., 389
Chaiyakunapruk, N., 192, 196
Chakrabarty, S., 162
Chakraborty, R., 351
Chalmers, J., 357
Chamberlin, C. L., 402, 404
Chambers, L., 52, 261
Chambless, L. E., 214
Chambliss, H. O., 383, 387
Chan, A.-W., 29
Chan, C. K., 195, 196
Chan, E. P., 189, 190
Chan, H., 297
Chan, M., 138
Chan, S. M., 194, 196
Chan, V. W. S., 157
Chan, W., 259
Chandrashekara, S., 129
Chang, A. B., 301
Chang, L., 332
Chang, Y., 224
Chao, A., 298
Chapman, C. R., 146, 147
Chapman, D. P., 352
Chapman, R. H., 65
Charlee, C., 52
Charles, S. T., 44
Charron-Prochownik, D., 72
Chase, A., 367
Chassin, L., 317

Chastain, D. C., 158
Chastek, B., 64
Chatkoff, D. K., 115
Chatters, L. M., 111
Chaturvedi, A. K., 247
Chaturvedi, N., 45
Chatzisarantis, N. L., 73
Chauvin, J., 300
Chayer, C., 259
Cheater, F., 44
Chei, C. L., 28
Chen, C. J., 297
Chen, C. M., 319, 320
Chen, E., 104, 128, 138
Chen, H. Y., 194, 196
Chen, I., 153, 157, 159
Chen, J., 141, 265, 402, 414
Chen, J. T., 404
Chen, J. Y., 194, 196
Chen, M., 272, 357
Chen, W. W., 414
Chen, Y., 382
Chen, Z., 141, 257
Cheng, A., 314
Cheng, B. M. T., 226
Cheng, E. M., 186
Cheng, T.-F., 392
Cheng, T. Y., 229, 297
Cheng, Y., 379, 386
Cheng, Y.-J., 78
Cherkin, D. C., 165, 191, 192, 193
Cherry, C., 273
Chesterman, J., 303
Chesterton, L. S., 166
Cheung, W. M., 189, 190
Chia, L. R., 67
Chialvo, D. R., 162
Chida, T., 268
Chida, Y., 66, 128, 134, 135, 222, 265, 276, 384, 387
Chiesa, A., 188, 190
Chinn, S., 305
Chipperfield, J. G., 48
Chipungu, S., 338
Chiuve, S. E., 226
Cholakians, E., 320
Chong, C. S., 189, 190
Chou, C.-P., 74
Chou, F., 272
Chou, P. S., 328, 330
Chou, R., 162
Chow, C. K., 214, 219
Christenfeld, N., 103
Christensen, B., 329
Christian, L. M., 129
Chu, M., 141
Chumbler, N. R., 261
Chung, M. L., 61, 65
Chung, T., 324
Chung, W. S. I., 297
Chu-Pak, L., 226
Chupp, G. L., 138, 267
Church, T., 65, 376, 386
Chyu, L., 186
Cibulka, N. J., 272
Cicognani, E., 112
Ciechanowski, P., 66
Ciesla, J. A., 65, 139
Cinciripini, P., 292
Cintron, A., 153
Cislak, A., 359
Claassens, L., 152
Clague, J., 292

Clapp-Channing, N. E., 220
Clare, L., 261
Clark, A. D., 410
Clark, A. E., 279
Clark, A. M., 228
Clark, C. G., 383, 387
Clark, K. M., 353
Clark, L., 159
Clark, L. A., 140
Clark, L. M., 70
Clark, L. T., 215
Clark, M. M., 305
Clark, N. M., 269
Clark, P. A., 276
Clark, R., 269, 406
Clarke, D., 259
Clarke, R., 162
Clark-Grill, M., 188
Claudino, A. M., 364
Claxton, A. J., 64
Claydon, L. S., 166
Cleary, M., 389
Cleeland, C. S., 162
Cleeman, J. I., 215
Cleland, J. A., 153
Clements, K. L., 168, 169
Clever, S. L., 54
Cline, R., 66
Clinton, W. J., 203, 206
Cloninger, L., 102
Clouse, R. E., 265
Clow, A., 103
Coast, J. R., 384, 387
Cobb, S., 43, 48
Cochran, J. E., 381, 387
Cody, M., 261, 407
Coe, C. L., 129
Coelho, J., 353
Coffman, C. J., 218
Coffman, J. M., 269
Cofield, M., 265
Cofino, J. C., 335
Cofta-Gunn, L., 414
Cofta-Woerpel, L., 411
Cofta-Woerpel, L. M., 290
Coghill, R. C., 157
Cohen, A., 218
Cohen, F., 49
Cohen, J., 64, 101, 306
Cohen, L. L., 56
Cohen, M. V., 205, 216
Cohen, N., 127
Cohen, S., 10, 44, 66, 99, 104, 129, 130, 131, 132, 133–134, 142, 249
Cohn, A., 298
Cohn, L., 138, 267
Colangelo, L. A., 219
Colbert, L. H., 380, 386
Colcombe, S. J., 385, 387
Colder, M., 116, 117
Colditz, G. A., 218, 237, 246, 264, 320, 379, 380, 386
Cole, B., 164
Cole, J. C., 195, 196
Cole, J. W., 34
Cole, P., 217
Cole, S. W., 134
Coleman, T., 304
Coles, S. L., 352
Coletta, R. D., 297
Colilla, S. A., 300
Collins, C. E., 359
Collins, E. M., 66

Collins, M. A., 318, 321
Collins, R. L., 275
Colloca, L., 21
Colner, W., 414
Comaty, J. E., 164, 332
Combs, A., 165
Commerford, P., 218
Cona, C., 198
Conger, J., 326
Congleton, C., 180
Conley, S. B., 357
Conn, D., 259
Conn, V. S., 381, 387
Connelly, M., 381, 386
Conner, M., 69, 72, 73, 76
Connolly, S. W., 293
Connors, G. J., 338
Constantino, M. J., 366
Cook, A. J., 158, 191, 193
Cook, B. J., 388
Cook, I. A., 189, 190
Cookson, W. O. C. M., 267
Cooley-Quille, M., 404
Coon, D. W., 261
Cooper, B., 375, 390
Cooper, C. L., 48
Cooper, H., 385
Cooper, M. J., 364
Cooper, N. J., 266
Cooper, V., 47
Corasaniti, M. T., 160, 161, 162
Corazzini, L. L., 21
Cordingley, J., 328
Corey, P. N., 54
Cornelisse, C. J., 238
Cornford, C. S., 49
Cornford, H. M., 49
Corrado, D., 389
Corrigan, J. M., 54
Cortez, D., 238
Cortina, L. M., 141
Cortón, E. S., 141
Costa, L. C. M., 158
Costa, L. O. P., 158
Costa, N. M., 101
Costa, P. T., 66, 410
Costa, T., 385
Costacou, T., 216
Costantini, A. S., 238
Costanza, M. E., 78
Costello, T. J., 290, 411
Coster, G., 52
Côté, F.-S., 238
Cottington, E. M., 106
Coughlin, J. A., 246
Coulter, I. D., 198
Counts, M., 52
Coupal, L., 306
Coupar, F., 184, 194, 196
Couper, J. W., 248
Courneya, K. S., 72, 74, 381, 386
Cournos, F., 131
Court, A., 364
Courtemanche, J., 190
Courtney, A. U., 268
Cousins, N., 173
Coussons-Read, M. E., 129
Covington, C. Y., 318
Covington, E. C., 151
Cowan, M. J., 228
Cowles, M., 100
Cox, B. J., 153
Cox, D. J., 265

Cox, K. L., 385, 387
Cox, N., 263
Coyle, J. R., 61
Coyne, J. C., 100, 139, 249, 250
Crabbe, J. C., 322, 323
Craciun, C., 79
Craig, A. D., 154
Craig, B. A., 380
Craig, C. L., 394
Craig, I. W., 140
Craig, R. G., 258
Cramer, J., 64
Cramer, J. A., 65, 266
Cramer, S., 412
Crane, C., 319
Cranos, C., 78
Creemers, M. C. W., 138
Crepaz, N., 115, 130, 277
Crerand, C. E., 357
Crimmins, E. M., 6, 259, 405
Crisp, A., 363
Crispo, A., 33
Critchley, J. A., 210, 211, 212, 303, 306
Crocker, T., 260
Croft, J. B., 210, 211, 352
Croft, P., 153, 160
Croghan, I. T., 305
Croghan, T. W., 60, 66
Crombez, G., 153, 154, 161, 162, 168
Cronan, T. A., 157
Cronenwett, L. R., 54
Cronin, E., 29
Crosby, R. D., 365
Cross, J. T., Jr., 162
Cross, T. H., 168, 169
Crowe, M., 259
Crowell, T. L., 273
Cruciani, R. A., 165
Cruess, D. G., 141, 277
Cruess, S., 277
Cruser, K., 304
Cuesta, A., 65
Cuite, C. L., 77
Cummings, D. E., 351
Cummings, S. R., 297
Cunha, M., 112
Cunning, D., 368
Cunningham, J. A., 328, 330
Curhan, G. C., 354, 355
Curlin, F. A., 20, 22
Curtin, J. J., 325
Cust, A. E., 380
Cutler, D. M., 400
Cutrona, C. E., 140
Czech, J., 260
Czernichow, S., 357
Czerniecki, J. M., 163

D

Dackor, J., 292
Da Costa, C., 179, 185, 186
Dagenais, S., 162
Dages, P., 261
D'Agostino, R. B., Sr., 200, 351, 354
Dalal, H. M., 229
Daley, A., 383, 387
Dal Maso, L., 245
Daly, J., 65
Damen, L., 191, 192, 193, 194
D'Amico, D., 133

Damjanovic, A. K., 129
Damschroder, L. J., 255
Danaei, G., 239, 241, 246, 252, 321
Daneman, D., 30
Danforth, E., Jr., 346
Daniels, M. C., 265
Daniels, N., 401
Daniels, S. R., 368
Dannecker, E. A., 153
Dans, T., 135, 212, 214, 215, 217
Dansinger, M. L., 228, 356
Dantzer, R., 127, 138, 140
Darbinian, J. A., 218
D'Arcy, Y., 165
Dare, C., 364
Darlington, A.-S. E., 56
Dasanayke, A. P., 258
Dasgupta, K., 214, 215, 216
da Silva, J. S., 297
Datta, S. D., 246
Daumann, J., 332
David, D., 357, 358
Davidson, K. W., 223, 227
Davidson, P., 229
Davidson, R. J., 21
Davidson, T. L., 353
Davies, D. L., 330
Davies, W. H., 137
Daviglus, M. L., 219, 221, 224
Davila, J., 139
Davis, B., 349
Davis, C., 388
Davis, C. C., 359
Davis, C. D., 243, 244
Davis, C. L., 385, 387
Davis, H., 136
Davis, J., 364
Davis, K. D., 349
Davis, M. C., 105, 138
Davis, R. B., 54, 183, 187, 381, 386
Davis, S. P., 298
Davis, T. C., 402
Davison, A., 183
Davoli, M., 329
Davydov, D. M., 189, 190
Daws, L. C., 353
Dawson, D. A., 328, 330
Dawson, D. V., 246
Day, H. E. W., 383
Day, N., 216, 320, 416
Day-Lally, C. A., 296
Daza, P., 414
Deandrea, S., 162
De Andrés, J., 166
Deary, I. J., 7
Deatrick, J. A., 256–257
Debanne, S. M., 259
DeBar, L., 369
DeBar, L. L., 29
De Benedittis, G., 184, 192, 194
de Bloom, J., 106
de Boer, M. R., 191, 193
de Brouwer, S. J. M., 138
de C. Williams, A. C., 158
Decaluwé, V., 368
De Civita, M., 65, 86
Decker, P. A., 305
DeCorby, K., 301
de González, A. B., 264
Dehle, C., 106
DeJong, G. M., 249
de Jong, J. R., 167, 169, 192, 194
De Jonge, N., 214

De Koning, H. J., 247
Delahanty, D. L., 76
Delahanty, J., 298
Delaney, H. D., 330
Delaney-Black, V., 318
de Leeuw, R., 133
DeLeo, J. A., 154
de Leon, M. J., 258
De Lew, N., 402
Delgaldo-Rodriques, M., 380, 386
Delmer, O., 141
DeLongis, A., 100, 139
Delvaux, T., 274
de M. Claudino, A., 364
DeMarce, J. M., 73
De Marzo, A. M., 238
Dembroski, T. M., 222
Demming, B., 324
Demoncada, A. C., 256
Demoto, Y., 156
Dempsey, A., 247
Denekens, J., 62
Denham, M., 103
Deniz, O., 133
Dennis, B., 218
Dennis, J., 238
Dennis, L. K., 246
de Nooijer, J., 78
de Oliveira, C., 217
Depue, R. A., 100
Derakhshan, M. H., 238
Derby, C., 257
Derhagopian, R. P., 249
de Ridder, D., 255, 256
Derogatis, L. R., 158
DeRubeis, R. J., 20
DeRue, D. S., 106
Desai, K., 187
Deschenes, M. R., 390, 391
DeSilva, M., 332
de Silva, V. C., 300
Desimone, M. F., 113, 114
Desnuelle, C., 157
Deters, C. A., 238
Detillion, C. E., 109
Dettenborn, L., 99
Deutscher, K., 25
de Vet, E., 78
Devilee, P., 238
Devlin, M. J., 388
Devlin, S. M., 198
DeVoe, J. E., 51
de Vreede, J., 306
DeVries, A. C., 109
De Vries, H., 292
de Vries, H., 292
de Vries, N. K., 78
de Vries, S., 103
DeWall, C. N., 148
Dewaraja, R., 101, 141
de Weerth, C., 106
Dewey, D., 133
de Wit, G. A., 408
Deyo, R. A., 21, 165, 191, 193
Dhabhar, F. S., 130, 140
Dhanani, N. M., 191
Diakogiannis, I., 314
Diamond, J. A., 218
Diamond, P., 61
Diaz, A., 114, 115, 130
DiCelmente, C., 298
Dickerson, F., 298
Dickerson, S. S., 110, 130

Dickinson, H. O., 329
DiClemente, C. C., 74, 75, 76, 224, 303
Diehr, P. K., 198
Dietz, P. M., 297
Dietz, W. H., 25
DiFranza, J., 292
DiIorio, C., 277
Dillard, J., 162, 198
Dillingham, T. R., 163
DiLorenzo, T., 265
DiMatteo, M. R., 52, 53, 60, 62, 64, 65, 66, 67, 83, 84
Dimidjian, S., 20
Dimitrov, S., 141
Dimsdale, J. E., 49, 222
Ding, E. L., 321
Ding, Y., 45
Dingwall, G., 320
DiNicola, D. D., 53, 83
Dionne, R. A., 154
di Sarsina, R., 186
Dishman, R. K., 383
Distefan, J. M., 292
Dittmann, M., 265
Dixon, J. B., 352
Dixon, K., 227
Dixon, L., 298
Doak, C. C., 403
Doak, L. G., 403
Dobbins, M., 301
Dobkin, P. L., 65, 86
Dobs, A. S., 198
Dobson, A., 299
Dobson, R., 242, 244
Dodd, S., 153
Doevendans, P. A., 214
Dogra, N., 255
Dohm, F.-A., 368
Dollard, K. M., 112
Dollard, M. F., 135
Dolor, R., 218
Domenico, E., III, 389
Donaghy, M. E., 383, 387
Donaldson, M., 54
Donenberg, G. R., 273
Donohue, K. F., 325
Donovan, J., 45
Doody, M. M., 239
Doody, R. S., 259
Dorenlot, P., 140
Dorer, D. J., 365
Dorn, J. M., 217
Dornbusch, S., 49
Dorr, N., 223
Dorwaldt, A. L., 303
Dosemeci, M., 380, 386
Doswell, W. M., 72
Doty, H. E., 45
Dougall, A. L., 130
Douglas, S. D., 141
Douketis, J. D., 359
Dovidio., J. F., 67
Doyle, W. J., 10, 44, 133
Drake, C. G., 238
Drapeau, A., 105
Dreer, L. W., 112
Dreisbach, J., 332
Dreon, D. M., 376
Dresler, C. M., 306
Drewnowski, A., 368
Driskell, J. E., 114, 115
Driskell, M.-M., 83
Drotar, D., 65

Drummond, D. C., 327
Drummond, J. A., 359
Dryden, J., 74
Dryden, T., 191
D'Souza, G., 247
Du, X. L., 237
Duangdao, K. M., 111
Dube, C. E., 50
Dube, S. R., 298
Dubois, S., 261
Ducharme, F. M., 269
Dudley, W. N., 224
Duerden, E. G., 190
Dufouil, C., 297
DuHamel, K. N., 192, 194
Duka, T. K., 320
Dunbar, H. F., 13
Dunbar-Jacob, J., 67
Duncan, A. E., 365
Duncan, G. H., 190
Dunckley, P., 149
Dunkel-Schetter, C., 100, 138
Dunn, A. L., 383, 387
Dunn, E. M., 48
Dunton, G. F., 61
Dupee, M. A., 83
Durán, M., 168, 169
Durán, R. E., 66
Durham, T. M., 275
Durkheim, E., 183
Durr-Holden, C. D. M., 319
Duscha, B. D., 391
Dusseldrop, E., 229
Dutra, L., 337
Duval, S., 381, 386
Dvorak, A., 328
Dwan, K., 29
Dyck, I., 338
Dye, C., 186
Dyer, A. R., 218
Dyment, S. J., 83
Dyson, M., 129
Dzurova, D., 328

E

Eaker, E. D., 220
Eakin, E. G., 394
Earll, L., 228
Easdon, C. M., 324
Easley, K. A., 382
Eaton, D. K., 290, 291, 294, 300, 356, 358, 365
Eaton, L., 273
Ebbeling, C. B., 263
Ebert, L., 102
Ebrahim, S., 82, 83, 220
Ebrecht, M., 129
Eccleston, C., 168, 411
Echwald, S., 264
Eckenrode, J., 49
Eckhardt, C. I., 319
Ecoffey, C., 192, 194
Eddy, K. T., 365
Edenberg, H. J., 322, 323
Edlund, C., 51
Edmundowicz, D., 224
Edwards, A. G. K., 250, 323
Edwards, C. L., 136, 153
Edwards, G., 312, 313, 323
Edwards, L. M., 105
Edwards, R., 293

Edwards, W. T., 163
Egbert, N., 415
Ege, M. J., 267
Eggert, J., 318
Egleston, B. L., 302
Egnatuk, C. M., 21
Ehde, D. M., 163
Ehrlich, G. E., 166
Eich, D., 185
Eisenbach, Z., 219
Eisenberg, D., 20
Eisenberg, D. M., 183
Eisenberg, M. E., 363
Eisenberg, M. J., 229
Eisenberger, N. I., 127, 148
Eisenmann, J. C., 380, 386
Ekeland, E., 381
Ekelund, U., 219
Ekholm, O., 328
Eklund, R., 100
Elbel, B., 30
Elgharib, N., 205, 216
Elias, J. A., 138, 267
Elifson, K. W., 273–274
Elkins, J. S., 410
Elks, C. E., 30
Ellard, D. R., 256
Elledge, S. J., 238
Eller, N. H., 99
Ellickson, P. L., 314
Elliott, C. H., 56
Elliott, J. O., 78
Elliott, P., 218
Elliott, R. A., 268, 269
Ellis, A., 168
Ellis, B. M., 54
Ellis, C., 135
Ellis, D. A., 65, 67
Ellis, L., 254, 261
Ellis, W., 157
Ellison, L., 162
Elsasser, G. N., 140, 228
Elswick, B. M., 381
Emanuel, A. S., 72
Emanuel, E. J., 20, 22, 408
Emanuel, L., 278
Emery, C. F., 250
Emmers-Sommer, T. M., 273
Emms, S., 219
Empana, J.-P., 278
Endler, N. S., 266
Endresen, G. K. M., 162
Endresen, I. M., 103
Engberg, J., 70
Engel, C. C., 114, 115
Engeland, A., 354, 355
Engels, E. A., 247
Engels, R. C. M. E., 293, 295
Engfeldt, P., 318
Engh, J. A., 337
England, L. J., 297
Engler, M. B., 219
Engler, M. M., 219
Engström, L.-M. T., 154
Engstrom, M., 338
Ensel, W. M., 384, 387
Enstrom, J. E., 299
Ephraim, P. L., 163
Epker, J., 153
Epstein, A. M., 402
Epstein, L. H., 352, 353
Erbas, B., 351
Erbaugh, J., 158

Erblich, J., 265
Erickson, K. I., 385, 387
Erikssen, J., 353
Ernst, E., 190, 191, 193, 195
Ernst, T., 332
Ernster, V. L., 297
Ertekin-Taner, N., 258
Erwin, P. J., 243, 244
Eslick, G. D., 195
Espelage, D. L., 108
Esser, G., 292
Esterman, A. J., 301
Estok, R., 264
Etherton, J. L., 158
Etnier, J., 194, 195, 196
Ettner, S. L., 7, 104
Etu, S. F., 349
Eurich, D. T., 60
Evans, B., 261
Evans, D., 48
Evans, G. W., 103
Evans, K., 261
Evans, M. A., 198
Evans, P., 103
Evans, P. C., 361
Evans, S., 402
Everett, B., 229
Everett, M. D., 382
Everitt, M., 326
Evers, A., 79
Everson, S. A., 136
Eves, F. F., 392
Ezekiel, J. E., 22
Ezzati, M., 220, 239, 241, 246, 252
Ezzo, J., 194, 196

F

Faden, R. R., 303
Faerden, A., 337
Faes, S., 81
Fafard, E., 238
Fagerstrom, K. O., 294
Fahey, J. L., 134
Fahey, T., 82, 83
Fahrbach, K., 264, 358
Fair, M. E., 238
Fairburn, C. G., 364, 368
Fairhurst, M., 149
Faith, M. S., 352
Falagas, M. E., 67
Falissard, B., 352
Falk, S., 198
Falkner, K. L., 217
Falzon, L., 65
Fang, C. V., 137
Fant, R. V., 294
Faravelli, C., 365
Farb, A., 389
Farley, J. J., 65
Farnham, P. G., 276
Farr, S. L., 297
Farran, C. J., 261
Farrar, W. B., 250
Farré, M., 20, 330
Farrell, D., 266
Farrell, S. P., 137
Fassino, S., 369
Fava, J. L., 358
Favier, I., 161
Federman, A., 402

Feenstra, T. L., 306, 408
Feighery, E. C., 293
Feinglos, M. N., 265
Feist, G. J., 36
Feist, J., 36
Feldman, E. A., 294
Feldman, P. J., 44
Feldman, R. S., 103, 104
Feldt, K., 157
Felson, R. B., 320
Feng, L., 195, 196
Feng, Y., 243, 244
Fenwick, J. W., 304
Ferguson, E., 74
Ferguson, J., 303
Ferguson, J. K., 183
Ferlay, J., 234
Fernandez, A., 408
Fernandez, E., 100
Fernandez, M. I., 66
Fernandez, R., 229
Fernandez, S., 60, 65
Fernandez-Berrocal, P., 116
Ferrando, L., 141
Ferrari, M. D., 161
Ferrence, R., 306
Ferri, M., 329
Ferris, T. G., 407
Feskens, E. J., 379, 386
Feuer, E. J., 162
Feuer, S., 298
Feuerstein, M., 256
Fichtenberg, C. M., 303
Fichter, M., 317
Fick, L. J., 192, 194
Fidler, J. A., 292
Field, R. W., 238
Fielder, R. L., 277
Fife-Schaw, C., 264, 265
Fifield, J., 138
Filion, K. B., 229, 357
Fillingim, R. B., 153, 154
Fillmore, M. T., 324
Finegood, D. T., 24
Fineman, N., 8
Fines, P., 401
Fink, P., 189, 190
Finkelstein, A., 51
Finlayson, G., 352
Finley, J. W., 243, 244
Finney Rutten, L. J., 65
Finniss, D. G., 21, 22
Fireman, B. H., 218
Firenzuoli, F., 195
Fischer, S., 365
Fischer, U., 317
Fishbain, D. A., 164
Fisher, C. A., 364
Fisher, J. D., 74
Fisher, M., 47
Fisher, W. A., 74
Fitzpatrick, A. L., 257, 258
Fitzpatrick, R., 364
Fjorback, L. O., 189, 190
Flanders, W. D., 296
Flaxman, P. E., 115
Flay, B. R., 301
Flegal, K. M., 24, 353, 355
Fleishman, S. B., 165
Fleming, A., 353
Fleming, P. L., 272
Fleshner, M., 127
Flicker, L., 385, 387

Flinn, M. V., 95
Flinois, A., 162
Floderus, B., 247
Flor, H., 159, 164
Flores, G., 52
Flores, L. Y., 146, 147
Floriani, V., 382
Flory, J. D., 223
Flower, K., 61
Flynn, B. S., 293, 303
Flynn, D. D., 335
Flynn, J., 265
Flynn, M. G., 380
Foa, E. B., 114, 115
Foets, M., 255
Fogel, J., 256
Foley, T. E., 383
Folkman, S., 97, 98, 100, 107, 108, 110, 111, 139, 256, 377
Folsom, A. R., 214
Foltin, R. W., 388
Foltz, V., 185
Fonseca, V., 61
Fontaine, T., 260
Fontan, G., 52
Foo, M.-D., 103
Foran, H., 319
Foran, K. A., 363
Forbes, G. B., 375
Ford, E. S., 210, 211, 415
Fordiani, J. M., 65
Fordyce, W. E., 21, 159, 167
Forey, B. A., 299
Forlenza, J. J., 128, 129
Foroud, T., 322, 323
Forouhi, N., 367
Forquera, R. A., 404
Forrester, K. K., 300
Forsman, M., 99
Försti, A., 238
Forsyth, M. R., 168, 169
Fortier, M. S., 394
Fortmann, A., 265
Fortmann, S. P., 293
Forys, K., 191, 193
Foster, B. D., 379, 386
Foster, J. K., 385, 387
Foster, N. E., 158
Foster, N. L., 260
Fouladi, R. T., 414
Foulon, C., 364
Fournier, J. C., 20
Fournier, M., 256
Fowler, S. L., 21
Fox, C. S., 351, 354
Fox, S. A., 194, 196
Fox, S. M., III., 389
Franceschini, N., 292
Francke, A. L., 260
Frank, E., 133, 197, 198
Frank, J., 292
Franklin, B. A., 382, 389, 390, 391
Franklin, T., 301
Franklin, V. L., 265
Franko, D. L., 365, 368
Franks, H. M., 111
Franks, M. M., 265
Franks, P. W., 219
Franzini, L., 237
Franzosi, M. G., 214, 218
Fraser, B, 349
Fraser, G. E., 410
Fratiglioni, L., 258, 259

Frattaroli, J., 116, 117, 228
Frederiksen, K., 247
Freedman, D. H., 185, 187, 198, 200
Freedman, D. M., 239
Freedman, D. S., 25
Freedman, L. S., 242
Freeman, E. L., 15
Freeman, L. E. B., 246
Freeman, M., 217
Freguson, T. F., 221
French, S. A., 293
Frenda, S., 228
Freud, S., 116
Freund, G. C., 138, 140
Freund, P. R., 168, 169
Frey, K. A., 52
Frey, M., 65, 67
Frey-Hewitt, B., 376
Frick, P. A., 71
Fried, L. P., 215, 219
Friedenreich, C. M., 380, 385
Friedlander, E., 22–23
Friedländer, L., 365
Friedlander, Y., 219
Friedman, H. S., 44, 66
Friedman, M., 205, 221
Friedmann, E., 110
Friedson, E., 49
Fries, J. F., 408
Frisina, P. G., 116, 117, 136, 222
Froberg, K., 380, 386
Frodi, A., 137, 265
Froelicher, E. S., 182, 189, 190
Froger, J., 157
Frone, M. R., 325
Froom, P., 306
Fu, R., 217
Fuchs, P. N., 154
Fuchs, V. R., 408
Fuertes, J. N., 52
Fuhrel, A., 273
Fuhrer, R., 259
Fujino, Y., 7
Fujiwara, Y., 137
Fukushima, M., 194
Fulkerson, J. A., 293
Fumal, A., 161, 167
Fung, T. T., 226
Furberg, A. S., 380, 386
Furberg, H., 292
Füredi, J., 365
Furlan, A. D., 191
Furnham, A., 186, 187
Furze, G., 47

G
Gaab, J., 115
Gaard, M., 245
Gable, S. L., 148
Gabriel, G., 316
Gabriel, R., 141
Gaertner, S. L., 67
Gaesser, G. A., 359
Gaffney, M., 228
Gagliese, L., 157
Gagnon, C. M., 153
Gail, M. H., 353, 355
Galdas, P. M., 44
Gallagher, B., 181
Gallagher, K. M., 72

Gallagher-Thompson, D., 261
Galland, L., 52
Gallegos-Macias, A. R., 66
Galli, A., 353
Gallo, L. C., 45, 104, 265
Galloway, G. P., 61
Galuska, D. A., 349, 356
Gambrell-Jones, J., 260
Gambrill, S., 270
Gamma, A., 185
Gan, T. J., 165
Gandevia, S. C., 153
Gandhi, T. K., 52
Gandini, S., 239
Gans, J. A., 65, 66, 83, 84
Gao, L., 321
Gao, X., 349, 357
Gao, Y., 20
Gapstur, S. M., 244
Garavello, W., 245
Garay, S. C., 376
Garber, C. E., 390, 391
Garber, M. C., 61
Garcia, G. E., 195, 196
García, J., 168, 169
Garcia, K., 79
García-Camba, E., 141
García-Sepulcre, M. F., 65
Gard, T., 180
Gardner, C. D., 179
Gardner, C. O., 139
Gardner, K. A., 140
Garfinkel, P. E., 349, 363
Garg, A. X., 84
Garn, H., 267
Garner, D. M., 349, 363
Garner, P., 84
Garofalo, R., 273
Garrison, M. E. B., 100
Garside, D., 224
Garssen, B., 247
Garssen, J., 219
Gaspar, T., 359
Gatchel, R. J., 153, 159, 165
Gatz, M., 44, 139
Gatz, S. L., 100
Gau, J., 367
Gauderman, W. J., 268
Gauthier, S., 260
Gaziano, J. M., 264
Gazmararian, J. A., 402
Geary, D. C., 95
Geers, A. L., 21
Geha, P. Y., 162
Geisser, M. E., 159
Geisser, M. S., 65
Gelbrich, G., 25
Gelernter, J., 131
Gelhaar, T., 112
Gellad, W. F., 66
Geller, P. A., 117
Gellert, M., 238
Gemmell, L., 303
Genao, I., 153, 157, 159
Genco, R. J., 217
Genest, J., 357
Gentilin, S., 115
Genuneit, J., 267
George, A., 383
George, S., 318, 320
Georges, J., 261
Gerrard, M., 80, 81, 292
Gervais, W. M., 128

Gestal-Otero, J. J., 134
Gettes, D. R., 141
Geurts, S., 106
Geurts, S. A. E., 106
Geyer, M. A., 335
Ghadirian, P., 238
Ghali, W. A., 220
Gianaros, P. J., 94, 223
Gibbons, F. X., 80, 81, 292
Gibbs, J. L., 46
Gibson, J., 162
Gibson, S. J., 159
Gidron, Y., 249
Gidycz, C. A., 413
Gielen, A. C., 78
Gielkens-Sijstermans, C. M., 306
Giese-Davis, J., 140, 250
Gilbert, M. T. P., 270
Gilbert, T. C., 52
Gildea, K. M., 97
Giles, M., 228
Giles, W. H., 34
Gillespie, C., 349
Gillies, C. L., 266, 401
Gillison, M. L., 247
Gilman, S. E., 368
Gilpin, E. A., 292, 293
Gil-Rivas, V., 102
Gima, A. S., 377
Ginsberg, J., 49
Giordani, P. J., 60
Girona, E., 65
Gitchell, J. G., 301, 304
Glahn, D. C., 61
Glantz, S. A., 303
Glanz, A., 74
Glaser, R., 129, 130, 140
Glasper, E. R., 109
Glassman, A. H., 228
Glasziou, P., 83
Glavin, P., 106
Gleason, J. A., 228, 356
Gleiberman, L., 222
Glennon, J. A., 346
Glimelius, B., 249
Glodzik-Sobanska, L., 258
Glueckauf, R. L., 261
Glynn, L. M., 100, 103
Glynn, R. J., 221, 320
Gmel, G., 316, 319
Go, A. S., 209, 218
Go, M.-H., 292
Gobrogge, K. L., 331
Godfrey, J. R., 227
Gödicke, R., 25
Godin, G., 81
Godtfredsen, N. S., 306
Gofer, D., 306
Goffaux, P., 149
Golberstein, E., 354, 355
Gold, D. R., 138, 268
Goldberg, J., 265
Goldberg, R., 298
Goldblatt, E., 301
Goldenberg, D. L., 191, 193
Golden-Kreutz, D. M., 250
Goldman, R., 262, 263
Goldring, M. B., 162
Goldring, S. R., 162
Goldschmidt, A. B., 368
Goldsmith, C., 318
Goldsmith, L. J., 52
Goldstein, A., 149

Goldstein, B. A., 249
Goldstein, M. S., 186
Goldston, K., 221, 227
Gomberg, E., 368
Gomuzzie, A. G., 378
Gonçalves, R. B., 297
Gonder-Frederick, L. A., 265
Gondoli, D. M., 365
Gonzaga, G., 95
Gonzalez, J. S., 66
Gonzalez, O., 268
Gonzalez, R., 139
González, V., 242
González-Cuevas, G., 331
Gooberman-Hill, R., 165
Good, M., 190, 193
Goode, A. D., 394
Goodin, S., 47
Goodpaster, B. H., 354, 355
Goodson, J. T., 183
Goodwin, D. G., 316
Goodwin, R. D., 44, 66, 153, 298
Goossens, M. E. J. B., 153, 154, 161, 162, 168
Gordon, D., 314
Gordon, D. B., 165
Gordon, J. R., 304, 324
Gordon, N., 168
Gori, L., 195
Gorin, A. A., 358
Gotham, H. J., 314
Gottdiener, J. S., 217
Gottfredson, L. S., 7
Gottheil, E., 250
Gotto, A. M., 226
Gøtzsche, P. C., 20, 21
Gouzoulis-Mayfrank, E., 332
Gowers, S., 363
Grady, D., 297
Grafton, K. V., 158
Graham, J. E., 129
Graham, K., 318, 319, 320, 326
Graig, E., 103
Gralla, O., 79
Grambow, S. C., 73
Granger, D. A., 95
Granlund, M., 257
Grant, B. F., 328, 330
Grant, J. A., 190
Graubard, B. I., 353, 355
Graves, J. V., 353
Gray, J. J., 349
Gray, L., 239
Gray-Donald, K., 306
Graziano, W. G., 117
Grazzi, L., 133
Greaves, L., 303
Green, C. R., 153
Green, H. D., 292
Green, N., 76, 302
Green, T., 273
Greenberg, E., 325
Greendale, G. A., 95
Greene, G., 367
Greene, S. A., 265
Greenfield, J. R., 357
Greenhouse, J. B., 66, 249
Greenlaw, R., 228
Greenley, R. N., 410
Greenlund, K. J., 221
Greenwood, B. N., 383
Greenwood, K. M., 178
Greer, D. S., 414
Gregg, E. W., 266

Gregory, J. W., 264
Greiner, J. W., 380, 386
Greve, K. W., 158
Greven, S., 135
Grey, M., 266
Griffin, J. A., 326
Griffin, K. W., 338
Griffin, P., 279
Griffing, S., 141
Griffith, J. L., 228, 356
Griffiths, M. D., 388
Griffiths, R., 229
Griffiths, R. R., 337
Grigsby, J., 332
Grigsby, P., 332
Grilo, C. M., 368, 369
Grimm, J. W., 261
Griswold, M. P., 134
Groenewegen, P. P., 103
Groesz, L., 367
Grogan, S., 44, 361
Grøholt, B., 320
Grønbæk, M., 7, 323
Grönberg, H., 238
Gross, C. R., 66
Gross, M. M., 323
Grossi, S. G., 217
Grossman, D., 246
Grossman, L. M., 325
Grossman, P., 189, 190
Grover, S. A., 306
Gruber, J., 51
Grubisich, S. A., 195, 196
Gruen, R., 100
Gruenewald, T. L., 94
Grum, C. M., 269
Grunau, R. E., 159
Grunberg, L., 325
Grundy, P., 407
Grundy, S. M., 215, 226
Grzywacz, J. G., 7, 104
Gual, A., 304
Guallar, E., 321
Guallar-Castillón, P., 353, 355
Guaragna, M., 191
Guck, T. P., 140, 228
Gueben, D., 157
Guelfi, J. D., 364
Guevara, J. P., 269
Guillén, J. E., 61
Guillot, J., 70
Guleria, R., 225
Gull, W. W., 361
Gulliford, K., 362
Gullion, C. M., 357
Gulliver, S. B., 304
Gumieniak, O., 266
Gunter, J. L., 257
Guo, Q., 74
Guo, X., 194
Guo, Z., 106, 219
Guralnik, J. M., 219
Guru, V., 214, 215, 216
Gurung, R. A. R., 94
Guski, R., 103
Gustafson, D. H., 249
Gustafson, E. M., 138
Gustafson, M. L., 52
Gustavsson, P., 238
Guthlin, D., 135
Gutierrez, K., 328
Gutiérrez-Fisac, J. L., 353, 355
Gwaltney, C. J., 70

Gwaltney, J. M., Jr., 10, 44, 133
Gyamfi, J., 30
Gyllenhammer, L., 116, 117

H

Ha, M., 239
Haahtela, T., 267, 268
Haak, T., 191, 193
Haan, J., 161
Haan, M. N., 257, 260
Haas, D. C., 228
Haas, J. S., 66
Haas, M., 191, 193
Hackett, T. P., 222
Hackl-Herrwerth, A., 329
Haddock, C. K., 24
Haden, S. C., 141
Hadjistavropoulos, T., 159
Haenle, M. M., 321
Hafdahl, A. R., 381, 387
Hagedoorn, M., 249
Hagen, K. B., 381
Hager, R., 228
Hagger, M. S., 48, 73
Haggerty, R. J., 49
Hagimoto, A., 303
Hagströmer, M., 391
Haig, A. J., 159
Haimanot, R. T., 161
Hains, A. A., 137
Hakala, P., 353
Haker, H., 185
Halberstadt, A. L., 335
Haldeman, S., 162
Hale, C. J., 108
Hale, S., 44
Haley, M., 12
Haley, W., 111
Hall, C. B., 257
Hall, C. R., 79
Hall, H. R., 272
Hall, J. A., 52
Hall, K. D., 24
Hall, M. A., 50
Hall, S., 183
Hallqvist, J., 263
Halm, E. A., 47, 64, 228
Halpern, P., 332
Halpin, H. A., 269
Ham, L. S., 326
Hamel, L. M., 394
Hamer, M., 135, 217, 265, 268, 384, 387, 388
Hamill-Ruth, R. J., 158
Hamilton-Barclay, T., 74
Hammen, C., 139
Hammond, D., 291
Hammond, K., 363
Hampson, S. E., 80, 264, 265
Hanewinkel, R., 292
Haney, T. L., 220, 222
Hanis, C., 351
Hanisch, R., 245
Hankey, B. F., 240
Hankinson, S. E., 320
Hanks, G. W., 165
Hanley, M. A., 163
Hanlon, C. A., 148
Hannigan, J. H., 318
Hannum, J. W., 108, 177
Hansen, Å. M., 99

Hansen, C. J., 384, 387
Hansen, K., 375
Hansen, K. B., 103
Hansen, L., 379, 386
Hansen, P. E., 99, 103, 247, 375, 384, 387
Hansmann, S., 255
Hanson-Turton, T., 52
Hanssen, P. F., 293, 295
Hanus, C., 353
Hanvik, L. J., 158
Hapke, U., 306
Harakeh, Z., 293, 295
Harboun, M., 140
Harburg, E., 222
Harder, B., 268
Hargreaves, D., 353
Hargreaves, M., 45
Hargrove, D. S., 15
Harkness, K. L., 139
Harman, J. E., 250
Harman, J. J., 277
Harnack, L. J., 347
Harper, C., 318, 332
Harper, T., 306
Harrell, W. A., 363
Harriger, J., 349, 361
Harrington, A., 175
Harrington, H., 140, 220
Harrington, J., 82
Harris, A. V. E., 62
Harris, J., 393
Harris, J. R., 351
Harris, M. I., 45
Harris, S. D., 248
Harris, T. B., 354, 355
Harris, T. R., 365
Harrison, B. J., 138
Harrison, P. J., 364
Harrisson, S., 292
Harter, J. K., 45, 106
Hartvigsen, G., 411
Hartz, A., 65
Hartz, A. J., 354
Hartzell, E., 365
Harvey, S. M., 274
Hasin, D. S., 102
Haskard, K. B., 64
Haskell, W. L., 182, 189, 190
Hasselbach, P., 247
Hasselblad, V., 306
Hastie, B. A., 153
Hatfield, J., 103
Hatsukami, D. K., 241
Hatzenbuehler, M. L., 102
Hausenblas, H. A., 388
Hausenloy, D. J., 379, 386
Hawken, S., 135, 212, 214, 215, 217, 218, 221
Hawkes, R. J., 191, 193
Hawkins, J., 290, 291, 300, 356, 358, 365
Hawkins, R. P., 249
Hawkley, L. C., 141, 220
Hay, P., 364
Hay, P. J., 364
Hay, P. P., 189, 190
Hayden, J., 191, 193
Hayes, S., 162
Hayes-Bautista, D. E., 402, 404
Hayes-Bautista, M., 402, 404
Hayley, S., 140
Haynes, R. B., 52, 60, 62, 65, 82, 84
Haynie, D. L., 70
Hays, R. D., 190, 193, 198
Haywood, J. R., 218

He, D., 181
Heady, J. A., 377
HealthGrades, 54, 410
Healy, K. E., 187
Heard-Costa, N. L., 351, 354
Hearn, W. L., 335
Hearnshaw, H., 62
Heath, C. W., Jr., 296
Heath, G. W., 392, 393–394
Heather, N., 330, 338
Heatherton, T. E., 363
Hebert, E., 70
Heckbert, S. R., 66
Heckman, C. J., 302
Hediger, K., 110
Heeren, T., 412
Heian, F., 381
Heijmans, M., 255
Heim, C. M., 141
Heimer, R., 273
Heinly, M. T., 158
Heinrich, K. M., 24
Heinrichs, N., 250
Heir, T., 353
Heisler, M., 64, 66
Heiss, G., 214
Helakorpi, S., 219
Held, C., 218
Helenius, H., 380, 386
Helfand, M. J., 217
Helgeson, V. S., 111, 112, 227, 249, 256
Helkala, E.-L., 258
Helmick, C. G., 162
Helweg-Larsen, M., 241
Hembree, E. A., 114, 115
Hemenway, D., 297
Hemminki, K., 238
Hemsing, N., 303
Henderson, B. E., 245
Henderson, K. A., 349
Henderson, L. A., 153
Henderson, M. D., 158
Hendriks, H. F. J., 321
Heneghan, C. J., 83
Henke-Gendo, C., 246
Henkin, Y., 228
Henley, S. J., 298, 306
Hennekens, C. H., 237, 389
Henningfield, J. E., 294
Hennings, S., 219
Henrard, J.-C., 140
Henriksen, J. E., 351
Henriksen, L., 293
Henriksen, T. B., 318
Henriksson, A., 247
Henry, E., 203, 227
Henschel, A., 345, 362
Henschke, N., 167
Henson, J. M., 412
Herbert, R., 218
Herbst, A., 381, 387
Herbst, J. H., 115, 130, 277
Herd, N., 304
Herman, C. P., 352, 353, 359, 361, 363, 365, 366
Hermann, D., 330
Hernán, M. A., 297
Hernández, A., 273, 402
Hernandez, B. Y., 247
Herrara, V. M., 103
Herrera, D., 153
Herrick, A., 273
Herring, M. P., 383
Herrmann, N., 259

Herrmann, S., 64, 65
Hertling, I., 328
Herzog, D. B., 365
Herzog, T., 76, 79
Hesselbrock, V., 365
Hession, M., 356
Hessling, R. M., 140
Hester, R. K., 330
Hetrick, S. E., 364
Hettema, J. E., 329
Hettige, S., 326
Heuser, I., 79
Hewitt, R. G., 65
Hextall, J., 129
Higgs, S., 294
Higuchi, K., 137
Hilbert, A., 368
Hilgard, E. R., 184
Hilgard, J. R., 184
Hill, J. O., 376, 386
Hill, M. D., 385
Hill, P. L., 66
Hiller-Sturmhöfel, S., 330
Hillmer-Vogel, U., 383
Hime, G. W., 335
Himmelstein, D. U., 50, 404, 406, 408
Hind, K., 381, 386
Hines, A., 249
Hingson, R., 412
Hirchman, L. A., 162, 198
Hiripi, E., 362, 368
Ho, E., 415
Hobel, C. J., 100
Hochbaum, G., 69
Hodgins, D., 328, 330
Hodgkins, S., 81
Hodgson, D., 128
Hoeger, R., 103
Hoeks, S. E., 226
Hoey, L. M., 249
Hoeymans, N., 7
Hoffman, B. M., 115, 385
Hoffman, C., 198
Hoffman, K. M., 295
Hoffmann, K., 353, 354
Hofmann, M. T., 302
Hogan, B. E., 222
Hogan, E. M., 364
Hogan, N. S., 256, 278
Hohmann-Marriott, B., 103
Holahan, C. J., 320, 321
Holahan, C. K., 320, 321
Holden, C., 332
Holder, J. S., 379, 386
Holder, R. L., 226, 378, 386
Holick, M. F., 246
Holl, R. W., 381, 387
Hollander, D., 70
Holley, H., 114, 115, 130
Hollis, J. F., 357, 358
Hollon, S. D., 20
Holm, N., 238
Holman, D., 181, 189, 190
Holman, E. A., 102, 111
Holmbäck, U., 352
Holmbeck, G. N., 410
Holmes, T. H., 99, 102, 398
Holst, C., 264
Holstad, M. M., 277
Holsti, L., 159
Holt-Lunstad, J., 220
Holtzman, D., 275
Hölzel, B. K., 180

Holzemer, W. L., 272
Hondros, G., 414
Honkoop, P. C., 133
Hood, C. J., 113, 114, 167
Hoogenveen, R. T., 306, 408
Hoorn, S. V., 220
Hootman, J. M., 162, 388
Hoover, R., 380, 386
Hope, T., 364
Hopkins, D. H., 392
Hopper, J. L., 351
Horacek, T., 367
Horan, J. J., 114, 115
Hord, H. G., 242, 243, 244
Horgen, K. B., 353, 370
Horn, W., 265
Horne, B. D., 216
Horne, R., 47, 64, 66
Hornik, R., 393
Horowitz, S., 194
Horsten, M., 105
Horton, E. S., 346
Houdeyer, K., 364
Houldin, A., 140
Houmard, J. A., 391
House, A., 260
House, J. S., 106, 354, 355
Houston, D. K., 359
Houts, P. S., 403
Hovey, K. M., 217
Howard, H. H., 24
Howe, G. W., 103
Howe, H. L., 240
Howze, E. H., 393–394
Hoyert, D. L., 3
Hrabosky, J. I., 368
Hróbjartsson, A., 20, 21
Hsiao, A.-F., 186, 198
Hsu, C., 192
Hsu, P., 402, 404
Hsu, R. T., 266
Hu, A. W., 111
Hu, B., 220, 386
Hu, F. B., 212, 217, 226, 264, 320, 354, 355, 379, 381, 386
Hu, G., 376, 386
Hu, P., 95
Hu, X., 161
Huang, B., 71, 328, 330
Huang, G., 407
Huang, J.-Q., 166
Huang, R.-C., 224
Hucklebridge, F., 103
Hudmon, K. S., 292
Hudson, J. I., 362, 368
Huebner, D. M., 105
Huebner, R. B., 329, 330
Hufford, D. J., 174
Hughes, J., 149, 218, 294, 304
Hughes, J. R., 302, 303
Hui, K.-K., 190, 193
Hukkelberg, S., 74
Hulbert-Williams, N., 250, 323
Hulme, C., 260
Hult, J. R., 111, 276
Hume, R. F., 318
Humphrey, L. L., 217
Humphreys, K., 410
Humphries, K. H., 214, 215, 216
Hunfeld, J. A. M., 56
Hunninghake, D. B., 215
Hunt, D., 217
Hunt, R. H., 166

Hunt, W. A., 304, 327, 330, 338
Hunter, A., 67
Hunter, D. J., 237, 246, 249
Huq, F., 335
Hurewitz, A., 116, 117
Hurley, J., 141
Hurley, S. F., 306
Hurling, R., 66
Hursting, S. D., 380, 386
Husten, C., 33
Hutchinson, A. B., 276
Hutchinson, M. R., 149
Hutchinson, R. G., 214
Huth, M. M., 190, 193
Huxley, R., 219, 264
Huy, N., 129
Hyde, J. S., 106
Hyde, R. T., 377, 386
Hyland, A., 304
Hyland, N., 64, 65
Hylton, J., 273
Hynan, L. S., 259, 260
Hyslop, T., 78

Iacovides, A., 314
Iacoviello, L., 217
Iadarola, M. J., 154, 157
Iagnocco, A., 166
Iannotti, R. J., 70
Ickovics, J. R., 277
Ide, R., 7
Ieropoli, S. C., 249
Iglesias, S. L., 113, 114
Igudin, I., 185
Ijadunola, K. T., 275
Ijadunola, M. Y., 275
Ilgen, D. R., 106
Ilies, R., 106
Im, C., 109
Imamura, M., 191
Imes, R. S., 50
Imhof, A., 321
Inaba, Y., 7
Inagaki, T. K., 127
Infante-Castañeda, C. B., 45
Ingersoll, K. S., 64
Inglis, N., 49, 50
Ingraham, B. A., 246
Iniguez, D., 402, 404
Innes, K. E., 194, 196, 197
Inoue, M., 28, 137
Intille, S. S., 61
Ioakeimidis, N., 217
Iodice, S., 239
Ionan, A. C., 140
Iqbal, R., 218
Iribarren, C., 218, 221
Irish, J., 295
Ironson, G., 65, 66, 71, 100, 114, 277
Irvin, E., 191
Irvin, J. E., 414
Irving, H., 318, 319, 320
Irwin, D. E., 46
Irwin, M. R., 127, 129, 130, 195, 196, 416
Isaacson, W., 232
Ishii, M., 71
Iskandar, S. B., 205, 216
Islam, S., 214, 218, 219

Islam, T., 268
Iso, H., 7, 28, 218
Israel, B., 265
Ito, T., 139
Ivanovski, B., 189, 190
Ivers, H., 48
Ives, D. G., 257
Iwamoto, D. K., 314

J

Jacka, F. N., 153
Jackson, A., 224
Jackson, G., 228
Jackson, J., 261
Jackson, K. M., 314
Jacobs, G. D., 113
Jacobsen, C., 265
Jacobson, E., 112, 167
Jacobson, M. P., 78
Jaddoe, V. W. V., 56
Jager, R. D., 297
Jagger, C., 401
Jagust, W., 257
Jahnke, R., 194, 195, 196
Jakicic, J. M., 376, 386
Jakobsson, R., 238
James, A., 342
James, P., 65
James, W. P. T., 349
Jämsä, T., 381, 386
Janicki, D., 112
Janicki, D. L., 136
Janicki-Deverts, D., 10
Janisse, J., 318
Jankowski, M. K., 131
Jansen, S., 261
Janssen, R. S., 275
Janssen, S. A., 153
Järup, L., 238
Jarvis, D., 305
Jarvis, M. J., 292
Jay, S. M., 56
Jayashree, K., 129
Jayawant, S. S., 61
Jeffery, R. W., 347, 359
Jefford, M., 249
Jeglic, E. L., 320
Jeifetz, M., 113, 114
Jelinski, S. F., 220
Jellinek, E. M., 323
Jemal, A., 233, 234, 236, 237
Jenkins, C. D., 221
Jenkins, E. F., 298
Jenkins, S., 41–42
Jenks, R. A., 294
Jennings, J. R., 223
Jensen, M. D., 264, 358
Jensen, M. P., 152, 157, 163, 192, 194
Jeon, C. Y., 381, 386
Jeon, Y.-J., 302
Jeste, D. V., 260
Jha, A. P., 180
Jiang, H., 238
Jiang, R., 298
Jiang, T., 353
Jick, H., 164, 297, 320
Jick, S. S., 297
Jin, L., 54
Jin, R., 141
Job, R. F. S., 103

Jochum, T., 317
Jockel, K.-H., 33
Johansen, C. B., 247
Johansson, B., 259
John, M., 64, 65, 198
John, U., 306
Johnson, A., 84
Johnson, A. K., 218
Johnson, B. T., 277
Johnson, C. A., 74, 293, 300
Johnson, C. H., 274
Johnson, E., 191, 193
Johnson, F., 349
Johnson, J. L., 83, 294, 391
Johnson, K. A., 298
Johnson, L. W., 216
Johnson, M. D., 106
Johnson, M. I., 191, 193
Johnson, R. J., 195, 196
Johnson, R. W., 127, 138, 140
Johnson, S. S., 83
Johnson, W. C., 298
Johnston, J. H., 114, 115
Johnston, L., 56
Johnston, L. D., 7, 290
Johnstone, E., 306
Joiner, T., 365
Jolanda, C. M., 382
Jolliffe, C. D., 169
Jolly, K., 229
Jonas, W. B., 21, 22
Jones, A. M., 380, 386
Jones, A. Y., 195, 196
Jones, B. Q., 220
Jones, D., 71
Jones, D. A., 356
Jones, D. L., 402
Jones, D. W., 214
Jones, G. N., 100
Jones, H. U., 216
Jones, K., 159
Jones, K. D., 157, 158
Jones, M., 368
Jones, M. E., 73
Jones, N. R., 300
Jones, P. J. H., 380
Jones, W. R., 363
Jordan, B. K., 102
Jorge, R., 259
Jorgensen, R. B., 228
Jorgensen, R. S., 222
Jorgensen, T., 295
Joseph, J., 72
Joseph, L., 185, 306, 357
Josephs, R. A., 325, 326
Joughin, N., 363
Jouven, X., 278
Judge, K., 303
Juliano, L. M., 337
Julien, R. M., 164, 332
Julius, H., 110
Julius, M., 222
Jump, R. L., 153
Juneau, M., 160
Juster, R. P., 94
Ju Wang, 292

K
Kabat, G. C., 299
Kabat-Zinn, J., 180, 194, 196

Kaciroti, N., 222
Kadowaki, T., 137
Kaell, A., 116, 117
Kagawa-Singer, M., 194, 196
Kahende, J. W., 297
Kahn, E. B., 393–394
Kahn, H. A., 377
Kahn, J., 191, 193
Kahokeher, A., 113, 114
Kaholokula, J. K., 67
Kalant, H., 335
Kalichman, S. C., 273, 274, 277
Kalish, R., 191, 193
Kalishman, N., 66
Kalsekar, A., 61
Kalten, M. R., 265
Kamarck, T. W., 99, 135, 136
Kambouropoulos, N., 325
Kamer, A. R., 258
Kamiya, J., 183
Kampert, J. B., 383, 387
Kaner, E. F. S., 329
Kann, L., 290, 291, 300, 356, 358, 365
Kanner, A. D., 100, 139
Kanning, M., 378
Kantarci, K., 257
Kantor, L. W., 329, 330
Ka'opua, L. S. I., 67
Kaplan, B., 256
Kaplan, B. H., 49
Kaplan, B. J., 188, 198
Kaplan, G. A., 136
Kaplan, R. M., 292, 400
Kaprinis, G., 314
Kaprio, J., 238
Kapsokefalou, M., 414
Kaptchuk, T. J., 20, 22–23, 187
Karageorghis, C., 388
Karam, E., 314
Karandish, M., 349
Karani, R., 382
Karavidas, M. K., 194, 196
Kardia, S. L. R., 292
Kargman, D. E., 215
Kark, J. D., 219
Karl, A., 164
Karlamangla, A. S., 6, 214, 220
Karoly, P., 157, 168, 169
Karon, J. M., 272
Karp, A., 259
Karp, I., 292
Karvinen, K. H., 74
Kasim, R., 338
Kasl, S. V., 43, 48
Katkin, E. S., 137
Kato, K., 44
Kato, M., 137
Katon, W. J., 66
Katsiaras, A., 354, 355
Katz, J., 158
Katz, M., 257
Katzper, M., 154
Kaufman, E., 66
Kaufman, M., 273
Kaufmann, R. B., 299
Kaur, S., 218
Kavan, M. G., 140, 228
Kavanagh, P., 83
Kavookjian, J., 381
Kawachi, I., 220, 221, 401
Kawamura, N., 101, 141
Kaya, M. D., 133
Kaye, J. A., 260

Kaye, W., 361, 362, 365
Kazinets, G., 303
Kazmi, K., 219
Keane, T. M., 64
Keefe, F. J., 151, 153, 159, 162
Keel, P. K., 362, 363, 364, 366, 367
Keeling, S., 278
Kehoe, T., 318, 319, 320
Keith, V., 186
Keller, A., 191, 193
Keller, M., 323
Kelley, F. J., 402
Kelley, G. A., 380
Kelley, J. M., 22–23
Kelley, K. S., 380
Kelley, K. W., 127, 138, 140
Kelly, B., 255
Kelly, C. N. M., 218
Kelly, J., 121
Kelly, J. A., 274
Kelly, J. F., 329
Kelly, K. M., 359
Kelly, K. P., 359
Kelly, M., 65
Kelly-Hayes, M., 220
Keltner, B., 402
Kemeny, M. E., 92, 94, 110, 130, 132, 134, 277
Kemp, B., 112
Kempen, G. I. J. M., 255
Kendall, L., 46
Kendler, K. S., 139
Kendzor, D. E., 290
Kennedy, C., 382
Kennedy, D. P., 292
Kent, C., 301
Kent, S., 65
Keogh, E., 115
Keppell, M., 56
Kerke, H., 379, 386
Kerlikowske, K., 297
Kerns, R. D., 15, 115, 158
Kerrigan, D., 121
Kerse, N., 52
Kersh, R., 30
Kershaw, T., 338
Kertesz, L., 29, 33
Kesmodel, U., 318
Kessler, R. C., 141, 256, 362, 368
Kesteloot, H., 218
Ketonen, M., 212
Ketterson, T. U., 261
Keuroghlian, A. S., 140
Keyes, K. M., 102
Keys, A., 345, 362
Keys, M., 256
Khamba, B. K., 325
Khan, C. M., 265
Khan, L. K., 25
Khan, M. I., 248
Kharbanda, R., 205
Khaw, K.-T., 216, 416
Kiazand, A., 179
Kickbusch, I., 414
Kiecolt-Glaser, J. K., 109, 129, 130, 140, 261
Kiefe, C. I., 214, 219, 220, 221
Kieffer, E., 265
Kiel, D. P., 381, 386
Kiess, W., 25
Ki Kim, J., 6
Kilgo, G., 168, 169
Kilpatrick, M., 70
Kim, A., 276
Kim, D., 220

Kim, D. S., 138
Kim, E., 247
Kim, H., 154
Kim, H. S., 111
Kim, J. S., 385, 387
Kim, K. H., 72
Kim, M. K., 181
Kim, S., 179
Kim, S. K., 138
Kim, Y., 302
Kim, Y. S., 138
Kimball, C. P., 13
Kinchen, S., 290, 291, 300, 356, 358, 365
King, A., 320
King, A. C., 65, 295, 296
King, C. D., 153, 154
King, C. R., 413
King, D., 335
King, J., 203, 227
King, K., 220
King, L., 295
King, N., 352
King, T. K., 305
Kinser, A. M., 382
Kipman, A., 364
Kipnis, V., 242
Kirchner, T. R., 320
Kirkeeide, R., 220
Kirsch, C., 191, 193
Kirsch, I., 184, 194, 196
Kirschbaum, C., 99
Kirschenbaum, D. S., 359
Kirtley, L.-G., 129
Kissane, D. W., 247
Kit, B. K., 24
Kittleson, M. J., 275
Kivimaki, M., 239
Kivipelto, M., 258
Kivlinghan, K. T., 95
Kiyohara, C., 297
Kjellström, T., 27
Klatsky, A. L., 320, 321
Kleber, H. D., 331
Klein, D. A., 388
Klein, D. J., 275
Klein, H., 273–274
Klein, L. C., 94, 95
Klein, M., 365
Klein-Hessling, J., 113, 114
Klimas, N., 277
Klimentidis, Y. C., 349
Klonoff, E. A., 105, 215
Klotz, U., 166
Kluger, R., 287–288
Klump, K. L., 362
Klusmann, V., 79
Knafl, K. A., 256–257
Knight, S. J., 278
Knoll, N., 79
Knopman, D. S., 257
Knottnerus, J. A., 167, 169
Knutson, K., 352
Knuttgen, H. G., 375
Ko, N.-Y., 274
Kobayashi, F., 349
Kobayashi, K., 186
Koçak, N., 133
Koch, D. S., 325
Kochanek, K. D., 7, 331
Koenig, H. G., 183
Koenig, W., 321
Koeppe, R. A., 21
Koes, B. W., 191, 192, 193, 194

Kofman, O., 137
Kohn, L. T., 54
Köhnke, M. D., 323
Kok, F. J., 298
Kokkotou, E., 22–23
Kolodziej, M. E., 222
Komaroff, A., 20
Kompier, M. A. J., 106
Kongkaew, C., 192, 196
Koomen, J. M., 68
Koopmans, G. T., 44
Kop, W. J., 135, 217
Koperdák, M., 365
Kopnisky, K. L., 134
Kopp, Z., 46
Kordonouri, O., 381, 387
Korpelainen, R., 381, 386
Koskenvuo, M., 353
Koski-Jännes, A., 328
Kosok, A., 330
Koss, M. P., 103
Kotrschal, K., 110
Kottke, T. E., 210, 211
Kottow, M. H., 23
Koulis, T., 292
Koutsky, L. A., 246
Koval, J. J., 295
Kowal, J., 394
Kozlenko, N., 111
Kozlowski, L. T., 301
Kraaimaat, F. W., 138
Kraaj, V., 229
Kraemer, H. C., 6, 250, 369
Krahn, D. D., 368
Kramer, J., 365
Krantz, D. S., 220
Krantz, G., 99
Krarup, L.-H., 379, 386
Kratzer, W., 321
Kraus, L, 325
Kravitz, R. L., 52, 53
Krebs, D. E., 381, 386
Kresevic, D., 190, 193
Kreuzer, M., 299
Krewski, D., 238
Kreyenbuhl, J., 298
Krieger, N., 404
Krikorian, R., 256
Krisanaprakornkit, T., 189, 190
Krisanaprakornkit, W., 189, 190
Krishna, S., 265
Krishnan, M., 326
Krishnan-Sarin, S., 303, 329
Krishnaswami, S., 354, 355
Kristal-Boneh, E., 306
Kriston, L., 189
Kritchevsky, S. B., 354, 355
Kroenke, C. H., 221
Krois, L., 51
Kromhout, D., 298
Krompinger, J., 180
Kronenfeld, J. J., 185, 186, 187, 190
Kröner-Herwig, B., 192, 194
Kronish, I., 65, 228
Kronmal, R. A., 215
Krueger, A. B., 45
Kruger, J., 356
Krupat, E., 52, 53
Krysta, J. H., 329
Kubetin, S. K., 358
Kübler-Ross, E., 278
Kubo, T., 7
Kubzansky, L., 227

Kubzansky, L. D., 221
Kudlur, S., 318
Kuendig, H., 326
Kuhajda, M. C., 168, 169
Kuhn, C. M., 222
Kuhnel, J., 106
Kujer, R. G., 249
Kuk, J. L., 359
Kulkarni, U., 356
Kuller, L. H., 224, 257, 258
Kumana, C. R., 226
Kumar, M., 277, 402
Kumar, S., 357
Kung, H. C., 3, 331
Kunisato, Y., 156
Kunst, A. E., 219, 290, 328
Kuntsche, S., 316
Kunz, C., 329
Kupelnick, B., 189, 190
Kuperman, S., 365
Kupper, S., 113, 114
Kupperman, J., 72, 74
Kurland, H., 182
Kurth, C. L., 368
Kurth, R., 164
Kurz, J., 153, 157, 159
Kutner, M. H., 382
Kuzik, R., 261
Kyngäs, H., 66
Kypri, K., 314
Kyrou, I., 357
Kyvik, K. O., 351

L

Laaksonen, M., 219
Laarhoven, A. I. M., 138
Laatikainen, T., 212
Labarthe, D. R., 210, 211
Laboy, A. F., 353
Lacey, J. H., 368
Lachman, M. E., 106
Laden, F., 246
Lafferty, W. E., 198
Lahelma, E., 352
Lai, D. T. C., 83
Laitinen, M. H., 258
Lake, J., 195, 197
Lakhani, R., 238
Lakka, T. A., 136, 376, 386
Lallukka, T., 352
Lalongo, N. S., 131
Lam, Z., 194, 196
Lambert, P. C., 266
Lamers, L. M., 44
Lamonte, M. J., 390, 391
Lamptey, P. R., 270
Lan, Y.-J., 238
Lanas, F., 135, 212, 214, 215, 217
Lancaster, K. L., 366
Lancaster, T., 76, 302, 303
Landers, D. M., 383, 387
Landers, J. E., 106
Lando, H. A., 295
Landolt, A. S., 192, 193
Landrine, H., 105, 215
Lang, A. R., 325
Lang, E. V., 192, 194
Lang, F. R., 277
Langa, K. M., 260
Lange, T., 141

Langer, E. J., 55, 109, 110
Langhorne, P., 184, 194, 196
Lannutti, P. J., 326
Lanotte, M., 21
Lansky, A., 275
Lantz, P. M., 354, 355
Laopaiboon, M., 189, 190
LaPelle, N., 78
LaPerriere, A., 277
López-Moreno, J. A., 331
Large, S., 49, 50
Largo-Wight, E., 414
Larkey, L., 194, 195, 196
Larsen, D., 106
Larson, E. B., 260
Larun, L., 381
Lash, S. J., 73
Laskowski, B., 129
Lasser, K. E., 404, 406, 408
Latendresse, S. J., 312
Latimer, R., 67
Latreille, B., 238
Lau, A. S., 111
Lau, D. T., 165
Lauber, C., 185
Laubmeier, K. K., 249
Laucht, M., 292
Laudenslager, M. L., 127, 129
Lauder, I. J., 226
Lauerman, J., 248
Laughlin, M. E., 377
Launer, L. J., 258
Laurenceau, J.-P., 221, 248
Laurent, M. R., 50
Laurin, D., 257
Lauritzen, T., 329
Lautenschlager, N. T., 385, 387
Lavagnino, L., 369
Lavallee, L. F., 116, 117
Laveda, R., 65
LaVeist, T. A., 404
Lavigne, J., 138
Lawler, P. R., 229
Lawrence, D., 298
Lawson, S. A., 404
Lawton, R. J., 72, 73
Lazarou, J., 54
Lazarus, R. S., 97, 98, 100, 101, 107, 108, 110, 139
Lazovich, D., 246
Leachman, S. A., 246
Leake, H., 47
Leanza, Y., 52
Leape, L. L., 54
Lear, S. A., 218
Leary, M. R., 148
Leavy, J. E., 392
Lebovits, A., 167, 190, 193
Lechner, S., 114, 115, 130, 249
Leddy, J. J., 352
Ledeboer, A., 149
Lee, C. M. Y., 357
Lee, C. S., 314
Lee, C.-W., 297
Lee, D. R., 323
Lee, E.-H., 302
Lee, H. H., 404
Lee, H. S., 338
Lee, I.-M., 379, 380, 386, 389, 390, 391
Lee, L., 74
Lee, L. M., 272
Lee, M. S., 181, 190, 193, 195
Lee, P., 323

Lee, P. N., 299
Lee, P. R., 323
Lee, R. E., 24
Lee, S., 255
Lee, T. H., 407
Lee, W. J., 380, 386
Leeks, K. D., 392
Leeuw, M., 153, 154, 161, 162, 168
Legedza, A. T. R., 183
le Grange, D., 364
Le Gros, V., 269
Lehman, D. R., 351, 353
Lehrer, P. M., 194, 196
Leigh, R., 385
Leineweber, C., 220
Leinsalu, M., 328
Leistner, D., 135
Lemaitre, R., 278
LeMaster, J. W., 381, 387
Lemer, C., 54
Lemos, K., 44
Lemstra, M., 338
Lennie, T. A., 61, 65
Lennon, L., 220
Lenssinck, M.-L. B., 191, 193
Leo, R. J., 189, 190
Leombruni, P., 369
Leon, A. S., 379, 380, 386
Leon, M. E., 306
Leonardi, M., 133
Leonardi Bee, J., 304
Leonido-Yee, M., 332
Le Parc, J.-M., 162
Lepore, S. J., 116, 117, 136, 222
Leppäluoto, J., 381, 386
Lepper, H. S., 60, 66
Leproult, R., 352
Lerman, C., 294
Leroux, B. G., 292
le Roux, P., 411
Lesage, A., 105
Lesch, O. M., 328
Leserman, J., 65, 141
Lestideau, O. T., 116, 117
Leucht, S., 329
Leuchter, A. F., 189, 190
Leung, D. P., 195, 196
Levenson, J. L., 134
Levenson, R. W., 325
Levenstein, S., 137
Leventhal, E. A., 44, 46
Leventhal, H., 44, 46, 47, 49, 64, 294
Lever, J. A., 261
Levi, F., 245
Levi, L., 131
Levin, B. E., 351
Levin, T., 247
Levine, J. M., 320
Levine, M. R., 168
Levinson, W., 54
Levy, D., 33, 211, 212, 218, 351, 354
Levy, M. L., 103
Levy, M. N., 210
Lew, J. F., 83
Lewin, R. J., 47
Lewis, B. P., 94
Lewis, C. A., 183
Lewis, C. E., 221
Lewis, C. S., 141
Lewis, D. C., 331
Lewis, E. T., 165
Lewis, J., 164
Lewis, J. E., 249

Lewis, M., 191, 193
Leyro, T. M., 337
Li, C., 415
Li, G., 266
Li, J. M., 54
Li, L., 186
Li, M.-D., 190, 193, 292
Li, P., 195, 196
Li, Q.-Z., 195, 196
Li, W., 220, 386
Liang, S., 186
Liang, X., 265
Liao, Y., 61
Lichtenstein, B., 275
Lichtenstein, P., 238
Lichter, E. L., 103
Lieberman, M. A., 249
Lieberman, M. D., 148
Liechty, J. M., 361
Ligier, S., 138
Ligot, J. S. A., Jr., 189, 190
Lillie-Blanton, M., 402
Lima, M. S., 364
Limburg, P. J., 243, 244
Lin, E. H. B., 66
Lin, I.-F., 215
Lin, N., 384, 387
Lin, V., 178, 179, 185, 186
Lin, Y., 47
Lincoln, K. D., 111
Lind, O., 65
Lindahl, M., 379, 386
Linde, K., 188, 189
Linden, D. E. J., 192
Linden, W., 222, 224
Lindsay, J., 257
Lindstrom, H. A., 259
Linet, M. S., 239
Linton, S. J., 153, 154, 161, 162, 168
Lints-Martindale, A. C., 159
Lippke, S., 26, 70, 79
Lipsey, T. L., 141
Lipton, R. B., 161
Liqing, Z., 109
Liria, A. F., 141
Lissner, L., 353
Lister, K. M., 359
Litten, R. Z., 327
Little, J., 238
Litz, B. T., 114, 115
Liu, H., 61
Liu, J., 61
Liu, K., 218, 219, 221
Liu, K. S., 70
Liu, L., 220, 386
Livermore, M. M., 106
Livingston, J. A., 320
Livneh, H., 109, 255, 256, 278
Ljungberg, J. K., 104
Llabre, M. M., 222
Lloyd-Jones, D. M., 209
Lloyd-Richardson, E., 292
Lloyd-Williams, M., 255
Lo, J. C., 218
Lobo, A., 321
Locher, J. L., 352
Lock, J., 6
Lock, K., 218, 242
Locke, J., 364
Loeser, J. D., 21
Lofgren, I. E., 414
Loftus, M., 89, 97, 98, 105, 106
Logan, D. E., 154

Loggia, M. L., 160
Logroscino, G., 226, 297
Loh, P., 214
Lohan, L., 88–89, 97, 98, 105, 106, 121
Lohaus, A., 113, 114
Lohr, K. N., 364, 366, 367
Lohse, B., 367
Loken, B., 393
Lokken, R. P., 381, 386
Loncaric, D., 112
Longabaugh, R., 338
Longman, R. S., 385
Loomis, J. S., 261
Lopez, A. D., 239, 241, 246, 252
Lopez, C., 115
Lopez, O. L., 257
López-García, E., 353, 355
Lopiano, L., 21
Lores Arnais, M. R., 113, 114
Loria, C. M., 358
Lo Sauro, C., 365
Loscalzo, M. J., 403
Lott, S. M., 109
Lotufo, P. A., 264
Louie, J. Y., 111
Louise, W., 175, 176
Loukissa, D. A., 261
Loving, T. J., 129
Low, C. A., 116, 117
Lowenfels, A. B., 239
Lowes, L., 264
Lowman, C., 327
Lowry, R., 294
Lu, Q., 116, 117
Lu, W., 131
Luben, R., 216, 416
Luben, R. N., 367
Lubin, J. H., 238
Luborsky, L., 140
Lucas, A. E. M., 410
Lucaspolomeni, M.-M., 192, 194
Luce, K. H., 368
Luchsinger, J. A., 258
Luckmann, R., 78
Luczynska, C., 305
Ludman, E., 66
Ludvigsson, J., 137, 265
Ludwig, D. S., 263
Lund, E., 245
Lundahl, B., 83, 329
Lundberg, U., 99
Luo, X., 161
Lupien, S. J., 94
Luqman-Arafath, T. K., 225
Lurie, N., 52, 53, 67
Lustig, A. P., 256
Lustman, P. J., 265
Luszczynska, A., 70, 359
Lutgendorf, S., 192, 194, 248, 250, 251, 277
Luthar, S. S., 312
Lutz, R. W., 65
Lycett, D., 306
Lydston, D., 71
Lynch, F., 369
Lynch, H. T., 238
Lynch, J. W., 136
Lyne, P., 264
Lynn, H., 138
Lyon, J. E., 77
Lytle, B. L., 220
Lyubomirsky, S., 116

Lyvers, M., 320
Lyytikäinen, P., 352

M

Mabuchi, K., 239
MacAllister, R. J., 205
MacCallum, R. C., 129, 261
MacCluer, J. W., 378
MacDonald, G., 148
MacDonald, T. K., 326
MacDougall, J. M., 222
Macedo, A., 20
Macefield, V. G., 153
Macera, C. A., 388
MacGregor, M. W., 227
Machan, J., 358
Macias, S. R., 66
Macie, C., 359
Maciejewski, P. K., 279
MacIntyre, P. D., 228
Mack, K. A., 275
Mackay, J., 211
MacKellar, D. A., 273, 275
Mackenbach, J. P., 219, 405
MacKenzie, B. A., 298
MacKenzie, E. J., 163
MacLean, D., 227
MacLeod, C. M., 325
Macleod, R., 278
MacPherson, H., 189, 190
Macrodimitris, S. D., 266
Maddox, T. M., 402
Madill, A., 256, 257
Madry, L., 141
Maenthaisong, R., 192, 196
Maes, S., 229
Magaret, A., 134
Magee, M., 353
Magill, M., 329
Magura, S., 329
Mah, J., 65
Mahajan, A., 361
Mahar, M., 408
Maher, C. G., 158
Mahon, M. J., 48
Maier, S. F., 127, 130, 149
Mainous, A. G., III, 52
Maisonneuve, P., 239
Maisto, S. A., 338, 412
Maizels, M., 166
Majdic, G., 344, 345, 350
Major, B., 105
Majundar, S. R., 60
Malarcher, A., 33, 34
Malarkey, W. B., 129
Malecka-Tendera, E., 263
Malhi, G. S., 189, 190
Malow, R. M., 115, 130, 277
Manchikanti, L., 165
Mancini, A. D., 279
Mandayam, S., 318
Mandel, J. S., 65
Mangels, A. R., 178
Manheimer, E., 191, 193
Manimala, M. R., 56
Manly, J., 258
Mann, D. M., 47, 64, 65
Mann, K., 329, 330
Mann, T. L., 79, 83
Manna, A., 188

Mannan, H. R., 306
Manne, S. L., 250
Manni, L., 191
Mannucci, E., 365
Manor, O., 219
Mansell, C., 65, 73
Manske, S., 301
Manson, J. E., 212, 217, 218, 237, 389
Manson, S. M., 67
Mant, D., 302, 303
Mantell, J. E., 270
Mantero-Atienza, E., 335
Manuck, S. B., 132, 133–134, 223
Manwaring, J. L., 368
Mao, J. J., 187
Mao, X., 134
Marchand, S., 149, 160
Marcus, B. H., 305
Marcus, D. A., 161
Marcus, M. D., 368
Margolis, R. D., 337
Marhefka, S. L., 65
Mariani, R. A., 195, 196
Mariotto, A. B., 162
Marisavljevich, D., 138
Markovitz, J. H., 221
Marks, G., 277
Marlatt, G. A., 304, 324, 329, 330–331
Marlowe, N., 133
Marmar, C. R., 141
Marmot, M. G., 239, 259, 297
Marques, L., 362
Marquié, L., 157
Marsee, M. A., 101
Marshall, J., 113
Marshall, P., 44
Marsland, A. L., 132, 133–134
Martelin, T., 219, 404
Martikainen, P., 404
Martin, A., 192, 193, 353
Martin, C. S., 324
Martin, M., 388
Martin, P. D., 44, 109
Martin, P. R., 168, 169, 331
Martin, R., 44, 46, 47, 49
Martin, T. M., 221
Martindale, D., 196
Martinez, F. D., 268
Martinez, O. P., 64, 65
Martins, I. J., 258
Martins, R. K., 83
Martire, L. M., 256
Marucha, P. T., 129
Mashal, N. M., 127
Masheb, R. M., 368, 369
Mason, J. W., 97
Mason, P., 156
Mason, R. A., 321
Masoomi, H., 358
Massarini, M., 26
Masse, L. C., 381, 386
Massman, P. J., 259
Masten, C. L., 148
Masters, K. S., 183, 411
Masui, S., 303
Masur, F. T., III, 64
Matacin, M., 305
Matarazzo, J. D., 12, 15
Mathers, M. I., 400, 401
Mathew, G., 318
Mathew, J., 218
Matis, T., 135
Matley, S. L., 46

Matsumoto, I., 318, 332
Matsuoka, H., 259
Matthews, A. M., 298
Matthews, J. P., 306
Matthews, K. A., 45, 104, 105, 135, 203, 214, 220, 221, 224
Matthies, E., 103
Mattlar, C.-E., 353
Matud, M. P., 112
Matyka, K., 357
Mau, M. K., 67
Maurer, D., 352
Mausbach, B. T., 74, 260
Mayeaux, R., 257, 258
Mayer, J., 412
Mayer, M., 267
Mayfield, D., 320
Maynard, L. M., 349
Mayo, R., 67
Mayo-Smith, M. F., 317
Mazas, C., 414
Mazerolle, L., 338
Maziak, W., 299
Mazur, A., 263
Mazure, C. M., 303
McAuley, E., 79, 385, 387
McAuley, J. H., 158
McBride, S. M., 316
McCabe, M. P., 363
McCaffrey, A. M., 183
McCaffrey, F., 136
McCall, G., 194, 196
McCallie, M. S., 113, 114, 167
McCarberg, B., 166
McCarl, L. A., 66
McCarter, D. F., 268
McCarthy, E. P., 190
McCarty, F., 224, 277
McCaskill, C. C., 265
McCauley, E., 256, 257
McCeney, K. T., 220
McClain, T., 246
McClave, A. K., 298
McClean, G. E., 351
McClelland, L., 363
McClure, J. B., 411
McColl, K. E. L., 238
McConnell, R., 268
McCoy, P., 359
McCracken, L. M., 168
McCrae, R. R., 66
McCullough, M. L., 226, 245
McCully, S. N., 72
McDaniel, S. H., 15, 411
McDonald, E. M., 78
McDonald, H. P., 62, 84
McDonnell, D. D., 303
McDowell, I., 257
McDowell, J. E., 385, 387
McEachan, R. R. C., 72, 73
McEwen, A., 294, 295
McEwen, B. S., 94, 95, 96, 140
McGee, D. L., 353, 354, 355
McGorry, P. D., 364
McGovern, F., 294
McGowan, B., 260
McGrady, A., 194, 196
McGrath, J., 214, 215, 216
McGregor, B. A., 250
McGuire, B. E., 158–159
McGuire, L., 129, 130, 261
McHugh, M. D., 364
McIntosh, C. N., 401

McIntosh, D. N., 102
McKay, D., 325
McKay, J. R., 140, 330
McKay, K. M., 411
McKechnie, R., 278
McKee, M., 218, 242
McKee, S. A., 303, 304
McKenna, M., 295
McKenzie, L. B., 78
McKeown, M. J., 148
McKinnon, E., 64, 65
McKnight-Eily, L. R., 298, 352
McLaughlin, M. A., 382
McLean, S., 150
McLellan, A. T., 331
McManus, V., 266
McMorris, C. A., 385
McNally, R. J., 141
McNeil, D. W., 83
McNeil, J. J., 306
McNeill, A., 304
McPherson, K., 24
McPherson-Baker, S., 66
McPhillips, T., 65, 66, 83, 84
McQuaid, E. L., 65, 73
Mcquillan, J., 138
McReynolds, C. J., 364
McRobbie, H., 294, 295
McSherry, W., 157, 159
McVey, D., 74
McWilliams, J. M., 51
McWilliams, L. A., 153
Meadows-Oliver, M., 138
Mechanic, D., 45
Mechoulam, R., 332
Medoff, D. R., 298
Meenagh, G., 166
Mehler, P. S., 366
Mehta, P., 394
Meichenbaum, D., 114, 168
Meijers-Heijboer, H., 238
Melamed, B. G., 256
Melamed, S., 306
Melander, A., 65
Melina, V., 178
Melotti, R., 305
Meltzer, D. O., 54
Melville, J., 330
Melzack, R., 146, 151, 154, 155, 156, 157, 158, 163, 164
Mendelson, J. E., 61
Mendelson, M., 158
Mendes, W. B., 110
Mensah, G. A., 211, 402
Merali, Z., 140
Mercado, A. M., 129
Mercante, J. P. P., 166
Mercken, L., 292
Merikangas, K. R., 141
Mermelstein, R., 99
Merrill, R. M., 228
Merritt, M. M., 136, 222
Merritt-Worden, T. A., 228
Mertz, C. K., 265
Messer, K., 293
Messier, S. P., 359
Messina, V., 178
Metzler, T., 141
Meulman, J., 229
Meunier, S. A., 168
Meyer, C., 306
Meyer, R. A., 146
Meyer, T., 383

Meyer, T. E., 237
Meyerowitz, B. E., 15
Meyers, J. E., 158
Meyrieux, A., 261
Mezzacappa, E. S., 137
Michael, K. C., 103
Michal, M., 192
Michaud, D. S., 238
Michie, S., 72, 228
Michultka, D., 191, 193
Mickelsen, O., 345, 362
Miczek, K. A., 324
Midtgaard, J., 381
Mieler, W. F., 297
Miettinen, O., 320
Miglioretti, D. L., 191, 193
Milam, J. E., 277
Milan, S., 277
Milat, A. J., 394
Miles, L., 380, 386
Miligi, L., 238
Milkie, M. A., 106
Miller, A., 352
Miller, D. B., 100
Miller, F. G., 20, 22
Miller, G. E., 104, 128, 129, 130, 132, 138, 216, 221, 256
Miller, J. W., 297
Miller, K., 52
Miller, L. G., 60, 61
Miller, M., 297
Miller, M. E., 359
Miller, M. R., 54
Miller, N. E., 183
Miller, P., 316
Miller, P. H., 385, 387
Miller, V. A., 65
Miller, W. R., 83, 329, 330
Miller, Y. D., 194, 196
Milligan, E. D., 149
Milling, L. S., 168, 184, 192, 193
Mills, N., 195, 196
Milne, B. J., 220
Milner, C. E., 184, 196
Milsom, I., 46
Mimiaga, M. J., 66
Mingote, C., 141
Miniño, A. M., 7, 331
Mislowack, A., 52
Mitchell, B. D., 378
Mitchell, H., 138
Mitchell, J. E., 366
Mitchell, M., 56
Mitchell, S. H., 298
Mitchell, W., 274
Mitrou, F., 298
Mittleman, M. A., 105, 220, 389
Miyazaki, T., 141
Mizrahi, R., 259
Mo, X., 265
Moak, Z. B., 109
Moats, C., 321
Mochly-Rosen, D., 321
Mock, J., 158, 368
Moeller, T., 381
Moen, P., 106
Moerman, D., 21
Moffitt, T. E., 140, 220
Mohammadpour-Ahranjani, B., 349
Mohebbi, M. H., 49
Moher, D., 29
Mohr, C., 325
Moja, L., 162

Mokdad, A. H., 268, 349
Moldovan, A. R., 357, 358
Molimard, M., 269
Moll, H. A., 56
Molloy, D. W., 261
Molloy, G. J., 67
Moltz, K., 65, 67
Mommers, M. A., 306
Monahan, J. L., 326
Mondon, S., 304
Mondraty, N., 361
Mongan, J. J., 407
Monroe, S. M., 99, 139
Mons, U., 290
Monshouwer, K., 293, 295
Montanari, M., 162
Montgomery, G. H., 192, 194, 265
Montplaisir, J., 352
Moodie, M. L., 24
Moore, J., 270
Moore, L. A., 67
Moore, L. L., 225
Moore, S., 325
Moorey, S., 249
Moos, B. S., 320, 321
Moos, R. H., 255, 320, 321, 410
Mora, P. A., 46
Moradi, T., 263
Moran, J., 64
Moreland, R. L., 320
Moreno, G., 331
Morenoff, J., 354, 355
Morgan, J. F., 363
Morgan, S. C., 195, 196
Morgan, W. P., 383, 387, 388
Morillo, L. E., 161
Morimoto, H. K., 129
Morita, T., 303
Morley, S., 158, 167
Morrell, J. S., 414
Morrill, B., 191, 193
Morris, J. C., 259
Morris, J. N., 377
Morris, R., 220
Morrison, C. D., 351
Morrison, E. L., 349
Morrison, R. S., 153
Mortensen, L. H., 7
Mortimer, J., 259
Moscone, F., 401
Moseley, J. B., 19, 23
Moser, D. K., 61, 65
Moser, J., 323
Moser, R., 249
Moser, R. P., 65
Mosimann, J. E., 349
Moskovich, J., 332
Moskowitz, J. M., 303
Moskowitz, J. T., 111, 256, 272, 276, 377
Mosley, P. E., 363
Moss-Morris, R., 249
Mostofsky, E., 223
Motivala, S. J., 138, 416
Motl, R. W., 383, 387
Mottillo, S., 216, 357
Moussavi, S., 66
Mouttapa, M., 293, 300
Mowery, P., 295
Moxham, T., 229
Moyer, A., 139
Moyer, C. A., 177
Mozaffarian, D., 218, 321

Muecke, M., 274
Mueller, C. W., 67
Mueser, K. T., 131
Muhajarine, N., 394
Mühlnickel, W., 164
Mukamal, K. J., 320
Müke, R., 297
Mulder, C., 364
Muldoon, M. F., 135
Müller, G., 25
Müller-Riemenschneider, F., 392
Mulvaney, C., 297
Mumma, M. T., 238
Munafò, M., 306
Munce, S., 140
Muñoz, R. F., 115
Munroe, K. J., 79
Muntner, P., 65
Murgraff, V., 81
Murphy, J. G., 27
Murphy, J. K., 136
Murphy, M., 306
Murphy, M. H., 226, 378, 386
Murphy, P., 158
Murphy, S., 407
Murphy, S. L., 3, 7, 331
Murray, C. J. L., 239, 241, 246, 252, 321
Murray, E., 50
Murray, J. A., 256, 278
Murtagh, E. M., 226, 378, 386
Murtaugh, M. A., 242, 244
Murthy, P., 318
Musante, L., 136
Must, A., 349
Mustanski, B. S., 273
Mustard, T. R., 62
Muthen, B. O., 315
Muthen, L. K., 315
Mutti, S., 295
Myers, C. D., 153
Myers, H. F., 137
Myers, J., 378
Myers, L. B., 248
Myers, T. C., 365
Mytton, O. T., 54
Myung, S.-K., 302, 303

N

Naar-King, S., 65, 67
Nahin, R. L., 174, 175, 176, 177, 178, 179, 180, 182, 184, 185, 186, 187, 195, 197
Naishadham, D., 233, 234, 236, 237
Najafi, F., 299
Nakamura, M., 303
Nakamura, Y., 146, 147
Nakazawa, T., 137
Naliboff, B. D., 134
Nanchahal, K., 218
Nannapaneni, U., 338
Nansel, T. R., 70
Napadow, V., 191
Naparstek, B., 190, 193
Naredo, E., 166
Nash, D. B., 52
Nash, J. M., 133, 168, 411
Nassiri, M., 100
Natale-Pereira, A., 50
Nathan, P. J., 138

Nausheen, B., 249
Navara, K., 368
Navarro, M., 331
Naylor, R. T., 113
Neal, J. J., 272
Neal, R. D., 250, 323
Neale, J. M., 133
Neaton, J. D., 224
Nebeling, B., 335
Nedeltcheva, A., 352
Neely, G., 104
Neff, R., 320
Negri, E., 245
Nehl, E., 72, 74
Neil, H. A. W., 219
Nelson, H. D., 297
Nelson, L. D., 349
Nelson, R. J., 130
Nemeroff, C. J., 46
Nes, L. S., 111
Ness, E. M., 218
Nestle, M., 349
Nestoriuc, Y., 192, 193
Netterstrøm, B., 99
Nettles, C. D., 129
Netz, Y., 383, 387
Neubauer, R., 317
Neubert, J. K., 154
Neudorf, C., 338
Neuman, R. J., 365
Neumark-Sztainer, D. R., 358, 361, 363
Neupert, S. D., 7, 104
Neve, M., 359
Nevill, A. M., 226, 378, 386
Neville, L. M., 394
Nevitt, M. C., 297
Newhouse, J. P., 51
Newlin, D. B., 325
Newman, J., 325
Newman, S. P., 82, 248
Newton, T. L., 109, 129
Ng, B. H. P., 189, 190
Ng, C. S., 194, 196
Ng, J. Y. Y., 229
Ng, M. K. C., 214
Ngandu, T., 258
Ng-Mak, D. S., 103, 104
Nguyen, L. T., 187
Nguyen, N. T., 358
Niaura, R., 137, 292
Nicassio, P. M., 15
Nichlas, B. J., 359
Nicholas, A. S., 357
Nicholas, M. K., 169
Nichols, W. P., 275
Nicholson, R. A., 168
Nickel, T., 135
Nicol, C. W., 218
Nicoll, R. A., 335
Nied, R. J., 382
Nielsen, G., 241
Nielsen, P. J., 381, 387
Nielsen, S. J., 356, 363
Nielsen, T. S., 103
Nielsen-Bohlman, L. T., 402
Niemann, L., 189, 190
Nieva, G., 304
Nigg, C. R., 26, 65, 76, 383, 387
Nikendei, C., 364
Nikolajsen, L., 164
Nilsson, J. L. G., 65
Niruntraporn, S., 192, 196

Nishimura, T., 194
Nissinen, A., 106, 213, 219, 376, 386
Niswender, K. D., 353
Nitzschke, K., 392
Nivison, M. E., 103
Noble, L. M., 82
Nocon, M., 378, 379, 392
Noda, M., 137
Noel, P. H., 255
Nohe, A., 246
Nolen-Hoeksema, S., 139
Norcross, J. C., 74, 75, 76, 224
Nordestgaard, B. G., 323
Nordheim, L. V., 381
Nordin, K., 249
Nordström, A., 386
Nori Janosz, K. E., 28
Norman, P., 48, 265
Norman, T. R., 138
Normand, A.-C., 267
Norris, C., 214, 215, 216
Norris, F. H., 141
North, S., 74
Northern, J. J., 359
Norton, W. E., 67
Nostlinger, C., 274
Nouwen, A., 66
Novack, D. H., 13
Novak, S., 292
Novins, D. K., 67
Novotni, A., 103
Nowson, C., 195
Numminen, P., 380, 386
Nunes, M., 166
Nunes, S. O. V., 129
Nunez-Smith, M., 292
Nusselder, W., 401
Nyberg, F., 33, 238
Nygård, J. F., 306

O

Oaten, M. J., 128
Obot, I., 326
O'Brien, C. P., 331
O'Brien, C. W., 249
O'Brien, L. T., 105
O'Brien, P. E., 352
O'Brien, W. H., 359
Obrocki, J., 335
O'Carroll, R. E., 74
Ocké, M. C., 298
Ockene, I., 266
O'Cleirigh, C., 65, 66
O'Connell, E., 412
O'Connor, D., 228
O'Connor, D. B., 110
O'Connor, D. W., 260
O'Connor, J. C., 138, 140
O'Connor, P. J., 383
O'Connor, R. J., 298
Odu, O. O., 275
Oei, T. P., 326
Oenema, A., 78
Offord, K. P., 305
Ogden, C. L., 24
Ogden, J., 74, 79
Ogedegbe, G., 60, 65
Ogeil, R. P., 326
Oguma, Y., 379, 386
Oh, K., 212

Oh, Y.-M., 138
O'Halloran, A., 299
O'Hara, B., 394
O'Hare, P., 338
O'Hea, E. L., 54
Ohno, Y., 297
Oja, P., 391
Okamoto, Y., 156
Okoli, C. T. C., 303
Okorodudu, A. O., 335
Okuda, M., 137
Okun, M. L., 129
Olander, E. K., 392
Oldenburg, R. A., 238
O'Leary, C. M., 318
O'Leary, K., 319
Olek, M. J., 297
Olendzki, B., 266
Olesen, J., 161
Oliker, S. J., 261
Olivardia, R., 363
Olmstead, M. C., 326
O'Loughlin, J., 292
Olsen, R., 65
Olsen, S. F., 318
Olshan, W., 65
Olshefsky, A. M., 403
Oluboyede, Y., 260
Olver, I. N., 248
Olver, J. S., 138
O'Malley, P. M., 7, 290
O'Malley, S., 329
Oman, R. F., 65
Ondeck, D. M., 153
O'Neal, H. A., 383, 387
O'Neal, K. K., 301, 338
Ong, K. K., 30
Onoda, K., 156
Onorato, I. M., 275
Operario, D., 7
Opitz, M., 383
Orav, E. J., 52
Orbell, S., 48, 81
Orchard, T., 215, 216
Orchowski, L. M., 413
Orford, J., 326
Orhan, A., 133
Orlando, M., 275, 314
Ormel, J., 255
Ørnbøl, E., 189, 190
Ornish, D., 228
Ortega, L. L., 304
Orth-Gomér, K., 105, 220
Ortner, C. N. M., 326
Osborn, C. Y., 402
Osborn, J. W., 224
Osborn, R. L., 256
Osborne, M. I., 388
Osei-Assibey, G., 357
Oshima, A., 303
Oskam, M.-J., 169
Ostelo, R. W. J. G., 167
Ostengen, R., 411
Ottaviani, C., 189, 190
Otto, A. D., 376, 386
Otto, M. W., 337
Ouimette, P., 117
Ôunpuu, S., 135, 212, 214, 215, 217, 218, 221
Overbeck, G., 192
Overvad, K., 353, 354
Oxman, M. N., 195, 196
Øystein, K., 7

Ozanne, S. E., 351
Ozer, E. J., 104, 141

P

Paasche-Orlow, M. K., 402
Pabst, A., 325
Pace, L., 335
Pace, T. W. W., 141
Padwal, R. S., 60
Paffenbarger, R. S., Jr., 377, 379, 386
Pagán, J. A., 51, 52, 186
Page, A. S., 380, 386
Pagliari, C., 265
Pagovich, O., 54
Pakalniskiene, V., 103
Palm, J., 322
Palmer, C. S., 187
Palmer, J. A., 153
Palmer, S. C., 250
Palmisano, G., 265
Palmores, A., 249
Palombaro, K. M., 381, 386
Paluch, A. E., 388
Pambianco, G., 216
Pan, T., 190, 193
Panagiotidis, P., 314
Panda, M., 153, 157, 159
Pandey, M. R., 217
Pandit, A. U., 402
Panos, G., 67
Pantalone, D. W., 277
Papacosta, O., 220
Papadaki, A., 414
Papadopoulos, A., 34
Papadopoulou, M., 314
Papas, R. K., 9, 13, 115, 153
Papies, E. K., 352
Paradis, G., 292
Paradis, S., 350
Parchman, M. L., 255
Parekh, P., 265
Parish, J. T., 52
Park, A., 315
Park, A. N., 404
Park, C.-H., 302
Park, E. R., 168
Park, J., 177
Parker, C. S., 60, 61
Parker, M., 259
Parker, R. M., 255, 402
Parkin, D. M., 234
Parks, J. W., 377
Parra, L. F., 100
Parraga, G., 228
Parrott, D. J., 319
Parschau, L., 78
Parsons, G. A., 220
Parsons, J. M., 46
Parsons, L., 332
Parton, E., 137
Pasanen, M., 153, 157, 159
Pasco, J. A., 153
Pascoe, E. A., 105, 109, 111
Passchier, J., 191, 192, 193, 194
Passin, W. F., 115, 130, 277
Patel, H., 332
Patel, R. S., 49
Patel, S. R., 416
Patra, J., 320, 321
Patrick, C. J., 325

Patrick, T. E., 72
Patten, C. A., 305
Patterson, D. R., 192, 194
Patterson, J., 367
Patterson, T. L., 74
Paty, J. A., 70
Paul, L., 52
Paull, T. T., 238
Paulozzi, L., 165
Pauly, M. V., 51, 52
Paun, O., 261
Pavlik, V. N., 259
Pavlin, D. J., 168, 169
Pawaskar, M., 61
Paxton, R. J., 383, 387
Payne, C. R., 27
Payne, D., 168
Payne, R., 153
Paynter, J., 293
Pearson, C. R., 277
Pearson, J., 29
Peay, E. R., 46
Peay, M. Y., 46
Pechacek, T. F., 33
Pedersen, A., 379, 386
Pedersen, A. F., 134
Pedersen, N. L., 44, 139, 259, 351
Pedersent, O., 264
Pederson, L. L., 294, 295
Peele, S., 325, 338
Peeters, A., 306
Peila, R., 258
Pekkarinen, H., 376, 386
Peleg, K., 332
Pelletier, K. R., 188
Pence, L. B., 152, 168, 169
Penedo, F. J., 66, 249
Penley, J. A., 111
Pennebaker, J. W., 115, 116, 117
Penner, L. A., 67
Pennington, K., 159
Pentz, M., 61
Penza-Clyve, S. M., 65, 73
Penzien, D. B., 167
Pepper, S., 304
Pereira, M. A., 349
Perella, C., 166
Perera, R., 83, 302, 303
Peres, M. F. P., 166
Peretti-Watel, P., 241
Perez, H. R., 50
Perkins, S. N., 380, 386
Perkins-Porras, L., 67
Perla, R. J., 401
Permutt, M. A., 263
Perram, S. W., 191, 193
Perraud, S., 261
Perrin, N., 29, 369
Perrine, N. E., 74
Perry, C. L., 361, 363
Perry, G. S., 352
Perry, K., 269
Perry, N. W., Jr., 15, 17
Pershagen, G., 238
Pert, C. B., 149, 150
Peruga, A., 300
Perugini, M., 66
Peterlin, B. L., 354, 355
Peters, J. M., 268
Peters, M. L., 167, 169, 192, 194
Petersen, A. V., 292
Petersen, K., 335
Petersen, S., 255

Petersen, S. R., 338
Peterson, A. L., 295
Peterson, C., 183
Peterson, C. B., 365
Peterson, D., 191, 193
Peterson, P. M., 414
Petit, D., 352
Petitto, J. M., 141
Petrelli, J. M., 65
Petrie, K. J., 135, 269
Petrilla, A. A., 65
Petronis, V. M., 249
Petry, N. M., 331
Petticrew, M., 249
Pettman, E., 177, 178
Peveler, R., 249
Peyrot, M., 66
Pezzin, L. E., 163
Pfeiffer, R. M., 247
Phelan, S., 45
Philis-Tsimkas, A., 265
Phillips, D. P., 103
Phillips, J. G., 326
Phillips, K., 81, 114, 115, 130
Phillips, K. A., 363
Phillips, K. M., 113, 114
Phillips, M. M., 27
Phillips, R. A., 218
Phillips, R. S., 183, 187, 190
Pho, L., 246
Picavet, H. S. J., 154
Pickup, J. C., 137, 264
Pickworth, W. B., 294
Pienaar, E., 329
Pierce, C., 64
Pierce, J. P., 292, 293
Pierò, A., 369
Pietiläinen, K. H., 347
Piette, J. D., 64, 66
Pike, J. L., 195, 196
Pike, K. M., 195, 365, 368
Pilkington, K., 194, 196, 198
Pillitteri, J. L., 301, 304
Pilote, L., 214, 215, 216
Pimlott-Kubiak, S., 141
Pineau, N., 353
Pinel, J. P. J., 351, 353
Pingitore, D., 12
Piotrowski, C., 158
Pischon, T., 349, 353, 354
Pisinger, C., 295, 306
Pi-Sunyer, F. X., 354, 355
Pitchenik, A. E., 270
Pittler, M. H., 190, 193, 195
Piyavhatkul, N., 189, 190
Plant, M. A., 316
Plant, M. L., 316
Plasqui, G., 381
Platz, E. A., 238
Pleasant, A., 414
Pleis, J., 49
Pliatsika, P. A., 67
Plotnick, L. P., 70
Plotnikoff, R. C., 74
Podolski, C.-L., 65, 67
Pohl, T., 135
Polder, J. J., 408
Pole, N., 141
Polich, J. M., 330
Polivy, J., 352, 353, 359, 361, 363, 365, 366
Pollack, M., 64
Pollard, M. S., 292
Pollart, S. M., 268

Polley, B. A., 357
Pollock, A., 184, 194, 196
Pollock, M. L., 389
Pomeranz, B. H., 54
Pomerleau, J., 218, 242
Pomerleau, O. F., 292
Ponieman, D., 47, 64
Pool, G. J., 154
Poole, H., 158
Pope, C., 332
Pope, H. G., Jr., 362, 363, 368
Pope, M., 301
Pope, S. K., 258
Popescu, D., 103
Popham, R. E., 313
Popkin, B., 349, 356
Popow, C., 265
Pories, W., 264, 358
Porte, M., 157
Portenoy, R. K., 165
Porter, J., 164
Portillo, C. J., 272
Porwal, M., 298
Poss, J. E., 80
Possemato, K., 117
Poston, W. S. C., 295
Potischman, N., 242
Pouchot, J., 162
Pouletty, P., 317
Poulin, M., 102
Poulos, C. X., 325
Poulter, M. O., 140
Poulton, R., 220
Powell, C., 148
Powell, J., 49, 50
Powell, K. E., 388, 393–394
Powers, M. B., 337
Powers, R. S., 106
Prakash, R., 385, 387
Prapavessis, H., 306
Prejean, J., 273
Presley-Cantrell, L. R., 352
Presnell, K., 367, 368
Pressman, S. D., 66
Presson, C. C., 317
Prestwich, A., 66
Price, D. D., 21, 153, 156, 184
Prictor, M., 84
Prigerson, H. G., 279
Primm, B. J., 141
Prince, M., 261
Prochaska, J. J., 65, 76
Prochaska, J. M., 83
Prochaska, J. O., 74, 75, 76, 83, 224
Pryor, D. B., 220
Psaty, B. M., 215, 258
Pukkala, E., 247
Puorro, M., 320
Purcell, D. W., 115, 130, 277
Purcell, R., 364
Purslow, L. R., 367
Puska, P., 212

Q

Qaseem, A., 162
Qin, Y., 83
Qiu, C., 258
Quadflieg, N., 317
Quartana, P. J., 249
Queffelec, L., 162

Quinn, D., 215
Quinn, J. F., 325
Quinn, J. R., 46, 47
Quirk, J., 46
Quist, M., 381
Qureshi, A. A., 246

R

Rabin, B., 10, 133–134
Rabin, C., 47
Raczynski, J. M., 27, 228
Radniz, C. L., 191, 193
Radstake, T. R. D. J., 138
Raffle, P. A. B., 377
Ragan, J., 116
Raggi, A., 133
Raghunathan, T., 278
Rahe, R. H., 99, 102, 398
Rahim-Williams, B., 153, 154
Rahim-Williams, F. B., 153
Rahkonen, O., 219, 352
Rains, J. C., 167
Rainville, P., 149, 160, 184, 190
Rainwater, D. L., 378
Rajan, K. B., 292
Rama, S. M., 115, 130, 277
Rambaut, A., 270
Ramel, J., 189, 190
Ramesh, M. N., 129
Rami, B., 265
Ramos, N., 116
Ramsay, S., 220
Ramsey, L. T., 393–394
Ramsey, M. W., 382
Ramskogler, K., 328
Ranavaya, M., 159
Ranchor, A. V., 249, 255
Rangarajan, S., 218
Ranke, A. H., 133
Rao, S. R., 320
Rapoff, M. A., 159
Rapoport, A. M., 354, 355
Rasheed, M., 249
Rashidi, A., 349
Rasinski, H. M., 21
Rasmussen, H. N., 66, 249
Rasmussen, S., 323
Ratanawongsa, N., 197, 198
Ratelle, S., 246
Raum, E., 389
Raunikar, R. A., 136
Rausch, D. M., 134
Ravaldi, C., 365
Rayburn, W. L., 52
Raynor, H. A., 353, 358
Rayworth, B. B., 363, 365
Rea, T., 278
Rea, T. D., 258
Read, J. P., 326
Reader, D. M., 263
Reagan, N., 254
Reas, D. L., 306, 369
Redd, W. H., 192, 194
Redmond, W. J., 149
Reece, J., 168, 169
Reed, B. R., 133
Reed, G. M., 12
Reed, G. W., 266
Reed, M., 195, 196
Reese-Smith, J. Y., 24

Reeves, M. M., 394
Regan, G. R., 24
Regidor, E., 328
Regoeczi, W. C., 104
Regueira, C., 134
Rehkopf, D. H., 404
Rehm, J., 306, 318, 319, 320, 321
Rehn, N., 316
Reich, A., 25
Reich, T., 365
Reiche, E. M. V., 129
Reid, C. M., 165
Reid, J., 324
Reilly, R. A., 414
Reilly, T., 276
Reinhold, T., 191, 193, 349
Reisine, S., 138
Reitz, C., 258
Reitzel, L. R., 290, 411
Ren, J., 316
Renard, E., 264
Rende, R., 292
Renner, B., 79
Reno, R. R., 69
Rentz, C., 256
Renz, H., 267
Resnicow, K., 224, 277
Rethorst, C. D., 383, 387
Reuben, A., 317
Reuber, M., 81
Reutenauer, E. L., 184
Reuter, T., 79
Revenson, T. A., 136, 222, 255, 256
Rexrode, K. M., 218, 221, 226, 264, 379, 386
Reyna, S. P., 216
Reynolds, K. A., 111, 256
Reynolds, K. D., 69
Reynolds, S. L., 111
Rhee, Y., 165
Rhodes, P., 272
Rhodes, R. E., 72, 74
Riazi, A., 137
Ribak, J., 306
Ribeiro-Dasilva, M. C., 153, 154
Ricciardelli, L. A., 363
Rice, D. P., 8
Rich, C., 413
Richards, M., 259
Richardson, A., 194, 196
Richardson, J., 194, 196, 198
Richardson, K. M., 115
Richardson, L., 238
Richardson, M. A., 64
Richardson, V. E., 278
Richman, J. A., 102
Richman, L. S., 105, 109, 111
Rico, C., 402, 404
Riddoch, C. J., 380, 386
Rieckmann, N., 228
Ries, L. A. G., 240
Rietveld, S., 68
Rigaud, D., 353
Rijken, M., 255
Riley, J. L., III, 153, 154
Rilling, J. K., 21
Rimm, A. A., 354
Rimm, E. B., 217, 297, 321
Ringdal, G. I., 250
Ringen, P. A., 337
Ringström, G., 44, 46, 48, 49
Rise, J., 74
Rissanen, A., 353
Ritchie, K., 400

Ritter, A., 338
Ritterband, L. M., 265
Rivers, P., 186
Rivis, A., 74
Rixt, H., 382
Robbins, L. B., 394
Roberts, B. A., 259
Roberts, B. W., 66
Roberts, C. G., 377
Roberts, D. A., 158
Roberts, J. E., 139
Roberts, J. W., 65
Roberts, L., 183
Roberts, S. O., 382
Roberts, W. O., 389
Robertson, R., 136, 222
Robine, J.-M., 400
Robins, L. N., 338
Robinson, D. E., 401
Robinson, J. P., 380
Robinson, L., 261
Robinson, L. R., 163
Robinson, M. E., 153
Robinson, R. G., 259
Robinson, S., 306
Robinson-Whelen, S., 129, 261
Robles, D. S., 363
Robles, T. F., 130, 140
Röder, C. H., 192
Rodgers, W. M., 79
Rodin, J., 55, 109, 110, 365
Rodrigue, J. R., 65
Rodriguez, A., 402
Rodriguez, B. L., 258
Rodriguez, D., 412
Rodriguez, J., 298
Rodríguez-Artalejo, F., 353, 355
Rodu, B., 217
Roe, S., 338
Roelofs, J., 167, 169, 192, 194
Roerig, J. L., 366
Roesch, S. C., 111, 249
Roesch, S. L., 249
Roesen, K., 168, 169
Roger, V. L., 209
Rogers, C., 194, 195, 196
Rogers, C. J., 380, 386
Rogers, R. D., 320
Rohde, P., 367
Rohsenow, D. J., 324
Roigas, J., 79
Rokkas, K., 217
Rolland, C., 356
Rollings, G., 145
Rollins, S. Z., 100
Rollman, G. B., 153
Rollnick, S., 83
Roman, A., 135
Roman, T. E., 319
Romano, J. M., 152
Rombouts, S., 338
Romero, A. J., 105
Romo, L., 364
Ronan, D. W., 112
Ronan, G. F., 112
Rones, R., 191, 193
Rönnemaa, T., 353
Ronnie, J., 49, 50
Rook, K. S., 265
Room, R., 320, 323
Rooney, B., 363
Rooney, K., 351
Roos, E., 219

Rorth, M., 381
Rosal, M. C., 78, 266
Rosario, M., 103, 104
Rose, J., 317
Rose, J. B., 154
Rose, J. P., 21
Rose, S., 326, 335
Roseman, J. M., 221
Rosen, A. B., 400
Rosen, C. S., 76
Rosenberg, E., 52
Rosenberg, H., 330
Rosenberg, M., 392
Rosenberg, N. L., 332
Rosenberg, S. D., 131
Rosenblatt, K., 247
Rosengren, A., 135, 214, 218, 219, 221
Rosengren, K. S., 195, 196
Rosenman, R. H., 205, 221
Rosenstock, I. M., 68, 69
Rosenthal, M., 78
Rosenthal, R., 140, 358
Rosenvinge, J. H., 363
Rosier, E. M., 157
Rosland, A., 265
Rösner, S., 329
Rosnick, C. B., 258
Rosomoff, H. L., 164
Rosomoff, R. S., 164
Rospenda, K. M., 102
Ross, J., 290, 291, 300, 356, 358, 365
Ross, M. J., 168, 169
Ross, R. K., 245
Rossen, R. D., 269
Rosser, B. A., 411
Rossingnol, M., 185
Rössler, W., 185
Rosso, A. L., 354, 355
Rossow, I., 320
Rotella, C. M., 365
Roter, D. L., 52
Roth, M., 186
Roth, R. S., 159
Rothenbacher, D., 321, 389
Rothman, A. J., 359, 411
Rothman, R. L., 402
Rothstein, H. R., 115
Rotskoff, L., 322
Rotter, J. B., 109
Rounds, J., 177
Rourke, K. M., 102
Routsong, T. R., 50
Rovio, S., 258
Rowan, J. S., 154
Rozanski, A., 227
Rozenberg, S., 185
Rozensky, R. H., 9, 13
Rozin, P., 352
Rózsa, S., 365
Ruan, W. J., 328, 330
Rubak, S., 329
Rubenstein, S., 349
Rubenstein, S. M., 191, 193
Rudd, R. R., 402
Rudich, A., 228
Rudy, T. E., 158
Ruehlman, L. S., 168, 169
Rugkåsa, J., 292
Ruiz, J. M., 219
Rumboldt, Z., 214
Rumpf, H.-J., 306
Rupley, D. C., 354
Ruppar, T. M., 381, 387

Rushford, N., 364
Rushing, O., 402
Russell, D. W., 80, 81, 140
Russo, J. E., 66
Russo, R., 160, 161, 162
Rutledge, P. C., 315
Rutten, G., 266
Rutten, L. J. F., 249
Rutter, P. D., 54
Ruzek, J. I., 115
Ryan, B., 168, 169
Ryan, C. J., 45
Ryan, G. W., 198
Ryan, S., 52, 412
Ryan-Wenger, N., 347
Rylander, R., 103
Ryu, H., 181

S

Saab, P. G., 222, 227, 228
Sääkslahti, A., 380, 386
Saartok, T., 154
Sabee, C. M., 50
Sabia, S., 297
Sacco, R. L., 215
Sachdev, P., 361
Sackett, D. L., 62
Sacks, G., 24
Sadowska, A., 261
Sáez, J., 65
Safran, D. G., 66
Safron, M., 359
Sage, R. E., 141
Saghafi, E. M., 256
Sagrestano, L. M., 275
Sahota, N., 62, 84
Sahyoun, N. R., 218
Saint-Jean, G., 402
Saito, E., 67
Saito, Y., 405
Salamonson, Y., 229
Salamoun, M., 314
Salans, L. B., 346
Salas-Lopez, D., 50
Salberg, A., 228
Sale, E., 338
Salem, J. K., 265
Sales, E., 114, 115
Salgueiro, M. F., 292
Sallis, J. F., 394, 412
Salomaa, V., 212, 213
Salonen, J. T., 136
Salzinger, S., 103, 104
Sambamoorthi, U., 183
Sambrano, S., 338
Samsa, G. P., 391
Samuelson, M., 194, 196
Sanabria-Ferrand, P.-A., 412
Sanandji, S., 61
Sanboek, A., 329
Sanborn, P. M., 294
Sanchez, M., 22–23, 412
Sanchez, O. A., 379, 380, 386
Sánchez del Rio, M., 161
Sánchez-Johnsen, L. A. P., 295, 296
Sancier, K. M., 181, 189, 190
Sanderman, R., 249, 255
Sanders, S., 261
Sanders, S. H., 152, 162, 167, 169
Sandford, J., 84

Sandhu, M. S., 367
Sandman, C., 100
Sandman, P. M., 77
Sandrik, L. L., 65
Sands, D. Z., 54
Sandvik, L., 353
Sanford, A. A., 50
Saperstein, S. L., 49
Saphire-Bernstein, S., 95
Sapolsky, R. M., 3, 220, 221
Saracino, M., 134
Sarason, I. G., 292
Sardinha, L. B., 380, 386
Sargent, J. D., 292
Saris, W. H., 379, 386
Sarvela, P. D., 275
Sasco, A. J., 299
Sattin, R. W., 382
Sattler, G., 358
Saules, K. K., 295
Saunders, T., 114, 115
Saunders, W. B., 220
Savage, E., 266
Savetsky-German, J., 381, 386
Sawyer, M. G., 298
Sayette, M. A., 320
Scalf, P. E., 385, 387
Scarpa, A., 141
Scarscelli, D., 328
Scavron, J., 266
Schaap, M. M., 290, 328
Schachter, S., 294, 301
Schachter, S. C., 190
Schaefer, C., 100, 139
Schaefer, E. J., 228, 356
Schaefer, J. A., 255
Schaffer, M., 320
Schaller, J., 255
Schaller, M., 128
Schare, M. L., 325
Schatzkin, A., 242
Schebendach, J., 388
Schechter, C. B., 218
Schedlowski, M., 132
Schéele, P., 238
Scheffler, R., 12
Scheiderman, N., 114
Scheier, M. F., 66, 249
Scheldeman, L., 12
Schell, L. M., 103
Schenck-Gustafsson, K., 105, 220
Schenker, S., 356
Scher, A. I., 354, 355
Schieman, S., 106
Schild, C., 318
Schillinger, D., 52
Schindler, L., 121
Schinkothe, D., 261
Schlatter, M., 250
Schleicher, N. C., 293
Schlenger, W. E., 102
Schlenk, E. A., 67
Schlesinger, C., 329
Schlicht, W., 378
Schmaltz, H. N., 220
Schmid, C. H., 189, 190, 191, 193
Schmidt, F., 381, 387
Schmidt, J. E., 133
Schmidt, L. A., 256, 278
Schmidt, M. H., 292
Schmidt, S., 189, 190
Schmidt, U., 364

Schmitz, K. H., 381, 386
Schmitz, N., 105
Schneider, A., 194, 196
Schneider, C. E., 50
Schneider, D. J., 216
Schneider, E. C., 402
Schneider, R. K., 134
Schneider, S., 70
Schneider, T. R., 97
Schneiderman, N., 228
Schnittker, J., 106
Schober, E., 265
Schoeller, D., 375
Schoenbaum, E., 277
Schoenbaum, M., 295
Schoenen, J., 161, 167
Schoenthaler, A., 60, 65
Scholz, U., 70, 79
Schommer, J., 66
Schork, M. A., 222
Schork, N. J., 131
Schousboe, K., 351
Schreck, M., 247
Schreiber, G. B., 368
Schreurs, K., 169, 255
Schroeder, C., 15
Schroeder, K., 82, 83
Schroeder, K. E. E., 131
Schroevers, M., 249
Schuckit, M. A., 337
Schuit, A. J., 379, 386
Schulenberg, J. E., 7, 290
Schull, W. J., 351
Schulz, K. F., 29
Schulz, R., 217, 249, 256, 278
Schulz, S., 317
Schulz, T. F., 246
Schulze, A., 290
Schulze, M. B., 353, 354
Schuman, P., 277
Schumann, A., 306
Schupf, N., 258
Schuster, D. V., 293, 300
Schutte, K. K., 320, 321
Schüz, B., 79
Schüz, N., 79
Schwab, K. O., 381, 387
Schwalm, D., 12
Schwartz, B. S., 161
Schwartz, D., 349
Schwartz, G. E., 13
Schwartz, J. E., 214, 220
Schwartz, J. S., 65
Schwartz, M. W., 351
Schwarzer, R., 70, 74, 75, 79
Schwarzfuchs, D., 228
Schwegler, A. F., 154
Schwind, K. M., 106
Sclafani, A., 353
Scolari, R., 403
Scott, B., 191, 193
Scott, C., 338
Scott, D. J., 21
Scott, J. A., 414
Scott, J. C., 297
Scott, T., 189, 190
Scott-Robertson, L., 388
Scott-Sheldon, L. A., 277
Scully, J. A., 101
Seals, B. F., 78
Searle, A., 100, 265
Sears, S. R., 394
Sebre, S., 103

Secher, N. J., 318
Secker-Walker, R. H., 303
Secretan, B., 306
Sedway, J. A., 364, 366, 367
Seegers, V., 352
Seeman, T., 6, 95
Seemann, E. A., 103
Segall, A., 48
Segerstrom, S. C., 111, 128, 129, 130, 132, 249
Segotas, M., 115
Seifert, T., 349
Seiffge-Krenke, I., 112
Seiler, E. M., 275
Seime, R. J., 158
Sel, S., 267
Selby, J., 297
Selik, R., 272
Selke, S., 134
Selker, H. P., 228, 356
Selkoe, D. J., 258
Seller, R., 52
Selmes, M., 261
Seltman, H., 249
Selye, H., 95
Semple, S. J., 74
Seniell, T., 12
Senjem, M. L., 257
Sensky, T., 168, 169
Seo, H. G., 302, 303
Seow, D., 260
Sepa, A., 137, 265
Sephton, S. E., 140
Sepulveda, M.-J., 407
Serdula, M. K., 349, 356
Serpa, L., 66
Serretti, A., 188, 190
Sesso, H. D., 379, 386
Seto, T. B., 67
Severens, J. L., 167, 169
Severson, H. H., 300
Shai, I., 228
Shanklin, S., 290, 291, 300, 356, 358, 365
Shannon, S., 188, 198
Shao, Y., 162
Shapiro, A. P., 137
Shapiro, D., 189, 190
Shapiro, J. R., 366, 367
Shapiro-Mendoza, C. K., 297
Sharma, A. M., 349
Sharma, M., 394
Sharp, D. J., 198
Sharp, J., 229
Sharp, L. K., 116, 117
Sharpe, L., 168, 169
Sharrett, A. R., 214
Shavlik, D. J., 410
Shaw, A. R. G., 198
Shaw, H., 367
Shea, M. K., 359
Shebilske, W. L., 97
Sheehy, R., 114, 115
Sheen, C., 311–312, 337, 338
Sheeran, P., 74, 76, 80, 81
Sheese, B. E., 117
Sheffield, D., 153
Sheffield, J., 100
Shekelle, P., 162
Shell, E. R., 268
Shelton, J. N., 67
Shelton, R. C., 20
Shelton, S., 295
Shen, B.-J., 137, 221
Shen, W.-H., 127

Shen, Z., 141
Shepherd, J., 226
Sheps, D. S., 135
Sher, K. J., 314, 315, 325
Sherman, D. K., 83, 111
Sherman, K. J., 191, 192, 193
Sherman, S. J., 317
Shernoff, M., 273
Sherry, D. D., 256, 257
Sherwood, L., 147, 149, 150
Sherwood, N. E., 359
Shi, L., 61
Shi, S., 166
Shi, Y., 194, 196
Shields, W. C., 78
Shiffman, S. S., 70, 135, 301, 304
Shih, J. H., 111
Shimabukuro, J., 259
Shimbo, D., 228
Shimizu, M., 110
Shimony, A., 357
Shinnick, P., 181
Shipley, M. J., 7, 239
Shiv, B., 21
Shlay, J., 246
Shmueli, A., 185
Shobha, A., 129
Shores, E. A., 158–159
Shrira, I., 103
Shriver, T., 375
Shue, V. M., 258
Shuval, J., 185
Siahpush, M., 304
Sichère, P., 162
Sidney, S., 219, 221
Sidorchuk, A., 263
Siegel, M., 299, 301
Siegel, R., 233, 234, 236, 237
Siegel, S., 56
Siegler, B., 262
Siegler, I. C., 220, 410
Siegman, A. W., 233
Siegrist, J., 135
Siemiatycki, J., 238
Sifakis, F., 273
Sifri, R., 78
Sigmon, S. T., 112
Sigurdson, A. J., 239
Sikora, P., 325
Silberstein, L., 365
Silberstein, S. D., 133
Silbret, M., 65
Silva, S. A., 292
Silver, R. C., 102, 111
Silvério, K. G., 297
Silverman, S. M., 88, 121
Sim, J., 166
Simmons, J. B., 83
Simon, D., 161
Simón, M. A., 168, 169
Simoni, J. M., 71, 277
Simonsick, E. M., 219, 354, 355
Simpson, S. H., 60
Simrén, M., 44, 46, 48, 49
Sims, E. A. H., 346
Sinco, B., 265
Singer, B. H., 214, 220
Singer, C. M., 260
Singer, J. P., 22–23
Singh-Manoux, A., 297
Singletary, K. W., 244
Sistla, S. C., 165
Sithole, F., 394

Sittlington, J., 292
Sitzer, D. I., 260
Sivenius, J., 136
Sjöström, M., 391
Skeer, M., 299
Skelly, J. M., 303
Skinner, B. F., 73
Skinner, T. C., 264, 265
Skinner, W., 301
Skipper, B., 66
Skirboll, L. R., 150
Skoluda, N., 99
Skoner, D. P., 10, 44, 133
Skybo, T., 347
Slater, J., 100
Slaughter, R., 272
Slaughter, V., 349, 361
Sleasman, J. W., 65
Slentz, C. A., 391
Sliwa, K., 135, 221
Sliwinski, M., 257
Sloan, F. A., 306
Slomkowski, C., 292
Slugg, R. M., 146
Small, B. J., 256, 258
Smedslund, G., 250
Smeele, I. J., 410
Smeenk, F. W. J. M., 410
Smeets, R. J., 167, 169
Smelt, A. H. M., 354
Smetana, G. W., 133, 161
Smile, S. R., 165
Smiles, R. V., 402
Smith, A. P., 133
Smith, B. J., 246, 301, 391
Smith, C., 195
Smith, C. A., 189, 190
Smith, D., 402
Smith, D. A., 218
Smith, D. G., 163
Smith, D. P., 6
Smith, E. E., 21
Smith, E. M., 127
Smith, G. D., 239, 354, 355
Smith, J., 349, 361
Smith, J. E., 194, 196, 198
Smith, K. M., 218
Smith, L. A., 135
Smith, L. J., 298
Smith, M. S., 256, 257
Smith, P., 137
Smith, P. C., 100
Smith, P. J., 385
Smith, R., 299
Smith, R. G., 249
Smith, S. J., 159, 162
Smith, T. W., 219
Smith-Warner, S. A., 65
Smolinski, M. S., 49
Smyser, M. S., 404
Smyth, J. M., 116, 117
Snaedal, J., 260
Sniehotta, F. F., 79
Snow, J. C., 62
Snow, V., 162
Snyder, C. R., 112
Snyder, P., 249
Snyder, S. H., 149
Sobel, B. E., 216
Sobell, L. C., 330

Sobell, M. B., 330
Soellner, R., 261
Soet, J., 277
Soffer, D., 332
Sokol, R. J., 318
Sola-Vera, J., 65
Soler, R. E., 392
Sollers, J. J., III, 136, 222, 223
Sololik, A., 21
Solomon, L. J., 293, 303
Song, G., 106, 219
Song, M.-Y., 198
Song, R., 273
Song, Z., 103
Sonnentag, S., 106
Sont, W. N., 238
Sood, A. K., 243, 244
Soole, D. W., 338
Sørensen, T. I. A., 306, 351
Sorkin, J. D., 34
Soroui, J. S., 402
Sotoodehnia, N., 278
Sours, J. A., 361
Southern, D., 220
Soyka, M., 329
Spagrud, L. J., 159
Spangler, D., 368
Sparling, P. B., 72, 74
Speck, O., 332
Speck, R. M., 381, 386
Spegman, A., 191, 193
Speizer, F. E., 218
Spence, J. C., 74
Spence, S. J., 228
Spencer, S. J., 215
Sper, S., 135
Spicer, P., 67
Spiegel, D., 140, 250
Spielmans, G. I., 183
Spierings, E. L. H., 133
Spilsbury, K., 47
Spira, T. J., 270
Spiro, A., 221
Spitzer, B. L., 349
Spraul, M., 348, 354
Spreeuwenberg, P., 103
Spring, B., 65, 76, 131
Springer, D., 353
Springer, J. F., 338
Sprugevica, I., 103
Spruijt-Metz, D., 61, 359
Squier, C., 297
Squillace, M., 113, 114
Sridhar, S., 166
Srinivasan, S. R., 25
Sri Vengadesh, G., 165
St. Peter, W. L., 66
St. Pierre, Y., 185
Stacey, P. S., 318
Staehelin Jensen, T., 164
Staessen, J. A., 209
Staff, J., 320
Stafford, R. S., 179
Stambul, H. B., 330
Stamler, J., 218, 224
Stamler, R., 224
Stampfer, M. J., 212, 217, 218, 237, 264, 354, 355, 379, 386
Standridge, J. B., 317, 318
Stanford, J. L., 247

Stanley, B., 320
Stanner, S. A., 218
Stansfeld, S. A., 140
Stanton, A. L., 112, 116, 117, 255, 256, 394
Stanton, J. M., 100
Starkstein, S. E., 259
Stason, W., 320
Stathopoulou, G., 337
Staton, L., 153, 157, 159
Stayner, L., 299
Stead, L. F., 302, 303
Stecker, R., 103
Steele, C. M., 215, 325, 326
Steenland, K., 299
Stefanadis, C., 217
Stefanek, M., 250
Stefanick, M. L., 376
Steffen, J. J., 388
Steffen, K. J., 366
Steffens, D. C., 410
Stegmaier, C., 321
Steifel, M. C., 401
Stein, M. B., 131
Stein, M. P., 378
Stein, P. K., 217
Stein, Z. A., 270
Steinbrook, R., 274
Steiner, H., 6
Steinhausen, H. C., 366
Stelfox, H. T., 52
Steliarova-Foucher, E., 234
Stephens, M. A. P., 265
Stephens, R. S., 73
Steptoe, A., 45, 66, 67, 135, 222, 268, 384, 387, 412
Sterk, C. E., 273–274
Sternberg, E. M., 138
Stetter, F., 113, 114
Stevens, L. C., 384, 387
Stevens, V. J., 29, 357, 358
Stevenson, C. E., 306
Stevenson, R. J., 128
Stewart, A., 364
Stewart, D. E., 140
Stewart, J. C., 136
Stewart, K. L., 191, 193
Stewart, L. K., 380
Stewart, S. T., 400
Stewart, W. F., 161
Stewart-Knox, B. J., 292
Stewart-Williams, S., 21
Steyn, K., 214
Stice, E., 367, 368
Stickney, S. R., 295
Stinson, F. S., 328, 330
Stockdale, S. E., 194, 196
Stockwell, T., 316
Stoff, D. M., 134
Stohler, C. S., 21
Stojanovich, L., 138
Stojek, M., 365
Stokes, B., 359
Stokols, D., 104
Stone, A. A., 45, 106, 116, 117, 133
Stone, G. C., 10
Stone, K. L., 297
Stoney, C. M., 136
Stoolmiller, M., 292
Storr, C. L., 131
Story, D. F., 178, 179, 185, 186

Story, M., 361, 363
Stotts, J., 367
Stout, R. L., 329, 338
Stowell, J. R., 129
Strachan, E., 134
Straif, K., 238, 306
Strasser, A. A., 294
Strathdee, S. A., 74
Strauman, T. A., 385
Straus, M. A., 413
Straus, R., 221
Straus, S. E., 174, 188
Strazdins, L., 109
Streitberger, K., 194, 196
Streltzer, J., 153
Streppel, M. T., 298
Strid, H., 44, 46, 48, 49
Striegel-Moore, R. H., 365, 368, 369
Strike, P. C., 67
Strine, T. W., 268
Stroebe, W., 352
Strong, C. A., 151
Strong, D. R., 298
Strong. W. G., 136
Stroud, C. B., 139
Stroud, L. R., 137
Strunk, R. C., 138
Strzeszynski, L., 303
Stuart, R., 405, 411
Stuart, R. B., 357
Studts, J. L., 162
Stuhr, J., 227
Stunkard, A. J., 351, 368
Stürmer, T., 247
Stussman, B. J., 197
Su, D., 186
Suarez, E. C., 222
Subramanian, S. V., 219, 404
Sufka, K. J., 156
Sugden, K., 140
Sullivan, K. A., 318
Sullivan, L. M., 220
Sullivan, M. J. L., 79, 168, 169
Sullivan-Halley, J., 245
Suls, J., 49, 141, 221, 223, 411
Sun, S., 103, 141
Sunday, S. R., 355
Sundblad, G. M. B., 154
Sundgot-Borgen, J., 363
Sundram, S., 320
Surwit, R. S., 265
Susser, I., 270
Susser, M., 34
Sutandar-Pinnock, K., 365
Sutcliffe, S., 238
Sutton, A. J., 266
Sutton, J., 65
Sutton, S., 74
Sutton-Tyrrell, K., 105, 135
Suurmeijer, T. P. B. M., 255
Svane, B., 220
Svansdottir, H. B., 260
Svensson, C., 65
Svetkey, L. P., 358
Swaim, R. C., 74
Swanson, K. S., 165
Sweeney, C. T., 294
Sweep, F. C. G. J., 138
Swinburn, B. A., 24
Swithers, S. E., 353

Sykes, E., 257
Syme, S. L., 31, 108
Symons Downs, D., 388
Sypeck, M. F., 349
Syrjala, K. L., 162
Szabo, A., 388
Szapary, P. O., 379, 386
Szekely, C. A., 258
Szomstein, S., 358

T

Tacker, D. H., 335
Tada, Y., 129, 261
Tafari, I., 402
Tahilani, K., 365
Taitel, M. S., 165
Takagi, K., 112
Takamatsu, S., 314
Takenaka, K., 139
Takkouche, B., 134
Talala, K., 219
Talamini, R., 245
Talbot, M., 19, 23
Tam, S. F., 229
Tamakoshi, A., 7
Tammi, A., 380, 386
Tamres, L. K., 112
Tan, J. O. A., 364
Tang, B. M. P., 195
Tang, J. L., 83
Tang, M. X., 258
Tang, S. S. K., 65
Tanigawa, T., 137
Tanofsky-Kraff, M., 366, 368
Tanuri, F. C., 166
Tanzi, R. E., 258
Tarbell, S., 15, 17
Tardon, A., 380, 386
Taris, T. W., 106
Tashman, L. S., 100
Tastekin, N., 162
Tatara, N., 411
Tate, D. F., 358
Tate, J. J., 184, 196
Taualii, M. M., 404
Taubman, S., 51
Tax, A., 140
Taylor, A., 129, 140, 384, 387
Taylor, A. E., 248
Taylor, B., 314, 320, 321
Taylor, C. B., 221
Taylor, D. H., Jr., 306
Taylor, E. N., 354, 355
Taylor, G. H., 229
Taylor, H. L., 345, 362
Taylor, J. E., 295
Taylor, L. K., 101
Taylor, N. J., 72, 73
Taylor, R., 299
Taylor, R. J., 111
Taylor, R. S., 229
Taylor, S. E., 94, 95, 104, 111, 277
Taylor-Piliae, R. E., 182, 189, 190
Teasdale, T. W., 351
Tedeschi, R. G., 279
Temple, J. L., 352
Templeton, D., 203

Tenenbaum, G., 100, 383, 387
Ten Have, T. R., 141
Tennen, H., 138, 249, 255, 256, 325
Teo, K. K., 217, 220, 386
Tepper, V. J., 65
Teramukai, S., 194
Terry, A., 388
Testa, M., 320
Thabane, L., 359
Thaw, J. M., 364
Thayer, J. F., 222, 223
Thebarge, R. W., 133
Theberge, N., 177
Theis, K. A., 162
Theobald, H., 318
Theodore, B. R., 154
Theorell, T., 220
Thiede, H., 273
Thielke, S., 405, 411
Thom, D., 52, 53
Thomas, J., 113, 114
Thomas, J. J., 363, 365
Thomas, M., 116
Thomas, S. A., 110
Thomas, W., 65
Thomasius, R., 335
Thompson, A., 405, 411
Thompson, D., 368
Thompson, E. A., 198
Thompson, J. K., 363
Thompson, M., 349
Thompson, O. M., 65
Thompson, P. D., 229, 389
Thompson, R., 265
Thompson, S. H., 363
Thompson-Brenner, H., 365
Thorburn, A. W., 349
Thorn, B. E., 152, 168, 169
Thorne, D., 50
Thornton, L. M., 250
Thorogood, A., 357
Thun, M. J., 240, 296, 298, 306
Thune, I., 245, 380, 386
Thuné-Boyle, I. C. V., 248
Tice, D. M., 141
Tice, T. N., 183
Tiebout, J., 115, 116, 117
Tietze, A., 99
Tilburt, J. C., 20, 22
Timberlake, N., 168, 169
Timmerman, K. L., 380
Timothy, B., 365
Tippetts, A. S., 319
Tleyjeh, I. M., 243, 244
Tobar, D. A., 385
Todaro, J. F., 221
Todd, J. E., 403
Todd, M., 325
Tolfrey, K., 380, 386
Tollefson, D., 329
Tolstrup, J. S., 323
Tomaka, J., 111
Tomar, S. L., 241
Tomfohr, L. M., 221
Tomich, P. L., 111, 256
Tominaga, K., 137
Tomita, T., 139
Tomporowski, P. D., 385, 387
Tong, V. T., 297
Tonigan, J. S., 329

Torchalla, I., 303
Torian, L., 272
Torpy, J. M., 218
Torres, A., 103
Torstveit, M. K., 363
Tosi, H., 101
Toubro, S., 264
Tousignant-Laflamme, Y., 160
Touw, D. J., 214
Tovian, S. M., 15, 404, 411
Townsend, A., 100
Tracey, I., 149
Tractenberg, R. E., 260
Tracy, R. P., 215, 217
Traeger, L., 249
Trafton, J. A., 165
Tran, C., 249
Trautner, C., 348, 354
Travis, L., 15
Travis, T., 320
Treacy, M., 292
Treanor, J. J., 10
Treasure, J., 363, 364, 366
Treede, R.-D., 148
Treiber, F. A., 136
Tremblay, A., 349
Trembley, R. E., 352
Treur, T., 365
Treutlein, J., 292
Treynor, W., 139
Tripodo, E., 166
Trivedi, M. H., 383, 387
Trockel, M., 221
Trost, A., 367
Troxel, W. M., 105
Truelsen, T., 379, 386
Trupp, R., 65
Tsai, A. G., 358, 359
Tsai, J., 415
Tsai, P.-S., 194, 196
Tsai, S. P., 297
Tsang, H. W. H., 189, 190, 195, 196
Tsang, W. W., 195, 196
Tsao, J. C. I, 190, 191, 193
Tsigos, C., 137
Tsiotra, P. C., 137
Tsoi, D. T., 298
Tsugane, S., 28, 137
Tsukayama, H., 197
Tsunaka, M., 189, 190
Tsuyuki, R. T., 60
Tuck, C., 215
Tucker, J. A., 27
Tucker, J. S., 292, 314
Tucker, O. N., 358
Tuna, H., 162
Tuomilehto, J., 213, 376, 386
Turk, D. C., 149, 151, 155, 156, 157, 158, 165, 166, 168
Turner, D. C., 110
Turner, H. M., 364
Turner, J., 255
Turner, J. A., 21
Turner, R. B., 10
Turner, R. J., 101
Turpin, R. S., 83
Turton, P., 198
Tverdal, A., 354, 355
Twamley, E. W., 260
Twenge, J. M., 109
Twicken, D., 181
Tybjærg-Hansen, A., 323
Tylka, T. L., 361, 363

Tynan, M., 299
Tyndall, J., 84
Tyree, P. T., 198
Tyrrell, D. A. J., 133

U

Ubel, P. A., 255
Udaltsova, N., 320, 321
Uellendahl, G., 112
Ullman, D., 198
Ulrich, C., 104
Umstattd, M. R., 326
Unger, E. R., 246
Unger, J. B., 74, 293, 300
Unger-Saldaña, K., 45
Upchurch, D. M., 186, 197
Updegraff, J. A., 72, 83, 94, 102, 111, 277
Urizar, G. G., 115
Usai, S., 133
Usdan, S. L., 326
Uusitalo, U., 258
Uvnäs-Moberg, K., 110
Uy, M. A., 103
Uzunca, K., 162

V

Vaarala, O., 137, 265
Vadiraj, H. S., 129
Vafa, M. R., 349
Vainionpää, A., 381, 386
Valdiserri, R. O., 275
Valente, T. W., 407
Valentin, V., 217
Valkonen, T., 404
Valleroy, L. A., 273
Valliere, W. A., 304
van Agt, H. M. E., 290
van Baal, P. H. M., 408
Vanbeek, M. J., 246
van Bockxmeer, F. M., 385, 387
Van Buyten, J.-P., 166
van Cauter, E., 352
van Dam, R. M., 357, 381, 386
Vandeberg, J. L., 378
Van der Does, A. J., 192, 194
van der Graaf, K., 326
Vander Hoorn, S., 239, 241, 246, 252
Van der Smagt, J., 214
van der Windt, D., 153, 160
van de Ven, V. G., 192
van Dillen, S. M. E., 103
Van Dyck, R., 192, 194
van Eijk, J. T., 382
van Elderen, T., 229
Van Ells, J., 352
van Furth, E. F., 368
Vangel, M., 180
van Hanswijck de Jonge, P., 368
van Jaarsveld, C. H. M., 292
van Kleef, M., 166
van Lindert, H., 7
van Middelkoop, M., 191, 193
Van Oyen, H., 401
VanPatter, M., 385, 387
van Reekum, R., 259
van Rossum, E., 382
Van Royen, P., 62

van Ryn, M., 45, 67
van Schayck, C. P., 410
van Strien, T., 359
Van Tilburg, M. A. L., 265
van Tulder, M. W., 167, 191, 193
Van Weert, J. C. M., 260
Van Winkle, L. C., 158
Van Wymelbeke, V., 353
van Zundert, J., 166
Varady, K. A., 380
Vargas, S., 114, 115, 130
Variyam, J. N., 403
Varnado-Sullivan, P. J., 364
Varney, J., 60
Varstala, V., 380, 386
Vartanian, L. R., 352
Vartiainen, E., 106, 212, 213, 219
Vase, L., 21
Vaskinn, A., 337
Vaughan, C., 298
Vavrek, D., 191, 193
Vazile-Tamsen, C., 320
Vecchi, S., 329
Vedhara, K., 128, 265, 276
Veehof, M. M., 169
Veeranna, H. B., 129
Vega, E., 162
Vega-Perez, E., 162
Veldtman, G. R., 46
Velicer, W. F., 76
Velligan, D. I., 61
Vemuri, P., 257
Venn, A., 299
Venner, P. M., 74
Venzke, J. W., 153
Veraldi, A., 238
Verbeeten, K. C., 30
Verghese, J., 257
Verhagen, A. P., 191, 192, 193, 194
Verhulst, F. C., 56
Verkaik, R., 260
Verkuilen, J., 195, 196
Verma, K. B., 248
Vermeire, E., 62
Vernon, S. W., 78
Verplanken, B., 81
Verreault, R., 257
Verschuren, W. M., 379, 386
Veugelers, P., 394
Vickers, K. S., 305
Vickers, T. J., 50
Victor, T. W., 161
Viikari, J., 380, 386
Viitanen, M., 258
Villalba, D., 326
Vincent, H. K., 194, 196, 197
Vineis, P., 238
Viner, R. M., 314
Virmani, R., 389
Virna, S., 267
Visscher, P. M., 351
Visser, M., 352
Vitaro, F., 352
Vitória, P. D., 292
Vitousek, K., 365
Vlachopoulos, C., 217
Vlaeyen, J. W., 153, 154, 161, 162, 167, 168, 169, 192, 194
Vlahov, D., 277
Voas, R. B., 319
Vogel, M. E., 411
Vogel, R. I., 246
Völker, C., 135

Volpato, S., 219
von Baeyer, C. L., 159
von Hertzen, L. C., 267, 268
Von Korff, M., 21, 165
von Strauss, E., 258
Vorchheimer, D., 228
Voss, A., 317
Voss, M. W., 385, 387
Vrshek-Schallhorn, S., 139
Vyas, P., 249

W

Waber, R. L., 21
Wachholtz, A., 183
Wada, D. R., 20
Wadden, T. A., 357, 358, 359
Wade, J. B., 153
Wade, S. L., 138
Wager, T. D., 21
Wagner, D. T., 106
Wagner, G. G., 277
Wahlberg, A., 188
Wahlberg, J., 137, 265
Waite-Jones, J. M., 256, 257
Wakefield, M., 393
Walach, H., 22, 189, 190
Walcher, T., 321
Wald, A., 134
Wald, H. S., 50
Waldhoer, T., 265
Waldrep, E., 115
Waldrop-Valverde, D., 402
Walen, H. R., 106
Walker, A. R. P., 351
Walker, B. B., 168
Walker, B. F., 351
Walker, D. R., 165
Walker, E. A., 265
Walker, F., 273
Walker, P., 61
Walker, S. S., 136
Wall, M. M., 361
Wall, P. D., 151, 152, 153, 154, 155–156, 163, 164
Wallace, R., 257, 260
Waller, A., 265
Waller, G., 368
Walls, H. L., 306
Wallston, K. A., 402
Walsh, B. T., 388
Waltenbaugh, A. W., 291, 295
Walter, H., 328
Walters, E. E., 141
Walters, S. T., 330
Wamala, S. P., 105
Wang, B., 65, 67
Wang, C., 189, 190, 191, 193
Wang, F., 52
Wang, H., 21
Wang, H.-W., 220
Wang, H.-X., 220, 259
Wang, J., 105, 114, 115, 209, 266, 368
Wang, M., 61
Wang, M.-C., 78
Wang, M.-Z., 238
Wang, Q., 265
Wang, S.-W., 111
Wang, T., 224
Wang, X., 220, 386
Wang, X.-R., 238
Wang, Y., 218

Wang, Z., 331
Wang, Z.-M., 238
Wansink, B., 27
Warburton, D. E. R., 218
Ward, C. H., 158
Ward, K. D., 221
Ward, L. C., 168, 169
Wardle, J., 292, 349, 412
Wareham, N., 216, 219, 416
Warner, R., 388
Warren, C. W., 300
Warren, E., 50
Warren, J. M., 359
Warren, L., 338
Warshaw, E. M., 246
Wasson, J., 263
Watabe, H., 238
Watanabe, T., 137
Waterman, P. D., 404
Waters, C. M., 182, 189, 190
Watkins, L. R., 127, 149
Watt, W., 217
Watts, S. E., 101
Waye, K. P., 103
Wayne, P. M., 381, 386
Webb, O. J., 392
Webb, T. L., 72
Weber, S., 366
Webster, A. C., 298
Webster, G. D., 148
Wechsler, H., 412
Weck, M. N., 321
Weech-Maldonado, R., 45
Weems, C. F., 101
Wegener, S. T., 163
Weidenhammer, W., 188
Weidner, G., 212, 214, 228, 406
Weil, A., 188, 198
Weil, C. M., 138
Weil, J. M., 404
Weinberger, A. H., 303
Weinberger, S. L., 136, 222
Weiner, H., 137
Weiner, M. F., 259, 260
Weingart, S. N., 54
Weinick, R. M., 402
Weinman, J., 47, 129, 269
Weinman, J. A., 135
Weinstein, N. D., 62, 74, 76, 77, 224, 241, 295
Weinstock, M. A., 246
Weinstock, R. S., 216
Weir, H. K., 240
Weiss, A., 66
Weiss, D. S., 141
Weiss, J. W., 293, 300
Weiss, R., 54
Weiss, S., 13, 71, 249
Weitz, R., 50, 51, 53, 174, 407, 408
Weizblit, N., 157
Welch, A., 216, 367, 416
Welk, G. J., 380, 386
Weller, I., 140
Wellman, R., 191, 193
Wells, J. C. K., 351
Wells, R. E., 190
Welsh-Bohmer, K., 385
Welty, T. K., 265
Wen, C., 297
Wen, M., 401
Wen, W., 362
Wendel-Vos, G. C., 379, 386
Wender, R., 78
Wenger, N. S., 186, 198

Wentworth, D., 224
Wenzel, S. E., 267
West, R., 292, 294, 295
West, S. G., 69
West, S. L., 301, 338
Westendorp, R. G. J., 226
Westert, G. P., 7
Westerterp, K. R., 381
Weston, P., 136, 222
Wetter, D. W., 411, 414
Whang, W., 221
Wheaton, A. G., 352
Wheaton, B., 101
Whelan, H. K., 228
Whetsel, T., 381
Whincup, P., 220
White, A., 191, 193, 367
White, C., III., 259, 260
White, C. M., 65
White, D., 81
White, K. S., 305
White, M. A., 368
White, M. J., 78
White, M. M., 293
White, R. O., 402
White, S., 402, 414
White, V. M., 249
White, W. L., 329
Whitehead, D., 100
Whitfield, K. E., 136, 406
Whitford, H. S., 248
Whitwell, J. L., 257
Whooley, M., 221
Wichman, H.-E., 33
Wichström, L., 320
Wickel, E. E., 380, 386
Wicklund, K. G., 247
Wider, B., 188
Wiebe, J. S., 111
Wiech, K., 149
Wiedemann, A. U., 79
Wiegand, F., 20
Wieseler-Frank, J., 149
Wilbert-Lampen, U., 135
Wilbourne, P. L., 329
Wilbur, J., 394
Wiley, J. A., 31, 416
Wilfley, D. E., 366, 368
Wilke, F., 335
Wilkin, H. A., 407
Wilkins, R., 401
Wilkinson, A., 301
Willaism, S. A., 64
Willems, P., 292
Willemsen, E. W., 183
Willett, W. C., 212, 217, 237, 264, 320, 379, 386
Williams, D. R., 7, 214, 220
Williams, G. D., 319
Williams, K. D., 148
Williams, L., 114, 115
Williams, L. J., 153
Williams, M. T., 242, 243, 244
Williams, P. G., 410
Williams, P. T., 376, 379
Williams, R. B., 220, 222
Williams, R. J., 363
Williams, S. L., 64
Williamson, D. A., 364
Williamson, D. F., 353, 355, 359
Willich, S. N., 191, 193, 349, 392
Willott, S., 44
Willoughby, D., 67
Wills, T. A., 109, 292

Wills-Karp, M., 138
Wilmore, J. H., 389
Wilsnack, R. W., 365
Wilsnack, S. C., 319, 365
Wilson, B., 157, 159
Wilson, C., 52
Wilson, D., 102
Wilson, G. T., 365, 369
Wilson, P. W. F., 351, 354
Wilson, S. L., 229
Wilson, V. B., 298
Wilz, G., 261
Wimberly, S. R., 248
Winblad, B., 259
Windsor, J. A., 113, 114
Winefield, A. H., 135
Wing, A. L., 377, 386
Wing, R. R., 357, 358
Wingard, D. L., 31
Wingo, P. A., 240
Winter, M., 412
Winter, W., 338
Winterling, J., 249
Wipfli, B. M., 383, 387
Wisborg, K., 318
Wise, A., 356
Wise, J., 210
Wiseman, C. V., 349, 355
Witherington, D., 349, 361
Witkiewitz, K., 329, 330–331
Witt, C. M., 191, 193
Wlasiuk, G., 270
Wobbes, T., 249
Wodey, E., 192, 194
Wohlheiter, K., 298
Wolcott, J., 54
Wolf, F. M., 269
Wolf, M. S., 402
Wolf, S. L., 382
Wolff, N. J., 56
Wolfgang, M. E., 320
Wolfson, M. C., 401
Wolin, K. Y., 380
Wonderlich, S. A., 365
Wong, M. D., 186
Woo, G., 276
Wood, D., 218
Wood, M. D., 326
Wood, P. D., 376
Wood, P. K., 314
Woodhouse, A., 163
Woodside, D. B., 363, 365
Woodward, C. K., 69
Woodward, H. I., 54
Woodward, M., 65, 264
Woody, P. D., 56
Woolhandler, S., 50, 404, 406, 408
Woollery, T., 33, 297
Woolrich, R. A., 364
Worden, J. K., 293
Worobey, M., 270
Worrall-Carter, L., 65
Wortman, C. B., 279
Wozniak, M. A., 34
Wright, B., 51
Wright, C. C., 158
Wright, J., 260
Wright, R., 138, 268
Wrubel, J., 276
Wu, J.-R., 61
Wu, M.-J., 383, 387
Wu, P., 29
Wu, T., 357

Wu, X., 292
Wurm, M., 221
Wyatt, G. E., 277
Wyatt, H. R., 376, 386
Wyden, P., 356

X

Xiao, J., 385, 387
Xiao, W., 247
Xie, B., 74
Xie, C., 214
Xin, L., 194, 196
Xu, J., 3, 7, 238, 331
Xu, Y., 65
Xue, C. C. L., 178, 179, 185, 186
Xutian, S., 175, 176

Y

Yabroff, K. R., 162
Yager, J., 369
Yager, S., 128
Yamagishi, K., 28
Yamamoto–Mitani, N., 261, 278
Yamashita, H., 197
Yan, L. L., 219, 221
Yan, Y., 380
Yanasak, N. E., 385, 387
Yang, H.-C. Y., 250
Yang, J., 141
Yang, X., 265
Yang, Y., 129, 195, 196
Yano, E., 238
Yanovski, J. A., 368
Yanovski, S. Z., 368
Yao, X, 62, 84
Yarborough, B. J., 29
Yardley, I. E., 54
Yardley, L., 72, 382
Yaroch, A. L., 65
Yasko, J., 249
Ye, X., 66
Yeager, K., 277
Yelin, E. H., 269
Yellon, D. M., 379, 386
Yerramsetti, S. M., 180
Yetgin, T., 226
Yi, H.-Y., 319
Yijn, Y.-M., 353
Yin, S., 402
Yinh, J., 191, 193
Ylvén, R., 257
Yoels, W. C., 352
Yong, H.-H., 304
Yoo, S. H., 138
Yoshimura, S., 156
Yoshino, A., 156
Young, E. H., 367
Young, G., 52
Young, K. A., 331
Young, K. M., 359
Young, L. R., 349
Younger, J., 138
Yu, B., 141
Yu, Y., 106
Yu, Z., 106, 219
Yuan, N. P., 103
Yucha, C., 194, 196
Yuhas, N., 260
Yung, K. K., 194, 196

YunJung, K., 292
Yusuf, S., 135, 212, 214, 215, 217, 218, 220, 386
Yusufali, A., 214

Z

Zaarcadoolas, C., 414
Zachariae, R., 134
Zacho, M., 381
Zack, J. A., 134
Zack, M., 325
Zagorski, B. M., 140
Zagummy, M. J., 291, 295
Zakhari, S., 321
Zakowski, S. G., 249
Zambon, P., 245
Zarkadoulia, E. A., 67
Zaslavsky, A. M., 402
Zautra, A. J., 10, 138
Zawada, A., 229
Zehnacker, C. H., 381, 386
Zeichner, A., 319
Zelenko, M., 6
Zell, B. L., 401
Zeltzer, L. K., 190, 193
Zemek, R., 269
Zerwic, J. J., 45
Zhan, C., 54
Zhan, P., 266
Zhang, A. L., 178, 179, 185, 186
Zhang, B., 279, 306
Zhang, G., 412
Zhang, S., 394
Zhang, X., 218, 295
Zhange, J., 175, 176
Zhao, G., 415
Zheng, G., 106, 219
Zhou, B., 194
Zhou, E. S., 249
Zhou, J.-H., 127
Zieball, R., 273
Ziegelmann, J. P., 70, 79
Ziegler, H., 389
Zielinski, J. M., 238
Ziginskas, D., 250
Zijlstra, G. A., 382
Zikmund-Fisher, B. J., 255
Zimmerman, E., 222
Zimmerman, M., 100
Zimmerman, R. S., 47
Zimmerman, T., 250
Zinberg, N. E., 317
Zive, M. M., 403
Zivian, M. T., 349
Zolnierek, K. B., 52
Zoorob, R., 162
Zorrilla, E. P., 140
Zubaid, M., 135, 221
Zubieta, J.-K., 21, 148
Zubin, J., 131
Zubrick, S. R., 298
Zucker, N., 265
Zucker, R., 159
Zuckerman, A., 256
Zuniga, M., 403
Zupancic, M. L., 361
Zvolensky, M. J., 298
Zweben, J. E., 337
Zyazema, N. Z., 67
Zylstra, R. G., 317, 318
Zywiak, W. H., 338

Subject Index

A

Abdominal fat, 354, 355
A-beta fibers, 146, 156
Absolute risks, 33, 35
Abstinence violation effect, 304, 394
Acceptance and commitment therapy (ACT), 168
Acetaminophen, 166
Acetylcholine, 90
Acquired immune deficiency syndrome. See AIDS
Acrolein, 287
ACT. See Acceptance and commitment therapy
ACTH. See Adrenocorticotropic hormone
Acupressure, 175–176, 178, 196
Acupuncture
    defined, 175
    limitations of, 196–197
    managing pain with, 175–176, 188–189, 190–191, 198
    reducing stress with, 191
Acute pain, 151, 156, 160
Addictions
    alcohol and drug, 312, 317
    bulimia and food, 366
    defined, 316
    exercise, 387–388
    smoking, 294
    12-step programs for, 329, 399
A-delta fibers, 146, 150, 155
Adherence
    age as factor in, 44, 65
    behavioral model of, 73
    behavioral strategies to improve, 82–84
    communication and, 53
    contingency contracts for, 83–84, 86
    cultural norms and, 67–68
    defining, 60, 61–62
    education to improve, 82
    emotional factors in, 65–66
    environmental factors and, 63–64, 66–68
    factors predicting, 63–68, 85
    gender as factor in, 65
    graduated regimen implementation, 83
    health action process approach, 78–79
    health belief model, 69
    health improvements with, 84
    improving, 82–84, 86
    interaction of factors, 68
    maintaining exercise programs, 391–394, 395
    managing HIV infection and, 274–276
    measuring, 60–61, 85
    medication packaging, 83, 84
    personality patterns and, 65
    planned behaviors theories, 71–73
    practitioner-patient interaction, 52
    precaution adoption process model, 76–78
    predicting relapses in, 70–71, 72, 73–74
    prompting individuals in, 83
    real-world profile on, 59–60
    reasons for lapses in, 62
    self-efficacy theory of, 69–71, 74
    severity of disease and, 64
    side effects and, 64
    social support for, 66–67
    suggested readings in, 86
    tailoring regimen to individual, 83, 86
    theories applying to, 69–71, 85–86
    theory of planned behavior, 71–73
    transtheoretical model, 75–76
    treatment complexity and, 64
    See also Predictors of adherence
Adolescents
    adherence for, 65
    alcohol use by, 316, 324
    asthma in, 267, 268, 269
    causes of death for, 4–5
    coping strategies among, 111–112
    diabetes in, 70, 263, 266, 381
    dieting and weight loss by, 356–359, 370
    drug use by, 335, 338
    eating disorders and, 364, 368, 369
    exercise benefits for, 380, 381, 382, 383–384, 385, 387–388
    overweight/obesity among, 356, 380
    pain sensitivity by gender, 153–154
    smokeless tobacco use by, 300
    smoking among, 290–295, 297, 300–301, 308, 404
    stress experienced by, 104–105, 142
    tobacco promotions to, 293
    See also Children
Adrenal cortex, 92, 94
Adrenal glands, 92–93
Adrenal medulla, 92
Adrenocortical response, 92
Adrenocorticotropic hormone (ACTH)
    pituitary release of, 92, 94, 118, 130
    stress mechanisms and, 130–131
Adrenomedullary response, 93
Adrenomedullary system, 94
Aerobic exercise, 374, 375
Afferent neurons, 146
Aflatoxin, 242
African Americans
    alcohol use by, 314
    cardiovascular reactivity among, 222
    effect of discrimination on, 136, 214
    health care disparities for, 402, 405
    inherent CVD risk factors of, 220
    pain perception by, 153–154
    percentage overweight and obese, 349
    See also Ethnicity
Age
    adherence and, 65
    alcohol use and, 315
    benefits of exercise and, 382
    mortality rates by, 4–5
    seeking health care and patient's, 44–45
    weight-related health risks and, 354
Aging
    Alzheimer's and, 257–258, 280, 321
    back pain and, 162
    CVD risks and, 213–214, 216
    distinguishing illness from signs of, 44–45
    health care for aging population, 406
    inherent cancer risks and, 237, 238
    mortality and, 3
Agoraphobia, 140
Agouti-related peptide, 344, 370
AIDS (acquired immune deficiency syndrome), 124–125, 270, 280
    epidemics of HIV and, 274–277
    incidence and mortality rates of, 270–272
    Kaposi's sarcoma and, 272
    symptoms of, 272
    transmission of HIV, 272–274
    See also HIV
Alameda County Study, 30–32, 108–109
Alarm reactions, 95, 96, 98
Alcohol
    benefits of, 320–321
    caffeine's effect with, 335
    cancer and, 244–245, 247, 251, 317–319
    cardiovascular system and, 318, 321
    cognitive-physiological theories of use, 325–326, 327–328
    consumption trends in, 312–316, 339
    direct hazards of, 317–319
    effects of, 316–321, 340
    expectancy and effects of, 324–325
    health risk checklist for, 311
    history of consumption, 312–313
    indirect hazards from, 319–320
    moderating intake of, 415, 416
    moral and medical models for drunkenness, 322–323
    potential for brain damage with, 332
    prevalence of consumption, 314–316
    real-world profile about, 311
    reasons for drinking, 322–327, 339
    social learning model of use, 326–327
    suggested readings on, 340
Alcohol abuse
    alcohol dependency syndrome, 323, 324, 327
    alcohol myopia, 325–326
    binge drinking, 314, 315, 321
    changing problem drinking, 328–331, 339–340
    cognitive-physiological theories and, 325–326, 339
    controlled drinking and, 330, 331
    disease model for alcoholism, 323–325, 327
    drinking and, 314–316
    liver cirrhosis, 317–318
    moral and medical models for drunkenness, 322
    relapses and, 330–331, 337–338, 340
    social learning model and, 326–327
    tolerance and dependency in, 317
Alcohol dehydrogenase, 316
Alcohol dependency syndrome, 323, 324, 327
Alcoholics Anonymous (AA), 328–329, 331

Alcoholism. *See* Alcohol abuse
Alcohol myopia, 325–326
Aldehyde dehydrogenase, 316
Aldehydes, 287
Alkalosis, 366
Allergies, 125–126
Allostasis, 94, 96
Allostatic load, 94, 97
Alternative medicine, 174
    See also Complementary and alternative
        medicine
Alveolar sacs, 286
Alzheimer's disease
    effect on family, 260–261, 280
    genetic predisposition toward, 258
    helping patients with, 260
    living with, 257–261, 380
    real-world profile of, 254
    risk factors and prevention for, 258–260
Amenorrhea, 362
American Medical Association, 177
American Psychological Association, 13
Amphetamines, 335
Amputation, 163
Anabolic steroids, 335–336
Anaerobic exercise, 374
Analgesia
    hypnosis for, 184
    prescription drugs for, 153, 154, 164–166
Anemia, 366
Anesthesia, 358
Aneurysms, 207
Anger
    cardiovascular disease (CVD) and, 221–222
    cardiovascular reactivity (CVR) and, 222
    hostility and, 221–222
    reducing, 226–227
    trait, 319
    Type A behavior and, 221–223
Angina pectoris, 206, 210, 229
Anorexia nervosa, 361–365
    binge-purge cycles and, 362
    comparing bulimia, binge eating, and, 368
    defined, 360–361
    health recommendations for, 368
    psychological factors in, 362–363
    real-world profile of, 342
    relapses in, 365
    suggested readings on, 370–371
    susceptibility to, 362–363
    treating, 363–365, 370
    types of, 362
ANS. *See* Autonomic nervous system
Antibodies, 124
Antigens, 124
Anus, 343, 344
Anxiety
    CVD and, 228
    exercise reducing, 383
    meditation and reducing, 188–189, 190
    reducing for hospitalized children, 56
    response to myocardial infarction, 228–229
    stress of hospitalization, 55
Anxiety disorders, 140–141, 142
Arteries
    blockage of, 207
    effect of high blood pressure on, 209
    function of coronary, 205
    role in cardiovascular system, 205
    smoking's effect on, 297

Arterioles, 204
Arteriosclerosis, 205
Arthritis
    pain of, 162, 164
    relaxation techniques for, 167
Asbestos, 238
Asian Americans
    alcohol use by, 314–316
    CAM therapies used by, 186
    health care disparities for, 404, 405
    lower reactivity of, 137
    percentage overweight and obese, 349
    See also Ethnicity
Aspirin, 165, 166
Asthma, 266–269, 280
    managing, 268–269
    stress and, 138
    triggers for, 268
Atheromatous plaques, 205
Atherosclerosis, 205, 206, 216
Atkins diet, 178–179, 356
Attitude
    views on weight and eating, 342
Autogenics training, 112–113
Autoimmune diseases, 126
Autonomic nervous system (ANS), 89–90, 95
    activation of adrenomedullary system,
        94–95
    effect of stress on, 121
    sympathetic and parasympathetic systems
        of, 89–90
    target organs of, 91
Aversion therapy, 329
Ayurveda, 176, 178, 179

B

Barbiturates, 333
B-cells, 121, 124, 125, 130
Beck Depression Inventory, 158, 160
Behavior
    anger and Type A, 221–223
    antismoking campaigns to change, 293, 301,
        303
    cancer risks and, 239–241, 247, 251
    changes with starvation, 345–346
    conditioning and reinforcing, 73
    hospital patient's role, 53–55, 57
    illness, 43–48
    lowering serum cholesterol, 226
    motivational interviewing to change, 83
    observing pain-related, 159, 160
    reciprocal determinism and, 69, 70
    reducing anger, 227
    reducing hypertension, 224–225, 230
    relating to disease, 142
    sick role, 43, 47, 48, 57
    smoking cessation, 224–227, 230
    stages of changing, 75–76
    stress and indulgent, 140
    theory of planned, 71–73
    See also Health-related behavior; Illness
        behavior
Behavioral cardiology, 227
Behavioral medicine, 13
Behavioral model of adherence, 60, 73, 76
Behavioral willingness, 80–81
Behavior modification

defined, 167
    for emotions linked to CVD risks,
        226–227
    improving adherence with, 83–84, 85
    managing pain with, 167–168
    pain management using, 166–169, 170
    weight loss with, 357
Beliefs
    adherence and, 65
    inventory of personal health, 19
    seeking health care and personal, 69
    See also Health belief model
Beta-carotene, 243
Bile salts, 344
Binge drinking, 314, 315, 318, 327
Binge eating, 367–369, 370
    characteristics of, 368
    compared with other eating disorders, 366,
        367, 368, 370
    health recommendations for, 368
    hypoglycemia and, 366
    treatments for, 369
Biofeedback, 183–184, 185
    effectiveness of, 191–192
    Raynaud's disease and, 194
Biomedical model, 9–10, 11
Biopsychosocial model, 10–11
    contributions of psychosomatic
        medicine, 12–13
    illustrated, 14
Blood circulation, 208, 210
Blood pressure, 207–210
    CVD risk and hypertension, 215
    hypertension and, 207–210
    lowering with CAM, 192, 197
    ranges of, 210
    stressors elevating, 136
    weight loss and lowering, 225–226, 230
Blood sugar, 263–266
BMI (body mass index)
    defined, 26
    defining obesity with, 348–349, 354
    mortality risks and, 252
Body fat
    anorexic preoccupation with, 362
    assessing obesity with, 348, 354
    exercise and, 376–377
    genetic tendency to store, 351, 354–355
    links with disease or mortality, 356
    setpoint and maintenance of, 350–351,
        352, 354
    studies on abdominal fat, 354
    See also Dietary fat
Body image
    eating disorders and, 361
    idealized thinness and, 349, 355,
        359–360
    men and attention on, 363
    self-esteem and regular exercise, 361, 367
    suggested readings on, 370
Body mass index. *See* BMI
Bone density loss, 381, 386
Brain
    alcohol use and effect on, 317–318
    blocking pain with endorphins, 149–150
    drug effects on, 332–333
    gate control theory of pain and, 155–156
    high blood pressure's effect on,
        208, 209
    reducing pain with opiates, 149, 164

response to emotional and physical pain, 148
somatosensory cortex, 147
Breast cancer
    alcohol consumption and, 244, 318
    decreasing death rates for, 234, 236
    genetic component of, 237–238
Bronchioles, 284, 285
Bronchitis, 284, 285
Bulimia, 360, 365–367, 370
    binge-purge cycles and, 362
    compared with other eating disorders, 368, 369
    defined, 360, 365
    harmfulness of, 366
    health recommendations for, 367
    historic occurrences of, 365
    prevalence of, 365–366
    psychological factors in, 365
    treatment for, 366–367
Burn treatment, 192, 194, 196, 199

C

Calories
    exercise and number burned, 376
    experimental starvation and intake of, 345–346
    maintaining weight and intake of, 344–345, 370
    overeating and, 346, 351, 353
CAM. See Complementary and alternative medicine
Cancer
    adequate drug dosages for, 164–166
    adjusting to diagnosis of, 248–249
    alcohol use and risks for, 243–245, 247, 251, 318–319
    behavioral risks for, 239–247, 251
    changing death rate for, 233–236, 251
    chronic pain and, 162, 164
    deaths related to smoking, 239–241, 247, 251, 297
    defined, 233
    diet and, 242–243, 244, 247, 251
    environmental risks and, 238–239, 251, 297
    exercise and protection against, 245, 380–381, 386
    foods protecting against, 242–243
    genetic predisposition toward, 233, 239
    immune surveillance theory and, 122
    inherent risk factors for, 237–238, 251
    medical treatments for, 248
    passive smoking and, 299–300, 308
    personal risk inventory for, 232
    psychological interventions, 250
    psychosocial risk factors in, 247
    psychological interventions for patients, 250
    real-world profile about, 232
    sedentary lifestyle and, 245, 251
    sexual behavior and, 246–247
    social support for patients of, 249–250, 251
    suggested readings on, 251–252
    types of, 236
    ultraviolet light exposure and, 245–246, 251
    understanding, 233, 250
    See also Risk factors for cancer

Capillaries, 204
Carcinogenic, 242
Carcinomas, 233
Cardiac arrhythmia, 364
Cardiac rehabilitation, 206
Cardiologists, 221
Cardiovascular disease (CVD)
    alternative treatments for, 194
    anger in, 221–222
    atherosclerosis, 205, 206, 321
    benefits of exercise on, 378–379, 384
    blood pressure and, 25, 208–209
    changing rates of, 210–212
    chocolate and, 219
    components of cardiovascular system, 203–210, 229
    coronary artery disease, 205–207, 210
    coronary heart disease, 206, 377
    declining death rates from, 210–211
    defined, 204
    exercise risks with, 388–389, 395
    glucose metabolism and, 216
    hypertension, 209–210, 215
    inflammation and, 217
    inventory of personal risks, 232
    lifestyle and, 218, 230
    lowering serum cholesterol, 226, 230
    myocardial infarction, 210
    obesity and, 212, 213, 218
    passive smoking and, 300, 308
    physiological conditions in, 215–217, 229
    preventing first heart attacks, 224–227
    psychosocial factors in, 219–220, 223, 229
    reactivity under stress, 136–137
    real-world profile of, 232
    reducing hypertension, 224–226, 230
    reducing risks of, 224–229, 230
    rehabilitating cardiac patients, 227–229
    risk factors in, 33, 212–223, 229–230
    smoking and, 217–218, 224, 230, 296–297
    stereotype threats and, 136–137
    stress, depression, and anxiety in, 221
    stress factors in, 135, 141
    suggested readings on, 230
    watching sports matches, 137
    weight and diet, 217–218
    See also Coronary heart disease; Myocardial infarction; Risk factors for CVD; Stroke
Cardiovascular reactivity (CVR), 222
    and anger, 222
Cardiovascular system, 203–210
    alcohol's effect on, 318, 321
    blood circulation in, 207–210
    coronary artery disease, 205–207
    exercise and health of, 377–380, 395
    functioning of coronary arteries, 205
    overview, 203, 210, 395
    risks of exercise with CVD, 389–390
    stroke, 207
    See also Cardiovascular disease
Case-control studies, 29, 30, 32
Cataclysmic events, 101–102, 107
Catecholamines, 93
Catharsis, 116
Causation
    beliefs about illness and, 47
    determining disease, 33–35, 38–39
CBT. See Cognitive behavioral therapy
Central control trigger, 156
Central nervous system (CNS), 89, 127

Cervical cancer, 246–247
C fibers, 146–147, 150, 155–156
Change as source of stress, 102–103
CHD (coronary heart disease), 206, 377
Checklists. See Personal health inventories
Chemotherapy, 248
Chewing tobacco, 300
Chi. See Qi
Children
    antismoking campaigns for, 301
    cancer among, 237
    chronic disease among, 257
    exercise and, 380
    HIV exposure at birth, 273
    hospitalization of, 55–56
    obesity among, 25, 359, 361
    passive smoking and, 299, 300, 308
    preventing drug abuse in, 338
    sexual abuse linked with bulimia, 365
    stress experienced by, 103, 104–105, 141
    See also Adolescents
Chiropractic treatment, 177, 179, 196
    effectiveness of, 191
Chocolate, 219
Cholecystokinin, 345
Cholesterol
    exercise and levels of, 379–380, 386
    HDL, 215–216, 226, 230, 379–380
    LDL, 215, 216, 226, 230, 379–380
Chronic disease, 3
    asthma and, 267–268, 280
    children and, 257
    cigarette smoking and, 33–35, 297
    determining cause of, 33–35, 38–39
    diabetes and, 262–264, 280
    facing death and, 277–279
    future management of, 410–411
    health expectancy and, 401
    HIV and AIDS, 270
    identifying risk factors for, 27–28
    impact of, 255–257, 279
    increases in, 3–8, 12
    living with Alzheimer's, 257–261, 280
    lowering risk of, 277
    real-world profile of, 255
    sick role behavior and, 48
    suggested readings on, 280
    treatment costs for, 9
    See also specific diseases
Chronic lower respiratory diseases, 284, 287
Chronic obstructive lung diseases (COLD), 267
Chronic recurrent pain
    arthritis, 162, 164
    cancer, 162, 164
    defined, 151, 156
    fibromyalgia, 162
    headache as, 161, 164
    hypnosis for, 192, 194
    low back pain, 161–162
    phantom limb pain, 163–164
    relaxation techniques for, 167
    syndromes and, 160, 170
    See also Managing pain; Pain
Cigarette smoking
    advertising and, 293
    chronic disease and, 31, 33–35, 297
    consumption rates for, 289, 295–296
    health consequences of, 296–298, 308
    history of, 288

Cigarette smoking *(continued)*
  See also Smoking
Cigars, 241, 287, 300
Cirrhosis, 317–318
Clinical trials, 29, 32
Cluster headaches, 161
CNS (central nervous system), 89, 127
Cocaine, 335, 336, 337
Cognitive behavioral therapy (CBT), 113–115, 117–118
  effectiveness of, 114–115, 168
  managing pain with, 168
  treating eating disorders with, 364, 367, 369
Cognitive functioning, better, 385
Cognitive-physiological theories of alcohol use, 325–326, 327–328
Cognitive therapy, 168, 170
COLD (chronic obstructive lung diseases), 267
Colon cancer, 243
Colorectal cancer, 236, 242
Complementary and alternative medicine (CAM), 174
  Ayurvedic medicine, 176–177, 179–180
  biofeedback, 183–184, 185
  chiropractic treatment, 177, 179, 187, 199
  conditions addressed with, 192, 194–195
  defined, 174
  diet and, 178–179, 199
  dietary supplements, 179, 200
  effectiveness of alternative treatments, 187–198
  energy healing, 182–183, 185, 198
  guided imagery, 180, 198
  homeopathy, 176–177
  hypnosis, 184–185, 192
  integrative medicine, 199
  inventory of personal health care preferences, 173
  limitations of, 195–197, 199
  massage, 177–178, 179, 199
  meditation and yoga, 180, 185
  mind-body medicine, 179–185, 198–199
  naturopathy, 179
  people who use, 185–187, 200
  practices and products for, 177–179, 199
  prayer and, 183
  qi gong, 181–182, 189–191, 198–199
  real-world profile of, 173–174
  reasons for seeking, 187
  suggested readings on, 200
  systems of, 174–177, 199
  tai chi, 182, 185, 190, 191, 194
  traditional Chinese medicine, 175–176
  treating anxiety, stress, and depression with, 188–189, 190
Complementary medicine, 174
Compliance. *See* Adherence
Condoms, 273, 274, 275
Contingency contracts for patients, 73, 83–84, 86
Continuum theories, 66, 68–74
  behavioral theory, 73
  critique of, 73–74
  health belief model, 69
  self-efficacy theory, 69–71
  summary of, 74
  theory of planned behavior, 71–73
Conscientiousness, 66
Control

coping and personal, 110–112
  perception of behavioral, 71
Control groups, 25, 26, 27
Controlled drinking, 330, 331
Coping
  defined, 98, 107
  hardiness and, 119
  personal control and, 109–110, 119
  progressive muscle relaxation for, 117
  resources influencing, 107–112
  social support and, 108–109, 119
  strategies for, 110–112, 119
Coronary artery disease, 205–207, 210
Coronary bypass, 206–207
Coronary heart disease (CHD), 206
  exercise and, 377–378, 386
  myocardial infarction, 206
  obesity and, 25
  prospective studies on weight and, 28
  See also Myocardial infarction
Correlational studies, 24–25, 28, 38
Correlation coefficient, 24
Cortisol
  defined, 92–93
  measuring, 99
  releasing, 94, 95
  stress and release of, 130–131
Costs. *See* Health care costs
Council of Chiropractic Education, 177
Cox-2 inhibitors, 166
Crack cocaine, 335
Crime
  alcohol consumption and, 319
  incidents affecting college students, 413–414
Cross-sectional studies, 24, 25, 38
Crowding, 104, 107
Cultivating healthier lifestyles
  adopting healthier behaviors, 415–416
  health psychology's role in, 415, 416, 417
  improving health expectancy, 400–401, 405
  increasing health literacy, 402, 403
  knowing effect of own choices, 414
  moderation and, 405
  reducing health disparities, 401–405
  understanding personal risks, 412–415
Cultural norms
  adherence and, 67–68
  attributing cause for disease and, 47
CAM therapy and, 186, 187
  defining health, 10
  differences in coping strategies, 111
  influencing perceptions of pain, 153
  See also Ethnicity
Curanderos, 51
CVD. *See* Cardiovascular disease
CVR (cardiovascular reactivity), 222
Cytokines, 127, 131, 142

D

Daily hassles, 99, 107, 118–119
  discrimination, 104, 105
  found in environment of poverty, 104, 107
  measuring stress of, 100, 101
  physical environment and, 103–104
  population density and crowding, 104, 107
  psychosocial environment and, 104–106
  urban press and, 103, 107

DARE, 338, 364
Dating violence, 413
Death
  adult and infant mortality, 7–8
  AIDS, 270, 272
  automobile crashes, 412–413
  chronic disease and, 278
  correlating education and mortality risks, 7
  declining rates from CVD, 211
  during exercise, 389–390
  facing, 277–279, 280
  grieving, 278–279, 280
  leading causes of, 3–5, 6
  lifestyle factors causing, 30
  nonadherence and, 73
  rates of cancer, 233–236, 251
  suicide, 413
Delirium tremens, 317
Delta alcoholism, 323
Dependence, 164
  alcohol dependency syndrome, 323, 324, 327
  alcohol misuse and, 317, 336–337
  barbiturate and tranquilizer, 333, 337
  drug, 165, 317, 336
  exercise, 388
  opiates and, 164
  table of psychoactive drug, 335
  tolerance, withdrawal, and, 317
Dependent variables, 26, 334
Depression
  Alzheimer's disease and, 259
  cataclysmic events and, 101–102
  CVD and, 221, 227
  defined, 382
  exercise's effect on, 382–383, 385
  linked to stress, 138–140, 141, 142
  reducing with meditation, 188–189
  response to myocardial infarction, 228
Diabetes mellitus
  alcohol's beneficial effect on, 321–322
  children and adolescents with, 263
  controlling with exercise, 381, 386–387, 395
  glucose metabolism and CVD, 216
  lifestyle adjustments for, 264
  living with, 262–264, 280
  stress and, 137, 265–266
  types of, 263
  yoga and, 194
Diagnosis
  adjusting to cancer, 248–249
  role in illness, 43
  sick role behavior following, 47–48, 49, 52–53
Diagnostic and Statistical Manual of Mental Disorders (DSM-IV-TR) (APA), 323, 362, 365, 382
Diaphragm, 284
Diastolic pressure, 208, 209
Diathesis-stress model, 131–132, 267
Diet
  adding dietary supplements to, 178–179, 195
  cardiac rehabilitation, 206
  Chinese medicine's view of, 176
  dietary cholesterol, 215, 216, 223
  food choices and CVD risks, 218
  improving health with, 178, 181, 183

links between cancer and, 239–240, 245, 247, 251
  obesity, weight gain and, 347
  recommendations for eating disorders, 368
  variety in and overeating, 353
  See also Dieting
Dietary fat
  cancer and high, 242, 245
  obesity and, 347, 353–354
  See also Body fat
Dietary supplements
  CAM use of, 178–179, 195
  and natural products, 178–179
  reducing CVD risks, 218, 219
Dieting, 355–360
  approaches to losing weight, 356–359
  behavior modification programs and, 357
  idealized thinness and, 349, 355, 359
  pros and cons of, 359, 360, 370
  suggested readings on, 370–371
  weight loss with exercise vs., 376
  See also Weight loss
Digestive system, 343–344, 369
Discrimination
  CVD among African Americans and, 214–215
  reactivity due to, 136
  stress generated by, 105–106
Disease
  adherence and severity of, 64
  biomedical models of, 9–10, 11
  changing patterns in death and, 3–8, 16
  components in concept of, 46–48, 49
  defined, 43, 48
  determining cause of, 33–35, 38–39
  diathesis-stress model of, 131–132
  emotions and psychosomatic, 12–13, 44
  ethnicity and income factors in, 5–7
  how people conceptualize, 46–48
  illness vs., 43–48
  role of stress in, 131–141
Disease model for alcoholism, 323–325, 327
Disulfiram, 329
Doctors. *See* Practitioners
Dopamine, 331
Dorsal horns, 146, 154–155
Dose-response relationship, 34, 35, 38
Double-blind research design, 22–23, 34
Drinking. *See* Alcohol; Alcohol abuse
Drug abuse
  cocaine and, 335, 336, 337
  effect on brain, 331
  FDA drug schedule, 333
  misuse and abuse of drugs, 336–337
  prevention strategies for, 338
  relapses in, 337, 339
  tolerance, dependence, addiction and, 317
  treating, 337–338, 340
Drugs
  acetaminophen, 166
  amphetamines, 335
  anabolic steroids, 335–336
  analgesic, 166, 169
  aspirin, 166, 169
  barbiturates, 333
  brain's response to, 331
  cocaine, 335
  Cox-2 inhibitors, 166

FDA classification of, 332, 333
  hazards of legal and illegal, 331–332
  health recommendations for, 333
  HIV risks with injection, 273, 275
  lowering serum cholesterol, 226
  managing pain with, 170
  marijuana, 332, 335, 336, 337
  misuse and abuse of, 336–337
  NSAIDs, 165–166
  opiates, 165, 333
  preventing and controlling use of, 338
  psychoactive, 331, 334, 336
  rates of use, 331
  real-world profile about, 311
  sedatives, 333
  stimulants, 335, 339
  suggested readings on, 340
  tolerance to, 316
  tranquilizers, 333
  treating eating disorders, 337–338, 367, 369
  weight regulation with, 350–351
  See also Drug abuse
DSM-IV-TR (APA), 362, 365, 382
Dying role, 278

E

Eating
  attitudes about, 342
  experimental overeating, 346, 350
  factors in maintaining weight, 344–346, 370
  food restriction strategies for weight loss, 357
  hormones involved in appetite and satiation, 345
  studies in experimental starvation, 345–346
  See also Binge eating; Diet; Overeating
Eating disorders, 360–369
  anorexia nervosa, 361–365, 370
  binge eating, 360, 361, 366, 367–369, 370
  body dissatisfaction and, 361
  bulimia, 365–367, 370
  cognitive behavioral therapy and, 364, 366, 369
  family violence and, 363
  health recommendations for, 368
  obligatory exercise and, 388
  real-world profile about, 342
  treating with Prozac, 364, 367, 369
  types of, 360
  See also specific disorders
Ecstasy, 335, 336
Education
  alcohol consumption and, 315–316
  college as positive health factor, 7
  CVD risks and level of, 218–219
  health care disparities and, 404–405
  improving adherence with, 82, 86
  profile for smokers, 290, 291
  successes in quitting smoking and, 303
Efferent neurons, 146
Electrolyte imbalance, 366
EMG (electromyography), 159, 184, 199
Emotion
  adherence and, 65
  adjusting to cancer diagnosis, 248–249

alcohol consumption and aggressive, 319–320
  anger's role in CVD, 221–222, 227
  arising from chronic disease, 256
  brain response to emotional pain, 148
  cancer incidence and repressed, 247
  as factor in health, 12–13, 44
  grieving death, 278–279, 280
  therapeutic disclosure of, 115–117
  See also Anger
Emotional disclosure, 115–117, 118
Emotion-focused coping, 110–111, 112
Emphysema, 284–285
Endocrine system
  defined, 90
  differences in nervous and, 91–92
  psychological and social factors affecting, 127
  See also Neuroendocrine system
Endorphins, 149–150
Energy healing, 182–183, 185, 199
Environmental factors
  cancer and, 239, 251, 296–297
  daily hassles, 103–104
  influencing adherence, 66–68
  passive smoking, 299, 300, 308
  pollution as, 103–104
  population density and crowding, 104, 107
  psychosocial stresses, 104–106
  vulnerability to stress related diseases, 131–132
Environmental tobacco smoke (ETS), 299, 300, 305
Epidemiologists, 27–28, 31
Epidemiology, 27–31
  prevalence and incidence in, 28, 33
  training and work of epidemiologists, 31
  value of, 38
Epinephrine, 93, 95, 99
Esophagus, 343
Essential hypertension, 209
Ethanol, 316
Ethical uses of placebo effect, 22
Ethnicity
  adherence and, 67–68
  alcohol use by, 314
  colorectal cancer deaths by, 236
  coping strategies and, 111–112
  discrimination and, 104–105, 136, 215
  exercise benefits with CVD risk, 378–379
  health-related behaviors and, 69, 77
  infant and adult mortality rate for, 5–7
  inherent cancer risk factors and, 237, 238
  life expectancy and, 7–8, 406
  overweight/obese individuals by, 349
  pain perception and, 153
  perceptions of illness and, 45
  rates of HIV infection by, 272
  reducing health disparities for all groups, 401–405
  smoker profiles by, 290, 295
  use of CAM therapy by, 185–187
  weight-related health risks and, 354
ETS (environmental tobacco smoke), 299, 300, 305
European Americans
  alcohol use by, 314–315
  pain perception by, 153
  percentage overweight/obese, 349
  reactivity due to discrimination, 136
  See also Ethnicity

Exercise
addiction to, 387–388
age and benefits of, 382
benefits of, 245, 380–385, 395
better cognitive functioning, 385
bone density loss prevention with, 381, 386
cancer prevention benefits of, 245
cardiovascular health and, 377–380, 395
Chinese medicine's view of, 176
cholesterol levels and, 379–380
controlling diabetes with, 381, 386, 395
death during, 389–390
decreasing depression with, 382–383, 387
gender and cardiovascular effects of, 379
hazards of, 385
increasing for adolescents, 380, 381, 389
injuries from, 388–389, 390, 412–414
obligatory, 388
personal health risks for, 373
physical fitness and, 375
preventing weight gain as ex-smoker, 305–306
psychological benefits of, 381–385
rates of coronary heart disease and, 377–378
recommendations for, 390–391, 395
reducing anxiety with, 383, 385
self-esteem and regular, 385
stress and, 385
sudden death during, 389
suggested readings for, 395–396
tai chi, 181, 182, 185
types of, 374, 376, 395
weight control and, 357–358, 375–376, 386
Exhaustion stage, 96
Expectations
placebos and positive, 20–22
studying control and experimental group, 25–26
Experimental designs
components of, 26
ex post facto, 26–27, 32, 38
placebos in, 37
Experimental groups, 25, 26, 27
Experimental overeating, 346, 350
Experimental starvation, 345–346
Experimental studies, 26, 27, 28
Ex post facto designs, 26–27, 32, 38
External locus of control, 109
Eysenck Personality Inventory, 247

F

Families
cancer risks of, 232, 237–238
caring for Alzheimer's patients, 260–261
eating disorders and violence in, 363
effect of chronic disease on, 256–257, 279
genetic tendency to obesity, 351, 354
grieving death of member of, 257, 278–279
problem drinking in, 328–331
stress and unsupportive, 106–107
Family Daily Hassles inventory, 100
Fear, 104, 107
Feces, 344
Fetal alcohol syndrome, 318, 319

Fibromyalgia, 162, 164, 168
Five Factor Model of personality, 66
Flavonoids, 219
Flexibility, 375
FMRI (functional magnetic resonance imaging), 148, 149
Food and Drug Administration (FDA), 29, 332, 333
Formaldehyde, 287
Framingham Heart Study, 211, 212, 215
Frequency of nonadherence, 63, 85
of symptoms, 45
Functional magnetic resonance imaging (fMRI), 148, 149
Function foods, 179
Future health challenges, 397–405
adapting to changing needs, 410–411
controlling rising costs, 407–408
future of health psychology, 411, 416
improving health expectancy, 400–401
importance of prevention, 408–410
increasing life expectancy, 400–401, 411
progress in health psychology, 405
reducing health disparities, 401–405

G

Gall bladder
alcohol consumption and stone prevention, 321
function in digestive system, 321
Gamma alcoholism, 323
GAS (general adaptation syndrome), 95–96, 98, 118
Gastric juices, 343
Gate control theory of pain, 155–156
Gender
adherence and practitioner's, 52–53
alcohol consumption and, 315–316
cardiovascular effects of exercise and, 379
cardiovascular reactivity and, 222
coping strategies and, 111–112
death from AIDS by, 272
illness behavior and, 53–58
as inherent CVD risk factor, 257–258
job-related stresses and, 128
neuroendocrine responses to stress and, 93
overweight and obese individuals by, 349
pain perception and, 153–154
profile for smokers by, 289, 290, 295
rates of HIV infection by, 272
use of CAM therapy by, 198
General adaptation syndrome (GAS), 95–96, 118
Genetic predisposition
Alzheimer's and, 257–261
cancer and, 232, 237–238
obesity and, 351–353, 354–355
problem drinking in families, 322–323
smoking and, 291–292, 296
Gestational diabetes, 263
Ghrelin, 344, 370
Glucagon, 262
Glucagon-like peptide 1, 345, 370
Gonads, 92
Graduated regimen implementation, 83
Granulocytes, 122

Grieving, 278–279, 280
Guided imagery, 180, 181, 190, 198

H

Harm reduction strategy, 338
Hassles and Uplifts Scale, 101
Hassles Scale, 100
HDL (high-density lipoprotein), 215–216, 226, 230, 379–380
Headaches
alternative therapies for, 190–191, 193–194
effectiveness of relaxation techniques for, 167
exercise and, 200
stress and, 133
types of chronic, 160, 161, 164
Health
behavioral medicine, 13
benefits of religion on, 183
changing views of, 3, 11, 17
cultural definitions of, 10
defined, 11, 42
development of health psychology, 13–14
education as positive factor in, 7
illness vs., 48–49
models of, 9–11
positive psychology's study of, 10–11
psychology's relevance in, 11–15
Health action process approach, 78–79
Health belief model, 69
critique of, 73–74
summary of, 74
Health care
challenges for aging populations, 405–411
distribution of funding for, 407–408
escalating costs of, 8–9, 11, 56
increase in HMOs, 407–408
innovative programs for elder, 401
personal preferences checklist, 173
psychologists' acceptance in, 12
psychosomatic medicine's contribution to, 12–13
reducing health disparities, 401–405
reluctance to seek, 41–42
seeking medical attention, 42–48, 57
suggested readings on, 417
See also Future health challenges
Health care costs
controlling, 407–408
income and health care standards, 404–405
life expectancy and, 405–408, 410
rising, 8–9, 11, 56, 57
suggested readings on, 417
treatment costs for chronic disease, 8–9
where money goes, 407–408
See also Insurance
Health care providers. See Practitioners
Health disparity
defined, 401
educational and socioeconomic, 404–405
racial and ethnic, 402, 404, 405
reducing, 401–405
Health expectancy
by nation, 402
increasing, 400–401, 416
life expectancy and, 400

Health literacy, 403, 415–416
Health maintenance organizations (HMOs), 15, 407–408
Health psychologists, 14–16
  duties of, 2
  training and work of, 15–16
Health psychology
  applying personally, 412–416
  contributing to Healthy People 2020 goals, 399, 416
  cultivating healthy lifestyle with, 414, 415, 416, 417
  defined, 13
  development of, 13–14, 16–17
  future of, 411–412, 416
  managing diabetes with, 266
  progress in, 405
  psychometrics' role in, 36–37, 38–39
  role of theories in research, 35–36, 39
  suggested readings in, 17
Health recommendations
  adopting healthier behaviors, 415–416
  alcohol and, 333
  drugs and, 333
  eating disorders and, 368
  making adherence pay off, 83
  smoking and, 305
Health research
  clinical trials, 35, 41
  determining cause of disease, 33–35, 38–39
  double-blind design of, 22–23, 24
  evaluating value of, 32
  examining your beliefs about, 19
  finding causal relationships to disease, 33–35
  informed consent and, 23
  meta-analysis techniques, 30, 38
  natural experiments, 28, 30, 32, 35, 38
  observational studies in, 28–29, 31, 34, 38
  placebo effect in, 21–24
  psychometrics in, 36–37, 39
  psychoneuroimmunology, 128–130
  questions in, 18
  randomized, controlled trials, 29, 32, 38
  reliability, 36–37, 39
  research methods in psychology, 24–28
  single-blind design, 22, 23, 37
  theoretical models in, 35–36, 39
  validity, 37, 100–101
  See also specific research and theories
Health risks. See Personal health inventories; Risk factors
Healthy People 2010, 4
Healthy People 2020
  health psychology's contribution to, 399, 416
  objectives of, 401, 405–406
Heart
  angina pectoris, 106, 210, 229
  coronary heart disease and, 206
  functioning of coronary arteries, 205
  illustrated, 205
  myocardium, 205
  preventing first heart attacks, 224–227
  See also Coronary heart disease
Hemorrhagic stroke, 207, 208
Heroin, 304, 332
Heterosexual transmission of HIV, 271, 274
High-density lipoprotein (HDL), 215, 321, 379–380

Highly active antiviral therapy (HAART), 275, 277
Hispanic Americans
  alcohol use by, 314–316
  health care disparities for, 404, 406
  pain perception by, 153
  percentage overweight and obese, 349
  vulnerability to PTSD, 141
  See also Ethnicity
HIV (human immunodeficiency virus), 124–125, 270–277, 280
  adherence to treatment for, 59
  epidemics of AIDS and, 270
  incidence and mortality rates of, 270–272
  injection drugs as risk factor in, 270, 273
  protective measures against, 275
  psychologist's role in managing, 274–277
  role of stress in, 127
  symptoms of, 272
  testing for, 275
  transmission of, 272–274, 277
  See also AIDS
HMOs (health maintenance organizations), 15, 407–408
Holistic health model, 10
Homeopathy, 176–177, 199
Hormones
  defined, 90
  effect of stress, 135
  involved in appetite and satiation, 345
  measuring, 98–99
Hospital patient's role, 53–55, 57
Hospitals, 53–56
  changes in care at, 53
  children and, 55–56
  cost of care at, 50–51, 56
  medical errors at, 54
  patient's role in, 53–55, 57
Hostility, 221–222
H. pylori
  alcohol's beneficial effect on, 321
  infection with, 137, 238–239
Human immunodeficiency virus. See HIV
Humoral immunity, 124
Hurricane Katrina, 101
Hydrocyanic acid, 287
Hygiene hypothesis for asthma, 267
Hypertension
  blood pressure ranges for stages of, 207–208, 209
  cardiovascular reactivity and, 222
  CVD risk and, 218
  defined, 135–136, 208, 209, 215
  reducing, 224–226
Hypnosis
  effectiveness of, 192
  managing pain with, 184–185
Hypoglycemia, 366
Hypothalamus, 350

Illegal drugs
  risks of, 331–332
  See also Drug abuse
Illness
  behavior and, 43–48

defined, 43
disease vs., 42–43, 48
immune system disorders and, 124–127
job-related stress and, 105
predicting from stress self-report, 100–101
seeking alternative treatments for, 187
sick role behavior, 43, 48, 53–54
Illness behavior diagnosis and, 43
  gender differences and, 44, 45–46
  hospital patient's role, 53–55, 57
  how people view disease, 46–48
  personality and, 44
  socioeconomic, ethnic, and cultural factors, 45
  symptoms and, 43–44
Immune deficiency, 124
Immune system, 121–127
  B- and T-cells, 121–122, 124, 125
  depression and immune function, 140
  disorders of, 124–127
  function of, 122–124
  interactions with nervous system, 127
  nonspecific responses of, 122–123, 127
  organs of, 121–122
  overview, 121, 142
  primary and secondary immune responses, 124, 126
  psychological and social factors affecting, 127
  specific responses of, 122, 124, 127
  stress and function of, 129–130
  weakened by stress, 127
Immunity, 124
  and stress, 120–142
Implementational intentions, 81
Incidence, defined, 27, 33
Income
  access to health care and, 57, 408
  adherence and, 66
  correlating health care standards and, 404
  CVD linked with low, 218–219
  health care standards and, 404
  influencing response to illness, 45
  life expectancy and, 5–7
  money as means to cope with stress, 108
Independent variable, 25–26
Induction, 184
Infant mortality rate, 7–8
Infectious disease
  cold, 10
  and stress, 133–135
Inflammation, 122
  cancer risks and chronic, 216–217
  function of, 122
  illustrated, 123
Informed consent, 23
Injuries
  exercise-related, 388–389, 390, 395
  understanding personal risk of, 412–414
Insensitivity to pain, 145
Insulin
  defined, 262
  function of, 369–370
  weight maintenance and, 344
Insurance
  access to health care and, 50–61
  CAM treatments and, 197
  role in nonadherence, 66
Integrative medicine, 197–198

INTERHEART study, 135
Interleukins, 127
Internal locus of control, 109
International health
    cardiovascular disease, 211–212
    CVD risks by gender and country, 213–214
    health care cost increases for, 408
    per capita care expenditures, 409
Internet, 49–50
Interneurons, 146
Ischemia, 206
Islet cells, 262
Isokinetic exercise, 374
Isometric exercise, 374
Isotonic exercise, 374

J

Japan Public Health Center-Based Study, 28

K

Kaposi's sarcoma, 246
Kidneys, 209, 210
Korsakoff syndrome, 318, 322

L

Lacto-vegetarian diet, 178
Laminae, 146–147
Lay referral network, 49, 57
LDL (low-density lipoprotein), 215, 218, 226,
    230, 379–380
LEARN diet, 356
Leptin, 344
Leukemia, 233
Leukocytes, 121
Life events, 99–100, 107, 118
    accuracy of self-reports of, 102–103
    defined, 99
    difficulty linking stress to, 132–133
    measuring stress of, 98–100, 101
Life expectancy, costs of greater, 405–412
    education and improved, 7
    health expectancy and, 400–401
    in the United States, 405–406
Life Skills Training program, The, 338
Lifestyle
    behavior and chronic disease, 12
    changing risk factors for CVD, 210–211
    cultivating healthy, 414, 415, 416, 417
    deaths related to, 2, 3
    effects of personal, 414
    factors in CVD, 218, 230
    identifying factors related to death,
        30–31
    lower cancer death rates and, 210–212
    optimistic bias and change in, 224
    real-world profile of healthier, 398
    stress related to, 135
    symptom and interference in, 45–46
    See also Cultivating healthier lifestyles;
        Sedentary lifestyle
Lipoproteins, 215

Liposuction, 358
Liver
    bile salt production in, 344
    cancer of, 236
    cirrhosis of, 317–318
Longitudinal studies, 24, 25, 27
Low back pain
    alternative therapies for, 191–192, 193–194
    chronic, 157, 160
    relaxation techniques for, 161–162
Low-density lipoprotein (LDL), 215, 218, 226,
    230, 379–380
Lung cancer
    decreasing deaths for, 234, 236
    increases in women's deaths for, 236
    linked to smoking, 239–241, 296
    passive smoking and, 299, 300
    risk factors for, 33
Lycopene, 218
Lymph, 121
Lymphatic system, 121
Lymph nodes, 121, 122
Lymphocytes, 121
Lymphoma, 233

M

Macrobiotic diet, 178
Macrophages, 122–123
Malignant cells, 251
Managing pain, 164–169
    acupuncture for, 175–176, 188–189,
        190–191, 198
    alternative therapies for, 189–192
    behavioral techniques for, 166–169, 170
    cognitive behavioral therapy for, 113–114,
        168
    drugs for, 164–166
    guided imagery for, 180, 181
    hypnosis for, 184–185, 192
    overview, 164
    surgery for, 166, 170
Marijuana, 332, 335, 336, 340
Massage, 177–179, 199
    Ayurvedic, 176
    pain management with, 192
    tui na, 176, 178, 182
Materia Medica, 176
McGill Pain Questionnaire (MPQ), 158, 160
Meaning-focused coping, 111, 112
Measurement
    adherence, 60–61, 85
    daily hassles, 100, 101
    hormones, 98–99
    life event stresses, 98–100, 101
    pain, 157–160, 170
    stress, 100, 101
Medicaid, 50, 56, 57
Medical advice
    getting and adhering to, 64, 65, 68, 73, 81
    reasons for not complying, 82–84, 86
Medical care
    choosing practitioners for, 51–53
    cost of hospital care, 50–51
    hospitals and, 53–56
    limited access to, 50–51
    medical errors at hospitals, 54
    receiving, 50–56, 57

Medical practitioners. See Practitioners
Medical qi gong, 181
Medicare, 50, 56, 57
Medication Event Monitoring System, 61
Medications. See Drugs
Meditation
    effectiveness of, 196
    reducing anxiety, stress, and depression with,
        187–188
    types of, 180
    uses for, 192, 194–195
Mediterranean diet, 243
Medulla, 149
Melanoma, 246
Memory loss, 259
Memory lymphocytes, 124
Men
    adherence of, 65, 88
    alcohol consumption by, 314, 316
    anorexia among, 363
    cardiovascular effects of exercise
        for, 379
    coping strategies for, 111–112
    death from AIDS, 270, 271
    identifying risk factors for, 31
    inherent CVD risk factors for, 213–215
    job-related stress for, 128
    marriage and social support for, 130
    mortality rates for CVD, 210–211
    neuroendocrine responses to stress, 95
    pain perception of, 153–154
    percentage of overweight/obese, 349
    rates of HIV infection for, 270, 271
    risk factors for smokers, 33, 240, 297
    seeking health care, 44
    smoking by, 289–291, 295
    stress and CVD, 135
    use of CAM therapy by, 186–187
Meridians, 175
Mesmerism, 184
Meta-analysis, 30, 38
Metabolic syndrome, 216
Metastasize, 233
Metropolitan Insurance Company weight
    charts, 362
Migraine headaches, 161
Mind-body medicine, 179–185
    biofeedback, 183–184, 185
    defined, 179, 199–200
    energy healing, 182–183
    hypnosis, 184–185, 192
    meditation and yoga, 180, 185
    overview, 179–180
    qi gong, 181–182, 181–182, 185
    tai chi, 182, 185, 190, 191, 194–195
    See also specific therapies
Mindfulness meditation, 180, 185, 198
MMPI (Minnesota Multiphasic Personality
    Inventory), 160
Model, 36
Moderation, 415
    management, 330
Morbidity, 31
Morphine, 332
Mortality
    alcohol and rate of, 320–321
    automobile crashes and, 412–413
    BMI and risks of, 353–354
    CVD death rates, 210–211
    exercise and, 373, 386

health practices and, 31
HIV and AIDS rates of, 270–272
lack of social support and, 66–67
quitting smoking and reduced rate
of, 306
rates for anorexics, 363–364
suicide and, 413–414
weight loss and risks of, 359–360
See also Death
Motivation, 49
Motivational interviewing, 83
Motivational phase, 78, 80
MPI (Multidimensional Pain Inventory), 158
MPQ (McGill Pain Questionnaire), 158
Muscle strength and endurance, 375
Myelin, 146
Myocardial infarction
defined, 206, 210
depression after, 228
resuming sex after, 228
Myocardium, 205, 206

N

Naltrexone, 329, 331
Narcotics Anonymous (NA), 337–338
NASPE (National Association for Sport and
Physical Education), 382
National Task Force on the Prevention and
Treatment of Obesity, 348, 354
Native Americans
alcohol use by, 314–316
health care disparities for, 404
See also Ethnicity
Natural disasters, 101–102
Natural experiments, 28, 30, 32, 38
Natural killer (NK) cells, 129
Naturopathy, 176, 177, 195
Negative reinforcement, 294–295
Neoplastic, 233
Nerves, 146
Nervous system
autonomic, 89–91
central, 89–90, 127
differences in endocrine and, 90–93
function of, 89
peripheral, 89–90
registering pain, 145–150, 170
stress effects on, 130–131
sympathetic and parasympathetic systems,
89–90
See also Autonomic nervous system;
Peripheral nervous system
Neuroendocrine system, 90–93
adrenal glands, 92, 93
gonads, 92
pancreas, 92
pituitary gland, 92–93
thyroid, 92
Neuromatrix, 163
Neuromatrix theory, 156
Neurons
activation in ANS, 90
afferent and efferent, 146
defined, 89
role in nervous system, 89
stroke's effect on brain, 205
Neuropeptide Y, 344, 370

Neurotransmitters, 89–90
defined, 89
dopamine, 292
drug effects on, 331
norepinephrine's role as, 90
perception of pain and, 149
Neuroticism, 44
Nicotine
addiction to, 285–286, 287
physiological effects of, 294
See also Smoking
Nicotine replacement therapy, 302
Nitric oxide, 287
NK (natural killer) cells, 121
Nocebo effect, 21
Nociceptors, 146
Noise, 103–104, 107
Nonadherence
frequency of, 61–62, 81
reasons for, 62, 63
Non-Hodgkin's lymphoma, 246
Nonmedical sources of health information
Internet, 49–50
lay referral network, 49, 57
Norepinephrine, 90, 93
NSAIDs (nonsteroidal antiinflammatory
drugs), 165
Nurses. See Practitioners
Nurses' Health Study, 237–238

O

Obesity
adolescents and, 349, 354
BMI as measure of, 348–349, 354
body fat and, 347–348, 354–355, 362
colorectal cancer and, 242
correlational studies on, 24–25
CVD risks and, 212, 213, 218
defining, 347–349
exercise and weight control, 26, 375–376, 377
fashion and weight, 349
genetic tendency to, 341, 354
health risks of, 353–354, 369–370
heart disease and, 25
increases in, 349
overeating and, 347, 350, 353–354
positive incentive model of, 351–353,
354–355
setpoint model of, 350–351, 352, 354
sleep deprivation and, 352
studies on, 355
See also Weight gain
Obligatory exercise, 388
Observational studies, 28–29, 31, 38
Oklahoma City bombings, 102
Oncologists, 248
Oncology, integrative, 198
Opiates, pain reduction with, 149–150
Optimistic bias
adherence and, 76
defined, 62
lifestyle changes and, 224
smoking and, 241, 295
Ornish diet, 178, 179, 199, 228
Osteoarthritis
alternative therapies for, 191, 197, 199
pain and, 162

Osteoporosis, 381–382, 386
Outcome expectations, 70, 78
Overeating
factors promoting, 353
obesity and, 347–354, 370
physiological effects of, 346
See also Binge eating
Overweight. See Obesity; Weight gain

P

Pain
acute, chronic, and prechronic, 151, 157
alternative therapies for, 189–192
arthritis, 162, 170
assessing, 144, 158–159
brain and, 147–149
cancer, 162
cultural perceptions of, 153
fibromyalgia, 162
gate control theory of, 155–156
gender and perception of, 153–154
guided imagery for managing, 180, 181
headache, 160, 161, 170
individual experiences of, 152–153
insensitivity to, 144
low back, 161–162
managing, 164–169, 170
meaning of, 150–156, 170
measuring, 157–160, 170
modulating, 149–150
neuromatrix theory of, 156
neurotransmitters and, 149
observing pain-related behavior,
159, 160
pain syndromes, 160–164, 170
phantom limb, 163–164
physiological measurements of, 159–160
placebo effect and reduced, 21–22
psychological and physical factors in, 151
reducing with opiates, 149–150
somatosensory system and, 146
specificity theory of, 154, 157
spinal cord and, 154–155
suggested readings on, 171
surgery for managing, 166, 169
theories of, 154–156
views of, 151
Pain inoculation, 168
Pain-prone personalities, 153
Pain questionnaires, 158
Pain syndromes, 160–164, 170
alternative treatments for, 189–192
arthritis, 162, 170
headache, 160, 161, 170
phantom limb pain, 163–164
related to cancer, 162
See also Chronic recurrent pain; and specific
syndromes
Pain traps, 167
Pancreas, 92
Pancreatic juices, 343
Parasympathetic nervous system, 89–90
Passive smoking, 299, 300, 308
Pathogens, 9
Patients
adapting to terminal illness, 277–278
age factor in seeking care, 44–45

Patients (continued)
communications with practitioners, 52
contingency contracts for, 83–84, 86
effect of chronic disease on, 255–256, 280
helping Alzheimer's, 260
psychological interventions for cancer, 250, 251
rehabilitating from CVD, 227–229
role of hospital, 53–55, 56
social support for cancer, 249–250
Peptide YY, 345, 370
Perceived Stress Scale (PSS), 99
Periaqueductal gray, 149–150
Periodontal disease, CVD, 297
Peripheral nervous system (PNS)
divisions of, 89–90
neural impulses and, 145–146
neuroendocrine system, 90–93
Peristalsis, 343
Persistence of symptoms, 46
Personal control, 109–110
Personal factors
adherence and, 65, 68
body image and eating disorders, 361–362
changing behavior patterns and, 73
choosing CAM treatments, 185–187
communicating with practitioners, 52
concept of disease, 65–66
effects of lifestyle on health, 140, 414
exercising control over life, 73–74
health care preferences and, 173
illness behavior and, 44
individual's experience of pain, 182–183
inventory of personal health risks, 54
perceiving stress, 96–97
personal control and coping, 109–110, 112
predicting adherence relapses, 69–71, 74
tailoring adherence regimen using, 83, 86
understanding personal health risks, 412–414
vulnerability to stress related diseases, 98, 131
Personal health inventories
adherence, 65
alcohol, 311
cancer, 232
CVD, 202
examining personal health beliefs, 19
exercise, 373
health care preferences, 173
personal health risks, 41
rating pain, 144
smoking, 283
stress, 88, 96–97, 100
weight and eating, 342
PET (positron emission tomography), 148
Phagocytosis, 122, 130
Phantom limb pain, 163–164
Pharynx, 318, 343
Physical activity. See Exercise
Physicians. See Practitioners
Physiology
alcohol's effect on, 316–321, 339
conditions contributing to CVD, 215–217, 229
of diabetes, 263–264

digestive system, 343–344, 369
effect of stress on, 130–131
functioning of coronary arteries, 205
immune system, 121–124
injuries from exercise, 388–389, 390, 412–414
measuring stress effects on, 98, 100–101, 118
overeating's effect on, 346, 351
physical factors of pain, 151–152
physiological measurements of pain, 159–160
respiratory system function, 284–285
smoking's effect on lungs, 285
starvation's effect on, 345–346
stress response and, 94–95, 118
Pipe smoking, 298–299, 308
Pituitary gland, 92, 94, 118
Placebo effect
case studies of, 19
double- and single-blind research design and, 22, 23, 37–38
informed consent and, 23
nocebo effects, 21
Placebos
defined, 20, 23
random use in clinical trials, 29
reduced pain and, 23
testing disease model of alcohol with, 325
use of, 37–38
Plasma cells, 124
PNI. See Psychoneuroimmunology
PNS. See Peripheral nervous system
Pollution as stressor, 103–104
Population density, 104
Positive incentive model of obesity, 351–353, 354–355
Positive psychology, 11
Positive reinforcement, 73
Positive reinforcers, 167
Positron emission tomography (PET), 148–149
Posttraumatic stress disorder (PTSD)
cataclysmic events and, 101–102, 107, 118–119
linked to stress, 141–142
Poverty
CVD increases linked with, 212
daily hassles and, 104, 107
health care availability and, 57
health-related behavior and, 48
life expectancy and, 6
Practitioners
choosing, 51–53
communications with, 52
dealing with patients with chronic disease, 255–256
patient adherence and interaction with, 52
personal characteristics of, 52–53
Prayer, 183
Precaution adoption process model, 76–78
critique of, 79–80
summary of, 61, 86
Prechronic pain, 151, 157
Predictive validity, 37
Predictors of adherence, 63–68
cultural norms, 67–68
environmental factors, 66–68
interaction of factors, 68
personal factors, 65–66

practitioner-patient interaction, 52
self-efficacy, 69–71
severity of disease, 64, 74
summary of research on, 68
treatment characteristics, 64
Pregnancy
alcohol's effect on fetus, 318–319
risks for women smokers, 296
Prescription drugs, 54
Prevalence, 27–28, 33
Prevention
Alzheimer's disease, 258–259
bone density loss, 381, 386
cancer, 243–245, 380, 385
CVD, 218–219, 224–227
drug abuse, 338
gallstone, 321, 322
primary and secondary, 410–411
relapses for smokers, 304, 305
weight gain for ex-smokers, 305–306
Primary afferents, 146
Primary appraisal, 97
Primary prevention, 410
Pritikin diet, 179
Probability, 73
Problem-focused coping, 111–112, 119
Progressive muscle relaxation, 112–113
Prohibition, 313, 382
Proinflammatory cytokines, 149
Project D.A.R.E., 301
Prospective studies
approaches for, 28
causation undetermined in, 33
defined, 32
Prostate cancer
decreasing death rates for, 236
psychosocial risks for, 238–239
Prozac, 364, 367, 369
Prudent diet, 226
PSS (Perceived Stress Scale), 99
Psychoactive drugs, 336
characteristics of, 334
effect on brain, 332
Psychological disorders and stress, 138–141, 142
Psychological factors
exercise and, 381–385
expectancy effects and, 22
in pain, 151–154
in stress, 97
Psychological tests for pain, 158–159
Psychologists
acceptance in health field, 12
helping people with HIV, 275–277
smoking interventions by, 302–303
training and work of health, 15–16
Psychometrics, 36–37, 38–39
Psychoneuroimmunology (PNI), 127–131
effect of stress on physiology, 130–131
history of, 127–128
overview, 131
relating behavior to disease, 142
research in, 128–130
Psychosocial stresses
CVD and, 219–220, 223, 229
daily hassles and, 104–106
Psychosomatic medicine, 12–13
Psychotherapy, treating alcoholism with, 329
PTSD. See Posttraumatic stress disorder

Punishment, 73
Purging, 366

Q

Qi, 175, 176
Qi gong, 176, 181–182
  pain control with, 189, 213
  reducing stress with, 189, 190
Quitting smoking, 301–303
  health benefits of, 306, 308
  preventing relapses, 304, 305
  weight gain and, 305–306, 309
  who succeeds in, 303–304, 308–309

R

Radiation, 248, 251
Randomized, controlled trials, 29, 32, 38
  dietary studies using, 243
  experimental studies and, 28
  testing alternative treatments with, 188
Rape, 413
Rating scales
  pain assessment, 157–158
  Social Readjustment Rating Scale, 99, 100,
    101, 102, 118, 132
  Visual Analog Scale, 157
Raynaud's disease, 194, 199
Reappraisals, 98
Reciprocal determinism, 69, 70
Recovery
  Alcoholics Anonymous and, 328–329, 331
  chemical treatments for, 329–330
  methods of alcoholism treatment and,
    328–330
  psychotherapy treatments in, 329
Rectum, 344
Reiki, 182, 185
Reinforcement, 73
Relapses
  adherence and, 70–71, 75, 76
  after weight loss, 358–359, 360
  anorexia recovery and, 365
  drug abuse, 337, 339
  frequency of nonadherence, 62
  preventing smoking, 304
  problems with alcohol, 330–331, 337–338,
    340
Relative risks, 33
Relaxation training, 117, 119
  effectiveness of, 113
  pain management with, 167, 170
  progressive muscle relaxation, 112–113
Reliability
  determining, 36–37, 39
  of stress measurements, 100–101
Religion, 180, 183
Research. *See* Health research
Resistance stage, 95–96
Respiratory system
  alcohol use and, 317
  chronic diseases of lower, 284, 287, 297
  functioning of, 284–285
  illustrated, 285
  smoking and, 285–287, 297, 308

Retrospective studies, 28–29, 31, 38
Rheumatoid arthritis
  defined, 138
  relaxation techniques and, 167
  stress as source of, 162, 164
  tai chi and, 181, 182
Risk factors
  absolute and relative, 33
  Alzheimer's, 258–260
  death during exercise, 389–390
  defined, 27, 33
  determining causation via, 33, 35
  identifying for chronic diseases, 30–31
  research identifying, 31–32
  understanding personal, 412–414
  See also Personal health inventories
Risk factors for cancer
  alcohol, 243, 247, 251, 317–319
  diet, 239–240, 245, 247, 251
  environmental risks, 239, 251, 296–297
  inherent, 237–238, 251
  lung cancer, 33–35
  psychosocial factors, 247
Risk factors for CVD
  changing lifestyle to lower, 210–212
  glucose metabolism and, 216
  inflammation and, 217
  inherent, 213–215
  obesity, 212, 213, 218
  physiological factors, 215–217, 229
  psychosocial factors, 219–220, 223, 229
  reducing risks of disease, 224–229, 230
  smoking and, 217–218, 224, 230,
    296–297
  weight and diet, 217–218
Rumination, 139, 222

S

Salivary glands, 343
Sarcomas, 233
Secondary appraisal, 97
Secondary hypertension, 209
Secondary prevention, 411
Sedatives, 333
Sedentary lifestyle, 394
  adding exercise to, 375
  asthma and, 268
  cancer risks with, 245, 247
  depression and, 382–383
Seeking and receiving health care, 42–48
  beliefs contributing to, 46–48
  cultural, ethnic, and socioeconomic
    views, 45
  gender differences in, 44
  how people view disease, 46–48
  medical information from nonmedical
    sources, 49–50
  overview, 57
  personal factors in, 44
  real-world profile on, 41–42
  symptom characteristics and, 45–46
Selenium, 243, 244
Self-care, 410, 411
Self-efficacy
  adherence and, 69–71, 78
  exercise maintenance and, 395
Self-esteem, 361, 367

Self-reports
  measuring pain with, 157–159
  stress, 100–101
Self-selection, 29
September 11 attacks, 102
Serotonin, 335
Serum cholesterol, 215–216, 218, 223, 226
Setpoint model, 350–351, 354, 370
Severity of symptoms
  adherence and, 64, 46
  seeking health care and, 65
Sexual behavior
  bulimia and sexual abuse, 365–367
  drinking and unprotected, 319, 326
  HIV infection and heterosexual contact, 273,
    275
  homosexual transmission of HIV, 272–274,
    277–278
  linked to cancer, 246–247
  resuming after myocardial infarction, 228
Shiatsu massage, 178
Sick role behavior
  defined, 43
  diagnosis and, 48, 49, 57
  hospital patients', 53–55, 57
Side effects, 64, 68
Single-blind design, 22, 23, 37–38
Skin
  pain receptors on, 146, 150
  skin cancer, 245–246
Sleep
  obesity and deprivation of, 351
  recommended amounts of, 416
Small intestine, 343–344, 369
Smokeless tobacco, 300, 308
Smokers
  advertising attracting, 293
  genetic predisposition of, 292, 296
  health recommendations for, 305
  nicotine addiction of, 294
  optimistic bias of, 241, 295
  preventing relapses by, 304, 305
  profiling, 289–290, 308
  quitting smoking, 301–303
  rates of cigarette consumption by, 289
  reinforcement for, 294–295
  social pressure on, 292
  successes in quitting, 303–304
  weight control motivating, 305–306, 309
  why they start, 291–292
  young people as, 290–291, 292–293, 308
Smoking
  advertising and, 293
  alcohol consumption and, 244
  cancer deaths related to, 239–241, 247, 251,
    297
  choosing to, 288–289
  chronic disease and, 31, 33–35, 297
  cigar and pipe, 298–299, 308
  consequences of, 296–298, 308
  CVD and, 217–218, 224, 230, 296–297
  dangerous components in, 285–287
  deaths from, 284
  deterring, 300–301
  effect on respiratory system, 285–287, 297, 308
  genetics and, 291–292, 296
  health benefits of quitting, 306, 308
  history of tobacco use and, 288
  nicotine addiction and, 294
  optimistic bias and, 241, 295

Smoking (continued)
  other health effects of, 297–298
  passive, 299, 300, 308
  personal health inventory for, 283
  profiling smokers and nonsmokers, 289–290, 308
  quitting, 301–303
  rates among young people, 290–291, 292–293, 308
  real-world profile on, 283
  reasons for starting, 291–292
  refraining from, 415
  reinforcement motivating, 294–295
  relapse prevention, 304, 305
  social pressure and, 292
  weight control with, 305–306, 309
Snuff, 241, 287
Social contacts, 108
Social coping, 111
Social isolation, 108
Social network, 108
Social Network Index, 31
Social pressure
  smoking and, 292
  social learning model of drinking, 326–327
Social Readjustment Rating Scale (SRRS), 99, 100, 101, 102, 118, 132
Social support
  boosting adherence with, 66–67
  cancer patients and, 249–250, 251
  college students' need for, 416
  CVD risk factors and, 221
  defined, 66–67
  drug abuse and, 337–338
  quitting smoking and, 301–303
  stress and, 108–109, 112
Somatic nervous system, 89
Somatosensory cortex, 147
Somatosensory system, 146
Specificity theory of pain, 154, 157
Spinal cord, 146–147, 150, 154–156
Spirituality and disease, 183
Spleen, 122
Spontaneous remission, 328
SRD (stress response dampening) effect, 325
SRRS (Social Readjustment Rating Scale), 99, 100, 101, 102, 118, 132
Stage theory, 278–279
State anxiety, 383
Steroids, 335–336
Stimulants, 335, 339
Stress
  alcohol myopia and, 325–326
  anxiety disorders and, 140–141, 142
  asthma and, 138
  behavioral interventions for, 112–117, 119
  caregiving and, 261
  cognitive behavioral therapy for, 113–115, 117–118
  college students and, 414
  coping with, 98, 107–112, 200
  CVD and, 135, 141, 221
  daily hassles and, 100, 101, 103–106, 107
  detecting with hormones levels, 98–99
  diabetes and, 137, 265–266
  diathesis-stress model, 131–132
  difficulty linking to life events, 132–138
  during sports matches, 135

  effect on lifestyle, 140
  emotional disclosure diffusing, 115–117, 118
  exercise's effect on, 383–384, 386
  factors in seeking care for, 44
  general adaptation syndrome and, 95–96, 98, 118
  headaches and, 133
  hypertension and, 135–136
  immune function lowered under, 129–130
  and immunity, 120–142
  infectious disease and, 133–135
  Lazarus's view of, 97–98
  life events and, 98–100, 101
  linking to disease, 132–138
  low back pain and, 157
  measuring, 100, 101
  nervous system and, 89–95
  personal control and, 109–110, 119
  personal hardiness and, 119
  physiological effects of, 89–95, 118, 130–131
  posttraumatic stress disorder, 101–102, 107, 118–119, 141–142
  produced by cataclysmic events, 101–102
  psychological disorders linked to, 138–141, 142
  psychological factors in, 97
  reactivity under, 136–137
  reducing with meditation, 188–189, 190
  relaxation training for, 113, 119
  reliability and validity of measurements, 100–101
  rheumatoid arthritis and, 162, 164
  role in disease, 131–141, 142
  self-report scales for evaluating, 100–101
  Selye's view of, 95–97, 98, 132
  sources of, 101–106, 119
  strategies for coping with, 111–112
  suggested readings, 119, 142
  theories explaining, 95–98, 118
  ulcers and, 137
  vulnerability and, 98
Stress-buffering hypothesis, 109
Stress in General Scale, 100
Stress inoculation training, 114
Stress management
  cognitive behavioral therapy for, 113–115, 117–118
  emotional disclosure for, 115–117, 118
  relaxation training for, 113, 119
  stress inoculation training, 114, 115
Stressors, 95
Stress response dampening (SRD) effect, 325
Stroke
  common, 208
  defined, 207
  effects of, 207
  hemorrhagic, 207, 208
  high blood pressure and, 208–209, 210
  inflammation and, 216–217
Subjective norms, 71–73
Subject variables, 26–27
Substantia gelatinosa, 146, 155
Suicide
  alcohol consumption and attempted, 319
  understanding risks of, 413–414
Suppressed anger, 222–223
Surgery
  managing pain with, 166, 170

  mesmerism and hypnosis as anesthetic for, 184
  placebo, 22–23
  types promoting weight loss, 358
Swedish Twin Registry, 247
Sympathetic nervous system, 89, 95, 99
Symptom Checklist-90, 158
Symptoms
  illness behavior and, 43–48
  influencing response to disease, 45–46
  when to seek care for, 42–43
Synaptic cleft, 89
Syndromes
  alcohol dependency, 323, 324, 327
  defined, 175
  fetal alcohol, 318, 319
  general adaptation, 95–96, 98, 118
  Korsakoff, 318, 322
  metabolic, 216
  See also Pain syndromes
Synergistic effects, 241
Systolic pressure, 208

T

Tai chi, 185, 190, 191, 194
  effectiveness of, 181, 182
  reducing stress with, 190–191, 194
Tars, 286
T-cells, 121–122, 124, 125
TCM. See Traditional Chinese medicine
Temperance, 313
TENS (transcutaneous electrical nerve stimulation), 166
Tension headaches, 161, 190–191
Text messaging, 82
Thalamus, 147
Theories
  defined, 36
  role in health psychology, 37, 39
  theoretical research models, 35–36
  See also specific theories
Theory of planned behavior, 71–73
  critique of, 73–74
  origin of, 45
  summary of, 74
Thermal biofeedback, 184
Thymosin, 121
Thymus, 121, 122
Thyroid, 92
Time lines for illness, 47
Tobacco
  cigar and pipe smoking, 298–299, 308
  cigarette consumption per person, 289
  health consequences of cigarettes, 296–298, 308
  history of use, 288
  passive smoking, 299, 300, 308
  smokeless, 300, 308
Tolerance
  defined, 317
  drug, 164
  table of psychoactive drug, 334
  tranquilizers and, 333
Tonsils, 122
Traditional Chinese medicine (TCM), 175–176, 176
  benefits found with, 195, 198–199

pain control with, 190–192
See also Acupuncture
Trait anxiety, 383
Tranquilizers, 333
Transcendental meditation, 180, 185
Transcutaneous electrical nerve stimulation
(TENS), 166
Transplant rejection, 126
Transtheoretical model, 75–76
Treatment effectiveness
of alternative therapies for pain, 189–192
of CAM for anxiety, stress, and depression,
188–189, 190
of cognitive behavioral therapy,
114–115, 168
of relaxation techniques for chronic
pain, 167
Treatments
adherence to complex, 64, 68
anorexia and, 363–365, 370
binge eating, 369
bulimia, 366–367
cancer, 248
changing problem drinking, 328–331,
339–340
drug abuse, 337–338, 340
graduated regimen implementation, 83
side effects of, 68
tailoring regimen for, 83, 86
Triglycerides, 215
Tui na massage, 176, 178, 182
Tumors, 233
12-step programs, 329, 399
Type A behavior, 221–223

U

Ulcers, 137
Ultraviolet light exposure, 245–246, 251
United Nations, 10
Uplifts Scale, 101
Urban press, 103, 107

V

Vaccination, 124, 134
Validity, 37, 100–101
Variables
independent and dependent, 26–27
subject, 26–27
VAS (Visual Analog Scale), 157
Vegetarian diet, 178
Veins, 204
Venules, 204
Violence
eating disorders and family, 363
fear and threats of, 104, 107

incidents among young people, 413–414
stress of, 104, 169
Vitamin D, 246
VLDL (very low-density lipoprotein), 215
Volitional phase, 78, 79
Vulnerability and stress, 98

W

Weekly Stress Inventory, 100
Weight
attitudes about, 342
body fat and, 347–348, 354–355, 362
charts of desirable, 362
controlling with smoking, 305–306, 309
dieting and, 355–359, 370
eating disorders and, 342, 360–369
exercise and control of, 357–358, 375–376,
386
experimental starvation studies,
345–346
factors in maintaining, 344–346, 370
fashion and, 349
growing occurrence of obesity, 349
health risks of obesity, 353–354, 369–370
idealized thinness and, 349, 355, 359–360
importance of maintaining healthy, 415–416
losing, 356–359
measuring obesity with BMI, 348–349, 354
obesity and CVD risks, 212, 213, 218
overeating, 346, 351, 353
positive incentive model of obesity, 351–353,
354–355
prospective studies on heart disease
and, 28
recommendations for eating disorders, 368
setpoint model of obesity, 350–351,
352, 354
sleep deprivation and obesity, 352
studies on obesity, 354–355
suggested readings on, 370–371
Weight charts, 362
Weight gain
diet and, 347
overeating and, 346, 351
quitting smoking and, 305–306, 309
See also Obesity
Weight loss
adolescents and, 356–359, 370
behavior modification for, 357
designing trials on effectiveness of, 29
drastic methods for, 357–358
exercise and, 357–358, 375–376
food
lowering blood pressure and, 225–226, 230
maintaining, 358–359, 360
methods for losing weight, 356–359
pros and cons of dieting, 359,
360, 370

surgeries for, 358
triggering anorexia nervosa, 361–365
See also Dieting; Eating disorders
Weight maintenance
calorie intake and, 356
factors promoting overeating, 353
idealized thinness and, 349, 355,
359–360
importance of healthy, 414, 415,
416, 417
maintaining weight loss, 358–359, 360
overeating and, 347–354
Well-year, 400
West Haven-Yale Multidimensional Pain
Inventory (WHYMPI), 158
WHO (World Health Organization),
10, 42, 48
Withdrawal, 324
Women
adherence of, 65, 88
alcohol consumption by, 314, 316
cardiovascular effects of exercise
for, 379
cervical cancer risks for, 246–247
characteristics of female physicians, 53
coping strategies of, 111–112
death from AIDS, 270, 271
effect of marital social support for, 109
HIV infection among, 270, 271
identifying risk factors for, 31
inherent CVD risk factors for,
213–215
job-related stress for, 128
mortality rates for CVD, 210–211
neuroendocrine responses to stress, 95
pain perception of, 153–154
percentage overweight/obese, 349
risk factors for smokers, 33, 297
seeking health care, 44
smoking by, 289–291, 295
stress factors and CVD, 135
use of CAM therapy by, 186–187
Work stresses, 106, 140
World Health Organization (WHO),
10, 42, 48
World Trade Center, 102

Y

Yang, 175
Yin, 175
Yoga, 176–177, 180, 189

Z

Zone diet, 178, 179, 199